Authors

Michael S. Bednar, MD
Professor and Chief of Hand Surgery,
    Department of Orthopaedic Surgery and
    Rehabilitation, Loyola University
    Medical Center, Maywood, Illinois
Hand Surgery

Randy Bindra, MD, FRCS
Professor, Department of Orthopaedic Surgery and
    Rehabilitation, Loyola University Medical Center,
    Maywood, Illinois
Hand Surgery

Scott D. Boden, MD
Director, The Emory Orthopaedics & Spine Center,
    Professor and Vice Chair, Department of Orthopaedic
    Surgery, The Emory University School of Medicine
CMO, CQO Emory University Orthopaedics & Spine
    Hospital, Staff Physician, Atlanta VA Medical Center,
    Georgia
Disorders, Diseases, and Injuries of the Spine

Loretta B. Chou, MD
Professor and Chief of Foot and Ankle Surgery,
    Department of Orthopaedic Surgery
    Stanford University School of Medicine,
    Stanford, California
Foot and Ankle Surgery

Brett A. Freedman, MD
LTC, MC, Chief, Spine and Neurosurgery Service,
    Landstuhl Regional Medical Center
Disorders, Diseases, and Injuries of the Spine

Bang H. Hoang, MD
Assistant Professor, Director, Multidisciplinary
    Sarcoma Center, Department of Orthopaedic Surgery,
    Chao Family Comprehensive Cancer Center,
    University of California, Irvine
Musculoskeletal Oncology

Omar Jameel, MD
Resident, Department of Internal Medicine, William
    Beaumont Hospital, Royal Oak, Michigan
Internal Medicine

Lee D. Kaplan, MD
Chief, Division of Sports Medicine, Associate Professor,
    Department of Orthopaedics, University of Miami
    Miller School of Medicine, Miami, FL
Sports Medicine

Mary Ann E. Keenan, MD
Chief, Neuro-Orthopaedics Surgery,
    Department of Orthopaedic Surgery,
    University of Pennsylvania School of
    Medicine, Philadelphia
Rehabilitation

Dann Laudermilch, MD
Graduate Medical Trainee, Department of Orthopedic
    Surgery, University of Pittsburgh, Pittsburgh,
    Pennsylvania
*Orthopedic Infections: Basic Principles of Pathogenesis,
    Diagnosis, and Treatment*

Terry R. Light, MD
Dr. William M. Scholl Professor and Chairman,
    Department of Orthopaedic Surgery and
    Rehabilitation, Loyola University Medical
    Center, Maywood, Illinois
Hand Surgery

Jeffrey A. Mann, MD
Alta-Bates Summit Medical Center, Oakland, California
Foot and Ankle Surgery

Richard L. McGough, III, MD
Chief, Division of Musculoskeletal Oncology,
    Associate Professor of Orthopaedic Surgery,
    Associate Professor of Surgery (Surgical Oncology),
    Co-Director, UPCI Sarcoma Program,
    University of Pittsburgh, Pittsburgh, Pennsylvania
*Orthopedic Infections: Basic Principles of Pathogenesis,
    Diagnosis, and Treatment*

Patrick J. McMahon, MD
McMahon Orthopedics & Rehabilitation,
    Adjunct Associate Professor, Bioengineering
    University of Pittsburgh, Pittsburgh, Pennsylvania
Sports Medicine; Rehabilitation

Samir Mehta, MD
Assistant Professor, Department of Orthopaedic Surgery,
    University of Pennsylvania School of Medicine, Chief,
    Orthopaedic Trauma & Fracture Service, Philadelphia
Rehabilitation

Gabrielle Peacher
Research Assistant, Department of Orthopedic Surgery,
Denver Health Medical Center
Denver, Colorado
Musculoskeletal Trauma Surgery

Charles A. Popkin, MD
Assistant Professor of Clinical Orthopaedic Surgery, Columbia University, College of Physicians and Surgeons, New York, NY
Sports Medicine

George T. Rab, MD
Professor, Department of Orthopaedic Surgery, University of California, Davis, Consultant, Shriners Hospitals for Children, Northern California
Pediatric Orthopedic Surgery

R. Lor Randall, MD, FACS
Professor of Orthopaedics, Director, Sarcoma Services Chief, SARC Lab, Huntsman Cancer Institute and Primary Children's Medical Center, University of Utah, Salt Lake City, Utah
Musculoskeletal Oncology

John M. Rhee, MD
Associate Professor, Orthopaedic Surgery, Emory Spine Center, Emory University, Atlanta, Georgia
Disorders, Diseases, and Injuries of the Spine

Steven D. K. Ross, MD
Clinical Professor, Department of Orthopaedic Surgery, University of California, Irvine, College of Medicine, Orange, California
Foot and Ankle Surgery

Jon K. Sekiya, MD
Larry S. Matthews Collegiate Professor of Orthopaedic Surgery, Associate Professor, MedSport–University of Michigan, Ann Arbor, Michigan
Adult Reconstructive Surgery

Harry B. Skinner, MD, PhD
Attending Physician, St. Jude Heritage Medical Group, Fullerton, California; Professor and Chairman, Emeritus, Department of Orthopedic Surgery, University of California, Irvine, College of Medicine
General Considerations in Orthopedic Surgery; Adult Reconstructive Surgery; Disorders, Diseases and Injuries of the Spine; Amputations

Douglas G. Smith, MD
Professor, Department of Orthopedics and Sports Medicine, University of Washington and Harborview Medical Center, Seattle, Washington
Amputations

Wade R. Smith, MD
Associate Professor of Orthopedic Surgery, University of Colorado School of Medicine, Denver, Colorado; Director of Orthopedic Surgery, Denver Health Medical Center, Denver, Colorado
Musculoskeletal Trauma Surgery

Phillip Stahel
Department of Orthopedic Surgery, University of Colorado School of Medicine, Denver, Colorado; Director of Orthopedic Surgery, Denver Health Medical Center, Denver, Colorado
Musculoskeletal Trauma Surgery

Takashi Suzuki, MD
Kitasato University Hospital, Kanagawa, Japan
Musculoskeletal Trauma Surgery

Bobby K. B. Tay, MD
Associate Professor, Department of Orthopaedic Surgery, University of California, San Francisco
Disorder, Diseases, and Injuries of the Spine

Russell Ward, MD
Fellow, American Academy of Orthopaedic Surgeons, Assistant Professor, Department of Surgery, Texas A&M University Health Science Center Sarcoma Services, Director, Department of Orthopedic Surgery, Scott and White Healthcare, Texas
Musculoskeletal Oncology

Kurt R. Weiss, MD
Assistant Professor of Orthopaedic Surgery Division of Musculoskeletal Oncology Director, Cancer/Stem Cell Lab, University of Pittsburgh, Pittsburgh, Pennsylvania
Orthopedic Infections: Basic Principles of Pathogenesis, Diagnosis, and Treatment

a LANGE medical book

CURRENT
Diagnosis & Treatment
in Orthopedics

DATE DUE

15/2/15		

GAYLORD   #3523PI   Printed in USA

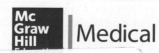

McGraw Hill | **Medical**

New York   Chicago   ...   don   Madrid   Mexico City
Milan   ...   ney   Toronto

Current Diagnosis & Treatment in Orthopedics, Fifth Edition

1 2 3 4 5 6 7 8 9 0   DOC/DOC   18 17 16 15 14 13

ISBN 978-0-07-159075-4
MHID 0-07-159075-7
ISSN: 1081-0056

This book was set in Minion Pro Regular by Cenveo® Publisher Services.
The editors were Brian Belval and Christina M. Thomas.
The production supervisor was Catherine H. Saggese.
Project management was provided by Vastavikta Sharma at Cenveo Publlisher Services.
The cover designer was Thomas De Pierro. Image Credit: © Kallista Images/Visuals Unlimited/Corbis.
RR Donnelley was printer and binder.

This book is printed on acid-free paper.

McGraw-Hill Education books are available at special quantity discounts to use as premiums and sales promotions or for use in corporate training programs. To contact a representative, please visit the contact us pages at http://www.mhprofessional.com.

To my daughters Lacey and Lauren, whose intelligence and beauty astonish me each and every day of my life. They have given me inspiration and motivation to complete this book.

Contents

Preface

This *Current Diagnosis and Treatment in Orthopedics* is the Fifth Edition of the Orthopaedic Surgery contribution to the Lange Current Series of books. It is surprising to realize that it has been 16 years since the first edition of this book. Much has changed in orthopedics since the first edition came out, but the goal of this book has not changed. It is intended to fill a need for a ready source of up-to-date information on disorders and diseases treated by orthopedic surgeons and related physicians. The format in this edition is unchanged from the previous edition: there is emphasis on the major diagnostic features of disease states, the natural history of the disease where appropriate, the workup required for definitive diagnosis, and finally, definitive treatment. The book focuses on orthopedic conditions, deemphasizing the treatment of the patient from a general medical viewpoint, except when it pertains to the orthopedic problem under consideration. Importantly, pathophysiology, epidemiology, and pathology are included when they assist in arriving at a definitive diagnosis or an understanding of the treatment of the disease or condition. In many conditions, such as infection or neoplasm, it is extremely important to understand the pathophysiology because the disease may be encountered at various time points in the progression of the disease.

This edition of *Current Diagnosis and Treatment in Orthopedics* is truly current. The entire book has been updated in its references to include only those references since 2005, except in cases where classic articles are necessary to refer back to major advances in understanding or treatment, or in situations where there has been little change in the subspecialization in orthopedics, such as rehabilitation. These selected references to the older literature represent landmarks in the advancement of the understanding of orthopedic diseases and conditions and serve as useful sources of the fundamental basis for understanding these diseases and conditions.

INTENDED AUDIENCE

The unique format of the Lange series textbooks allows readers of many levels of understanding to derive benefit from the information.

Students will find that the book encompasses virtually all aspects of orthopedics that they will encounter in classes and as subinterns in major teaching institutions. Residents and house officers can use the book as a ready reference covering the majority of disorders and conditions in emergency and elective orthopedic surgery. Despite its small size, it is truly comprehensive. Because of the organization of the book on a subspecialty basis, review of individual chapters will provide house officers rotating on subspecialty orthopedic services with an excellent basis for further in-depth study.

For emergency room physicians, especially those with medical backgrounds, the text provides an excellent resource in managing orthopedic problems seen on an emergent basis. Similarly, family practice, pediatricians, general practitioners, and internists will find the book particularly helpful in the referral decision process and as a resource to explain disorders to patients. Finally, practicing orthopedic surgeons, particularly those in subspecialties of orthopedics, will find the book a helpful resource in reassuring them that their treatment in areas outside their subspecialty interest is current and up-to-date.

ORGANIZATION

The book is structured similarly to the structure of orthopedic surgery. Natural subspecialization has occurred in orthopedic surgery over the years, which has resulted in some overlap in anatomic areas. This has resulted in the book having some overlap and some artificial division of subjects. Because of the primarily subspecialization structure, the reader is encouraged to read entire chapters or, for more discrete topics, go directly to the index for information. For example, the house officer rotating on the pediatric orthopedic service would find reading the pediatric chapter to be a prudent method of developing a baseline knowledge in pediatric orthopedic surgery. Knee problems, however, might be best approached by looking in the sports medicine chapter or in the adult reconstruction chapter, since these areas overlap, mostly in age of patient.

The first chapter introduces aspects of interest in the perioperative care of the orthopedic patient, including social aspects of the patient/physician relationship. This is a new addition and is an outgrowth of the importance of outcomes in orthopedics. Management of orthopedic problems arising from trauma is covered in Chapter 2, while Chapter 3 deals with sports medicine with an emphasis on the knee and shoulder. Chapter 4 covers all aspects of spine surgery, including infection of the spine, degenerative spinal problems, spinal deformity, and spinal trauma.

Chapter 5 provides comprehensive coverage of tumors in orthopedic surgery, including benign and malignant soft-tissue and hard-tissue tumors. Adult joint reconstruction, including the disorders that lead to joint reconstruction, are covered in Chapter 6. In Chapter 7, infections, with their special implications for orthopedic surgery, are covered. Chapter 8 discusses foot and ankle surgery, and Chapter 9, hand surgery. Chapter 10 covers diseases in orthopedics unique to children. The final two chapters deal with amputation and all aspects of rehabilitation fundamental to orthopedic surgeons in returning patients to full function.

OUTSTANDING FEATURES

Illustrations have been carefully selected to maximize their benefits in pointing out orthopedic principles and concepts. The effect of changes in imaging technology on optimal diagnostic studies is emphasized, including cost-effectiveness.

Bone and soft tissue tumor differential diagnoses are simplified by comprehensive tables that categorize tumors by age, location, and imaging characteristics. The molecular basis of the current understanding of tumor etiology is expanded.

Concise, current, and comprehensive treatment of the basic sciences underlying the understanding of orthopedic surgery is provided in individual chapters, where pertinent.

NEW TO THIS EDITION

- Information on shoulder evaluation has been widely expanded, including tables to elucidate the diagnosis of shoulder problems.
- Advances in treatment of back pain, including disk replacement, are included.
- The latest on molecular biology of neoplasms has been expanded in the musculoskeletal tumor section.
- Surgical management of osteoporosis, including techniques such as kyphoplasty and vertebroplasty, and information on shoulder replacement have been widely expanded.
- Guidelines for predicting function, such as ambulatory capability after spinal cord injury, are updated.
- New materials in orthopedics that are making changes in the way replacement arthroplasty is performed are included.
- Hip conditions amenable to arthroscopic treatments are discussed.
- The latest information on important growth factors in orthopedics is elucidated with their current usage.

We are pleased to be able to say, with the concurrence of our coauthors, that these new features added to the information in the previous edition make this edition a significant improvement over the last.

General Considerations in Orthopedic Surgery

Harry B. Skinner, MD, PhD

Orthopedic surgery encompasses the entire process of caring for the surgical patient, from diagnostic evaluation to the preoperative evaluation and through the postoperative and rehabilitative period. Although the surgical procedure itself is the key step toward helping the patient, the preliminary and follow-up care can determine whether the surgery is successful.

DIAGNOSTIC WORKUP

▶ History and Physical Exam

Although it may seem obvious, the history and physical exam are still important in the evaluation of the patient. Every office visit is a history and physical exam, whether a new or a return visit. The completeness of the history and physical has assumed new importance in view of the complexities required for compliance with federal regulations. Regulations require that a chief complaint be specified, and this must be clearly defined because it determines the direction for the rest of the history and physical. The history must address the key features of the problem, both to elucidate the medical problem and to cover the subsidiary requirements for billing purposes. The social history and past medical history are similarly important because they change billing codes without necessarily affecting outcome or success of care. The physical again must cover the essentials necessary for diagnosis, and frequently the confirmation of the diagnosis is based on physical exam, but such considerations as skin condition and blood supply must be documented, despite the fact that this process is also part of the surgical evaluation. The next step is imaging and laboratory exams. The most important point here is to use the most cost-effective examination possible while keeping patient safety, satisfaction, and convenience in mind.

▶ Imaging Studies
A. Roentgenography

Roentgenography is still the most cost-effective and most important initial diagnostic test in the orthopedist's armamentarium.

Almost every patient should have a radiograph prior to going to a more sophisticated imaging study. Certain situations are obvious; for example, a 68-year-old man with knee pain should have standing, flexed-knee posteroanterior (PA), lateral, and merchant plain film views taken. If those views show normal joint spaces, consideration of intraarticular pathology, such as a degenerative meniscus tear, can be worked up with magnetic resonance imaging (MRI). The normal views usually ordered are as follows:

1. **Neck pain—**
   No history of trauma, more than 4 weeks' duration.
   Younger than 35 years: anteroposterior (AP) lateral, odontoid.
   Older than 35 years: obliques.
   History of trauma: flexion/extension laterals (obtain on first visit).

2. **Thoracic spine pain and tenderness—**
   Younger than 40 years, no reason to suspect malignancy: AP and lateral (if history of trauma, or possibility of osteoporosis on first visit, otherwise at 4 weeks).
   Consider cervical (C)-spine as a source of referred pain to thoracic (T)-spine if no tenderness in T-spine.

3. **Lumbar (L)-sacral (S)-spine—**
   Younger than 40 years, no reason to suspect malignancy after 4 weeks' duration of the pain. With significant trauma, at first visit, or possible malignancy (ie, weight loss, malaise, fatigue): AP, lateral.
   Add obliques for chronic low back pain (ie, spondylolisthesis).

4. **Hips—**
   AP pelvis, lateral of affected hip.
   Consider lumbar-sacral (L-S) series if pain is in the buttock rather than in the groin.

5. **Knees—**
   Older than 40 years or history of meniscectomy: Rosenberg, lateral, and sunrise films. Merchant views are similar to sunrise. The Rosenberg view is a 10-degree down

shot of the PA of the knees while standing at 45 degrees of flexion.

For other knees: AP, lateral, and sunrise.

In the child, up to age 16, consider a pelvis film with the complaint of knee pain and negative physical exam referable to the knee.

6. **Femur, tibia, humerus, forearm**—AP and lateral are indicated for trauma, palpable lesions, or suspected tumors.

7. **Ankle**—AP lateral and mortise.

8. **Foot**—AP, lateral, and oblique for routine evaluation.

9. **Shoulder**—AP, axillary, scapular Y, and outlet views.

10. **Elbow**—AP and lateral (true lateral).

11. **Hand/wrist**—

 Hand: PA and lateral.

 Wrist: PA, lateral, and oblique

 For suspected instability: clenched fist PA in radial and ulnar deviation.

Follow-up radiographs are obtained when a change in the radiographic findings is expected. Remember that bone changes occur slowly, so radiographic changes take a comparable length of time. Radiographs are obtained in view of the clinical picture. For example, closed treatment of a distal radius fracture would not be expected to show changes because of healing for a minimum of 2 weeks. However, displacement of the fracture could occur sooner. Hence, radiographs to show displacement might be obtained at 1 week and 2 weeks. If no displacement is observed, the fracture position could be considered stable, and the next films might be obtained at 6 weeks—the earliest time healing might be observed. Similarly, closed treatment of an adult tibia fracture might be followed with radiographs at 2-week intervals, checking for displacement and healing, whereas a tibia fracture treated with an intramedullary rod might be followed at monthly intervals to check for healing.

B. Magnetic Resonance Imaging

This imaging modality is very useful, but like electron beam computed tomography (CT), MRI is sometimes too revealing. This method should be reserved for clarifying a particular problem. Frequently in orthopedics, a bony lesion can be localized with a radiograph or bone scan, which then provides a focus for the MRI. MRI is useful for some bony lesions, such as osteonecrosis, tumors, fatigue fractures, and osteomyelitis. It is also helpful in some soft-tissue problems, such as knee meniscus tears and shoulder rotator cuff tears. Distortion of the magnetic field by metallic implants may limit the usefulness of MRI studies of conditions such as total knee or hip replacement, or fracture fixation devices. MRI should not be used when the diagnosis can be made with a less expensive test. For example, the use of the MRI

in knee studies in patients older than 45 years should always be preceded by plain films of the knee, as noted earlier. An MRI of an arthritic knee adds little additional information because the meniscus and anterior cruciate ligament are likely to be damaged from the arthritic process already. However, the MRI can be very helpful in determining soft-tissue extension of tumors or infection.

The advent of new portable MRI units that perform limited studies with more resolution adds a new dimension to their use. These can provide data on the progression of disorders such as rheumatoid arthritis or osteomyelitis in a timely and cost-effective way. The possibility of osteomyelitis in the bones adjacent to ulcers on the foot is easily determined with this test because it shows the changes, typically edema, in the bone with osteomyelitis. A bone scan usually does not have the resolution to distinguish the inflammatory response in the soft tissue from the bony involvement. Osteomyelitis should be treated much differently from a soft-tissue ulcer, which does not affect the bone.

C. Computed Tomography

The CT scan is an extremely important imaging modality for examining bony lesions such as fractures. Frequently, plain films provide some information about the fracture of interest, but the CT scan provides the three-dimensional information that can only otherwise be determined from the integration of the plain films in the surgeon's mind. The CT scan adds significantly to the management of such fractures as tibial plateaus, scapular fractures, ankle fractures, and cervical and lumbar spine fractures, as well as many others. Furthermore, nonunions of fractures, with or without fixation, can be identified and followed with CT scans. Again, if little information can be gained that cannot be already discerned from the plain films, the CT scan only adds expense and patient inconvenience. The spiral CT makes imaging with this modality less expensive and much more rapid. The CT scan is also now the method of choice for determining whether a pulmonary embolus (PE) has occurred. Again, a CT for this indication is easier on the patient, more accurate, and less invasive than angiography.

D. Technetium-99m Bone Scan

The bone scan finds many uses in orthopedic surgery. Keep in mind that the bone scan labels the osteoblast activity with the radioactive tracer, technetium-99; thus, bone formation activity is recorded, and little or no bone resorption activity is noted. Any disorder that results in increased bone formation, therefore, results in a "hot" bone scan. This means that a disorder such as multiple myeloma may not show up on a bone scan because only osteoclastic activity is involved in the majority of lesions. This test is helpful in discerning loose total hip and total knee prostheses, however, even though the findings are nonspecific. It is very helpful in examining probable benign bone lesions because a cold bone scan largely rules out an aggressive process such as a malignancy. The bone scan is also helpful in diagnosing any disorder of unknown origin when there is pain localized to a particular region. A cold bone scan implies that the problem is a soft-tissue one, whereas a hot bone scan points to a region that may benefit from MRI.

▶ Laboratory Exams

The two most important laboratory exams are for C-reactive protein and the erythrocyte sedimentation rate. These two tests indicate whether an inflammatory process, malignancy, or rheumatologic disorder is a diagnostic consideration. If these tests are negative, systemic causes of a complaint can frequently be ruled out. In that situation, a more localized disorder should be identified. The next most important test is the complete blood count, which provides the general indication of the patient's health, revealing information about anemia, infectious processes, and so on. The next most useful laboratory test for the orthopedic surgeon is the synovial fluid analysis. This test typically should include a culture and sensitivity. If there is any concern about infection, a cell count, differential, protein, and glucose measurement should be performed. Crystals should be looked for because they indicate chondrocalcinosis or gout. Elevated protein and reduced glucose levels suggest infection. The final factor that should be considered with any major surgery is the patient's nutritional status, which is evaluated with several tests, including lymphocyte count and levels of prealbumin, albumin, zinc, and serum iron transferrin. In addition, the Mini Nutritional Assessment is a nursing tool to screen elderly individuals at risk of malnutrition.

▶ Educating and Informing Patients and Their Families

Surgical procedures in orthopedics have varying degrees of difficulty and importance, ranging from a relatively simple claw toe correction to the performance of a multilevel complex spinal fusion. After the decision to employ surgery as a therapeutic modality is made, it is important to help the patient completely understand what to expect before, during, and after surgery. This process, which the legal profession calls **informed consent**, has the more important purpose of ensuring the patient's cooperation and satisfaction.

To comply with the requirements of the legal profession and accrediting organizations, such as the Joint Commission on Accreditation of Healthcare Organizations (JCAHO), the surgeon must provide an explanation of the risks, prognosis, alternatives, and complications that might be encountered. The risks should be reviewed in some detail for the general risks encountered in typical orthopedic surgical procedures. The risks and the complications that occur in surgery are intimately associated and thus must be dealt with together. The alternatives are sometimes straightforward. For example, a patient with an open fracture has a high risk of infection if not adequately treated with irrigation, debridement,

and antibiotics. Thus, in such a situation, any reasonable and prudent person would consent to the procedure. The choice between alternatives can become significantly more subtle, however. For example, it is possible that a choice must be made between two different procedures or between a particular procedure and no procedure. In this situation, the surgeon must consider the psychosocial and physical attributes of the patient so as to assist him or her in making this decision. For example, consider men, both 75 years of age, with severe degenerative disease in the right knee noted on radiograph. One individual is now at the point where he cannot play golf, a situation that is reducing his physical exercise and a number of his social outlets. The other individual leads a relatively sedentary lifestyle, seldom walks more than a block, and obtains cardiorespiratory exercise by swimming, an activity in which his knee does not bother him. The surgeon should recommend knee replacement to one individual but not the other. At the same time, both men must be offered the alternatives, which include continued nonsteroidal anti-inflammatory medicine, bracing, sleeping medication, and analgesics.

Patients with an active lifestyle are becoming much more concerned about what will happen to them in the postoperative period, including how soon they can safely travel, when they can work, and when they will be fully able to take care of themselves. They are also concerned about what social services are available to help them if they cannot care for themselves fully. The surgeon must be prepared to address these questions and also advise patients with lower extremity or spinal problems about when they will be able to walk. In the same manner, after procedures on the hand or upper extremity, patients must be advised about when they will be able to use the hand. Advising the patient of these situations before surgery can prevent unexpected surprises in the postoperative period.

The patient should also be informed about the range of expectations for ambulation or use of the upper extremity because individuals vary in their response to surgery. For example, patients should be advised that after surgery on the hip or knee, they will need a walker for a few days, move to crutches, and typically be done with the crutches in the range of 2–4 weeks. They will use a cane before 6 weeks and be done with the cane before 3 months. Patients' response to surgery is somewhat unpredictable, so conservative estimates on the length of medication use, pain, restricted driving, and so on are prudent. Patients should be cautioned about travel after surgery, particularly with lower extremity injuries, because of the risk of deep venous thrombosis (DVT). In such cases, discourage (for the first 6–12 weeks) plane trips longer than an hour and extended car trips made without stopping perhaps every 45 minutes. Anti-inflammatory medication (to reduce platelet adhesion) or anticoagulants should be recommended if such travel is unavoidable.

A. Explaining the Procedures

An essential part of the patient's presurgical preparation and postsurgical cooperation is knowing what to expect at every step in the process. Nuances become important in the process of explaining the surgical procedures and their implications. For example, scheduling a bunion procedure 2 weeks prior to a patient's participation in her daughter's wedding could upset the patient if she fails to realize that she will be unable to wear the shoes she purchased for the event. Similarly, lifestyle considerations can affect the decision-making process in cases of medial gonarthrosis, in which the choice between a unicompartmental knee replacement and a high tibial osteotomy could be influenced by whether the patient plays tennis and holds a physically strenuous job or, alternatively, whether the patient is sedentary and works behind a desk most of the day.

B. Reviewing the Risks and Possible Complications

Reviewing the perioperative risks is important for all patients and optimally should be done well in advance and then repeated closer to the time of surgery. Some patients require more detailed explanations, particularly if their relatives have undergone surgery in the past and had a problem with anesthesia or a complication such as a PE or infection. Based on the patient's responses to explanations, the health care team members need to alter their approach to reach a balance between inadequately informing the patient and inducing unnecessary alarm that could make the patient refuse to undergo a procedure judged to be both beneficial and necessary.

Risk is a poorly understood concept in our culture. Some situations are considered to be higher in risk than they actually are. Some risks are understood better than others. It can help the patient to understand if these risks are put in perspective. The risks can be surprisingly high or low but still disturbing to the patient. For example, many people have moved away from California to avoid an earthquake or refuse to fly commercial aircraft because of the risk, not realizing that the risk of death is 10–100 times higher while driving a car (Table 1–1). This lack of understanding of the risk can contribute to significant differences in the perception of liability associated with these activities. For example, the death benefit from a commercial airline accident might reach several million dollars per passenger, whereas death in an automobile accident might have no death benefit at all. Thus, the *perception* of risk is very important and must be clarified in the patient's mind. Similarly, patients can understand and accept having a myocardial infarction after a major surgery because they can clearly see the strain on the heart from the surgery. However, they are not nearly as understanding of a lower extremity paralysis that can result from the epidural anesthetic for that surgery. The explanation of risks must be individualized for each patient. The patient with a previous myocardial infarction is clearly different from the healthy 20-year-old (see Table 2–1). Across-the-board rates of problems do not translate into direct risks for the individual patient.

Table 1–1. Rates of death and complications associated with common activities.

Death or Complication	Percentage
Death (from MI after previous MI)	1
Major bleed (7 days, warfarin, INR 2.65)	0.02
GI ulcer/bleed perforation (naproxen 6 months)	1
Paralysis (from epidural)	0.02
Death (frequent flying professor/year)	0.001
Death (automobile/year)	0.016
Earthquake in California/per year	0.00018

GI, gastrointestinal; INR, international normalized ratio; MI, myocardial infarction.

Although all procedures carry some risks, the incidence and type of risks and complications vary with the surgical procedure as well as with the patient's age and general health. Potential problems are listed and discussed here in alphabetical order.

1. Amputation—The potential problem of amputation is seldom of acute concern except in cases of significant trauma. The topic of amputation can frequently be discussed with the risk of infection because ischemia and infection can increase the risk of amputation.

2. Anesthesia—One of the major risks in orthopedic surgery is associated with anesthesia, not because complications of anesthesia are frequent but because they can be devastating. Death occurs at a rate of approximately 1 in 200,000 patients undergoing elective anesthesia. Other complications include, but are not limited to, the following: nerve damage and paraplegia from nerve blocks, headaches from dural leaks following use of spinal anesthetics, aspiration of stomach contents, and cardiac problems, including ischemia and arrhythmias. The surgeon should discuss these problems with the patient only in general terms, allowing the anesthesiologist to provide the most detailed explanations.

3. Arthritis—Virtually any procedure that enters a joint, other than to replace it, has the potential to cause damage to that joint. In some instances, as in an intraarticular fracture, the surgery will likely lessen the risk of arthritis. Even in these instances, the patient should be told that the risk of damage is still real because the joint surface healing will not result in a normal cartilage surface.

4. Blood loss—Patients should be given a reasonably accurate estimate of blood loss as well as the opportunity to donate autologous blood prior to surgery. Designated donor blood is probably not safer but gives the patient who receives it a sense of security. The use of erythropoietin can elevate preoperative hemoglobin (Hgb) levels in selected cases and thereby reduce postoperative homologous blood transfusion needs. Other alternatives include the use of intraoperative blood salvage for reinfusion (OrthoPAT, Sure-Trans, Constavac). The use of erythropoietin is generally accepted by Jehovah's Witness patients, whereas the autologous reinfusion acceptance is variable. To help minimize blood loss during surgery, the patient's use of nonsteroidal anti-inflammatory drugs (NSAIDs) should be discontinued approximately 2 weeks before surgery. Discontinuation of NSAIDs can significantly compromise comfort and incite rheumatoid flares in many patients who rely on these drugs. To minimize the risk, newer cyclooxygenase-2 (COX-2) inhibitor NSAIDs may be used as a substitute during this period; no platelet disorder or bleeding time derangement occurs with these drugs because they do not affect platelet function or inhibit thromboxane A_2.

5. Blood vessel damage—Arterial and venous damage take on greater significance as the size of the vessel increases and the arterial supply becomes more calcified with age and vascular disease. Patients generally understand this, but it must be emphasized where appropriate. Hip and knee replacement puts unusual strains on the femoral and popliteal vessels, from positioning, and may damage calcified arteries.

6. Deep venous thrombosis/pulmonary embolism—Virtually all lower extremity and spine procedures in orthopedics involve some risk of DVT, which should be explained to the patient. As many as 40–60% of patients who undergo a relatively high-risk procedure such as total hip arthroplasty develop DVT if not receiving thromboprophylaxis. The risk of PE is much less, however, and is in the range of 0.3% for fatal emboli. This rate of fatal PE is approximately a 10-fold increase over the rate of fatal PE in the U.S. population in men older than 65 years. The risks associated with other procedures may be lower. In any case, the patient should be reassured that prevention procedures commensurate with risk will be undertaken.

7. Fracture—Many procedures in orthopedic surgery carry the risk of a bone fracture. Some procedures, such as uncemented hip replacement, present a higher risk for this complication, but virtually any orthopedic procedure could result in fracture of a bone. The patient must be informed of the risk in relation to the probability of the occurrence of such a problem.

8. Infection—The risk of infection in orthopedic surgery ranges from near zero in procedures such as arthroscopy to several percent in open fracture surgery. The problem of infection should be emphasized in proportion to risk. For example, if a diabetic patient is to undergo knee replacement,

he or she should not only be assured that all steps will be taken to prevent infection (eg, administration of prophylactic antibiotics, use of ultrafiltration of air, or ultraviolet lights in the operating room) but should also be told of the various techniques that would be considered if infection occurred. These options include debridement, prosthesis removal, gastrocnemius flap, reinsertion, arthrodesis, and amputation. The common use of external fixation devices for fracture care is accompanied by the frequent problems associated with pin care. The patient and family should be informed about the problems caused by percutaneous devices to prevent the presumption that something has gone wrong. Skin problems are frequently associated with infection but may arise from other causes, such as adjacent scars compromising the blood supply to a surgical flap. Older patients and individuals who are smokers, have diabetes and/or obesity, or have wounds on the distal lower extremity are at increased risk. In such cases, the patient may be warned that delayed healing or necrosis of the skin edges may occur.

9. Loss of reduction—Although fracture care continues to improve, displacement of hardware or fracture fragments may necessitate a second procedure. The explanation of this risk should be individualized, based on the type of fracture. Loss of reduction may contribute to delayed union or nonunion of fractures. These problems may occur despite optimal care by the orthopedic surgeon. Poor vascular supply or smoking can be a factor leading to nonunion. The rate of nonunion is site dependent but is only a few percent.

10. Nerve damage—Certain procedures are associated with nerve damage, although the damage is usually minor. For example, medial parapatellar incisions on the knee cause some numbness from cutting the infrapatellar branch of the saphenous nerve. The patient should be informed in advance if some degree of minor nerve damage is anticipated in association with the particular surgical procedure being pursued and should also be informed of the risks of unexpected nerve damage that accompany all surgical procedures.

C. Prognosis

The patient's prognosis is intimately related to the procedure. However, certain guidelines may be given. The expected time off work or time away from activities is important to the patient and depends on the patient's occupation, age, and available sick leave. The bank president with more control over her agenda will be able to return to work activities sooner than the day laborer. Driving is an important activity for many people, and limitations placed by a procedure can determine how much postoperative assistance a patient will need.

    The patient should be given reasonable expectations about range of motion, strength, possible disability, and when these should return to normal, if at all. Furthermore, walking or writing ability, ability to use a computer keyboard, and the time to expect to be able to do such activities may be appropriate for some patients. Again, these have to be individualized for each patient and determined for each home situation.

D. Keeping the Patient and Family Informed

Immediately before elective surgery, the surgeon can help comfort the patient and family by meeting them in the preoperative area and appearing relaxed, well rested, and positive about the outcome of the surgery. Giving the family a good estimate of the surgery time is important, but they should also be reassured that delays do not necessarily indicate the occurrence of complications that are detrimental to the patient. If the family members wish to be notified about delays, they should be encouraged to leave instructions about where they can be contacted. When surgery is completed and the patient is no longer at risk of untoward accidents such as aspiration during extubation, a member of the surgical team should apprise the family of the outcome. At this time, it is appropriate to emphasize particular concerns to the family, such as the need to continue vigilance for infection in a diabetic patient who has undergone foot surgery.

Geerts WH, Bergqvist D, Pineo GF, et al: Prevention of venous thromboembolism. Antithrombotic and thrombolytic therapy, ACCP Evidence-Based Clinical Practice Guidelines (8th Edition). *Chest* 2008;133(Suppl):381S. [PMID: 18574271]

Johnson BF, Manzo RA, Bergelin RO, Strandness DE Jr: Relationship between changes in the deep venous system and the development of the postthrombotic syndrome after an acute episode of lower limb deep vein thrombosis. A one- to six-year follow-up. *J Vasc Surg* 1995;21:307. [PMID: 7853603]

Lilienfeld DE: Decreasing mortality from pulmonary embolism in the United States, 1979–1996. *Int J Epidemiol* 2000;29:465. [PMID: 10869318]

Lilienfeld DE, Godbold JH: Geographic distribution of pulmonary embolism mortality rates in the United States, 1980 to 1984. *Am Heart J* 1992;124:1068. [PMID: 1529881]

McKee MD, DiPasquale DJ, Wild LM, et al: The effect of smoking on clinical outcome and complication rates following Ilizarov reconstruction. *J Orthop Trauma* 2003;17:663. [PMID: 14600564]

Mini Nutritional Assessment. Available at: http://www.mna-elderly.com/forms/MNA_english.pdf.

Nosanchuk JS: Quantitative microbiologic study of blood salvaged by intraoperative membrane filtration. *Arch Pathol Lab Med* 2001;125:1204. [PMID: 11520273]

Schneider D, Lilienfeld, DE: The epidemiology of pulmonary embolism: racial contrasts in incidence and in-hospital case fatality. *J Natl Med Assoc* 2006;98:1967. [PMID: 17225843]

Sweetland S, Green J, Liu B, et al: Duration of the magnitude of the postoperative risk of venous thromboembolism in middle aged women: prospective cohort study. *BMJ* 2009;339:b4583. [PMID: 19959589]

Warner C: The use of the orthopaedic perioperative autotransfusion (OrthoPAT) system in total joint replacement surgery. *Orthop Nurs* 2001;20:29. [PMID: 12025800]

SURGICAL MANAGEMENT

▶ Preoperative Care

A. The Team Approach

Inclusion of nurses, residents, anesthesiologists, and other members of the surgical team in the planning process can improve the efficiency and therefore affect the outcome of a surgical procedure. Good estimates of the length of the operative procedure and of the patient's anticipated blood loss and muscle relaxation requirements minimize the risks from anesthesia and surgery. Reviewing the site of the operation and assessing the need for any special supplies and equipment, such as prostheses, lasers, or fracture tables, also contribute to efficiency and optimal results. Special care must be exercised by all members of the operative team to prevent "wrong side" surgery. It is now a JCAHO standard to have the surgical team "mark" the surgical site.

B. Preparing and Positioning the Patient

Once the patient is in the operating room, every effort should be made to make him or her comfortable. A calm, efficient, and professional demeanor by everyone involved is necessary both before and after anesthesia is induced. If the anesthesiologist indicates that placement of the anti-thromboembolic hose, intermittent pneumatic compression stockings, or tourniquets will improve efficiency, these can be put in place prior to induction. Placement of arterial lines, central lines, and Foley catheters should be done after the patient is anesthetized, if possible. Location of the operating table must be adjusted to ensure good lighting, optimize the efficiency of the surgeon and staff, and allow for maintenance of surgical sterile technique.

Positioning of the patient is the responsibility of both the surgeon and the anesthesiologist to facilitate the operation and to ensure the patient's safety. A perfectly executed operation can be marred by a nerve palsy that results from the failure to pad a remote area appropriately. If the patient is placed in the lateral decubitus position, the peroneal nerve at the knee and the brachial plexus of the downside shoulder girdle must be protected. During shoulder surgery, the surgeon must take care to avoid stretching the patient's brachial plexus or cervical nerve roots while attempting to maximize the operative field. Similarly, the patient's shoulder should not be abducted past 90 degrees, and joints with contractures should not be forced into unusual positions. These precautions are particularly necessary in treating rheumatoid patients or older osteoporotic patients. Injury to the extremities and loss of lines can be avoided by careful planning and synchronization when positioning patients into the lateral decubitus position or prone position.

▶ C. Use of Antibiotics

Except in cases in which concern about infection requires unambiguous cultures to be obtained, prophylactic antibiotics have been mandated to be started within 1 hour prior to skin incision by JCAHO. A first- or second-generation cephalosporin antibiotic is considered appropriate for orthopedic procedures. JCAHO has also mandated that prophylactic antibiotics be stopped within 24 hours of orthopedic surgery.

D. Use of a Tourniquet

A tourniquet can be extremely helpful in some procedures and is practically mandatory for others. The tourniquet stops the flow of blood to and from an extremity. To achieve this, the pneumatic tourniquet is inflated to a pressure that must be significantly higher than the arterial pressure because the pressure is dissipated in the soft tissue underneath the tourniquet.

1. Tourniquet size and placement—The tourniquet should be wide enough for the extremity while still permitting adequate exposure of the extremity. Particularly in cases involving surgery on muscles that cross the elbow or knee, the tourniquet should be placed as proximal as possible to ensure the muscles have adequate stretch to permit full joint motion. When a tourniquet is used on a large extremity with a great deal of adipose tissue, care must be taken to ensure that the tourniquet does not slip distally, which could result in wrinkles in the tourniquet and localized pressure on the skin. Slippage can be prevented by applying 5-cm (2-in) adhesive tape to the skin in a longitudinal direction below the cast padding placed under the tourniquet.

2. Tourniquet time and pressure—The effects of tourniquets on tissues are a combination of time and pressure on individual structures. Neural and muscle tissue are most sensitive, with deleterious effects arising from direct pressure to structures and from distal ischemia.

Several considerations are involved in the selection of the level of tourniquet pressure. First, the level must be low enough to avoid pressure damage to sensitive neural structures but high enough so the pressure around the arterial supply to the extremity is greater than systolic pressure (Figure 1–1). Second, if the patient's blood pressure is labile, a margin of safety is usually necessary. The 2009 Association of Perioperative Registered Nurses (AORN) recommendation is to use a graduated increment in pressure above the measured occlusion pressure. Thus, the incremental increases are 40, 60, and 80 mm Hg for occlusion pressures of <130, 131–190, and >190 mm Hg, respectively. The measured occlusion pressure is defined as the pressure at which arterial flow to an extremity is stopped. If the tourniquet is on an extremity with a great deal of adipose tissue, higher pressures may be necessary to achieve adequate pressure at the artery to stop blood flow. Tourniquets should be calibrated and can be tested with an independent pressure measurement device or alternatively calibrated by palpation of the pulse and gradual elevation of pressure until the pulse disappears.

Complications will arise if tourniquets are used at high pressure for too long. The effects can sometimes be mitigated by using wider cuffs and curved cuffs, which allow for higher and

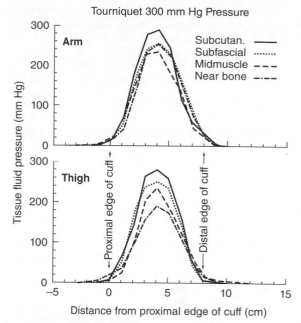

▲ **Figure 1–1.** Distribution of tissue fluid pressure at four depths beneath pneumatic tourniquet with cuff pressure of 300 mm Hg applied on arms (top) and thighs (bottom). Values represent means for six limbs on each graph. (Reproduced, with permission, from Hargens AR, McClure AG, Skyhar MJ, et al: Local compression patterns beneath pneumatic tourniquets applied to arms and thighs of human cadavers. *J Orthop Res* 1987;5:247.)

more uniform pressure below the tourniquet. A rule of thumb is that tourniquet pressures should not be elevated for longer than 2 hours, and less time is preferable. In a canine study of the muscle tissue distal to the tourniquet, investigators found that 90-minute tourniquet times with 5 minutes between reinflation minimized the ischemic damage. This finding points to the need for efficiency in performing surgical procedures under tourniquet. After tourniquet release, reflex hyperemia and edema are frequently encountered, making closure more difficult. Exsanguination with an Esmarch bandage prior to tourniquet inflation facilitates emptying of large veins of the thigh and arm, although it is not recommended to use an Esmarch in trauma cases. Careful exsanguination may help prevent DVT, especially when reinflation of the tourniquet is planned.

Barwell J, Anderson G, Hassan A, Rawlings I: The effects of early tourniquet release during total knee arthroplasty: A prospective randomized double-blind study. *J Bone Joint Surg Br* 1997;79:265. [PMID: 9119854]

Classen DC, Evans RS, Pestotnik SL, et al: The timing of prophylactic administration of antibiotics and the risk of surgical wound infection. *N Engl J Med* 1992;326:281. [PMID: 1728731]

Fernandez AH, Monge V, Garcinuno MA: Surgical antibiotic prophylaxis: effect in postoperative infections. *Eur J Epidemiol* 2001;17:369. [PMID: 11767963]

Hargens AR, McClure AG, Skyhar MJ, et al: Local compression patterns beneath pneumatic tourniquets applied to arms and thighs of human cadavers. *J Orthop Res* 1987;5:247. [PMID: 3572594]

Idusuyi OB, Morrey BF: Peroneal nerve palsy after total knee arthroplasty. Assessment of predisposing and prognostic factors. *J Bone Joint Surg Am* 1996;78:177. [PMID: 8609107]

Noordin S, McEwen JA, Kragh JF Jr, et al: Current concepts review: surgical tourniquets in orthopaedics. *J Bone Joint Surg Am* 2009;91A:2958. [PMID: 19952261]

Ostman B, Michaelsson K, Rahme H, Hillered L: Tourniquet-induced ischemia and reperfusion in human skeletal muscle. *Clin Orthop Relat Res* 2004;418:260. [PMID: 15043128]

Pedowitz RA, Gershuni DH, Botte MJ, et al: The use of lower tourniquet inflation pressures in extremity surgery facilitated by curved and wide tourniquets and an integrated cuff inflation system. *Clin Orthop Relat Res* 1993;287:237. [PMID: 8448950]

Sapega AA, Heppenstall RB, Chance B, et al: Optimizing tourniquet application and release times in extremity surgery. *J Bone Joint Surg Am* 1985;67: 303. [PMID: 3968122]

Wakai A, Winter DC, Street JT, Redmond PH: Pneumatic tourniquets in extremity surgery. *J Am Acad Orthop Surg* 2001;9:345. [PMID: 11575914]

▶ Operative Care

The surgical team should make every effort to work efficiently during the period between the administration of anesthesia and the conclusion of the final steps of preoperative preparation, which may take from 10 to 30 minutes or longer. It is in the best interests of the patient to minimize the time between onset of anesthesia and the beginning of surgery.

A. Incision Sites and Approaches

Although the surgical wound "heals side-to-side, not end-to-end," the incorrect placement or the excessive length of a surgical incision for a given procedure only serves to increase surgical trauma to the patient, slow the healing process, and lengthen the rehabilitation period. If there is any doubt about the surgical incision site, roentgenographic examination should be considered. Use of an image intensifier should be considered in obese patients or in patients with previous surgery and retained hardware.

The incision should be made perpendicular to the skin, generally longitudinally, and with a sharp knife. In tumor biopsies, longitudinal incisions are always made. The approach by the surgeon through the subcutaneous fatty layer is variable and depends on the location on the body. In most areas, sharp dissection with a knife through the subcutaneous tissue to the fascial layer is indicated. In the upper extremity and in areas where cutaneous nerves can be troublesome if injured, blunt dissection is used because cutaneous nerves travel in the fatty tissue. Many surgeons prefer blunt dissection with scissors used to spread tissue perpendicular to the wound. Hemostasis is obtained layer by layer. Subcutaneous fat usually is not dissected from the skin, because this might devascularize it.

Surgeons must be extremely careful with the skin, making sure to avoid crushing it when forceps are used. The skin should never be clamped, nor should it be excessively stretched. A larger incision is much better for the skin than extreme tension. Care of the soft tissues includes keeping them moist, avoiding excessive retraction, and being especially careful of neurovascular bundles. Nerves suffer damage from both traction and compression. Nerve palsies and paresthesias can spoil an otherwise well-performed operation in the eyes of both the surgeon and the patient. Care of the cartilage includes keeping it moist because drying has a deleterious effect.

Surgical approaches that go through internerve planes, such as between the deltoid and the pectoralis major, should be used to avoid denervation of muscles. The splitting of muscles in the surgical approach should also be avoided because splitting is generally more traumatic and more likely to denervate the muscle. This rule does not always apply in tumor surgery because it is important to keep tumor cells in a single compartment.

B. Orthopedic Instruments and Drains

It is mandatory that tools be sharp at all times because the sharpness enables the surgeon to avoid the excessive pressure that creates problems by plunging into the depths of the wound. When an osteotome or elevator is needed, the concurrent use of a hammer is preferred because achieving exact control is possible by the strength and number of hammer taps, whereas control is difficult to achieve by pushing on an osteotome. With drill points and power saws, the sharpness of the instruments should be maintained to reduce necrosis secondary to heating and to facilitate the operation. Unless using a drill guide, the surgeon should start drilling bone in a perpendicular direction even though the final direction may be at some angle to the direction of the bone. This prevents slipping off the desired bone entry point. Holes in long bones are stress concentration sites. Care should be taken to minimize the likelihood and degree of stress concentration by rounding holes and using drill holes to terminate saw cuts (Figure 1–2). When holes were made in bone, especially in the lower extremity, the patient should be advised against torsional loading.

Obtaining hemostasis in bone can be troublesome, and the use of microcrystalline collagen is preferred to bone wax because of the foreign body response. Postoperative bleeding is common from bony surfaces. Despite the traditional use of drains by surgeons, evidence is accumulating that at least for some operations, such as total hip or total knee replacement, wound drainage may not be necessary and may lead to increased blood loss. If drains are used, they should be secured to prevent accidental removal and should be large

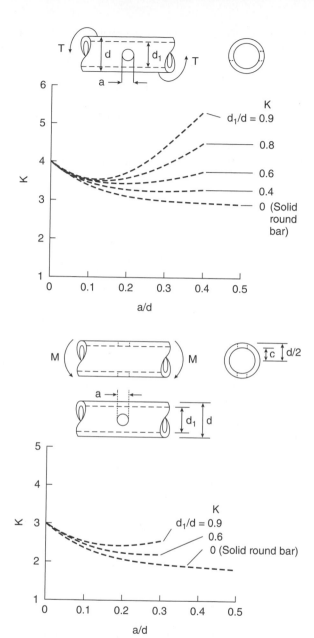

▲ **Figure 1–2.** Stress concentration factors for torsion (top) or bending (bottom) of a round bar or tube with a transverse hole, where a = the size of the hole; d = the outside diameter of the tube; d_1 = the inside diameter of the tube; K = the stress concentration factor, defined as the factor by which stress is increased by the hole; M = the bending moment; and T = the torsional load. (Modified and reproduced, with permission, from Peterson RE: *Stress Concentration Factors: Charts and Relations Useful in Making Strength Calculations for Machine Parts and Structural Elements.* New York, NY: Wiley; 1974.)

enough to prevent clogging by clot formation. Drains are generally removed within 48 hours of surgery unless they are used to eliminate dead space.

C. Closure and Dressing

Wound closure should be done quickly and efficiently to minimize total operative and anesthesia time. It should also be accomplished carefully to avoid damage to the skin. When a previous scar is entered, it is sometimes worthwhile to remove scar tissue from the edge of the skin, as well as from the subcutaneous tissue, to provide a more vascular area for healing. Meticulous subcutaneous wound closure is necessary to avoid tension on the skin in many areas on the extremities. Four-throw square knots are important for knot security, especially when plans call for use of continuous passive motion machines or early motion, which may apply repetitive stress to the wound before it heals. Barbed sutures, while eliminating knots, may not be as strong in maintaining tissue apposition. Tissue adhesives are an advent in wound closure. One study found sutures were significantly better than adhesives for minimizing dehiscence of incisions, although the adhesives generally resulted in a more cosmetic wound.

Dressings should be padded with cotton or gauze to discourage the formation of hematomas. Closed wound suction drainage does not change outcome and is associated with a higher infection rate and higher transfusion rate in total knee arthroplasty. Tape should be avoided when possible because it sometimes causes allergic reactions, and also the combination of wound swelling and shear from the tape can lead to blistering and other problems.

Batra EK, Franz DA, Towler MA, et al: Influence of surgeon's tying technique on knot security. *J Appl Biomater* 1993;4:241. [PMID: 10146307]

Brown MD, Brookfield KF: A randomized study of closed wound suction drainage for extensive lumbar spine surgery. *Spine* 2004;29:1066. [PMID: 15131430]

Coulthard P, Esposito M, Worthington HV, et al: Tissue adhesives for closure of surgical incisions. *Cochrane Database Syst Rev* 2010;2:CD004287. [PMID: 20464728]

Hazarika S, Bhattacharya R, Bhavikatti M, Dawson M: A comparison of post-op haemoglobin levels and allogeneic blood transfusion rates following total knee arthroplasty without drainage or with reinfusion drains. *Acta Orthop Belg* 2010;76:74. [PMID: 20306968]

Minnema B, Vearncombe M, Augustin A, et al: Risk factors for surgical site infections following primary total knee arthroplasty. *Infect Control Hosp Epidemiol* 2004;25:477. [PMID: 15242195]

Ong CC, Jacobsen AS, Joseph VT: Comparing wound closure using tissue glue versus subcuticular suture for pediatric surgical incisions: a prospective randomized trial. *Pediatr Surg Int* 2002;18:553. [PMID: 12415411]

Torcchia AM, Aho HN, Sobol G: A re-exploration of the use of barbed sutures in flexor tendon repairs. *Orthopedics* 2009;32:10. [PMID: 19824603]

POSTOPERATIVE CARE

▶ Inpatient Care

Postoperative care begins in the postanesthesia room and is the same for both inpatients and outpatients. It is imperative that the orthopedic surgeon takes an active and early role in the treatment of the postoperative patient, including pain management, blood management, and DVT prophylaxis. As soon as practicable, neurologic and vascular evaluation of the operated area should be made. Sensory and motor exam of the pertinent upper or lower extremity nerves should be documented as soon as practical. Early vascular surgery consultation is indicated if pulses are absent or diminished. The wound site should be checked for excessive drainage, and, when appropriate, compartment syndrome should be considered. The general medical condition of the patient, although primarily the concern of the anesthesiologist, should be evaluated to be sure the anesthesiologist is aware of special concerns regarding the individual patient.

During the subsequent postoperative period, orthopedic aspects of care are relatively routine for most procedures. The main responsibility of the orthopedic surgeon is the evaluation of the vascular and neural status of the extremities affected by the surgery, as well as pain control and vigilance for disorders such as DVT or PE. The frequency of postsurgical examinations depends on the clinical setting. Hourly examinations may be necessary in the face of a potential compartment syndrome, although daily examinations are usually adequate. Epidural morphine analgesia may significantly mute or alter the pain picture in a compartment syndrome, making accurate clinical evaluation difficult, if not impossible, in the immediate postoperative period.

A. Pain Management

Pain management is a major issue in the United States. There has been a concern that patients are undermedicated and not achieving adequate pain control. The public has embraced this concept, resulting in litigation and disciplinary action by state medical boards for undermedication. Physicians traditionally were seen as being reluctant to prescribe narcotic medication as a result of concerns that they would be disciplined by state medical boards. This concept has led to a major initiative by the JCAHO to address pain control as a patient "right." JCAHO mandates that pain control be a factor in the total evaluation of the patient and pain evaluation be performed as the fifth vital sign. The scale used is the numeric scale from 0 to 10, similar to the visual analogue scale, with 0 being no pain and 10 being unbearable pain. Patients typically have no real standards upon which to assign their pain scores, resulting in frequent use of a "10" score, or higher. This scale can be explained to the patient in more understandable terms as follows: 1–3 is "nuisance" pain, 4–6 is "distracting" pain, 7–9 is "disabling" pain, and 10 is "worst possible pain." This more functional

scale is easier to use by the patient. Acceptable pain levels are defined as 4 and below.

Pain is a very subjective sensation that is an emotional response to the process of nociception: the sum of four separate components beginning with tissue damage, which results in the first component, transduction to a nerve impulse. The next component is transmission to the spinal cord, where the third component occurs: modulation. This modulated signal is then perceived in the cerebral cortex (perception). Pain perception depends on culture, ethnicity, and gender. It is nonlinear, in that a stimulus two times higher does not necessarily result in twice the pain. Pain perception is also based on patient expectations. Studies show that preoperative patient education can reduce patients' pain after major (eg, total knee arthroplasty [TKA]) orthopedic surgery.

Traditional postoperative pain management included the administration of intravenous (IV) or intramuscular narcotic analgesics until oral narcotics were able to control the pain. Patient-controlled analgesia (PCA) is now a mainstay. In this system, morphine is usually used as the analgesic and typically administered IV at a rate of 1 mg/h with a patient-controlled dose of 1 mg, which can be administered as often as every 10 minutes. Doses can be increased or decreased to tailor the dose to the patient. Dosing at this level can result in depressed respiration in some patients. However, more cautious dosing can result in insufficient pain relief that can stress the heart, leading to myocardial ischemia in some patients. Other problems can result from traditional pain management with narcotics. Patient rehabilitation can be delayed; nausea, vomiting, constipation, hallucinations, and disorientation can result in lengthened hospital stay and patient dissatisfaction.

Alternative postoperative analgesic methods have been utilized. These include epidural and intrathecal administration of local anesthetics and analgesics on a continuous and one-shot basis. These methods have the potential of providing significant pain relief but must be balanced against the alternatives available and the drawbacks that each presents. The one-shot method of adding morphine to the spinal or epidural anesthetic provides pain relief for a limited time, usually on the order of 12–24 hours, although a longer acting form of morphine (DepoDur) has come on the market for single-injection epidural use, providing pain relief for up to 48 hours. It has the additional problem of limiting additional narcotic analgesia by other routes because overdosing may be possible. Long-term use of continuous epidural or intrathecal analgesia poses the problem of inhibiting rehabilitation. Nurses and physical therapists tend not to mobilize patients with catheters into the spinal canal, and in some hospitals, these patients are mandated to go to the intensive care unit. Nerve blocks and injections into joint cavities are limited by the length of action of the local anesthetic agent. Nerve blocks must address all nerves to an area to control postoperative pain. Hence, studies show best results with a longer-term effect achieved by the use of pumps that provide a continuous anesthetic flow into the joint or body cavity, with some designs allowing an intermittent bolus for more pain relief. These pumps typically use a long-acting agent such as bupivacaine (0.25% or 0.5%) and infuse at the rate of 2 or more mL/h. Ropivacaine is reported to have vasoconstrictive properties and less cardiotoxicity than bupivacaine, although at a higher cost. Studies suggest damage to chondrocytes from exposure to local anesthetics such as lidocaine, bupivacaine, and ropivacaine, with possibly even a single injection. Thus, treatment of postoperative pain with infusions or infusion pumps should be reserved for total joint replacements or incision sites unconnected to a joint.

In the past, nonnarcotic pharmacologic treatment of acute postoperative pain was largely restricted to ketorolac, which can be administered by the IV or intramuscular (IM) route in the patient who is restricted in oral intake. Although ketorolac is an effective analgesic, demonstrated through reduction in the need for morphine, it also increases the perioperative blood loss due to its COX-1 activity on platelets. After oral intake is permitted, other NSAIDs can be used for analgesics. Neither ketorolac nor other NSAIDs play a routine role in the acute pain management for most orthopedic surgical patients because of the effect these drugs have on the platelets and subsequent blood loss. The availability of COX-2–selective NSAIDs has opened up the possibility of using these drugs as major analgesics for postoperative pain control, without fear of bleeding problems. These drugs act to reduce the need for narcotics with improved pain relief and decreased narcotic side effects. On the horizon are new COX-2 drugs that can be administered parenterally, and these drugs may be of major assistance in the management of early postoperative pain. Such a drug is parecoxib, which is the prodrug for valdecoxib (available in Europe, but not available in the United States). The use of highly specific COX-2 inhibitors as analgesics came into question with the withdrawal of rofecoxib and valdecoxib from the market because of concern over increased cardiovascular events with long-term use. At this time, other less specific NSAIDs may be considered as alternatives (celecoxib, diclofenac, meloxicam, etodolac) because their effect on platelet function is minimal.

Other analgesics and techniques do not get sufficient recognition for their role in pain control. Acetaminophen is thought to be a central prostaglandin synthase inhibitor and thereby achieves significant relief of pain. It can be tolerated in doses up to 4 g/day, and because it does not act in the same pathway as narcotics, its effect is additive to that of morphine or other narcotics and can reduce the requirement for narcotics. Another analgesic that should be used more often for analgesia is tramadol. This analgesic has very low abuse potential but provides significant analgesia, acting through inhibition of norepinephrine reuptake as well as a weak μ-agonist (similar to morphine) action. Again this mechanism of action is additive to that of traditional opioids and acetaminophen in its analgesic effect.

Glucocorticoids are naturally increased in periods of stress such as surgery and are provided exogenously for those patients with suppressed adrenal function. One study showed an increase in cortisol production of 17-fold after TKA, but no such increase after knee arthroscopy. Divided doses of approximately 200 mg of hydrocortisone (8 days normal production) are typically prescribed for such patients. High doses (20 mg) of dexamethasone (equivalent to 400 mg of hydrocortisone) reduce the early postoperative pain in tonsillectomy patients. Although such doses may reduce postoperative nausea, swelling, and pain, as well as create a feeling of well-being, an increased susceptibility to infection may result from longer term dosing. Short courses of relatively high doses of glucocorticoids may be beneficial in reducing postoperative pain. Other methods of pain control may be indirect, such as controlling swelling and pain through hemostasis and cold therapy. Hemostasis may be achieved through the use of bone wax on cancellous bone or through the use of fibrin glue. Vasoconstriction from cold therapy can reduce swelling and also have a direct effect on nociceptive transduction.

A comprehensive approach to pain management can lead to beneficial effects. Multimodal analgesic regimens are suggested using several analgesics that address different points in the nociception process. Combinations of medications can include narcotics, acetaminophen, tramadol, COX-2 inhibitors, and local anesthetics administered through the use of pain pumps. Peripheral nerve blocks and subarachnoid morphine blocks can assist in control of pain in the early postoperative period. Injections of local anesthetics and steroids into the pericapsular tissues can also be helpful. Consideration should be given to administering medications in the preanesthesia room to preempt the pain of surgery. This can also assist in diminishing peripheral sensitization that occurs with tissue damage. In addition to pharmacologic interventions, patient education can reduce preoperative anxiety, reducing pain and increasing satisfaction.

Bianconi M, Ferraro L, Traina GC, et al: Pharmacokinetics and efficacy of ropivacaine continuous wound instillation after joint replacement surgery. Br J Anaesth 2003;91:830. [PMID: 14633754]

Chu CR, Coyle CH, Chu CT, et al: In vivo effects of a single intra-articular injection of 0.5% bupivacaine on articular cartilage. J Bone Joint Surg 2010;92A:599. [PMID: 20194318]

Cook P, Stevens J, Gaudron C: Comparing the effects of femoral nerve block versus femoral and sciatic nerve block on pain and opiate consumption after total knee arthroplasty. J Arthroplasty 2003;18:583. [PMID: 12934209]

Grishko V, Xu M, Wilson G, Pearsall AW 4th: Apoptosis and mitochondrial dysfunction in human chondrocytes following exposure to lidocaine, bupivacaine, and ropivacaine. J Bone Joint Surg 2010;92A:609. [PMID: 20194319]

Hartrick CT, Hartrick KA: Extended release epidural morphine (DepoDur): review and safety analysis. Expert Rev Neurother 2008;8:1641. [PMID: 18986234]

Kuritzky L, Weaver A: Advances in rheumatology: coxibs and beyond. *J Pain Symptom Manage* 2003;25(Suppl2):s6. [PMID: 12604153]

Leopold SS, Casnellie MT, Warme WJ, et al: Endogenous cortisol production in response to knee arthroscopy and total knee arthroplasty. *J Bone Joint Surg Am* 2003;85:2163. [PMID: 14630847]

Mallory TH, Lombardi AV Jr, Fada RA, et al: Pain management for joint arthroplasty: preemptive analgesia. *J Arthroplasty* 2002;17:129. [PMID: 12068423]

Parvizi J, Porat M, Gandhi K, et al: Postoperative pain management techniques in hip and knee arthroplasty. *Instr Course Lect* 2009;58:769. [PMID: 19385585]

Rasmussen S, Kramhøft MU, Sperling KP, Pedersen JH: Increased flexion and reduced hospital stay with continuous intraarticular morphine and ropivacaine after primary total knee replacement: open intervention study of efficacy and safety in 154 patients. *Acta Orthop Scand* 2004;75:606. [PMID: 15513495]

Sinatra RS, Torres J, Bustos AM: Pain management after major orthopedic surgery: current strategies and new concepts. *J Am Acad Ortho Surg* 2002;10:117. [PMID: 11929206]

Sjoling M, Nordahl G, Olofsson N, Asplund K: The impact of preoperative information on state anxiety, postoperative pain and satisfaction with pain management. *Patient Educ Couns* 2003;51:169. [PMID: 14572947]

B. Deep Venous Thrombosis/Pulmonary Embolus

DVT, a potentially life-threatening disorder, frequently accompanies orthopedic surgery. It is much more of a problem for total joint replacements, spine surgery, and lower extremities immobilized after surgery, but can occur without surgery in patients having arthroscopy or cast treatment for fractures or even Achilles tendon ruptures. This is one of the expected risks after surgery and cast treatment. It is such an important issue that since 2006, JCAHO has mandated that hospitalized patients be screened and treated to prevent DVT. Venous thromboembolic phenomenon can result in three problems: postphlebitic (or postthrombotic) syndrome, nonfatal PE, and fatal PE. It is necessary to put the risks of PE into appropriate perspective because, contrary to prevailing assumptions in the public and among orthopedic surgeons, PE can occur without surgery (Table 1–2). The risk of having a PE depends on a number of risk factors, including age, weight, the presence of varicose veins, immobility, smoking, previous DVT, joint replacement, the season of the year, estrogen therapy, and the location. There is an uncertain relationship between DVT and the probability of having a PE. Obviously one cannot have a PE without having a clot, but which clots are likely to break off and become emboli and which ones will cause problems are still unresolved issues. It is thought that thigh clots are more important than calf clots because of their size and the potential damage they can do. It is generally conceded, however, that DVT is a marker for PE, and that is the surrogate variable used to determine the effectiveness of treatment of PE. A nonfatal

Table 1–2. Rates of complications associated with total hip replacement at the Mayo Clinic.

Complication	Percentage
Death (overall)	0.5
Myocardial infarction	0.5
Pulmonary embolism	0.4
Deep venous thrombosis	1.1

Reproduced, with permission, from Mantilla et al: Poster presented at the American Academy of Orthopaedic Surgeons Annual Meeting; 2001.

PE can cause cor pulmonale, but this is thought to be an unlikely circumstance, and it is speculated that nonfatal PE would result in a residual effect in the range of 0.1–0.01% of cases. DVT itself is thought to be a significant problem that results in incompetence of the valves in the deep veins of the calf and thigh. This results in persistent edema, which can progress to brawny edema and ulceration over time. However, many things are thought to cause these changes in addition to DVT. There is an uneven geographic distribution of fatal PE without surgery in the United States, with the West Coast census region having the lowest fatal PE rate. The rate of fatal PE increases with age, although age may simply be a marker for health and activity level. The rate of fatal PE in the general population older than 65 years is in the range of 0.03%, whereas approximate total joint PE rates are typically approximately 0.3%. Thus, there is a 10-fold increase in risk of having a fatal PE with a total hip or knee replacement.

Three classes of drugs can be used for chemoprophylaxis of DVT in the United States: warfarin (the vitamin K inhibitor), the low-molecular-weight heparins (dalteparin, enoxaparin, and similar drug fondaparinux), and the platelet aggregation inhibitors (aspirin, naproxen, other NSAIDs). Each approach has its advantages and disadvantages. Sodium warfarin has a slow onset of action, sometimes taking several days to reach therapeutic levels, but its oral route of administration is convenient. However, monitoring of the prothrombin time is necessary to ensure appropriate therapeutic levels. The low-molecular-weight heparins do not affect the prothrombin time or the partial thromboplastin time but do affect factor IIa and Xa levels. These do not have to be monitored because the medications are given in standard doses. These medications are provided parenterally. Both warfarin and the low-molecular-weight heparins are associated with bleeding problems. Aspirin, naproxen, and other NSAIDs have proponents who recommend them because of their relative safety, but they are probably not effective in prevention of DVT. Mechanical means of preventing DVT include compression hose and intermittent pneumatic compression. These have recently been demonstrated to be as efficacious as chemoprophylaxis.

The American College of Chest Physicians regularly performs and publishes meta-analyses of the data available on DVT with updated recommendations. Generally, for orthopedic indications after high-risk surgery, warfarin with an international normalized ratio (INR) of 2–3, a low-molecular-weight heparin starting 12–24 hours after surgery, and elastic stockings and intermittent pneumatic compression are useful as supplemental protection against DVT. The recommended period is a minimum of 7 days. Occasionally, use of heparin or vena cava filters is recommended in high-risk situations. Table 1–3 lists the current recommendations.

The community standard in orthopedic surgery probably differs somewhat from that recommended by the American College of Chest Physicians. Newer orthopedic literature seems to suggest that warfarin is the drug of choice but with lower INR values. However, the choice of prophylactic agent is made by the doctor and the patient and is influenced by their interpretation of the risk of thromboembolism and bleeding problems.

Both warfarin and heparin, either low-molecular-weight (LMWH) or regular, have problems that can cause catastrophic side effects in rare cases. Warfarin can cause skin necrosis and venous limb gangrene syndromes unrelated to the operative site. Heparin can induce thrombocytopenia. This is apparently an immunoglobulin G (IgG) antibody formation that occurs 5–10 days after starting heparin

(including LMWH) and can result in a hypercoagulable state that can result in serious problems of coagulation in unintended areas. Some new agents are becoming available, some of which are on the market at the time of this writing but are not indicated for DVT prophylaxis. These drugs are related to the antithrombin drug produced by leeches. Two of these are desirudin and bivalirudin, and they are indicated for anticoagulation in the presence of heparin-induced thrombocytopenia.

In addition, dabigatran is an antithrombin drug that may soon be available for DVT prophylaxis as an oral prescription (presently available in Europe). Another drug, rivaroxaban, an oral factor Xa inhibitor, is approved for use in Canada and Europe and has been recommended for approval in the United States by a Food and Drug Administration advisory panel. A pentasaccharide (fondaparinux) is approved for DVT prophylaxis and acts in a manner similar to heparin.

1. Diagnosis—DVT is diagnosed with ultrasound in the postsurgical patient with calf swelling or with Homan's sign in the appropriate clinical setting. Several risk factors can be elicited from the history to increase the suspicion of DVT. These include immobilization, lower extremity or pelvic surgery (in the previous 4 weeks), previous history of DVT, and history of cancer. Ultrasound is a reliable, noninvasive screen for DVT of the lower extremity veins and has replaced the venogram as the gold standard for diagnosing DVT. Testing for PE has also evolved. In nonsurgical

Table 1–3. Recommendations for management of DVT prophylaxis for high-risk orthopedic patients.

Procedure	Grade	Recommendation
THA/TKA	1A	LMWH started 12–24 h after surgery
		Or
	1A	Fondaparinux 2.5 mg started 6–24 h after surgery
		Or
	1A	Warfarin started immediately after surgery (target INR 2.5, range 2.0–3.0)
		Or
	1B	Optimal use of intermittent pneumatic compression (for TKA only)
Hip fractures	1A	Fondaparinux
	1B	LDUH
	1B	LMWH
	1B	Warfarin (as above)
Trauma	1A	LMWH (when safe to use)
	1B	GCS and IPC until LMWH is safe
Acute SCI	1B	LMWH (when hemostasis is evident)
	1A	GCS and IPC (high bleeding risk; pharmacologic thromboprophylaxis contraindicated)

GCS, graduated compression stockings; IPC, intermittent pneumatic compression; LDUH, low-dose unfractionated heparin; LMWH, low-molecular-weight heparin; SCI, spinal cord injury; THA, total hip arthroplasty; TKA, total knee arthroplasty; 1A Grade, clear risk/benefit ratio based on randomized trials without important limitations; 1B Grade, same as 1A but with inconsistent results or methodologic flaws.
Derived from Geerts WH, Bergqvist D, Pineo GF, et al: Prevention of venous thromboembolism. Antithrombotic and thrombolytic therapy, ACCP Evidence-Based Clinical Practice Guidelines (8th Edition). *Chest* 2008;133(Suppl):381S.

patients, D-dimer can be helpful in the diagnosis of PE, and the risk of PE continues for weeks after surgery, so there may be a role for it in the late postoperative period. Previously, ventilation/perfusion scans were the standard method, followed by pulmonary angiography, if the probability was intermediate. Now spiral CT is quite reliable but is still only reported to be 70% sensitive and 91% specific. In outpatients with a normal ultrasound and a normal lung scan, spiral CT has only a 7% false-positive rate and 5% false-negative rate. Furthermore, evidence from a preliminary study suggests that fibrin monomer discriminates between total hip arthroplasty patients with PE and those without PE. The D-dimer was also higher in PE patients but not significantly until 7 days postoperatively.

Colwell CW: The ACCP guidelines for thromboprophylaxis in total hip and knee arthroplasty. *Orthopedics* 2009;32 (12 Suppl):67. [PMID: 20201479]

Colwell CW, Froimson MI, Mont MA, et al: Thrombosis prevention after total hip arthroplasty: a prospective, randomized trial comparing a mobile compression device with low-molecular-weight heparin. *J Bone Joint Surg Am* 2010;92A:527. [PMID: 20194309]

Freedman KB, Brookenthal KR, Fitzgerald RH Jr, et al: A meta-analysis of thromboembolic prophylaxis following elective total hip arthroplasty. *J Bone Joint Surg Am* 2000;82:929. [PMID: 10901307]

Geerts WH, Pineo GF, Heit JA, et al: Prevention of venous thromboembolism: the Seventh ACCP Conference on Antithrombotic and Thrombolytic Therapy. *Chest* 2004;126:338S. [PMID: 15383478]

Hong MS, Amanullah AM: Heparin-induced thrombocytopenia and thrombosis. *Rev Cardiovasc Med* 2010;11:13. [PMID: 20495512]

Johnson BF, Manzo RA, Bergelin RO, Strandness DE Jr: Relationship between changes in the deep venous system and the development of post thrombotic syndrome after an acute episode of lower limb deep vein thrombosis: a one- to six-year follow-up. *J Vasc Surg* 1995;21:307. [PMID: 7853603]

Lilienfeld DE: Decreasing mortality from pulmonary embolism in the United States, 1979–1996. *Int J Epidemiol* 2000;29:465. [PMID: 10869318]

Lilienfeld DE, Godbold JH: Geographic distribution of pulmonary embolism with mortality rates in the United States, 1980–1984. *Am Heart J* 1992;124:1068. [PMID: 1529881]

Mont MJ, Eurich DT, Russell DB, et al: Post-thrombotic syndrome after total hip arthroplasty is uncommon. *Acta Orthop* 2008;79:794. [PMID: 19085497]

Nazarian RM, Van Cott EM, Zembowicz A, Duncan LM: Warfarin-induced skin necrosis. *J Am Acad Dermatol* 2009;61:325. [PMID: 19615543]

Perrier A, Howarth N, Didier D, et al: Performance of helical computed tomography in unselected outpatients with suspected pulmonary embolism. *Ann Intern Med* 2001;135:88. [PMID: 11453707]

Rafee A, Herlikar D, Gilbert R, et al: D-dimer in the diagnosis of deep vein thrombosis following total hip and knee replacement: a prospective study. *Ann R Coll Surg Engl* 2008;90:123. [PMID: 18325211]

Schneider D, Lilienfeld DE: The epidemiology of pulmonary embolism: racial contrasts in incidence and in-hospital case fatality. *J Natl Med Assoc* 2006;98:1967. [PMID: 17225843]

Stevenson M, Scope A, Holmes M, et al: Rivaroxaban for the prevention of venous thromboembolism: a single technology appraisal. *Health Technol Assess* 2009;13(Suppl 3):43. [PMID: 19846028]

Turpie AG, Gallus AS, Hoek JA: A synthetic pentasaccharide for the prevention of deep-vein thrombosis after total hip replacement. *N Engl J Med* 2001;344:619. [PMID: 11228275]

▶ Outpatient Care

Economic realities today mandate earlier discharge from the hospital after some procedures and after outpatient surgery in procedures previously done on an inpatient basis. This trend suggests that patients must take more responsibility for their care, and surgeons must provide outpatient access for patients previously treated as inpatients. The indications for discharge have broadened just as the reasons for admission have narrowed. The reasons for keeping a postoperative patient in the acute-care setting are few. The main indications for hospitalization are pain control requiring parenteral narcotics, presence of hemodynamic instability, a need for traction, or a need for frequent physician observation (drains, infection, etc.). Even extended administration of IV antibiotic therapy is not an adequate reason for an acute-care stay. Thus timing of follow-up visits is important to ensure that the patient is not only unnecessarily inconvenienced but also does not suffer delayed recognition of a complication. In most cases, the first visit should be for suture removal (10–14 days). Again, economic realities mandate a 90-day follow-up as part of the global surgical fee. Follow-up for a total hip replacement patient might be at 2 weeks, 6 weeks, and 12 weeks after surgery. Longer or shorter intervals may be necessary, depending on how the patient is progressing and how much external support the patient is receiving (physical therapy, home nurse visits, home caregivers, and home environment). Joint-replacement patients should be followed up at least yearly on a permanent basis after the first 5 or so years. The American Academy of Orthopedic Surgeons recommends prophylactic antibiotics for joint-replacement patients for procedures such as dental cleaning in which bacteremia may occur for life, especially when immune compromise is likely (eg, diabetes or renal transplant).

Long-term follow-up for patients with plates, screws, pins, rods, or other fracture devices is not typically necessary after healing of the fracture and rehabilitation of the affected muscles and joints. Antibiotic prophylaxis is not necessary for these patients. In cases of painful hardware, removal may be indicated after healing. Removal of hardware in older (more than 75 years) patients is generally not indicated. In younger (less than 50 years), active patients, hardware removal may be justified to reduce the stress concentration or stress shielding effects of the metal devices to prevent fracture prophylactically. An adequate period (12 weeks or more, depending on activity) of stress protection, especially in torsion, is indicated to reduce the risk of fracture through defects incurred by the bone during removal of hardware. For a detailed discussion of rehabilitation, see Chapter 12, "Rehabilitation".

Pacheco RJ, Buckley S, Oxborrow NJ, et al: Gluteal compartment syndrome after total knee arthroplasty with epidural postoperative analgesia. *J Bone Joint Surg Br* 2001;83:739. [PMID: 11476317]

Richards H, Langston A, Kulkarni R, Downes EM: Does patient controlled analgesia delay the diagnosis of compartment syndrome following intramedullary nailing of the tibia? *Injury* 2004;35:296. [PMID: 15124799]

Yang J, Cooper MG: Compartment syndrome and patient-controlled analgesia in children- analgesic complication or early warning system. *Anaesth Intensive Care* 2010;38:359. [PMID: 20369773]

▶ Blood Loss and Replacement

Because blood replacement is now a complicated issue, it is fortunate that not all orthopedic procedures require blood replacement. In California, the surgeon is obligated to give the patient a brochure from the state that describes the blood management options available to the surgeon and the patient when blood transfusion is likely after surgery. Patient involvement in the decision on how to manage blood loss is certainly a good idea.

The data on when to transfuse are conflicting, however, and generally the decision is based on the physician's clinical assessment to determine the need for transfusion. This uncertainty is reflected in the variability in the postoperative transfusion "trigger," as shown by the percentages of patients receiving blood varying from 16 to 87% for total hip arthroplasty and 12 to 87% for TKA in one study; it should be noted that these rates also reflect differences in blood loss for these procedures at various hospitals. Blood volume is approximately 7–8% of body weight, or approximately 5 L in a 70-kg individual. Normal individuals can be resuscitated from acute blood losses of up to 25% with crystalloid/colloid. Greater blood losses can be tolerated if the euvolemic state is maintained, but transfusion should be considered. The status of the clotting system must be monitored in the acute blood loss phase to prevent accelerated blood loss. Blood loss in the postoperative subacute phase can be managed with volume replacement and evaluation of symptomatology to determine the need for transfusion of red cell mass. Patients at risk of stroke or myocardial infarction or those with decreased cardiac output may need transfusion at higher hemoglobin levels. Younger (less than 50 years), healthier patients may tolerate lower hemoglobin levels unless they have postural hypotension, tachycardia, dizziness, or fainting.

A. Criteria for Blood Transfusion

The decision to transfuse in the immediate postoperative period is predicated on numerous factors, including age, medical condition and cardiac status, estimated blood loss, projected blood loss, availability of blood (autologous, designated donor, or bank), and the patient's perception of risk. Consideration of all factors argues against transfusion in the younger (less than 50 years) or healthier patient until the patient has a hematocrit level of 20–22% or has symptoms that include tachycardia, early and postural hypotension, and dizziness or fainting. Older (more than 60 years) patients at risk of stroke or myocardial infarction would be candidates for transfusion at higher hematocrit levels or with a lower threshold of symptoms.

B. Strategies for Minimizing the Risks Associated With Blood Transfusion

Blood loss is an inevitable part of surgery. With the realization that the banked blood supply is at low risk, but still at risk, of containing infectious agents, strategies to minimize the risk of transmission have been developed.

An obvious method of accomplishing this goal is to reduce blood loss. Anesthetic techniques to reduce mean arterial blood pressure can reduce blood loss by reducing the time of surgery as well as the actual blood loss. The patient has to be counseled to avoid antiplatelet drugs in the period prior to surgery. These medications include baby aspirin and clopidogrel but also all of the ubiquitous NSAIDs that are in over-the-counter analgesics, cough and cold remedies, and arthritis medications. In the operative period, topical agents such as bone wax, Gelfoam and similar collagen products, thrombin, tranexamic acid and aminocaproic acid (antifibrinolytics), and fibrin glue should be considered. Tranexamic acid can be administered IV or locally to help control bleeding. Surgical technique should be efficient and meticulous to reduce time and therefore blood loss. The patient should be positioned to minimize venous pressure and blood loss, such as closing a total knee in flexion or positioning a postoperative total knee in flexion to reduce blood loss.

Presurgical banking of autologous blood by the patient (with or without hematopoietic growth factors), immediate preoperative autodonation by hemodilution, and salvage of the patient's intraoperative and postoperatively lost blood with infusion of either washed or unwashed red cells can reduce the patient's exposure to the risks of designated donor blood or homologous banked blood. The problems with autologous blood begin with the cost, but there are other issues. Older (more than 70 years) patients sometimes do not tolerate the anemia from donation. Perhaps the greatest risks are bacterial contamination and clerical error, in which a patient gets a potentially fatal ABO-incompatible unit instead of his or her own. Autologous blood that is not used is discarded and not put into the general blood bank pool.

Preoperative hemodilution has the cost associated with the operating room time to draw off the blood and that of the anesthesiologist in supervising the process. Preoperative hematocrit can be boosted through parenteral erythropoietin, which can minimize the effect of surgical blood loss. Erythropoietin is estimated to cost $900 per unit of blood saved, which is more than the cost of autologous blood at $300–400/unit. Furthermore, there may be risks with abnormally high hematocrits. Thus, it is only considered when there is little other choice, such as for surgery on Jehovah's Witnesses who refuse transfusions.

Despite initial resistance and continued questions about cost-effectiveness by blood bank officials, autologous blood donation has achieved considerable acceptability from patients, physicians, and blood bank administrators. There are disadvantages of autologous donation that counterbalance the obvious advantages of eliminating transfusion-related disease and incompatibility. These are possible bacterial contamination of the blood, perioperative anemia with increased risk of transfusion, administrative error resulting in blood incompatibility from receiving the wrong blood, cost, and wastage of autologous blood that is not used. Blood can be stored for 35 days or can be frozen as a red cell mass for up to 1 year, but loss in viability of the red cells occurs with both storage methods. Use of autologous blood can eliminate the need for banked blood for many but not all orthopedic patients. Some patients, for example, have marginal laboratory test results (eg, Hgb level of 10 g/dL and hematocrit level of 30%) that preclude their predonation of blood. The ability of patients to predonate blood and the amount of blood donated can sometimes be increased through the use of recombinant human erythropoietin therapy. Injections can be given twice weekly and may result in a higher red cell mass collected and a higher hematocrit level at the time of hospital admission. Although expensive, this therapy can be of benefit to patients, especially those who have blood types that are difficult to match or have religious beliefs that conflict with the practice of receiving blood from others.

Red blood cells can be salvaged by suction in the operating room or collected via surgical drains in the recovery room. Adequate loss of blood must be present to make these procedures cost effective. Blood salvage is probably effective (absolute reduction in risk of receiving an allogeneic red cell transfusion, 21%, with a saving of 0.68 units of allogeneic blood per patient) in minimizing perioperative allogeneic transfusion, but should be reserved for cases with high expected blood loss (ie, greater than 2 units), patients with low starting hemoglobins, and/or Jehovah's Witness patients who will accept intraoperative salvage. The salvaged blood is generally washed to remove cell debris, fat, and bone fragments. Newer filtration techniques permit the transfusion of blood collected from drains without the washing process.

Bezwada HP, Nazarian DG, Henry DH, Booth RE Jr: Preoperative use of recombinant human erythropoietin before total joint arthroplasty. *J Bone Joint Surg Am* 2003;85:1795. [PMID: 12954840]

Carless PA, Henry DA, Moxey AJ, et al: Cell salvage for minimizing perioperative allogeneic blood transfusion. *Cochrane Database Syst Rev* 2010;4:CD001888. [PMID: 20393932]

Gombotz H, Rehak PH, Shander A, Hofmann A: Blood use in elective surgery: the Austrian benchmark study. *Transfusion* 2007;47:1468. [PMID: 17655591]

Goodnough LT: Autologous blood donation. *Crit Care* 2004;8 (Suppl 2):S49. [PMID: 15196325]

Keating EM, Ritter MA: Transfusion options in total joint arthroplasty. *J Arthroplasty* 2002;17:125. [PMID: 12068422]

Strumper D, Weber EW, Gielen-Wijffels S, et al: Clinical efficacy of postoperative autologous transfusion of filtered shed blood in hip and knee arthroplasty. *Transfusion* 2004;44:1567. [PMID: 15504161]

Zohar E, Ellis M, Ifrach N, et al: The postoperative blood-sparing efficacy of oral versus intravenous tranexamic acid after total knee replacement. *Anesth Analg* 2004;99:1679. [PMID: 15562053]

ETHICS IN ORTHOPEDIC SURGERY

Ethics in medicine started with Hippocrates and was codified by Thomas Percival in 1803, with the publication of his Code of Medical Ethics. This was extended by the American Medical Association in 1847 and has undergone several revisions over time. Ethics basically define the standards of conduct of honorable or moral behavior by the physician. Many areas of medical ethics, such as abortion or artificial insemination, have little to do with orthopedics. Although many areas of ethics are more restrictive than the law, litigation and legislation have in some cases become the standard by which orthopedists have to abide, with tighter constraints than ethics alone would place. Although ethics as a field is too broad a subject for a text such as this, certain areas that impinge on orthopedics are addressed here.

▶ Clinical Trials

A particularly difficult ethical area is the clinical research study. Although many of these are now more than adequately controlled by institutional review boards (IRBs), the federal government's Office for Human Research Protections, and sponsors of research, the single practitioner in a small orthopedic group is still at risk of performing human, or even animal, research without appropriate ethical controls. The three main areas for concern are the use of ionizing radiation for exams that are not clinically indicated, the use of patient or third-party-payer funds for exams that are not clinically indicated, and the use of patient data in a manner that does not maintain confidentiality. Certainly, ionizing radiation can be used, even for control subjects, if adequate IRB review and patient/subject consent are obtained. This must be done in a formal manner. However, the use of third-party-payer funds for research or revealing patient confidentiality is never ethical. Performing unindicated studies (laboratory, radiographs) at patient expense is certainly unethical. Also, patient confidentiality is fundamental to the doctor–patient relationship. The Health Insurance Portability and Accountability Act (HIPAA) changed the way physicians have to look at confidentiality. Verbal, written, and electronic privacy must be maintained in the office and hospital setting. Patient data have to be closely controlled with care taken regarding personal data assistants, scraps of paper with patient identifiers and data, and roentgenographic images. Photos or slides of football injuries in the public domain may be acceptable for presentation, although in some situations, this may not be true. Certainly, photos or slides of radiographs with patient identifiers for professional presentations or publications cannot be used without written patient permission. The electronic medical record will produce many potential areas that might violate HIPAA regulations, especially with local area networks that permit laptop access in an entire office or building.

The typical orthopedic clinical research study is a retrospective review of a surgeon's cases. This model of research is considered to be of modest value by researchers doing multicenter, randomized, controlled, double-blind studies, but until the funding is found to do this type of study on something as common as knee replacement, retrospective reviews will have to serve as the database for decision making. This is especially true for low-volume procedures. These types of studies raise several issues. The main issues are paying for the study (not through patient or third-party funds), maintaining patient confidentiality, and conflict of interest. The first two issues can be resolved by IRB oversight, and private practitioners are advised to obtain that help from their hospital. Conflict of interest has at least two aspects. Physicians may be consultants or designers of the prosthesis or drug and have a financial interest in the success of the product, and they have ego invested in their surgery, that is, they do not want to look like "bad" surgeons and hence may be hesitant to report poor results. Furthermore, they may be professors and need to demonstrate clinical research publications as part of promotion requirements or simply want to "advertise" their abilities through publication. The latter aspects are implied conflicts of interest but are probably as important as a financial conflict. The potential financial conflict should be disclosed to the patient and to other parties such as the hospital and to the journal of publication. Surgeons have an ethical obligation to share medical advances, and presenting surgeons' results with a procedure certainly meets that standard.

▶ Gifts From Industry

The concept that gifts from industry may affect the choice of medication, prosthesis, and so on, is of concern. Generally, the guidelines recommended by the American Medical Association allow gifts, other remuneration, subsidies for meetings, and so on, if the primary purpose is education or of benefit to the patient. Gifts should be of minimal value and related to the physician's work. The pharmaceutical and orthopedic manufacturers are now self-regulated by industry organizations regarding the type of meetings that they can sponsor. Meetings directly sponsored by the company are only allowed to discuss "label" applications of the drug or device, whereas continuing medical education credit courses, which can only be done through an educational institution, can discuss "off-label" uses of products. Payment for travel costs, lodging, and honoraria to attend such meetings is considered inappropriate unless the physician is performing a service, such as faculty duties or consulting. Although it seems unlikely that a physician would change his or her prescribing practice based on a free meal, the appearance of impropriety is important and should be kept in mind.

Cartwright JC, Hickman SE, Bevan L, Shupert CL: Navigating federalwide assurance requirements when conducting research in community-based care settings. *J Am Geriatr Soc* 2004;52:1567. [PMID: 15341563]

Council on Ethical and Judicial Affairs: *Code of Medical Ethics: Current Opinions with Annotations* (2000–2001 edition). Chicago: American Medical Association; 2000.

Epps CH: Ethical guidelines for orthopedists and industry. *Clin Orthop* 2003;412:14. [PMID: 12838046]

Healy WL Peterson RN: Department of Justice investigation of orthopedic industry. *J Bone Joint Surg* 2009;91A:1791. [PMID: 19571103]

Laskin RS, Davis JP: The use of a personal digital assistant in orthopaedic surgical practice. *Clin Orthop* 2004;421:91. [PMID: 15123932]

Oyama L, Tannas HS, Moulton S: Desktop and mobile software development for surgical practice. *J Pediatr Surg* 2002;37:477. [PMID: 11877671]

Pancoast PE, Patrick TB, Mitchell JA: Physician PDA and the HIPAA privacy rule. *J Am Med Inform Assoc* 2003;10:611. [PMID: 14631929]

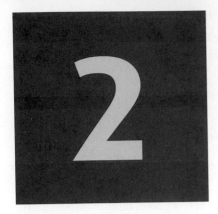

Musculoskeletal Trauma Surgery

Wade R. Smith, MD, FACS

Philip F. Stahel, MD, FACS

Takashi Suzuki, MD

Gabrielle Peacher, MD

THE HIGH COST OF MUSCULOSKELETAL TRAUMA

Injury has become a major cause of death and disability globally. Trauma is the leading cause of death for people age 1–34 years of all races and socioeconomic levels and the third leading cause of death for all age groups. Traumatic motor vehicle accidents (MVAs) are the leading cause of traumatic death. Approximately 1.3 million people die on the world's roads every year. Over 20 million people sustain nonfatal injuries. In 2010, death from road traffic accidents was the ninth cause of all deaths; it is estimated to be the fifth leading cause of death by 2030, resulting in 2.4 million fatalities per year. The economic impact of MVAs is approximately $230 billion in the United States and €180 billion in the European Union. The global losses due to road traffic injuries are estimated to be $518 billion, and these injuries cost governments between 1 and 3% of their gross national product. Low-income and middle-income countries account for $65 billion, which is more than they receive in development assistance.

Gunshot injuries are the third cause of all injury-related deaths in the United States. There are 60,000–80,000 nonfatal gunshot wounds annually in the United States. In 2006, 30,896 persons died from firearm injuries in the United States, with estimated lifetime medical costs over $2 billion.

Trauma is the leading cause of death and disability in children, accounting for some 11 million hospitalizations, 150,000 disabilities, and 15,000 deaths every year in the United States. Although direct costs of pediatric trauma exceed $8 billion per year, indirect costs to families and society are impossible to estimate but undoubtedly substantial.

With an unprecedented increase in population and life expectancy, age-related musculoskeletal conditions such as fragility fractures and sports-related ligamentous injuries are now more common than ever, even in the elderly population. Approximately 1.6 million hip fractures occur worldwide each year. By 2050, this number is expected to increase three- or fourfold. In 2005 in the United States, over 2 million osteoporotic fractures cost $17 billion.

Both natural and man-made disasters have caused hundreds of thousands of deaths and disabilities in the past 20 years, and the World Health Organization estimates an overall increase over the next two decades. Although true mass casualty situations are rare, the earthquake in Haiti in 2010 left 300,000 injured behind. These situations require highly organized trauma systems for optimal outcomes.

While considering the cost of musculoskeletal injuries, effects on the patient, the family, and society in general should be considered. Practitioners should keep in mind that there are direct expenditures for diagnosis, treatment, and rehabilitation, and also indirect economic costs associated with lost labor and diminished productivity.

Dougherty PJ, Vaidya R, Silverton CD, Bartlett C, Najibi S: Joint and long-bone gunshot injuries. *J Bone Joint Surg Am* 2009;91:980-997. [PMID: 20415399]

Galano GJ, Vitale MA, Kessler MW, Hyman JE, Vitale MG: The most frequent traumatic orthopaedic injuries from a national pediatric inpatient population. *J Pediatr Orthop* 2005;25:39-44. [PMID: 15614057]

Gullberg B, Johnell O, Kanis JA: World-wide projections for hip fracture. *Osteoporos Int* 1997;7:407-413. [PMID: 9425497]

Heron M, Hoyert DL, Murphy SL, Xu J, Kochanek KD, Tejada-Vera B: Deaths: final data for 2006. *Natl Vital Stat Rep* 2009;57:1-134. [PMID: 19788058]

Mathers CD, Loncar D: Projections of global mortality and burden of disease from 2002 to 2030. *PLoS Med* 2006;3:e442. [PMID: 17132052]

Peden M, Scurfield R, Sleet D, et al: *World Report on Road Traffic Injury Prevention*. Geneva, Switzerland: World Health Organization; 2004.

THE HEALING PROCESS

▶ Bone Healing

Bone is a unique tissue among all musculoskeletal tissues because it heals by the formation of normal bone, as opposed to scar tissue. In fact, it is considered a nonunion when a bone heals by a fibroblastic response instead of by bone formation.

Fracture healing can be divided into primary and secondary healing. In primary healing, the cortex attempts to reestablish itself without the formation of callus (osteonal or haversian healing). This occurs when the fracture is anatomically reduced, the blood supply is preserved, and the fracture is rigidly stabilized by internal fixation. Secondary fracture healing results in the formation of callus and involves the participation of the periosteum and external soft tissues. This fracture healing response is enhanced by motion and is inhibited by rigid fixation.

Fracture healing can be conveniently divided, based on the biologic events taking place, into the following four stages:

1. Hematoma formation (inflammation) and angiogenesis
2. Cartilage formation with subsequent calcification
3. Cartilage removal and bone formation
4. Bone remodeling

Initially, there is *hematoma* formation followed by an inflammatory phase characterized by an accumulation of mesenchymal cells around the fracture site. These mesenchymal cells differentiate into chondrocytes or osteoblasts. Growth factors and cytokines derived mainly from platelets are essential for angiogenesis, cellular chemotaxis, proliferation, and differentiation. Growth factors induce mesenchymal cells and osteoblasts to produce type II collagen and proteoglycans. Platelet-derived growth factor (PDGF) recruits inflammatory cells at the fracture site. Bone morphogenetic proteins (BMPs) are osteoinductive mediators inducing metaplasia of mesenchymal cells into osteoblasts. Interleukin (IL)-1 and IL-6 recruit inflammatory cells to the fracture site. Periosteum is the main source of mesenchymal cells. In high-energy fractures where the periosteum has been compromised, stem cells originate from the circulation and the surrounding soft tissues.

Low oxygen tension, low pH, and movement favor the differentiation into chondrocytes; high oxygen tension, high pH, and stability predispose toward osteoblast stimulation. In the presence of mechanical instability, fractures heal by the process of endochondral ossification—bony callus formation is preceded by a *cartilaginous template.*

Chondrocytes and fibroblasts produce a semirigid soft callus that is able to provide a mechanical support to the fracture, as well as act as a template for the bony callus that will later supersede it. The most active stage of osteogenesis, also known as primary bone formation, is characterized by high levels of osteoblast activity and the formation of mineralized bone matrix, which arises directly in the peripheral callus in areas of stability. Mineralization causes chondrocyte degeneration, hypertrophy, and finally apoptosis. The phase of mineralized callus leads to a state in which the fracture site is enveloped in a polymorphous mass of mineralized tissues consisting of calcified cartilage, woven bone made from cartilage, and *woven bone* formed directly. The woven-bone mineralized callus has to be replaced by lamellar bone arranged in osteonal systems to allow the bone to resume its normal function. In order for bridging new hard callus to form, the insecure soft callus is gradually removed, concomitant with revascularization. The new bone is known as *hard callus,* and it is typically irregular and underremodeled.

The final stage of fracture repair, also referred to as secondary bone formation, encompasses the *remodeling* of the woven bone hard callus into the original cortical and/or trabecular bone configuration. The key cell type involved with the resorption of mineralized bone is the osteoclast, which is a large, multinucleated cell formed by fusion of monocytes. Osteoblasts are mononuclear and are responsible for the accretion of bone.

Macrophage colony-stimulating factor (M-CSF) and receptor activator of nuclear factor-κB ligand (RANKL) are two principal cytokines secreted by osteoblasts that are critical for the induction, survival, and competency of osteoclasts.

▶ Cartilage Healing

Articular cartilage consists of extracellular matrix (ECM) and chondrocytes. The ECM is formed by water (65–80%), collagen (95% type II), and proteoglycans (chondroitin sulfate and keratan sulfate). Collagen in the ECM provides form and tensile strength. Proteoglycans and water give the cartilage stiffness, resilience, and endurance.

Chondrocytes are sparse in the adult cartilage, which is not a vascularized tissue. Their nutrition comes from the synovial fluid, and adequate circulation of the fluid through the spongelike cartilage matrix is crucial. The low baseline metabolic rate and small cell-to-matrix ratio of chondrocytes also diminish the reparative capacity of articular cartilage. Motion of the joint is responsible for most of the circulation. Rigid internal fixation of articular fractures and early weight bearing of immobilized joints allow cyclical compression of the cartilage and circulation of the synovial fluid. If the defect in the cartilage does not go through the calcified plate, the body attempts repair with hyaline cartilage. This may be seen at superficial articular cartilage lesions. Chondral fissures, flap tears, and chondral defects are loss of segmental cartilage. They have a limited, short chondrocytic reparative response. If the calcified plate is violated, as in osteochondral lesions, the subchondral capillaries bring an inflammatory reaction, which fills the defect with granulation tissue and, eventually, fibrocartilage. The quality of this fibrocartilage can be improved by passive or active motion of the joint. Basic and clinical research has shown the potential of artificial matrices, growth factors, perichondrium, periosteum, transplanted chondrocytes, and mesenchymal stem cells to stimulate the formation of cartilage in articular defects.

Tendon Healing

Tendons are specialized structures that allow muscles to extend their contractile action. Tendons consist of long bundles of collagen scattered with relatively inactive fibrocytes. These cells are nourished by the synovial fluid secreted by the one-cell-thick synovial membrane that covers the tendon (endotenon) and the parietal surface of the sheath (epitenon). The flexor tendons are covered by a richly vascularized adventitia (paratenon).

Muscle Healing

Type 1 fiber, known as *slow twitch, slow oxidative,* or *red* muscle, has a slow speed of contraction and the greatest strength of contraction. It functions aerobically and, therefore, is fatigue-resistant. Type 2 fiber, known as *fast twitch* or *white* muscle, is subdivided into two types, according to metabolic activity level: fiber that functions by oxidative and glycolytic metabolism (type 2A) and fiber that is largely glycolytic (type 2B). Both subtypes of white fast-twitch muscles are fatigable but have high strength of contraction and high speed of contraction. Traumatic injury to muscle can occur from a variety of mechanisms, including blunt trauma (muscle contusion), laceration, and strains resulting from excessive stretching or ischemia. Recovery occurs through a process of degeneration and regeneration, with new muscle cells arising from undifferentiated cells. In addition to muscle regeneration, laceration repair requires reinnervation of denervated muscle areas. Muscle contusion frequently results in hematoma. The normal repair process includes an inflammatory reaction, formation of connective tissue, and muscle regeneration. Blunt trauma may result in myositis ossificans and may cause decreased function.

Orthopedic surgeons should be aware of atrophy of muscle tissue due to immobilization and lack of activity. Loss of muscle weight initially occurs rapidly and then tends to stabilize, and loss of strength occurs simultaneously. Resistance to fatigue diminishes rapidly.

Nerve Healing

Multiple nerve fibers combine to form a fascicle surrounded by perineurium. Multiple fascicles are surrounded by epineurium. Nerves fall into patterns of monofascicular, oligofascicular, and polyfascicular structures. The size and distribution of fascicles change as a function of length, reflecting greater or lesser nerve fibers in each fascicle. Increasing distance from the nerve injury to the distal point of innervation reduces the likelihood of recovery. Other factors include the length of the damage to the nerve, the technical ability of the surgeon, and the length of time prior to repair. Nerves can be damaged in many ways, including stretching, and ischemic damage may occur at elongation of 15%.

Nerve injuries are rated from 1 to 5 degrees; however, Mackinnon introduced a sixth-degree injury to describe a mixed nerve injury that combines the other degrees of injury. First-degree injury is the least severe and equivalent to neurapraxia. Second-degree injury is equivalent to axonotmesis, with degeneration of the axon; recovery is complete. Third-degree injury is the same as second-degree injury with the addition of loss of continuity of the endoneurial tube. Despite the continuity of the nerve trunk, because of extensive degeneration of the fascicles, fourth-degree injuries may require excision of the damaged segment, with reapproximation or grafting of the nerve ends to achieve a functional outcome. Fifth-degree injury involves complete loss of continuity of the nerve trunk. Surgical repair is required to achieve restoration of function.

The outcome of recovery is much more optimistic for children than adults, and the prognosis diminishes with age.

Browne JE, Branch TP: Surgical alternatives for treatment of articular cartilage lesions. *J Am Acad Orthop Surg* 2000;8:180. [PMID: 10874225]

Buckwalter JA: Articular cartilage injuries. *Clin Orthop Relat Res* 2002;402:21-37. [PMID: 14620787]

Jackson DW, Scheer MJ, Simon TM: Cartilage substitutes: overview of basic science and treatment options. *J Am Acad Orthop Surg* 2001;9:37. [PMID: 11174162]

Lee SK, Wolfe SW: Peripheral nerve injury and repair. *J Am Acad Orthop Surg* 2000;8:243. [PMID: 10951113]

Mackinnon SE, Dellon AL: *Surgery of the Peripheral Nerve.* New York: Thieme; 1988.

Robinson LR: Role of neurophysiologic evaluation in diagnosis. *J Am Acad Orthop Surg* 2000;8:190. [PMID: 10874226]

ORTHOPEDIC ASSESSMENT AND MANAGEMENT OF MULTIPLY INJURED PATIENTS

A thorough understanding of the pathophysiology of trauma is essential for prompt diagnosis and timely treatment of musculoskeletal injuries. Sound therapeutic principles improve the overall outcome for the patient and optimize the utilization of limited health care resources.

Life-Threatening Conditions: The ABCs of Trauma Care

A systematic approach is required in all cases. The patient is assessed, and treatment priorities are established according to the type of injury, stability of vital signs, and mechanism of injury. In a severely injured patient, treatment priorities are dictated by the patient's overall condition, with the first goal being to save life and preserve the major functions of the body. Assessment consists of four overlapping phases:

1. Primary survey (ABCDE)
2. Resuscitation
3. Secondary survey (head-to-toe evaluation and history)
4. Definitive care

This process identifies and treats life-threatening conditions and can be remembered as follows:

Airway maintenance (with cervical spine protection)

Breathing and ventilation

Circulation (with hemorrhage control)

Disability (neurologic status)

Exposure and environmental control (undress the patient but prevent hypothermia)

A brief overview of the treatment of polytrauma patients, with special emphasis on the orthopedic aspects, follows.

A. Airway

Great care should be taken while assessing the airway. The cervical spine should be carefully protected at all times and not be hyperextended, hyperflexed, or rotated to obtain a patent airway. Any patient with a blunt injury above the clavicle should be considered at risk for cervical spine injury. The airway should be rapidly assessed for signs of obstruction, foreign bodies, and facial, mandibular, or tracheal/laryngeal fractures. A chin lift or jaw thrust maneuver should be used to establish an airway. A Glasgow Coma Score of 8 or less, decreased mental status, severe pulmonary injury, facial fracture, or laryngeal injury is an indication for the placement of a definitive airway.

B. Breathing

The trauma surgeon should evaluate the patient's chest. Adequate ventilation requires not only airway patency but also adequate oxygenation and carbon dioxide elimination. Remember that the following four conditions, if present, must be addressed emergently:

1. Tension pneumothorax
2. Flail chest with pulmonary contusion
3. Open pneumothorax
4. Massive hemothorax

C. Circulation

Hemorrhage is the principal cause of preventable postinjury death. Postinjury hypotension is considered hypovolemic in origin until proven otherwise. Level of consciousness, skin color, and pulses are simple to assess and reliably mirror the hemodynamic status of the patient, especially if recorded serially. Fractures of the femur or pelvis can cause major blood loss, which can severely compromise survival. (See sections on pelvic and femoral fracture.)

D. Disability (Neurologic Status)

The Glasgow Coma Score (see Chapter 12, "Rehabilitation") should be used to assess neurologic status; it is quick, simple, and predictive of patient outcome. An even simpler way to monitor central neurologic status is to remember the mnemonic AVPU and check if the patient is Alert and oriented, or responds to Vocal stimuli, or responds only to Painful stimuli, or is Unresponsive.

E. Exposure and Environmental Control

For a thorough examination of lacerations, contusions, abrasions, swelling, and deformities, the patient should be completely disrobed. This also prevents further displacement of fractures and minimizes the risk of overlooking significant problems. Hypothermia must be avoided because cardiac function may be affected, especially when there is decreased blood volume.

F. Care of Patient Before Hospitalization

As a general rule, the following measures should be taken for patients with fractures:

1. The joints above and below the fracture should be mobilized and adequate immobilization of the cervical spine should be obtained to prevent further damage to the neurovascular elements and limit hemorrhage.
2. Splints can be improvised with pillows, blankets, or clothing.
3. Immobilization does not need to be absolutely rigid.
4. Apply gentle in-line traction to realign the extremity when there is severe angulation.
5. Overt bleeding should be tamponaded with available dressings and firm pressure.
6. Tourniquets should be avoided, unless the patient's life is in danger from extremity bleeding.

▶ Orthopedic Examination

A. History

An adequate assessment of the conditions in which the injury was sustained is crucial. Information from paramedics, patient relatives, and bystanders should be recorded. Obtain the following information according to injury mechanism:

1. MVA: speed; direction (T bone, rollover, etc.); patient location in the vehicle, impact location, postimpact location of the patient (if ejection, determine distance); internal and external damage to the vehicle; restraint use and type.
2. Falls: distance of the fall; landing position.
3. Crush: weight of the object, site of the injury, duration of weight application.

4. Explosion: blast magnitude; patient distance from the blast: primary blast injury (force of the blast wave); secondary blast injury (projectiles).

5. Vehicle-pedestrian: type of vehicle, site of collision, speed.

Environmental exposure, comorbidity (diabetes, coronary artery disease, etc.), use of steroids, prehospital care, and observations at the accident scene should be determined. Estimated bleeding, open wounds, deformity, motor and sensory function, and delays in extrication or transport are recorded.

B. General Examination

The clinical orthopedic examination requires assessment of the axial skeleton, pelvis, and extremities. The extent of this examination depends on the patient's overall central neurologic status. Swelling, hematomas, and open wounds are assessed visually in the undressed patient. It is obligatory to palpate the entire spine, pelvis, and each joint. Examination soon after trauma may precede telltale swelling in joint or long bone injuries. In the unresponsive patient, only crepitation and false motion may be discerned. The pelvic examination is important; however, if the patient is hemodynamically unstable, manipulation of the pelvis should be avoided in order to prevent increased bleeding.

C. Neurologic Examination

The neurologic examination of the extremities should be documented to the fullest extent possible, in light of the patient's mental status, because it is central to subsequent decision making. This examination includes delineation of sensory function in the major nerves and dermatomes in the upper and lower extremities. Perianal sensation is also important. A normal neurologic examination does not rule out cervical spine injuries; it only makes them less likely. Particularly important when there is spinal cord injury or suspected injury are the reflexes of the anal "wink" and bulbocavernosus muscle. Other spinal reflexes (ie, of the biceps and triceps muscles, of the knee and ankle, and the Babinski reflex) are important in "fine-tuning" the neurologic examination. (These are discussed more fully in Chapter 4, "Disorders, Diseases, and Injuries of the Spine.")

D. Muscle Examination

Motor examination can be difficult because of pain or impaired mental status, but even in such cases, useful and relatively complete information can be obtained. One must be sure to evaluate all upper and lower extremity motion. Hematoma, ecchymosis, and dermabrasions should be noted for an underlying muscle injury. Muscle strength grading is desirable, but demonstration of a minimum of volitional control (even if withdrawal to painful stimuli) is important in verifying the presence of intact central sensory-motor integration.

▶ Imaging Studies

Radiologic assessment follows the same general hierarchy as the clinical assessment. The severely injured polytrauma patient requires plain films of the chest, abdomen, *and* pelvis to indicate sources of respiratory and circulatory compromise. The second level of examination requires the cervical spine cross-table lateral view. The information obtained from this film dictates treatment and the need for any further evaluation of the cervical spine. In the hemodynamically unstable patient, the anteroposterior (AP) pelvis film is sufficient to make immediate treatment decisions. Complementary pelvis films can be obtained later.

Subsequent evaluation is dependent on clinical findings. Any long bone or joint with a laceration, hematoma, angulation, or swelling must undergo roentgenographic evaluation. Any long bone fracture requires complete evaluation of the joints proximal and distal to the fracture. At the minimum, two views of the extremities are needed, usually the AP and lateral views. The use of focused assessment sonography in trauma (FAST) has also become an extension of the physical examination of the trauma patient. Coordination of more sophisticated studies with other trauma specialties (eg, neurosurgery or urology) is necessary to allow cardiorespiratory monitoring of the patient while efficiently performing these studies.

▶ "Clearing" the Cervical Spine

The ATLS (Advanced Trauma Life Support) protocol mandates that all patients are presumed to have a cervical spine injury until proven otherwise. The objective of cervical spine clearance is to establish that an injury does not exist. If there is a change in orientation from one cervical spine level to another, then cervical fracture, jumped facets, or dislocation should be suspected. Immobilization in a cervical collar should be initiated until the secondary evaluation has been made. In the conscious and responsive patient, swelling or tenderness on physical examination of the cervical spine is readily apparent. In the unconscious patient, cervical spine injuries can go undetected, and a careful physical examination must be performed with heavy reliance on radiographic evaluation.

The essential radiographs for evaluation of the cervical spine include AP views, lateral views, and an open-mouth odontoid view. It is essential to be able to see to the top of T1. If this level is not visualized through these conventional views, the inclusion of oblique view and swimmer's view, which is a lateral cervical spine radiograph with the arm abducted and elevated, only slightly improves the sensitivity and, therefore, has been deemed cost-inefficient.

On the open-mouth view, the lateral masses of C1 should line up with the body of C2. The amount of total overhang

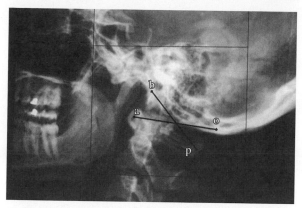

▲ **Figure 2–1.** Powers ratio: a – anterior arch of atlas, b – basion, p – posterior arch of atlas, o – opisthion. The ratio of bp:oa should be approximately 0.77 in the normal population. Anterior occipitoatlantal dislocation is present when the Powers ratio is greater than 1.15.

of C1 over C2 should be less than 7 mm. On the lateral view, the anterior border of the bodies of the cervical segments should be an arc. The distance from the basion to the posterior arch of C1 divided by the distance from the opisthion to the anterior arch of C1 should be less than 1 (Powers ratio) (Figure 2–1). A basion to odontoid tip distance greater than 10 mm in children and 5 mm in adults indicates craniocervical dislocation, a potentially fatal injury. The posterior border of the anterior arch of C1 should be within 2–3 mm of the anterior border of C2. There should be no diastasis of the spinous processes, and the joints and facet joints should all be visible. In the obtunded patient, computed tomography (CT) and/or magnetic resonance imaging (MRI) scan is necessary to delineate soft-tissue injuries. Although CT is sensitive in the identification of osseous abnormalities, it has not been shown to have the same level of accuracy as MRI in detecting an isolated ligamentous injury. MRI is not indicated for primary cervical spine clearance imaging procedures. MRI requires extensive time to perform, interferes with the patient's monitoring equipment, and is expensive. MRI is most useful in the patient for whom other imaging modalities are not consistent with the neurologic presentation.

In the case of neurologic deficit, careful evaluation of the neurologic status is important, and immediate decompression-stabilization must be considered.

▶ Immediate Management of Musculoskeletal Trauma

The orthopedic injuries in the polytrauma patient are seldom truly emergency situations, except for those involving neural or vascular compromise. For example, fracture-dislocation of the ankle or knee resulting in distal ischemia justifies immediate attempts at reduction to minimize the sequelae of ischemia. A more subtle situation requiring emergent treatment would be dislocation of the hip in which vascular compromise of the femoral head, avascular necrosis, may result. Arterial bleeding from an open fracture should be treated immediately with pressure to minimize blood loss. Other bone and joint injuries, although urgent, may be approached in a more deliberate manner.

Orthopedic surgeons must be aware that management of traumatic injuries requires consideration of the entire patient as well as the entire extremity.

▶ Complications

There is ample evidence to indicate that the early treatment of fractures in a multiply injured patient has a significant effect on the risk of the subsequent development of respiratory complications. Traumatic injury leads to systemic inflammation as a normal response to injury. Extent of injury, hypoxia, consequent surgeries, and blood loss may impair the balance existing between the beneficial effects of inflammation and the potential for the process itself to cause and aggravate tissue injury, leading to acute respiratory distress syndrome (ARDS) and multiple organ failure (MOF). Early fracture fixation allows early mobilization, which is beneficial to prevent pulmonary complications. Definitive or lengthy surgery, however, causes further complications.

A. Acute Respiratory Distress Syndrome and Multiple Organ Failure

ARDS is used to describe the respiratory failure associated with evidence of multiple organ dysfunction, which occurs in patients after high-energy injury. The lung is prominently targeted in the early stages, but if the patient survives, features of cardiac, gastrointestinal, renal, hepatic, hematologic, and cerebral failure become apparent as part of the syndrome of MOF. Massive tissue injury activates the immunologic system and releases inflammatory mediators, with subsequent disruption of the microvasculature of the pulmonary system. Some acute orthopedic procedures have been shown to similarly activate the immune system. The incidence of ARDS after major trauma is probably between 5 and 8%, with mortality between 3 and 40% of cases. Postinjury MOF is the most significant cause of late trauma mortality.

Fat embolism syndrome (FES) is a unique manifestation of ARDS caused by the release of marrow fat into the circulation. Embolism occurs in over 95% of patients after fracture and invariably during reamed nailing of fractures. However, only 1–5% of patients develop severe pulmonary compromise and FES. This syndrome may also occur in nonfracture situations involving pressurization of the medullary canal of long bones. Cardinal pulmonary signs of ARDS and FES are refractory hypoxemia, not correctable by high-dose oxygen therapy (60–100%), associated with the development of a characteristic "snowstorm" appearance in both lung fields on chest radiography. A characteristic petechial rash is found in 60% of patients with FES, and neurologic features are encountered in over 80%, including the development of an acute confusional state or a focal neurologic deficit.

B. Atelectasis

Atelectasis, or localized collapse of alveoli, is a frequent postoperative complication because of patient immobilization. Combined with respiratory depression due to analgesia, significant hypoxemia can result, and onset may be relatively rapid. This may be a source of postoperative fever in the early recovery phase. Occasionally, radiograph examination, showing collapse of areas of the lung, will confirm the diagnosis. By encouraging coughing and deep breathing, using incentive spirometry, and, in resistant cases, using respiratory therapy, resolution can be expected.

C. Pulmonary Embolism and Deep Venous Thrombosis

Pulmonary embolism (PE) is the third most common cause of death in trauma patients who survive after the first day. The trauma patient is at a 13-fold increased risk of venous thromboembolism (VTE). There are several factors associated with increased risk of VTE in a trauma patient (Table 2–1). Patients at high risk for PE are those with deep venous thrombosis (DVT) in the lower extremities and pelvic veins. Clinically significant PE usually arises from the large veins proximal to the knee. Prevention of DVT in the venous system in this area reduces the risk of PE. Various strategies used to accomplish this include drug therapy with low-dose heparin, low-molecular-weight heparin, pentasaccharide, or sodium warfarin and mechanical prophylaxis with intermittent pneumatic compression devices or inferior vena cava filters in high-risk patients with contraindications to pharmacologic prophylaxis.

Clinical diagnosis of DVT is unreliable. Definitive diagnosis is made with venography, duplex ultrasound scanning, impedance plethysmography, or CT or MRI venography. Prevention appears to be the best strategy because even routine surveillance screening in a trauma population is cost-ineffective and does not appear to lower the overall rate of PE.

PE is suspected in the orthopedic patient suffering an onset of tachypnea and dyspnea usually more than 5 days after an inciting event. The patient frequently reports chest pain and can often point to the painful area. On physical examination, tachycardia, cyanosis, and pleural friction rub can be noted. Arterial blood gas studies demonstrate hypoxemia, although this is a nonspecific finding. Use of the D-dimer is unreliable in the early trauma patient but may be useful later in the recovery period. Definitive diagnosis is best made with CT angiogram. Perfusion ventilation scanning is less invasive and may help determine whether there is a high or low probability of PE. Single-slice spiral CT has become the reference standard for imaging acute PE in clinical practice. The negative predictive value of a normal spiral CT approaches 98%.

Treatment involves pulmonary support and heparin therapy. The natural history of treated PE is gradual lysis of the emboli, with the return of flow through the pulmonary arterial tree. The natural history of proximal DVT involves recanalization and arborization to bypass the clot. Patients may suffer from postphlebitic syndrome characterized by chronically painful swelling in the extremity.

D. Compartment Syndrome

The term *compartment syndrome* refers to pathologic developments in a closed space in the body caused by buildup of pressure. Most commonly, such compartments are circumscribed by fascia and incorporate one or more bones. Pressure rises from edema or bleeding within the compartment, compromising circulation to the contents of the compartment over a period, and can result in necrosis of muscle and damage to nerves.

Compartment syndrome may result from a fracture; a soft-tissue injury; a vascular injury causing ischemia, necrosis, and edema; or a burn. Failure to redistribute pressure through postural changes results in ischemia of the area under pressure because of collapse of capillaries.

The diagnosis of compartment syndrome must be considered in the postoperative or posttrauma patient who has pain out of proportion to that expected from the inciting injury. As the pain worsens, it can become totally unresponsive to narcotic medication. Subsequent to fracture or injury, pain with passive stretching of involved muscles is also a subjective finding and must be differentiated from pain arising from the original injury.

The five P's (pulselessness, paresthesia, paresis, pain, and pressure) characteristic of compartment syndrome are helpful, but not diagnostic. Pulses are poor indicators of compartment syndrome as they generally remain intact until late.

Patients with equivocal clinical findings or those at high risk but without a reliable clinical examination (eg, those

---

Table 2–1. Factors that increase the risk for developing venous thromboembolism (VTE) in trauma patients.

1. Obesity
2. Age >55 years
3. Spinal cord injuries
4. Major thoracolumbar spinal fractures
5. Major pelvic and lower extremity fractures
6. History of prior VTE
7. Major abdominal surgery
8. Multiple trauma with ISS >16
9. Admission to ICU with immobilization for ≥4 days
10. Malignancy

ICU, intensive care unit; ISS, Injury Severity Score.

who are comatose, have psychiatric problems, or are under the influence of narcotics) should have compartmental pressure measurements.

Intracompartmental pressure readings within 30 mm Hg or less of the diastolic blood pressure are indications for fasciotomy. Prior to fasciotomy, circular dressings, including casts, should be removed, and the patient should be observed for a short period for signs of improvement. Positive clinical findings may justify fasciotomy despite normal pressures. Late fasciotomy may result in muscle damage or possible necrosis, with resulting risk of infection.

Although compartment syndrome can occur in almost any portion of the body, young patients who have a tibia fracture or patients with a high-energy forearm fracture are at particular risk. In the forearm, an extensile volar incision to permit complete release, including the carpal tunnel distally and the lacertus fibrosus proximally, is necessary. Dorsally, a longitudinal incision is used. In the calf, two incisions are used to release the four compartments of the leg. The anterior and lateral compartments are decompressed using a longitudinal incision approximately over the anterior intermuscular septum. Posteromedially, a second incision is used to approach the superficial and deep posterior compartments. While single and limited incision approaches have been described, these may be unreliable and have a higher incidence of iatrogenic nerve injury in trauma patients.

E. Heterotopic Bone Formation

Clinically significant heterotopic ossification occurs as a consequence of trauma in perhaps 10% of cases and may cause pain or joint motion restriction even to the point of ankylosis. Trauma patients without head injuries frequently manifest heterotopic ossification on radiograph 1–2 months following trauma; if the ossification is clinically significant, resection may be indicated when the bone has matured as indicated by radiographs and bone scan. This can take up to 18 months to achieve.

Resection is accomplished by removing the entire piece of heterotopic bone. Selected patients may benefit from low-dose radiation (7 Gy) and oral indomethacin for 3–6 weeks. In acetabular fractures, a focused single dose of radiation may be better than oral indomethacin. Heterotopic bone is a much more common occurrence in patients with head injuries. This is believed to result from release of humeral modulators that have not yet been characterized. Further discussion of this topic can be found in Chapter 12, "Rehabilitation."

▶ Classification of Open Fractures: Gustilo and Anderson Classification

The Gustilo and Anderson classification, the most popular and generally accepted classification of open fractures, uses three grades and divides the third most severe grade into three subtypes (Table 2–2). The prevalence of wound infection increases with the increase in grade of open injury.

Table 2–2. Gustilo-Anderson classification for open fractures.

Type I		Clean wound <1 cm, inside-out perforation, little or no contamination, simple fracture pattern.
Type II		Skin laceration >1 cm, surrounding soft tissue without signs of contusion, vital musculature, moderate-to-severe fracture instability.
Type III		Extensive soft tissue damage, wound contamination, exposed bone, marked fracture instability due to comminution or segmental defects.
	IIIA	Adequate soft-tissue coverage of the fractured bone after surgical debridement.
	IIIB	Exposed bone with periosteal stripping, requiring flap coverage.
	IIIC	Any open fracture with associated arterial injury requiring vascular repair.

Open fractures resulting from natural disasters, highly contaminated or comminuted, independent of wound size, are automatically classified as grade III open fractures.

The magnitude of soft-tissue and bony injuries complicates the decision making between immediate amputation and reconstruction in the lower extremity. Despite the advent of microvascular surgery, prosthetic replacements are a viable alternative to a poorly functioning, insensate lower extremity. Long years of reconstruction to achieve union without infection, multiple operations, and emotional trauma should be considered in the decision making of salvage versus amputation.

▶ Early Total Care

The desirability of early fracture stabilization in multiply injured patients has become well established. Benefits of timely and aggressive treatment include decreased rates of mortality, primarily due to reductions in ARDS and MOF. In a classic study by Bone et al, 178 patients with femoral fractures were entered into an early fixation group (treatment within 24 hours) or a delayed fixation group (treatment after 48 hours). The incidence of pulmonary complications, such as ARDS, fat embolism, or pneumonia, was higher, the hospital stay was longer, and the intensive care unit requirements increased when femoral fixation was delayed. A follow-up, retrospective, multicenter study of 676 patients who had an Injury Severity Score greater than 18 and major pelvic or long-bone injuries treated with early fixation within 48 hours revealed a lower mortality rate for patients whose fractures were stabilized early.

▶ Damage Control Orthopedics

Controversy exists regarding the appropriate timing of orthopedic intervention for specific subsets of severely injured patients, particularly those with head injury or systemic hypotension. Long bone fracture fixation with reamed intramedullary rods, in particular, may cause intraoperative hypotension or an increased release of inflammatory mediators with deleterious results in specific patients.

The multiply injured patient's immunologic system is stimulated or primed after trauma (first event). Subsequent resuscitation, hemorrhage, blood products, hypotension, and surgery (second event) may produce an exaggerated systemic inflammatory response syndrome (SIRS), potentially leading to ARDS or MOF. Activated neutrophils are the principal effector of the inflammatory response, releasing active oxygen species, which damage the vascular endothelium. Bone marrow contents pushed to the systemic circulation during reaming and nailing can activate neutrophils, leading to SIRS in polytrauma patients, particularly during the first 96 hours after trauma. Damage control orthopedics (DCO) aims to decrease the additional surgical trauma through external fixation and secondary definitive surgery. Several studies demonstrated that conversion of an external fixator to a reamed intramedullary nail is safe and effective if performed within 2 weeks. Alternatives to modify the inflammatory response are currently under investigation. Tuttle et al showed that DCO is a safer initial approach that helps to reduce blood loss and significantly decrease the initial operative exposure. Additionally, in 2008, Parekh et al demonstrated that temporary bridging fixation and planned conversion to internal fixation of periarticular knee fractures resulting from high-energy injury avoid the risk of potential local soft-tissue damage of early internal fixation.

▶ Soft-Tissue Injuries and Traumatic Arthrotomies

Lacerations of the extremities can result in neural or vascular compromise to an extremity and may also cause traumatic arthrotomies. Compromise of the sterility of any joint requires surgical debridement of that joint. For many joints, arthroscopic irrigation and debridement will minimize trauma and improve the return to function. All complete tendon lacerations of the hand, except for those of the palmaris longus, should be repaired. In the foot, extrinsic tendons are repaired to prevent late imbalance or loss of function. Muscle belly injuries generally require surgical debridement because their subfascial location makes simple irrigation difficult. Laceration involving only the muscle belly usually requires no surgical repair. Frequently, however, muscle belly laceration involves the continuation of the origin or the insertion tendon of the muscle. In this case, optimal function is obtained by reattaching the lacerated ends.

In most cases, immediate treatment of open fractures and lacerations consists of surgical debridement. Debridement removes nonviable tissue. Generally, care should be taken to remove only tissue that is necrotic. Skin edges should

be debrided, as should dead muscle and the surface of any contaminated fat or fascia. Soft-tissue attachments to bone should be maintained whenever possible. Fragments of bone, particularly cortical bone, without attachment, should be removed from the wound. Prior to formal debridement, it is appropriate to splint fractures and cover open wounds with sterile wet dressings. Antibiotic therapy is begun immediately, usually with a cephalosporin bactericidal antibiotic. Tetanus prophylaxis is administered if needed. Antibiotic therapy is continued based on the clinical course.

Although it is acceptable practice to leave any wound open, grade I wounds may be closed completely. Following effective operative debridement, grade II wounds may be treated in a similar fashion, with close initial follow-up. Primary closure of grade III wounds is rarely performed. Patients with massive wounds should be returned to the operating room within 48 hours and then every 48 hours until the wound is completely clean and granulating. Smaller wounds that are left open may be closed safely at 3–5 days.

▶ Flaps and Soft-Tissue Coverage for Open Trauma

Because of extensive soft-tissue damage involved, type IIIB and IIIC open fractures require aggressive surgical management for wound coverage. These wounds may be treated by regional or free flap reconstruction. With the advent of microsurgical techniques for skin, muscle, and fascia transplantation, the treatment of large soft-tissue trauma has changed, and local rotational flaps, fasciocutaneous flaps, or free tissue transfer can be used successfully. Despite the classic study by Godina favoring immediate free flap reconstruction within the first 48 hours after trauma, controversy still exists for the timing for reconstruction. The requirement for this procedure is radical debridement of the zone of injury, similar to the way one would resect a tumor.

If radical debridement is not performed, then flap reconstruction should be delayed until soft tissues have healed at the margins and there is no sign of infection. The use of free flaps gives an overall improved outcome by bringing a new source of vascularity to a compromised extremity, preventing infection and simultaneously providing soft-tissue coverage.

There are many sites that can be harvested for flaps. The most common and hardiest flaps include fasciocutaneous flaps from the latissimus dorsi, gracilis, serratus anterior, and rectus abdominis muscles. These are suitable for medium- to large-size wounds in a variety of locations. Additionally, there are a host of smaller tissue transfers designed for more specific uses that have advantages in the matching of defect to donor and minimizing problems at the donor site.

A recent innovation in wound management is vacuum-assisted closure (VAC) therapy. The VAC system exposes the wound bed to negative pressure in a closed system. The stretching stimulus is transformed into microchemical forces that promote wound healing through increased cell division and proliferation, angiogenesis stimulation, and local increase of growth factors. Also, edema fluid is removed from the extravascular space, eliminating the extrinsic cause of microcirculatory alteration and improving local blood supply. Although this device does not replace the need for surgical debridement, it may avoid the need for a free tissue transfer in patients with large traumatic wounds. Additional orthopedic indications include the treatment of infected wounds after debridement, war wounds, and fasciotomy closures.

Gunshot Wounds

Gunshot wounds to the musculoskeletal system result in complex soft-tissue lesions, fractures that are often comminuted, and related nerve, artery, and tendon involvement. A gunshot wound near a major joint should also be suspected of penetrating the joint. Optimum treatment of fractures caused by gunshots relies on an appreciation of the kinetic energy of injury, direction, caliber, and distance. Differences between high-velocity (>2000 ft/s) and low-velocity (<2000 ft/s) weapons and civilian and military settings for these wounds are also important. Additional characteristics are the efficiency of energy transfer, including deformation and fragmentation, kinetic energy, stability, profile of entrance, path through the body, and biologic characteristics of the tissues. In general, kinetic energy associated with an injury is calculated by the formula, $E = M/2 \times V^2$, where M equals mass and V equals velocity. Along with the characteristics of the tissue penetrated, velocity and missile mass are the determinants of resultant type and amount of tissue damage. Velocity is more important than mass, doubling the velocity quadruples the kinetic energy. Shotguns are technically low-velocity weapons, but shotgun injuries are different from single gunshot wounds, because the weight of the shot causes an increase in the kinetic energy, resulting in a more severe injury.

In gunshot wounds and high-velocity missiles, shock waves, laceration and crushing, and cavitation result in tissue damage. Shock waves can produce injury in areas that are relatively distant from the direct path of the missile. Cavitation is an important mechanism of tissue damage in high-velocity injuries. The subatmospheric pressure in the cavity sucks contaminants in from both ends. Missile wound tracks close to a major vessel may be associated with occult vascular injury despite normal pulses. Doppler ultrasound is indicated when a vascular injury is suspected. Retained bullet or a fragment in the synovial fluid within a joint can cause lead toxicity.

The majority of low-velocity gunshot wounds can be managed with local wound care and outpatient treatment. The wound should be left open for drainage. If the fracture requires surgical treatment, antibiotic prophylaxis is recommended.

The use of immediate fixation by either internal or external fixator means is controversial. On the one hand, the danger of treatment of these open fractures with foreign material is a deterrent for immediate stabilization. However, in grossly unstable injuries, treatment that would be used for other open fractures appears to be reasonable in selected cases. The use of temporary external fixation as a bridge from the injury to definitive fracture stabilization has become a popular means of initially stabilizing the fracture.

High-velocity and shotgun fractures require surgical irrigation, appropriate debridement, and at least 24–48 hours of intravenous antibiotic treatment. Vascular injuries should be explored and repaired after prompt fracture stabilization. Distal neurologic deficit alone is not an indication for exploration, as it often resolves without surgical intervention and is due to a blast neurapraxia.

Multiple Trauma Patient Scoring Systems

Several classification systems have been used to try to stratify multiple injured patients and to determine severity of injuries. The classification systems serve as a guide for both patient treatment and eventual outcomes. The Revised Trauma Score (RTS) was developed to help with patient triage. The scores for systolic blood pressure and respiratory rate are separated into five domains with each assigned a point value from 0 to 4. These scores are added to the Glasgow Coma Score (GCS) to yield an RTS. The GCS is the most accepted score for traumatic brain injury. This scale ranges from 3 to 15, with 15 being normal. Evaluation is based on three sections: eye movement, verbal response, and motor response. In the United States, the American College of Surgeons' guidelines direct patients with a GCS of 11 or less to a designated trauma center.

The Abbreviated Injury Scale (AIS) divides injuries into nine body regions and stratifies the injuries from minor to fatal on a 6-point scale. These scores take into account life-threatening aspects of injuries, anticipated permanent impairment, treatment, and injury pattern.

The Injury Severity Score (ISS) is the sum of the squares of the highest AIS scores in the three most severely injured body regions, which are chosen from head or neck, face, chest, abdomen, extremities or pelvic girdle, and external (skin). Multiple-trauma patients are defined as patients with an ISS greater than or equal to 14. A good prognosis is associated with an ISS of less than 30, whereas an ISS greater than 60 is usually fatal.

Factors at the time of injury that have a bearing on the decision to amputate include status of the opposite leg, the time of limb ischemia, and the age of the patient. Many of these factors have been accounted for by Johansen et al, who have defined a Mangled Extremity Severity Score (MESS). The MESS was previously used as a predictor of eventual amputation; however, recent studies have shown the MESS and other scoring systems to be inaccurate in predicting the functional outcome for mangled limb patients (Table 2–3).

Table 2–3. Factors in evaluation of the mangled extremity severity score (MESS) variables.

	Points
A. Skeletal and soft-tissue injury	
Low energy (stab; simple fracture; "civilian" gunshot wound)	1
Medium energy (open or multiple fractures, dislocation)	2
High energy (close-range shotgun or "military" gunshot wound, crush injury)	3
Very high energy (above plus gross contamination, soft-tissue avulsion)	4
B. Limb ischemia[a]	
Pulse reduced or absent but perfusion normal	1
Pulseless; paresthesia, diminished capillary refilling	2
Cool, paralyzed, insensate, numb	3
C. Shock	
Systolic blood pressure almost >90 mm Hg	0
Hypotensive transiently	1
Persistent hypotension	2
D. Age	
<30 years	0
30–50 years	1
>50 years	2

[a]Score doubled for ischemia more than 6 hours.

Anglen JO: Wound irrigation in musculoskeletal injury. *J Am Acad Orthop Surg* 2001;9:219. [PMID: 11476531]

Bartlett CS: Ballistic and gunshot wounds: effects on musculoskeletal tissues. *J Am Acad Orthop Surg* 2000;8:21. [PMID: 10666650]

Biffl WL, Smith WR, Moore EE, et al: Evolution of a multidisciplinary clinical pathway for the management of unstable patients with pelvic fractures. *Ann Surg* 2001;233:843. [PMID: 11407336]

Bone LB, McNamara K, Shine B, Border J: Mortality in multiple trauma patients with fractures. *J Trauma* 1994;37:262. [PMID: 8064927]

Bosse MJ, Mackenzie EJ, Kellam JF, et al: A prospective evaluation of the clinical utility of the lower-extremity injury-severity scores. *J Bone Joint Surg Am* 2001;83-A:3-14. [PMID: 11205855]

Dickson K, Watson TS, Haddad C, Jenne J, Harris M: Outpatient management of low-velocity gunshot-induced fractures. *Orthopedics* 2001;24:951. [PMID: 11688773]

Giannoudis PV, Pountos I, Pape HC, Patel JV: Safety and efficacy of vena cava filters in trauma patients. *Injury* 2007;38:7-18. [PMID:17070525]

Godina M: The tailored latissimus dorsi free flap. *Plast Reconstr Surg* 1987;80:304. [PMID: 3602183]

Gustilo RB, Anderson JT: Prevention of infection in the treatment of 1025 open fractures of long bones. *J Bone Joint Surg Am* 1976;58:453. [PMID: 773941]

Hammert WC, Minarchek J, Trzeciak MA: Free-flap reconstruction of traumatic lower extremity wounds. *Am J Orthop* 2000;29:22. [PMID: 11011776]

Hildebrand F, Giannoudis P, Krettek C, Pape HC: Damage control: extremities. *Injury* 2004;35:678. [PMID: 15203308]

Johansen K, Daines M, Howey T, et al: Objective criteria accurately predict amputation following lower extremity trauma. *J Trauma* 1990;30:568. [PMID: 2342140]

Mendelson SA, Dominick TS, Tyler-Kabara E, et al: Early versus late femoral fracture stabilization in multiply injured pediatric patients with closed head injury. *J Pediatr Orthop* 2001;21:594. [PMID: 11521025]

Mullett H, Al-Abed K, Prasad CV, O'Sullivan M: Outcome of compartment syndrome following intramedullary nailing of tibial diaphyseal fractures. *Injury* 2001;32:411. [PMID: 11382428]

Pape HC, Tornetta P 3rd, Tarkin I, Tzioupis C, Sabeson V, Olson SA: Timing of fracture fixation in multitrauma patients: the role of early total care and damage control surgery. *J Am Acad Orthop Surg* 2009;17:541-549. [PMID: 19726738]

Parekh AA, Smith WR, Silva S, et al: Treatment of distal femur and proximal tibia fractures with external fixation followed by planned conversion to internal fixation. *J Trauma* 2008;64: 736-739. [PMID: 18332816]

Perrier A, Howarth N, Didier D, et al: Performance of helical computed tomography in unselected outpatients with suspected pulmonary embolism. *Ann Intern Med* 2001;135:88. [PMID: 11453707]

Pierce TD, Tomaino MM: Use of the pedicled latissimus muscle flap for upper-extremity reconstruction. *J Am Acad Orthop Surg* 2000;8:324. [PMID: 11029560]

Schoepf UJ: Diagnosing pulmonary embolism: time to rewrite the textbooks. *Int J Cardiovasc Imaging* 2005;21:155-163. [PMID: 15915948]

Stannard JP, Riley RS, McClenney MD, et al: Mechanical prophylaxis against deep-vein thrombosis after pelvic and acetabular fractures. *J Bone Joint Surg Am* 2001;83-A:1047. [PMID: 11451974]

Tuttle MS, Smith WR, Williams AE, et al: Safety and efficacy of damage control external fixation versus early definitive stabilization for femoral shaft fractures in the multiple-injured patient. *J Trauma* 2009;67:602-605. [PMID: 19741407]

Van Belle A, Büller HR, Huisman MV, et al: Effectiveness of managing suspected pulmonary embolism using an algorithm combining clinical probability, D-dimer testing, and computed tomography. *JAMA* 2006;295:172. [PMID: 16403929]

PRINCIPLES OF OPERATIVE FRACTURE FIXATION

Fractures occur when one or more types of stress, in excess of failure strength, are applied to bones. Fractures may occur from axial loading (tension, compression), bending, torsion (a twisting force), or shearing. The type of failure and mechanism of injury may be helpful in determining fracture treatment. Examples of these are shown in Figure 2–2.

▶ Biomaterials Used in Fracture Fixation

Operative fracture fixation requires strength and flexibility of the fixation materials. Metal implants made of stainless steel and titanium offer high stiffness and strength, good

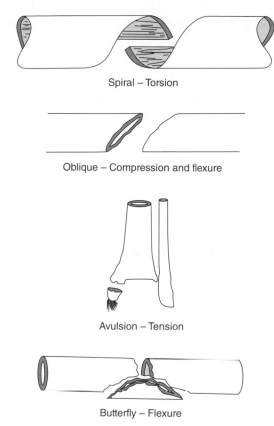

Spiral – Torsion

Oblique – Compression and flexure

Avulsion – Tension

Butterfly – Flexure

▲ **Figure 2–2.** Mechanisms of failure of bones.

ductility, and are biologically well tolerated. Titanium alloy and stainless steel both may be contoured to fit irregularities without compromising stability in bone surfaces at the time of surgery. They provide adequate strength and fatigue resistance to permit fracture healing to occur. The elastic modulus of titanium is half that of stainless steel, resulting in half the flexural rigidity in plates of equal size. The modulus measures the material stiffness and its ability to resist deformation when a force is applied. Ductility is the property of a material that undergoes significant plastic deformation before failure. An example of a ductile material is stainless steel.

▶ Biomechanical Principles of Fracture Fixation

Fracture healing requires specific sufficient biologic and mechanical conditions. This is provided by blood supply, mediator and hormonal stimuli, and a certain degree of immobilization. By compression of two anatomically reduced fracture fragments, absolute stability can be achieved. Lag screw, compression plate fixation, and tension band techniques are examples of absolute stability. If there is some motion between fracture fragments that is compatible with fracture healing, this is called relative stability and promotes indirect bone healing, resulting in callus. Motion should be below strain level of tissue repair. Intramedullary nails, bridge plates, and external fixators are examples of devices that provide indirect healing.

A. Screws

Screws are the most common and basic form of fixation. They are generally used to function as lag screws, locking or nonlocked plate screws, and positioning screws. They can be used alone or with a plate. The locking head screws have a head with a thread that engages with the reciprocal head of the plate hole. Lag screw technique is a powerful way to compress a fracture plane providing absolute stability. This can be achieved by fully or partially threaded screws. An example of a positioning screw is a screw placed between the tibia and fibula in the presence of a syndesmotic injury.

B. Titanium and Stainless Steel Rods

Regardless of the localization or the type of the fracture, the most important feature in application of an intramedullary nail is the entry point. Current literature supports "gentle" reaming to be superior and safe compared with unreamed technique. One must pay attention to the general condition of a patient especially with the multiply injured patients. Insertion of a femoral nail may exacerbate pulmonary injury in the polytrauma patient with chest injury. Many available nail options for the femur, tibia, and humerus are on the market. Current techniques recommend that all nails be statically locked.

C. Bone Plate

The placement of a plate on a bone has a significant bearing on its function. Optimal placement of a plate is on the tension side of the bone, so that the bone will be placed in compressive loading as a result of muscle action. This stimulates healing and minimizes the stresses on the plate.

The conventional plate and screw system requires substantial bone exposure for access for open reduction and internal fixation. The surgeon-contoured plate is compressed onto the bone with screws resulting in anatomic reduction and absolute stability. The compressive forces acting on the bone–plate interface can compromise the blood supply and hence the healing process. The low contact dynamic compression (LCDC) plate was developed to reduce the bone–plate contact surface area.

Locking plates or internal fixators use a system where the screw head threads into the plate hole, thereby locking the plate just above the bone to minimize contact surface area and compressive forces. The locked screws in the plate also act as a second bone cortex, and therefore self-tapping unicortical screws can be used. This achieves relative stability and therefore promotes callus formation at the fracture site.

During fixation, the working length of the plate and screws should be kept in mind with the aim of increasing the working length of the plate and reducing the number of screws used in order to facilitate callus.

D. External Fixation

External fixation is an important treatment modality for musculoskeletal injuries. The basic principles are that pins are placed within the musculoskeletal system proximal and distal to the zone of injury. These pins are then placed on an external frame, a frame outside the confines of the bone and soft-tissue envelope, to stabilize fractures. These devices can be useful as temporary treatment for musculoskeletal injuries or as definitive treatment, depending on their location and the type of bone and soft-tissue trauma. In the upper extremity, they play a significant role in treating comminuted distal radius fractures.

For the pelvis, rapidly applied external fixation with compression for pelvic injuries can stabilize the pelvis, reduce blood loss, be of assistance in initial resuscitation, and in some cases provide definitive treatment of such injuries.

For femur and tibia fractures, external fixation may provide excellent and safe initial or provisional stabilization, which can then be converted to intramedullary fixation for definitive care.

External fixators are frequently used as provisional treatment for grade III open fractures with segmental bone loss and large soft-tissue injuries of the upper and lower extremity.

▶ Bone Substitutes Used in Fracture Fixation

A. Autogenous Bone Grafting

Autologous bone grafting is the gold standard for management of bone defects and nonunion due to a combination of osteogenic, osteoinductive, and osteoconductive properties. Different types of autologous bone grafts have variable properties associated with structural anatomy. Cancellous grafts are most commonly harvested from the iliac crest. These have a history of success despite variable complication rates. However, with the recently developed reamer-irrigator-aspirator (RIA) system, large quantities of autologous bone graft can be harvested from the femoral and tibial medullary cavities with minimal morbidity.

B. Osteoconductive Graft Substitutes

Hydroxyapatite and tricalcium phosphate are inorganic structural bone graft substitutes that are primarily osteoconductive. They provide scaffold for new bony growth and do not stimulate bone formation. These materials can be injected into fracture sites, such as the distal radius and calcaneus, to provide stabilization from compressive loads. If they are combined with growth factors (eg, BMPs), they may also show osteoinductive and osteogenic properties.

C. Donor Bone Allografts

Allograft bone grafting, which is the transfer of bone between two genetically dissimilar individuals of same species, is used primarily to support mechanical loads and resist failure at sites where structural support is desired. The greatest concern with using allograft materials is the possibility of viral disease transmission. Several methods may be used to process allograft bone, including low-dose (<20 kGy) irradiation, physical debridement, ultrasonic or pulsatile water washes, ethanol treatment, and antibiotic soaking. Sterilization treatments, such as irradiation and ethylene oxide, are known to compromise these qualities to some extent, with ethylene oxide perhaps being worse than irradiation. Freeze-dried bone is convenient for storage at room temperature but must be sterilized secondarily with ethylene oxide. Because ethylene oxide is unable to penetrate to the depths of large pieces, secondary sterilization of large structural allografts is safer with radiation. The accepted dosage of gamma radiation is 2.5 mrad, but even this dose may not be sufficient to eradicate the human immunodeficiency virus. However, allograft bone usage with the current sterilization technique has been shown to be safe and effective for specific indications.

D. Osteoinductive Agents

BMPs have been identified as important components of musculoskeletal repair for bone and cartilage growth. With recent advances in molecular biology and recombinant DNA techniques, rhBMP-7 and rhBMP-2 have been used in clinical trials. These proteins can potentially be coupled with a collagen matrix and the addition of blood products from the patient to stimulate bone healing. Current usage includes spine fusion, tibial nonunions, and open tibia grafting.

Demineralized bone matrix (DBM) is another osteoinductive agent containing decalcified bone treated to reduce the potential for an immunogenic host reaction and transmission of infection. The resulting product is a biologic scaffold with some remaining growth factors (BMPs). This has the potential to impart a greater osteoconductive effect than standard allograft, as the growth factors have not been exposed by demineralization in the latter.

Belthur MV, Conway JD, Jindal G, et al: Bone graft harvest using a new intramedullary system. *Clin Orthop Relat Res* 2008;466:2973-2980. [PMID: 18841433]

Centers for Disease Control and Prevention: Update: allograft-associated bacterial infections—United States, 2002. *MMWR Morb Mortal Wkly Rep* 2002;51:207. [PMID: 11922189]

Cobos JA, Lindsey RW, Gugala Z: The cylindrical titanium mesh cage for treatment of a long bone segmental defect: description of a new technique and report of two cases. *J Orthop Trauma* 2000;14:54. [PMID: 10630804]

El Maraghy AW, El Maraghy MW, Nousiainen M, et al: Influence of the number of cortices on the stiffness of plate fixation of diaphyseal fractures. *J Orthop Trauma* 2001;15:186. [PMID: 11265009]

Kurdy NG: Serology of abnormal fracture healing: the role of PIIINP, PICP, and BsALP. *J Orthop Trauma* 2000;14:48. [PMID: 10630803]

Laurencin C, Khan Y, El-Amin SF: Bone graft substitutes. *Expert Rev Med Devices* 2006;3:49. [PMID: 16359252]

Radomisli TE, Moore DC, Barrach HJ, et al: Weight-bearing alters the expression of collagen types I and II, BMP 2/4 and osteocalcin in the early stages of distraction osteogenesis. *J Orthop Res* 2001;19:1049. [PMID: 11781004]

Spinella-Jaegle S, Roman-Roman S, Faucheu C, et al: Opposite effects of bone morphogenetic protein-2 and transforming growth factor-beta I on osteoblast differentiation. *Bone* 2001;29:323. [PMID: 11595614]

Wagner M: General principles for the clinical use of the LCP. *Injury* 2003;34(Suppl 2):B31-B42. [PMID: 14580984]

Zlotolow DA, Vaccaro AR, Salamon ML, Albert TJ: The role of human bone morphogenetic proteins in spinal fusion. *J Am Acad Orthop Surg* 2000;8:3. [PMID: 10666648]

▼ I. TRAUMA TO THE UPPER EXTREMITY

SHOULDER AND ARM INJURIES

▶ Anatomy and Biomechanical Principles

A. Bony Anatomy

1. Humeral shaft—The humeral shaft extends from the level of the insertion of the pectoralis major muscle proximally to the supracondylar ridge distally. The upper portion of the shaft is cylindrical and then becomes more flattened in an anteroposterior direction as it proceeds distally. Medial and lateral intermuscular septae divide the arm into anterior and posterior compartments. In the anterior compartment reside the biceps brachii, coracobrachialis, and brachialis muscles, along with the neurovascular bundle coursing along the medial border of the biceps with the brachial artery and vein and the median, musculocutaneous, and ulnar nerves. In the posterior compartment reside the triceps brachii muscle and the radial nerve. Understanding the insertions of the muscle forces around the humerus helps explain the tendency for fractures to displace in predictable patterns, based on the influence of these muscles (Figure 2–3).

2. Shoulder girdle—The shoulder girdle is a complex arrangement of bony and soft-tissue structures. The glenoid cavity is a shallow socket, approximately one third the size of the humeral head. Stability of the joint depends on capsule, ligament, and muscle. A redundant capsule allows for motion.

3. Proximal humerus—The proximal humerus contains the humeral head, lesser and greater tuberosities, bicipital groove, and proximal humeral shaft. The anatomic neck lies at the junction of the head and the tuberosities. The surgical neck lies below the greater and lesser tuberosities. The major blood supply to the humeral head is through the ascending branch of the anterior humeral circumflex artery, which penetrates the head at the bicipital groove and becomes the arcuate artery. Important structures that lie in the vicinity of the shoulder joint include the brachial plexus and axillary artery, which are anterior to the coracoid process of the scapula and humeral head. Nerves innervating muscles around the shoulder include the axillary, suprascapular, subscapular, and musculocutaneous nerves. Fractures of the anatomic neck have a poor prognosis because of complete disruption of the blood supply to the head. Surgical neck fractures are common, and with these, the blood supply to the head is preserved. Within the bicipital groove lies the biceps tendon, which is covered by the transverse humeral ligament. The greater tuberosity provides attachment for the supraspinatus, infraspinatus, and teres minor muscles. The lesser tuberosity contains the attachment of the subscapularis muscle. The neck-shaft angle measures an average of 135 degrees, and the humeral head is retroverted an average of 30 degrees.

The rotator cuff consists of four muscles: the subscapularis, supraspinatus, infraspinatus, and teres minor muscles. The teres major is not a rotator cuff muscle. The cuff muscles serve as depressors of the humeral head to allow the deltoid to efficiently abduct the humerus. The infraspinatus and teres minor are external rotators, while the subscapularis is an internal rotator of the humerus. Two other important muscles in this region are the deltoid and the pectoralis major muscles. These muscles, along with the rotator cuff, cause predictable displacement of fractures around the proximal humerus. Additionally, injury to the rotator cuff, independent of injuries to the insertion of the tuberosities, may be encountered and need to be considered when evaluating the shoulder.

B. Nerve Supply

Injuries to the nerves around the shoulders occur with fractures and dislocations. The brachial plexus and axillary artery can also be injured with anterior shoulder dislocations.

The most important evaluation consists of a neurovascular examination after injury around the arm and shoulder girdle. The radial nerve is commonly injured in humeral shaft fractures, particularly at the junction of the middle and distal third (Holstein-Lewis fracture). Careful evaluation of radial nerve sensory and motor function is critical. Evaluation should include sensation of the dorsal web space between the thumb and index finger, independent digital extension, and wrist extension.

Around the shoulder girdle, fractures of the proximal humerus and fracture-dislocations can on occasion result in axillary nerve and artery injuries. An axillary nerve injury from proximal humeral fracture or fracture-dislocation would result in paralysis of the deltoid muscle and anesthesia over the "badge" region at the lateral proximal arm.

FRACTURES AND DISLOCATIONS AROUND THE SHOULDER

- *The second most common fractures of the upper extremity.*
- *Incidence sharply increases in the elderly.*
- *Eighty-five percent of fractures can be treated nonoperatively.*

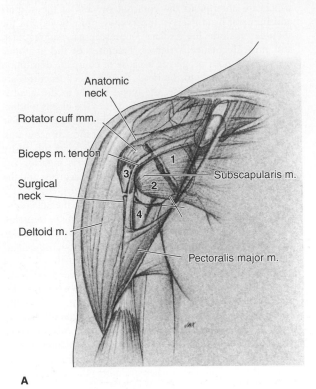

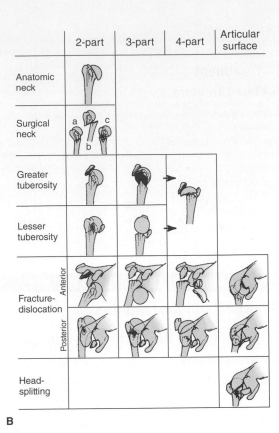

A

B

▲ **Figure 2–3. A:** Muscle insertions on humerus and fracture displacement. **B:** Neer four-part classification of displaced fractures. (Reproduced, with permission, from Rockwood CA, Green DP, Bucholz RW, et al, eds: *Fractures in Adults,* 4th ed. Philadelphia: Lippincott; 1996.)

▶ Classification

An extension of Codman's observations, Neer introduced the concept of "parts" based on the epiphyseal growth centers that collectively compose the proximal humerus. Displaced parts then include the anatomic neck, surgical neck, or tuberosities. Segments are considered to be displaced if they are separated by more than 1 cm or angled more than 45 degrees from the normal anatomic position. Other categories include fracture-dislocations and head-splitting injuries. The relationship of the humeral head to the displaced parts in the glenoid, as well as the blood supply, is also taken into consideration.

▶ Clinical Findings

Young people sustain these injuries in high-energy accidents, whereas fractures in older patients are usually from lower energy mechanisms. Clinical presentation is usually with pain, swelling, and ecchymosis.

Radiographic evaluation is a cornerstone for diagnosis and planning of treatment. The recommended series of radiographs is the so-called Neer trauma series, which consists of

(1) an AP view, (2) a lateral view in the scapular plane, and (3) a Velpeau modified axillary view. The lateral radiograph in the scapular plane is the tangential Y-view of the scapula. The combination of three of these views allows evaluation of the shoulder joint in three separate perpendicular planes. The axillary view is important for evaluating the glenoid articular surface and the relationship of the humeral head anteriorly and posteriorly. On occasion, other studies, including CT scanning for detailing bony anatomy, may be necessary.

Rotator cuff injuries can be expected with fractures of the tuberosities, but can also result from strictly soft-tissue injuries such as shoulder dislocations. Evaluation of the integrity of the rotator cuff may be difficult in the acute setting. Ultrasound, MRI, arthrogram, or arthroscopy may be valuable in making this diagnosis.

Axillary artery injuries, although uncommon, generally result from fractures or fracture-dislocations in which a medial bone spike injures or penetrates the axillary artery. The index of suspicion is high if the arm shows significant color differences compared with the uninjured arm. Pulses should be palpated and evaluated by Doppler studies. In late diagnosis, the outcome is determined by the neurologic morbidity, even though the results of acute vascular reconstruction are good.

▶ Treatment

A. Closed Treatment

Approximately 85% of proximal humerus fractures are minimally displaced or nondisplaced and can be treated nonoperatively with a sling for comfort and early motion exercises. The mainstay of closed treatment is initial immobilization and then early motion. Physical therapy or physician-directed exercises are essential and should be started at 7–10 days if possible. Monitoring of the exercises is important to prevent a program that is either too conservative (thus causing unnecessary contractures) or too aggressive (leading to displacement, with excessive pain and swelling).

B. Surgical Treatment

Techniques useful for the smaller percentage of fractures include closed reduction and percutaneous pinning, intramedullary nails, tension band, open reduction and internal fixation (ORIF) with either conventional plates or locking plates, and hemiarthroplasty. Locking plates provide angular stability and a favorable bone–implant interface for comminuted and osteoporotic fractures.

Hemiarthroplasty remains a useful option for older patients with anatomic neck and head-splitting fractures. Good bone quality and simple fracture patterns are essential to make use of the minimal soft-tissue dissection in the closed reduction and percutaneous pinning method. In younger patients, ORIF may be possible even in comminuted fractures.

The age of the patient, quality of the bone, fracture pattern, and amount of comminution are all important considerations in developing a treatment plan.

C. Two-Part Anatomic Neck Fractures (ICD-9:812.01)

Two-part anatomic neck fractures are rare. No single optimal method of management has been established. Closed reduction is difficult because controlling the articular fragment, which is usually rotated and angulated within the joint capsule, is difficult. The fragment can be preserved in a young patient (<40 years old) with ORIF with pins or interfragmentary screws. It may be difficult to obtain adequate screw purchase without violating the articular surface. Additionally, the prognosis for head survival is poor because the blood supply is usually completely disrupted. In general, prosthetic hemiarthroplasty provides the most predictable result in the elderly (>75 years old).

D. Two-Part Greater Tuberosity Fractures (ICD-9:812.03)

Greater tuberosity fractures generally displace posteriorly and superiorly because of traction by the supraspinatus muscle. This is often associated with anterior glenohumeral dislocation. It is appropriate to attempt closed reduction, which may result in an acceptable position for the greater tuberosity. Neer has reported that displacement of the fragment by more than 1 cm is pathognomonic of a rotator cuff defect. The result of fracture healing in this position is subacromial impingement, with limitation of forward elevation and external rotation. In one series, ORIF is recommended if displacement is greater than 5 mm with some references recommending ORIF with greater than 3 mm displacement in the high-performance athlete because impingement symptoms may develop. A variety of methods, including screws, pins, wires, and suture, can be used to repair the greater tuberosity. Treatment of this condition should be directed at rotator cuff repair as well as bony reconstruction. Percutaneous pinning tends to be inadequate for preventing redisplacement of greater tuberosity fractures.

E. Two-Part Lesser Tuberosity Fractures (ICD-812.00)

If the displaced fragment (usually medially by subscapularis) is small, closed reduction of this rare injury is satisfactory. This fracture may be associated with posterior dislocation and may be treated by closed reduction in the acute setting. The position of immobilization in this case would be either neutral or slight external rotation. Larger fragments may require internal fixation.

F. Two-Part Surgical Neck Fractures (ICD-9:812.01)

In these conditions, both tuberosities remain attached to the head, and the rotator cuff in general remains intact. The diaphysis is often displaced anteromedially by the pull of the pectoralis major muscle. Reduction may be blocked by interposition of the periosteum, biceps tendon, or deltoid muscle, or by buttonholing of the shaft in the deltoid, pectoralis major, or fascial elements. One attempt at closed reduction is advisable; if this fails, operative intervention is recommended. If, on the other hand, the reduction is successful, percutaneous pinning under fluoroscopic control may be an excellent choice for the reducible but unstable fracture (Figure 2–4). If open reduction is required to remove displaced soft tissues, internal fixation can be accomplished by means of percutaneous pinning or intramedullary fixation in conjunction with a tension band wiring technique. In the osteoporotic patient, wire or suture material for tension banding can be passed through the soft tissues and the rotator cuff, which may be superior to bone for fixation.

Another technique for internal fixation uses intramedullary devices such as Enders nails or Rush rods, which can be inserted through a limited deltoid-splitting incision; however, the control of rotational alignment is poor. For elderly (>75 years old) or debilitated patients, this may be the best solution to achieve overall alignment with minimal surgical morbidity.

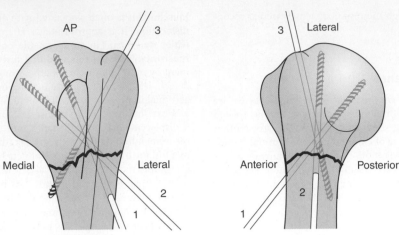

▲ **Figure 2–4.** Pinning of the unstable surgical neck fracture. AP, anteroposterior. (Reproduced, with permission, from Fu FH, Smith WR, eds: Percutaneous pinning of proximal humerus fractures. *Oper Tech Orthop* 2001;11:235.)

G. Three-Part and Four-Part Fractures (ICD-9:812.00)

Optimal treatment of three- and four-part fractures of the proximal part of the humerus in patients with poor bone quality is controversial. ORIF of these fractures has generally produced unsatisfactorily high rates of complications such as avascular necrosis and malunion. Avascular necrosis in three-part fractures has been reported to be as high as 27%. The Atlas Orthogonal (AO) buttress plate has had significant complications, including a high rate of avascular necrosis related in part to extension of soft-tissue displacement and dissection, superior placement of the plate with secondary impingement, loss of plate and screw fixation, malunion, and infections. Recent studies with locking plates show improved fracture stability and healing. Screws, which lock into the plate, may decrease pullout in osteoporotic fractures. In the less active or elderly (>75 years old) patient, the accepted method of treatment is hemiarthroplasty, particularly because the avascular necrosis rate may be as high as 90% and the bone is usually osteoporotic. Appropriate prosthesis level and humeral retroversion, as well as the attachment of greater and lesser tuberosities, are critical in achieving a good result. Repair of any rotator cuff defects is necessary to prevent proximal migration of the humeral component as well as loss of rotator cuff power. With postoperative rehabilitation, generally good pain relief can be expected; however, function is usually limited.

H. Fracture-Dislocations

Fracture-dislocations require reduction of the humeral head, and their management is generally based on the fracture pattern. These injuries usually produce impression defects or head-splitting fractures, with concomitant posterior dislocation. Management is determined by the size of the impression defect and the time of persistent locked dislocation. Fractures of less than 20% will generally be stable with closed reduction and can be treated with immobilization in external rotation for 6 weeks to restore long-term stability. If the defect is 20–50%, however, transfer of the lesser tuberosity with the subscapularis tendon into the defect by open means is indicated. With impression fractures of greater than 50% or chronic dislocations, hemiarthroplasty may be the best treatment. If concomitant glenoid destruction is present, total shoulder arthroplasty may be required.

Eberson CP, Ng T, Green A: Contralateral intrathoracic displacement of the humeral head. *J Bone Joint Surg Am* 2000;82-A:105. [PMID: 10653090]

Helmy N, Hintermann B: New trends in the treatment of proximal humerus fractures. *Clin Orthop Relat Res* 2006;442:100. [PMID: 16394747]

Hintermann B, Trouillier HH, Schafer D: Rigid internal fixation of fractures of the proximal humerus in older patients. *J Bone Joint Surg Br* 2000;82-B:1107. [PMID: 11132267]

Naranja RJ, Iannotti JP: Displaced three- and four-part proximal humerus fractures: evaluation and management. *J Am Acad Orthop Surg* 2000;8:373. [PMID: 11104401]

Palvanen M, Kannus P, Niemi S, Parkkari J: Update on the epidemiology of proximal humerus fractures. *Clin Orthop Relat Res* 2006;442:87. [PMID: 16394745]

Ruch DS, Glisson RR, Marr AW, et al: Fixation of three-part proximal humeral fractures: a biomechanical evaluation. *J Orthop Trauma* 2000;14:36. [PMID: 10630801]

Steinmann SP, Moran EA: Axillary nerve injury: diagnosis and treatment. *J Am Acad Orthop Surg* 2001;9:328. [PMID: 11575912]

Thanasas C, Kontakis G, Angoules A, Limb D, Giannoudis P: Treatment of proximal humerus fractures with locking plates: a systematic review. *J Shoulder Elbow Surg* 2009;18:837-844. [PMID: 19748802]

HUMERAL SHAFT FRACTURE (ICD-9:812.21)

- *Account for 3–5% of all fractures.*
- *More than 90% can be managed nonsurgically.*
- *Traumatic and/or iatrogenic radial nerve injury is common.*

Fractures of the shaft of the humerus usually result from a direct blow, a fall, an automobile injury, or a crushing injury. Missiles from firearms or shell fragments may pierce the arm and cause an open fracture. Other indirect means of injury, such as a fall on an outstretched upper extremity or violent muscle contracture, can cause midshaft fractures.

▶ Classification

Fractures are classified according to whether they are open or closed and according to the level of the fracture in relation to the insertions of the pectoralis major and deltoid muscles. Characteristics of fracture and associated injury are also factors.

▶ Clinical Findings

Clinical signs and symptoms include a shortened extremity with crepitus and pain at the diaphysis of the humerus. Confirmation should be obtained by radiographs in two planes. Both the shoulder and elbow joints should be thoroughly evaluated, clinically and radiographically, as should the neurovascular status.

▶ Treatment

A. Closed Treatment

The majority of these fractures do well with nonoperative methods with high union rates. Nonoperative methods include traction by hanging casts, functional bracing, Velpau dressings, and skeletal traction. Cast bracing appears to be the most effective closed treatment.

The musculature of the upper arm will accommodate 20 degrees of anterior angulation, 30 degrees of varus angulation, and 3 cm of shortening without apparent deformity and functional loss.

1. Hanging cast—Treatment with a hanging cast involves placement of the arm in a cast and correcting the fracture by the weight of cast. This treatment requires weekly radiographic evaluations. Patients with a large body habitus may develop more significant angulation at the time of healing with this technique, compared with slimmer patients. The vertical position must be maintained even at night. Spiral, comminuted, and oblique fractures have additional advantages of large fracture surfaces for ready healing. Transverse fractures may have more difficulty in healing. One risk of this treatment is distraction of the fracture site and eventual nonunion.

2. Coaptation splint—A TU-shaped coaptation splint with cuff and collar is another method for initial treatment of humerus fractures. It gives greater stabilization but less distraction than a hanging arm cast, so it is indicated for minimally shortened fractures and short oblique or transverse fractures that may displace in hanging cast.

3. Functional bracing—Functional cast braces are typically applied 2 weeks after the injury following the initial treatment with a hanging cast or a coaptation splint. During this period, swelling has subsided. The sleeve is ready-made or custom-made from thermoplastic splinting materials and fixed with Velcro straps that can be adjusted to achieve the appropriate level of compression. A collar and cuff may be used to support the forearm, but sling application may result in varus angulation. Repeat graphs are checked, and healing is expected in 8–12 weeks.

4. External fixation—External fixation is applicable to the humerus in the case of burns, gunshot wounds, or severe comminuted open injuries with defects of skin, bone, or soft tissue. Other indications may include osteitis and infected nonunion. Complications include pin tract infections, nonunion, and neurovascular injury.

B. Open Treatment

Special circumstances may merit ORIF. Selected segmental fractures, inadequate closed reduction, "floating" elbow, bilateral humeral fractures, open fractures, multiple trauma, pathologic fractures, and trauma with associated vascular injuries requiring exploration may benefit from internal fixation. Recent advances in internal fixation techniques and instrumentation have led to an expansion of surgical indications for such fractures. There are three general forms of internal fixation: (1) compression plate and screw fixation using the AO techniques, with posterior, modified lateral, and anterolateral surgical approaches; (2) intramedullary nailing, which is especially useful in osteopenic bone, segmental, and pathologic fractures; and (3) percutaneous humeral bridge plating with minimal incision as described by Livani and Belangero. In multiply injured patients, humeral stabilization, permitting mobilization, pulmonary toilet, and pain control may be beneficial. The incidence of radial nerve palsy with acute fracture is about 16%; however, current literature does not recommend operative fixation and nerve exploration in these injuries.

Blum J, Janzing H, Gahr R, et al: Clinical performance of a new medullary humeral nail: antegrade versus retrograde insertion. *J Orthop Trauma* 2001;15:342. [PMID:11433139]

Chapman JR, Henley MB, Agel J, et al: Randomized prospective study of humeral shaft fracture fixation: intramedullary nails versus plates. *J Orthop Trauma* 2000;14:162. [PMID: 10791665]

Cox MA, Dolan M, Synnott K, et al: Closed interlocking nailing of humeral shaft fractures with the Russell-Taylor nail. *J Orthop Trauma* 2000;14:349. [PMID: 10926243]

Livani B, Belangero WD: Bridging plate osteosynthesis of humeral shaft fractures. *Injury* 2004;35:587. [PMID: 15135278]

McCormack RG, Brien D, Buckley R, et al: Fixation of fractures of the shaft of the humerus by dynamic compression plate or intramedullary nail. *J Bone Joint Surg Br* 2000;82-B:336. [PMID: 10813165]

Orthoteers. Available at: http://www.orthoteers.co.uk/Nrujp~ij33lm/Orthcrps.htm

Pickering RM, Crenshaw AH Jr, Zinar DM: Intramedullary nailing of humeral shaft fractures. *Instr Course Lect* 2002;51:271. [PMID: 12064112]

Sarmiento A, Zagorski JB, Zych GA, et al: Functional bracing for the treatment of fractures of the humeral diaphysis. *J Bone Joint Surg Am* 2000;82:478. [PMID: 10761938]

Strothman D, Templeman DC, Varecka T, et al: Retrograde nailing of humeral shaft fractures: a biomechanical study of its effects on the strength of the distal humerus. *J Orthop Trauma* 2000;14:101. [PMID: 10716380]

Ziran BH, Belangero W, Livani B, Pesantez R: Percutaneous plating of the humerus with locked plating: technique and case report. *J Trauma* 2007;63:205. [PMID: 17622893]

INJURIES AROUND THE ELBOW

- *Intercondylar fractures are the most common fracture pattern.*
- *CT scan with three-dimensional reconstruction is helpful for preoperative planning.*
- *ORIF is the choice of treatment in the majority of cases.*

▶ Anatomy and Biomechanical Principles

On cross-section, the humerus is circular at the midshaft but flared and flattened at the distal end. The distal humerus consists of an arch formed by two condyles. Articular surface of the condyles: capitellum, on the lateral, and trochlea medial to it, articulates with radial head and proximal ulna, respectively. The ulnohumeral joint allows the flexion extension of the joint, and the radiocapitellar joint allows forearm rotation. The proximal ulna, which articulates with the trochlea, contains the olecranon process posteriorly, the coronoid process anteriorly, and the sigmoid or semilunar notch. The trochlea has a 300-degree arc of cartilage. The medial column diverges from the humeral shaft at a 45-degree angle, and the lateral column diverges at a 20-degree angle.

The triceps has a broad tendinous insertion into the olecranon posteriorly; anteriorly, the brachialis inserts on the coronoid process and the tuberosity of the ulna. The radial head lines up in its lesser sigmoid, or radial notch, with the annular ligament surrounding it. Medial to the trochlea, the medial epicondyle locates and the medial collateral ligament and flexor-pronator group of muscles attach here. The most important portion of the medial or ulnar collateral ligament is the anterior portion, which attaches to a small process on the medial surface of the coronoid. The supinator-extensor muscle group attaches to the lateral epicondyle, which is slightly proximal and lateral to the capitellum.

With the elbow in 90 degrees of flexion, the medial condyle, lateral condyle, and olecranon form a palpable triangle. These boney landmarks are important when assessing the elbow for fractures, dislocations, or effusions. Effusions can be discerned by swelling between the lateral epicondyle and the olecranon.

The ulnar nerve passes through the cubital tunnel at the medial column of the elbow and must be appropriately assessed following injury. The ulnar nerve enters the anterior forearm by traveling between the two heads of the flexor carpi ulnaris.

A complete neurovascular examination of the radial, median, ulnar, and anterior and posterior interosseous nerves should be done before and after treatment.

DISTAL HUMERUS FRACTURES

- *Account for 30% of elbow fractures.*
- *Treatment similar to other intraarticular fractures.*

1. Intercondylar-T or -Y Fractures (ICD-9:812.49)

Intercondylar humerus fractures are among the most challenging fractures treated by the orthopedic surgeon. The usual mechanism of injury is axial loading of the ulna in the trochlear groove. Studies have demonstrated increasing numbers of these injuries in the older (>60 years) population. It is critical to assess the integrity of the medial and lateral column for reconstructible bone fragments and the degree of comminution.

▶ Classification

Jupiter and Mehne classified distal humerus fractures into intraarticular and extraarticular patterns. Intraarticular fractures are divided into the following types:

1. Single column: Divided into medial or lateral
2. Bicolumnar: Divided into TT, TY, TH, lambda, or multiplane pattern
3. Capitellum fractures
4. Trochlea fractures

Extraarticular fractures are classified into intracapsular and extracapsular (Table 2–4).

▶ Treatment

Treatment options include bracing, ORIF, total elbow arthroplasty (TEA), elbow arthrodesis, and distal humerus replacement. It is difficult to achieve and maintain the fracture reduction by casting, and prolonged immobilization leads to stiffness and ankylosis of the adult elbow joint. Nonsurgical management of distal humerus fractures is mainly reserved for medically unstable older patients, those with limited arm function (eg, paralysis), and some nondisplaced fractures.

Table 2–4. The Jupiter and Mehne classification of distal humerus fractures.

I. Intraarticular fracture
  A. Single-column fractures
    1. Medial
      a. High
      b. Low
    2. Lateral
      a. High
      b. Low
    3. Divergent
  B. Bicolumn fractures
    1. T pattern
      a. High
      b. Low
    2. Y pattern
    3. H pattern
    4. Lambda pattern
      a. Medial
      b. Lateral
    5. Multiplane pattern
  C. Capitellum fractures
  D. Trochlear fractures
II. Extraarticular intracapsular fractures
  A. Transcolumn fractures
    1. High
      a. Extension
      b. Flexion
      c. Abduction
      d. Adduction
    2. Low
      a. Extension
      b. Flexion
III. Extracapsular fractures
  A. Medial epicondyle
  B. Lateral epicondyle

Reproduced, with permission, from Browner BD, Levine A, Jupiter J, et al, eds: *Skeletal Trauma,* 2nd ed. New York: WB Saunders; 1998.

With modern hardware and techniques, ORIF is preferred for most fractures. Surgical exposure is through a transolecranon approach (ie, either transverse osteotomy or chevron osteotomy). Triceps-sparing and triceps-splitting posterior approaches have also been shown to be effective.

The intraarticular fracture fragments should be anatomically restored with lag screw fixation of periarticular fragments and stable attachment of the metaphysis to the diaphysis with small fragment contoured plates. When possible, dual plate fixation should be used.

2. Fracture of the Humeral Condyles

Both medial and lateral condyles can be disrupted. These fractures can correspond with the ossification centers of the distal humerus.

▶ Lateral Condylar Fracture (ICD-9:812.42)

Lateral column fractures are single-column injuries and are divided into "low" and "high." Low fractures have the lateral wall of the trochlea attached to the main mass of the humerus and are generally stable, whereas high fractures involve a majority of the trochlea and are unstable. "Low" and "high" correspond to Milch type I and II injuries, respectively. Stable internal fixation with early range of motion is generally recommended for displaced fractures.

▶ Medial Condylar Fracture (ICD-9: 812.43)

Medial condyle fractures are similarly single-column injuries with low fractures (Milch type I) involving a portion of the trochlea, with preservation of the trochlear ridge, and are generally stable. In high medial condyle fractures (Milch type II), the lateral trochlear ridge is included with the fracture portion.

Both fractures, if displaced, should be treated with ORIF and early range of motion.

3. Fracture of the Epicondyles (ICD-9:812.43)

Although lateral epicondylar fractures are rare, medial epicondylar fractures are fairly common, especially among children or adolescents. They commonly present as avulsion fractures. Treatment depends on the amount of displacement. If displacement is minimal, then closed reduction is appropriate. A displaced fracture may require percutaneous pinning or open reduction. Elbow instability is not generally a problem; however, irritation of the ulnar nerve can result. Early motion seems to be important for restoration and ultimate function. If a displaced fracture results in ulnar symptoms or is itself symptomatic, the fragment can be excised at a later date.

ELBOW DISLOCATION

- *Posterior dislocation is the most common.*
- *Simple dislocations are those without fracture.*

Dislocations of the elbow occur when loads are placed on the structures about the elbow that exceed the intrinsic stability provided by the anatomic shape of the joint surfaces and soft-tissue constraints. These are potentially limb-threatening, as vascular compromise is a possible sequela. Expeditious reduction of the elbow joint is the goal of treatment.

Elbow dislocations are characterized according to direction of the distal bone. Isolated radial head dislocation is rare; it is usually accompanied by an ulnar fracture (Monteggia fracture). When combinations of dislocations with concomitant fractures occur, treatment of the combined injury is usually dictated by the treated fracture. Adequate fracture care will usually cause secondary reduction of the dislocation.

▶ Posterior Elbow Dislocations (ICD-9:832.02)

Posterior dislocations are the most common type (80%) of elbow dislocations, resulting from an axial force applied to the extended elbow. Both collateral ligaments are disrupted, whether the dislocation is posteromedial or posterolateral.

Diagnosis is made by clinical examination and verified by radiograph to rule out associated fractures. The extremity is typically shortened and the elbow held slightly flexed.

Treatment is initiated after documenting the neurovascular examination. Anesthesia, either injected locally into the joint or administered intravenously, is necessary. Traction on the extremity with correction of the medial or lateral displacement usually produces reduction with a "clunk." The elbow is put through a range of motion to ensure that reduction has been obtained and that there is no soft-tissue or bony mechanical blockage to motion. The elbow is generally splinted in flexion and pronation to maintain stability. Postreduction radiographs are necessary to rule out occult fracture.

▶ Anterior Elbow Dislocations (ICD-9:832.01)

Anterior dislocations are relatively rare. Soft-tissue damage is typically severe. Treatment is similar to that for posterior dislocations, except that the method of reduction is reversed.

▶ Medial and Lateral Elbow Dislocations (ICD-9:832.03 and 832.04)

The radius and ulna may be displaced medially or laterally. Some semblance of joint motion may be present with lateral dislocations, as the ulna may be displaced into the groove between the trochlea and the capitellum. The anteroposterior radiograph is diagnostic. Medial or lateral force is used, after attempting to distract the joint surfaces, to reduce these dislocations.

▶ Isolated Ulnar Dislocations

Isolated ulnar dislocations occur when the humerus pivots around the radial head, causing the coronoid process to be displaced posterior to the humerus or the olecranon anterior to the humerus. The more common injury is posterior dislocation, which causes cubitus varus deformity of the forearm. Traction in extension and supination reduces the ulna.

▶ General Treatment Procedures

A. Early Treatment

The elbow is tested for stability to varus and valgus stress and to pronation and supination. Stable dislocations are splinted for comfort at 90 degrees of flexion, and motion is instituted as soon as possible, generally within a few days. Maintenance of reduction is necessary, and radiographs should be taken periodically if any doubt exists. Immobilization does not guarantee maintenance of reduction. Unstable reductions

are rare. Immobilization for longer periods may be necessary in these cases, as a stiff but stable elbow is preferable to an unstable elbow. The lateral ulnar collateral ligament injury is the cause of recurrent instability.

Uncomplicated elbow dislocations have a favorable long-term prognosis. A loss of extension of 5–10 degrees compared with the contralateral elbow can be expected following this injury. Posterolateral dislocation has been associated with persistent valgus instability in some patients, which is associated with a worse overall clinical result.

B. Delayed Treatment

Late reduction of elbow dislocations can be accomplished with closed techniques for up to several weeks from the time of injury. Dislocations left untreated for longer periods generally require open reduction techniques. Better function with less flexion contracture after open reduction of posterior dislocations is obtained by lengthening the triceps tendon.

C. Elbow Dislocation and Coronoid Fracture (ICD-9:813.12 for coronoid fracture)

An elbow dislocation and associated fracture of the coronoid process increase the risk of recurrent and chronic instability. The size of the coronoid fragment varies from a small marginal fragment (Reagan-Morrey type I) to a larger fragment (Reagan-Morrey type II), or includes the insertion of the anterior bundle of the medial collateral ligament (Reagan-Morrey type III). The decision to fix a coronoid fracture should be made based on elbow stability. Even small rim fractures may require surgical fixation if instability is present after repair of associated fractures. When there is greater than 50% loss of coronoid, fixation is mandatory according to the cadaver studies. Interfragmentary screws can be used to fix a large fragment. Otherwise, a pullout technique can be used.

D. Elbow Dislocation With Radial Head and Coronoid Fractures

Denominated the terrible triad of the elbow, these injuries are difficult to treat, and the reported results have been poor. The most common problems after these lesions are recurrent and chronic instability, stiffness, posttraumatic arthrosis, and pain. Appropriate treatment should include ORIF of the coronoid fracture and/or repair of the anterior capsule, ORIF or replacement of the radial head, and repair of the lateral ligament complex. Residual instability after treatment represents an indication for medial collateral ligament repair and/or application of a hinged external fixator.

Bailey CS, MacDermid J, Patterson SD, et al: Outcome of plate fixation of olecranon fractures. *J Orthop Trauma* 2001;15:542. [PMID: 11733669]

Eygendaal D, Verdegaal SH, Obermann WR, et al: Posterolateral dislocation of the elbow joint. *J Bone Joint Surg Am* 2000; 82-A:555. [PMID: 10761945]

Hak DJ, Golladay GJ: Olecranon fractures: treatment options. *J Am Acad Orthop Surg* 2000;8:266. [PMID: 10951115]

Mckee MD, Wilson T, Winston L, et al: Functional outcome following surgical treatment of intraarticular distal humeral fractures through a posterior approach. *J Bone Joint Surg Am* 2000;82-A:1701. [PMID: 11130643]

Paramasivan ON, Younge DA, Pant R: Treatment of nonunion around the olecranon fossa of the humerus by intramedullary locked nailing. *J Bone Joint Surg Br* 2000;82-B:332. [PMID: 10813164]

Popovic N, Rodriguez A, Lemaire R: Fracture of the radial head with associated elbow dislocation: results of treatment using a floating radial head prosthesis. *J Orthop Trauma* 2000;14:171. [PMID: 10791667]

Pugh DMW, Wild LM, Schemitsch EH, et al: Standard surgical protocol to treat elbow dislocations with radial head and coronoid fractures. *J Bone Joint Surg Am* 2004;86:1122. [PMID: 15173283]

Sanchez-Sotelo J, Romanillos O, Garay EG: Results of acute excision of the radial head in elbow radial head fracture-dislocations. *J Orthop Trauma* 2000;14:354. [PMID: 10926244]

Schneeberger AG, Sadowski MM, Jacob HA: Coronoid process and radial head as posterolateral rotatory stabilizers of the elbow. *J Bone Joint Surg Am* 2004;86-A:975. [PMID: 15118040]

Wainwright AM, Williams JR, Carr AJ: Interobserver and intraobserver variation in classification systems for fractures of the distal humerus. *J Bone Joint Surg Br* 2000;82-B:636. [PMID: 10963156]

FRACTURE OF THE RADIAL HEAD (ICD-9:813.05)

- *Accounts for 15–25% of all elbow fractures.*
- *The radial head is the secondary restraint to valgus stability of elbow.*
- *Associated injuries are common.*

The radial head is seated in the lesser sigmoid notch and has contact axially with the capitellum of the distal humerus. Radial head fractures are generally caused by longitudinal loading from a fall on an outstretched hand; dislocation of the elbow is another cause.

▶ Clinical Findings

One generally describes these fractures based on their location, percentage of articular involvement, and amount of displacement. Radiographs in the anteroposterior and lateral projections show the injury. The fat pad sign is usually present on the lateral projection (Figure 2–5).

▶ Classification

Mason proposed a classification scheme for radial head fractures: Type I is a nondisplaced fracture; type II is a fracture that is displaced, usually involving a single large fragment;

type III is a comminuted fracture; and type IV is a fracture associated with an elbow dislocation (Figure 2–6).

▶ Treatment

For type I fractures, nonoperative treatment with early motion can generally produce a good outcome.

The treatment of type II fractures is controversial. For fractures with near-normal motion, less than 2 mm step-off, and without associated injury, nonsurgical treatment is indicated.

Type II fractures with associated injuries that may compromise elbow stability or fractures with a mechanical block to full motion after injection of anesthetic into the elbow joint are indications for ORIF. ORIF can be performed with pins, articular screws, or Herbert screws. Implants should be placed into the nonarticular safe zone to avoid impingement on the sigmoid fossa of the ulna. The safe zone corresponds to the lateral 100-degree arc with the forearm in neutral rotation.

The result of ORIF is less predictable when there is more than one fragment in type II fractures, and limitation of forearm rotation not attributable to implant prominence can be expected.

Early excision with immediate motion is recommended for type III fractures with no associated elbow instability, coronoid fracture, wrist pain, or distal radioulnar joint injury. If any of these conditions exist, then current literature recommends placement of a metallic radial head prosthesis. Replacement of the radial head becomes most important when there is evidence of the Essex-Lopresti injury (longitudinal disruption of interosseous membrane, distal radioulnar joint injury, and radial head fracture/dislocation). Some suggest that replacement of the radial head should be considered in healthy, active patients even if the elbow and forearm are stable. Antuna et al showed that radial head resection in young patients with isolated fractures without instability yields satisfactory results in greater than 90% of cases after 15 years of follow-up. Broberg and Morrey noticed a 92% incidence of arthrosis 10 years after fracture-dislocation treatment without repair or replacement of the radial head.

1. Capitellar Fractures (ICD-9:812.44)

Capitellar fractures frequently accompany and result from the same mechanism that causes radial head fractures. The medial collateral ligament, the interosseous ligament, and the distal radioulnar joint may also be injured. Various levels of injury, from cartilage damage to large osteochondral portions of the capitellum, can occur from impaction of the radius against the capitellum. Low-grade radial head fractures create higher-grade cartilage lesions as the intact radial head can cause more damage to the capitellum. Shearing forces can result in more significant injuries: an osteochondral injury or complete fracture (type 1 or Hahn-Steinthal), an articular-cartilage-only injury (type 2 or Kocher-Lorenz), a comminuted fracture (type 3), or a fracture line extending into the trochlea (Hahn-Steinthal II). CT reconstructions are

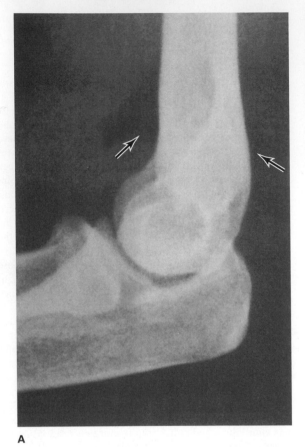

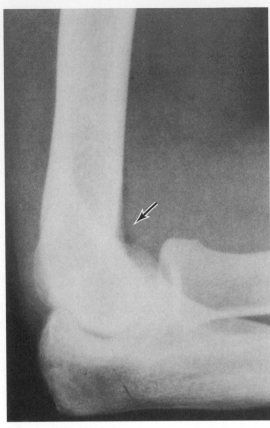

A   **B**

▲ **Figure 2–5.** Positive fat pad sign on lateral radiograph of elbow. This finding indicates that fluid is in the elbow joint. In the acute setting, the fluid is blood, most commonly from a fracture.

useful to further delineate the fracture and for surgical planning. Osteochondral pieces can be overlooked or confused with bone chips from radial head fractures.

▶ Treatment

Today, anatomic reduction and early motion compose the standard treatment for these injuries, whether obtained by open or closed means. Open reduction is performed through a lateral approach between the anconeus and extensor carpi ulnaris.

OLECRANON FRACTURES (ICD-9:813.01)

- *Tension band is the gold standard treatment for transverse fractures.*
- *Hardware-related problems are common.*

Olecranon fractures compose approximately 10% of all fractures around the elbow. Fractures of the olecranon commonly occur with a direct blow, generally resulting in comminuted fractures, or as an avulsion injury with triceps

contracture. Contraction of the triceps often results in transverse or short oblique types of fractures.

▶ Clinical Findings

Radiographic evaluation consists of a true lateral radiograph of the elbow, and classifications or descriptions generally analyze the fracture based on the percentage of articular surface involved in the fractured proximal fragment. This factor, the amount of comminution, the fracture angle, intraarticular step-off, the degree of displacement, and patient comorbidities and functional demands are all critical in evaluating the injury and selecting the appropriate treatment.

▶ Treatment

Methods of treatment vary from closed treatment to ORIF. Nondisplaced fractures or fractures with less than 2 mm displacement and an intact extensor mechanism should be immobilized in a long arm cast with the elbow in 90 degrees of flexion.

Type I

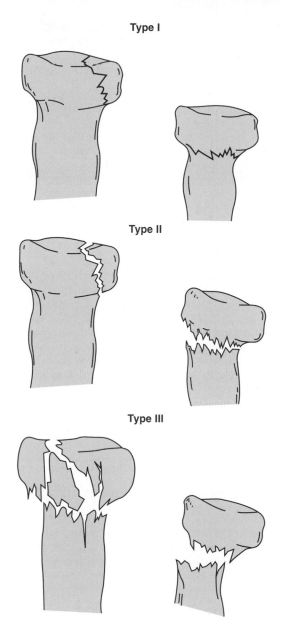

Type II

Type III

▲ **Figure 2–6.** Mason classification of radial head fractures. (Reproduced, with permission, from Browner BD, Levine A, Jupiter J, et al, eds: *Skeletal Trauma*, 2nd ed. New York: WB Saunders; 1998.)

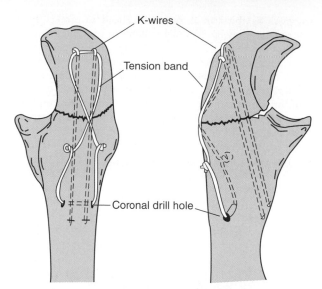

▲ **Figure 2–7.** Tension band technique for fixation of olecranon fractures. (Reproduced, with permission, from Browner BD, Levine A, Jupiter J, et al, eds: *Skeletal Trauma*, 2nd ed. New York: WB Saunders; 1998.)

a neutralization plate. Wire protrusion and pain frequently result and may necessitate removal of the hardware.

For the significantly comminuted fractures, or oblique fractures distal to the midpoint of the trochlear notch, a low-profile, limited contact compression plate can be applied to the dorsal surface of the ulna. Selected comminuted fractures may be treated by selective bony excision or complete excision of the fragment followed by reattachment of the triceps. All these treatments generally can be accompanied with early protected range-of-motion exercises.

FOREARM SHAFT FRACTURES (ICD-9:813)

- *Incidence is greater in men than in women.*
- *Patients should be treated within intraarticular fracture principles.*
- *Volkmann ischemia and compartment syndrome are devastating complications.*

In general, any fracture requires evaluation both clinically and radiographically of a joint above and joint below the fracture. It is not uncommon for fractures of the midshaft of the forearm to have significant consequences to either the wrist or elbow.

1. Isolated Fracture of the Ulna (Nightstick Fracture) (ICD-9:813.22)

The most common injury mechanism is from a direct blow. Isolated ulna fractures are commonly known as nightstick

Displaced transverse or short oblique fractures generally are best treated with ORIF. The optimal method for treating this fracture is tension banding with two longitudinal K-wires placed across the fracture site and stabilized with a figure-of-8 wire loop (Figure 2–7). More oblique fractures can be treated with interfragmentary screws with fractures as the arm is raised overhead to protect from injury. They may be classified as stable or unstable. Unstable fracture are those that have more than 50% displacement, more than 10 degrees of angulation, involve the proximal third, or have associated instability at the proximal or the distal radioulnar joint (DRUJ). The time to union is about 3 months, with union achieved with cast immobilization and early mobilization of the wrist and elbow. Excellent results have been achieved using a functional brace for isolated ulnar fractures. With displaced fractures, ORIF is the choice of treatment. Current recommendations include fixation with a 3.5-mm dynamic or limited contact compression plate with six to eight cortices of fixation proximal and distal to the fracture. Nonunion, delayed union, and radioulnar synostosis with or without operation are not rare complications. Loss of forearm rotation and refracture after hardware removal are other important complications.

2. Isolated Radial Shaft Fractures (ICD-9:813.21)

A fracture anywhere along the length of the radius with or without associated ulnar fracture with injury to the DRUJ is defined as a Galeazzi fracture. Injuries associated with the DRUJ include ulnar styloid fractures, radial shortening of more than 5 mm, and DRUJ dislocation.

▶ Treatment

ORIF with plate fixation is recommended in adult patients to ensure a reasonable chance of restoration of the DRUJ. After ORIF of the radial shaft through a volar Henry approach using compression plating, the DRUJ should be carefully inspected. If it is unstable, pinning in a position of stability (usually full supination) is required. If it is frankly dislocated and cannot be reduced closed and maintained by closed or percutaneous means, then open stabilization with repair of associated ligaments or removal of interposed soft tissue is mandatory.

3. Monteggia Fracture (ICD-9:813.03)

▶ Classification of Fractures

In 1814, Monteggia of Milan described an injury involving fracture of the proximal third of the ulna, with anterior dislocation of the radial head. This definition was extended by Bado to include the entire spectrum of these fractures with associated radial head dislocations, regardless of the direction of dislocation. They are classified in the following way:

Type 1: Fracture of the ulnar diaphysis with anterior angulation and anterior dislocation of the radial head (60% of cases)

Type 2: Fracture of the ulnar diaphysis with posterior angulation or posterior or posterolateral dislocation of the radial head (15% of cases)

Type 3: Fracture of the ulnar metaphysis, with lateral or anterolateral dislocation of the radial head (20% of cases)

Type 4: Fracture of the ulna and radius at the proximal third, with anterior dislocation of the radial head (5% of cases)

Other authors have noted that type 3 fractures may be more common than type 2 fractures, but all agree that type 1 lesions are the most common.

It is important to perform an adequate neurovascular examination at the time of evaluation. Albeit rare, the radial and/or median nerve and the posterior and/or anterior interosseous nerve can be injured in conjunction with Bado type 2 and 3 fractures. The index of suspicion must be high because radial head dislocation may be missed if appropriate radiographs are not obtained and scrutinized.

▶ Treatment

Closed treatment is usually satisfactory for children, but ORIF is the treatment of choice for Monteggia lesions in an adult. Optimal results require early diagnosis, rigid internal fixation of the fractured ulna, complete reduction of the dislocated radial head, and immobilization for approximately 6 weeks to allow healing with sufficient stability. Internal fixation is best performed with a compression plate technique. The radial head can often be completely reduced by closed means once the ulnar fracture is reduced and rigidly fixed. If this is not possible, open reduction is required; attention should be paid to the relationship between the annular ligament, the lateral epicondyle, and the radial head. Entrapment of the soft tissues is the most common reason for inability to obtain concomitant closed radial head reduction at the time of ORIF of the ulna.

4. Fractures of Both the Radius and Ulna (ICD-9:813.23)

Fractures of both the radius and ulna (both-bones fractures) usually result from high-energy injuries. These fractures are usually displaced because of the force required to produce such an injury. Careful neurovascular examination and adequate radiographs to show both the wrist and the elbow are mandatory.

▶ Treatment

Treatment of choice for both-bones fractures is ORIF. The volar Henry approach should be used for radius repair, between the flexor carpi radialis and brachioradialis, with the ulna approached subcutaneously. ORIF offers the best chance of restoring the normal positions of the radius and ulna, which is critical to forearm function and, in particular, pronation and supination. For fractures of the proximal half of the radius, the dorsal Thompson approach can be used; however, the risk of iatrogenic injury to the posterior interosseous nerve is increased. Technical points to be considered include minimal subperiosteal stripping only of the fracture site. The plates can be placed on top of the periosteum to preserve the blood supply as much as possible. A 3.5-mm dynamic compression plate or limited-contact compression plate can be used for AO/ASIF compression plating. The recent development and implementation of locked intramedullary nail systems provide an effective alternative to plating. Bone grafting can be used for severely comminuted fractures with significant bone loss. Only the skin is closed so as not to cause compartment syndrome or Volkmann contracture.

Many authors recommend plate fixation for Gustilo type I, II, and IIIA open both-bones fractures. Use of an external fixator is a viable alternative, however, particularly if severe open wounds are present with skin and soft-tissue loss as in Gustilo type IIIB and IIIC injuries.

Catalano LW 3rd, Barron OA, Glickel SZ: Assessment of articular displacement of distal radius fractures. *Clin Orthop Relat Res* 2004;423:79-84. [PMID: 15232430]

Chung KC, Spilson SV: The frequency and epidemiology of hand and forearm fractures in the United States. *J Hand Surg Am* 2001;26:908. [PMID: 11561245]

Dell'Oca AA, Tepic S, Frigg R, et al: Treating forearm fractures using an internal fixator. *Clin Orthop Relat Res* 2001;389:196. [PMID: 11501811]

Iqbal MJ, Abbas D: Distal radioulnar synostosis following K-wire fixation. *Orthopedics* 2001;24:61. [PMID: 11199355]

Qidwai SA: Treatment of diaphyseal forearm fractures in children by intramedullary Kirschner wires. *J Trauma* 2001;50:303. [PMID: 11242296]

Ruch DS, Vallee J, Poehling GG, Smith BP, Kuzma GR. Arthroscopic reduction versus fluoroscopic reduction in the management of intraarticular distal radius fractures. *Arthroscopy* 2004;20:225. [PMID: 15007310]

Wei SY, Born CT, Abene A, et al: Diaphyseal forearm fractures treated with and without bone graft. *J Trauma* 1999;46:1045. [PMID: 10372622]

FRACTURES AND DISLOCATIONS OF THE DISTAL AND MID-FOREARM

▶ Anatomy and Biomechanical Principles

The distal radius has three articular components (Figure 2–8): distally the scaphoid and lunate fossae, which allow articulation with the scaphoid and the lunate bones, respectively; the sigmoid notch, which allows articulation with the ulna medially. Between the scaphoid and the lunate fossa is a ridge that corresponds with the scapholunate interval. This entire surface is covered with articular cartilage. The radial styloid allows attachment of the brachioradialis tendon. Also, it is the origin of several important wrist ligaments, including the radial scapholunate and radial lunocapitate ligaments.

The third articular component of the distal radius is the sigmoid notch. This convex structure allows the radius to rotate around the distal ulna. The distal ulna itself has an ulnar styloid, which contains attachments to the triangular fibrocartilage complex, including the meniscus homolog,

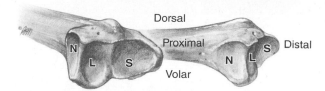

▲ **Figure 2–8.** Articular components of the distal radius. L, lunate articular surface; N, sigmoid notch; S, scaphoid articular surface. (Reproduced, with permission, from Green DP, Hotchkiss RN, Pederson WC, eds: *Operative Hand Surgery*, 4th ed. New York: WB Saunders; 1999.)

the volar and dorsal ulnar carpal ligaments, and the ulnar collateral ligament at the wrist. The concave elliptical distal radius is oriented in the sagittal plane with an average of 11 degrees of volar tilt. In the frontal plane, the average radial inclination is 23 degrees. Radial length is measured from the tip of the radial styloid to the ulnar articular surface and averages 13 mm.

In addition to the bony surfaces, the articular cartilage, joint capsule, and wrist ligaments, there are other soft tissues within the distal forearm and wrist. On the dorsal surface, six dorsal compartments contain wrist and digital extensor tendons (Figure 2–9). On the volar surface reside the contents of the carpal tunnel, with nine flexor tendons and the median nerve. On the ulnar surface, the flexor carpi ulnaris tendon can be palpated near its insertion on the pisiform. The boundaries of the ulnar tunnel, or Guyon's canal, are the volar carpal ligament and transverse carpal ligament, the hook of the hamate radially, and the pisiform ulnarly. Guyon's canal contains the ulnar artery and nerve. The ulnar shaft remains fixed in its rotation at the ulnohumeral joint, and the radius rotates around the ulna in pronation and supination. The radius has a lateral bow that is crucial to the maintenance of full pronation and supination.

The interosseous membrane in the interosseous space connects the shafts of the radius and ulna. The central portion is thickened and has been shown to be important in force transmission between the radius and ulna. Origins of flexor and extensor muscles are located along the anterior and posterior surfaces of the radius, ulna, and interosseous membrane.

Berger RA: The anatomy of the ligaments of the wrist and distal radioulnar joints. *Clin Orthop Relat Res* 2001;383:32. [PMID: 11210966]

Blazar PE, Chan PS, Kneeland JB, et al: The effect of observer experience on magnetic resonance imaging interpretation and localization of triangular fibrocartilage complex lesions. *J Hand Surg Am* 2001;26:742. [PMID: 11466652]

Cober SR, Trumble TE: Arthroscopic repair of triangular fibrocartilage complex injuries. *Orthop Clin North Am* 2001;32:279. [PMID: 11331541]

Freeland AE, Geissler WB: The arthroscopic management of intraarticular distal radius fractures. *Hand Surg* 2000;5:93. [PMID: 11301502]

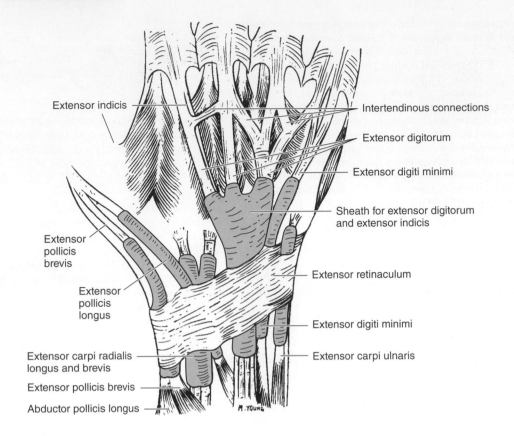

Extensor indicis

Intertendinous connections

Extensor digitorum

Extensor digiti minimi

Sheath for extensor digitorum and extensor indicis

Extensor pollicis brevis

Extensor pollicis longus

Extensor retinaculum

Extensor digiti minimi

Extensor carpi radialis longus and brevis

Extensor carpi ulnaris

Extensor pollicis brevis

Abductor pollicis longus

A

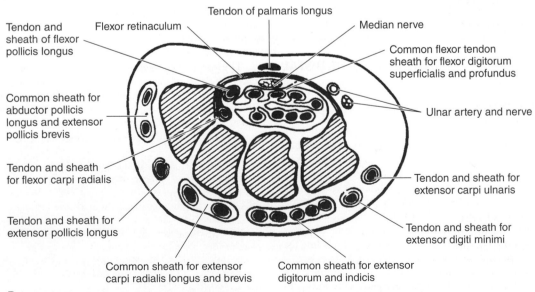

Tendon of palmaris longus

Flexor retinaculum

Median nerve

Tendon and sheath of flexor pollicis longus

Common flexor tendon sheath for flexor digitorum superficialis and profundus

Common sheath for abductor pollicis longus and extensor pollicis brevis

Ulnar artery and nerve

Tendon and sheath for flexor carpi radialis

Tendon and sheath for extensor pollicis longus

Tendon and sheath for extensor carpi ulnaris

Tendon and sheath for extensor digiti minimi

Common sheath for extensor carpi radialis longus and brevis

Common sheath for extensor digitorum and indicis

B

▲ **Figure 2–9. A:** Dorsal section of the wrist, showing the six dorsal compartments of the extensor tendons. **B:** Cross section of the wrist, showing the tendons, arteries, and nerves. (Reproduced, with permission, from Jenkins DB: *Hollinshead's Functional Anatomy of the Limbs and Back,* 6th ed. New York: WB Saunders; 1991.)

Gupta R, Bozenthka DJ, Osterman AL: Wrist arthroscopy: principles and clinical applications. *J Am Acad Orthop Surg* 2001;9:200. [PMID: 11421577]

Lindau T, Adlercreutz C, Aspenberg P: Peripheral tears of the triangular fibrocartilage complex cause distal radioulnar joint instability after distal radial fractures. *J Hand Surg Am* 2000;25:464. [PMID: 10811750]

McGinley JC, D'addessi L, Sadeghipour K, Kozin SH: Mechanics of the antebrachial interosseous membrane: response to shearing forces. *J Hand Surg Am* 2001;26:733. [PMID: 11466651]

Nakamura T, Takayama S, Horiuchi Y, Yabe Y: Origins and insertions of the triangular fibrocartilage complex: a histological study. *J Hand Surg Br* 2001;26:446. [PMID: 11560427]

Poitevin LA: Anatomy and biomechanics of the interosseous membrane: its importance in the longitudinal stability of the forearm. *Hand Clin* 2001;17:97. [PMID: 11280163]

DISLOCATION OF THE RADIOCARPAL JOINT

Dislocation of the radiocarpal joint is usually accompanied by significant carpal-ligamentous injury or fracture. Treatment of these injuries involves restoration of the bony architecture through immediate closed reduction, if possible; elective closed reduction; ORIF; or a combination of these procedures. Associated fractures, such as transscaphoid perilunate or distal radius fracture associated with carpal dislocation, should be treated with ORIF. Ligamentous repair should be performed at this time (see Chapter 9, "Hand Surgery"). Median nerve evaluation is mandatory, and surgical exploration is indicated if a dense neuropathy is present.

DISTAL RADIUS AND ULNA INJURIES

- *Account for approximately 14% of all fractures.*
- *Most common osteoporotic upper extremity fracture.*
- *Fall on outstretched hand is the most common injury mechanism.*

1. Distal Radius and Ulna Fracture (ICD-9:813.40)

In 1814, Abraham Colles described the distal radius fracture as a "silver fork deformity"—volarly angulated, dorsally displaced, with loss of radial inclination and resultant radial shortening. In contrast, the *Smith fracture,* or *reverse Colles fracture,* is a dorsally angulated fracture of the distal radius, with the hand and wrist displaced volarly with respect to the forearm. The fracture may be extraarticular, intraarticular, or a part of a fracture-dislocation involving the wrist. *Barton fracture* is a fracture-dislocation with an intraarticular fracture in which the carpus and a rim of the distal radius are displaced together (Figure 2–10). The *Chauffeur's fracture* is a radial styloid fracture, described initially in car drivers operating automobiles, which required hand cranking to start. When the engine engaged, the crank would "kick back," and the Chauffeur's fracture would result.

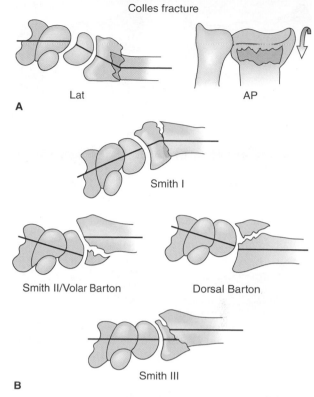

▲ Figure 2–10. Schematic drawings of Colles fracture **(A)** and Smith and Barton fractures **(B)**. AP, anteroposterior. (Reproduced, with permission, from Green DP, Hotchkiss RN, Pederson WC, eds: *Operative Hand Surgery,* 4th ed. New York: WB Saunders; 1999.)

▶ Fracture Classification

In modern day fracture care, the emphasis has shifted from "named" fractures to anatomic descriptions of the injury.

No one fracture classification system is comprehensive in describing all important variables of distal radius fractures.

The Frykman classification categorizes fractures by the presence or absence of an ulnar styloid fracture and by whether fracture lines are extraarticular, intraarticular involving the radiocarpal joint, intraarticular involving the DRUJ, or intraarticular involving both the radiocarpal joint and DRUJ (Figure 2–11).

The AO classification and its derivative, the OTA fracture classification system, are the most comprehensive systems currently used to classify distal radius fractures. Broadly, distal radius fractures are separated into three groups: extraarticular (type A), partial articular (type B), and complete articular (type C). Within these are subclassifications that relate to the particular amount of displacement and comminution (Figure 2–12). These subclassifications are primarily used for research.

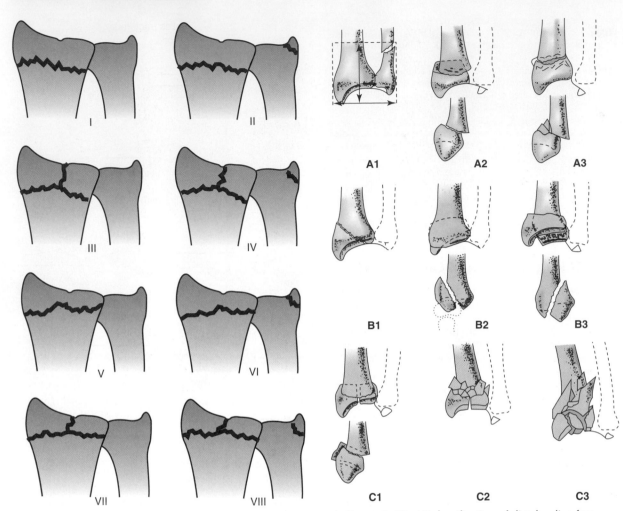

▲ **Figure 2–11.** Classification of distal radius fractures according to Frykman. (Reproduced, with permission, from Green DP, Hotchkiss RN, Pederson WC, eds: *Operative Hand Surgery*, 4th ed. New York: WB Saunders; 1999.)

▲ **Figure 2–12.** AO classification of distal radius fractures. **A:** Extraarticular metaphyseal fracture. Junction of the metaphysis and diaphysis is identified by the "square" or T method (greatest width on frontal plane of distal forearm; illustrated in **A1**). **A1:** Isolated fracture of distal ulna. **A2:** Simple radial fracture. **A3:** Radial fracture with metaphyseal impaction. **B:** Intraarticular rim fracture (preserving the continuity of the epiphysis and metaphysis). **B1:** Fracture of radial styloid. **B2:** Dorsal rim fracture (dorsal Barton fracture). **B3:** Volar rim fracture (reverse Barton 5 Goyrand-Smith type 2, Letenneur). **C:** Complex intraarticular fracture (disrupting the continuity of the epiphysis and metaphysis). **C1:** Radiocarpal joint congruity preserved; metaphysis fractured. **C2:** Articular displacement. **C3:** Diaphyseal-metaphyseal involvement. It should be considered that injury of the distal radioulnar joint is possible in any of these fractures. (Reproduced, with permission, from Green DP, Hotchkiss RN, Pederson WC, eds: *Operative Hand Surgery*, 4th ed. New York: WB Saunders; 1999.)

Another useful classification that addresses intraarticular fractures is that popularized by Melone (Figure 2–13). The Melone classification describes four major fracture components including the shaft, radial styloid, and dorsal and volar medial fragments. Often, the lunate fossa is fractured into dorsal and volar components, with the scaphoid fossa a separate component. Four-part articular fractures can have varying degrees of displacement and comminution.

▶ **Treatment**

Treatment of distal radius fractures should be influenced by fracture pattern and bone quality with a goal of restoring normal alignment and articular congruity. Patients' activity

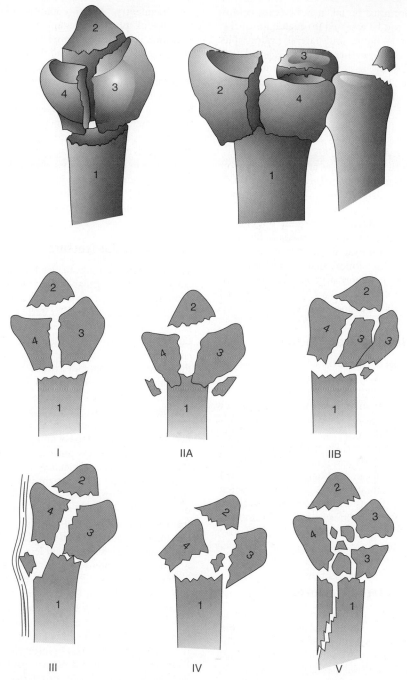

▲ **Figure 2–13.** Intraarticular fracture classification of Melone. (Reproduced, with permission, from Green DP, Hotchkiss RN, Pederson WC, eds: *Operative Hand Surgery,* 4th ed. New York: WB Saunders; 1999.)

level and comorbidities must be taken into account. Most distal radius fractures can be assessed through high-quality posteroanterior (PA), oblique, and lateral radiographs. The normal alignments as measured in the AP and lateral radiographs of the wrist are as follows: radial inclination, 22 degrees; volar tilt, 11–12 degrees; and radial length, 11–12 mm. Additional factors to consider are fracture displacement, intraarticular components, angulation, and degree of comminution; age of the patient; and functional level. Additional imaging techniques can be used to assess complex fracture patterns, including CT scan for preoperative planning of intraarticular fractures and MRI to rule out injuries to the carpal ligaments (eg, lunotriquetral and scapholunate ligament) or to the triangular fibrocartilage complex.

Surgery is indicated in patients with an open fracture or those with an inherently unstable fracture pattern (generally defined by at least three of the following criteria as discussed by Lafontaine et al: initial dorsal angulation of more than 20 degrees, initial shortening of more than 5 mm, more than 50% dorsal comminution, an intraarticular fracture, or an age of more than 60 years with an associated ulnar fracture), a shear fracture, or a fracture dislocation of the wrist.

A. Extraarticular Nondisplaced Fractures

Extraarticular nondisplaced fractures can be treated with cast immobilization for 4–6 weeks until fracture healing occurs, followed by mobilization with an off-the-shelf brace. Radial length and angulation are generally not fully restored with closed reduction techniques. Small amounts of radial shortening can lead to increased load in the lunate fossa, distal ulna, and triangular fibrocartilage. In most low-demand patients, however, this treatment can be successful, and functional wrist motion can be obtained. If shortening is significant, midcarpal instability may occur. Another potential problem is DRUJ arthrosis and ulnar carpal abutment, which may necessitate later reconstruction. In minimally displaced fractures, a rapid cast conversion to a supportive splint (2 or 3 weeks) and early mobilization can be safely done and may yield improved outcomes.

B. Extraarticular Displaced Fractures

Closed reduction should be attempted on extraarticular displaced fractures. If radial length and volar tilt are restored, then a sugar tong splint or long arm cast can be effective in holding the reduction. If the reduction is not adequate by closed means, then an external fixator (for ligamentotaxis) and percutaneous pins (to manipulate the fracture) may be necessary. Although current trends are toward plating via a volar approach with specialized locking plates, new low-profile plate designs make the dorsal approach a reliable option. Major drawbacks of dorsal plating are tendon irritation and joint stiffness. Recent studies indicate that locked plates and early postoperative range of motion may provide improved long-term results.

Percutaneous pin fixation can be an effective adjunct to cast treatment or external fixation. It can be intrafocal or interfragmentry. Arthroscopically assisted reduction can be a useful tool for assessing articular reduction. Loss of reduction is a potential complication in older patients. Also, granuloma formation around the pin can be seen.

External fixation is an effective way to handle distal radius fractures. With external fixation, there is the additional advantage of not devascularizing bony fragments and not creating a surgical wound. Use of indirect traction on fracture fragments, taking advantage of "ligamentotaxis" via the fixator pins, can be effective. In cases of open fractures, an external fixator can facilitate wound care. External fixation is effective in preventing loss of reduction and length in situations where there is comminution of bone. Complications with external fixation include pin tract infection, superficial radial nerve neuropathy, pin loosening, and stiffness.

C. Intraarticular Fractures

The treatment of intraarticular fractures aims to restore the congruity of the articular surface and the anatomic axis of the distal radius in order to improve the outcome. ORIF is the treatment of choice. For volar Barton fractures, the treatment of choice is the volar buttress plate. The only contraindications to this treatment are cases with excessive comminution such that ORIF will fail to achieve a stable bony construct. In these situations, use of an external fixator as a distractor and neutralization device is generally indicated. Using a fluoroscopy unit to visualize the fracture will help ascertain that both articular alignment and overall radial length have been adequately restored with external fixation. Minor adjustments as necessary can be effectively done with adjunct percutaneous pins. These maneuvers may fail to achieve the appropriate articular alignment, particularly if some healing has already occurred or if the displacement is severe. In this case, ORIF should be performed. Justification for aggressive treatment of distal radius fractures in young patients (<60 years) comes from several studies. The goal should be articular step-off less than 2 mm, radial shortening less than 4 mm, dorsal tilt less than 15 degrees, volar tilt less than 20 degrees, and loss of radial inclination less than 10 degrees. Arthroscopically assisted repair of distal radius fractures has been advocated. Intraarticular step-off and associated injuries such as triangular fibrocartilage, scapholunate, and lunotriquetral tears, as well as osteochondral lesions, can be accurately assessed. Some authors advocate bone grafting in the acute treatment of comminuted fractures. In intraarticular fractures, external fixation can be used, but reductions are difficult to maintain without percutaneous pins or internal fixation.

2. Distal Radioulnar Joint Dislocation (ICD-9:833.01)

The distal ulna transmits significant loads to the forearm through the distal ulna via the triangular fibrocartilage complex. Even minor disruptions of the precise anatomic relationships between the distal radius and ulna and ulnar carpus result in pain syndromes. The DRUJ can be dislocated by a variety of mechanisms, including low- and high-energy trauma. These are associated with disruption of the ulnar soft-tissue triangular fibrocartilage complex, including the articular disk and associated ligaments. There should be a high index of suspicion in order to diagnose this lesion because radiographs that are not taken in the perfect lateral orientation will tend to look relatively normal. A displaced fracture at the ulnar styloid base indicates a high risk of distal radioulnar instability. In the presence of forearm and elbow fracture-dislocations, further evaluation of the radioulnar joint is mandatory.

▶ Clinical Findings

The clinical examination is key, with identification of the DRUJ surface anatomy and clinical evaluation of the joint. The amount of stability should be carefully assessed and compared with that of the opposite wrist. The patient should position the wrist to reproduce the pain. With the hand pronated, the examiner tries to displace the ulnar head, applying a dorsal to volar load 4 cm proximal to the DRUJ ("piano key test"). Little resistance to ballottement and volar movement of the ulna head corresponds to a positive piano key test. Subluxation is much more common than anterior or posterior dislocation. Limitation of pronation and supination, or pain associated with such motion, would be expected in such a situation. Palpation of the sixth extensor compartment during resisted pronation is useful to identify any subluxation. The other common cause of DRUJ problems is rheumatoid arthritis.

▶ Treatment

Dorsal dislocation, or subluxation, should be treated by reduction of the ulnar head into the sigmoid fossa and placement of the forearm in full supination. The arm should be immobilized in supination, which requires a long arm cast or splint. Volar dislocation is relatively rare and is usually stable after reduction. If dorsal or volar dislocation or subluxation of the distal ulna cannot be reduced with manipulation in the outpatient setting, closed treatment can be attempted under anesthesia. If this fails, open reduction and soft-tissue reconstruction may be necessary. If this is performed, a retinacular flap may be used to transpose the extensor carpi ulnaris to a more dorsal position to stabilize the distal ulna, as has been described for Darrach reconstruction of the joint.

3. Malunion of Distal Radius

Malunion of the distal radius can have a variety of negative consequences. Alteration of the biomechanical function of the wrist may lead to weakness, limitation of motion, and midcarpal instability. Associated DRUJ arthrosis may be present, as well as ulnocarpal abutment. Also, rotational deformity is common with angulated malunions. CT of both wrists can be used to identify and measure malrotation preoperatively.

▶ Treatment

The treatment of choice in such a situation, if conservative treatment fails, is reconstructive surgery. Fernandez has elegantly described the strategy. An osteotomy of the radius with iliac crest bone grafting and plate fixation is performed (Figure 2–14).

The DRUJ must be addressed and, depending on the degree of subluxation or arthrosis, may require closed reduction, open reduction, or reconstruction using the Darrach or Sauve-Kapandji procedure (Figure 2–15). In the Sauve-Kapandji

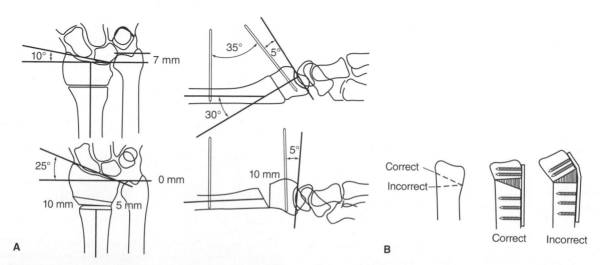

▲ **Figure 2–14.** Open wedge osteotomy of the distal radius with iliac crest bone graft and plate fixation. (Reproduced, with permission, from Green DP, Hotchkiss RN, Pederson WC, eds: *Operative Hand Surgery*, 4th ed. New York: WB Saunders; 1999.)

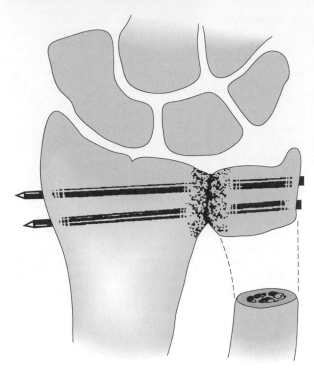

▲ **Figure 2–15.** Suave-Kapandji reconstruction of the distal radioulnar joint. (Reproduced, with permission, from Green DP, Hotchkiss RN, Pederson WC, eds: *Operative Hand Surgery,* 4th ed. New York: WB Saunders; 1999.)

procedure, instead of distal ulnar resection as in the Darrach procedure, transverse segmental resection of the ulnar metaphysis is followed by creation of an arthrodesis of the distal ulna to the radius, using the resected bone as grafting material. Forearm rotation occurs through the ulnar metaphyseal pseudoarthrosis. Additionally, restoration of the radial length may be difficult with manipulation alone. Useful adjuncts to achieve restoration of appropriate length and orientation in severe malunion include use of laminar spreaders to distract the proximal and distal fragments of the radius after osteotomy. Alternatively, an external fixator may prove useful in helping to achieve appropriate length after osteotomy.

If the distal radius has settled into a position of shortening and significant angulatory deformity but the fracture is not yet fully healed, osteotomy for early or "nascent" malunion is justified. The advantage of taking down a nascent malunion is that the operation is technically simpler to perform, shortens the time of disability, and leads to better long-term results. Additionally, the DRUJ can be restored more reliably in these early reconstructions than when osteotomy is required for established malunion. The latter often requires adjunctive DRUJ reconstruction with Darrach resection, Sauve-Kapandji procedure, hemiresection, or matched resection arthroplasty.

Abboudi J, Culp RW: Treating fractures of the distal radius with arthroscopic assistance. *Orthop Clin North Am* 2001;32:307. [PMID: 11331543]

Antuña SA, Sánchez-Márquez JM, Barco R: Long-term results of radial head resection following isolated radial head fractures in patients younger than forty years old. *J Bone Joint Surg Am* 2010;92:558. [PMID: 20194313]

Carter PB, Stuart PR: The Sauve-Kapandji procedure for post-traumatic disorders of the distal radio-ulnar joint. *J Bone Joint Surg Br* 2000;82:1013. [PMID: 11041592]

Chhabra A, Hale JE, Milbrandt TA, et al: Biomechanical efficacy of an internal fixator for treatment of distal radius fractures. *Clin Orthop Relat Res* 2001;393:318. [PMID: 11764365]

Jakob M, Rikli A, Regazzoni P: Fractures of the distal radius treated by internal fixation and early function. *J Bone Joint Surg Br* 2000;82-B:341. [PMID: 10813166]

Ladd AL, Pliam NB: The role of bone graft and alternatives in unstable distal radius fracture treatment. *Orthop Clin North Am* 2001;32:337. [PMID: 11331546]

Lafontaine M, Hardy D, Delince P: Stability assessment of distal radius fractures. *Injury* 1989;20:208. [PMID: 2592094]

Margaliot Z, Haase SC, Kotsis SV, et al: A meta-analysis of outcomes of external fixation versus plate osteosynthesis for unstable distal radius fractures. *J Hand Surg* 2005;30:1185. [PMID: 16344176]

May MM, Lawton JN, Blazar PE: Ulnar styloid fractures associated with distal radius fractures: incidence and implications for distal radioulnar joint instability. *J Hand Surg Am* 2002;27:965. [PMID: 12457345]

Medoff RJ: Essential radiographic evaluation for distal radius fractures. *Hand Clin* 2005;21:279. [PMID: 16039439]

Nalbantoglu U, Gereli A, Kocaoglu B, Aktas S, Turkmen M: Capitellar cartilage injuries concomitant with radial head fractures. *J Hand Surg Am* 2008;33:1602. [PMID: 18984344]

Orbay JL, Fernandez DL: Volar fixed-angle plate fixation for unstable distal radius fractures in the elderly patient. *J Hand Surg Am* 2004;29:96. [PMID: 14751111]

Penzkofer R, Hungerer S, Wipf F, von Oldenburg G, Augat P: Anatomical plate configuration affects mechanical performance in distal humerus fractures. *Clin Biomech* 2010;25:972. [PMID: 20696508]

Rogachefsky RA, Lipson SR, Applegate B, et al: Treatment of severely comminuted intraarticular fractures of the distal end of the radius by open reduction and combined internal and external fixation. *J Bone Joint Surg Am* 2001;83-A:509. [PMID: 11315779]

Schneeberger AG, Ip W, Poon T, et al: Open reduction and plate fixation of displaced AO type C3 fractures of the distal radius: restoration of articular congruity in eighteen cases. *J Orthop Trauma* 2001;15:350. [PMID: 11433140]

Simic PM, Robison J, Gardner MJ, Gelberman RH, Weiland AJ, Boyer MI: Treatment of distal radius fractures with a low-profile dorsal plating system: an outcomes assessment. *J Hand Surg Am* 2006;31:382. [PMID: 16516731]

Stoffel K, Cunneen S, Morgan R, Nicholls R, Stachowiak G: Comparative stability of perpendicular versus parallel double-locking plating systems in osteoporotic comminuted distal humerus fractures. *J Orthop Res* 2008;26:778. [PMID: 18203185]

Viso R, Wegener EE, Freeland AE: Use of a closing wedge osteotomy to correct malunion of dorsally displaced extraarticular distal radius fractures. *Orthopedics* 2000;23:721. [PMID: 10917249]

II. TRAUMA TO THE LOWER EXTREMITY

PELVIC FRACTURES AND DISLOCATIONS

- *Pelvic fractures are potentially life-threatening injuries with high mortality rates.*
- *Most are caused by MVAs and falls from height.*
- *A multidisciplinary approach is necessary to reduce mortality and disability.*
- *Pelvic ring fractures account for 3% of all fractures.*

▶ Mechanism of Injury

Four patterns of injury are responsible for pelvic fractures. *Anteroposterior compression* results in external rotation of the hemipelvis and rupture of the pelvic floor and anterior sacroiliac ligaments. *Lateral compression* creates compression fractures of the sacrum and disruption of the posterior sacroiliac ligament complex. The sacrospinous and sacrotuberous ligaments remain intact, limiting the instability. In high-energy lateral compression injuries, the contralateral hemipelvis can be pushed in external rotation, as seen in rollover or crush injuries. *Combined external rotation-abduction* is common in motorcycle accidents, and the deforming forces are transmitted through the femur. The fourth pattern is a *shear force* vector resulting from fall from heights, where the grade of translational instability is variable.

▶ Clinical Findings

Knowledge of the injury mechanism is of prime importance to estimate the outcomes; the physical examination includes inspection of the skin, perineum, and rectum. Closed degloving injuries (Morel-Lavallée) should be properly identified. Palpation of the pelvic bony landmarks, including posterior palpation of the sacrum and sacroiliac joint, should be done, but anteroposterior and lateral iliac wing compression maneuvers to assess stability should be performed only once or avoided in hemodynamically unstable patients because excessive manipulation can increase bleeding by mobilizing the initial clotting. Rectovaginal examination is mandatory in all cases to identify open fractures. Bony spikes protruding through the mucosa contaminate the fracture hematoma. Associated injuries should also be systematically sought: lower urinary tract injuries, distal vascular status, and a thorough recorded neurologic examination.

An initial AP pelvic radiograph as per ATLS protocol is examined to evaluate the pelvic ring as a possible cause of shock. Following successful resuscitation, AP pelvis radiography should be obtained. When the patient is hemodynamically stabilized, inlet and outlet views and, if acetabular fractures are suspected, obturator or iliac oblique views should be ordered. Actual displacement of the symphysis pubis can also be evaluated by stress views under general anesthesia. CT scan is essential to further define the fracture pattern. Vascular and urologic imaging may also be required.

▶ Treatment

Most pelvis fractures treated by orthopedic surgeons are stable injuries, and management of these low-energy fractures generally requires nonsurgical treatment. On the contrary, management of unstable pelvic injuries requires a systemic approach in a multidisciplinary manner. Thus, in the hemodynamically unstable patient, the ATLS protocol should be followed. Hemorrhage and shock are the primary causes of death due to pelvic fracture. The cornerstones of successful treatment include identification of a significant pelvic injury; rapid resuscitation; hemorrhage control (using angiography or pelvic packing); assessment and treatment of associated injuries; and mechanical stabilization in selected cases. Initial resuscitation started with 2 L of crystalloid should be followed by packed blood cells, fresh frozen plasma, and platelets in a 1:1:4 ratio. A pelvic binder or sheet can be used to stabilize the unstable pelvis temporarily. After ruling out other sources of bleeding by chest and spine radiography and focused abdominal sonography for trauma (FAST), an external fixation device (pelvic clamp and/or anterior external fixator) should be applied. Pelvic packing and/or arterial angiography should be executed according to the protocol of the trauma center. If the patient's hemodynamic status stabilizes, the need for definitive versus temporizing mechanical fixation of the pelvis should be determined. Anterior fixation may involve anterior plating of the pubic symphysis or maintaining the external fixation device in place, which does not provide posterior stability and can potentially increase displacement of the fractured pelvis in vertical unstable fracture configuration. It usually resists stresses imposed by sitting but not those from weight bearing, and further internal fixation is often required at a later stage. Posterior fixation (either surgical or CT-guided percutaneous fixation) is usually deferred until a later time.

In open pelvic fractures, which account for 2–4% of all pelvic fractures, early surgical intervention using a multidisciplinary approach should be undertaken. Seventy-two percent of open pelvic fractures are grade III open wounds and should be appropriately treated. The definitive method of stabilization of open pelvic fractures remains controversial. Internal fixation can be done when no gross contamination is present. Otherwise, external fixation is preferred when fecal or environmental contamination is present. If the fecal content contacts the open wound, colostomy is indicated.

A. Associated Injuries

1. Hemorrhage—Most of the bleeding associated with pelvic ring fractures usually comes from the small to medium-sized veins in the surrounding soft tissues and from the bone itself. Arterial injuries causing significant bleeding occur only in about 10% of pelvic fractures. After blunt trauma, the most common pelvic arteries injured are the superior gluteal and internal pudendal arteries. CT scans can be used to detect arterial bleeding before angiography but should be postponed until the patient is hemodynamically stable for transfer. Embolization can be used to prevent arterial bleeding. Pelvic packing helps tamponade the bleeding by increasing the intrapelvic pressure. Surgery for repair or bypass is urgently required if there is a distal ischemia.

2. Thrombosis—Pelvic fractures increase the risk of venous thromboembolic problems in trauma patients. DVT is seen not only in distal calf veins, but also in pelvic venous plexus. Magnetic venous venography is more advantageous than duplex color ultrasound to detect pelvic thrombosis. Guidelines for prophylaxis are controversial, and one should consider the benefits, risks, and cost of different treatment options. Early administration of low-molecular-weight heparin (LMWH) may decrease the incidence of symptomatic pulmonary emboli. More trauma centers now use intermittent pneumatic compression after trauma and temporary vena cava filters in severely traumatized patients with contradictions to pharmacologic prophylaxis (heparin, warfarin, or LMWH).

3. Neurologic injury—Neurologic injuries are common, and the frequency increases with complexity of the fractures. Up to 40% of unstable pelvic injuries may have neurologic injuries. After unstable vertical shear sacral fractures, the incidence rises to 50%. L5 and S1 are the most common affected roots. It is of paramount importance that a thorough neurologic examination is performed and recorded as soon as possible, searching for sensory or motor deficits in the distribution of sciatic, femoral, obturator, pudendal, or superior gluteal nerves. Peripheral nerve injuries have, overall, a better prognosis than root injuries. Partial nerve injuries also have a better outcome than complete ones. Most of the lesions are of the neurapraxia type, with favorable outcome. It is still accepted that nearly 10% have clinically significant permanent neurologic sequelae.

4. Urogenital injuries—Urogenital injuries are common and occur in as many as 24% of adults with pelvic fractures. Males have twice the urethral injury incidence than females because of the anatomic disadvantage. In males, these injuries should be suspected in a patient who is unable to void, who has gross hematuria at the meatus, swelling or hematoma of the perineum or penis, or a "high-riding" or "floating" prostate at digital rectal examination.

Additionally in female patients, vaginal bleeding, labial edema, blood at the meatus, and urinary leak per rectum can be clinical signs of possible urethral injury. Blind insertion of a Foley catheter may cause extension of a partial tear into a complete tear, may increase the extent of a hemorrhage, or may introduce an infectious agent into a previously sterile hematoma, so a retrograde (ascending) urethrogram should be obtained before insertion. When a partial or complete urethral disruption is diagnosed, a suprapubic cystotomy should be performed.

1. Injuries to the Pelvic Ring (ICD-9:808.41-42-43-49, 808-2)

Injuries that are stable do not deform under normal physiologic forces, whereas unstable injuries are characterized by their type of displacement, such as vertically unstable or horizontally unstable.

From the anatomic standpoint, the posterior sacroiliac ligamentous complex is the single most important structure for pelvic stability. Injuries involving the pelvic ring in two or more sites create an unstable segment. The integrity of the posterior sacroiliac ligamentous complex will determine the degree of instability. Inlet and outlet views and CT scanning are necessary imaging techniques to make this determination. When intact, the hemipelvis will be rotationally unstable but vertically stable. When disrupted, the hemipelvis will be both rotationally and vertically unstable.

▶ Classification and Treatment

Tile devised a dynamic classification system based on the mechanism of injury and residual instability (Table 2–5).

Table 2–5. The Tile classification of pelvic ring disruptions.

Type A: Stable, posterior arch intact
A1: Posterior arch intact, fracture of innominate bone (avulsion)
 A1.1 Iliac spine
 A1.2 Iliac crest
 A1.3 Ischial tuberosity
A2: Posterior arch intact, fracture of innominate bone (direct blow)
 A2.1 Iliac wing fractures
 A2.2 Unilateral fracture of anterior arch
 A2.3 Bifocal fracture of anterior arch
A3: Posterior arch intact, transverse fracture of sacrum caudal to S2
 A3.1 Sacrococcygeal dislocation
 A3.2 Sacrum undisplaced
 A3.3 Sacrum displaced

Type B: Incomplete disruption of posterior arch, partially stable, rotation
B1: External rotation instability, open-book injury, unilateral
 B1.1 Sacroiliac joint, anterior disruption
 B1.2 Sacral fracture
B2: Incomplete disruption of posterior arch, unilateral, internal rotation (lateral compression)
 B2.1 Anterior compression fracture, sacrum
 B2.2 Partial sacroiliac joint fracture, subluxation
 B2.3 Incomplete posterior iliac fracture
B3: Incomplete disruption of posterior arch, bilateral
 B3.1 Bilateral open-book
 B3.2 Open-book, lateral compression
 B3.3 Bilateral lateral compression

Type C: Complete disruption of posterior arch, unstable
C1: Complete disruption of posterior arch, unilateral
 C1.1 Fracture through ilium
 C1.2 Sacroiliac dislocation and/or fracture dislocation
 C1.3 Sacral fracture
C2: Bilateral injury, one side rotationally unstable, one side vertically unstable
C3: Bilateral injury, both sides completely unstable

Reproduced, with permission, from Browner BD, Levine A, Jupiter J, et al, eds: *Skeletal Trauma,* 2nd ed. New York: WB Saunders; 1998.

Type A: Fractures that involve the pelvic ring in only one place and are stable.

Type A1: Avulsion fractures of the pelvis that usually occur at muscle origins (eg, the anterosuperior iliac spine [sartorius], anteroinferior iliac spine [direct head of the rectus femoris], and ischial apophysis [hamstring muscles]). These fractures occur most often in the adolescent, and conservative treatment is usually sufficient. On rare occasions, symptomatic nonunion occurs and is best dealt with surgically.

Type A2: Stable fractures with minimal displacement. Isolated fractures of the iliac wing without intraarticular extension usually result from direct trauma. Even with significant displacement, bony healing is to be expected, and therefore, treatment is symptomatic. On rare occasions, the soft-tissue injury and accompanying hematoma may heal with significant heterotopic ossification.

Type A3: Obturator fractures. Isolated fractures of the pubic or ischial rami are usually minimally displaced. The posterior sacroiliac complex is intact, and the pelvis is stable. Treatment is symptomatic, with bed rest and analgesia, early ambulation, and weight bearing as tolerated.

Type B: Fractures that involve the pelvic ring in two or more sites. They create a segment that is rotationally unstable but vertically stable.

Type B1: Open-book fractures occur from anteroposterior compression. Unless the anterior separation of the pubic symphysis is severe (>6 cm), the posterior sacroiliac complex is usually intact and the pelvis relatively stable. Significant injury to perineal and urogenital structures is often present and should always be looked for. One should remember that fragment displacement at the time of injury might have been significantly more than what is apparent on radiograph. For minimally displaced symphysis injuries, only symptomatic treatment is needed. The same applies for the so-called straddle (four rami) fracture. For more displaced fracture-dislocations, reduction is done by lateral compression using the intact posterior sacroiliac complex as the hinge on which "the book is closed." Reduction can be maintained by external or internal fixation. "Closing the book" decreases the space available for hemorrhage. It also increases patient comfort, facilitates nursing care, and allows earlier mobilization, which is beneficial to the polytrauma patient.

Type B2 and B3: Lateral compression fractures. A lateral force applied to the pelvis causes inward displacement of the hemipelvis through the sacroiliac complex and the ipsilateral (B2) or, more often, contralateral pubic rami (B3, bucket-handle type). The degree of involvement of the posterior sacroiliac ligaments will determine the degree of instability. The posterior lesion may be impacted in its displaced portion, affording some relative stability. The hemipelvis is infolded, with overlapping of the symphysis. Major displacement requires manipulation under general anesthesia. This should be done soon after injury because disimpaction becomes difficult and hazardous after the first few days. Reduction can be maintained with external or internal fixation, or both. External fixation alone decreases pain and makes nursing care easier but is not strong enough for ambulation if the fracture is unstable posteriorly.

Type C: Fractures that are both rotationally and vertically unstable. They often result from a vertical shear mechanism, like a fall from a height. Anteriorly, the injury may fracture the pubic rami or disrupt the symphysis pubis. Posteriorly, the sacroiliac joint may be dislocated, or there may be a fracture in the sacrum or in the ilium immediately adjacent to the sacroiliac joint, but there is always loss of the functional integrity of the posterior sacroiliac ligamentous complex. The hemipelvis is completely unstable. Three-dimensional displacement is possible, particularly proximal migration. Massive hemorrhage and injury to the lumbosacral nerve plexus are common. Indirect radiologic clues of pelvic instability should be looked for such as avulsion of the sciatic spine or fracture of the ipsilateral L5 transverse process. Reduction is relatively easy, with longitudinal skeletal traction through the distal femur or the proximal tibia. If chosen as definitive treatment, traction should be maintained for 8–12 weeks. Bony injuries heal quicker than ligamentous injuries. External fixation alone is insufficient to maintain reduction in highly unstable fractures, but it may help control bleeding and eases nursing care. ORIF is often required. The surgical technique is demanding, and there is a significant risk of complications. It is best left to experienced pelvic surgeons.

▶ Complications

Long-term complications of unstable pelvic ring disruptions are more frequent and disabling than once thought. If anatomic restoration of anatomic bony alignment cannot be achieved and maintained, complications such as pain, leg-length discrepancy, and residual gait abnormalities can be seen. The overall nonunion rate is around 3%. Chronic low back pain and sacroiliac pain are frequent and seen in up to 50% of cases on long-term follow-up. Changes in voiding pattern, altered defecation, and sexual dysfunction are common after sacral fractures or sacroiliac dislocations.

2. Fractures of the Acetabulum (ICD-9:808.0)

The acetabulum results from the closure of the Y or triradiate cartilage and is covered with hyaline cartilage.

Fractures of the acetabulum occur through direct trauma on the trochanteric region or indirect axial loading through the lower limb. The position of the limb at the time of impact (rotation, flexion, abduction, or adduction) will determine the pattern of injury. Comminution is common.

▶ Anatomy

The acetabulum appears to be contained within an arch. It is supported by the confluence of two columns and enhanced by two walls. The posterior column is the strongest one and where more space is available for fixation. It begins at the dense bone of the greater sciatic notch and extends distally through the center of the acetabulum to include the ischial spine and ischial tuberosity. The inner surface forms the posterior wall, and the anterior surface forms the posterior articular surface of the acetabulum. The anterior column extends from the iliac crest to the symphysis pubis. The anterior column rotates 90 degrees just above the acetabulum as it descends. The medial part of the anterior column is the true pelvic brim. The quadrilateral plate is the medial structure preventing medial displacement of the hip and is an independent structure between the two columns. The acetabular dome or weight-bearing area extends from the bone posterior to the anterior inferior iliac spine to the posterior column.

▶ Classification

Letournel has classified acetabular fractures based on the involved column. Fractures may involve one or both columns in a simple or complex pattern.

Proper fracture classification requires good-quality radiographs. Two oblique views (Judet views) taken 45 degrees toward and away from the involved side complement the standard AP view of the pelvis. The obturator (internal) oblique view is obtained by elevating the fractured hip 45 degrees from the horizontal. This view shows the anterior column (iliopectineal line) and the posterior lip of the acetabulum, and the iliac wing is perpendicular to its broad surface. In this view, the spur sign can be identified in 95% of cases of both-column fractures (type C), and it corresponds to the area of the iliac wing above the acetabular roof. The iliac (external) oblique view is obtained by elevating the nonfractured hip 45 degrees. This view best shows the posterior column (ilioischial line), including the ischial spine, the anterior wall of the acetabulum, and the full expanse of the iliac wing. In addition, inlet and outlet pelvic views can be complementary if any doubt about pelvic ring compromise is present.

CT scanning gives further information on the fracture pattern, the presence of free intraarticular fragments, and the status of the femoral head and the rest of the pelvic ring.

Letournel has classified acetabular fractures into 10 different types: five simple patterns (one fracture line) and five complex patterns (the association of two or more simple patterns) (Figure 2–16). This is the most widely used classification system, as it allows the surgeon to choose the appropriate surgical approach.

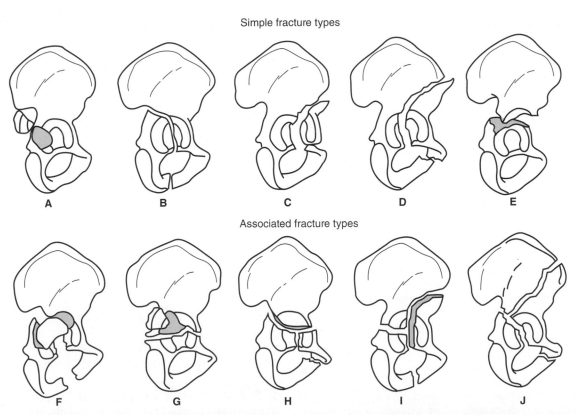

Simple fracture types

Associated fracture types

▲ **Figure 2–16.** Letournel classification of acetabular fractures. (Reproduced, with permission, from Canale ST, ed: *Campbell's Operative Orthopaedics,* 9th ed. Philadelphia: Lippincott; 1998.)

Treatment

The goal of treatment is to attain a spherical congruency between the femoral head and the weight-bearing acetabular dome and to maintain it until bones are healed. As with other pelvic fractures, acetabular fractures are frequently associated with abdominal, urogenital, and neurologic injuries, which should be systematically sought and treated. Significant bleeding can be present and should be addressed as soon as possible. Examination of the knee ligaments and vascular status of the extremities is mandatory. A careful neurologic examination is necessary. Sciatic nerve compromise occurs in 20% of cases. The peroneal branch is often involved. The femoral nerve and superior gluteal nerve are also susceptible to injury during trauma or surgery. Prophylaxis and surveillance for DVT should be started soon after trauma.

The stabilized patient should be put in longitudinal skeletal traction through a distal femoral or proximal tibial pin pulling axially in neutral position. A trochanteric screw for lateral traction is contraindicated, because it will create a contaminated pin tract and thus preclude possible further surgical treatment. Postreduction radiographs are obtained. In general, a displaced acetabular fracture is rarely reduced adequately by closed methods. If the reduction is judged acceptable, traction is maintained for 6–8 weeks until bone healing is evident. Another 6–8 weeks is necessary before full weight bearing can be attempted. Surgical indications include intraarticular displacement of 2 mm or more, an incongruous hip reduction, marginal impaction of more than 2 mm, or intraarticular debris. The choice of approach is of primary importance, and sometimes more than one approach will prove necessary. Acetabular surgery uses extensile approaches and sophisticated reduction and fixation techniques and is best performed by trained pelvic surgeons. Other surgical indications include free osteochondral fragments, femoral head fractures, irreducible dislocations, or unstable reductions.

Complications

Complications inherent to the injury include posttraumatic degenerative joint disease, heterotopic ossification, femoral head osteonecrosis, DVT, and other complications related to conservative treatment. Surgery is performed to prevent or delay osteoarthritis but increases the possibility of complications such as infection, iatrogenic neurovascular injury, and heterotopic ossification. When the reduction is stable and fixation is solid, the patient can be mobilized after a few days with non–weight-bearing ambulation, and weight bearing may begin as early as 6 weeks. Most pelvic surgeons now routinely use postoperative prophylactic anticoagulation and heterotopic bone formation prophylaxis with irradiation or indomethacin, or both.

American College of Surgeons, Committee on Trauma: *Advanced Trauma Life Support for Doctors: Student Course Manual*, 7th ed. Chicago: American College of Surgeons; 2008.

Bellabarba C, Ricci WM, Bolhofner BR: Distraction external fixation in lateral compression pelvic fractures. *J Orthop Trauma* 2000;14:475. [PMID: 11083609]

Carlson DA, Scheid DK, Maar DC, et al: Safe placement of S1 and S2 iliosacral screws: the vestibule concept. *J Orthop Trauma* 2000;14:264. [PMID: 10898199]

Grotz MRW, Allami MK, Harwood P, Pape HC, Kretekk C, Giannoudis PV: Open pelvic fractures: epidemiology, current concepts of management and outcome. *Injury* 2005;1:1. [PMID: 15589906]

Hak DJ, Smith WR, Suzuki T: Management of hemorrhage in life-threatening pelvic fracture. *J Am Acad Orthop Surg* 2009;17:447. [PMID: 19571300]

McCormick JP, Morgan SJ, Smith WR: Clinical effectiveness of the physical examination in diagnosis of posterior pelvic ring injuries. *J Orthop Trauma* 2003;17:257. [PMID: 12679685]

Saterbak AM, Marsh JL, Nepola JV, et al: Clinical failure after posterior wall acetabular fractures: the influence of initial fracture patterns. *J Orthop Trauma* 2000;14:230. [PMID: 10898194]

Slobogean GP, Lefaivre KA, Nicolaou S, O'Brien PJ: A systematic review of thromboprophylaxis for pelvic and acetabular fractures. *J Orthop Trauma* 2009;23:379. [PMID: 19390367]

Switzer JA, Nork SE, Routt ML: Comminuted fractures of the iliac wing. *J Orthop Trauma* 2000;14:270. [PMID: 10898200]

Tornetta P: Displaced acetabular fractures: indications for operative and nonoperative management. *J Am Acad Orthop Surg* 2001;9:18. [PMID: 11174160]

Tötterman A, Glott T, Madsen JE, Røise O: Unstable sacral fractures: associated injuries and morbidity at 1 year. *Spine* 2006;31:E628. [PMID: 17545913]

HIP FRACTURES AND DISLOCATIONS

- *Globally, 6.3 million hip fractures are estimated by year 2050.*
- *Primarily occur in older patients over 55 years.*
- *Fall from standing height is the main cause of injury.*
- *Almost all hip fractures are treated surgically.*
- *One-year mortality after femoral neck and intertrochanteric fracture exceeds 14–36%.*

Anatomy and Biomechanical Principles

The hip joint is the articulation between the acetabulum and the femoral head. The trabecular pattern of the femoral head and neck, and that of the acetabulum, is oriented to optimally accept the forces crossing the joint. Calcar femorale is the dense bone oriented in posteromedial portion of the femoral shaft under the lesser trochanter that supports the force transfer from the neck to the shaft.

The total force acting across the joint is 2.5 times body weight when standing on one leg and five times body weight when running. Using a cane in the opposite hand reduces the force to body weight when standing on that leg.

1. Femoral Neck Fractures (ICD-9:820.0)

Femoral neck fractures occur in the intracapsular region between the trochanters distally and the head proximally.

Main arterial blood supply of the neck comes from an extracapsular ring of vessels formed by the ascending branch of the lateral circumflex artery anteriorly and medial circumflex artery posteriorly. These fractures are classified as subcapital, transcervical, and basicervical. The latter acts more like an intertrochanteric fracture. These fractures are generally low-energy injuries in the elderly population; however, they are more often seen as high-energy injuries at young ages. The typical patient is a female who had a falling incident and presents with a painful hip, with shortened and externally rotated extremity on physical examination. Stress fractures of the femoral neck can also occur and should be excluded in young athletes. These fractures may be difficult to diagnose. Physical examination, as well as the initial radiographs, may be normal. Repeat radiographs, radionuclide imaging, and MRI may be necessary to confirm the diagnosis. Plain AP view and a cross-table lateral view of the involved hip are indicated to diagnose and classify the fracture. Bone scans can be false negative in the acute phase.

Classification

The Garden classification for acute fractures is the most widely used system:

Type 1: Valgus impaction of the femoral head

Type 2: Complete but nondisplaced

Type 3: Complete fracture, displaced less than 50%

Type 4: Complete fracture displaced more than 50%

This classification is of prognostic value for the incidence of avascular necrosis: The higher the Garden number, the higher the incidence. The benefits of either skeletal or skin traction are unclear prior to definitive treatment. Traction may offer comfort in some patients but does not improve overall outcome.

Stable Femoral Neck Fractures

These include stress fractures and Garden type 1 and 2 fractures. Nonsurgical treatment should be reserved for patients with extreme medical risks for surgery.

The Garden type 1 fracture is impacted in valgus position and is usually stable. Impaction must be demonstrated on both AP and lateral views. The risk of displacement is nevertheless significant; most surgeons recommend prophylactic internal fixation with screws or sliding hip screw to maintain reduction and allow earlier ambulation and weight bearing.

Unstable Femoral Neck Fractures

Treatment is directed toward preservation of life and restoration of hip function, with early mobilization. This is best attained by rigid internal fixation or primary arthroplasty as soon as the patient is medically prepared for surgery. In general, the younger the patient, the greater the effort is justified to save the femoral head. More studies are in favor of

an urgent intervention in a young patient to protect the head viability. Necessity of a capsulotomy to decompress the joint is controversial. In the elderly patient, surgical options are either ORIF or primary arthroplasty. Gjertsen et al showed that hemiarthoplasty for displaced femoral neck fractures in the elderly resulted in fewer reoperations, less pain, and higher satisfaction rates than internal screw fixation in 4335 patients from the Norwegian Hip Fracture Register.

Treatment

A. Internal Fixation

The fracture is reduced under fluoroscopic imaging as anatomically accurately as possible. Gentle manipulation is usually sufficient. Rarely, open reduction may be necessary before fixation. Open reduction, if performed, should be approached anteriorly because this results in less disruption of blood supply than a posterior approach. The most accepted method is fixation with three screws (in an inverted triangle manner with one screw in the posteroinferior of the neck). Sliding hip screw or plate should be placed with center-apex distance within 25 mm. An additional screw is inserted superior or posteroinferior in order to control the rotational forces. The patient can usually be mobilized the following day, and weight bearing is allowed according to the stability of the construct.

B. Primary Arthroplasty

Arthroplasty is reserved for elderly displaced fractures, particularly for Garden type 4 fractures, in which avascular necrosis is highly probable, and for Garden type 3 fractures that cannot be satisfactorily reduced or for femoral heads with preexisting disease. Recent studies indicate that a lower rate of reoperations and better outcomes are expected after total hip arthroplasty versus hemiarthroplasty.

Complications

The most common sequelae of femoral neck fractures are loss of reduction with or without hardware failure, nonunions or malunions, and avascular necrosis of the femoral head. This latter complication can appear as late as 2 years after injury. According to different series, the incidence of avascular necrosis varies from 0 to 15% for Garden type 1 fractures, 10 to 25% for type 2 fractures, 25 to 50% for type 3 fractures, and 50 to 100% for type 4 fractures. Secondary degenerative joint disease appears somewhat later. The most disabling complication, infection, is fortunately rare.

2. Trochanteric Fractures (ICD-9:820.2)

Lesser Trochanter Fracture (ICD-9:820.20)

Isolated fracture of the lesser trochanter is rare. When it occurs, it is the result of the avulsion force of the iliopsoas muscle. Rarely, a symptomatic nonunion may require fragment fixation or excision.

Greater Trochanter Fracture (ICD-9:820.20)

Isolated fracture of the greater trochanter may be caused by direct injury or may occur indirectly as a result of the activity of the gluteus medius and gluteus minimus muscles. It occurs most commonly as a component of intertrochanteric fracture.

If displacement of the isolated fracture fragment is less than 1 cm and there is no tendency to further displacement (as determined by repeated radiographic examinations), treatment may be bed rest until acute pain subsides. As rapidly as symptoms permit, activity can increase gradually to protected weight bearing with crutches. Full weight bearing is permitted as soon as healing is apparent, usually in 6–8 weeks. If displacement is greater than 1 cm and increases on adduction of the thigh, extensive tearing of surrounding soft tissues may be assumed, and ORIF is indicated. Tension band wiring is the preferred technique.

Intertrochanteric Fractures (ICD-9:820.21)

- *Approximately 50% of all hip fractures.*
- *Older age, female gender, osteoporosis, history of fall, and gait abnormalities are risk factors.*

By definition, these fractures usually occur along a line between the greater and the lesser trochanter. They typically occur at a later age than do femoral neck fractures. They are most often extracapsular and occur through cancellous bone. Bone healing within 8–12 weeks is the usual outcome, regardless of the treatment. Nonunion and avascular necroses of the femoral head are not significant problems.

Clinically, the involved extremity is usually shortened and can be internally or externally rotated. If there is comminution in the calcar (posteromedial cortex) or the fracture line extends through the subtrochanteric region, the fracture is considered unstable. Reverse oblique fractures, where the course fracture line is proximal-medial to distal-lateral, are extremely unstable. A wide spectrum of fracture patterns is possible, from the nondisplaced fissure fracture to the highly comminuted fracture with four major fragments (head and neck, greater trochanter, lesser trochanter, and femoral shaft). The Muller/AO system is useful in classifying intertrochanteric femur fractures and has gained more popularity in recent years (Figure 2–17).

The selection of definitive treatment depends on the general condition of the patient and the fracture pattern. Rates of illness and death are lower when the fracture is internally fixed, allowing early mobilization. Operative treatment is indicated as soon as the patient is medically able to tolerate surgery. Overall mortality decreases if surgery can be performed within 48 hours. Initial treatment in the hospital should be by gentle skin traction to minimize pain and further displacement. Skeletal traction as the definitive treatment is rarely indicated and is fraught with complications such as pressure sores, DVT and PE, deterioration of mental

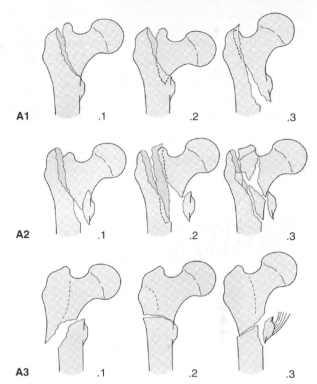

▲ **Figure 2–17.** Muller/AO system for intertrochanteric femur fracture classification. (Reproduced, with permission, from Browner BD, Levine A, Jupiter J, et al, eds: *Skeletal Trauma,* 2nd ed. New York: WB Saunders; 1998.)

status, and varus malunion. When surgery is contraindicated, it may be preferable to mobilize the patient as soon as pain permits and accept the eventual malunion or nonunion.

The great majority of these fractures are amenable to surgery. The goal is to obtain a fixation secure enough to allow early mobilization and provide an environment for sound fracture healing in a good position. Reduction of the fracture is usually accomplished by closed methods, using traction on the fracture table, and monitored using fluoroscopic imaging. Internal fixation can be obtained by dynamic hip screw (DHS), intramedullary (IM) nail, and side plate. Fixation with IM nail has biomechanical advantages over DHS, especially for the unstable fracture patterns. Early full weight bearing, return to preinjury activity, decrease in blood loss, insertion through small incision, and shorter surgery time also make IM nailing favorable. While inserting the hip screw, the screw should be centrally positioned in the head, and the distance of the lag screw to the apex of the femoral head on both AP and lateral radiographic views should be within 25 mm. Reverse oblique fractures should be treated as subtrochanteric fractures. Although generally it is not the primary option for fixation, calcar replacement arthroplasty may be an option for patients with preexisting arthritic change who have poor bone quality or for salvage procedures. General complications include infection, hardware failure, loss of reduction, nonunion, irritation bursitis over the tip of the sliding screw, and dislocation for prosthetic implants.

3. Traumatic Dislocation of the Hip Joint

- *Usually results from a high-energy trauma.*
- *Occurs with or without acetabular fracture.*
- *Eighty-five percent are posterior dislocations.*
- *Concomitant femur, knee, and patella fractures are common.*

▶ Posterior Hip Dislocation (ICD-9:835.01)

Usually the head of the femur is dislocated posterior to the acetabulum when the thigh is flexed, for example, as may occur in a head-on automobile collision when the knee is driven violently against the dashboard. Posterior dislocation is also a complication of hip arthroplasty, especially with the posterior approach.

The significant clinical findings are shortening, adduction, and internal rotation of the extremity. Anteroposterior, lateral, and, if fracture of the acetabulum is demonstrated, oblique radiographic projections (Judet views) are required. Common associated injuries include fractures of the acetabulum or the femoral head or shaft and sciatic nerve injury. The head of the femur may be displaced through a tear in the posterior hip joint capsule. The short external rotator muscles of the femur are commonly lacerated. Fracture of the posterior margin of the acetabulum can create instability.

If the acetabulum is not fractured or if the fragment is small, reduction by closed manipulation is indicated. Reduction should be achieved as soon as possible, under general anesthesia with maximum muscle relaxation, preferably within the first few hours after injury. The incidence of avascular necrosis of the femoral head increases with time until reduction. The main feature of reduction is traction in the line of deformity followed by gentle flexion of the hip to 90 degrees with stabilization of the pelvis by an assistant. While manual traction is continued, the hip is gently rotated into internal and then external rotation to obtain reduction (Allis method).

The stability of the reduction is evaluated clinically by ranging the extended hip in abduction and adduction and internal and external rotation. If stable, the same movements are repeated in 90 degrees of hip flexion. The point of redislocation is noted, the hip is reduced, and an AP radiograph of the pelvis is obtained. Soft-tissue or bone fragment interposition will be manifested by widening of the joint space as compared to the contralateral side. Irreducible dislocations, nonconcentric reductions, open dislocations, dislocations with ipsilateral femoral neck fractures, and dislocations that redislocate after reduction despite hip extension and external rotation (usually because of associated posterior wall fracture of the acetabulum) are indications for immediate ORIF if necessary. Most authors agree that a widened joint space on radiograph, despite a stable reduction, is also an indication for immediate arthrotomy. Others prefer obtaining a CT scan first to further delineate the incarcerated fragments and associated injuries before surgery. Recent studies support the use of hip arthroscopy as a safer alternative to arthrotomy for managing loose bodies.

Minor fragments of the posterior margin of the acetabulum may be disregarded, but larger displaced fragments are not usually successfully reduced by closed methods. ORIF with screws or plates is indicated.

Postreduction treatment will vary according to the type of initial surgery and the extent of the injury. Some period of skin or skeletal traction may be beneficial after strictly soft-tissue injury with a stable concentric reduction. Gradual weight bearing starting with crutch ambulation follows this period, progressing to full weight bearing at 6 weeks. Securely fixed fractures are treated as soft-tissue injuries, but weight bearing is allowed when radiologic signs of bone healing are present. When fixation is tenuous, skeletal traction for 4–6 weeks or hip spica immobilization may be necessary.

Complications include infection, avascular necrosis of the femoral head, malunion, posttraumatic degenerative joint disease, recurrent dislocation, and sciatic nerve injury. Avascular necrosis occurs because of the disruption of the retinacular arteries providing blood to the femoral head. Its incidence increases with the duration of the dislocation. It can occur as late as 2 years after the injury. MRI studies enabling early diagnosis and protected weight bearing until revascularization has occurred are recommended. Sciatic nerve injury is present in 10–20% of patients with posterior hip dislocation. Although usually of the neurapraxia type, these lesions leave permanent sequelae in about 20% of cases. The rare patient who is neurologically intact before reduction but has a deficit after reduction should be explored surgically to see if the nerve has been entrapped in the joint. Associated injuries also, on rare occasions, include fracture of the femoral head. Small fragments or those involving the non–weight-bearing surface should be ignored if they do not disturb hip mechanics; otherwise, they should be excised. Large fragments of the weight-bearing portion of the femoral head should be reduced and fixed if at all possible.

▶ Anterior Hip Dislocation (ICD-9:835.03)

- *Accounts for 10–15% of hip fracture dislocations.*
- *Occurs when the hip is extended and externally rotated at the time of impact.*

Usually, the femoral head remains lateral to the obturator externus muscle but can be found rarely beneath it (obturator dislocation) or under the iliopsoas muscle in contact with the superior pubic ramus (pubic dislocation).

The hip is classically flexed, abducted, and externally rotated. The femoral head is palpable anteriorly below the inguinal flexion crease. AP and transpelvic lateral radiographic projections are usually diagnostic.

Closed reduction under general anesthesia is generally successful. Here also the surgeon must ensure a concentric reduction, comparing both hip joints on the postreduction AP radiograph. The patient starts mobilization within a few days when pain is tolerable. Active and passive hip motion, excluding external rotation, is encouraged, and the patient is usually fully weight bearing by 4–6 weeks. Skeletal traction or spica casting may rarely be useful for uncooperative patients.

4. Rehabilitation of Hip Fracture Patients

There has been an increased interest in the psychosocial outcomes of patients with hip fractures. The goal of rehabilitation after hip injuries is to return the patient as rapidly as possible to the preinjury functional level. Factors influencing rehabilitation potential include age, mental status, associated injuries, previous medical status, myocardial function, upper extremity strength, balance, and motivation.

For the rare patient treated conservatively, rehabilitation focuses early on preventing stiffness and weakness of the other extremities and, eventually, on mobilizing the patient out of bed when pain is tolerable. Because the great majority of these injuries are now treated with internal fixation or prosthetic replacement, rehabilitation efforts are focused toward early range of motion, muscle strengthening, and weight bearing. Early full weight bearing as tolerated is encouraged for patients with prosthetic replacements, cemented or not, and for patients with stable fixation of an intertrochanteric fracture to allow compression of the fracture fragments. Most authors now agree that the same applies for femoral neck fractures with stable internal fixation, although some still prefer partial weight bearing until radiologic evidence of bone healing is present to prevent hardware failure. When internal fixation does not provide stable fixation of the fracture fragments, supplemental protection may be added with a spica cast or brace; however, it is highly undesirable in elderly patients. Otherwise, restricted range of motion or weight bearing may be allowed according to the surgeon's specifications.

Ahn J, Bernstein J: Fractures in brief: intertrochanteric fractures. *Clin Orthop Relat Res* 2010;468:1450. [PMID: 20195807]

Bernstein J, Ahn J: In brief: fractures in brief: femoral neck fractures. *Clin Orthop Relat Res* 2010;468:1713. [PMID: 20224957]

Conn KS, Parker MJ: Undisplaced intracapsular hip fractures: results of internal fixation in 375 patients. *Clin Orthop Relat Res* 2004;421:249. [PMID 15123955]

Cooper C, Campion G, Melton LJ 3rd: Hip fractures in the elderly: a world-wide projection. *Osteoporos Int* 1992;2:285. [PMID: 1421796]

Foulk DM, Mullis BH. Hip dislocation: evaluation and management. *J Am Acad Orthop Surg* 2010;18:199. [PMID: 20357229]

Gjertsen JE, Vinje T, Engesaeter LB, et al: Internal screw fixation compared with bipolar hemiarthroplasty for treatment of displaced femoral neck fractures in elderly patients. *J Bone Joint Surg Am* 2010;92:619. [PMID: 20194320]

Gotfried Y: Percutaneous compression plating of intertrochanteric hip fractures. *J Orthop Trauma* 2000;14:490. [PMID: 11083611]

Gruson K, Aharonoff GB, Egol KA, et al: The relationship between admission hemoglobin level and outcome after hip fracture. *J Orthop Trauma* 2002;15:39. [PMID: 11782632]

Jaglal S, Lakhani Z, Schatzker J: Reliability, validity and responsiveness of the lower extremity measure for patients with a hip fracture. *J Bone Joint Surg Am* 2000;82-A:955. [PMID: 10901310]

Kaplan K, Miyamoto R, Levine BR, Egol KA, Zuckerman JD: Surgical management of hip fractures: an evidence-based review of the literature. II: intertrochanteric fractures. *J Am Acad Orthop Surg* 2008;16:665. [PMID:18978289]

Kenny AM, Joseph C, Taxel P, Prestwood KM: Osteoporosis in older men and women. *Conn Med* 2003;67:481. [PMID: 14587128]

Miyamoto RG, Kaplan KM, Levine BR, Egol KA, Zuckerman JD: Surgical management of hip fractures: an evidence-based review of the literature. I: femoral neck fractures. *J Am Acad Orthop Surg* 2008;16:596. [PMID: 18832603]

Parker MJ, Handoll HH: Pre-operative traction for fractures of the proximal femur. *Cochrane Database Syst Rev* 2001;3:CD000168. [PMID 11686954]

Parker MJ, Handoll HH, Bhargara A: Conservative versus operative treatment for hip fractures. *Cochrane Database Syst Rev* 2000;4:CD000337. [PMID 11034683]

Rosen JE, Chen FS, Hiebert R, Koval KJ: Efficacy of preoperative skin traction in hip fracture patients: a prospective randomized study. *J Orthop Trauma* 2001;15:81. [PMID: 11232658]

Sahin V, Karakaş ES, Aksu S, Atlihan D, Turk CY, Halici M: Traumatic dislocation and fracture-dislocation of the hip: a long-term follow-up study. *J Trauma* 2003;54:520. [PMID: 12634533]

FEMORAL SHAFT FRACTURES

- *Fractures between 5 cm distal to the lesser trochanter and 5 cm proximal to the adductor tubercle.*

- *Closed intramedullary nailing is the standard of care for most of the fractures.*

- *Associated orthopedic injuries are common.*

1. Diaphyseal Fractures (ICD-9:813.20)

Fracture of the shaft of the femur usually occurs as a result of severe trauma. Indirect force, especially torsional stress, is likely to cause spiral fractures that extend proximally or, more commonly, distally into the metaphyseal regions. Most are closed fractures; open fracture is often the result of compounding from within.

▶ Clinical Findings

Extensive soft-tissue injury, bleeding, and shock are commonly present with diaphyseal fractures. The most significant features are severe pain in the thigh and deformity of the lower extremity. Hemorrhagic shock may be present, as multiple units of blood may be lost into the thigh, though only moderate swelling may be apparent. Careful radiographic examination in at least two planes is necessary to determine the exact site and configuration of the fracture pattern. The hip and knee should be examined and radiographs obtained to rule out associated injury. Concomitant ipsilateral femoral neck fractures may occur up to 9% of patients and must be suspected and evaluated as ipsilateral ligamentous and meniscal injury of the knee.

Injuries to the sciatic nerve and the superficial femoral artery and vein are uncommon but must be recognized promptly. Hemorrhagic shock and secondary anemia are the most important early complications. Later complications include those of prolonged recumbency, joint stiffness, malunion, nonunion, leg-length discrepancy, and infection.

▶ Classification

Classically, the fracture is described according to its location, pattern, and comminution. Winquist has proposed a comminution classification that is now widely used.

Type 1: Minimal or no comminution at the fracture site, stable after intramedullary nailing

Type 2: Fracture with comminution leaving at least 50% of the circumference of the two major fragments intact

Type 3: Fracture with comminution of 50–100% of the circumference of the major fragments; nonlocked intramedullary nails do not afford stable fixation

Type 4: Fracture with completely comminuted segmental pattern with no intrinsic stability

▶ Treatment

Treatment depends on the age and medical status of the patient as well as the site and configuration of the fracture.

A. Closed Treatment

This remains a treatment option for some skeletally immature patients. Depending on the age of the pediatric patient and the amount of initial displacement at the fracture site, treatment may consist of immediate immobilization in a hip spica cast. In the adult, closed treatment of femoral shaft fractures is rarely indicated. Malalignment and joint stiffness are frequent. Other rare complications are pressure sores due to prolonged recumbency and DVT.

B. Operative Treatment

Reamed, locked, antegrade intramedullary nailing through the piriformis fossa is the gold standard for the treatment for most of the cases. Intramedullary fixation of femoral shaft fractures allows early mobilization of the patient (within 24–48 hours if the fracture fixation is stable), which is of particular benefit to the polytraumatized patient; more anatomic alignment; improved knee and hip function by decreasing the time spent in traction; and a marked decrease in the cost of hospitalization.

Although open nailing procedures have been described, intramedullary fixation is routinely performed closed. Utilization of the novel fluted reamer designs and use of sharp reamers help to avoid thermal necrosis and excessive fat embolization. Despite the theoretic damaging effect of reaming on the fracture healing, reaming allows use of a larger diameter and stronger implant, improves rotational control, and has been shown to reduce the rate of nonunion.

Closed nailing decreases the chance of infection by decreasing the amount of soft-tissue dissection necessary. In most cases, static interlocking should be used to provide rotational control and to prevent shortening of the bone at the fracture site. Dynamic interlocking screws are used at only one end of the nail, and this allows axial compression at the fracture site. Reamed interlocked nailing is recommended for most grade 1, 2, and 3a open fractures. Temporary bony stability may be achieved with external fixation devices when there is extensive soft-tissue loss associated, as in grade 3b and 3c open fractures.

Because of technical problems (eg, choice of a rod length) during the surgery, complications like malalignment or shortening may occur. Nonunions are rare, and one should always suspect deep infections if considered. Infections, leg-length discrepancy, and heterotrophic ossification are other complications after this procedure. The rod may be removed after healing is complete, usually at 12–16 months. Retrograde nailing may be beneficial in some multiply injured trauma patients and morbidly obese and pregnant patients.

Flexible intramedullary rods of the Ender type do not provide sufficient stability in the adult; however, they are routinely used in the pediatric population. Plates and screws require significant soft-tissue dissection and opening of the fracture hematoma and are usually reserved for special cases such as ipsilateral femoral neck and diaphyseal fractures. External fixation remains indicated in some open fractures. In polytrauma patients, initial external fixation may be indicated when early intramedullary nailing (first 24 hours after trauma) might be potentially hazardous due to hemodynamic instability or head or chest trauma. It has also recently gained acceptance as treatment for closed femoral shaft fractures in children to allow earlier mobilization and decreased hospital stays. The distal fragment pins should always be inserted with the knee in flexion to avoid quadriceps tenodesis that will prevent knee flexion. Superficial pin tract infection is common but rarely involves the bone.

2. Subtrochanteric Fractures (ICD-9:822.22)

- *Between lesser trochanter and a point 5 cm distal to the lesser trochanter.*
- *Frequent site of pathologic fracture.*

Subtrochanteric fractures occur below the level of the lesser trochanter and are usually the result of high-energy trauma in young to middle-aged adults. They are often comminuted, with distal or proximal extension toward the greater trochanter. The patient usually presents with a swollen painful proximal thigh with or without shortening or malrotation. If the lesser trochanter is intact, the proximal fragment will tend to displace in flexion, external rotation, and abduction because of the unopposed pull of the iliopsoas and abductor muscles.

Recent reports suggest there may be a correlation between bisphosphonate use and low-energy subtrochanteric fractures that radiographically present atypically as transverse or slightly oblique, with medial beaking and marked thickening of the lateral cortex. These fractures typically heal late and necessitate surgical intervention.

The Russell and Taylor classification (Figure 2–18) is a treatment-based classification system that incorporates involvement of the piriformis fossa. Type Ia Russell-Taylor fractures do not involve the piriformis fossa, with the lesser trochanter attached to the proximal fragment. These fractures may be treated with a first-generation intramedullary nail. Type Ib fractures do not involve the piriformis fossa; however, the lesser trochanter is detached from the proximal fragment. These fractures require a second-generation nail, with screw fixation into the head and neck. Type II fractures have fracture extension into the piriformis fossa and are best treated with a sliding hip screw or fixed angle plate.

In the vast majority of cases, internal fixation (by closed or open methods) is now widely favored. Temporary skeletal traction will maintain femoral length until the definitive surgical procedure can be performed. A variety of devices are available.

Fixation can be obtained with first-generation intramedullary nails, "gamma nails," intramedullary hip screws, or a variety of cephalomedullary nails or blades and long side plates based on the fracture pattern.

Postoperative activity depends on the adequacy of internal fixation. If fixation is solid, an agile cooperative patient can be out of bed within a few days after surgery and ambulating on crutches with toe-touch weight bearing on the affected side. The fracture is usually healed at 3–4 months, but delayed union and nonunion are not uncommon. Hardware failure is not uncommon. Repeat internal fixation with autogenous bone grafting is then the treatment of choice.

Black DM, Kelly MP, Genant HK, et al: Bisphosphonates and fractures of the subtrochanteric or diaphyseal femur. *N Engl J Med* 2010;362:1761. [PMID: 20335571]

Brumback RJ, Virkus WW: Intramedullary nailing of the femur: reamed versus nonreamed. *J Am Acad Orthop Surg* 2000;8:83. [PMID: 10799093]

Das De S, Setiobudi T, Shen L, Das De S: A rational approach to management of alendronate-related subtrochanteric fractures. *J Bone Joint Surg Br* 2010;92-B:679. [PMID: 20436006]

Dora C, Leunig M, Beck M, et al: Entry point soft tissue damage in antegrade femoral nailing: a cadaver study. *J Orthop Trauma* 2001;15:488. [PMID: 11602831]

Giannoudis PV, MacDonald DA, Matthews SJ, et al: Nonunion of the femoral diaphysis. *J Bone Joint Surg Br* 2000;82-B:655. [PMID: 10963160]

Herscovici D, Ricci WM, McAndrews P, et al: Treatment of femoral shaft fracture using unreamed interlocked nails. *J Orthop Trauma* 2000;14:10. [PMID: 10630796]

Nowotarski PJ, Turen CH, Brumback RJ, et al: Conversion of external fixation to intramedullary nailing for fractures of the shaft of the femur in multiply injured patients. *J Bone Joint Surg Am* 2000;82-A:2000. [PMID: 1085909]

Ostrum RF, Agarwal A, Lakatos R, et al: Prospective comparison of retrograde and antegrade femoral intramedullary nailing. *J Orthop Trauma* 2000;14:496. [PMID: 11083612]

Patton JT, Cook RE, Adams CI, et al: Late fracture of the hip after reamed intramedullary nailing of the femur. *J Bone Joint Surg Br* 2000;82-B:967. [PMID: 11041583]

Ricci WM, Bellabarba C, Lewis R, et al: Angular malalignment after intramedullary nailing of femoral shaft fractures. *J Orthop Trauma* 2001;15:90. [PMID: 11232660]

Ricci WM, Bellabarba C, Evanoff B, et al: Retrograde versus antegrade nailing of femoral shaft fractures. *J Orthop Trauma* 2001;15:161. [PMID: 11265005]

Scalea TM, Boswell SA, Scott JD, Mitchell KA, Kramer ME, Pollak AN: External fixation as a bridge to intramedullary nailing for patients with multiple injuries and with femur fractures: damage control orthopedics. *J Orthop Trauma* 2004;18(8 Suppl):S2. [PMID: 15472561]

Shepherd LE, Shean CJ, Gelalis ID, et al: Prospective randomized study of reamed versus undreamed femoral intramedullary nailing: an assessment of procedures. *J Orthop Trauma* 2001;15:28. [PMID: 11147684]

Tornetta P, Tiburzi D: Antegrade or retrograde reamed femoral nailing. *J Bone Joint Surg Br* 2000;82-B:652. [PMID: 10963159]

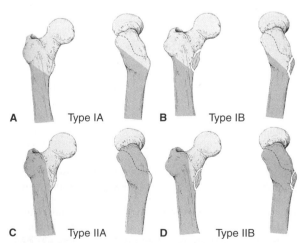

▲ Figure 2–18. Russell and Taylor classification of subtrochanteric femur fractures. (Reproduced, with permission, from Browner BD, Levine A, Jupiter J, et al, eds: *Skeletal Trauma,* 2nd ed. New York: WB Saunders; 1998.)

A   Type IA   **B**   Type IB

C   Type IIA   **D**   Type IIB

Tornetta P, Tiburzi D: Reamed versus nonreamed antero-grade femoral nailing. *J Orthop Trauma* 2000;14:15. [PMID: 10630797]

Tornetta P 3rd, Kain MS, Creevy WR: Diagnosis of femoral neck fractures in patients with a femoral shaft fracture. Improvement with a standard protocol. *J Bone Joint Surg Am* 2007;89:39. [PMID: 17200308]

PATELLAR INJURIES

- *Largest sesamoid bone in the body.*
- *Straight leg test is mandatory to assess extensor mechanism.*
- *Severe hemarthrosis is common.*

1. Transverse Patellar Fracture (ICD-9:822.0)

Transverse fractures of the patella (Figure 2–19) are the result of an indirect force, usually with the knee in flexion.

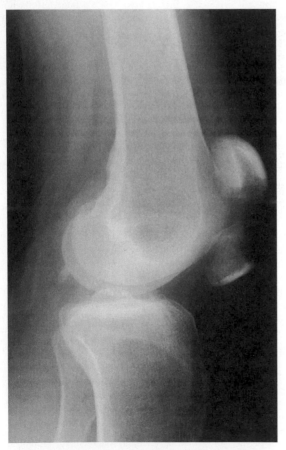

▲ **Figure 2–19.** Transverse fracture of the patella. (Reprinted from Canale ST, ed: *Campbells Operative Orthopaedics*, 9th ed. Vol. 3. Copyright 1998, Mosby, with permission from Elsevier.)

Fracture may be caused by sudden voluntary contraction of the quadriceps muscle or sudden forced flexion of the leg with the quadriceps contracted. The level of fracture is commonly in the middle. Associated tearing of the patellar retinacula depends on the force of the initiating injury. The activity of the quadriceps muscle causes upward displacement of the proximal fragment, the magnitude of which depends on the extent of the retinacular tear.

▶ Clinical Findings

Swelling of the anterior knee region is caused by hemarthrosis and hemorrhage into the soft tissues overlying the joint. If displacement is present, the defect in the patella can be palpated, and active extension of the knee is lost. A straight leg raise may be preserved if the retinaculum is intact.

▶ Treatment

Nondisplaced fractures can be treated with a walking cylinder cast or brace for 6–8 weeks followed by knee rehabilitation. Open reduction is indicated if the fragments are displaced more than 3 mm or if articular step-off is more than 2 mm. The fragments must be accurately repositioned to prevent early posttraumatic arthritis of the patellofemoral joint. If the minor fragment is small (no more than 1 cm in length) or severely comminuted, it may be excised and the quadriceps or patellar tendon (depending on which pole of the patella is involved) sutured directly to the major fragment. Whenever possible, internal fixation of anatomically reduced fragments should be done, allowing early motion of the knee joint. This is best achieved by figure-of-8 tension banding over two longitudinal parallel K-wires or cannulated screws. Accurate reduction of the articular surface must be confirmed by lateral radiographs taken intraoperatively.

2. Comminuted Patellar Fracture (ICD-9:822.0)

Comminuted fractures of the patella are usually caused by a direct force. Severe injury may cause extensive destruction of the articular surface of both the patella and the opposing femur.

If comminution is not severe and displacement is insignificant, immobilization for 8 weeks in a cylinder extending from the groin to the supramalleolar region is sufficient.

Severe comminution can often be treated with ORIF with addition of a cerclage wire, but on rare occasions, excision of the patella with repair of the defect by imbrication of the quadriceps expansion is the only viable alternative. Excision of the patella can result in decreased strength, pain in the knee, and general restriction of activity. No matter what the treatment, high-energy injuries are frequently complicated by chondromalacia patella and patellofemoral arthritis.

3. Patellar Dislocation (ICD-9:836.3)

Acute traumatic dislocation of the patella should be differentiated from episodic recurrent dislocation, because the latter condition is likely to be associated with occult organic lesions. When dislocation of the patella occurs alone, it may be caused by a direct force or activity of the quadriceps, and the direction of dislocation of the patella is almost always lateral. Spontaneous reduction is apt to occur if the knee joint is extended. If so, the clinical findings may consist merely of hemarthrosis and localized tenderness over the medial patellar retinaculum. Gross instability of the patella, which can be demonstrated by physical examination, indicates that injury to the soft tissues of the medial aspect of the knee has been extensive. Balcarek et al found that 98.6% of the patients who had lateral patella dislocations also had medial patellofemoral ligament injuries, with a complete tear in 51.4% of cases and injuries most frequently localized at the femoral attachment site.

Reduction is maintained in a brace or cylinder cast with the knee in extension for 2–3 weeks. Isometric quadriceps exercises are encouraged. Physical therapy should be initiated to maximize the strength of the vastus medialis. Dynamic bracing may be helpful. Recurrent episodes require operative repair for effective treatment.

4. Tear of the Quadriceps Tendon (ICD-9:727.65)

Tear of the quadriceps tendon occurs most often in patients over the age of 40. Apparent tears that represent avulsions from the patella occur in patients with renal osteodystrophy or hyperparathyroidism. Preexisting attritional disease of the tendon is apt to be present, and the causative injury may be minor.

Swelling is caused by hemarthrosis and extravasation of blood into the soft tissues. The patient is unable to extend the knee completely. Radiographs may show a bony avulsion from the superior pole of the patella if a small flake of bone is avulsed from the superior pole of the patella.

Operative repair is recommended for complete tear. Postoperative immobilization should be encouraged in a walking cylinder cast or brace for 6 weeks, at which time knee mobilization is started.

5. Tear of the Patellar Tendon (ICD-9:727.66)

The same mechanism that causes tears of the quadriceps tendon, transverse fracture of the patella, or avulsion of the tibial tuberosity may also cause the patellar ligament to tear. The characteristic finding is proximal displacement of the patella. A bony avulsion may be present adjacent to the lower pole of the patella if the tear takes place in the proximal patellar tendon.

Operative treatment is necessary for a complete tear. The ligament is resutured to the patella, and any tear in the quadriceps mechanism is repaired. The extremity should be immobilized for 6–8 weeks in a cylinder cast extending from the groin to the supramalleolar region. Guarded exercises may then be started.

Balcarek P, Ammon J, Frosch S, et al: Magnetic resonance imaging characteristics of the medial patellofemoral ligament lesion in acute lateral patellar dislocations considering trochlear dysplasia, patella alta, and tibial tuberosity-trochlear groove distance. *Arthroscopy* 2010;26:926. [PMID: 20620792]

Jutson JJ, Zych GA: Treatment of comminuted intraarticular distal femur fractures with limited internal and external tensioned wire fixation. *J Orthop Trauma* 2000;14:405. [PMID: 1100141])

Meyer RW, Plaxton NA, Postak PD, et al: Mechanical comparison of a distal femoral side plate and a retrograde intramedullary nail. *J Orthop Trauma* 2000;14:398. [PMID: 11001413]

Stahelin T, Hardegger F, Ward JC: Supracondylar osteotomy of the femur with use of compression. *J Bone Joint Surg* 2000; 82-A:712. [PMID: 10819282]

Woo SL, Vogrin TM, Abramowitch SD: Healing and repair of ligament injuries in the knee. *J Am Acad Orthop Surg* 2000;8:364. [PMID: 11104400]

DISTAL FEMUR FRACTURES (ICD-9:821.23)

- *Account for 7% of all femur fractures.*
- *Important to distinguish between supracondylar and articular fractures.*
- *Increasingly seen as periprosthetic fractures.*

These fractures involve the distal 10–15 cm of the femur and are usually seen as low-energy fractures in the elderly and high-energy fractures in young patients. The distal fragment is usually rotated into extension from traction by the gastrocnemius muscle. The distal end of the proximal fragment is apt to perforate the overlying quadriceps and may penetrate the suprapatellar pouch, causing hemarthrosis. The distal fragment may impinge on the popliteal neurovascular bundle, and an immediate thorough neurovascular examination is mandatory. Absence or marked decrease of pedal pulsations is an indication for immediate reduction. If this fails to restore adequate circulation, an arteriogram should be obtained immediately and the vascular lesion repaired as indicated. Injuries to the tibial or peroneal nerves are less frequent. Treatment should be aimed at restoring the mechanical axis, anatomic reduction of the articular surface, and early knee range of motion.

A temporary spanning external fixation can be used to stabilize the fracture in polytrauma patients. Two pins can be rapidly allocated in the femoral shaft and two additional pins in the tibial shaft. ORIF can be safely done in the first 2 weeks when the patient has been hemodynamically stabilized without increasing the risk of infection, provided that no infection at the pin sites has occurred. Complex trauma of the knee encompasses a distal supra- or intercondylar femoral fracture combined with a proximal tibial fracture (floating knee); a supra- or intercondylar femoral fracture with a second- or third-degree closed or open injury; or a complete knee dislocation and possible associated neurovascular injuries. Because of the complexity of injury and multidisciplinary team approach, this subset of patients is better treated in level 1 trauma centers.

Most extraarticular fractures are best treated with internal fixation: fixed-angle plates, locking plates using minimally invasive percutaneous plate osteosynthesis (MIPPO) techniques, or retrograde intramedullary nailing. Skeletal traction treatment is reserved for patients for whom surgery is contraindicated.

As for any intraarticular fracture, maximal functional recovery of the knee joint requires anatomic reduction of the articular components and restitution of the mechanical axis. Closed reduction of displaced fragments is almost never successful. Displaced intraarticular fractures usually require ORIF with a variety of methods including dynamic compression screws, AO buttress plating, and less invasive stabilization system (LISS), with or without MIPPO.

According to the configuration of the articular fragments, displaced T- or Y-type fractures of the distal femoral epiphysis are best treated by open reduction. Even if the fracture heals in anatomic position, joint stiffness, pain, and posttraumatic arthritis are not uncommon outcomes.

Isolated fractures of the lateral or medial femoral condyles are rare and usually associated with ligament injury. They usually result from varus or valgus stress to the knee joint. Fractures of the posterior portion of one or the other condyle in the frontal plane can also be seen (Hoffa fracture).

ORIF is usually indicated and requires anteroposterior lag screws. Associated ligamentous ruptures are repaired as needed. If fixation is solid, postoperative immobilization is kept at a minimum, and the patient can start moving the knee joint early. Weight bearing is usually allowed at 3 months when clinical and radiologic evidence of bone healing is present.

INJURIES AROUND THE KNEE

▶ Anatomy and Biomechanical Principles

The knee is a modified synovial hinge joint formed by three bones: the distal femur, the proximal tibia, and the patella. It is often divided into three compartments: medial, lateral, and patellofemoral.

The distal femoral diaphysis broadens into two curved condyles at the metaphyseal junction. Each condyle is convex and articulates distally with its corresponding tibial plateau. Their articular surfaces join anteriorly to articulate with the patella. Posteriorly, they remain separate to form

the intercondylar notch. The lateral condyle is wider in the sagittal plane (preventing lateral patella displacement) and extends further proximally. The medial condyle is narrower but extends further distally. This difference in length of both condyles allows for the distance between both knees, when weight bearing, to be smaller than the distance between both hips. Both condylar surfaces form a horizontal plane parallel to the ground and create an anatomic angle (physiologic valgus position) of 5–7 degrees with the femoral shaft. Normally, the centers of the hip, knee, and ankle joints are all aligned to form a mechanical angle of 0 degrees. The supracondylar area of the femur is defined as the distal 9 cm. Fractures proximal to this are considered femoral shaft fractures and carry a different prognosis.

As for the distal femur, the proximal tibia widens proximally at the diaphyseal-metaphyseal junction to form the medial and lateral tibial plateaus (condyles). There is a 7- to 10-degree slope from anterior to posterior of the tibial plateaus. The tibial eminence, with its medial and lateral spines, separates both compartments and is the attachment for the cruciate ligaments and the menisci. Distal to the joint itself, the tibia has two prominences: the tibial tubercle anteriorly, where the patellar tendon attaches, and Gerdy's tubercle anterolaterally, where the iliotibial band inserts. Posterolaterally, the under surface of the tibial condyle articulates with the fibular head to form the proximal tibiofibular joint.

The patella is the biggest sesamoid bone in the body. It lies within the substance of the quadriceps tendon. The distal third of the under surface is nonarticular and provides attachment for the patellar tendon. The proximal two thirds articulates with the anterior surface of the femoral condyles and is divided into medial and lateral facets by a longitudinal ridge. The area of contact at the patellofemoral joint varies according to the degree of knee flexion. On each side of the patella are the medial and lateral retinacular expansions formed by fibers of the vastus medialis and vastus lateralis muscles. These expansions bypass the patella to insert directly on the tibia. When intact, they can allow active knee extension even in the presence of a fractured patella. The blood supply to the patella is derived from anastomosis of the genicular vessels from the distal pole proximally. Avascular necrosis of a proximal fracture fragment is not uncommon.

The main plane of motion of the knee is flexion and extension, but physiologically, internal and external rotation, abduction and adduction (varus and valgus), and anterior and posterior translations also occur. The intrinsic bony configuration of the joint affords little stability. A complex soft-tissue network provides joint stability under physiologic loading. It includes passive stabilizers, such as medial and lateral collateral ligaments, medial and lateral menisci, anterior and posterior cruciate ligaments, and joint capsule, and active stabilizers, such as the extensor mechanism, the popliteus muscle, and the hamstrings with their capsular expansions. All these soft-tissue components work together in an extremely complex and finely tuned way to prevent excessive displacement of the joint surfaces throughout the full arc of motion under physiologic loading. When abnormal stresses that exceed the soft tissues' ability to resist them are transmitted across the joint, an infinite range of injuries can occur. These may be isolated or combined, partial or complete, and may or may not be associated with bony injuries. An accurate diagnosis, although sometimes difficult, is essential before the appropriate treatment can be decided upon.

LIGAMENTOUS INJURIES

- *Associated injuries to bone, cartilage, and menisci are common.*
- *Knowledge of the mechanism of injury is of paramount importance, as certain injury patterns may be anticipated.*
- *Grade 1 and 2 medial collateral injuries can be treated conservatively.*

An efficient clinical examination is sometimes difficult, because patients guard examinations due to pain in the acute phase and these are generally young muscular athletes with a large lower extremity, but clinical examination is essential and will usually provide key diagnostic information.

Plain radiographs are of limited benefit. They will show fractures, bony avulsions at ligament attachment sites, or capsular avulsions.

MRI is now by far the imaging tool of choice for ligamentous injuries of the knee, with an accuracy rate above 95%. Diagnostic arthroscopy is now reserved for cases when MRI is inconclusive or the surgeon is fairly sure that surgical treatment of a lesion will be necessary.

1. Medial (Tibial) Collateral Ligament Injury (ICD-9:844.1)

This ligament normally resists valgus angulation at the knee joint. It is the most commonly seen isolated ligament injury and generally seen in the young athletic population. A history of abduction injury, often with an external torsional component, is usually obtained. Examination reveals tenderness over the site of the lesion and often some knee effusion. When compared with the contralateral knee, valgus stressing with the knee flexed at 20–30 degrees will show exaggerated laxity at the joint line, signaling a complete tear. The subjective gapping on the medial joint line during valgus applied force at 30 degrees of knee flexion is used for grading these injuries (Table 2–6). Stress radiographs can, on rare occasions, be useful in confirming the diagnosis.

Grade 1 and 2 sprains (incomplete) are treated with protective weight bearing in a hinged brace or cast to prevent further injury while healing progresses. Grade 3 sprains (complete) are rarely isolated. Known associated injuries, such as medial meniscus damage, anterior cruciate ligament

Table 2–6. Subjective gapping of the medial joint line during valgus applied force at 30 degrees of knee flexion.

Grade	Gapping
1	3-5 mm
2	6-10 mm
3	>10 mm

(ACL) tear, or lateral tibial plateau fractures, should be systematically ruled out. Most surgeons now favor conservative treatment of isolated grade 3 medial collateral ligament tears in a long leg hinged-knee brace for 4–6 weeks. Concomitant ACL injuries determine the success of treatment for these injuries.

2. Lateral (Fibular) Collateral Ligament Injury (ICD-9:844.0)

This ligament originates from the lateral femoral condyle and inserts on the fibular head. It is the primary static varus stabilizer of the knee joint. Isolated injuries are extremely rare. Most often, there is a combination of varying degrees of injury to the posterolateral corner (PLC), which includes the biceps tendon, posterolateral capsule, popliteus tendon, and iliotibial band. Associated ACL and posterior cruciate ligament injuries are more common than isolated injuries. Injury to the peroneal nerve can be seen. Pain and tenderness are present over the lateral aspect of the knee, usually with some intraarticular effusion. A through physical examination combined with plain x-ray and MRI is paramount for diagnosis. ACL and posterior cruciate ligament reconstructions often fail in the presence of an unrecognized fibular collateral or PLC injury. Varus stress radiographs are useful for detecting these injuries. In severe injuries, there is abnormal laxity on varus stressing at 0 and 30 degrees of flexion, compared with the other knee.

When there is an avulsion of the fibular head and this fragment is of sufficient size, internal fixation with a screw gives excellent results. Most injuries require operative treatment. Immediate repair or primary reconstruction in the acute setting gives better results than late reconstruction.

3. Anterior Cruciate Ligament Injury (ICD-9:844.2)

This ligament originates at the posteromedial aspect of the lateral femoral condyle and inserts near the medial tibial spine. Because it is composed of at least two distinct fiber bundles, part of it remains taut throughout the normal flexion-extension arc of motion. It prevents anterior translation (gliding) of the tibia under the femoral condyles. Isolated injuries are frequent, especially with hyperextension mechanism, as seen in skiers, volleyball players, or basketball players. Valgus, flexion, external rotation injury results in damage to the medial collateral ligament, medial meniscus, and ACL (the terrible triad). When the tear is complete, it most often occurs within the substance of its fibers. Rarely, bony avulsion at the femoral or tibial attachment will be seen on plain radiograms. Associated medial collateral ligament, medial meniscus, posteromedial capsule, and even posterior cruciate ligament injuries are more common.

▶ Clinical Findings

The patient usually recalls the mechanism of injury and classically feels a popping or snapping sensation in the knee. A moderate effusion usually accumulates during the first few hours. The only clinical finding in acute ACL deficiency may be a positive Lachman test, which is the anterior drawer test performed with 20–30 degrees of knee flexion. The classic drawer test, done with the knee flexed at 90 degrees and the foot resting on the table, is not as reliable. The injured knee should always be compared with the uninjured contralateral knee. In chronic ACL deficiency, secondary restraints have stretched out and other clinical signs, such as the pivot shift and the active drawer sign, become more apparent.

▶ Treatment

Despite the fact that ACL reconstruction does not prevent osteoarthritis, ACL deficiency causes knee pain, functional impairment, and an increased risk of meniscus tear and early knee osteoarthritis. Although surgical reconstruction is indicated in most instances, functionally stable knees can be managed conservatively with rehabilitation therapy and bracing. Patients who remain unacceptably unstable after conservative treatment can still benefit from delayed reconstructive surgery. When bony avulsions from the femur or tibia are present, surgical repair is indicated, as bone-to-bone healing and good long-term results have been demonstrated. Primary repair of the ligament stumps without reconstruction is likely to fail. Arthroscopically assisted reconstruction with the middle third of the patellar tendon or harvest of an autogenous hamstrings graft gives excellent results. Recently, there has been a trend to perform anatomic double-bundle repairs and single-bundle reconstruction through an anteromedial portal.

4. Posterior Cruciate Ligament Injury (ICD-9:844.2)

The posterior cruciate ligament is a broad thick ligament that extends from the lateral aspect of the medial femoral condyle posteriorly and inserts extraarticulary over the back of the tibial plateau approximately 1 cm below the joint line. It resists posterior translation (gliding) of

the tibia under the femoral condyle. It usually ruptures after a posteriorly directed force on the proximal tibia as is sometimes seen in dashboard injuries. Posterior cruciate ligament ruptures can also occur as the end stage of severe hyperextension injuries.

▶ Clinical Findings

The posterior drawer test will be positive, as will the sag test, showing posterior sagging of the tibia with the knee flexed to 90 degrees compared with the opposite side. As for the ACL, the rupture may be at the bone–ligament junction or more often in the middle substance of the ligament.

▶ Treatment

Most isolated posterior cruciate ligament tears can be treated successfully with conservative treatment with rehabilitation (ie, reducing inflammation, strengthening extensor mechanism, regaining knee motion, and gradual return to sports within 3–6 weeks). If the posterior tibial translation compared with that of the contralateral knee is over 10 mm, there is associated PLC injury and surgical treatment is recommended.

5. Meniscal Injury (ICD-9:836.0, 1, 2)

The meniscus is a fibrocartilage that allows a more congruous fit between the convex femoral condyle and the flat tibial plateau. Both medial and lateral menisci are attached peripherally and have a central free border. They are wedge-shaped and thicker at the periphery. The medial meniscus is C-shaped, and the lateral meniscus is O-shaped, with both anterior and posterior horns almost touching medially. They are vascularized only at their peripheral third. Tears involving that vascularized portion have a better repair potential. The menisci spread the load more uniformly on the underlying cartilage, thus minimizing point contact and wear. They are secondary knee stabilizers but are more important in the ligament-deficient knee.

▶ Clinical Findings

Tears can be secondary to trauma or attrition. The medial meniscus is more often involved. Symptoms include pain, swelling, a popping sensation, and occasionally locking and giving way. Examination usually reveals nonspecific medial or lateral joint-line pain, and occasionally grinding or snapping can be felt with tibial torsion and the knee flexed to 90 degrees (McMurray sign). Radiographs are of minimal value but may rule out other disorders; MRI has replaced contrast arthrography as the diagnostic tool of choice.

▶ Treatment

Initial conservative management with immobilization, bracing, protective weight bearing, and exercises can give good results. Arthroscopic evaluation and treatment are recommended for recurrent or persistent locking, recurrent effusion, or disabling pain. If the tear is large enough and in the vascularized portion, repair should be attempted. For other tears, the affected area should be removed, leaving as much as possible of the healthy meniscus. Routine total meniscectomy has been abandoned because of the high incidence of subsequent arthritis.

6. Chondral and Osteochondral Injuries (ICD-9:733.92)

The hyaline articular cartilage is avascular and has no intrinsic capability to repair superficial lacerations. Deep injuries involve the bone in the subchondral plate, and extrinsic repair occurs first with a fibrin clot replaced by granulation tissue, which is then transformed to fibrocartilage. Repetitive injury can cause abnormal motion with shearing stresses that can loosen chondral or osteochondral fragments. Compression injuries to the cartilage can lead to posttraumatic chondromalacia.

▶ Clinical Findings

Chondral injuries usually give nonspecific symptoms that mimic meniscal injury. Plain radiographs will often reveal a loose body if the osteochondral fragment is big enough. Tunnel views and patellar tangential views can be helpful in visualizing fragments. Although it can miss the delaminating injuries, superficial flap tears, and surface fibrillations, MRI is the optimal diagnostic tool for articular lesions. However, arthroscopy remains the most accurate diagnostic procedure.

▶ Treatment

Debridement, fixation of the osteochondral fragment, bone marrow stimulation, which is excision of the free fragment, debridement of the donor site, microfracture or drilling of the underlying subchondral bone to promote fibrin clot formation, mosaicplasty, and autologous chondrocyte implantation with or without using a scaffold are the most common treatment options. Selection of the treatment depends on the age of the patient, size of the defect, skeletal maturity, and presence of adequate subchondral bone. After the surgery, gaining preoperative function usually takes months depending on the extent of the articular damage.

7. Knee Dislocation (ICD-9:836.5)

Traumatic dislocation of the knee is a rare injury that often results from high-energy trauma but may occur from low-energy injuries in the elderly. It is classified according to the direction of displacement of the tibia: anterior, posterior, lateral, medial, or rotatory. Complete dislocation can occur only after extensive tearing of the supporting ligaments and soft tissues. Injury to the neighboring neurovascular bundle is common and should be looked for systematically.

▶ Treatment

Knee dislocations require prompt reduction. This is most easily accomplished in the emergency room by applying axial traction on the leg. Rarely, reduction can only be obtained under general anesthesia. The role of angiography is controversial. If pulses and ankle-brachial pressure index are normal, the limb is closely observed. Studies have shown that the isolated presence of abnormal foot pulses is not sensitive enough to detect a surgical vascular injury. Furthermore, one study demonstrated no vascular injury in any of their traumatic knee dislocations with initial normal vascular examination. Angiograms can be useful in the limb with obvious vascular injury but should not delay treatment. Any vascular injury should be repaired as soon as possible. Ischemia of more than 4 hours implies a poor prognosis for salvage of a functional limb. Prophylactic fasciotomies should be performed at the time of vascular repair to prevent compartment syndrome caused by postrevascularization edema.

Most authors now agree that surgical repair of all ligaments is indicated in relatively young (<50 years) active patients. Early reconstructions yield better results. Open dislocations, irreducible dislocations, and popliteal artery damage necessitate immediate surgical treatment.

Intensive quadriceps and hamstring rehabilitation is necessary to minimize functional loss. The need for a brace for strenuous activities may be permanent.

PROXIMAL TIBIA FRACTURES (ICD-9:823.0)

1. Tibial Plateau Fractures (ICD-9:823.00)

- *Tibia plateau represents a spectrum of intraarticular injuries with a wide variety of injury patterns.*
- *Regardless of the treatment choice, posttraumatic osteoarthritic changes are common.*

Proximal tibia plateau fractures account for 1% of all fractures. Lateral tibial plateau fractures account for 60% of plateau fractures. Like other metaphyseal fractures, impaction injury creates a void of structural bone loss. These fractures commonly result from axial loading, combined with varus and valgus force. Associated meniscal and ligamentous injuries are common. Using MRI, Gardner et al showed that 91% of patients had evidence of lateral meniscus pathology, 44% had medial tears, 57% had ACL injuries, and 68% had pathology in the posterolateral corner. A thorough neurovascular evaluation should also be recorded as high-energy fractures and fracture-dislocations can be associated with a popliteal artery injury.

▶ Classification

Many different classification systems have been proposed, none with universal acceptance. The most widely used

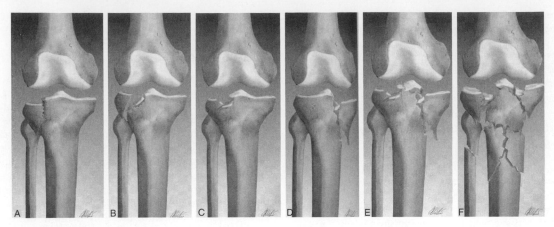

▲ **Figure 2–20.** Schatzker classification of tibial plateau fractures: **A**, type I: lateral split; **B**, type II: lateral split depression; **C**, type III: lateral depression; **D**, type IV: medial plateau; **E**, type V: bicondylar; **F**, type VI: bicondylar with separation of metaphysis from diaphysis. (Reproduced, with permission, from Rockwood CA, Green DP, Bucholz RW, et al, eds: *Fractures in Adults,* 4th ed. Philadelphia: Lippincott; 1996.)

system is the Schatzker classification: type I, split fracture of the lateral plateau; type II, split-depression of the lateral plateau; type III, depression of the lateral plateau; type IV, medial plateau fracture; type V, bicondylar fracture; and type VI, a fracture with metaphyseal-diaphyseal dissociation (Figure 2–20). Proper classification is based on quality radiographs, including oblique views if necessary. CT and three-dimensional CT have become an important adjuvant for preoperative planning and evaluating postoperative reductions. MRI is useful for the identification of associated soft-tissue injuries.

▶ Treatment

The goal of treatment is to restore the anatomic contours of the articular surface, facilitate soft-tissue healing, and prevent knee stiffness. Both closed and open treatment can achieve these goals. The choice will depend on multiple factors, including the patient's age and general medical condition, the degree of displacement and comminution of the fracture, associated local soft-tissue and bony injuries, local skin condition, residual knee stability, and fracture configuration.

Closed treatment with a functional brace is appropriate for minimally displaced fractures with stable ligaments. Varus and valgus laxity at full extension is a poor prognostic sign for closed treatment. Articular step-offs of 3 mm or less and condylar widening of 5 mm or less can be treated conservatively. Lateral or valgus tilt up to 5 degrees is well tolerated. Medial plateau fractures with any significant displacement should be surgically stabilized due to the propensity for further displacement. Bicondylar fractures with any medial displacement, valgus tilt of more than 5 degrees, or significant articular step-off should be surgically stabilized. Immediate range of motion is usually encouraged with protected weight bearing at 8–12 weeks. Noncomminuted fractures can undergo closed reduction with fluoroscopic imaging and percutaneous screw placement.

ORIF with plates and screws remains an effective operative treatment. Reduction should be as anatomically precise as possible, and fixation should be solid enough to allow early mobilization. More recently, minimally invasive plate osteosynthesis (MIPO) is being used in the treatment of these injuries. Bone defects should be grafted with autograft, allograft, or structural graft substitutes. Early range of motion is allowed according to the stability of the construct. Open surgery should only be undertaken when the soft tissues are minimally swollen; for unstable fractures, temporary external fixation with delayed definitive surgery has been shown to be safe and effective.

External monolateral or ring fixator can be used for provisional and definitive treatment depending on the clinical situation and experience of the surgical team. The proximal pin in the tibia must be no closer than 14 mm to the joint line to prevent septic arthritis. Hybrid and ring external fixators have been found to be useful for bicondylar injuries with severe soft-tissue trauma.

Bai B, Kummer FJ, Sala DA, et al: Effect of articular step-off and meniscectomy on joint alignment and contact pressures for fractures of the lateral tibial plateau. *J Orthop Trauma* 2001;15:101. [PMID: 11232647]

Bedi A, Feeley BT, Williams RJ 3rd: Management of articular cartilage defects of the knee. *J Bone Joint Surg Am* 2010;92:994. [PMID: 20360528]

Cain EL, Clancy WG: Treatment algorithm for osteochondral injuries of the knee. *Clin Sports Med* 2001;20:321. [PMID: 11398361]

Chen FS, Rokito AS, Pitman MI: Acute and chronic posterolateral rotatory instability of the knee. *J Am Acad Orthop Surg* 2000;8:97. [PMID: 1075373]

Collinge CA, Sanders RW: Percutaneous plating in the lower extremity. *J Am Acad Orthop Surg* 2000;8:211. [PMID: 10951109]

Fanelli GC, Stannard JP, Stuart MJ, et al: Management of complex knee ligament injuries. *J Bone Joint Surg Am* 2010;92:2235. [PMID: 20844167]

Gardner MJ, Yacoubian S, Geller D, et al: The incidence of soft tissue injury in operative tibial plateau fractures: a magnetic resonance imaging analysis of 103 patients. *J Orthop Trauma* 2005;19:79. [PMID: 15677922]

Geller J, Tornetta P 3rd, Tiburzi D, et al: Tension wire position for hybrid external fixation of the proximal tibia. *J Orthop Trauma* 2000;14:502. [PMID: 11083613]

Griffin LY, Agel J, Albohm MJ, et al: Noncontact anterior cruciate ligament injuries: risk factors and prevention strategies. *J Am Acad Orthop Surg* 2000;8:141. [PMID: 10874221]

Kumar A, Whittle AP: Treatment of complex (Schatzker type VI) fractures of the tibial plateau with circular wire external fixation: a retrospective case review. *J Orthop Trauma* 2000;14:339. [PMID: 10926241]

Larsson S, Bauer TW: Use of injectable calcium phosphate cement for fracture fixation: a review. *Clin Orthop Relat Res* 2002;395:23. [PMID: 11937863]

Levy BA, Dajani KA, Whelan DB, et al: Decision making in the multiligament-injured knee: an evidence-based systematic review. *Arthroscopy* 2009;25:430. [PMID: 19341932]

Lundy DW, Johnson KD: "Floating knee" injuries: ipsilateral fractures of the femur and tibia. *J Am Acad Orthop Surg* 2001;9:238. [PMID: 11476533]

Matava MJ, Ellis E, Gruber B: Surgical treatment of posterior cruciate ligament tears: an evolving technique. *J Am Acad Orthop Surg* 2009;17:435. [PMID: 19571209]

Ranawat A, Baker CL 3rd, Henry S, Harner CD: Posterolateral corner injury of the knee: evaluation and management. *J Am Acad Orthop Surg* 2008;16:506. [PMID: 18768708]

Stevens DG, Beharry R, McKee MD, et al: The long-term functional outcome of operatively treated tibial plateau fractures. *J Orthop Trauma* 2001;15:312. [PMID: 11433134]

Wijdicks CA, Griffith CJ, Johansen S, Engebretsen L, LaPrade RF: Injuries to the medial collateral ligament and associated medial structures of the knee. *J Bone Joint Surg Am* 2010;92:1266. [PMID: 20439679]

Yacoubian SV, Nevins R, Sallis J, et al: Impact of MRI on treatment plan and fracture classification of tibial plateau fractures. *J Orthop Trauma* 2002;16:632. [PMID 12368643]

▶ **Complications**

Early complications of tibia plateau fracture management include infection, DVT, compartment syndrome, loss of reduction, and hardware failure. Late complications include residual instability and posttraumatic degenerative joint disease that may require total knee replacement arthroplasty or arthrodesis.

2. Tibial Tuberosity Fracture (ICD-9:823-02)

Tibial tuberosity fractures can occur with a violent quadriceps muscle contraction causing avulsion of the tibial tuberosity. When the fracture is complete, the extensor mechanism is disrupted and active knee extension is impossible.

Although conservative treatment of a nondisplaced avulsion fracture with a cylinder cast in extension for 6–8 weeks will allow it to heal, rigid screw fixation permits earlier knee mobilization. Closed or open reduction with internal fixation is recommended for all fractures displaced by 5 mm or more.

3. Tibial Eminence (Spine) Fracture (ICD-9:823.80)

A tibial eminence fracture occurs as an isolated injury or as part of the comminution of tibial plateau fractures. The isolated type of injury occurs mostly in the pediatric population. Meniscal, capsular, or collateral ligament or osteochondral injuries are seen in up to 40% of patients.

Meyers has classified this lesion into three types. Nondisplaced type 1 can be treated nonsurgically with a cylinder cast with the knee in extension for 6 weeks. Type 2 is displaced in the anterior margin and can be treated nonsurgically if anatomic reduction is achieved with a cast. Type 3 fractures should be surgically fixed. Permanent or absorbable sutures, K-wire, or screws can be used for fixation. When associated with other fractures of the tibial plateau, the tibial eminence fragment usually keeps its attachment to the anterior cruciate ligament, and anatomic reduction with rigid fixation should be obtained.

TIBIA AND FIBULA INJURIES

- *Tibia fracture is the most common long bone fracture.*
- *Due to the subcutaneous location of the anteromedial tibia, open fractures occur in high incidence.*
- *The treating physician must be aware of the clinical signs of compartment syndrome.*

▶ **Anatomy**

The tibial diaphysis is straight and triangular in cross-section. Its anteromedial border and anterior crest are palpable throughout the entire length of the bone and are useful landmarks for closed reduction techniques and cast molding with pressure relief, as are the palpable fibular head, distal third of the fibula, medial malleolus, and patellar tendon. The distal half of the leg has more tendons and less muscle than the proximal half, and thus soft-tissue coverage and blood supply of the distal tibia are more precarious than in the proximal portion. The fibula transmits approximately one sixth of the axial load from the knee to the foot and the tibia five sixths.

From a surgical standpoint, the leg is divided into four fascial compartments. A compartment is defined by the unyielding boundaries, such as bone and fascia, enclosing a group of muscles. The anterior compartment is limited medially by the tibia, posteriorly by the interosseous membrane, laterally by the fibula, and anteriorly by the crural fascia. The anterior compartment contains the tibialis anterior, extensor hallucis longus, extensor digitorum longus, and peroneus tertius muscles, responsible for ankle and toe extension, as well as the anterior tibial artery and the deep branch of the peroneal nerve. The lateral compartment contains the peroneus brevis and longus muscles responsible for ankle flexion and foot eversion and the superficial branch of the peroneal nerve. The superficial posterior compartment contains the gastrocnemius, soleus, plantaris, and popliteus muscles and the sural nerve. The deep posterior compartment is enclosed by the tibia, the interosseous membrane, and the deep transverse fascia and contains the tibialis posterior, flexor hallucis longus, flexor digitorum longus muscles, and posterior tibial and peroneal arteries and the tibial nerve.

1. Tib-Fib Fractures (ICD-9:823.22)

Fractures of the tibial or fibular diaphysis are the result of direct or indirect trauma, with some of these injuries being open fractures. A thorough assessment of the surrounding soft tissues is mandatory. One must remember that the size of the skin wound does not necessarily correlate with the amount of underlying soft-tissue damage. A 1-cm skin laceration can be associated with an extensive muscle and periosteal injury, making the fracture a Gustilo grade III instead of I, with a much poorer prognosis. Also, closed tibia fractures can be associated with significant soft-tissue injury. In 1982, Tscherne and Oestern classified the soft-tissue injury in ascending order of severity (grades 0–3):

Grade 0: Soft-tissue damage is absent or negligible.

Grade 1: There is a superficial abrasion or contusion caused by fragment pressure from within.

Grade 2: A deep contaminated abrasion is present associated with localized skin or muscle contusion from direct trauma. Impending compartment syndrome is included in this category.

Grade 3: The skin is extensively contused or crushed, and muscular damage may be severe. Subcutaneous avulsions, compartment syndrome, and rupture of a major blood vessel associated with a closed fracture are additional criteria.

When the fracture is displaced, the clinical diagnosis is usually evident. All compartments should be palpated, and a thorough distal neurovascular examination should be recorded.

Radiographs in the AP and lateral projections are taken of the entire leg, including the knee and ankle joints. Oblique views are sometimes necessary. Fractures of the distal end of the tibia (pilon or plafond fractures) can be better visualized with CT scanning.

▶ Fibula Diaphysis Fractures (ICD-9:823.21)

Isolated fibula fractures can be associated with other injuries of the leg, such as fracture of the tibia or fracture-dislocation of the ankle joint. One should pay particular attention to the medial malleolus to rule out deltoid ligament rupture or medial malleolus fracture. Isolated fibula fracture can be the result of a direct blow; however, it can also coincide with syndesmosis disruption. If reduction of the mortise is congruent, radiographic follow-up is needed to ensure maintenance of reduction.

▶ Tibia Diaphyseal Fractures (ICD-9:823.20)

Isolated fractures of the tibial diaphysis are usually the result of torsional stress. There is a tendency for the tibia to displace into varus angulation because of an intact fibula.

Fractures of both the tibia and fibula are more unstable, and displacement can recur after reduction. The fibular fracture usually heals independently of the reduction achieved. The same does not apply to the tibia. There is some controversy as to what is an acceptable reduction of a tibial shaft fracture in the adult. The following criteria are generally accepted: apposition of 50% or more of the diameter of the bone in both AP and lateral projections, no more than 5 degrees of varus or valgus angulation, 5 degrees of angulation in the anteroposterior plane, 10 degrees of rotation, and 1 cm of shortening. It is assumed that fracture healing in an unacceptable position (ie, malunion) will affect the mechanics of the knee or ankle joint and possibly lead to premature degenerative joint disease.

Acceptable reduction can be obtained in one of many ways, and this is another area of ongoing controversy: closed versus open treatment. The goal of any treatment is to allow the fracture to heal in an acceptable position with minimal negative effect on the surrounding tissues or joints. Closed reduction is obtained under general anesthesia if necessary, and the patient is immobilized in a long leg non–weight-bearing cast. If radiographs at 2 weeks show acceptable alignment, the patient can be transitioned to a Sarmiento type fracture brace with full weight bearing.

If acceptable and stable reduction cannot be obtained by closed means, common options for surgical treatment include early definitive fixation or delayed stabilization after provisional splinting or external fixation. A reamed intramedullary nail is the recommended treatment for most displaced closed and Gustilo type I–IIIA fractures. External fixation is used as temporary fixation until soft-tissue management permits definitive nailing. Intramedullary nails are placed percutaneously under fluoroscopic control without opening the fracture site. Dynamic or static interlocking can be achieved with transfixing screws on both ends of the nail, and this maintains length and provides rotational control.

ORIF with plates and screws is rarely performed for tibial shaft fracture. MIPPO may be used as if there is distal or proximal fracture extension prohibiting nailing. This technique avoids exposure of the fracture and decreases soft-tissue dissection, devascularization of the bone, risk of infection, and delayed union.

Fracture of the Distal End of the Tibia (ICD-9:823.80, 823.82)

- *Protecting the soft-tissue envelope while restoring the artic-ular surface and the alignment of the tibia are the primary goals of the treatment.*
- *Postoperative complications are common.*

Also referred to as *pilon* or *plafond* fractures, these fractures involve the distal articular surface of the tibia at the tibiotalar joint. As for any intraarticular fracture, the goal of treatment is to restore an anatomic articular surface. This can be difficult and sometimes impossible. Closed reduction of displaced fractures is almost never successful, and external fixation spanning the injury, with or without ORIF of the fibula, can be initially performed. Once soft-tissue swelling subsides, ORIF can be safely undertaken. Bone graft can be added to metaphyseal defects to support the articular surface. When the fracture is so comminuted that internal fixation is impossible, an attempt at indirect reduction by ligamentotaxis should be done, with or without an ORIF of the fibular fracture to restore length, closed reduction, and external fixation of the tibia. This can usually restore normal contours and alignment of the distal leg and make an even-tual tibiotalar fusion easier should disabling posttraumatic arthritis occur. Primary ankle fusion is an alternative for severely comminuted fractures.

Surgical incisions through hemorrhagic blisters should be avoided. Healing is likely to be slow, and weight bearing should be carefully started only when radiologic evidence of bone healing is present. Postoperative pain, stiffness, and swelling can be seen in almost 25% of patients. Failure of healing is higher than 5% after primary procedures.

Compartment Syndrome (ICD-9:958.62)

Compartment syndrome is a frequent concern in tibia fractures and is caused by increased pressure in any of the four closed osteofascial spaces, compromising circulation and perfusion of the tissues within the involved compart-ment. Nerves and muscle tissue are particularly susceptible. Compartment syndrome can occur in crush injuries without fractures and in open fractures. The hallmark of compart-ment syndrome is severe pain out of proportion to the injury. The pain is increased with passive stretch to the leg muscles.

Fasciotomies should be performed emergently and are performed through lateral and medial incisions in the skin and fascia of all four compartments. Compartment pressure measurements may be used preoperatively but are not man-datory if the diagnosis is clear. Debridement of all necrotic tissue is imperative. The wounds are left open, possibly with a wound VAC system, and then treated by delayed primary closure or split-thickness skin grafting within 5 days. Delaying treatment of any compartment syndrome by more than 6–8 hours can lead to irreversible nerve and muscle damage.

Complications

Complications are common after tibia and fibula fractures and include infection, malunion, nonunion, muscle contrac-tions, and chronic pain.

A. Delayed Union or Nonunion

The tibia, particularly its distal third, is prone to delayed union or nonunion due to lower blood flow and muscle coverage. This occurs more frequently in high-energy, open, and segmental fractures. Pain and motion at the fracture are noted to be present more than 6 months after injury. Radiographs show the persistence of the fracture line with or without callus. Sclerosis and flaring of the bone ends char-acterize the hypertrophic nonunion, whereas osteopenia and thinning of the fragments are seen in atrophic nonunions. Early weight bearing is thought to stimulate bone healing. If nonunion develops, rigid fixation with or without bone grafting (atrophic nonunion) will be required to achieve healing. Electrical stimulation, ultrasound, and shock waves have limited efficacy but may achieve union in selected cases.

B. Malunion

Malunion may lead to premature degenerative joint disease. Corrective osteotomies may be required. When associated with shortening, multiple-plane correction and lengthening can be obtained after corticotomy and external fixation with ring-type fixation devices, which allow progressive correc-tion of the deformity.

C. Infection

Infection of the tibia following open fracture or surgical treatment remains the most severe complication, especially when associated with nonunion. Perioperative prophylactic antibiotic therapy and adequate debridement and irrigation of open fractures are not always successful in preventing this complication. Aggressive utilization of early muscle transfers to increase the local blood supply has significantly improved the overall results of treatment. However, amputation may be required and is a viable functional alternative.

D. Complex Regional Pain Syndrome (Reflex Sympathetic Dystrophy) (ICD-9:337.20)

Complex regional pain syndrome is a fortunately rare complication of unknown cause. It is characterized by pain out of proportion to the original injury. Swelling, pain, and vasomotor disturbances are the hallmarks of this syndrome.

Gradual increase in weight bearing and early joint mobilization will minimize the occurrence of this complication. Chemical or surgical sympathetic blockade may be helpful for the more severe forms of this disease.

E. Other Complications

Posttraumatic arthritis is a frequent occurrence after pilon fractures or as a complication of tibial shaft malunion. Joint stiffness and ankylosis may occur after prolonged immobilization. Soft-tissue injuries, including those of nerve, vessels, or muscles, have been discussed in the compartment syndrome section. Sequelae may include dropfoot and claw toe deformities and may require further soft-tissue or bone procedures.

Blauth M, Bastian L, Krettek C, et al: Surgical options for the treatment of severe tibial pilon fractures: a study of three techniques. *J Orthop Trauma* 2001;15:153. [PMID: 11265004]

Bozic V, Thordarson DB, Hertz J: Ankle fusion for definitive management of non-reconstructable pilon fractures. *Foot Ankle Int* 2008;29:914. [PMID: 18778670]

Finkemeier CG, Schmidt AH, Kyle RF, et al: A prospective, randomized study of intramedullary nails inserted with and without reaming for the treatment of open and closed fractures of the tibial shaft. *J Orthop Trauma* 2000;14:187. [PMID: 10791670]

Fulkerson EW, Egol KA: Timing issues in fracture management: a review of current concepts. *Bull NYU Hosp Jt Dis* 2009;67:58. [PMID: 19302059]

Gopal S, Majumder S, Batchelor AG, et al: Fix and flap: the radical orthopaedic and plastic treatment of severe open fractures of the tibia. *J Bone Joint Surg Br* 2000;82-B:959. [PMID: 11041582]

Hernigou P, Cohen D: Proximal entry for intramedullary nailing of the tibia. *J Bone Joint Surg Br* 2000;82-B:33. [PMID: 10697311]

Keating JF, Blachut PA, O'Brien PJ, et al: Reamed nailing of Gustilo grade-IIIB tibial fractures. *J Bone Joint Surg Br* 2000;82-B:1113. [PMID: 11132268]

Larsen LB, Madsen JE, Hoiness PR, Ovre S: Should insertion of intramedullary nails for tibial fractures be with or without reaming? A prospective, randomized study with 3.8 years' follow-up. *J Orthop Trauma* 2004;18:144. [PMID: 15091267]

LeBus GF, Collinge C: Vascular abnormalities as assessed with CT angiography in high-energy tibial plafond fractures. *J Orthop Trauma* 2008;22:16. [PMID: 18176160]

Lin J, Hou SM: Unreamed locked tight-fitting nailing for acute tibial fractures. *J Orthop Trauma* 2001;15:40. [PMID: 11132268]

Nassif JM, Gorczyca JT, Cole JK, et al: Effect of acute reamed versus unreamed intramedullary nailing on compartment pressure when treating closed tibial shaft fractures: a randomized prospective study. *J Orthop Trauma* 2000;14:554. [PMID: 11149501]

Tscherne H, Lobenhoffer P: A new classification of soft-tissue damage in open and closed fractures. *Unfallheilkunde* 1982;85:111. [No PMID]

Samuelson MA, McPherson EJ, Norris L: Anatomic assessment of the proper insertion site for a tibial intramedullary nail. *J Orthop Trauma* 2002;16:23. [PMID: 11782628]

Sarmiento A, Latta LL: 450 closed fractures of the distal third of the tibia treated with a functional brace. *Clin Orthop Relat Res* 2004;428:261. [PMID: 15534552]

Thordarson DB: Complications after treatment of tibial pilon fractures: prevention and management strategies. *J Am Acad Orthop Surg* 2000;8:253. [PMID: 10951114]

Vives MJ, Abidi NA, Ishikawa SN, et al: Soft tissue injuries with the use of safe corridors for transfixion wire placement during external fixation of distal tibia fractures: an anatomic study. *J Orthop Trauma* 2001;15:555. [PMID: 11733671]

Zelle BA, Bhandari M, Espiritu M, et al: Treatment of distal tibia fractures without articular involvement: a systematic review of 1125 fractures. *J Orthop Trauma* 2006;20:76. [PMID: 16424818]

Ziran BH, Darowish M, Klatt BA, Agudelo JF, Smith WR: Intramedullary nailing in open tibia fractures: a comparison of two techniques. *Int Orthop* 2004;28:235. [PMID: 15160254]

FOOT AND ANKLE INJURIES

A thorough physical examination should compare the injured extremity to the uninjured contralateral side (looking for ecchymosis, swelling, or deformity), palpating carefully all points of tenderness, stressing the different joints when indicated, and assessing the neurovascular status. Associated injuries and certain systemic disorders (particularly diabetes and peripheral vascular disease) should be identified. An appropriate radiographic evaluation is mandatory. AP and lateral views are standard. Oblique and special views are requested according to clinical suspicion. Although some fracture patterns are still best delineated by conventional tomography, CT scanning with three-dimensional rendering has recently proved to be valuable, especially for ankle and calcaneal fractures. Radionuclide imaging is helpful to identify occult injuries and stress fractures. MRI is gaining popularity and is particularly helpful in diagnosing soft-tissue damage to the tibialis posterior tendon or gastrocnemius muscle, osteochondral fractures, and avascular necrosis.

ANATOMY AND BIOMECHANICAL PRINCIPLES

The foot is a complex, highly specialized structure that permits weight bearing in a smooth, energy-conserving pattern; thus, when planning treatment of an injured foot, delicate balance between soft tissues and bones should be addressed. High-energy injuries, such as crush injuries, generally have a poorer prognosis, even if the bones are anatomically reduced. Scarring of soft tissues, particularly specialized tissues like the heel fat pad or the plantar fascia, prevents normal function and is often painful.

Embryologically, the foot develops from proximal to distal into three functional segments: the tarsus, metatarsus, and phalanges. Anatomically, it is divided into the hindfoot (talus and calcaneus), the midfoot (navicular, cuboid, and three cuneiforms), and the forefoot (five metatarsals and 14 phalanges). Besides skin, vessels, and nerves, the soft tissues include extrinsic tendons, intrinsic musculotendinous units, a complex network of capsuloligamentous structures, and some uniquely specialized tissues such as fat pads.

The bones, ligaments, and muscles of the foot actively maintain the integrity of the three arches of the foot. The two longitudinal arches aid in weight bearing and absorbing the forces during motion. The transverse arch helps with the movements of the foot. The plantar aspect of the foot is divided into four layers, each containing different muscles and tendons, from superficial to deep.

These 28 bones, 57 articulations, and extrinsic and intrinsic soft tissues work harmoniously as a unit resembling functionally a ball and socket to allow walking, running, jumping, and accommodation of irregular surfaces with a minimal expense of energy.

Restoration of the complex relationship between bone and soft-tissue structures is often challenging, but is the goal of treatment of foot injuries.

FRACTURES COMMON TO ALL PARTS OF THE FOOT

1. Stress Fractures

Also known as *fatigue* or *march* fractures, stress fractures are commonly seen in young active adults involved in vigorous and excessive exercise. These are fractures of bones due to repetitive loading rather than a single traumatic event. Fracture occurs when damage from cyclical loading of a bone overwhelms its physiologic repair capacity. A high longitudinal arch and excessive forefoot varus are intrinsic precipitating factors. Sites of fracture are most frequently the metatarsals and the calcaneus, but fatigue fractures can be found anywhere.

▶ Clinical Findings

Incipient pain of varying intensity at rest is then accentuated by walking. Swelling and point tenderness are likely to be present. Depending on the stage of progress, radiographs may be normal or may show an incomplete or complete fracture line or only extracortical callus formation that can be mistaken for osteogenic sarcoma. Radionuclide imaging, CT, and MRI can be helpful for occult fractures. CT is also helpful to differentiate incomplete and complete fractures. Persistent unprotected weight bearing may cause arrest of bone healing and even displacement of the fracture fragment.

▶ Treatment

Treatment is by protection in a short leg cast, walking boot, or a heavy stiff-soled shoe. Weight bearing is restricted until pain has subsided and restoration of bone continuity is confirmed radiographically, usually within 3–4 weeks. Because of the high risk of displacement and nonunion, early surgical management is proposed for high-risk stress fractures in the elite athlete.

2. Multiple High-Energy Injuries

Violent forces applied to the foot may cause more extensive damage than initially appreciated. High-energy fractures are often open, and the basic principles of open fracture management should be applied.

▶ Treatment

The objectives of treatment are to preserve circulation and sensation (particularly of the plantar region), maintain a plantigrade position of the foot, prevent or control infection, preserve plantar skin and fat pads, preserve gross motion of the different joints (both actively and passively), achieve bone union, and, ultimately, preserve fine motion. Fasciotomies of the severely injured foot may be necessary to avoid compartment syndromes and their serious sequelae.

Early stabilization of multiple fractures and dislocations will simplify wound management. This can be accomplished through external fixation or internal fixation with K-wires, plates, or screws. Early soft-tissue coverage with local or free flaps is also beneficial.

3. Neuropathic Joint Injuries and Fractures

Fractures and other foot disorders often present in the patient with Charcot arthropathy. Neuropathic fractures are frequently seen with diabetes. Other rare causes are tabes dorsalis, syringomyelia, peripheral nerve injury, and leprosy.

The potential for bone healing is normal if no other comorbidities exist. It has been found, however, that healing of fractures is often delayed in this patient group. Protection, rest, and elevation can result in union without deformity. ORIF is sometimes necessary. Rarely, arthrodesis is indicated; however, the rate of nonunion is higher than for normal joints.

ANKLE FRACTURES AND DISLOCATIONS

- *Among the most common injuries treated by orthopedic surgeons.*
- *Recognizing and treating syndesmotic injury are important for a successful outcome.*

▶ Anatomy and Biomechanical Principles

The ankle joint itself is limited to one plane of motion: plantarflexion and dorsiflexion in the sagittal plane. With incorporation of the motion of the subtalar joint (which allows for inversion and eversion in the coronal plane), the foot is able to move in a complex and varied arc in relationship to the leg.

The inner and distal articular surfaces of the distal tibia and fibula form the ankle mortise (a uniplanar hinge joint). The ankle mortise serves as the "roof" over the talus. The articular portions of the lateral and medial malleoli serve as constraining buttresses to allow for controlled plantarflexion and dorsiflexion in the ankle mortise. This geometric configuration resists rotation of the talus in the ankle mortise. Further constraint and stability are provided by ligaments and the soft tissue surrounding the ankle joint. The syndesmotic ligament is composed of four ligaments of which the posterior inferior tibiofibular ligament is the thickest and strongest and connects the tibia to the fibula at the level of the tibial plafond. The bony architecture of the mortise also provides some constraint to posterior subluxation of the talus. This is provided by the cup-shaped tibial plafond and the slightly increased width of the talar dome anteriorly as compared with posteriorly.

The distal tibia also serves to absorb the compressive loads and stress placed on the ankle. The internal trabecular pattern of the bone helps transmit, diffuse, and resorb the compressive forces. Cross-sectional studies have shown that reduced activity and old age lead to resorption of cancellous bone, thereby decreasing the compressive resistance of the distal tibia.

Fracture-dislocations of the ankle are frequently referred to as *bimalleolar* (fractures of the medial and lateral malleoli) or *trimalleolar* (fractures of the medial, lateral, and posterior malleoli). Fracture of the lateral malleolus with complete rupture of the deltoid ligament or fracture of the medial malleolus with complete disruption of the syndesmosis and a proximal fibular shaft fracture (Maisonneuve fracture) are also considered bimalleolar fractures on a functional basis.

▶ Classification

The purpose of any classification scheme is to provide a means to better understand the extent of injury, describe an injury, and determine a treatment plan. Presently, the two most widely used classification schemes for describing ankle fractures are the Lauge-Hansen and Weber-Danis classifications.

In 1950, Lauge-Hansen described a classification system based on mechanism of injury that described over 95% of all ankle fractures (Figure 2–21 shows a comparison of the

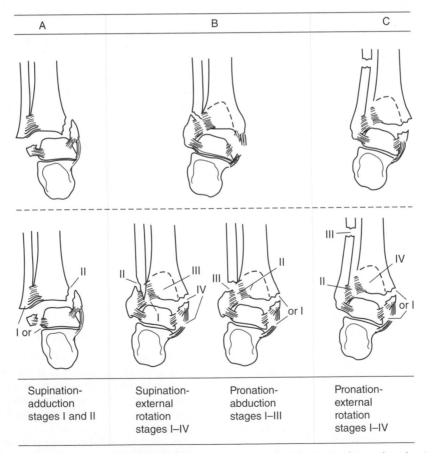

▲ **Figure 2–21.** Comparison of Lauge-Hansen and Weber-Danis ankle classifications. (Reproduced, with permission, from Browner BD, Levine A, Jupiter J, et al, eds: *Skeletal Trauma,* 2nd ed. New York: WB Saunders; 1998.)

Weber-Danis and Lauge-Hansen schemes). By stressing freshly amputated limbs in combinations of supination, pronation, adduction, abduction, and external rotation, he was able to describe nearly all fracture patterns. Pronation and supination refer to the position of the patient's foot at the instance of injury, while adduction, abduction, and external rotation refer to the vector of the force that is applied. Thus, four mechanisms of injury were described for ankle fractures: (1) supination adduction, (2) supination-external rotation, (3) pronation abduction, and (4) pronation-external rotation. Lauge-Hansen later added a fifth type of injury, the pronation dorsiflexion injury, in order to include a mechanism for tibial plafond fractures. This fifth type is caused by a compression-type axial loading injury.

The Weber-Danis classification is much simpler and is based on anatomy rather than mechanism as it relates to the level at which the fibular fracture occurs.

Type A: Fracture in which the fibula is avulsed distal to the joint line. The syndesmotic ligament is left intact, and the medial malleolus is either undamaged or is fractured in a shear-type pattern.

Type B: Spiral fracture of the fibula beginning at or near the level of the joint line and extending in a proximal-posterior direction up the shaft of the fibula. Parts of the syndesmotic ligament complex can be torn, but the large interosseous ligament is usually left intact so that no widening of the distal tibiofibular articulation occurs. Complete syndesmotic disruptions, however, can result from this fracture pattern. The medial malleolus can either be left intact or sustain a transverse avulsion fracture. If the medial malleolus is left intact, there can be a tear of the deltoid ligament. Avulsion fracture of the posterior lip of the tibia (posterior malleolus) can also occur.

Type C: Fracture of the fibula proximal to the syndesmotic ligament complex, with consequent disruption of the syndesmosis. Medial malleolar avulsion fracture or deltoid ligament rupture is also present. Posterior malleolar avulsion fracture can also occur.

The AO classification represents an alpha-numeric system based on the Weber-Danis classification.

▶ Treatment

Four criteria should be met for the optimal treatment of ankle fractures: (1) dislocations and fractures should be reduced as soon as possible; (2) all joint surfaces must be precisely restored; (3) the fracture must be held in a reduced position during the period of bony healing; and (4) joint motion should be initiated as early as possible. If these treatment goals are met, a good outcome can be expected, keeping in mind that disruption of the articular cartilage results in permanent damage.

Previous studies have demonstrated that the ankle has the thinnest articular cartilage but the highest ratio of joint congruence to articular cartilage thickness of any of the large joints. This suggests that loss in congruity of the ankle joint following fracture will be poorly tolerated and lead to post-traumatic arthritic changes. Thus, it is important to obtain anatomic reduction of the articular surfaces of the ankle after a fracture. A lateral talar shift of as little as 1 mm will decrease surface contact at the tibiotalar joint by 40%.

Initial treatment of ankle fractures should include immediate closed reduction and splinting, with the joint held in the most normal position possible to prevent neurovascular compromise of the foot. An ankle joint should never be left in a dislocated position. If the fracture is open, the patient should be given appropriate intravenous antibiotics and taken to the operating room on an urgent basis for irrigation and debridement of the wound, fracture site, and ankle joint. The fracture should also be appropriately stabilized at this time.

When performing ORIF of ankle fractures, several principles must be followed. It is important to gently handle the soft tissues about the ankle so as to minimize the risks of infection and wound-healing problems. In the treatment of bimalleolar and trimalleolar fractures, the lateral malleolus should usually be reduced and fixed first. This has two benefits: (1) it helps to correctly restore the original limb length, and (2) because of the strong ligamentous connections between the lateral malleolus and talus (anterior and posterior talofibular ligaments), initial fixation of the lateral malleolus will correctly position the talus in the mortise. When performing ORIF of the medial malleolus, it is important to remove any soft tissue or periosteum interposed in the fracture site. It is also preferable to fix the medial malleolus with either two cancellous-type lag screws or by tension banding principles to achieve interfragmentary compression.

The necessity for fixation of the posterior malleolar fragment is dependent on several factors. After the lateral and medial malleolar fractures have been internally fixed, ligamentotaxis often will anatomically reduce the posterior malleolar fragment. If this fragment represents less than 25% of the articular surface of the tibial plafond and there is less than 2 mm of displacement, internal fixation is not always required. If the fragment does not reduce on the intraoperative radiograph with ligamentotaxis, or if the fragment represents more than 25% of the articular surface, most authors agree that it should be internally fixed. Several methods have been described for this, using either direct fixation posteriorly via the posterolateral approach or by lag screw from anterior to posterior.

Following surgery, the limb is placed in a bulky sterile dressing with plaster splints from the ball of the foot to the proximal calf to allow for wound healing. The ankle is kept in neutral position to prevent equinus deformity. After the sutures are removed at 2 weeks, the surgeon must decide whether to begin early mobilization of the ankle joint. If the patient is reliable and stable fixation was achieved at the time of surgery, then early range of motion may be initiated, keeping the patient on crutches and not allowing weight bearing. If there is a question about patient reliability or stability of fixation, the limb can be placed in a short leg cast for added protection. Usually at 6 weeks, all immobilization is discontinued and weight bearing is slowly advanced. Physical therapy often helps promote ankle motion, strengthening, and regained ankle proprioception.

Brockwell J, Yeung Y, Griffith JF: Stress fractures of the foot and ankle. *Sports Med Arthrosc* 2009;17:149. [PMID: 19680111]

Egol KA, Dolan R, Koval KJ: Functional outcome of surgery for fractures of the ankle. *J Bone Joint Surg Br* 2000;82-B:246. [PMID: 10755435]

Egol KA, Pahk B, Walsh M, Tejwani NC, Davidovitch RI, Koval KJ: Outcome after unstable ankle fracture: effect of syndesmotic stabilization. *J Orthop Trauma* 2010;24:7. [PMID: 20035171]

Hess F, Sommer C: Minimally invasive plate osteosynthesis of the distal fibula with the locking compression plate: first experience of 20 cases. *J Orthop Trauma* 2011;25:110. [PMID: 21245715]

Horisberger M, Valderrabano V, Hintermann B: Posttraumatic ankle osteoarthritis after ankle-related fractures. *J Orthop Trauma* 2009;23:60. [PMID: 19104305]

Manjoo A, Sanders DW, Tieszer C, MacLeod MD: Functional and radiographic results of patients with syndesmotic screw fixation: implications for screw removal. *J Orthop Trauma* 2010;24:2. [PMID: 20035170]

Miller AN, Paul O, Boraiah S, Parker RJ, Helfet DL, Lorich DG: Functional outcomes after syndesmotic screw fixation and removal. *J Orthop Trauma* 2010;24:12. [PMID: 20035172]

Moore JA Jr, Shank JR, Morgan SJ, Smith WR: Syndesmosis fixation: a comparison of three and four cortices of screw fixation without hardware removal. *Foot Ankle Int* 2006;27:567. [PMID: 1691920]

Stark E, Tornetta P 3rd, Creevy WR: Syndesmotic instability in Weber B ankle fractures: a clinical evaluation. *J Orthop Trauma* 2007;21:643. [PMID: 17921840]

Tornetta P: Competence of the deltoid ligament in bimalleolar ankle fractures after medial malleolar fixation. *J Bone Joint Surg* 2000;82-A:843. [PMID: 10859104]

Wikerøy AK, Høiness PR, Andreassen GS, Hellund JC, Madsen JE: No difference in functional and radiographic results 8.4 years after quadricortical compared with tricortical syndesmosis fixation in ankle fractures. *J Orthop Trauma* 2010;24:17. [PMID: 20035173]

HINDFOOT FRACTURES AND DISLOCATIONS

1. Talus Fractures (ICD-9:825.21)

- *Second in frequency among all tarsal fractures after calcaneus fractures.*
- *Sixty percent of the talus is covered with articular cartilage.*

Fractures of the talus commonly occur either through the body or the neck. Talar neck fractures represent almost 50% of all talus fractures. The blood supply enters the talar neck area and is tenuous. Fractures and dislocations may disrupt this vascularization, causing delayed healing or avascular necrosis. CT is essential for exact assessment and classification of the fracture and preoperative planning for every talus fracture.

▶ Fractures of the Neck of the Talus

The most common mechanism of talar neck fracture is hyperdorsiflexion with an axial load causing impingement between the talar neck and tibia. The most widely used classification, which relies on the degree of initial dislocation and number of affected joints, has been described by Hawkins:

Type 1: Nondisplaced vertical fracture

Type 2: Displaced and dislocation or subluxation at the subtalar joint

Type 3: Displaced and dislocation or subluxation at the subtalar and tibiotalar joints

Type 4: Essentially type 3 injuries with talonavicular subluxation or dislocation (Figure 2–22)

This classification is of prognostic value for avascular necrosis of the body: 0–13% for type 1 fractures, 25–50% for type 2 fractures, 80–100% for type 3 fractures, and 100% for type 4 fractures.

Complications of talar neck fractures include infection, delayed union or nonunion, malunion, and osteoarthritis of the tibiotalar and subtalar joints.

Treatment of talar fractures is aimed at minimizing the occurrence of these complications. Type 1 fractures are best treated with a non–weight-bearing below-knee cast for 6–8 weeks until clinical and radiologic signs of healing are present.

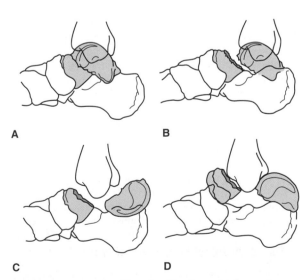

▲ **Figure 2–22.** Hawkins classification of talar neck fractures. (Reproduced, with permission, from Coughlin MJ, Mann RA, eds: *Surgery of the Foot and Ankle,* 7th ed. New York: WB Saunders; 1999.)

Closed reduction is first attempted for type 2 fractures, and if this is successful in attaining anatomic alignment, treatment is as for a type 1 fracture. In about 50% of cases, closed reduction is unsuccessful, and ORIF with K-wires, pins, or screws is indicated. Closed reduction of type 3 and 4 fractures is almost never successful; ORIF is the rule. The postoperative regimen is the same as above. Progressive weight bearing will be allowed after fracture union if there is no avascular necrosis of the body. Within 6–8 weeks, a subchondral lucency seen in the dome of the talus ("Hawkins sign") is possible only if the talar body is vascularized. The absence of the Hawkins sign, however, does not predict the occurrence of avascular necrosis in histologic and MRI-based studies.

Fractures of the Body of the Talus

Talus body fractures occur mainly due to shear and axial compression forces, and they are intraarticular and involve the surfaces of both the tibiotalar and subtalar joints.

Fractures of the body of the talus are generally categorized as follows:

Type 1: Osteochondral fracture

Type 2: Coronal, sagittal, or horizontal fracture

Type 3: Posterior process fracture

Type 4: Lateral process fracture

Type 5: Crush fracture of the body

Treatment of talar body fractures is based on restoring joint integrity of both the tibiotalar and subtalar joints. Minimally displaced fractures of the talar body are not likely to cause disability if immobilization is continued until union is restored. Associated fractures of the malleoli, talar neck, and calcaneus occur frequently. AP, mortise, lateral, and Broden (45 degrees internal oblique) views aid radiographic assessment of the injury and enable the quantification of articular surface involvement and displacement. CT is recommended in all talar body fractures to assess comminution and associated fractures.

Open anatomic reduction and internal fixation via a two-incision approach, lateral and medial, should be the choice of treatment. Fixation may also allow earlier motion. Medial malleolar osteotomy can be performed over the more comminuted side of the talar body side to allow direct access to the fracture fragments. If reduction is not anatomic, delayed healing of the fracture may follow, and posttraumatic arthritis is a likely sequela. If this occurs, arthrodesis of the ankle or subtalar joints may be necessary to relieve painful symptoms in the long term.

Osteochondral Fractures of the Talar Dome

Any chronic pain after ankle sprain should raise the suspicion of osteochondral lesions. A history of trauma may not always be present.

Initial radiograph evaluation often does not demonstrate these lesions. CT and MRI have been used successfully as imaging modalities, but they are not as sensitive and specific as arthroscopy.

Classic staging performed by Berndt and Harty is based on the appearance on the plain radiographs:

Stage 1: Localized compression

Stage 2: Incomplete separation of the fragment

Stage 3: Completely detached but nondisplaced fragment

Stage 4: Completely detached, displaced fracture

Others proposed classification systems are based on MRI, CT, and existence of a cystic component. A cyst around the lesion is accepted as a bad prognostic factor.

Symptomatic stage 1, 2, and 3 lesions are usually initially treated conservatively with immobilization and restricted weight bearing. Healing is monitored radiographically with AP and mortise views. Lesions that fail conservative treatment and all stage 4 lesions require surgical treatment. Reduction and pinning or fixation with screws and excision with or without drilling have been recommended. Arthroscopic management seems to give as good a result as arthrotomy, with fewer complications. Degenerative disease of the tibiotalar joint is a frequent long-term complication.

Subtalar Dislocation (ICD-9:837)

Subtalar dislocation, also called *peritalar* dislocation, is the simultaneous dislocation of the talocalcaneal and talonavicular joints. Inversion injuries result in medial dislocations (85%), whereas eversion injuries result in lateral dislocations (15%). Anterior and posterior dislocations are rare.

Prompt, gentle, closed reduction under sedation is usually successful. Immobilization in a non–weight-bearing short leg cast for 6 weeks is usually satisfactory. Soft-tissue interposition, particularly of the posterior tibial tendon, may prevent closed reduction. Open reduction, with or without internal fixation, is then indicated.

Total Dislocation of the Talus (Extrusion Injury)

This injury usually results from high-energy trauma, and most dislocations are open dislocations. Despite adequate prompt reduction and thorough wound debridement, the complication rate is extremely high, including persistent infection and avascular necrosis.

2. Calcaneus Fractures (ICD-9:825.0)

- *The most common tarsal fracture.*
- *Approximately 75% involve an intraarticular component.*
- *Wound dehiscence and infection are the most common postoperative complications.*

The most common mechanism of fracture is high-energy axial loading driving the talus downward. Ten percent of calcaneal fractures are associated with compression fractures of the thoracic or lumbar spine, and 5% are bilateral. Comminution and impaction are common features.

▶ Clinical Findings

A. Symptoms and Signs

Pain is usually significant but may be masked by associated injuries. Swelling, deformity, and blistering of the skin occur frequently during the first 36 hours as a result of the severe damage to surrounding soft tissues. The heel pad in particular is a highly specialized fatty structure that acts as a hydraulic cushion. Major disruptions of the heel pad lead to persistent pain and deformity and can produce poor functional results despite adequate bony healing.

B. Imaging Studies

Initial radiographs include three views: anteroposterior, lateral, and axial projection (Harris view). Disruption of Böhler's angle and the angle of Gissane can be determined from initial radiographs (Figure 2–23). Oblique and Broden views are useful to demonstrate subtalar joint incongruity. CT scanning is the diagnostic tool of choice and will further delineate fracture patterns and occult injuries.

C. Classification

Various classification systems for calcaneus fractures have been advocated. In general, calcaneus fractures can be divided into intraarticular and extraarticular fractures. Intraarticular fractures are frequently (80%) associated with worse outcomes than extraarticular fractures. Sanders has developed a classification system for intraarticular fractures based on coronal CT images (Figure 2–24). This classification has been found to be useful in both treatment and prognosis. Type I fractures are nondisplaced articular fractures. Type II fractures are two-part fractures of the posterior facet and are divided into A, B, and C based on the location of the fracture line. Type III fractures are three-part fractures with a centrally depressed fragment, also divided into A, B, and C. Type IV fractures are four-part articular fractures with extensive comminution. The

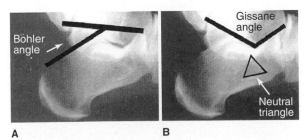

▲ **Figure 2–23.** Böhler angle (**A**) and Gissane angle (**B**), indicating normal anatomic landmarks. (Reproduced, with permission, from Coughlin MJ, Mann RA, eds: *Surgery of the Foot and Ankle,* 7th ed. New York: WB Saunders; 1999.)

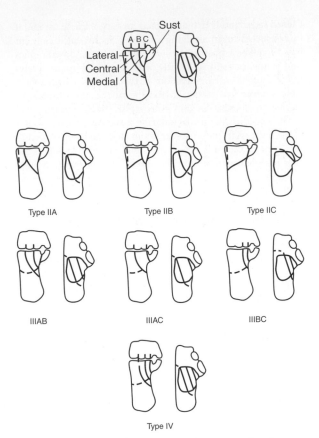

▲ **Figure 2–24.** Sanders computed tomography classification of calcaneus fractures. Sust, sustentaculum. (Reproduced, with permission, from Coughlin MJ, Mann RA, eds: *Surgery of the Foot and Ankle,* 7th ed. New York: WB Saunders; 1999.)

Essex-Lopresti classification describes the "joint depression–type" and the "tongue-type" fractures.

1. Nondisplaced fractures—These fractures (eg, Sanders type I) are successfully treated by nonoperative management with protected weight bearing for 6–8 weeks, until clinical and radiographic signs of healing are present.

2. Tongue-type fractures—This fracture pattern (Figure 2–25) splits the tuber in the axial plane and involves the subtalar joint. The pull of the achilles tendon displaces the dorsal fragment cranially.

3. Joint depression—This fracture pattern (Figure 2–26) creates a separate fragment of the posterior facet with joint incongruity.

4. Comminuted fractures—Some fracture patterns create such comminution and impaction that they defy classification. They all have in common significant soft-tissue injury and subtalar joint incongruity.

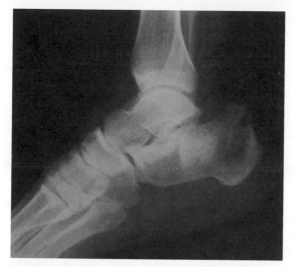

▲ **Figure 2–25.** Tongue-type fracture of the calcaneus showing involvement of the subtalar joint.

▶ Treatment

Treatment of displaced intraarticular fractures remains controversial. As already stated, the final outcome can depend on soft-tissue as well as bony healing.

Prospective large-scale studies out of Canada have revealed excellent clinical outcomes by conservative treatment even for displaced intraarticular fractures. Heavy smoking, severe peripheral vascular disease, and poorly controlled diabetes are considered to be relative contraindications for surgery. The extent of varus displacement in the axial plane (Harris heel view) appears to guide operative management more than the extent of joint depression in the posterior facet.

Some surgeons advocate early closed manipulation of displaced intraarticular fractures to at least partially restore the external anatomic configuration of the heel region. Internal fixation with percutaneous pins may be performed. This is particularly successful for noncomminuted tongue-type fracture patterns. An axial pin is inserted in the tongue fragment, which is then disimpacted and reduced. The pin is then pushed further to stabilize the fracture (Essex-Lopresti technique). ORIF with pins, screws, or plates, with or without bone grafting, has gained acceptance. The aim of ORIF is to restore Böhler's angle and improve heel alignment out of varus through stable fixation. Immediate surgery is associated with a high incidence of wound healing complications. Therefore, a 10- to 14-day delay in surgical fixation is recommended to decrease the risk of wound breakdown and infection. The "wrinkle test" should be positive prior to surgery. More recently, concerns surrounding the complications of wound healing have encouraged the use of minimally invasive approaches. Few authors advocate primary subtalar arthrodesis for severely comminuted fractures.

Fractures of the sustentaculum represent rare injuries that are usually caused by a high-energy trauma. This fracture should be suspected in patients with a history of eversion injury and pain below the medial malleolus. The injury is mainly diagnosed by CT scan. Displaced sustentaculum fractures may require surgical fixation through a medial approach.

Fractures of the anterior process are usually caused by forced inversion of the foot and must be differentiated from midtarsal and ankle sprains. The firmly attached bifurcate ligament avulses a bony flake from the anterior process. Maximal tenderness and swelling occur midway between the tip of the lateral malleolus and the base of the fifth metatarsal. A lateral oblique radiograph will demonstrate the fracture line.

Fractures of the medial process give origin to the abductor hallucis and part of the flexor digitorum brevis muscle and can be avulsed in eversion-abduction injuries.

▶ Complications

The most significant complications are postoperative wound breakdown and infection. Posttraumatic degenerative arthritis is a relatively common long-term complication requiring subtalar fusion or triple arthrodesis. The rate of wound complications after ORIF has been reported to be as high as 30–50%. Other complications include compartment syndrome, nerve entrapment syndromes (medial or lateral plantar branches and sural nerve, either from posttraumatic or postsurgical scarring), peroneal tendon injury, heel pad pain, exostosis, and malunion. Compartment syndrome is present in 10% of patients and should be excluded during the examination.

Allmacher DH, Galles KS, Marsh JL: Intra-articular calcaneal fractures treated nonoperatively and followed sequentially for 2 decades. *J Orthop Trauma* 2006;20:464. [PMID: 16891937]

Attiah M, Sanders DW, Valdivia G, et al: Comminuted talar neck fractures: a mechanical comparison of fixation techniques. *J Orthop Trauma* 2007;21:47. [PMID: 17211269]

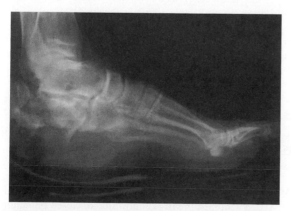

▲ **Figure 2–26.** Joint depression-type fracture of the calcaneus. The posterior facet is a separate fragment.

Benirschke S: Calcaneal fractures: to fix or not to fix. Opinion: open reduction internal fixation. *J Orthop Trauma* 2005;19:356. [PMID: 15891548]

Buckley R: Calcaneal fractures: to fix or not to fix. Opinion: nonoperative approach. *J Orthop Trauma* 2005;19:357. [PMID: 15891549]

Buckley RE: Evidence for the best treatment for displaced intraarticular calcaneal fractures. *Acta Chir Orthop Traumatol Cech* 2010;77:179. [PMID: 20619108]

Buckley RE, Tough S: Displaced intra-articular calcaneal fractures. *J Am Acad Orthop Surg* 2004;12:172. [PMID: 15161170]

Della Rocca GJ, Nork SE, Barei DP, Taitsman LA, Benirschke SK: Fractures of the sustentaculum tali: injury characteristics and surgical technique for reduction. *Foot Ankle Int* 2009;30:1037. [PMID: 19912711]

Early JS: Talus fracture management. *Foot Ankle Clin* 2008;13:635. [PMID: 19013400]

Gardner MJ, Nork SE, Barei DP, Kramer PA, Sangeorzan BJ, Benirschke SK: Secondary soft tissue compromise in tongue-type calcaneus fractures. *J Orthop Trauma* 2008;22:439. [PMID: 18670282]

Lim EV, Leung JP: Complications of intraarticular calcaneal fractures. *Clin Orthop Relat Res* 2001;391:7. [PMID: 11603691]

Longino D, Buckley RE: Bone graft in the operative treatment of displaced intraarticular calcaneal fractures: is it helpful? *J Orthop Trauma* 2001;15:280. [PMID: 11371794]

Marsh JL, Saltzman CL, Iverson M, Shapiro DS: Major open injuries of the talus. *J Orthop Trauma* 1995;9:371. [PMID: 8537838]

McGahan PJ, Pinney SJ: Current concept review: osteochondral lesions of the talus. *Foot Ankle Int* 2010;31:90. [PMID: 2006772]

Rammelt S, Zwipp H: Calcaneus fractures: facts, controversies and recent developments. *Injury* 2004;35:443. [PMID: 15081321]

Rammelt S, Zwipp H: Talar neck and body fractures. *Injury* 2009;40:120. [PMID: 18439608]

Sanders DW, Busam M, Hattwick E, Edwards JR, McAndrew MP, Johnson KD: Functional outcomes following displaced talar neck fractures. *J Orthop Trauma* 2004;18:265. [PMID: 15105747]

Swanson SA, Clare MP, Sanders RW: Management of intra-articular fractures of the calcaneus. *Foot Ankle Clin* 2008;13:659. [PMID: 19013401]

Tezval M, Dumont C, Sturmer KM: Prognostic reliability of the Hawkins sign in fractures of the talus. *J Orthop Trauma* 2007;21:538. [PMID: 17805020]

Verhagen RA, Maas M, Dijkgraaf MG, Tol JL, Krips R, van Dijk CN: Prospective study on diagnostic strategies in osteochondral lesions of the talus. Is MRI superior to helical CT? *J Bone Joint Surg Br* 2005;87:41. [PMID: 15686236]

MIDFOOT FRACTURES AND DISLOCATIONS

1. Navicular Fractures (ICD-9:825.22)

▶ Avulsion Fractures

Avulsion fractures of the tarsal navicular may occur as a result of severe midtarsal sprain and require neither reduction nor elaborate treatment. Avulsion fracture of the tuberosity near the insertion of the posterior tibialis tendon is uncommon and must be differentiated from a persistent ununited apophysis (accessory navicular) from the supernumerary sesamoid bone, or os tibiale externum. Dorsal lip avulsions also occur.

▶ Body Fractures

Body fractures occur either centrally in a horizontal plane or, more rarely, in a vertical plane. They are occasionally characterized by impaction. Noncomminuted fractures with displacement of the dorsal fragment can be reduced. Closed manipulation by strong traction on the forefoot and simultaneous digital pressure over the displaced fragment can restore normal position. If a tendency to redisplace is apparent, this can be counteracted by temporary fixation with a percutaneously inserted Kirschner wire. Non–weight-bearing immobilization in a cast or splint is required for a minimum of 6 weeks. Comminuted and impacted fractures cannot be anatomically reduced in a closed manner. Where fragments involve more than 25% of the bone, ORIF may be required to prevent dorsal subluxation of the navicular fragment. Bone graft may be used for depressed areas. Some authorities offer a pessimistic prognosis for comminuted or impacted fractures. It is their contention that even though partial reduction has been achieved, posttraumatic arthritis supervenes, and that arthrodesis of the talonavicular and naviculocuneiform joints will be ultimately necessary to relieve painful symptoms.

▶ Stress Fractures (ICD-9:733.95)

The navicular is also a frequent site of fatigue fracture in runners. CT or radionuclide imaging is often necessary to make the diagnosis. Six weeks in a non–weight-bearing short leg cast is usually required for fracture healing.

2. Cuneiform and Cuboid Bone Fractures (ICD-9:825.23, 825.24)

Because of their relatively protected position in the midtarsus, isolated fractures of the cuboid and cuneiform bones are rarely encountered. Avulsion fractures occur as a component of severe midtarsal sprains. Extensive fractures usually occur in association with other injuries of the foot and often are caused by severe crushing. A "nutcracker" fracture is a compression fracture of the cuboid and, when associated with lateral column shortening, can be treated by lateral column lengthening, ORIF, and bone grafting.

3. Midtarsal Dislocations (ICD-9:838.12)

Midtarsal dislocation through the naviculocuneiform and calcaneocuboid joints, or more proximally through the talonavicular and calcaneocuboid joints (Chopart's joint), may occur as a result of a twisting injury to the forefoot. Fractures of varying extent of adjacent bones are frequently associated.

When acute treatment is administered, closed reduction by traction on the forefoot and manipulation is generally effective. If reduction is unstable and displacement tends to recur upon release of traction, stabilization for 4 weeks by percutaneously inserted Kirschner wires is recommended.

FOREFOOT FRACTURES AND DISLOCATIONS

1. Metatarsal Fractures and Dislocations

Fracture of the metatarsals and dislocation of the tarsometatarsals are frequently caused by a direct crushing or indirect twisting injury to the forefoot. With severe trauma, circulation may be compromised from injury to the dorsalis pedis artery, which passes between the first and second metatarsals.

▶ Metatarsal Shaft Fractures (ICD-9:825.25)

Undisplaced fractures of the metatarsal shafts cause only temporary disability, unless failure of bone healing occurs. Displacement is rarely significant when the first and fifth metatarsals are not involved because they act as internal splints. These fractures can be treated with a hard-soled shoe with partial weight bearing or, if pain is marked, a short leg walking cast.

For displaced fractures of the shaft, it is of paramount importance to correct angulation in the longitudinal axis of the shaft. Residual dorsal angulation causes prominence of the metatarsal head on the plantar surface. The concentrated local pressure may produce a painful skin callus. Residual plantar angulation of the first metatarsal will transfer weight to the heads of the second and third metatarsals. After reduction of angular deformity, a cast should be well molded to the plantar surface to minimize recurrence of deformity and support the transverse and longitudinal arches. If significant angulation or intraarticular displacement persists, open or closed reduction and internal fixation should be considered.

▶ Metatarsal Neck and Head Fractures (ICD-9:825.25)

Fractures of the metatarsal "neck" are close to the head but remain extraarticular. Dorsal angulation is common and should be reduced to avoid reactive skin callus formation from pressure on the plantar skin. Intraarticular fractures of the metatarsal heads are rare. Even when they heal in a displaced position, some remodeling occurs and the functional outcome is surprisingly good. The indications for open reduction with or without internal fixation remain controversial.

Closed reduction of metatarsal fractures is best achieved by applying traction (Chinese finger traps) to the involved toes. Reduction is evaluated with intraoperative radiographs, and if judged unacceptable, ORIF with K-wires or plates and screws is indicated. Unstable reductions should also undergo percutaneous pinning under fluoroscopic imaging.

▶ Tarsometatarsal (Lisfranc) Dislocations (ICD-9:838.25)

Lisfranc injuries have traditionally been associated with high-energy trauma such as motor vehicle collisions and industrial accidents, but recently there is an increased incidence of such energy resulting from low-energy trauma such as athletic activity. These injuries are often overlooked following an athletic injury or in a polytrauma patient, so a high index of suspicion is necessary for proper diagnosis.

The base of the second metatarsal is recessed proximally to the base of the other metatarsals in a cleft between the first and third cuneiforms, thus "locking" the joint. Whereas primary stabilization is provided by bony skeleton, the strong ligamentous attachments provide substantial stability to the Lisfranc joint. The ligament structures are divided into plantar, dorsal, and interosseous components, with plantar being the strongest. The medial border of the fourth metatarsal and the cuboid should align on the 30-degree oblique view, and on the lateral view, the superior border of the metatarsal base should be aligned with the superior border of the medial cuneiform. For subtle injuries, MRI, CT, or stress x-rays may be useful.

Three commonly occurring patterns of this injury are identified: total incongruity, partial incongruity, and divergent (Figure 2–27).

With nondisplaced injuries, cast immobilization with limited weight bearing can be used. Generally a short-leg cast for 6 weeks is followed by 6 weeks in a walking cast until the pain and tenderness subside.

More than 2 mm of displacement between the first and second metatarsal bases compared with the contralateral foot is indication for operative treatment. Achieving anatomic reduction is the key to successful treatment, and if this cannot be achieved by closed means, open reduction is indicated. Reduction can be secured with screws, bioabsorbable screws, plates, or a suture endobutton, which has recently gained popularity.

Failure to diagnose the injury or malreduction may cause posttraumatic arthritis, which is the most common complication after Lisfranc injuries. Other common complications are complex regional pain syndrome, symptomatic hardware, and incomplete reduction or loss of reduction.

▶ Fracture of the Base of the Fifth Metatarsal (ICD-9:825.25)

This is the most common of all metatarsal fractures. Three distinct patterns occur: (1) avulsion fracture of a variably sized portion of the tuberosity (styloid process) that may, on rare occasions, involve the joint between the cuboid and the fifth metatarsal; (2) acute Jones fracture involving the intermetatarsal joint (located at the metaphyseal-diaphyseal junction); and (3) transverse fracture of the proximal metatarsal diaphysis.

Avulsion fractures usually occur after adduction injury to the forefoot. The peroneus brevis muscle may pull and displace the fractured fragment proximally. A hard-soled shoe, cast brace, or elastic wrapping for 3 weeks is often successful for treatment, and bony healing rarely fails to occur. Symptomatic nonunions, displacement of more than 2 mm, and more than 30% involvement of the cubometatarsal joint

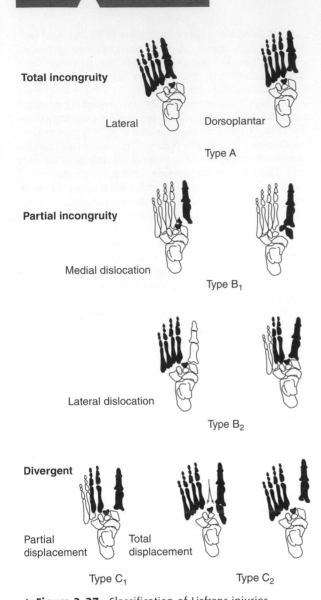

Total incongruity

Lateral   Dorsoplantar

Type A

Partial incongruity

Medial dislocation

Type B₁

Lateral dislocation

Type B₂

Divergent

Partial   Total
displacement   displacement

Type C₁   Type C₂

▲ **Figure 2–27.** Classification of Lisfranc injuries. (Reproduced, with permission, from Coughlin MJ, Mann RA, eds: *Surgery of the Foot and Ankle,* 7th ed. New York: WB Saunders; 1999.)

should be treated surgically. Symptomatic small fragments can be excised.

Acute Jones fractures are best treated in a non–weight-bearing cast for 6–8 weeks. Some authors recommend acute ORIF of Jones fractures in the high-performance athlete. Proximal diaphyseal fractures, or "chronic Jones fractures," are most probably secondary to fatigue failure. Again, conservative treatment in a non–weight-bearing short leg cast for 6 weeks will usually bring healing of the

fracture. Nonunions do occur (due to the poor inherent blood supply) and are often symptomatic. If there is no evidence of bone healing at 12 weeks, internal fixation and bone grafting are recommended. Treatment of proximal metatarsal shaft fractures is similar to that for Jones fractures.

2. Fractures and Dislocations of the Phalanges of the Toes

Fractures of the phalanges of the toes are most commonly caused by a direct force such as a crush injury. Spiral or oblique fractures of the shaft of the proximal phalanges of the lesser toes may occur as a result of an indirect twisting injury. The injury should be assessed in terms of deformity, soft-tissue injury, and neurovascular status and also radiographically.

▶ Treatment

Comminuted fracture of the proximal phalanx of the great toe, alone or in combination with fracture of the distal phalanx, is a disabling injury. Because wide displacement of fragments is not likely, correction of angulation and support by a splint usually suffice. A weight-bearing removable cast boot may be useful for relief of symptoms arising from associated soft-tissue injury. Spiral or oblique fracture of the proximal or middle phalanges of the lesser toes can be treated adequately by binding the involved toe to the adjacent uninjured toe (buddy taping). Comminuted fractures of the distal phalanx are treated as soft-tissue injuries.

Dislocation of the metatarsophalangeal joints and dislocation of the proximal interphalangeal joints usually can be reduced by closed manipulation. These dislocations are rarely isolated and usually occur in combination with other injuries to the forefoot.

3. Fracture of the Sesamoids of the Great Toe (ICD-9:825.20)

Fractures of the sesamoid bones of the great toe are rare but may occur as a result of a crushing injury. These injuries must be differentiated from a bipartite sesamoid by comparing radiographs of the contralateral uninvolved foot.

▶ Treatment

Undisplaced fractures require no treatment other than a hard-soled shoe or metatarsal bar. Displaced fractures may require immobilization in a walking boot or cast, with the toe strapped in flexion. Persistent delay of bone healing may cause disabling pain arising from arthritis of the articulation between the sesamoid and the head of the first metatarsal. If conservative modalities have been exhausted, excision of the sesamoid may be necessary; however, this should be a last resort treatment.

Brin YS, Nyska M, Kish B: Lisfranc injury repair with the TightRope device: a short-term case series. *Foot Ankle Int* 2010;31:624. [PMID: 20663431]

Chuckpaiwong B, Queen RM, Easley ME, Nunley JA: Distinguishing Jones and proximal diaphyseal fractures of the fifth metatarsal. *Clin Orthop Relat Res* 2008;466:1966. [PMID: 18363075]

DeOrio M, Erickson M, Usuelli FG, Easley M: Lisfranc injuries in sport. *Foot Ankle Clin* 2009;14:169. [PMID: 19501801]

Desmond EA, Chou LB: Current concepts review: Lisfranc injuries. *Foot Ankle Int* 2006;27:653. [PMID: 16919225]

Haapamaki V, Kiuru M, Koskinen S: Lisfranc fracture-dislocation in patients with multiple trauma: diagnosis with multidetector computed tomography. *Foot Ankle Int* 2004;25:614. [PMID: 15563381]

Porter DA, Duncan M, Meyer SJ: Fifth metatarsal Jones fracture fixation with a 4.5-mm cannulated stainless steel screw in the competitive and recreational athlete: a clinical and radiographic evaluation. *Am J Sports Med* 2005;33:726. [PMID: 1572227]

Richter M, Wippermann B, Krettek C, et al: Fractures and fracture dislocations of the midfoot: occurrence, causes and long-term results. *Foot Ankle Int* 2001;22:392. [PMID: 11428757]

Vorlat P, Achtergael W, Haentjens P: Predictors of outcome of non-displaced fractures of the base of the fifth metatarsal. *Int Orthop* 2007;31:5. [PMID: 16721621]

Zwitser EW, Breederveld RS: Fractures of the fifth metatarsal; diagnosis and treatment. *Injury* 2010;41:555. [PMID:19570536]

▶ Complex Regional Pain Syndrome (CRPS) (ICD-9:337.20)

This is defined as an abnormal reaction to injury characterized by burning pain, mechanical and thermal allodynia (pain caused by a stimulus that is normally not painful), hyperalgesia, stiffness, vasomotor changes, swelling, and osteoporosis of the affected limb. It is classified into two types depending on the presence of nerve lesion following the injury. Type 1 (formerly reflex sympathetic dystrophy) is associated with pain out of proportion to the initial injury, hyperesthesia, restricted mobility and movement disorder, skin changes (color, texture, and temperature), edema, patchy osteoporosis, and spreading symptoms to become more diffuse. Type 2 (formerly causalgia) includes the features of type 1 with an identified nerve lesion. CRPS can be precipitated by trauma, infection, myocardial infarction, stroke, surgery, and spinal cord disorders or sometimes without obvious cause. The pathophysiology is not fully understood, but damage to the nervous control of the affected part has been speculated. There is an increased incidence in people aged 40–60 years. Women are affected three times more often than men. Early diagnosis is the key to try to prevent chronic changes (muscle wasting and contractures) and can be made based on history and examination. Investigations include x-rays, bone scans, nerve conduction studies, and thermography. The cause, if identified, should be treated.

Clinically, reflex sympathetic dystrophy has three stages that are not completely distinct from one another. During the first, or early, stage, a burning or aching pain may be present and may be increased by external stimuli. Vasospasm that affects the color and temperature of the skin may also occur. The second stage generally develops at approximately 3 months. Pain is more severe, and this stage is characterized by significant edema, cold glossy skin, and joint limitations. Radiographs may reveal diffuse osteopenia. The third, or atrophic, stage is marked by progressive atrophy of skin and muscle and significant joint contractures.

Sudeck atrophy is a radiographic term that is extended to a clinical condition. Spotty rarefaction is distinguished from generalized diffuse atrophy of bone and may occur 6–8 weeks after the onset of symptoms. *Shoulder-hand syndrome* is a variation of this phenomenon that often occurs with upper extremity disorders. Stiffness is characteristic, both at the shoulder and at the wrist and hand level.

Because the cause is unclear, the recommended treatment is an aggressive program of physical therapy modalities to help with soft-tissue sensitivity; prevention or treatment of joint contractures can also be useful. Progressive loading of the extremity and progressive resistance-type exercises can also be of benefit in the appropriate setting.

FAILURE OF FRACTURE HEALING

There are many reasons why a fracture might not heal. The optimal time for healing depends on the bone in question, location of the fracture, the nature of the injury, and the quality of the soft tissues.

Generally, a fracture has united when there is radiographic evidence of bony bridging of the fracture on at least three cortices on orthogonal projections. Clinical criteria, such as absence of motion and resolution of pain at the fracture site, while helpful, are much less sensitive in confirming that a fracture has healed.

▶ Nonunion of Fracture (ICD-9:733.82)

According to the Food and Drug Administration, *delayed union* of a long bone is defined as a fracture that has not gone on to full bony union after 6 months. Delayed union is represented by evident cessation of periosteal new bone formation before union has been achieved.

Nonunion is less well defined. Clearly, a fracture that fails to show progressive evidence of healing over a 4- to 6-month period can be considered a nonunion. One can immediately declare a fracture with a 2-in bony defect, for example, a nonunion, as one knows that bony reconstitution will not occur spontaneously if this fracture is simply left immobilized.

Nonunion corresponds to scar formation in which the rate of endosteal and periosteal osteogenesis is zero or low and outweighed by bone resorption, with sclerosis of the medullary canal at the fracture surfaces. If the periosteum is active and there is no bridging despite new bone formation, the result is hypertrophic nonunion. If no new bone formation is taking place, the morphology will be atrophic.

A. Reasons for Nonunion

The two most common reasons are lack of adequate blood supply at the fracture site and inadequate stabilization of the fracture. Soft-tissue interposition at the fracture site, fractures stabilized in an unacceptable amount of distraction, metabolic abnormalities, initial displacement of fracture fragments, whether the fracture is open or closed, the patient's age, comorbidities and nutritional status, medication use (eg, steroids, anticoagulants), smoking, and infection are other variables affecting fracture healing. Infection at the fracture site does not in and of itself preclude a fracture from healing, but it can be a contributing cause to the development of nonunion. Rosen has outlined the known causes of nonunion (Table 2–7).

Certain areas of the skeleton (distal tibial diaphysis, scaphoid, subtrochanteric femoral region, and proximal diaphysis of the fifth metatarsal) are more prone to developing nonunion, even when appropriate treatment is rendered. Fracture pattern also plays a role in the development of nonunion. Segmental fractures of long bones are much more prone to nonunion, as are fractures with large "butterfly" fragments, because of devascularization of the intermediary segment.

Table 2–7. Causes of nonunion.

1. Excessive motion: inadequate immobilization
2. Diastasis of fracture fragments
   a. Soft-tissue interposition
   b. Distraction from traction or internal fixation
   c. Malposition
   d. Loss of bone
3. Compromised blood supply
   a. Damage to nutrient vessels
   b. Stripping or injury to periosteum and muscle
   c. Free fragments; severe comminution
   d. Avascularity because of internal fixation devices
4. Infection
   a. Bone death (sequestrum)
   b. Osteolysis (gap)
   c. Loosening of implants (motion)
5. General: age, nutrition, steroids, anticoagulants, radiation, burns, predisposure to nonunion
6. Distraction from traction or internal fixation

Adapted and reproduced, with permission, from Rosen H: Treatment of nonunions: general principles. In: Chapman MW, ed: *Operative Orthopedics,* 2nd ed. Philadelphia: Lippincott; 1988.

B. Classification of Nonunions

Nonunions have been classified according to their radiologic characteristics. The most widely used classification is that developed by Weber and Cech, who classified nonunion of long bones as being either hypertrophic or atrophic. They used standard radiographs and strontium isotope studies to differentiate these two categories. *Hypertrophic nonunions* have viable bone ends, whereas *atrophic nonunions* have nonviable bone ends. This differentiation has importance both in prognosis and in determining appropriate treatment. They further subdivided hypertrophic nonunions into "elephant's foot type," "horse's foot type," and oligotrophic nonunions (Figure 2–28). As a generalization, those nonunions with better blood supply and some degree of micromotion at the fracture site develop more callus, while those with no motion, excess motion, or distraction and a less rich blood supply produce less callus.

C. Complications of Nonunion

Grossly mobile hypertrophic or atrophic nonunions that are left untreated for an extended period often develop into a pseudarthrosis (false joint) (Figure 2–29). There is an actual synovial-lined capsule enveloping the bone ends. Synovial fluid is present in the cleft. As a joint now exists between the ununited bone ends, surgical intervention is the only treatment option available.

D. Treatment

The degree of shortening or deformity of the affected limb and the joints above and below the nonunion must be evaluated to determine their function and motion. One must also determine the general health of the patient as well as the degree of functional impairment the patient is actually experiencing. This is especially important because some patients are actually asymptomatic and therefore do not warrant treatment. Treatment must also be tailored in the sick or elderly (>70 years) because these patients may not be able to safely tolerate surgical intervention.

1. Stimulation of osteogenesis by external forces— It is now known that several pathways exist to stimulate healing of nonunion. The pathways can be divided into the type of force required to stimulate osteogenesis. These inductive forces can be categorized as mechanical, electrical, and chemical and can be applied with varying success both operatively and nonoperatively.

A. MECHANICAL FORCES—Cyclic mechanical force of ambulation while the fracture reduction is maintained with an external support is the presumed mechanism with which fracture healing is achieved without surgical intervention. Sarmiento has shown that the use of functional bracing incorporated with weight bearing can lead to union of documented tibial nonunions.

Mechanical forces can also be generated by surgical means. Mechanical stabilization of a long bone nonunion

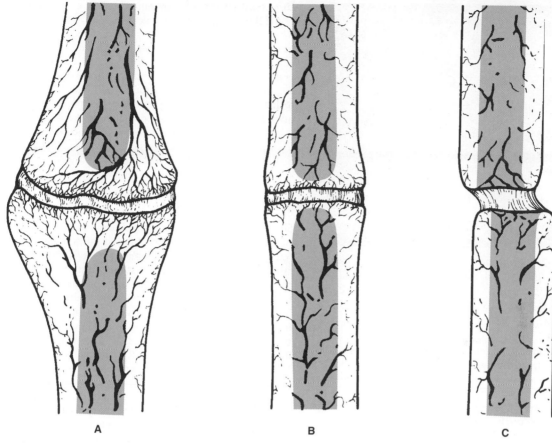

▲ **Figure 2–28.** Weber and Cech's subclassification of hypertrophic nonunions: elephant's foot (**A**); horse's foot (**B**); and oligotrophic (**C**). (This can often resemble atrophic nonunion and is hard to distinguish.) (Reprinted, with permission, from Browner BD, Levine A, Jupiter J, et al, eds: *Skeletal Trauma,* 2nd ed. New York: WB Saunders; 1998.)

can be achieved either by placement of an intramedullary rod or compression plating. The rod works by providing mechanical stabilization of the fracture, hence allowing for cyclic axial loading of the limb without shearing forces caused by weight bearing. The compression plate provides stability as well as immediate rigid compression across the fracture fragments. These forms of treatment are often all that is necessary in elephant's foot-type nonunions.

B. ELECTRICAL STIMULATION—Studies generated by Fukada and Yasuda led to the development of electrical bone growth stimulators for clinical application in the treatment of delayed union and nonunion. Electrical fields have been shown to stimulate the inactive chondrocytes and mesenchymal cells in the nonunion site to "turn on" and produce bone that results in healing. Surgically implanted devices have the disadvantage of implantation, removal, and infection, so shorter application time would be advantageous. Current opinion is to use combined magnetic fields applied over fracture sites.

c. Biologic enhancement—Chemical modulators also play an important role in promoting nonunion healing. Application of autogenous cancellous bone graft (most frequently obtained from the iliac crest) is a potent stimulator of fracture healing. Because a rigid nonunion will heal with autogenous bone grafting alone and no internal fixation, it is apparent that chemical modulators from the grafted cancellous bone are responsible for stimulating the healing response. There has been recent intense interest in determining the growth factors present in this cancellous bone responsible for "turning on" the healing process. Some surgeons have even reported success by obtaining bone marrow via a large-bore needle from the iliac crest and injecting this into the nonunion site. In the future, it is likely that the humoral modulator responsible will be isolated, synthesized in sufficient quantities by genetic engineering techniques, and simply injected into nonunion clefts to attain union.

2. Atrophic nonunions—Atrophic nonunions are not as easily treated as hypertrophic nonunions, and fewer

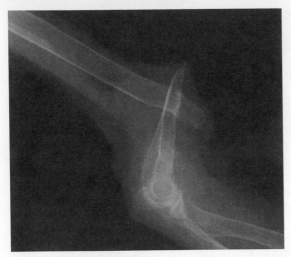

▲ **Figure 2–29.** Fourteen-year-old distal humeral pseud-arthrosis left untreated in an 89-year-old woman. All motion about the elbow is occurring through the pseud-arthrosis, as the elbow is ankylosed.

treatment options are available. Electrical stimulation and nonoperative treatment methods have not been effective. The treatment most commonly used, and most successfully, is "freshening up" of the avascular bone ends, combined with rigid internal fixation and autogenous bone grafting. This same procedure is used in treating pseudarthroses.

The Ilizarov method has also shown great success in the treatment of complex hypertrophic and atrophic nonunions, sometimes in combination with autogenous bone grafting. This method allows not only for achievement of bony union but also for treatment of any accompanying deformity, segmental bone loss, or shortening that may be present.

▶ Malunion of Fracture (ICD-9:733.81)

A fracture that has healed with an unacceptable amount of angulation, rotation, or overriding that has resulted in shortening of the limb is defined as malunion. Shortening is better tolerated in the upper than the lower extremity, and angulatory deformities are better tolerated in bones such as the humerus than in the femur or tibia. Hence, no absolute guidelines can be given as to an acceptable versus an unacceptable malunion. Generally, shortening greater than 1 in is poorly tolerated in the lower extremity. Smaller discrepancies, however, are well treated with just a shoe lift in most situations. When the degree of deformity is sufficient to cause pain (eg, caused by walking on the side of the foot secondary to varus malunion of the distal tibia) or impair normal function, surgical correction of the malunion is indicated.

When correction of malunion is undertaken, proper preoperative planning is imperative. Determination of the true plane of deformity is essential in planning for the surgical correction. One must determine the true mechanical axis of the limb to determine the actual site of deformity. If an osteotomy is performed, the surgeon must decide whether to use a closing wedge (where a wedge of bone is removed) or an opening wedge (where a wedge of autogenous or allograft bone is added). This is important, as it will alter the limb length. If the limb is already short, the surgery should also include a limb-lengthening procedure. Proper fixation and often autogenous cancellous bone grafting should be incorporated to ensure that the osteotomy heals, because converting a malunion to a nonunion is only worsening an already bad situation. Special care must be paid to treatment of the soft tissues to prevent wound breakdown and infection.

▶ Ilizarov Method

Since its introduction in Kurgan, Siberia, in 1951 by Gavril A. Ilizarov, the Ilizarov apparatus and the concepts of distraction osteogenesis have dramatically revolutionized the application of the principles of external fixation in the management of bony defects, nonunions, malunions, pseudarthroses, and osteomyelitis. Ilizarov realized that healing and neogenesis both required a dynamic state, which could occur in either controlled distraction or compression. This dogma is a function of many principles that Ilizarov classified into three categories: biologic, clinical, and technical. Important biologic concepts include preservation of endosteal and periosteal blood supply via low-energy corticotomy and stable fixation. A 5- to 7-day latency and a distraction rate of 1 mm/day in three or four divided increments follow the osteotomy. At the termination of distraction, neutral fixation is required to allow maturation, calcification, and strengthening of the new bone. In essence, the technique fools the body into believing it is a child again, with the corticotomy site acting as a physis. Ilizarov fixation prevents shearing forces but permits axial micromotion with postoperative weight bearing, which enhances bone formation. From a technical viewpoint, the Ilizarov method relies on the use of an extremely rigid (in all planes except the axial loading plane), extremely versatile external fixator, employing K-wire fixation under tension. It is this "tension stress" phenomenon of gradually controlled distraction of bone ends at the corticotomy site that makes possible the limb lengthening or osteogenesis required in bone transport. Neogenesis of the accompanying soft tissues, including vessels, nerves, muscle, and skin, also occurs. Likewise, because of the dynamic nature of the apparatus, constant high loads of compression can be maintained across fracture sites to help stimulate fracture healing. A hyperemic state exists during distraction osteogenesis, with abundant neovascularization in the distraction gap. The overall blood flow to the affected limb is also increased up to 40%.

The most important parts of circular fixators are rings and rods. Ring diameter and the distance between the rings affect the stability. Small-diameter rings are more stable; however, a general rule is to leave 2 cm of space between the ring and skin circumferentially to allow for possible limb swelling. Rings that are far apart and connected with long rods will be less stable. Ideally, four connecting rods between the rings and at least two points of fixation or wires per ring are required. Two diameters of wires are used: 1.5 mm in small children and in upper extremities in adults, and 1.8 mm (twice as stiff in bending) in lower extremities in adults and adolescents. Beaded wires (olive wires) are used for bony transport, as well as to provide for rigidity of fixation, to prevent unwanted translation of the bone on the frame. An appropriately applied frame on the lower extremity should allow full weight bearing on the limb, irrespective of the extent of the bony defect present. This cyclic axial loading of the affected limb is a crucial element of the Ilizarov method.

Clinical principles such as the geometry of the apparatus once it is constructed, adjustment of the rate of transport, and wound care directly affect the outcome of the procedure. The initial operation for the application of the apparatus is only one small part in the whole treatment scheme. The construct should be as safe and comfortable as possible because the apparatus is worn for an extended period of time. Pin tract infections are common and must be addressed aggressively with oral antibiotics and local pin care.

With the incorporation of hinges, plates, rods, and other elements, correction of a deformity can be accomplished in any plane. Hence, the apparatus has become an increasingly useful tool in the treatment of congenital, acquired, and posttraumatic limb deformities, as well as nonunion and malunion. What makes this treatment method unique is that all problems affecting a limb can be managed with the application of one apparatus.

Bhandari M, Guyatt GH, Tong D, et al: Reamed versus nonreamed intramedullary nailing of lower extremity long bone fractures: a systematic overview and meta-analysis. *J Orthop Trauma* 2000;14:2. [PMID: 10630795]

Einhorn TA, Lee CA: Bone regeneration: new findings and potential clinical applications. *J Am Acad Orthop Surg* 2001;9:157. [PMID: 11421573]

Goldstein C, Spraque S, Petrisor BA: Electrical stimulation for fracture healing: current evidence. *J Orthop Trauma* 2010; 24(Suppl 1): S62. [PMID: 20182239]

Hak DJ, Lee SS, Goulet JA: Success of exchange reamed intramedullary nailing for femoral shaft nonunion or delayed union. *J Orthop Trauma* 2000;14:178. [PMID: 10791668]

Henson P, Bruehl S: Complex regional pain syndrome: state of the art update. *Curr Treat Options Cardiovasc Med* 2010;12:156. [PMID: 20842553]

Hupel TM, Weinberg JA, Aksenov SA, Schemitsch EH: Effect of unreamed, limited reamed, and standard reamed intramedullary nailing on cortical bone porosity and new bone formation. *J Orthop Trauma* 2001;15:18. [PMID: 11147683]

Ilizarov GA: The significance of the combination of optimal mechanical and biological factors in the regenerate process of transosseous synthesis. In: Abstracts of First International Symposium on Experimental, Theoretical, and Clinical Aspects of Transosseous Osteosynthesis Method Developed in Kniekot, Kurgan, USSR, September 20–23, 1983.

Ilizarov GA: *Transosseous Osteosynthesis.* New York: Springer-Verlag; 1992.

Katsenis D, Bhave A, Paley D, et al: Treatment of malunion and nonunion at the site of an ankle fusion with the Ilizarov apparatus. *J Bone Joint Surg Am* 2005;87:302. [PMID: 15687151]

Lowenberg DW, Randall RL: The Ilizarov method. In: Braverman MH, Tawes RL, eds: *Surgical Technology International II.* San Francisco: Surgical Technology International; 1993.

Marsh D: Concepts of fracture union, delayed union, and nonunion. *Clin Orthop Relat Res* 1998;355S:S22. [PMID: 9917623]

Paley D, Maar DC: Ilizarov bone transport treatment for tibial defects. *J Orthop Trauma* 2000;14:76. [PMID: 10716377]

Spiegelberg B, Parratt T, Dheerendra SK, Khan WS, Jennings R, Marsh DR: Ilizarov principles of deformity correction. *Ann R Coll Surg Engl* 2010;92:101. [PMID: 20353638]

Weresh MJ, Hakanson R, Stover MD, et al: Failure of exchange reamed intramedullary nails for ununited femoral shaft fractures. *J Orthop Trauma* 2000;14:335. [PMID: 11029556]

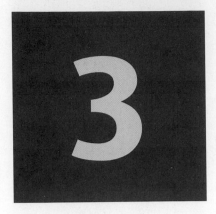

Sports Medicine

Patrick J. McMahon, MD

Lee D. Kaplan, MD

Charles A. Popkin, MD

INTRODUCTION

Sports medicine developed in the 1970s as an orthopedic specialty focusing on competitive athletes. Today, sports medicine includes the overall care of athletes from many skill levels. Increasingly, care of recreational athletes has risen to that common for professional athletes. In addition to the musculoskeletal system, care includes the cardiovascular and pulmonary systems and also focuses on training techniques, nutrition, and women's athletics. This wide range of care requires a multidisciplinary team of medical personnel, including athletic trainers, physical therapists, cardiologists, pulmonologists, orthopedic surgeons, and general practitioners.

▼ KNEE INJURIES

▶ Anatomy

The bones of the knee are the distal femur, the proximal tibia, and the patella. These bones depend on supporting ligaments, the joint capsule, and the menisci to provide stability for the joint.

A. Menisci and Joint Capsule

The menisci, or semilunar cartilages, are C-shaped fibrocartilaginous disks in the knee that provide shock absorption, allow for increased congruency between joint surfaces, enhance joint stability, and aid in distribution of synovial fluid.

The medial and lateral menisci provide a concave surface with which the convex femoral condyles can articulate. If the menisci are not present, the convex femoral condyles articulate with the relatively flat tibial plateaus, and the joint surfaces are not congruent. This decreases the surface area of contact and increases the pressure on the articular cartilage of the tibia and femur, which may lead to rapid deterioration of the joint surface. The medial meniscus is firmly attached

to the joint capsule along its entire peripheral edge. The lateral meniscus is attached to the anterior and posterior capsule, but there is a region posterolaterally where it is not firmly attached (Figure 3–1). Therefore, the medial meniscus has less mobility than the lateral meniscus and is more susceptible to tearing when trapped between the femoral condyle and tibial plateau. The lateral meniscus is larger than the medial meniscus and carries a greater share of the lateral compartment pressure than the medial meniscus carries for the medial compartment.

B. Ligaments

Within the knee, the anterior cruciate ligament (ACL) travels from the medial border of the lateral femoral condyle to its insertion site anterolateral to the medial tibial spine. This ligament prevents anterior translation and rotation of the tibia on the femur (Figure 3–2). The posterior cruciate ligament (PCL) prevents posterior subluxation of the tibia on the femur. It runs from the lateral aspect of the medial femoral condyle to the posterior aspect of the tibia, just below the joint line (Figure 3–3). On the medial side, the medial collateral ligament has superficial and deep portions (Figure 3–4), which stabilize the knee to valgus stresses. The lateral collateral or fibular collateral ligament runs from the lateral femoral condyle to the head of the fibula. It is the main stabilizer against varus stress (Figure 3–5). The lateral collateral ligament is part of the posterolateral "complex" or "corner" of the knee that also resists external rotation. An important component is the popliteofibular ligament, present in 90% of knees, that runs from the tendon of the popliteus muscle to the styloid on the posterior fibular head.

▶ History and Physical Examination

A. General Approach

The history of a knee injury may be obtained by asking the patient the questions listed in Table 3–1. The physical examination begins with observation of the patient's gait. The

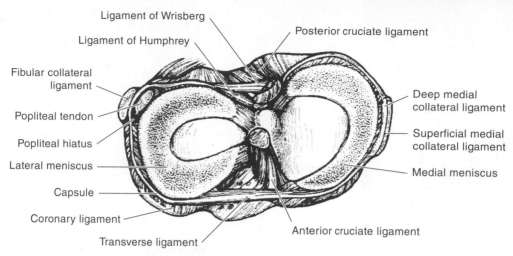

▲ **Figure 3–1.** The medial and lateral menisci with their associated intermeniscal ligaments. Note: The lateral meniscus is not attached in the region of the popliteus tendon. (Reproduced, with permission, from Scott WN: *Ligament and Extensor Mechanism Injuries of the Knee: Diagnosis and Treatment.* New York: Mosby-Year Book; 1991.)

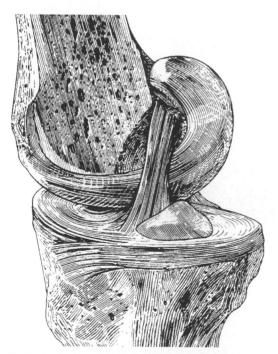

▲ **Figure 3–2.** Drawing of the anterior cruciate ligament with the knee in extension, showing the course of the ligament as it passes from the medial aspect of the lateral femoral condyle to the lateral portion of the medial tibial spine. (Reproduced, with permission, from Girgis FG, Marshall JL, Monajem A: The cruciate ligaments of the knee joint: anatomical, functional, and experimental analysis. *Clin Orthop Relat Res* 1975;106:216.)

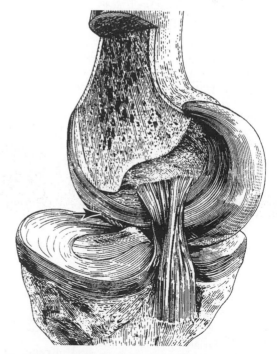

▲ **Figure 3–3.** Drawing of the posterior cruciate ligament, showing the course of the ligament as it passes from the lateral aspect of the medial femoral condyle to the posterior surface of the tibia. (Adapted, with permission, from Girgis FG, Marshall JL, Monajem A: The cruciate ligaments of the knee joint: anatomical, functional, and experimental analysis. *Clin Orthop Relat Res* 1975;106:216.)

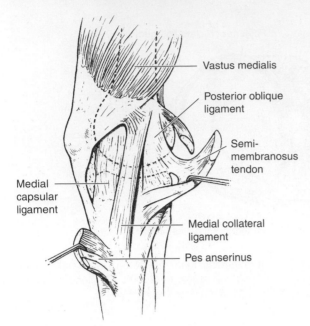

▲ Figure 3-4. Medial capsuloligamentous complex. (Reproduced, with permission, from Feagin JA Jr: *The Crucial Ligaments*. New York: Churchill Livingstone; 1988.)

uninjured knee is then examined as a basis of comparison with the injured knee. Any swelling or effusion should be noted. A small effusion will cause obliteration of the recesses on the medial and lateral aspects of the patellar tendon; with a larger effusion, diffuse swelling is present in the region of the suprapatellar pouch. Then, a fluid wave can be palpated on the sides of the patella. Active and then passive range of motion is tested carefully. The knee is palpated to define areas of localized tenderness. The joint lines are located at the level of the inferior pole of the patella when the knee is flexed to 90 degrees.

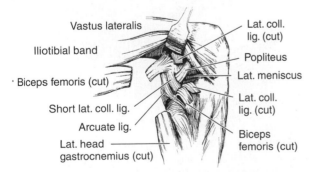

▲ Figure 3-5. The lateral supporting structures of the knee. (Reproduced, with permission, from Rockwood CA Jr, Green DP, Bucholz RW, et al: *Fractures in Adults*, 2nd ed. New York: Lippincott; 1984.)

Table 3-1. History of a knee injury.

Did an injury occur?	Yes: possible ligament tear or meniscus tear. No: overuse problem or degenerative condition.
Was it a noncontact injury?	Yes: often the ACL is the only ligament torn.
Was it a contact injury?	Yes: possible multiple ligament injuries, including ACL and MCL, ACL and LCL, ACL, PCL, and a collateral ligament.
Did the patient hear or feel a pop?	Yes: a pop often occurs with ACL tears.
How long did it take to swell up?	Within hours: often an ACL tear. Overnight: often a meniscus tear.
Does the knee lock?	Yes: often a meniscus tear flipping into and out of the joint.
Does it buckle (trick knee)?	Yes: not specific; may arise from quadriceps weakness, trapped meniscus, ligament instability, or patella dislocating.
Is climbing or descending stairs difficult?	Often patellofemoral problems.
Are cutting maneuvers difficult?	ACL tear.
Is squatting (deep knee bends) difficult?	Meniscus tear.
Is jumping difficult?	Patellar tendinitis.
Where does it hurt?	Medial joint line: medial meniscus tear or medial compartment arthritis. MCL: MCL sprain. Lateral joint line: lateral meniscus tear, injury, iliotibial band tendinitis, popliteus tendinitis.

ACL, anterior cruciate ligament; LCL, lateral collateral ligament; MCL, medial collateral ligament; PCL, posterior cruciate ligament.

B. Ligament Laxity Evaluation

To determine varus and valgus stability, the patient's foot is held between the examiner's elbow and hip. This leaves both hands free to palpate the joint (Figure 3-6). Stability should be determined at both full extension and 30 degrees of knee flexion. Grading of laxity is based on the amount of opening of the joint (grade 1, 0–5 mm; grade 2, 5–10 mm; and grade 3, 10–15 mm). Laxity in full extension to varus or valgus angulation is an ominous sign that indicates disruption of key ligamentous structures. If significant valgus laxity is present in full extension, the posteromedial capsule and medial collateral ligament are torn. With varus laxity in full extension, the posterolateral capsular complex is torn, in addition to the lateral collateral ligament. With either varus or valgus laxity

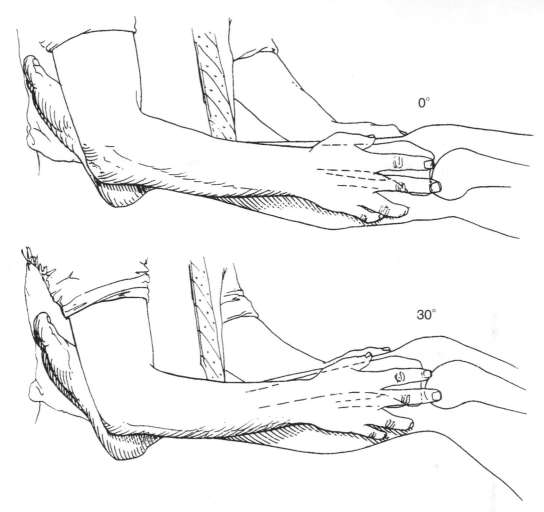

0°

30°

▲ **Figure 3–6.** The collateral ligaments being tested in extension and 30 degrees of flexion with the foot held between the examiner's elbow and hip. (Reproduced, with permission, from Feagin JA Jr: *The Crucial Ligaments.* New York: Churchill Livingstone; 1988.)

at full extension, ACL and PCL tears are likely. At 30 degrees of flexion, the posterior capsule and cruciate ligaments are relaxed and the medial and lateral collateral ligaments are isolated. Pain with varus or valgus stress is more suggestive of ligament damage than a meniscus tear.

C. Lachman Test

The Lachman test is the most sensitive test for ACL tears. It is done with the knee flexed at 20 degrees, stabilizing the distal femur with one hand and pulling forward on the proximal tibia with the other hand (Figure 3–7). With an intact ligament, minimal translation of the tibia occurs and a firm end point is felt. With a torn ACL, more translation is noted, and the end point is soft or mushy. The hamstring

muscles must be relaxed during this maneuver to prevent false-negative findings. Comparison of the injured and uninjured knees is essential.

D. Anterior Drawer Test

The anterior drawer test is done with the knee at 90 degrees of flexion and is not as sensitive as the Lachman test but serves as an adjunct in the evaluation of ACL instability (Figure 3–8). With the patient supine and the knee flexed to 90 degrees (hip flexed to about 45 degrees), the foot is restrained by sitting on it and the examiner's hands are placed around the proximal tibia. Then, while the hamstrings are felt to relax and the tibia is pulled forward, the displacement and the end point are evaluated.

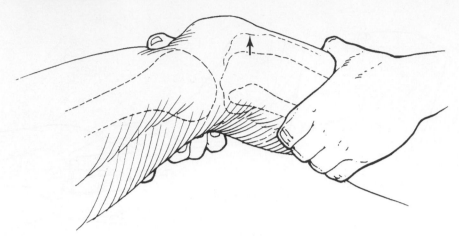

▲ **Figure 3–7.** Lachman test. (Reproduced, with permission, from Feagin JA Jr: *The Crucial Ligaments*. New York: Churchill Livingstone; 1988.)

E. Losee Test

The pivot shift phenomenon demonstrates the instability associated with an ACL tear. Once demonstrated, it is often difficult to repeat because the patient may find this maneuver uncomfortable and will guard against having it done again.

As described by Losee, a valgus and internal rotation force is applied to the tibia (Figure 3–9). Starting at 45 degrees of flexion, the lateral tibial plateau is reduced. Extending the knee causes the lateral plateau to subluxate anteriorly with a thud at about 20 degrees of flexion. It reduces quietly at full extension. Many other ways of doing this test have been described, but the phenomenon and significance of the different tests are similar.

F. Posterior Drawer Test

The posterior drawer test evaluates the integrity of the PCL. It is performed with posterior pressure on the proximal tibia with the knee flexed at 90 degrees and (Figure 3–10). Normally, the tibial plateau is anterior to the femoral condyles, and a "step-off" to the tibia is palpated when the

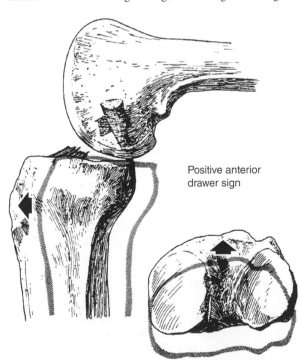

Positive anterior drawer sign

▲ **Figure 3–8.** A positive anterior drawer test signifying a tear of the anterior cruciate ligament. (Reproduced, with permission, from Insall JN: *Surgery of the Knee*. New York: Churchill Livingstone; 1984.)

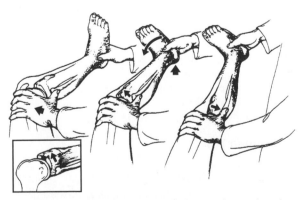

▲ **Figure 3–9.** The Losee pivot shift test. (Reproduced, with permission, from Scott WN: *Ligament and Extensor Mechanism Injuries of the Knee: Diagnosis and Treatment*. New York: Mosby-Year Book; 1991.)

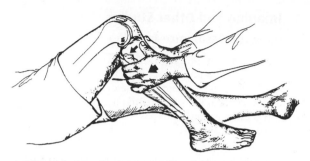

▲ **Figure 3–10.** The posterior drawer test is done in the same fashion as the anterior drawer test, except that the examiner exerts a posterior force. (Reproduced, with permission, from Scott WN: *Ligament and Extensor Mechanism Injuries of the Knee: Diagnosis and Treatment.* New York: Mosby-Year Book; 1991.)

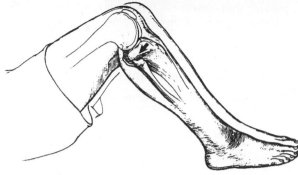

▲ **Figure 3–11.** The posterior sag seen in posterior cruciate disruption. (Reproduced, with permission, from Scott WN: *Ligament and Extensor Mechanism Injuries of the Knee: Diagnosis and Treatment.* New York: Mosby-Year Book; 1991.)

thumb is slid down the femoral condyles. With a PCL injury, sagging of the tibial plateau may be appreciated, and no step-off is palpated (Figure 3–11). An associated contusion on the anterior tibia suggests a PCL injury.

G. McMurray Test

With the McMurray test, forced flexion and rotation of the knee will elicit a clunk along the joint line if there is a meniscus injury (see Figure 3–12). Found in less than 10%

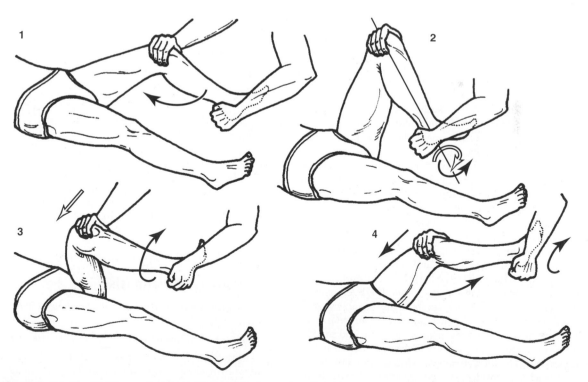

▲ **Figure 3–12.** The McMurray test to produce click. (Reproduced, with permission, from American Academy of Orthopaedic Surgeons: *Athletic Training and Sports Medicine*, 2nd ed. Burlington, MA: Jones and Bartlett; 1991.)

of patients with a meniscus injury, joint line pain with the McMurray test is much more common.

Arthroscopic Examination

A. Indications for Knee Injuries

Indications for arthroscopic examination in the knee include the following:

1. Acute hemarthrosis
2. Meniscus injuries
3. Loose bodies
4. Selected tibial plateau fractures
5. Patellar chondromalacia and/or malalignment
6. Chronic synovitis
7. Knee instability
8. Recurrent effusions
9. Chondral and osteochondral fractures

Today, a specific diagnosis of the type of knee injury can usually be made with a history, physical examination, and appropriate imaging studies. With an examination under anesthesia and arthroscopic evaluation, a specific diagnosis can be confirmed, expanded, or revised, and treatment can be rendered as needed.

B. Technique

Examination under anesthesia is very helpful in diagnosing ligament injuries and instability. It should be performed before the beginning of the procedure, before preparing and draping the extremity. For diagnostic arthroscopy, the knee joint is distended with irrigating fluid (usually saline or lactated Ringer solution), which washes away blood and debris from the joint. A lateral portal for the arthroscope is placed about a thumb's breadth above the joint line and just lateral to the patellar tendon. The medial portal is placed at about the same level, but just medial to the patellar tendon for introducing arthroscopic tools such as a probe. One approach to the general inspection of the joint is to start in the suprapatellar pouch. Loose bodies and plicas are sought. The patellofemoral joint is then inspected and observed for tracking problems and cartilage damage. The lateral gutter and the popliteus tendon are examined by flexion and valgus stress to the leg, prior to entering the medial compartment. The medial meniscus is probed using a nerve hook through the medial portal. The intercondylar notch, including the ACL, is inspected. The lateral compartment is then examined in a similar manner. Documentation of findings and procedures performed is important and may be done by videotape, photographs, and diagrammatic sketches. With assessment of the pathologic changes, treatment can be initiated, such as debridement and repair of meniscus tears, removal of loose bodies, or ACL reconstruction.

Imaging and Other Studies

A. Magnetic Resonance Imaging

Magnetic resonance imaging (MRI) is a powerful technique for evaluation of the knee joint. While the diagnosis is usually evident from the history and physical examination, MRI can be used to confirm the suspected injury. Other times, when a physical examination is not possible because of pain or the diagnosis remains elusive, MRI can aid in proper diagnosis. The specificity, sensitivity, and accuracy of MRI are greater than 90% for the medial and lateral menisci and the ACL and PCL. Therefore, MRI is often appropriate for ruling out the need for diagnostic arthroscopic examination. It is less helpful for the diagnosis of problems in knees with previous surgery.

B. Imaging Studies

Roentgenographic examination of the knee is indicated in the evaluation of traumatic injury. In cases of minimal trauma, radiographs may not be needed if the injury proves to be self-limited. Arthrographic examination can be helpful in patients who are unable to undergo MRI because of claustrophobia, metal in the body that may be dislodged, or other contraindications.

C. Laboratory Tests

Laboratory tests may be helpful in ruling out nonmechanical disorders such as inflammatory arthritis, as described in Chapter 6.

Behairy NH, Dorgham MA, Khaled SA: Accuracy of routine magnetic resonance imaging in meniscal and ligamentous injuries of the knee: comparison with arthroscopy. *Int Orthop* 2009;33:961. [PMID: 18506445]

Kramer DE, Micheli LJ: Meniscal tears and discoid meniscus in children: diagnosis and treatment. *J Am Acad Orthop Surg* 2009;17:698. [PMID: 19880680]

Meserve BB, Cleland JA, Boucher TR: A meta-analysis examining clinical test utilities for assessing meniscal injury. *Clin Rehabil* 2008;22:143. [PMID: 18212035]

Sanders TG, Miller MD: A systematic approach to magnetic resonance imaging interpretation of sports medicine injuries of the knee. *Am J Sports Med* 2005;33:131. [PMID: 15611010]

MENISCUS INJURY

Essentials of Diagnosis

- *Acute tears occur after axial loading combined with rotation.*
- *Sensation of clicking or catching of the knee with motion.*
- *Positive joint line tenderness, effusion, and a positive McMurray test are important physical exam findings.*
- *MRI can help classify location and morphology.*

Meniscal injuries are the most common reason for arthroscopy of the knee. The medial meniscus is more frequently torn than the lateral meniscus because the medial meniscus is securely attached around the entire periphery of the joint capsule, whereas the lateral meniscus has a mobile area where it is not attached. Meniscus injury is rare in childhood, occurs in the late teens, and peaks in the third and fourth decades. After the age of 50, meniscus tears are more often the result of arthritis than trauma.

▶ Clinical Findings

Acute traumatic tears of the menisci are often caused by axial loading combined with rotation. Patients typically report pain and swelling. Patients with smaller tears may have a sensation of clicking or catching in the knee. Patients with larger tears in the meniscus may complain of locking of the knee as the meniscus displaces into the joint and/or femoral notch. Loss of knee motion with a block to extension may result from a large bucket-handle tear. In acute tears involving an associated ACL injury, the swelling may be more significant and acute. ACL injuries often involve a lateral meniscus tear as the lateral compartment of the knee subluxates forward trapping the lateral meniscus between the femur and tibia.

Conversely, chronic or degenerative tears of the menisci often present in older patients (>40 years old) with the history of an insidious onset of pain and swelling with or without an acute increase superimposed. Often, no identifiable history of trauma is obtained, or the inciting event may be quite minor such as a bending or squatting motion.

The most important physical examination findings in the knee with a meniscus tear are joint line tenderness and an effusion. Other specialized tests include the McMurray, flexion McMurray, and Apley grind tests. The McMurray test is performed with the patient lying supine with the hip and knee flexed to about 90 degrees. While one hand holds the foot and twists it from external to internal rotation, the other hand holds the knee and applies compression (Figure 3–12). A positive test is one that elicits a pop or click that can be felt by the examiner when the torn meniscus is trapped between the femoral condyle and tibial plateau. A variation of this test is the flexion McMurray, in which the knee is held as for the McMurray test. To test the medial meniscus, the foot is externally rotated and the knee maximally flexed. A positive test occurs when the patient experiences pain over the posteromedial joint line as the knee is gradually extended. The Apley grind test requires placing the patient prone with the knee flexed to 90 degrees. The examiner applies downward pressure to the sole of the foot while twisting the lower leg in external and internal rotation. A positive test results in pain at either joint line.

In addition to the above, physical examination of the entire leg is essential. Assessing hip range of motion and irritability is useful, especially in children, as referred pain from the hip to the knee area is common. Examining for quadriceps atrophy and the presence of a knee effusion should also be done. Measurement of range of motion may reveal a loss of the normal knee extension. Assessing for tenderness of the femoral condyles, joint lines, tibial plateaus, and patellofemoral joint may give clues as to a possible osteochondral lesion, meniscus lesion, fracture, or chondrosis, respectively. Ligamentous testing including varus and valgus stress testing at full extension and 30 degrees of flexion and Lachman, anterior drawer, and posterior drawer testing should be done to assess stability.

▶ Tear Classification

Meniscal tears can be classified either by etiology or by their arthroscopic and MRI appearance. Etiologic classification divides tears into either acute tears (excessive force applied to an otherwise normal meniscus) or degenerative tears (normal force applied to a degenerative structure).

Classification should describe the tear location and its associated vascularity, morphology, and stability. Tear location is described by its location in the anteroposterior plane (anterior, middle, or posterior) and its circumferential location with respect to its vascularity. The common vascular zones include the most peripheral red/red zone near the meniscocapsular junction, the intermediate red/white zone, and the most central white/white zone. As tears occur more centrally, the healing rate is lower because of a decreased blood supply. Tears can also occur at the meniscal root, which is the attachment of the meniscus to the tibia.

Tear morphology describes the orientation of the tear within the meniscus and includes vertical or horizontal longitudinal, radial (transverse), oblique, and complex (including degenerative) tears (Figure 3–13). Most acute tears in younger patients are vertical longitudinal or oblique tears, while complex and degenerative tears occur more commonly in older patients. Vertical longitudinal, or bucket-handle tears, can be complete or incomplete and usually start in the posterior horn and continue anteriorly a variable distance. Large tears can cause significant mobility of the torn meniscal fragment, allowing it to displace into the femoral notch and cause a locked knee (Figure 3–14). This more commonly occurs in the medial meniscus, possibly owing to its decreased mobility. Oblique tears commonly occur at the junction of the middle and posterior thirds. They are often smaller tears, but the free edge of the tear can catch in the joint and cause symptoms of catching. Complex or degenerative tears occur in multiple planes, are often located in or near the posterior horns, and are more common in older patients with degenerative menisci. Horizontal longitudinal tears are often associated with meniscal cysts. They usually start at the inner margin of the meniscus and extend toward the meniscocapsular junction. They are thought to result from shear stresses and, when associated with meniscal cysts,

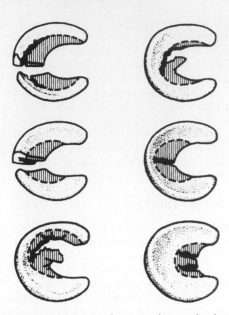

▲ Figure 3–13. Patterns of meniscal tears: bucket-handle, flap, horizontal cleavage, radial, degenerative, and double radial tear of a discoid meniscus.
(Reproduced, with permission, from Scott WN: *Arthroscopy of the Knee*. New York: WB Saunders; 1990.)

occur in the medial meniscus and cause localized swelling at the joint line.

▶ Treatment and Prognosis

Small stable meniscus tears often become asymptomatic and do not need to be treated surgically. Those causing persistent symptoms should be assessed with the arthroscope. Before the importance of the meniscus was understood and arthroscopy became available, the meniscus was often removed, even when normal. We now attempt to remove only the torn portion of the meniscus or repair the meniscus, if possible.

During arthroscopy, the meniscus can be visualized and palpated with a probe. The inner two thirds of the meniscus is avascular and often requires resection when torn. The remaining meniscus is smoothed and contoured to prevent further tearing from a jagged edge. Return to full function may be expected in 6–8 weeks.

Tears in the peripheral third of the meniscus, if small (<15 mm), may heal spontaneously because there is a blood supply in this portion of the adult meniscus. Larger tears need to be repaired because those who undergo meniscectomy at a young age are at risk of early osteoarthritis. These changes were first described by Fairbanks and include flattening of the femoral condyle, joint space narrowing, and osteophyte formation. Therefore, every effort should be made to preserve the meniscus.

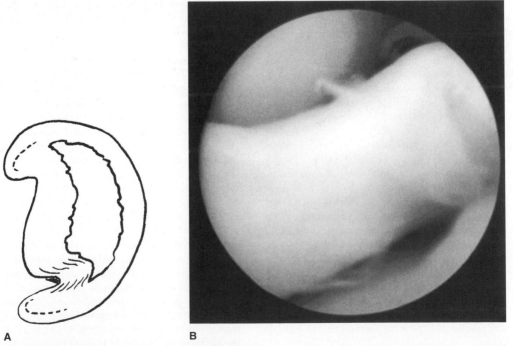

A   B

▲ Figure 3–14. A: Diagram of a typical bucket-handle tear of the medial meniscus. **B:** Arthroscopic view of a bucket-handle fragment displaced into the intercondylar notch. (Reproduced, with permission, from McGinty JB: *Operative Arthroscopy*. Baltimore: Raven Press, 1991.)

A. Partial Meniscal Resection

Partial meniscectomy has a 90% rate of good or excellent results in patients without knee instability or osteoarthritis. A major advantage over meniscus repair is a short recovery period. However, results diminish over time, and osteoarthritis occurs with over 10 years of follow-up. Medial meniscus tears generally do better than lateral tears after partial resection, and an intact meniscal rim and those with normal articular cartilage and normal knee stability are associated with a better prognosis.

B. Meniscus Repair

Most surgeons will attempt a meniscus repair rather than a partial meniscectomy in young, active individuals. Other commonly accepted criteria for meniscus repair include a complete vertical longitudinal tear greater than 15 mm in length, a tear within the peripheral 10–30% of the meniscus (ie, within 3–4 mm of the meniscocapsular junction), a peripheral tear that can be displaced toward the center of the plateau with a probe, the absence of secondary meniscus degeneration, and a tear in a patient undergoing concurrent ligament or articular cartilage repair.

Multiple factors affect the success of meniscus repair. Although no absolute age limit exists, patients younger than 40 years are thought to have a better chance for healing. Knees with associated ligamentous instability, particularly ACL instability, have inferior rates of meniscus healing because of abnormal meniscus stresses from tibiofemoral instability. The location of the tear and the time lapsed from injury to treatment are also important. Acute tears located in the peripheral red/red or red/white zone have better healing capability than chronic tears located in the red/white or white/white zones. Tears 5 mm or more from the periphery are considered avascular (white zone), whereas those between 3 and 5 mm are variable in vascularity (red/white), and tears in the peripheral 3 mm are considered vascular (red). In areas with marginal vascularization, abrasion of the meniscocapsular junction or use of a fibrin clot may be performed. It is thought that a vascular pannus forms from the abraded tissue that aids in healing. Finally, the stability of the meniscus repair is a factor, with vertical mattress sutures generally considered the gold standard in meniscus repair. It is generally believed that the superiority of vertical mattress over horizontal mattress sutures is from the vertical mattress sutures capturing the strong peripheral, circumferential fibers of the meniscus.

Meniscus repair is more successful when done at the same time as ACL reconstruction. Then it is successful up to 90% of the time compared to approximately 50% success in patients with intact ACLs who had meniscus repairs. Many of the meniscus tears that occur with an ACL tear are amenable to repair. Then stabilizing the knee with ACL reconstruction protects the repaired meniscus from abnormal knee motion and has more success than if the knee is left unstable.

Types of repairs include the traditional open repair and arthroscopic repairs that can be done with inside-out, outside-in, or all-inside techniques. Inside-out and outside-in repairs are usually done with sutures and require a mini-incision and securing of the meniscus to the capsule with sutures. The all-inside technique has many device options, including sutures and various devices. Regardless of the type of repair chosen, adequate preparation of the tear site is required. The tear edges should be debrided or abraded with a shaver or rasp to stimulate bleeding. Restoration of biomechanical function is encouraged by anatomic apposition of the tear edges to ensure good healing potential.

1. Open meniscal repair—Open repair of meniscus tears has been shown to have successful long-term results. The technique involves making a small incision through the subcutaneous tissue, capsule, and synovium to directly visualize the tear. Open repair is most useful in peripheral or meniscocapsular tears, often occurring in conjunction with open repair of a collateral ligament injury or a tibial plateau fracture. Follow-up studies of 10 years or longer have shown survival rates of repaired menisci of 80–90%, in part influenced by the peripheral nature of the tear and the associated hemarthrosis present in ligament tears or fracture repair cases.

2. Arthroscopic meniscal repair

A. INSIDE-OUT MENISCAL REPAIR—Arthroscopic inside-out meniscus repairs are performed using long needles introduced through cannula systems with attached absorbable or nonabsorbable sutures passed perpendicularly across the tear from inside the knee to a protected area outside the joint capsule. These sutures are able to obtain consistent perpendicular placement across the meniscus tear, which gives this method an advantage over other repair techniques. Improved suture placement is gained at the expense of possible neurovascular injury from passing the needle from inside the knee to outside the joint. This technique requires a posteromedial or posterolateral incision to protect the neurovascular structures and safely retrieve the exiting needles. Because surgeons are able to place vertical mattress sutures, the best biomechanical construct for meniscus repair, this technique remains the gold standard for many surgeons. Numerous retrospective and prospective studies using second-look arthroscopy or arthrography to evaluate healing of the meniscus repairs have consistently shown rates of 70–90% in isolated repairs, and greater than 90% when done in conjunction with an ACL reconstruction. This technique is ideal for posterior and midposterior horn tears. There is difficulty in passing needles in mid to anterior horn meniscus tears.

B. OUTSIDE-IN MENISCAL REPAIR—The arthroscopic outside-in repair was developed in part to decrease the neurovascular risk associated with the inside-out technique. The outside-in technique involves passing a needle from outside the joint, across the tear, and into the joint. Two options then exist for repair of the meniscus tear. One option is then to retrieve the suture through an anterior portal, tie a knot outside the knee joint, and then bring the knot back in through the anterior portal placing the knot against the reduced meniscus body fragment. A second option is to use parallel needles and retrieve the suture through the second needle. This can be done using a suture relay. A knot is then tied outside the joint over the capsule. This method is useful for tears in the anterior horn or body of the menisci, but does not work for tears in or near the posterior horn. Results of the outside-in technique using MRI, arthrography, or second-look arthroscopy to assess healing have shown complete or partial healing; between 74% and 87% of meniscus repairs have been successful. As expected, more posterior horn tears and tears in unstable knees did worse.

C. ALL-INSIDE MENISCAL REPAIR—The popularity of the all-inside repairs has increased with the introduction of numerous devices and techniques to ease the technique. They do not require accessory incisions, thereby saving operative time, and they avoid more technical arthroscopic techniques required in other types of repairs. However, repairs with some devices have not been as successful as those with traditional techniques. Success rate is 60–90%, and some have found results comparable to traditional techniques, but there are complications including devices that have migrated from their original position, broken fragments, foreign-body reactions, inflammation, chronic effusions, and articular cartilage injuries.

Recent biomechanical studies have found repair with some of these devices to have properties equivalent to vertical mattress sutures. But there is considerable variation with the type of device. What remains to be known, however, is the meniscus repair strength needed for optimal meniscus healing.

C. Meniscal Transplantation

An alternative to leaving the patient with a meniscus-deficient knee, and almost certain early osteoarthrosis, is meniscus transplantation. This technique yields satisfactory results in about two thirds of patients. In the future, biologic scaffolds may enable menisci to be regenerated after meniscectomy.

Ahn JH, Wang JH, Yoo JC: Arthroscopic all-inside suture repair of medial meniscus lesion in anterior cruciate ligament–deficient knees: results of second-look arthroscopies in 39 cases. *Arthroscopy* 2004;20:936. [PMID: 15525926]

Hommen JP, Applegate GR, Del Pizzo W: Meniscus allograft transplantation: ten-year results of cryopreserved allografts. *Arthroscopy* 2007;23:388. [PMID: 17418331]

Metcalf MH, Barrett GR: Prospective evaluation of 1485 meniscal tear patterns in patients with stable knees. *Am J Sports Med* 2004;32:675. [PMID: 15090384]

Salata MJ, Gibbs AE, Sekiya JK: A systematic review of clinical outcomes in patients undergoing meniscectomy. *Am J Sports Med* 2010;38:1907. [PMID: 20587698]

Shelbourne KD, Dersam MD: Comparison of partial meniscectomy versus meniscus repair for bucket-handle lateral meniscus tears in anterior cruciate ligament reconstructed knees. *Arthroscopy* 2004;20:581. [PMID: 15241307]

Steenbrugge F, Verstraete K, Verdonk R: Magnetic resonance imaging of the surgically repaired meniscus: a 13-year follow-up study of 13 knees. *Acta Orthop Scand* 2004;75:323. [PMID: 15260425]

Stone KR, Adelson WS, Pelsis JR, Walgenbach AW, Turek TJ: Long-term survival of concurrent meniscus allograft transplantation and repair of the articular cartilage: a prospective two- to 12-year follow-up report. *J Bone Joint Surg Br* 2010;92:941. [PMID: 20595111]

▶ CPT Codes for the Meniscus

27403 Arthrotomy with meniscus repair, knee

29868 Arthroscopy, knee, surgical; meniscal transplantation (includes arthrotomy for meniscal insertion), medial or lateral

29870 Arthroscopy, knee, diagnostic, with or without synovial biopsy (separate procedure)

29880 Arthroscopy, knee, surgical; with meniscectomy (medial and lateral, including any meniscal shaving)

29881 Arthroscopy, knee, surgical; with meniscectomy (medial or lateral, including any meniscal shaving)

29882 Arthroscopy, knee, surgical; with meniscus repair (medial or lateral)

29883 Arthroscopy, knee, surgical; with meniscus repair (medial and lateral)

KNEE FRACTURE

Articular cartilage injuries of the knee are infrequent, and there must be a high index of suspicion to detect them. MRI and arthroscopy are very helpful with these injuries, especially pure articular cartilage injuries, where radiographs will be normal.

1. Osteochondral Lesions

▶ Essentials of Diagnosis

- *Patients usually present with vague, poorly localized complaints of knee pain.*
- *Classic location is the posterolateral aspect of the medial femoral condyle.*
- *Involvement is bilateral in up to 25% of cases, so examine both knees.*
- *Effusion, crepitus, and an antalgic gait are possible findings on exam.*
- *Radiographs and MRI can be helpful in determining the location and size of the lesion.*

▶ Osteochondral Fracture

There is much confusion about the nomenclature and etiology of juvenile and adult osteochondral lesions (OCL) of the knee, also called osteochondritis dissecans. Inflammatory, ossification abnormalities and avascular necrosis have all been considered etiologies of this condition. However, basic science, histopathology, and vascular studies do not support any of them. The term "osteochondral injuries" has been used to describe injuries ranging from acute osteochondral fractures to pure chondral injuries. Currently, OCLs are defined as potentially reversible idiopathic lesions of subchondral bone, resulting in delamination or fragmentation with or without destruction of the overlying articular cartilage. OCLs are subdivided into juvenile and adult forms depending on the presence of an open distal femoral physis. In children, a combination of etiologies is now thought to be responsible for OCLs. For example, a stress fracture may develop in the subchondral bone of the distal femoral condyle. Such an injury may provoke further vascular compromise, which results in injury to the subchondral bone that was initially covered with normal articular cartilage. Loss of support from the subchondral bone may result in damage to the overlying articular cartilage. The vast majority of adult OCLs are thought to have arisen from a persistent juvenile OCL, although new lesions in adults are possible as well.

Both adult and juvenile OCLs that do not heal have the potential for further sequelae, including degenerative osteoarthritis. Juvenile OCLs, defined as knees with an open physes, generally have a better prognosis than adult lesions. The classic location of an OCL is the posterolateral aspect of the medial femoral condyle, which accounts for 70–80% of all OCLs. Lateral condyle OCLs are seen in 15–20% of patients, and patellar involvement ranges from 5–10%. The increased use of MRI and arthroscopy over the past decade may have resulted in greater recognition of OCLs.

▶ Clinical Findings

A common presentation of a patient with an OCL is aching and activity-related anterior knee pain that is poorly localized. Pain may worsen with stair climbing or running. Patients with stable OCLs do not have mechanical symptoms or knee instability. Mechanical symptoms are more common in patients with unstable or loose OCLs. Patients may limp, and knee swelling may be present. Tenderness with palpation of the femoral condyle may be observed with various degrees of knee flexion. Loss of range of motion or quadriceps atrophy may be noted in more long-standing cases.

It is important to identify patients with unstable lesions. There may be crepitus and pain with range of motion, and an effusion is typically present. Involvement is bilateral in up to 25% of cases, so both knees should be evaluated regardless of symptoms. Initial evaluation should include anteroposterior, lateral, and tunnel views of both knees. The goal of plain radiographs is to exclude any bony pathology, evaluate the physes, and localize the lesion. Lesion location and an estimation of size can be determined as described by Cahill. MRI may be helpful in diagnosis and can give an estimation of the size of the lesion (prognosis is better for small lesions), the condition of the overlying cartilage and underlying

subchondral bone, the extent of bone edema, the presence of any loose bodies, and assessment of OCL stability. Four MRI criteria have been identified on T2-weighted images to assess OCL stability: a line of high signal intensity at least 5 mm in length between the OCL and underlying bone, an area of increased homogeneous signal at least 5 mm in diameter beneath the lesion, a focal defect of 5 mm or more in the articular surface, and a high signal line traversing the subchondral plate into the lesion. A high signal line is the most common sign in patients found to have unstable lesions that are most likely to fail nonoperative treatment. MRI is helpful with these injuries, especially pure articular cartilage injuries, where radiographs will be normal or may result in false-positive findings of fragment loosening. Arthroscopy remains the gold standard in evaluation of these lesions.

Equivocal prognostic value has been found in the use of intravenous gadolinium in OCLs. Technetium bone scans were initially proposed to monitor the presence of healing. However, because MRI eliminates the ionizing radiation and increased time required in bone scanning, bone scanning is not widely used.

▶ Treatment and Prognosis

Prognosis is good for the immature child. Nonoperative management should be pursued in those with a stable OCL and open physes. The goal of nonoperative treatment is to obtain a healed lesion before physis closure so as to prevent early-onset osteoarthritis. Even if patients are within 6–12 months of physeal closure, a trial of nonoperative treatment is warranted.

Because failure of the subchondral bone precedes failure of the overlying articular cartilage, most orthopedists recommend some sort of activity modification. Debate exists whether activity modification should include the use of cast or brace immobilization. The tenet of nonoperative treatment is to reduce the activity level where pain-free activities of daily living are possible. However, there is no optimal immobilization protocol available in the literature.

Patients should be non–weight bearing or partial weight bearing with crutches for 3–6 weeks or until they are pain free. Repeat radiographs are obtained at approximately 6-week intervals. Physical therapy with full weight bearing may be initiated once patients are pain free. Physical therapy should focus on low-impact quadriceps and hamstring strengthening. If patients remain asymptomatic up to at least 3 months after the diagnosis was made, activity may be slowly advanced to higher impact activities such as running or jumping. Any recurrence of symptoms or any progression of the OCL on plain radiographs should prompt a return to non–weight bearing and possible immobilization for a longer period. Obvious patient frustration and lack of compliance (especially in adolescents) is common, and a full discussion of the risks and benefits of nonoperative or operative treatment is required.

Operative treatment should be considered in the following instances: (1) loose bodies, (2) an unstable OCL, (3) persistence of symptoms despite nonoperative treatment in a compliant patient, (4) worsening appearance on imaging studies, and (5) near or complete epiphyseal closure. Goals of operative treatment should include achievement of a stable osteochondral fragment that maintains joint congruity and allows early range of motion.

For stable lesions with an intact articular surface, arthroscopic drilling of the lesions is preferred. This creates channels for potential revascularization through the subchondral bone plate. Options include transarticular drilling and transepiphyseal drilling. Radiographic healing and relief of symptoms can be expected in 80–90% of patients with open physes. This decreases to 50–75% in those with closed physes.

Patients with partially unstable lesions such as a flap lesion should be managed by the status of the subchondral bone. If present, fibrous tissue between the lesion and subchondral bone should be debrided. If significant subchondral bone loss has occurred, it can be filled with autogenous bone graft prior to fixation of the OCL. If the OCL has sufficient bone such that an anatomic fit into its donor site is possible, fixation should be attempted. Various fixation methods have been described including Herbert or cannulated screws and bioabsorbable screws or pins, but there are complications with these treatments. Complications include devices that have migrated from their original position, broken fragments, foreign-body reactions, inflammation, chronic effusions, and articular cartilage injuries.

Simple excision of the larger fragments has shown poor results with more rapid progression of radiographic osteoarthritic changes. For lesions greater than 2 cm^2, drilling or microfracture methods that depend on replacement of the defect with fibrocartilage have yielded poor results with worsening osteoarthritis over time. For these larger lesions, cartilage transplantation has been tried. Disadvantages of autologous osteochondral plugs or mosaicplasty include donor site morbidity and incongruent articular fit. Advantages include good fixation of the patient's own tissue. Another option is autologous chondrocyte implantation, which involves harvesting of the patient's chondrocytes, proliferating them over time, and then reimplanting the chondrocytes. Advantages include use of the patient's own tissue and lessened donor site morbidity. Longer-term results in young adult patients show successful clinical results in up to 90% for both procedures. However, additional larger and longer-term follow-up studies are needed.

Cepero S, Ullot R, Sastre S: Osteochondritis of the femoral condyles in children and adolescents: our experience over the last 28 years. *J Pediatr Orthop B* 2005;14:24. [PMID: 15577303]

Crawford DC, Safran MR: Osteochondritis dissecans of the knee. *J Am Acad Orthop Surg* 2006;14:90. [PMID: 16467184]

Detterline AJ, Goldstein JL, Rue JP, et al: Evaluation and treatment of osteochondritis dissecans lesions of the knee. *J Knee Surg* 2008;21:106. [PMID: 18500061]

Gomoll AH, Farr J, Gillogly SD, Kercher J, Minas T: Surgical management of articular cartilage defects of the knee. *J Bone Joint Surg Am* 2010;92:2470. [PMID: 20962200]

Vasiliadis HS, Wasiak J: Autologous chondrocyte implantation for full thickness articular cartilage defects of the knee. *Cochrane Database Syst Rev* 2010;10:CD003323. [PMID: 20927732]

▶ CPT Codes for Osteochondral Lesions

27415 Osteochondral allograft, knee, open

29850 Arthroscopically aided treatment of intercondylar spine(s) and/or tuberosity fracture(s) of the knee, with or without manipulation; without internal or external fixation (includes arthroscopy)

29866 Arthroscopy, knee, surgical; osteochondral autograft(s) (eg, mosaicplasty) (includes harvesting of the autograft[s])

29867 Arthroscopy, knee, surgical; osteochondral allograft (eg, mosaicplasty)

29874 Arthroscopy, knee, surgical; for removal of loose body or foreign body (eg, osteochondritis dissecans fragmentation, chondral fragmentation)

29877 Arthroscopy, knee, surgical; debridement/shaving of articular cartilage (chondroplasty)

29879 Arthroscopy, knee, surgical; abrasion arthroplasty (includes chondroplasty where necessary) or multiple drilling or microfracture

29885 Arthroscopy, knee, surgical; drilling for osteochondritis dissecans with bone grafting, with or without internal fixation (including debridement of base of lesion)

29886 Arthroscopy, knee, surgical; drilling for intact osteochondritis dissecans lesion

29887 Arthroscopy, knee, surgical; drilling for intact osteochondritis dissecans lesion with internal fixation

KNEE LIGAMENT INJURY

Knee injuries occur during both contact and noncontact athletic activities. Advances in the diagnosis and treatment of ligament injuries have allowed athletes at all levels of ability to return to sports at their preinjury level of activity. The ligaments and menisci of the knee work in concert with one another, and frequently more than one structure is damaged when an acute injury occurs.

Ligament injuries are graded as follows: grade 1, stretching of the ligament with no detectable instability; grade 2, further stretching of the ligament with detectable instability, but with the fibers in continuity; and grade 3, complete disruption of the ligament.

▶ Anatomy

Knee stability requires proper functioning of four ligaments. These ligaments include the ACL, the PCL, the medial collateral ligament (MCL), and the lateral collateral ligament (LCL). There are also several accessory or secondary stabilizers of the knee. Secondary stabilizers of the knee include the menisci, iliotibial band, and biceps femoris. These secondary stabilizers become more important when a primary stabilizer is injured.

The MCL is the primary static stabilizer against valgus stress at the knee. The MCL originates from the central sulcus of the medial epicondyle. The sulcus of the C-shaped medial epicondyle is located anterior and distal to the adductor tubercle. The MCL is made up of three main static medial stabilizers of the knee. This includes the superficial MCL, the posterior oblique ligament, and the deep capsular ligament.

The LCL is the primary static stabilizer against varus stress at the knee. The LCL originates from the lateral epicondyle. This is the most prominent point of the lateral femoral condyle. The LCL insertion is on the styloid process of the fibular head, which projects superiorly from the posterolateral fibular head. The LCL joins with the arcuate ligament, the popliteus muscle, and the lateral head of the gastrocnemius to form a lateral arcuate complex to control statically and dynamically varus angulation and external tibial torsion. The iliotibial band and biceps femoris also contribute to stability on the lateral aspect of the knee.

The ACL is the primary static stabilizer of the knee against anterior translation of the tibia with respect to the femur. The ACL originates from the posteromedial surface of the lateral femoral condyle in the intercondylar notch. The ACL inserts on the tibial plateau just medial to the anterior horn of the lateral meniscus about 15 mm posterior to the anterior edge of the tibial articular surface. The blood supply to the ACL and PCL is the middle geniculate artery. Both the ACL and PCL are covered by a layer of synovium, making these ligaments intraarticular and extrasynovial.

The PCL is the primary static stabilizer of the knee against posterior translation of the tibia with respect to the femur. The PCL originates from the posterior aspect of the lateral surface of the medial femoral condyle in the intercondylar notch. The PCL inserts on the posterior aspect of the tibial plateau in a central depression just posterior to the articular surface. The insertion extends distally along the posterior aspect of the tibia for up to 1 cm in length. The PCL is a complex structure consisting of two major bands: the anterolateral and posteromedial bands. The anterolateral band is tight in flexion and loose in extension. The posteromedial band is loose in flexion and tight in extension. The cross-sectional area of the anterolateral band is twice as large as the posteromedial band. The meniscofemoral ligaments, the ligaments of Wrisberg and Humphrey, are the third component of the PCL. The meniscofemoral ligaments travel from the posterior horn of the lateral meniscus to the posteromedial femoral condyle.

Differential Diagnosis of Knee Instability

The differential diagnosis of acute or chronic knee instability can involve any of the knee ligaments and/or the structures of the posterolateral corner. There are often combinations of ligament injuries in addition to injuries of secondary stabilizing structures such as the menisci. The history and mechanism of injury are valuable information, if available. Similarly, the location of pain can help to narrow the diagnosis. Clearly, however, a thorough physical examination helps to distinguish which ligaments have been injured. Additionally, imaging studies are often obtained to confirm clinical suspicions and to evaluate for occult injuries.

Fanelli GC, Orcutt DR, Edson CJ: The multiple-ligament injured knee: evaluation, treatment and results. *Arthroscopy* 2005;21:471. [PMID: 15800529]

Micheo W, Hernández L, Seda C: Evaluation, management, rehabilitation, and prevention of anterior cruciate ligament injury: current concepts. *PM R* 2010;2:935. [PMID: 20970763]

1. Medial Collateral Ligament Injuries

▶ Essential of Diagnosis

- *Occurs after a valgus stress to the knee or noncontact rotational injury.*
- *Medial knee pain and instability at 30 degrees of flexion is diagnostic; consider ACL or PCL injuries in addition if opening at full extension with a valgus stress.*
- *Chronic injuries may have calcification at the insertion of the MCL on the medial femoral condyle.*
- *MRI can be helpful in confirming diagnosis and helping to rule out concomitant meniscal injury.*

▶ Symptoms (History)

How and when the patient was hurt are important parts of the history. Lower-grade MCL injuries typically occur in a noncontact external rotational injury, whereas higher-grade injuries generally involve lateral contact to the thigh or upper leg. Other important pieces of historical information include the location and presence of pain, instability, timing of swelling, and sensation of a "pop" or tear. Surprisingly, grade I and II injuries are often more painful than complete MCL rupture. Immediate swelling should make one suspicious for an associated cruciate ligament injury, fracture, and/or patellar dislocation.

A prior history of knee injuries or instability should always be sought when evaluating a new knee injury.

▶ Signs (Physical Examination)

MCL injuries are evaluated with a complete knee examination to evaluate for any other coexisting injuries. This is especially true with ACL and PCL evaluation because an injury to either of these ligaments would significantly change the treatment. Given the frequency of coexisting patellar dislocations in MCL injuries, palpation of the patella and the medial parapatellar stabilizing ligaments should be performed in addition to patellar apprehension testing.

Medial joint line tenderness along the course of the MCL is typical at the location of the tear. Laxity to valgus stresses is assessed by the amount of medial joint space opening that occurs at 30 degrees of flexion. It is important to stress the knee at 30 degrees of flexion because with the knee in full extension the posterior capsule and PCL will stabilize the knee to valgus stress. This stability to valgus stress in full extension could mislead the examiner to believe that the MCL is intact. Zero opening is considered normal, with 1-4 mm indicating a grade I injury, 5–9 mm indicating a grade II injury, and 10–15 mm indicating a complete or grade III injury. Additionally, grade I and II injuries typically have a firm end point, whereas a grade III injury tends to have a soft end point to valgus stress.

▶ Imaging Studies

A. Radiographs

A series of knee radiographs should be obtained in any patient with a suspected significant knee injury. Radiographs should be inspected for acute fracture, lateral capsular avulsion (Segond fracture; see section on ACL imaging), loose bodies, Pellegrini-Stieda lesion (MCL calcification), and evidence of patellar dislocation. Stress radiographs should be obtained in patients prior to skeletal maturity to rule out an epiphyseal fracture.

B. MRI

MRI is useful for confirming MCL injury and identifying the site of injury. It is also useful to detect the presence of meniscal and other injuries to the knee. Relative indications for an MRI include an uncertain ACL status despite multiple examinations, evaluation of a suspected meniscal tear, or preoperative evaluation for a planned MCL reconstruction or repair.

C. Special Tests

An examination under anesthesia can be valuable when physical examination is unreliable because of the patient guarding the knee. Diagnostic arthroscopy can also be used to evaluate for coexistant pathology. However, both of these diagnostic methods have largely been replaced by MRI.

▶ Treatment (Nonsurgical and Surgical)

Treatment of an isolated MCL injury is generally nonoperative with protection against valgus stress and early motion. Grade I and grade II injuries can be placed in either a cast or a brace and bear weight as tolerated. Generally, knee motion is started within the first week or two, and full recovery is usually achieved more rapidly with early knee range of motion.

Grade III injuries are a bit more controversial. Several authors have shown increased instability in grade III tears treated nonsurgically, although most of these studies did not exclude knees with multiligamentous injuries. Comparison of isolated grade III MCL tears treated with surgical reconstruction versus nonsurgical management showed that the nonsurgical treatment group enjoyed better results in both subjective scoring and earlier return to activity.

The exception to the current trend of nonsurgical treatment of grade III injuries is in the setting of a multiligamentous knee injury. In this setting, particularly with a distal tibial avulsion of the MCL, nonsurgical treatment has not fared nearly as well as in isolated MCL injuries. MCL repair in the acute setting can include a primary repair, with shortening if needed, of the torn ligament. Similarly, avulsion fragments are treated with reduction and fixation in the acute setting. Primary repairs can be reinforced with autograft or allograft tissues if the remaining MCL is insufficient for a stand-alone repair. Chronic reconstructions also often include autograft or allograft tissue reconstruction.

Traditionally, casting or operative treatment of MCL injuries significantly limited an early return to range-of-motion exercises. With the addition of functional bracing and early motion to a nonsurgical treatment protocol, motion and strengthening of the knee can occur at an early stage while the ligament is protected from valgus stress. As knee motion improves, isotonic strengthening exercises are introduced. As the strength of the extremity improves, the intensity of functional rehabilitation increases accordingly.

▶ Complications

With nonsurgical treatment becoming the standard of care, complications associated with an MCL injury have decreased. The main complication of nonsurgical therapy is residual valgus laxity or medial knee pain. Radiographs may show residual calcification of the MCL (Pellegrini-Stieda lesion). Potential surgical complications include arthrofibrosis, infection, damage to the saphenous nerve or vein, or recurrent valgus laxity.

▶ Results/Return to Play

In general, good outcomes can be achieved with nonsurgical treatment and rehabilitation of isolated MCL injuries. Return to professional football after nonsurgical treatment of isolated MCL injuries is 98%.

Azar FM: Evaluation and treatment of chronic medial collateral ligament injuries of the knee. *Sports Med Arthrosc* 2006;14:84. [PMID: 17135952]

Robinson JR, Bull A, Thomas R, et al: The role of the medial collateral ligament and posteromedial capsule in controlling knee laxity. *Am J Sports Med* 2006;34:1815. [PMID: 16816148]

Robinson JR, Sanchez-Ballester J, Bull AM, et al: The posteromedial corner revisited. An anatomical description of the passive restraining structures of the medial aspect of the human knee. *J Bone Joint Surg Br* 2004;86:674. [PMID: 15274262]

Stannard JP: Medial and posteromedial instability of the knee: evaluation, treatment, and results. *Sports Med Arthrosc* 2010; 18:263. [PMID: 21079506]

2. Lateral Collateral Ligament Injuries

▶ Essentials of Diagnosis

- *Patients may complain of lateral knee pain and a varus thrust with daily activity.*
- *Varus stress to the knee with opening at 30 degrees of flexion is diagnostic for an isolated LCL injury.*
- *Frequently part of a multiligamentous injury to the knee.*
- *There is a high incidence of peroneal nerve injury; document neurovascular status to the involved extremity.*
- *MRI should be obtained as a useful adjunct to help diagnose posterolateral corner injuries.*

▶ Symptoms (History)

The most consistent symptom of an acute LCL injury is lateral knee pain. However, the symptoms of lateral and posterolateral instability are quite variable and depend on the severity of injury, patient activity level, overall limb alignment, and other associated knee injuries. For example, a sedentary individual with minimal laxity and overall valgus alignment will have few, if any, symptoms. However, if LCL laxity is combined with overall varus alignment, hyperextension, and an increased activity level, symptoms will be quite pronounced. These patients may complain of lateral joint line pain and a varus thrust of their leg with everyday activities. This is often described as the knee buckling into hyperextension with normal gait.

▶ Signs (Physical Examination)

Patients with an LCL and/or posterolateral corner injury often also have additional ligamentous injuries to the knee. Therefore, a thorough knee examination should be performed to evaluate for coexistant knee pathology. Additionally, a careful neurovascular examination should be performed as the incidence of neurovascular injury, particularly peroneal nerve injury, has been reported in 12–29% of posterolateral knee injuries.

The integrity of the LCL is assessed by placing a varus stress, with the knee in full extension and 30 degrees of flexion. Baseline varus opening is widely variable and should be compared to the contralateral leg. The average baseline for varus opening is 7 degrees. Exam findings with an isolated LCL injury should include varus laxity at 30 degrees of flexion and no instability in full extension. This is due to the stabilizing effect that the intact cruciate ligaments provide in full extension.

It is important to note that a significant posterolateral knee injury can be present without significant varus laxity. The most useful test to evaluate for posterolateral instability is the dial test. This is done by externally rotating each tibia and noting the angle subtended between the thigh and the foot. The dial test is performed at 30 and 90 degrees of flexion with a significant difference being an angle 5 degrees or greater than the contralateral leg. Injury to the posterolateral capsule alone is confirmed with greater external rotation at 30 degrees, an isolated PCL at 90 degrees, and to both structures when there is greater rotation at 30 and 90 degrees compared to the uninjured leg.

▶ Imaging Studies

A. Radiographs

A series of knee radiographs should be obtained in any patient with a suspected knee injury. Radiographs should be inspected for acute fractures, lateral capsular avulsion (Segond fracture; see section on ACL imaging), loose bodies, fibular head avulsions, and evidence of patellar dislocation. With chronic posterolateral instability, degenerative changes of the lateral compartment are often noted. Lateral joint space narrowing with osteophytes and subchondral sclerosis can be seen. Stress radiographs can help to better quantify the amount of varus angulation present.

B. MRI

MRI is often a useful adjunct for diagnosing posterolateral corner and LCL injuries in the severely injured knee. As mentioned earlier, this posterolateral injury can often go unnoticed during an initial evaluation, and MRI findings can refocus the examination to the posterolateral structures. Pain and guarding at the time of injury can often obscure posterolateral injury, and MRI can prove to be an extremely valuable adjunct in diagnosis.

C. Special Tests/Examinations

1. Reverse pivot shift test—This test involves starting with the knee flexed to 90 degrees. While the knee is extended, the leg is loaded axially with a valgus stress applied to the knee and the foot is held in external rotation. A palpable shift is noted as the tibia reduces from its posteriorly subluxed position as the knee is extended.

2. External rotation recurvatum test—This test is performed with the patient supine and the hip and knee fully extended. The leg is lifted off the bed by the toes. Hyperextension, varus instability, and external rotation of the tibial tubercle occurs with adequate quadriceps relaxation in a patient with posterolateral instability.

3. Posterolateral drawer test—A standard posterior drawer test (see section on PCL physical examination) is performed with the tibia in internal rotation, neutral, and externally rotated positions. With posterolateral injury, the magnitude of the posterior drawer displacement will be greatest with external tibial rotation.

4. Examination under anesthesia—An examination while the patient is relaxed under general anesthetic is extremely useful, particularly in the acute setting. If the patient with a multiligamentous knee injury is taken to the operating room, this is an excellent opportunity to examine the knee without guarding to improve the accuracy of the examination.

▶ Treatment

A. Nonsurgical

Isolated LCL ligament injuries, as noted earlier, are rare injuries. However, in the case of an isolated LCL ligament injury with grade II or less magnitude, a period of immobilization from 2–4 weeks followed by a quadriceps strengthening program will usually yield good results. Grade III injuries often have better results with surgical treatment. The combination of delayed diagnosis along with an uncertain natural history of posterolateral instability makes the treatment of these injuries a challenge.

B. Surgical

LCL and posterolateral ligament injuries, as discussed earlier, rarely occur in isolation. Therefore, other injuries must also be considered in the treatment plan of the multiligamentous knee injury. Ideally, the posterolateral and LCL injuries are diagnosed in the acute setting. This allows the preferred surgical treatment of a primary repair of the injured structures with augmentation as needed. Primary repair is generally only feasible in the first few weeks following the knee injury.

The knee with chronic posterolateral instability will often require ligamentous reconstruction or advancement to reconstitute a static restraint to varus stresses. The key biomechanical concept of any lateral ligamentous reconstruction is that the isometric point of the LCL lies between the fibular head and the lateral epicondyle. Therefore, regardless of the graft material used to reconstruct the lateral ligamentous complex, a portion of the graft must pass between the lateral femoral epicondyle and the fibular head.

To improve the success rate of reconstruction of chronic lateral ligamentous instability, a proximal tibial valgus osteotomy may be performed to decrease the stress on the lateral structures of the knee.

▶ Rehabilitation

The rehabilitation of the knee after posterolateral reconstructions or repairs is largely guided by associated injuries to the ACL or PCL. It is generally necessary, however, to limit weight bearing for at least 6 weeks and protect the lateral structures with a brace for at least 3 months.

▶ Complications

The peroneal nerve runs just posterior to the fibular head. It is important to isolate the peroneal nerve prior to any lateral knee exposure to minimize the complication of a peroneal nerve injury.

▶ Results

If injuries to the posterolateral corner of the knee are diagnosed and repaired acutely, the results are good for restoration of varus stability and return to play. Chronic posterolateral corner injury reconstructions also perform well when an isometric lateral reconstruction is achieved.

Laprade RF, Engebretsen L, Johansen S, et al: The effect of a proximal tibial medial opening wedge osteotomy on posterolateral knee instability. *Am J Sports Med* 2008;36:956. [PMID: 18227230]

Markolf KL, Graves BR, Sigward SM, et al: Effects of posterolateral reconstructions on external tibial rotation and forces in a posterior cruciate ligament graft. *Bone Joint Surg Am* 2007;89:2351. [PMID: 17974876]

Ranawat A, Baker C 3rd, Henry S, et al: Posterolateral corner injury of the knee: evaluation and management. *J Am Acad Orthop Surg* 2008;16:506. [PMID: 18768708]

Rios CG, Leger RR, Cote MP, Yang C, Arciero RA: Posterolateral corner reconstruction of the knee: evaluation of a technique with clinical outcomes and stress radiography. *Am J Sports Med* 2010;38:1564. [PMID: 20445013]

3. Anterior Cruciate Ligament Injuries

▶ Essentials of Diagnosis

- *Mechanism is either noncontact deceleration/rotation injury or contact injury with valgus force to an extended knee.*
- *Patients often hear a "pop." They note feelings of instability and the knee giving out with twisting activities.*
- *Substantial knee effusion is present within first 12 hours after injury.*
- *There is a high incidence of associated injuries, including meniscus tears.*
- *Lachman is most sensitive test for diagnosis; pivot shift or Losee test helps evaluate rotational instability.*
- *Segond sign (avulsion of the anterolateral capsule of the tibia) may be seen on plain radiographs.*
- *MRI is helpful to confirm diagnosis and verify any additional concomitant injuries.*

▶ Symptoms (History)

The mechanism of injury should be elicited in any knee injury evaluation. This can guide the examination to additional structures that may also be injured. ACL injury can occur in a variety of ways; however, a few mechanisms predominate. The most common noncontact ACL injury mechanism involves a deceleration and rotational injury during running, cutting, or jumping activities. The most common contact injury involves either hyperextension and/or valgus forces to the knee by a direct blow.

ACL injury is often associated with a "pop" heard by the patient at the time of injury. This piece of history is not ACL specific, however. Upon return to competition, the patient will often notice instability of the knee or describe the knee "giving out" with twisting activities. Substantial knee swelling secondary to a hemarthrosis typically occurs within the first 4–12 hours following the injury.

▶ Signs (Physical Examination)

With the above history obtained and a proper physical examination, an ACL tear should be able to be diagnosed without any additional tests. A complete examination of the knee should be performed to evaluate for any other associated injuries. The uninjured knee is examined first to familiarize the patient with the knee examination.

The Lachman test is the most useful test for anterior laxity of the knee. The Lachman test is performed with the knee in 20–30 degrees of flexion as an anterior force is applied to the tibia while the other hand stabilizes the distal femur. The degree of anterior translation and the presence and character of an end point are assessed. The laxity is graded based on comparison to the uninjured contralateral knee. Grade 1 laxity is 1–4 mm of increased translation. Grade 2 laxity is 5–9 mm of increased translation. Grade 3 laxity is more than 10 mm of translation as compared to the injured contralateral knee.

The anterior drawer test is another test to evaluate anterior tibial translation. This is performed with the knee in 90 degrees of flexion as an anterior force is applied to the tibia. This test is less sensitive than the Lachman test.

In the acute setting of an ACL tear, there is often a window where an accurate examination can occur before extensive knee swelling and guarding inhibit examination. Aspiration of a hemarthrosis can help to decrease pain and improve the quality of the examination in the acute setting as well.

The pivot shift test (Losee test) is performed to test the rotational instability associated with an ACL tear. The test is based on the lateral tibial plateau subluxing anteriorly with extension and reduction of the lateral compartment with flexion. The most effective method of achieving this result is by flexing the knee with an axial load from full extension with valgus stress at the knee and internal rotation of the tibia. The reduction of the subluxation should occur at approximately 30 degrees of flexion. MCL injury and some meniscal tears may produce a false-negative test.

The pivot shift test is considered the most functional test to evaluate knee stability after ACL injury. An examination under anesthesia is also often useful in obtaining a more accurate pivot shift test. This can be useful in a patient with an unclear history of instability and an equivocal examination in the office.

▶ Imaging Studies

Plain radiographs of the knee should be obtained to rule out fractures about the knee. The Segond fracture, as discussed earlier, is an avulsion of the anterolateral capsule of the tibia. Before skeletal maturity, an avulsion of the tibial insertion of the ACL can also be seen radiographically. Following radiographs, an MRI is the most useful examination for an evaluation of associated injuries. Although generally not needed for diagnosis of an ACL tear, MRI can diagnose an ACL tear with 95% or better accuracy. Bone bruises of the lateral femoral condyle and lateral tibial plateau are noted in up to 80% of ACL injuries.

▶ Special Studies

Instrumented laxity evaluations can augment the physical examination and provide an objective baseline for future comparison. The most commonly used arthrometer, the KT-1000 (MEDmetric, San Diego, CA), uses a series of standard forces to measure anterior translation of the tibia with the knee in 20–30 degrees of flexion similar to the Lachman test.

▶ Treatment

A. Nonsurgical

Rehabilitation following an isolated ACL injury should include an effort to regain knee motion and strengthen the muscles about the knee. Returning to activities that produce episodes of instability is discouraged. Once motion and strength have been restored, a gradual return to activities can be attempted to determine the functional level that can be attained without instability.

Nonoperative management with rehabilitation after an ACL injury generally yields poor results in patients who return to competitive activities. Significant episodes of instability resulting in pain, swelling, and disability occur in about 80% of individuals who participate in sporting activities such as tennis, football, and soccer. These episodes of instability are thought to place the menisci and articular cartilage of the knee at risk for further injury (Figure 3–15).

B. Surgical

The decision to surgically reconstruct an ACL tear is individualized and based on the patient's desire to return to competition, age, accompanying degenerative changes, and objective and subjective knee instability. For example, a young, active patient with continued desire to compete in cutting and jumping sports with both objective and subjective knee instability may be best treated with surgical reconstruction. On the other hand, an older patient with some degenerative arthritis of the knee and minimal desire for continued competitive athletics and no subjective instability would be much more suited to nonsurgical care.

Early in the history of ACL surgery, primary repairs of the ligament were found to do poorly. This gave way to ligament reconstruction using a variety of graft materials. Everything from synthetics to autograft and allograft tissues

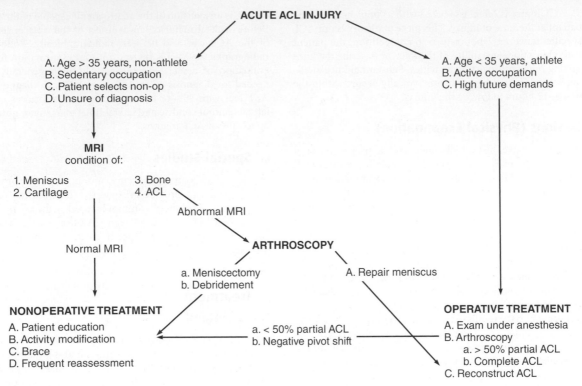

ACUTE ACL INJURY

A. Age > 35 years, non-athlete
B. Sedentary occupation
C. Patient selects non-op
D. Unsure of diagnosis

A. Age < 35 years, athlete
B. Active occupation
C. High future demands

MRI
condition of:

1. Meniscus   3. Bone
2. Cartilage   4. ACL

Abnormal MRI

Normal MRI

ARTHROSCOPY

a. Meniscectomy   A. Repair meniscus
b. Debridement

NONOPERATIVE TREATMENT

A. Patient education
B. Activity modification
C. Brace
D. Frequent reassessment

a. < 50% partial ACL
b. Negative pivot shift

OPERATIVE TREATMENT

A. Exam under anesthesia
B. Arthroscopy
   a. > 50% partial ACL
   b. Complete ACL
C. Reconstruct ACL

▲ **Figure 3–15.** Flow chart that summarizes the current management of acute anterior cruciate ligament (ACL) injuries. MRI, magnetic resonance imaging. (Reproduced, with permission, from Marzo JM, Warren RF: Results of nonoperative treatment of anterior cruciate ligament injury: changing perspectives. *Adv Orthop Surg* 1991;15:59.)

has been used for reconstruction of the ACL. Over time, autograft bone-patellar tendon-bone, semitendinosus/gracilis hamstring autograft, and allograft bone-patellar tendonbone constructs have proven to be the most commonly used grafts and have been successful for ACL reconstructions.

The goal of ACL reconstruction is to reproduce the strength, function, and location of the intact ACL. Recently, there have been some articles challenging the results seen after single-bundle reconstruction. They point to instability in up to 30% of patients and only a 60–70% return to sport. Therefore, in an effort to replicate the normal anatomy and try to improve outcomes after ACL surgery, the doublebundle reconstruction has been advocated. This technique attempts to take advantage of the anatomy of the native ACL, which is composed of two bundles: anteromedial (AM) and posterolateral. The AM bundle is thought to provide stability to anteroposterior movement, and the posterolateral bundle provides rotational control. Advocates of the double-bundle reconstruction point to its ability to resist rotatory loads and mimic normal knee kinematics more closely. Biomechanical and some level I studies have demonstrated a benefit in objective rotational stability, but a clear clinical improvement has not been proven versus traditional single-bundle

reconstruction. Double-bundle versus single-bundle reconstruction of the ACL remains a controversial and highly debated topic. Regardless of whether single-bundle or doublebundle reconstruction is used, the focus should be on attempting to restore the normal anatomy of the ACL with the position and placement of the tunnels.

1. Single bundle—Once a graft of adequate strength is selected, the location of placement of the graft is of utmost importance. The graft is generally passed through a bone tunnel in the tibia and a bone tunnel through the femur. The intraarticular placement of the tibial tunnel is generally in the center of the native ACL stump just in front of the PCL origin and just medial to the center of the notch in the coronal plane for a single-bundle reconstruction (Figures 3–16 and 3–17).

Once the graft is in place, the proper tension and fixation of the graft must occur to achieve a successful ACL reconstruction. Establishing proper tension in the graft is important. A lax ACL graft may not restore stability to the knee, and an overtightened graft may cause failure of the graft or limit knee range of motion. Fixation of the graft is achieved through a variety of measures. The most common method

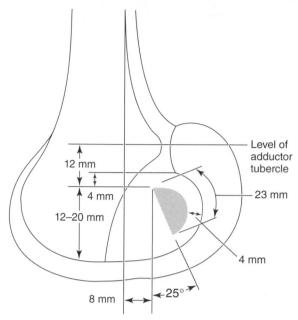

▲ **Figure 3–16.** Drawing of the medial surface of the right lateral femoral condyle showing the average measurements and body relations of the femoral attachment of the anterior cruciate ligament. (Reproduced, with permission, from Arnoczky SP: Anatomy of the anterior cruciate ligament. *Clin Orthop Relat Res* 1983;172:19.)

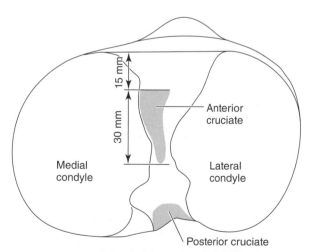

▲ **Figure 3–17.** The upper surface of the tibial plateau to show average measurements and relations of the tibial attachments of the anterior cruciate ligament. (Reproduced, with permission, from Girgis FC, Marshall JL, Monajem A: The cruciate ligaments of the knee joint: anatomical, functional, and experimental analysis. *Clin Orthop Relat Res* 1975;106:216.)

involves placing an interference screw up the bone tunnel that captures the graft in the tunnel. The graft can also be fixed via sutures tied over various devices located on the outer cortex of the tunnels.

2. Double bundle—There are a couple differences to point out with the double-bundle reconstruction. First, an accessory AM portal is required in addition to the AM and anterolateral portals normally required for a knee arthroscopy. This portal becomes crucial for drilling accurately the femoral-sided tunnels, especially the AM femoral tunnel. Furthermore, special attention is taken to examine the tear pattern, which helps in locating the native locations of the AM and posterolateral bundles. Measuring the width/length of the insertions is also important because an ACL insertion less than 12 mm is extremely difficult technically to perform. Care must also be taken to ensure that there is at least a 2-mm bridge of bone between the two tunnels or the risk of convergence of the tunnels becomes very high. The recommended grafts by the authors at Pittsburgh are two tibialis anterior or posterior allograft tendons. Fixation on the femoral side is done with EndoButtons (Smith and Nephew endoscopy) and on the tibial side with interference screws. The grafts are tensioned at 0–15 degrees for the posterolateral bundle and 45–60 degrees for the AM bundle.

▶ **Complications**

Although ACL reconstruction often results in a successful outcome, there are several complications that can occur. One of the most common complications is a loss of knee motion. This is minimized by obtaining and maintaining full knee extension immediately following surgery. Knee flexion exercises are begun as soon as possible postoperatively, with a goal of 90 degrees by 1 week after surgery. Additionally, patellar mobilization is performed in an attempt to minimize patellofemoral scarring. Another common complication of ACL reconstruction is anterior knee pain. The exact etiology of this pain is unclear. However, it is thought that patellar tendon autograft harvest may increase the incidence of patellofemoral pain. Less common complications (<1%) include patellar fracture, patellar tendon rupture, and quadriceps tendon rupture depending on the graft harvest site.

▶ **Results/Return to Play**

The goal of any rehabilitation protocol for an ACL reconstruction is to return the patient to the full desired level of activity in as short amount of time as possible while avoiding any complications or setbacks. Through improved surgical techniques and accelerated rehabilitation protocols, most studies have shown a 90% or better return to play and patient satisfaction. Patients generally are able to return between 4 and 6 months postoperatively, with some professional athletes returning successfully to competition in 3 months. Specific criteria for return to sports vary from institution to institution, with a combination of functional testing, subjective reporting, and clinical examination contributing to the decision. In general, the criteria for return to sports include full range of motion, KT1000 testing within 2–3 mm of the uninjured knee, ≥85% quadriceps strength and full hamstring strength, and functional testing within 85% of the contralateral leg.

Herrington L, Wrapson C, Matthews M, et al: Anterior cruciate ligament reconstruction, hamstring versus bone-patella tendon-bone grafts: a systematic literature review of outcome from surgery. *Knee* 2005;12:41. [PMID: 15664877]

Järvelä T, Moisala AS, Sihvonen R, et al: Double-bundle anterior cruciate ligament reconstruction using hamstring autografts and bioabsorbable interference screw fixation: prospective, randomized clinical study with 2 year results. *Am J Sports Med* 2008;36:290. [PMID: 17940145]

Laxdal G, Kartus J, Hansson L, et al: A prospective randomized comparison of bone-patellar tendon-bone and hamstring grafts for anterior cruciate ligament reconstruction. *Arthroscopy* 2005;21:34. [PMID: 15650664]

Prodromos CC, Fu FH, Howell SM, et al: Controversies in soft-tissue anterior cruciate ligament reconstruction: grafts, bundles, tunnels, fixation and harvest. *J Am Acad Orthop Surg* 2008;16:376. [PMID: 18611995]

4. Posterior Cruciate Ligament Injuries

▶ Essentials of Diagnosis

- *Most common mechanisms of injury are a direct blow to the anterior tibia with the knee flexed or a fall into the ground with the foot plantar flexed.*
- *Patients complain of knee pain, swelling, and stiffness.*
- *Physical examination may show positive posterior drawer, Godfrey, and reverse pivot shift tests.*
- *Must perform thorough knee exam because concomitant injuries are common with PCL injury (posterolateral corner, meniscus).*
- *Imaging studies should include plain radiographs as well as confirmatory MRI. Radiographs are helpful in chronic setting of PCL to assess patellofemoral and medial compartment arthritis.*

▶ Symptoms (History)

When evaluating a patient for a PCL injury, it is important to obtain the mechanism of injury, the severity of the injury, and any potential associated injuries. In contrast to an ACL tear, it is rare for patients with PCL injuries to report hearing a "pop" or report any feelings of subjective instability. More commonly, patients will complain of knee pain, swelling, and stiffness.

The presentation of a patient with a subacute or chronically injured PCL can range from asymptomatic to significant instability and pain. Patients with significant varus alignment or injury to the lateral structures of the knee will often complain of feelings of instability and giving way. There are a few characteristic mechanisms of PCL injury that differ significantly from the mechanism of ACL injuries. One of the most common mechanisms of PCL injury is the "dashboard" injury during which the anterior tibia sustains a posteriorly directed force from the dashboard with the knee in 90 degrees of flexion. Sports injuries to the PCL result from an outside force or blow, in contrast to the typical deceleration twisting mechanism of an ACL injury. The most common methods of a sports PCL injury include a direct blow to the anterior tibia or via a fall onto the flexed knee with the foot in plantar flexion. The most common mechanism for isolated PCL injury in the athlete is a partial tear associated with hyperflexion of the knee. Additionally, significant multiligamentous knee injuries with PCL tears can be seen after a varus or valgus stress is applied to the hyperextended knee.

▶ Signs (Physical Examination)

As with other ligamentous injuries, a thorough knee examination is necessary. Specific cues to injury to the PCL on initial inspection include abrasions or ecchymosis around the proximal anterior tibia and ecchymosis in the popliteal fossa. Assessment for meniscal damage and associated ligamentous injury should be performed. Evaluation of ACL laxity in the presence of an acute PCL injury is challenging due to the lack of a stable reference point to perform a Lachman or anterior drawer test.

Examination of the PCL in the acutely injured knee can be challenging. Despite increased awareness of the injury, many PCL injuries go undiagnosed in the acute setting. The most accurate clinical test of PCL integrity is the posterior drawer test. The knee is flexed to 90 degrees with the patient supine and a posteriorly directed force is applied to the anterior tibia. The amount of posterior translation and the presence and character of the end point are noted. The extent of translation is assessed by noting the change in the distance of the step-off between the AM tibial plateau and the medial femoral condyle. The tibial plateau is approximately 1 cm anterior to the medial femoral condyle on average. However, the contralateral knee must be examined to establish a baseline.

Another test for examination of the PCL is the posterior sag or Godfrey test. This test involves flexing the knee and hip and noting the posterior pull of gravity creating posterior "sag" of the tibia on the femur. An adjunct to this test involves watching for a reduction of this subluxation with active quadriceps contraction.

The reverse pivot shift is the analog to the pivot shift in the evaluation of an ACL injury. This is performed by placing a valgus stress on the knee with the foot externally rotated. The knee is then extended from 90 degrees of flexion, and a palpable reduction of the posterolateral tibial plateau is noted between 20 and 30 degrees of flexion.

It is extremely important to evaluate the posterolateral structures of the knee in the setting of a suspected PCL injury. Injury to the posterolateral structures has been reported to occur in up to 60% of PCL injuries.

▶ Imaging Studies

A. Radiographs

Given the magnitude of the forces required to injure the PCL, plain radiographs of the knee are essential to evaluate for bony injuries, dislocation, or evidence of other associated injuries. Subtle posterior subluxation on the lateral radiograph may also indicate PCL injury. Stress posterior drawer radiographs and contralateral comparisons may also increase the sensitivity for detecting PCL injuries with plain radiographs. In the chronic setting of PCL injury, radiographs are useful to assess for patellofemoral and medial compartment degenerative changes that can occur over time.

B. MRI

Although plain films are necessary and useful in the evaluations of these injuries, MRI has become the diagnostic study of choice for the knee with a presumed PCL injury. MRI has been reported to be 96–100% sensitive at diagnosing PCL tears. Equally or more importantly, MRI is extremely valuable in its ability to detect associated injuries. This is particularly important in diagnosing posterolateral corner injuries because these can often be missed on the initial clinical examination. In multiligamentous knee injuries, MRI can also be of use in assessing the ACL as clinical examination of the ACL is challenging in the setting of a complete PCL tear.

C. Special Studies

In the setting of a chronic isolated PCL tear, pain in the medial and patellofemoral compartments is generally evaluated with radiographs. If these are normal, some surgeons will proceed with a bone scan to evaluate for increased uptake in these areas. Areas under increased stress demonstrate increased uptake on the bone scan before signs of advanced arthritis occur on radiographs. This subset of patients may benefit from a PCL reconstruction to decrease the stress and delay osteoarthritis.

▶ Treatment

There is significant controversy in the treatment of isolated PCL injuries. There are multiple factors that must be evaluated in the decision to treat a complete PCL rupture. The patient's age, activity level, expectations, and associated injuries must be taken into account. The literature on operative versus nonsurgical treatment of these injuries can be difficult to interpret, and there are no long-term follow-up studies of randomized patient groups.

A. Nonsurgical

Rehabilitation of the PCL injured knee is often largely dependent on the associated injuries sustained by the knee. This is particularly true with the commonly associated posterolateral corner injury. Therefore, we will focus on the rehabilitation of the isolated PCL injured knee. Regaining motion and strength are the two key objectives of a rehabilitation program. Obtaining full quadriceps strength is essential for achieving the optimal result with nonsurgical treatment. The initial treatment is aimed at keeping the tibia reduced under the femur and minimizing tension on the injured PCL. With partial injuries (grade I and II), the prognosis is quite good, and early motion with weight bearing is the usual course of therapy. In a complete PCL tear, most will keep the knee immobilized in extension to protect the posterolateral structures. Early strengthening exercises focus on quadriceps strength with quadriceps sets, straight leg raises, and partial weight bearing in extension.

Overall, most patients benefit from nonsurgical treatment of a PCL tear. Despite objective findings of instability that are often noted on examination, most patients subjectively are satisfied with the function of the knee. Bracing is generally ineffective in controlling PCL laxity clinically.

The main subjective complaint with chronic PCL insufficiency, however, is pain rather than instability. A PCL-deficient knee with posterior tibial subluxation places significantly increased stresses on the patellofemoral and medial compartments of the knee. In one series where patients with PCL injuries were followed with serial radiographs, 60% of patients displayed some degenerative changes of the medial compartment.

B. Surgical

Surgical management of PCL injuries are broken down into avulsion fractures, isolated acute PCL injuries, multiligamentous injuries, and chronic PCL insufficiency. Avulsion fractures of the PCL are rare fractures. If nondisplaced, these injuries are treated nonsurgically. If significantly displaced, these fractures are generally treated with open reduction and internal fixation.

Isolated PCL injuries are generally still treated with nonsurgical care by the majority of surgeons at this time. However, it has been shown that nonoperative care of these injuries is not without consequences. Although subjective results in these patients are good in the short term, many continue to have objective instability and display degenerative arthritic changes over time. A follow-up of PCL-deficient knees at an average of 15 years after injury found that 89% of patients had persistent pain and half had chronic effusions. All patients in this group showed degenerative changes when followed for 25 years. Therefore, given the risks of continued instability and the potential of an increased chance of arthritic changes, surgical reconstruction of the PCL is a reasonable choice.

Initially, surgical care of complete PCL tears consisted of a primary repair of midsubstance tears. The objective stability of these repairs was generally disappointing. Current reconstruction methods generally involve routing either autograft or allograft tendons through bone tunnels to reconstruct the PCL in an anatomic fashion. Although there are several different methods of reconstructing the PCL, the two main categories of PCL reconstruction consist of single- and double-bundle repairs. Classically, reconstructions of the PCL anatomically replicated the anterolateral bundle of the native PCL with a single-bundle reconstruction. As problems were noted with recurrence of posterior laxity in the postoperative period, a double-bundle technique was derived to reconstruct both the anterolateral and posteromedial bundles of the native PCL. The advantages of the double-bundle technique are thus far theoretical, and there is no long-term clinical follow-up demonstrating the superiority of a double-bundle reconstruction at this time.

The severe instability noted with PCL injuries associated with multiligamentous knee injuries makes the argument for ligament reconstruction more compelling in this patient population. Many of the studies involving PCL reconstruction in these complex knee injuries have involved primary repair attempts. Although subjective results were generally good, residual excessive, objective laxity was very common following repairs. More recently, ligament reconstructions with allograft and autograft have become the dominant method of PCL reconstruction in this challenging patient population.

Complications

The most common complication following PCL reconstruction is the return of objective posterior laxity on physical examination. This does not present as subjective laxity, however, and patient satisfaction remains high despite objective laxity. Acute PCL reconstructions in the setting of a multiligamentous knee repair/reconstruction can result in arthrofibrosis with extensive postoperative scarring.

Results/Return to Play

Even with nonsurgical management of a PCL injury, the prognosis for a functional recovery and return to competition is very good. A strong quadriceps muscle and extensor mechanism can significantly compensate for PCL laxity. Athletes should spend a minimum of 3 months in rehabilitation before attempting a return to competition. However, a subset of patients experience significant instability with a grade III PCL injury that does not allow a return to competition. This subset of patients may benefit from PCL reconstruction.

On the other hand, the prognosis for a PCL tear associated with a multiligamentous knee injury is guarded with respect to return to play. Although prompt recognition of a multiligamentous injury and appropriately timed treatment, reconstruction, and rehabilitation are essential for optimal recovery, these injuries are such that a significant percentage of patients will not be able to return to full competition.

Jung TM, Lubowicki A, Wienand A, Wagner M, Weiler A: Knee stability after posterior cruciate ligament reconstruction in female versus male patients: a prospective matched-group analysis. *Arthroscopy* 2011;27:399. [PMID: 21168303]

Li G, Papannagari R, Li M, et al: Effect of posterior cruciate ligament deficiency on in vivo translation and rotation of the knee during weightbearing flexion. *Am J Sports Med* 2008;36:474. [PMID: 18057390]

Lien OA, Aas EJ, Johansen S, Ludvigsen TC, Figved W, Engebretsen L: Clinical outcome after reconstruction for isolated posterior cruciate ligament injury. *Knee Surg Sports Traumatol Arthrosc* 2010;18:1568. [PMID: 20571763]

McAllister DR, Petrigliano FA: Diagnosis and treatment of posterior cruciate ligament injuries. *Curr Sports Med Rep* 2007;6:293. [PMID: 17883964]

▶ CPT Codes for Ligament Injuries to the Knee

27405 Repair, primary, torn ligament and/or capsule, knee; collateral

27407 Repair, primary, torn ligament and/or capsule, knee; cruciate

27409 Repair, primary, torn ligament and/or capsule, knee; collateral and cruciate ligaments

27427 Ligamentous reconstruction (augmentation), knee; extraarticular

27428 Ligamentous reconstruction (augmentation), knee; intraarticular (open)

27429 Ligamentous reconstruction (augmentation), knee; intraarticular (open) and extraarticular

27552 Closed treatment of knee dislocation; requiring anesthesia

27556 Open treatment of knee dislocation, includes internal fixation, when performed; without primary ligamentous repair or augmentation/reconstruction

27557 Open treatment of knee dislocation, includes internal fixation, when performed; with primary ligamentous repair

27558 Open treatment of knee dislocation, includes internal fixation, when performed; with primary ligamentous repair, with augmentation/reconstruction

27570 Manipulation of knee joint under general anesthesia (includes application of traction or other fixation devices)

29850 Arthroscopically aided treatment of intercondylar spine(s) and/or tuberosity fracture(s) of the knee, with or without manipulation; without internal or external fixation (includes arthroscopy)

29875 Arthroscopy, knee, surgical; synovectomy, limited (eg, plica or shelf resection) (separate procedure)

29876 Arthroscopy, knee, surgical; synovectomy, major, two or more compartments (eg, medial or lateral)

29884 Arthroscopy, knee, surgical; with lysis of adhesions, with or without manipulation (separate procedure)

29888 Arthroscopically aided anterior cruciate ligament repair/augmentation or reconstruction

29889 Arthroscopically aided posterior cruciate ligament repair/augmentation or reconstruction

5. Patella Dislocation

▶ Essentials of Diagnosis

- *Almost always a lateral dislocation.*
- *Pain, swelling, and tenderness over medial border of the patella and apprehension with knee flexed and patella pushed laterally.*
- *Check hypermobility of the contralateral knee for comparison.*
- *Look for osteochondral fragment on radiographs.*

Dislocation of the patella is a potential cause of acute hemarthrosis and must be considered when evaluating a patient with an acute knee injury. The injury occurs when valgus force and external rotation of the tibia are applied to a flexed leg. It is most common in females in the second decade of life.

▶ Clinical Findings

The patella almost always dislocates laterally. The patient may notice the patella sitting laterally or might say that the rest of the knee has shifted medially. It is unusual to see actual dislocation of the patella except at the time of injury. Reduction occurs when the knee is extended.

Examination will demonstrate tenderness over the medial retinaculum and adductor tubercle, which is the origin of the medial patellofemoral ligament. The patient will also have pain and apprehension when the patella is pushed laterally with the knee slightly bent. Radiographs, including an axial patellar view, should be obtained to determine whether there are osteochondral fractures. Often, a small fleck of bone is avulsed by the capsule on the medial aspect of the patella. This is not intraarticular and does not require removal. A displaced osteochondral fracture will require excision or internal fixation. Examination of the uninjured knee is recommended to determine whether there are predisposing factors for dislocation, such as patella alta, genu recurvatum, increased Q angle, and patellar hypermobility. Patella alta, or high-riding patella, is identified by measuring the length of the patellar tendon and dividing by the length of the patella. The upper limit of normal is 1.2. The Q angle is formed by a line through the patellar tendon intersecting a line from the anterior superior iliac spine in the center of the patella. A normal Q angle is about 10 degrees, with a range of about plus or minus 5 degrees. Patients with generalized hypermobility have increased extension of the knee, or genu recurvatum, which in effect gives them patella alta. They also often have hypermobility of all the capsular ligamentous

structures, including the static stabilizers of the kneecap, giving them significant patellar hypermobility.

▶ Treatment and Prognosis

A wide variety of treatment options have been recommended for patellar dislocations, including immediate mobilization and strengthening exercises, immobilization in a cylinder cast for 6 weeks followed by rehabilitation, arthroscopy with or without retinacular repair, surgical repair of the torn retinaculum, or immediate patellar realignment.

Treatment is based on which predisposing factors are present. Little is lost by functional treatment, similar to the treatment of isolated MCL sprains, which is often successful. If dislocation recurs, realignment may be performed. A long-term study showed that patients treated surgically for patellar malalignment problems had a higher incidence of osteoarthritis than those treated nonoperatively.

Buchner M, Baudendistel B, Sabo D, et al: Acute traumatic primary patellar dislocation: long-term results comparing conservative and surgical treatment. *Clin J Sport Med* 2005;15:62. [PMID: 15782048]

Gerbino PG, Zurakowski D, Soto R, et al: Long-term functional outcome after lateral patellar retinacular release in adolescents: an observational cohort study with minimum 5 year follow-up. *J Pediatr Orthop* 2008;28:118. [PMID: 18157056]

Smith TO, Davies L, Chester R, Clark A, Donell ST: Clinical outcomes of rehabilitation for patients following lateral patellar dislocation: a systematic review. *Physiotherapy* 2010;96:269. PMID: 21056161]

▶ CPT Codes for Patellar Dislocations

27340 Excision, prepatellar bursa

27420 Reconstruction of dislocating patella (eg, Hauser-type procedure)

27422 Reconstruction of dislocating patella, with extensor realignment and/or muscle advancement or release (eg, Campbell, Goldwaite-type procedure)

27524 Open treatment of patellar fracture, with internal fixation and/or partial or complete patellectomy and soft-tissue repair

27562 Closed treatment of patellar dislocation; requiring anesthesia

27566 Open treatment of patellar dislocation, with or without partial or total patellectomy

27570 Manipulation of knee joint under general anesthesia (includes application of traction or other fixation devices)

29435 Application of patellar tendon bearing cast

29873 Arthroscopy, knee, surgical; with lateral release

29874 Arthroscopy, knee, surgical; for removal of loose body or foreign body (eg, osteochondritis dissecans fragmentation, chondral fragmentation)

KNEE TENDON INJURY

Ruptures of the quadriceps and patellar tendons usually result from a tremendous eccentric contraction of the quadriceps muscle, as may occur when an athlete stumbles and tries not to fall. Both types of ruptures are more common in patients with underlying disorders of the tendon.

1. Rupture of the Quadriceps Tendon

▶ Essentials of Diagnosis

- *Occur in patients older than 40 years.*
- *Patient will be unable to extend the knee.*
- *The quadriceps will retract proximally if left untreated.*

Quadriceps tendon ruptures occur most frequently in patients over 40 years old. Biopsies of fresh rupture sites showed local degenerative changes already present, consistent with the theory that normal tendons do not rupture. Rarely the injury occurs bilaterally and is often associated with gout, diabetes, or steroid use. When it does occur bilaterally with only a small amount of trauma, the diagnosis may be difficult to make because of the small amount of swelling or symptoms of injury.

The cardinal symptom is inability to extend the knee. When extension is attempted, a gap develops in the suprapatellar region. The patella rides at a slightly lower level, and the anterior border of the femoral condyles may be palpated.

Acute complete quadriceps tendon ruptures should be paired surgically. If left untreated, proximal migration and scarring of the quadriceps muscle will occur. Direct-end repair produces excellent results. Neutralizing the forces across the repair is difficult, and immobilization in extension is recommended. Repair of ruptures more than 2 weeks old may be difficult and may require quadriceps lengthening, muscle or tendon transfers, or a combination of these procedures.

West JL, Keene JS, Kaplan LD: Early motion after quadriceps and patellar tendon repairs: outcomes with single-suture augmentation. *Am J Sports Med* 2008;36:316. [PMID: 17932403]

2. Rupture of the Patellar Tendon

▶ Essentials of Diagnosis

- *Typically occurs in patients younger than 40.*
- *Patella alta on radiographs.*
- *Inability to extend the knee.*

Rupture of the patella tendon occurs more frequently in patients less than 40 years old. The patient cannot actively extend the knee, the patella is high-riding, and a defect is palpable beneath the patella. Surgical repair is the treatment of choice. The tendon, along with the medial and lateral retinaculum, should be sewn end to end. A stress-relieving wire may be placed around the patella and through the tibial tubercle. The wire should be removed in 6–8 weeks. Chronic patellar tendon ruptures are very hard to treat. The quadriceps must be freed up from the femur and the patella pulled down to the proper location. The gracilis and semitendinosus tendons can be used to substitute for the patellar tendon.

The extensor mechanism may also be disrupted at the inferior pole of the patella where the patellar tendon originates. This usually occurs in a child aged between 8 and 12 years. The distal pole of the patella plus a large sleeve of articular cartilage is pulled off (Figure 3–18). This may be easily misdiagnosed if the fragment of bone is small. Reestablishment of an intact extensor mechanism is necessary. With displaced fractures, open reduction and internal fixation with tension band wiring are recommended.

Brooks P: Extensor mechanism ruptures. *Orthopedics* 2009;32:9. [PMID: 19751001]

▶ CPT Codes for Tendon Ruptures

27380 Suture of infrapatellar tendon; primary

27381 Suture of infrapatellar tendon; secondary reconstruction, including fascial or tendon graft

27385 Suture of quadriceps or hamstring muscle rupture; primary

27386 Suture of quadriceps or hamstring muscle rupture; secondary reconstruction, including fascial or tendon graft

27430 Quadricepsplasty

KNEE PAIN

Pain in the knee region is a very common complaint of athletes. If there is no history of an acute injury, then overuse is commonly the cause. The patient is often able to point to the area of pain. The history of activity must be obtained as well as overall evaluation of the extremities.

1. Anterior Knee Pain

▶ Patellofemoral Disorders

A. Essentials of Diagnosis

- *Pain with activity involving stairs or hills.*
- *Commonly involves young females.*
- *Check Q angle, femoral anteversion, patellar mobility, and quadriceps strength and tone.*
- *On radiographs, look for valgus alignment of knee, OCLs, and patella alta.*

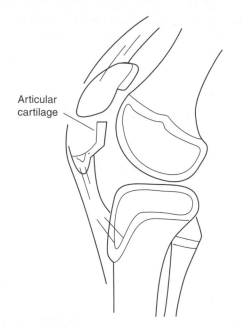

Articular cartilage

A

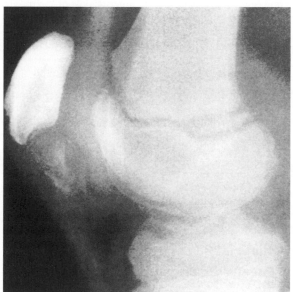

B

▲ **Figure 3–18.** Sleeve fracture of the patella. **A:** A small segment of the distal pole of the patella is avulsed with a relatively large portion of the articular surface. **B:** Lateral radiograph of the knee with a displaced sleeve fracture of the patella. Note that the small osseous portion of the displaced fragment is visible, but the cartilaginous portion is not seen. (Reproduced, with permission, from Rockwood CA Jr, ed: *Fractures in Children*, 3rd ed. Philadelphia: Lippincott; 1991.)

B. Clinical Findings

1. Symptoms and signs—This is a common complaint and is frequently bilateral. It is most common in females during the second decade of life. The patellofemoral joint is often the source of pain. Entities such as chondromalacia patella, patellofemoral arthralgia, and lateral patellofemoral compression syndrome are diagnostic considerations.

Patellar pain is often felt when going up or down hills or stairs, and there may be complaints of instability during walking, running, or other sports activities. These activities may create a joint reaction force of several times the body weight on the patella with each step. Swelling is seldom a complaint. If the pain is in one knee only, the patient may alter the way of climbing and descending stairs so that the affected leg is kept straight and each step leads with the same foot. This strategy significantly decreases the joint reaction force on the patellofemoral joint.

Many of these problems arise because the patellofemoral joint is semiconstrained, especially in the range of 0–20 degrees of flexion, and the constraint increases as flexion increases. The degree of constraint is also dependent on a number of other factors, including the angle of the sulcus of the femur, the presence or absence of patella alta, and the generalized ligamentous laxity of the patient. In addition, femoral anteversion and increased Q angle (Figure 3–19) may lead to increased instability of the patellofemoral joint. This lack of constraint may predispose the patella to frank dislocation, although subluxation is a much more common finding. The degree of congruity is anatomically variable and may lead to high-contact stresses caused by anatomic configuration and static and dynamic constraints on the patella. Increased pressure may cause pain and patellofemoral osteoarthritis.

On physical examination of the patient with patellofemoral subluxation, minimal findings in relation to complaints may be present. Occasionally, crepitance, a crackling or clicking sound, is found with flexion and extension. Quadriceps strength, tone, and bulk are usually reduced. Pain may be elicited at a particular angle of flexion by putting the knee through its range of motion with resistance. Subluxation may often be diagnosed with the apprehension sign, a rapid contraction of the quadriceps when the patella is passively moved laterally.

2. Imaging studies—Roentgenographic examination will frequently show a valgus angulation of the knee on anteroposterior views. Occasionally, patella alta may be identified on the lateral view, and tangential views of the patella at various knee flexion angles will reveal a lack of contact of the medial facet of the patella with the medial facet of the trochlear groove of the femur. Lateral subluxation of the patellofemoral joint may also be observed.

This syndrome with a normal roentgenographic examination is frequently called chondromalacia patellae, or with subluxation identified on radiograph, it is referred to as patellofemoral subluxation. A more accurate term would

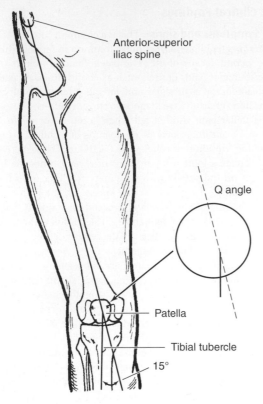

▲ **Figure 3–19.** Q angle and valgus angulation. (Reproduced, with permission, from American Academy of Orthopaedic Surgeons: *Athletic Training and Sports Medicine*, 2nd ed. Burlington: Jones and Bartlett; 1991.)

be patellofemoral arthralgia, because patellofemoral subluxation was probably present prior to the onset of pain and because chondromalacia patellae (softening of the patellar cartilage) is an arthroscopic or pathologic diagnosis. Patellofemoral arthralgia is a clinical diagnosis.

C. Treatment

1. Chondromalacia patellae—Initially, treatment is conservative, with the intent of improving quadriceps strength and stamina to stabilize the patellofemoral joint. Weight loss is prescribed to decrease the stress on the patellofemoral joint; reduction in loading the knee in the flexed position also accomplishes pressure reduction. Knee orthotics may be beneficial. When subluxation and fear of dislocation are major concerns, an orthotic that limits extension of the knee may be beneficial because the patella becomes inherently more stable with knee flexion. Nonsteroidal anti-inflammatory medication may be beneficial.

2. Patellofemoral arthralgia—Only when conservative treatment has been exhausted is surgical treatment considered. Alteration in the alignment of the patellofemoral joint may

be beneficial in patellofemoral arthralgia. Lateral retinacular release followed by a period of conservative treatment will be beneficial in some cases. Distal realignment may be necessary to achieve appropriate alignment and reduction in pain in those cases with an abnormality such as valgus knee or increased femoral anteversion.

3. Patellofemoral compression syndrome—With lateral patellofemoral compression syndrome, there is tenderness along the lateral facet of the patella or along the femoral condyle. Without cartilage damage, an effusion is rarely present. Treatment includes decreasing the activity level, including avoiding hills or step aerobics. Ice massage, quadriceps and hamstring stretching, and short-arc quadriceps exercises against resistance are recommended to strengthen the vastus medialis obliquus muscle without aggravating the pain. Patellar supports or neoprene sleeves may also be helpful. Most patients will respond to this regimen and gradually resume their activities. The role of releasing a contracted lateral patellofemoral retinaculum is controversial.

4. Patellar tendinitis—Patellar tendinitis, or jumper's knee, is seen in basketball and volleyball players. Tenderness along the tendon, usually at the inferior pole of the patella, is noted. Treatment with ice and avoiding jumping usually suffice. In refractory cases, debridement of mucinous degenerative material from the tendon may be successful.

D. Prognosis

The prognosis for jumper's knee is quite good. The condition is often persistent but self-limiting. The patient can always alleviate the symptoms by avoiding the activities that cause the problem.

Collado H, Fredericson M: Patellofemoral pain syndrome. *Clin Sports Med* 2010;29:379. [PMID: 20610028]

2. Lateral Knee Pain

▶ Iliotibial Band Friction Syndrome

A. Essentials of Diagnosis

- *Lateral knee pain.*
- *Commonly affects runners and cyclists.*
- *Tenderness over lateral epicondyle and positive Ober test.*

Lateral knee pain that is not located on the joint line may result from iliotibial band friction syndrome. This is a form of bursitis caused by rubbing of the iliotibial band against the lateral epicondyle. Tenderness over the lateral epicondyle at about 30 degrees of flexion when the knee is being extended is indicative of this diagnosis. The Ober test, with abduction and then adduction of the leg, can also demonstrate the tightness of the iliotibial band when the patient is in a lateral decubitus position and the hip is hyperextended. Runners and cyclists are commonly afflicted. Crossover gait or running on banked terrain is thought to be a causative factor.

Treatment involves decreasing the athlete's activities, ice massage, stretching of the iliotibial tract, and use of a lateral wedge orthotic in patients with heel varus. Running on flat terrain and changing the gait pattern may be helpful. In cyclists, lowering the seat height so the full extension of the knee is not reached and adjusting the pedals so that the toes are not internally rotated should help. Steroid injections are infrequently needed, and release of the inflamed portion of the iliotibial band is seldom necessary. As for other overuse syndromes of the knee, the prognosis is good.

Hariri S, Savidge ET, Reinold MM, Zachazewski J, Gill TJ: Treatment of recalcitrant iliotibial band friction syndrome with open iliotibial band bursectomy: indications, technique, and clinical outcomes. *Am J Sports Med* 2009;37:1417. [PMID: 19286912]

Lavine R: Iliotibial band friction syndrome. *Curr Rev Musculoskelet Med* 2010;3:18. [PMID: 21063495]

▶ Other CPT Codes for the Knee

27305 Fasciotomy iliotibial band

27310 Arthrotomy, knee, with exploration, drainage, or removal of foreign body

27412 Autologous chondrocyte implantation, knee

27552 Closed treatment of knee dislocation; requiring anesthesia

27570 Manipulation of knee joint under general anesthesia (includes application of traction or other fixation devices)

29870 Arthroscopy, knee, diagnostic, with or without synovial biopsy (separate procedure)

29871 Arthroscopy, knee, surgical; for infection, lavage and drainage

29874 Arthroscopy, knee, surgical; for removal of loose body or foreign body (eg, osteochondritis dissecans fragmentation, chondral fragmentation)

29875 Arthroscopy, knee, surgical; synovectomy, limited (eg, plica or shelf resection) (separate procedure)

29876 Arthroscopy, knee, surgical; synovectomy, major, two or more compartments (eg, medial or lateral)

29877 Arthroscopy, knee, surgical; debridement/shaving of articular cartilage (chondroplasty)

29884 Arthroscopy, knee, surgical; with lysis of adhesions, with or without manipulation (separate procedure)

▼ ANKLE OR FOOT PAIN

Evaluation of foot and ankle injuries is described in Chapter 8. Injury specific to athletics includes chronic Achilles tendonitis, heel pain, plantar fasciitis, and posterior tibial syndrome.

▶ Clinical Findings

Achilles tendonitis is a frequent complaint in runners. This may result from a contracted gastrocsoleus, or hyperpronation may cause overpulling of the medial insertion. Additionally, there may be a bony prominence on the superior-posterior aspect of the calcaneus, causing retrocalcaneal bursitis.

Heel pain is a common problem in runners and is difficult to treat because of the uncertainty as to cause. Theories include painful heel spurs, bursitis, fat-pad atrophy, stress fracture, plantar fasciitis, or entrapment of the terminal branches of the posterior tibial nerve.

Many patients have pain localized in the posteromedial surface of the foot just distal to the attachment of the plantar fascia to the calcaneus (plantar fasciitis). This pain is often most severe on initially getting up in the morning and decreases as the day goes on.

Posterior tibial syndrome occurs in runners with hyperpronation. As the longitudinal arch flattens out, the posterior tibial musculotendinosis unit elevates the flattened arch and has abnormal strain placed upon it.

▶ Treatment

Treatment depends on the cause of the injury but includes decreasing running activities, using a heel lift, and performing stretching exercises. If hyperpronation is thought to be the cause, an orthotic may be used. Steroid injections are not recommended as they could lead to weakening and subsequent rupture of the tendon.

Surgical intervention for chronic Achilles tendinitis or retrocalcaneal bursitis is rarely necessary. This would be done to remove areas of fibrosis or calcium within the tendon and possibly some bone from the posterior process of the calcaneus. The treatment for plantar fasciitis includes rest, ice massage, and possibly anti-inflammatory medications. A small shock-absorbing type of heel cup often is helpful, and a steroid injection may be given in recalcitrant cases. Acute rupture of the plantar fascia may occur. The pain is usually quite sharp and may cause significant disability for 6–12 weeks.

Hyperpronation may also cause fibular stress fractures. A semirigid orthosis may be recommended for this to decrease the amount and angular velocity of pronation. Using an orthosis while running actually increases the work of running, but if it decreases abnormal stresses in those who hyperpronate, it may be quite helpful.

Hanlon DP: Leg, ankle, and foot injuries. *Emerg Med Clin North Am* 2010;28:885. [PMID: 20971396]

Mizel MS, Hecht PJ, Marymont JV, et al: Evaluation and treatment of chronic ankle pain. *Instr Course Lect* 2004;53:311. [PMID: 15116624]

Simpson MR, Howard TM: Tendinopathies of the foot and ankle. *Am Fam Physician* 2009;80:1107. [PMID: 19904895]

CPT Codes for the Ankle and Foot

27650 Repair, primary, open or percutaneous, ruptured Achilles tendon

27652 Repair, primary, open or percutaneous, ruptured Achilles tendon; with graft (includes obtaining graft)

27654 Repair, secondary, Achilles tendon, with or without graft

27675 Repair, dislocating peroneal tendons; without fibular osteotomy

27676 Repair, dislocating peroneal tendons; with fibular osteotomy

27810 Closed treatment of bimalleolar ankle fracture (eg, lateral and medial malleoli, or lateral and posterior malleoli or medial and posterior malleoli); with manipulation

27814 Open treatment of bimalleolar ankle fracture (eg, lateral and medial malleoli, or lateral and posterior malleoli, or medial and posterior malleoli), includes internal fixation, when performed

28119 Ostectomy, calcaneus; for spur, with or without plantar fascial release

28445 Open treatment of talus fracture, includes internal fixation, when performed

29894 Arthroscopy, ankle surgical; with removal of loose body

29895 Arthroscopy, ankle surgical; synovectomy, partial

29897 Arthroscopy, ankle surgical; debridement, limited

29898 Arthroscopy, ankle surgical; debridement, extensive

▼ OTHER INJURIES OF THE LOWER BODY

Many disorders seen while caring for athletes may be difficult to diagnose with certainty. The differential diagnosis must be carefully made to rule out more severe injuries. Often, a period of rest followed by gradual return to activities is the best treatment. During convalescence, application of ice packs, stretching exercises, and gradual strengthening of the injured limb will facilitate return to sports activities.

OVERUSE SYNDROMES OF THE LOWER EXTREMITIES

Many athletes such as runners, cyclists, aerobics enthusiasts, volleyball players, and basketball players have developed painful disorders of the lower extremities without an acute injury. History taking is very important, and the examiner should ask specific questions about the circumstances in which the discomfort occurs. In a runner, for example, the examiner should ask whether there was an increase in the distance run or a change in the running surface, at what

point the pain was felt, and what home remedies have been tried before the runner sought advice from a physician.

The physical examination should include not only the affected area but also evaluation of the back, pelvis, leg lengths, genu varum or valgum, femoral and tibial torsion, and cavus or flatfoot deformities. The presence of hamstring and heel cord contracture should be determined, and the gait pattern should be observed. Running shoes should be inspected for wear patterns, which may be quite helpful.

1. Muscle Strains

▶ Essentials of Diagnosis

- *Classically involves muscles that span two joints (gastrocnemius).*
- *Patient will feel muscle "grab," localized pain in the involved area.*
- *Eccentric forces thought to be causative factors.*

Muscle strains of the lower extremity are frequent and disabling muscle injuries, with strain of the distal muscle tendon junction being most common. Muscles may stretch to about 125% of their resting length before tearing. Strains are graded as mild, moderate, and severe, based on the degree of pain, spasm, and disability that the strain causes. A severe strain would be complete disruption of the muscle, with a palpable defect and balling up of the muscle proximally.

Despite the frequency of muscle strains and the disability they produce, there is little scientific information on their pathologic basis. Muscles susceptible to more stretching are more susceptible to strains. In the lower extremity, the muscles most frequently injured are the hamstring, quadriceps, and gastrocnemius muscles. These muscles all cross two joints, and they may be unable to resist full stretching across both joints. The most powerful muscles are more likely to be strained, and strains are more common in "explosive" type athletics. Eccentric contraction (muscle contraction while the muscle is lengthening) is often thought to be causative in muscle strains.

▶ Clinical Findings

The diagnosis is relatively easy. Often the athlete will feel the muscle "grab" while he or she is accelerating. There is localized tenderness over the muscle and pain on stretching of the muscle. Because the two joint muscles are most frequently involved, the muscles should be stretched over both of the joints during examination.

▶ Treatment and Prognosis

The treatment of muscle strains should begin with ice in the immediate postinjury period. Flexibility and strength should be regained prior to return to activity. This may take many months, and if the patient returns to activity too early, there may be a setback to the level of the original injury.

Strengthening of the muscles might make them less susceptible to being torn. It is commonly believed that flexibility will help prevent muscle strains, but there are conflicting reports regarding this.

Askling CM, Tengvar M, Saartok T, et al: Proximal hamstring strains of stretching type in different sports: injury situations, clinical and magnetic imaging characteristics and return to sport. *Am J Sport Med* 2008;36:1799. [PMID: 18448581]

Fousekis K, Tsepis E, Poulmedis P, Athanasopoulos S, Vagenas G: Intrinsic risk factors of non-contact quadriceps and hamstring strains in soccer: a prospective study of 100 professional players. *Br J Sports Med* 2011;45:709. [PMID: 21119022]

2. Shin Pain

► Essentials of Diagnosis

- *Pain over the anterior tibia.*
- *Associated with increase in training or activity level.*
- *Radiographs will be negative for fracture.*

► Clinical Findings

A. Shin Splints

The term "shin splints" is widely used for shin pain, but it is not a diagnostic term. A more specific diagnosis should be made if possible. Shin splints are usually defined as pain associated with activity in the beginning of training after a relatively inactive period. The pain and tenderness are usually located over the anterior compartment and disappear in 1–2 weeks as the athlete becomes conditioned to the exercise. Care must be taken to differentiate shin splints from stress fractures of the tibia, which cause more localized pain and have many more potential complications if not cared for properly.

B. Medial Tibial Syndrome

Medial tibial syndrome is also seen in runners, occurring along the medial border of the distal tibia. After 3–4 weeks, some hypertrophy of the cortical bone and periosteal new bone formation may be seen on radiograph. It is thought to be either a periosteitis or possibly an incomplete stress fracture. The pull of the tibialis posterior muscle from its origin on the tibia and posterior tibial tendinitis are also thought to be possible causes.

► Treatment

Treatment for shin splints and medial tibial syndrome is rest and resumption of athletic activities in a graduated fashion.

3. Stress Fractures

► Essentials of Diagnosis

- *Localized pain after increase in training or activity.*
- *Plain radiographs often normal initially; MRI and bone scan are better diagnostic tests.*

Stress fractures may occur in the pelvis, femoral neck, tibia, navicular, and metatarsals. They are usually the result of a significant increase in training and activity. In the female athlete, a triad of eating disorders resulting in poor nutrition, osteoporosis, and amenorrhea are associated with a higher prevalence of stress fractures.

The history is important in differentiating stress fractures from infection or neoplasm, particularly when there is a finding on radiographs. Plain radiographs are normal at first. MRI and technetium bone scans are the best diagnostic tests. If symptoms persist for over a month, radiographs may become positive.

Treatment of stress fractures involves rest and avoidance of high-impact activities until healing has occurred. This includes resolution of the tenderness and signs of fracture healing on plain radiographs. Continuous activity with stress fractures may lead to complete fractures. Patients must be made aware of this and all the complications that may develop with a complete fracture.

Feingold D, Hame SL: Female athlete triad and stress fractures. *Orthop Clin North Am* 2006;37:575. [PMID: 17141015]

Fredericson M, Jennings F, Beaulieu C, et al: Stress fractures in athletes. *Top Magn Reson Imaging* 2006;17:309. [PMID: 17414993]

Rauh MJ, Macera CA, Trone DW, et al: Epidemiology of stress fracture and lower-extremity overuse injury in female recruits. *Med Sci Sports Exerc* 2006;38:1571. [PMID: 16960517]

4. Exertional Compartment Syndromes

► Essentials of Diagnosis

- *Recurrent claudication/pain during exertional activity and relieved by rest.*
- *Measure compartment pressures while exercising on treadmill (pressures >30 mm Hg 1 minute after exercise or >20 mm Hg 5 minutes after exercise, or absolute values >15 mm Hg while resting are consistent with this diagnosis).*

Exertional compartment syndromes may result from muscle hypertrophy within the confining osseofascial compartment. As the muscles hypertrophy and the amount of edema within the compartment increases, the blood supply to the nerves and muscles within the involved compartment is diminished, and the pressure continues to increase.

The syndrome presents as recurrent claudication during exertional activity and is relieved by rest. After exercise, the findings of localized pain, pain on passive motion, and hypesthesia are indicative.

Treatment consists of activity modification including gradual onset of training. If unsuccessful, compartment pressures may be measured while the patient is exercising on a treadmill, and if the pressures are elevated, surgical fasciotomy is usually effective.

Shah SN, Miller BS, Kuhn JE: Chronic exertional compartment syndrome. *Am J Orthop* 2004;33:335. [PMID: 15344575]

Tucker AK: Chronic exertional compartment syndrome of the leg. *Curr Rev Musculoskelet Med* 2010;3:32. [PMID: 21063498]

CPT Codes for Overuse Injuries

20950 Monitoring of interstitial fluid pressure (includes insertion of device, eg, wick catheter technique, needle manometer technique) in detection of muscle compartment syndrome

27187 Prophylactic treatment (nailing, pinning, plating or wiring) with or without methylmethacrylate, femoral neck and proximal femur

27600 Decompression fasciotomy, leg; anterior and/or lateral compartments only

27601 Decompression fasciotomy, leg; posterior compartment(s) only

27602 Decompression fasciotomy, leg; anterior and/or lateral, and posterior compartment(s)

27759 Open treatment of tibia fracture by intramedullary implant

27892 Decompression fasciotomy, leg; anterior and/or lateral compartments only, with debridement of nonviable muscle and/or nerve

27893 Decompression fasciotomy, leg; posterior compartment(s) only, with debridement of nonviable muscle and/or nerve

27894 Decompression fasciotomy, leg; anterior and/or lateral, and posterior compartment(s), with debridement of nonviable muscle and/or nerve

28485 Open treatment of metatarsal fracture, includes internal fixation, when performed, each

CONTUSIONS AND AVULSIONS OF THE LOWER BODY

1. Contusion to the Quadriceps Muscle

Essentials of Diagnosis

- *History of direct trauma.*
- *Peripheral calcification on radiographs (as opposed to parosteal osteosarcoma, which has central calcification).*

Clinical Findings

A severe contusion to the quadriceps muscle (charley horse) is disabling, results in prolonged inactivity, and frequently occurs in football players. With significant bleeding into the muscle, there is inhibition of movement. Rarely, a compartment syndrome will occur.

Myositis ossificans may occur after these injuries. It may be apparent 2–4 weeks after the injury. Radiographically and histologically, myositis ossificans may be similar to parosteal osteosarcoma; therefore, the history of contusion is very important. Radiographs should be obtained after such a contusion to minimize myositis ossificans being confused with cancer.

Treatment and Prognosis

Quadriceps contusions should be treated with elevation of the leg and the hip and knee flexed to tolerance to minimize bleeding. After a few days, the knee can be moved with continuous passive motion or "drop-and-dangle," gravity-assisted exercises. For the latter, the patient is seated on a table high enough to keep the feet off the floor. The patient then hooks the uninjured foot behind the ankle of the injured leg. The uninjured leg extends the knee of the injured leg, and gravity flexes the injured knee. Average length of disability for mild contusions is 2 weeks, and length for severe contusions is 3 weeks.

If heterotopic ossification is present, no specific treatment is recommended other than treatment for the contusion. Normal function may be obtained, but the recovery period is longer. Because early surgery may cause exacerbation of the heterotopic ossification, it should be avoided. There have also been recent animal studies examining the benefit of suramin, an antifibrotic agent that has been shown to help muscle regeneration and improved healing. While these initial results are encouraging, further studies are needed before suramin gains widespread clinical use after contusions.

Cooper DE: Severe quadriceps muscle contusions in athletes. *Am J Sports Med* 2004;32:820. [PMID: 15090402]

Kary JM: Diagnosis and management of quadriceps strains and contusions. *Curr Rev Musculoskelet Med* 2010;3:26. [PMID: 21063497]

CONTUSIONS ABOUT THE HIP AND PELVIS

Clinical Findings

Contusions about the pelvis and hip region may be very painful and disabling. Because of the subcutaneous location of the iliac crests and the greater trochanters, these regions are at risk in contact sports.

A contusion over the greater trochanter may cause persistent bursitis, tenderness directly over the greater trochanter, and increased pain with adduction of the leg. Females are more prone to trochanteric bursitis because of their broader pelvis.

A hip pointer is a very painful contusion over the iliac crest that occurs from many contact sports. It must be differentiated from an avulsion fracture in a child, and a tear of the muscle aponeurosis in an adult. Profuse bleeding may occur and can be very painful.

Treatment and Prognosis

For contusion over the greater trochanter, treatment consists of ice applications and decreased activities. Padding may be helpful to prevent recurrent injuries. The prognosis is good. For hip pointer injuries, initial treatment with ice is helpful. Protective pads are useful in preventing these injuries and returning the athlete to activities sooner.

AVULSION OF THE TIBIAL TUBERCLE

Essentials of Diagnosis

- *Adolescent athletes between 14 and 16 years of age.*
- *Result of a forceful contraction by quadriceps against a fixed tibia.*
- *Significant swelling and tenderness over the tubercle; palpable defect with substantial displacement.*
- *Patient will not be able to actively extend the knee.*
- *Radiographs will be helpful to determine amount of displacement and guide treatment course.*

Clinical Findings

Tibial tubercle avulsions occur in adolescent athletes, most often in males aged between 14 and 16 years. They result from a powerful contraction of the quadriceps muscle against a fixed tibia. This can occur by forced passive flexion of the knee against a powerful quadriceps contraction, as in an awkward landing at the end of a jump or fall. Avulsion of the tubercle may occur with either a sudden acceleration or deceleration of the knee extensor mechanism. The patellar tendon must pull hard enough to overcome the strength of the growth plate, the surrounding perichondrium, and the adjacent periosteum.

Swelling and tenderness are located over the proximal anterior tibia. A tense hemarthrosis may be present. A palpable defect in the anterior tibia is associated with a much-displaced avulsion. Proximal migration of the patella occurs, and the patella may seem to float off the anterior aspect of the femur. The knee is held flexed; with displaced fractures, the patient is unable actively to extend the knee.

Watson-Jones defined three types of avulsion fractures, which were subsequently refined as the following three types (Figure 3–20): type 1 fracture, in which the fracture line lies across the secondary center of ossification at the level of the posterior border of the patellar ligament; type 2 fracture, in which a separation breaks out at the primary and secondary ossification centers of epiphysis; and type 3 fracture, in which the separation propagates upward through the main portion of the proximal tibial epiphysis. The degree of displacement depends on the severity of injury to the surrounding soft-tissue moorings. A lateral radiograph with the tibia slightly internally rotated is the best view to see the fracture and the degree of displacement.

Differential Diagnosis

Osgood-Schlatter disease, or osteochondrosis of the tuberosity of the tibia, should not be confused with acute avulsion of the tibial tubercle. In the former, the patient is usually between 11 and 15 years of age and is involved in athletics. Pain is located at the tibial tubercle, and it has usually been present intermittently over a period of several months. Walking on a flat surface is not difficult, but ascending or

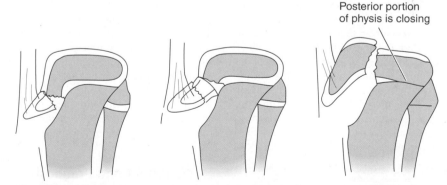

▲ **Figure 3–20.** Classification of avulsion fractures of the tibial tubercle. Type 1 fracture (**left**) across the secondary ossification center at level with the posterior border of the inserting patellar ligament. Type 2 fracture (**center**) at the junction of the primary and secondary ossification centers of the proximal tibial epiphysis. Type 3 fracture (**right**) propagates upward across the primary ossification center of the proximal tibial epiphysis into the knee joint. This fracture is a variant of the Salter-Harris III separation and is analogous to the fracture of Tillaux at the ankle because the posterior portion of the physis of the proximal tibia is closing. (Reproduced, with permission, from Odgen JA, Tross RB, Murphy MJ: Fractures of the tibial tuberosity in adolescents. *J Bone Joint Surg Am* 1980;62:205.)

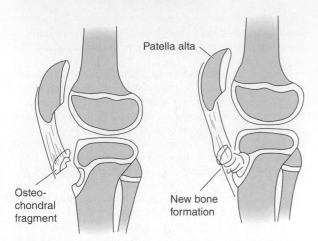

Patella alta

Osteo-
chondral
fragment

New bone
formation

▲ **Figure 3–21.** Development of Osgood-Schlatter lesion. (**Left**) Avulsion of osteochondral fragment that includes surface cartilage and a portion of the secondary ossification center of the tibial tubercle. (**Right**) New bone fills in the gap between the avulsed osteochondral fragment and the tibial tubercle. (Reproduced, with permission, from Rockwood CA Jr, ed: *Fractures in Children*, 3rd ed. Philadelphia: Lippincott; 1991.)

descending stairs causes difficulty. Radiograph examination shows slight separation of the tibial tubercle with new bone formation beneath it (Figure 3–21).

Treatment recommendations vary from decreasing the amount of running and jumping, but continuing participation in athletics, to cylinder cast immobilization for a short period of time. The long-term prognosis is excellent. While symptoms are often present for 2 years, early short-term cast immobilization may shorten this period of discomfort to 9 months. In most children, casting is not necessary. Explaining the benign nature of the problem to both the patient and the parents, reassuring them that the long-term prognosis is good, and modifying activities usually allow continued participation in athletics. Hamstring stretching and ice massage will hopefully decrease symptoms during the time needed for maturation of the tibial tubercle. The pain will go away when the tubercle unites with the tibia. In a very small number of cases, chronic pain will be present if the ossicle fails to unite. Painful ossicles in the adult are successfully treated with simple excision.

▶ Treatment

Full function of the extensor mechanism is necessary, and therefore, treatment of tibial tubercle avulsion fractures is aimed at this goal. If the fracture is minimally displaced and the patient is able to fully extend the knee against gravity, nonoperative treatment is acceptable. A cylinder cast should be applied with the knee extended and worn for 4 weeks. Active range of motion and strengthening exercises should

then commence. At 6 weeks, quadriceps exercises against resistance are initiated. For displaced fractures, open reduction and internal fixation are recommended, with screws if the piece or pieces are large enough. If rigid fixation of large fragments is obtained, early active flexion and passive extension may be initiated. If a tenuous repair is obtained, protection in a cast is advisable.

▶ Prognosis

Because the injury occurs in children who are close to skeletal maturity, meaningful growth abnormalities at the proximal tibial physis do not occur. Return to activities is allowed after the athlete develops quadriceps mass and strength equal to the contralateral side.

Abalo A, Akakpo-numado KG, Dossim A, Walla A, Gnassingbe K, Tekou AH: Avulsion fractures of the tibial tubercle. *J Orthop Surg* 2008;16:308. [PMID: 19126896]

▶ CPT Codes for Tibial Tubercle Avulsion

27418 Anterior tibial tubercleplasty

27530 Closed treatment of proximal tibial fracture (including tubercle)

27535 Open treatment of tibial fracture, proximal (plateau); unicondylar, includes internal fixation, when performed

AVULSIONS ABOUT THE PELVIS

▶ Clinical Findings

In the skeletally immature athlete, the apophysis, or growth plate where the muscle attaches to bone, is the weak link in the bone-muscle-tendon unit. Therefore, just as the growth plate is prone to breaking in children's fractures, the bony origin of muscles may be pulled off. This most commonly occurs in athletes between 14 and 25 years of age. Comparison radiographs may be helpful to make sure the avulsion fracture is not just a normal anatomic variant. In the pelvis, this may occur at the iliac crest (abdominal muscles), anterior superior iliac spine (sartorius origin), anterior inferior iliac spine (rectus femoris origin), ischial tuberosity (hamstring origin), and lesser trochanter of the femur (iliopsoas insertion).

▶ Treatment and Prognosis

Symptomatic care with a few days of rest followed by ambulation with crutches for about a month is recommended. It is usually 6–10 weeks before athletic activities may be resumed. Long-term athletic activity will probably not be affected. Open reduction and internal fixation have not shown superior results and therefore are usually not warranted. Abundant calcification may occur in the ischial tuberosity region and may be the cause of chronic bursitis and pain. Excision of the exuberant callous should cure this problem. Another indication for surgery is a painful fibrous nonunion, which also may be cured with excision of the fragment.

Sanders TG, Zlatkin MB: Avulsion injuries of the pelvis. *Semin Musculoskelet Radiol* 2008;12:42. [PMID: 18382943]

▼ SHOULDER INJURIES

The shoulder is the third most commonly injured joint during athletic activities, after the knee and the ankle. Sports-related injuries of the shoulder may result from a direct traumatic event or repetitive overuse. Any activity that requires arm motion, particularly overhead arm motion such as throwing, may stress the soft tissues surrounding the glenohumeral joint to the point of injury. The shoulder is the most mobile joint in the body partly, as a result of minimal containment of the large humeral head by the shallow and smaller glenoid fossa. The tradeoff for this mobility is less structural restraint to undesirable and potentially damaging movements. Thus, a fine balance must be struck to maintain full range of shoulder motion and normal glenohumeral joint stability.

▶ Anatomy

A. The Bony Articulation of the Glenohumeral Joint

The glenohumeral joint is a modified ball-and-socket joint. The glenoid fossa is a shallow inverted, comma-shaped, articular surface one fourth the size of the humeral head. The articular surface of the humeral head is retroverted approximately 30 degrees relative to the transverse axis of the elbow. Because the scapula is oriented anterolaterally about 30 degrees on the thorax, relative to the coronal plane of the body, the glenoid fossa matches the humeral head retroversion. So with the arm relaxed at the side, the glenoid fossa matches the humeral head retroversion. With shoulder motion, the scapula also moves so that the glenoid accommodates changing humeral head positions. As a result, the humeral head is centered in the glenoid throughout most shoulder motions. When this centered position is disturbed, instability may result.

B. The Clavicle and Its Articulations

The clavicle articulates medially with the sternum at the sternoclavicular joint and laterally with the acromion of the scapula at the acromioclavicular joint. The clavicle rotates on its long axis and acts as a strut, serving as the only bone connecting the appendicular upper extremity to the axial skeleton.

C. The Glenohumeral Joint Capsule, Ligaments, and Labrum

The thin redundant joint capsule has almost twice the surface area of the humeral head to allow large range of joint motion. Different regions of the joint capsule provide stability at different joint positions. With the arm at the side, the superior portion of the capsule is taut and the inferior portion is lax. With overhead elevation, this relationship reverses.

There are folds or thickenings visible on the inside of the capsule with the shoulder at the side, which have been termed glenohumeral ligaments. Traditionally the anterior capsule has been described as being composed of the superior, middle, and inferior glenohumeral ligaments (Figure 3–22). While use of the term "ligament" is generally

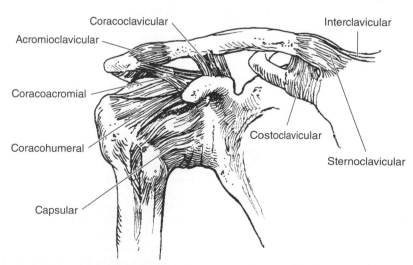

▲ **Figure 3–22.** Ligaments about the shoulder girdle.

accepted, it needs some clarification. Ligaments are soft-tissue structures that connect bones. They are most commonly band-like with parallel collagen fibers running between their insertion sites and have clearly defined edges, such as the MCL of the knee. The glenohumeral capsule as a whole may be considered a sheetlike ligament connecting the humerus and the scapula. The collagen fibers are not organized in a parallel fashion, the margins of the folds are indistinct, and functional study does not indicate it to have "band-like" properties. This may be the reason that the "ligaments" of the anterior capsule have been described with variable prevalence; different authors have had varying success in identifying them. Also, with the shoulder in abduction and external rotation, even the most consistently reported fold in the anteroinferior capsule, the anterior band of the inferior glenohumeral ligament, is often indistinct. While terminology may be currently causing confusion in anatomic, biomechanical, and clinical studies, there is little doubt that different regions of the capsule have differing roles in joint function, and this understanding has resulted in improved outcomes for shoulder injuries.

The capsule inserts into the glenoid labrum and onto the glenoid bone. The glenoid labrum acts not only as an attachment site for the capsuloligamentous structures but also as an extension of the articular cavity. Its presence deepens the glenoid socket by nearly 50%, and the triangular cross-section of the labrum acts as a chock-block to help prevent subluxation.

D. The Shoulder Musculature

The muscles around the shoulder may be divided into three functional groups: glenohumeral, thoracohumeral, and those that cross both the shoulder and elbow.

1. Glenohumeral muscles—Four muscles compose the rotator cuff: the supraspinatus, subscapularis, infraspinatus, and teres minor. The supraspinatus has its origin on the posterosuperior scapula, superior to the scapular spine. It passes under the acromion, through the supraspinatus fossa, and inserts on the greater tuberosity with an extended attachment of fibrocartilage. The supraspinatus is active during the entire arc of scapular plane abduction; paralysis of the suprascapular nerve results in an approximately 50% loss of abduction torque. The infraspinatus and the teres minor muscles originate on the posterior scapula, inferior to the scapular spine, and insert on the posterior aspect of the greater tuberosity. Despite their origin below the scapular spine, their tendinous insertions are not separate from the supraspinatus tendon. These muscles function together to externally rotate and extend the humerus. Both account for approximately 80% of external rotation strength in the adducted position. The infraspinatus is more active with the arm at the side, while the teres minor activates mainly with the shoulder in 90 degrees of elevation. The subscapularis muscle arises from the anterior scapula and is the only muscle to insert on the lesser tuberosity. The subscapularis is

the sole anterior component of the rotator cuff and functions to internally rotate and flex the humerus. The tendinous insertion of the subscapularis is continuous with the anterior capsule so that both provide anterior glenohumeral stability.

The deltoid is the largest of the glenohumeral muscles. It covers the proximal humerus on a path from its tripennate origin at the clavicle, acromion, and scapular spine to its insertion midway on the humerus at the deltoid tubercle. Abduction of the joint results from activity of the anterior and middle portions. The anterior portion is also a forward flexor. The posterior portion does not abduct the joint, but instead adducts and extends the humerus. The deltoid is active throughout the entire arc of glenohumeral abduction; paralysis of the deltoid results in a 50% loss of abduction torque. The deltoid muscle can fully abduct the glenohumeral joint with the supraspinatus muscle inactive.

The teres major muscle originates from the inferior angle of the scapula and inserts on the medial lip of the bicipital groove of the humerus, posterior to the insertion of the latissimus dorsi. The axillary nerve and the posterior humeral circumflex artery pass inferior to the subscapularis muscle and the inferior glenohumeral joint capsule, and then inferior to the teres minor muscle through the quadrilateral space also bordered by the teres major, the triceps, and the humerus. The teres major muscle contracts with the latissimus dorsi muscle, and the two muscles function as a unit in humeral extension, internal rotation, and adduction.

2. Thoracohumeral muscles—The pectoralis major and the latissimus dorsi muscles are powerful movers of the shoulder and, hence, contribute to the joint force that in turn usually stabilizes the glenohumeral joint. The pectoralis major muscle arises as a broad sheet of two distinct heads with the lowermost fibers of the sternal head inserting most proximally on the humerus.

Muscles that have origin on the thorax contribute to glenohumeral stability and may have roles in instability as well. When the shoulder is placed in horizontal abduction, similar to the apprehension position, the lowermost fibers of the sternal head of the pectoralis major muscle are stretched to an extreme. Because anterior instability also occurs from forcible horizontal abduction of the shoulder, the humeral head can be pulled out of the glenoid by passive tension in the pectoralis major and latissimus dorsi muscles.

3. Biceps brachii muscle—Both heads of the biceps brachii muscle have their origin on the scapula. The short head originates from the coracoid and, with the coracobrachialis muscle, forms the conjoined tendon. The long head of the biceps has its origin just superior to the articular margin of the glenoid from the posterosuperior labrum and the supraglenoid tubercle and is inside the synovial sheath of the glenohumeral joint. It traverses the glenohumeral joint, passing over the anterior aspect of the humeral head to the bicipital groove where it exits the joint under the transverse humeral ligament.

Its origin on the scapula and insertion of the radius leaves the long head of the biceps brachii muscle with potential for function at both the shoulder and the elbow. Its function at the elbow has been well established to include both flexion and supination. Long considered a depressor of the humeral head, the role of the active biceps has been recently questioned as electromyographic studies have shown that there was little or no activity of the biceps when elbow motion was controlled. This does not preclude a passive role or an active role associated with elbow motion, as tension in the tendon may then contribute to glenohumeral joint stability.

E. The Neurovascular Supply

The axillary artery traverses the axilla, extending from the outer border of the first rib to the lower border of the teres minor muscle, forming the brachial artery. The axillary artery lies deep to the pectoralis muscle, but is crossed in its midregion by the pectoralis minor tendon, just before the tendon inserts on the coracoid process. The axillary vein travels with the axillary artery, and branches of the axillary artery supply most of the shoulder girdle. The brachial plexus consists of the ventral rami of the fifth through eighth cervical nerves and the first thoracic nerve. This network of nerve fibers begins with the joining of the ventral rami proximally in the neck and continues anteriorly and distally, crossing into the axillary region obliquely underneath the clavicle at about the junction area of the distal one third and proximal two thirds. Clavicular fractures in this area have the potential of injuring the brachial plexus. The plexus then lies inferior to the coracoid process, where its cords form the peripheral nerves that continue down the arm. Muscles of the shoulder girdle are supplied by the nerves arising at all levels of the brachial plexus.

Moore SM, Stehle JH, Rainis EJ, McMahon PJ, Debski RE: The current anatomical description of the inferior glenohumeral ligament does not correlate with its functional role in positions of external rotation. *J Orthop Res* 2008;26:1598. [PMID: 18524007]

Rispoli DM, Athwal GS, Sperling JW, Cofield RH: The anatomy of the deltoid insertion. *J Shoulder Elbow Surg* 2009;18:386. [PMID: 19186076]

▶ History and Physical Examination

A. General Approach

The history of shoulder complaints must include age, arm dominance, location, intensity, duration, temporal occurrence, aggravating and alleviating factors, radiation of discomfort, physical activity level, occupation, and the mechanism of injury. Previous responses to treatments will help to characterize their efficacy and establish a pattern of disease or injury progression. The physical examination begins with the patient undressing so that both shoulders are fully exposed. Patients should be examined first in the standing position. The surface anatomy should be checked for asymmetry, atrophy, or external lesions. The supraspinatus and infraspinatus fossae are especially important to examine for atrophy. The area of pain should be pointed out by the patient prior to the physician manipulating the shoulder to avoid hurting the patient unnecessarily. A thorough neurovascular examination of the upper extremity should be performed.

B. Shoulder Range of Motion

1. Types of movement—Many terms may be used to describe movements of the shoulder joint (Figure 3–23). Flexion occurs when the arm begins at the side and elevates in the sagittal plane of the body anteriorly. Extension occurs when the arm starts at the side and elevates in the sagittal plane of the body posteriorly. Adduction occurs when the arm moves toward the midline of the body, with abduction occurring as the arm moves away from the midline of the body. Internal rotation occurs when the arm rotates medially, inward toward the body, and external rotation occurs as the arm rotates laterally or outward from the body. Horizontal adduction occurs as the arm starts at 90 degrees of abduction and adducts forward and medially toward the center of the body, and horizontal abduction happens as the arm starts at 90 degrees of abduction and moves outward, away from the body. Elevation is the angle made between the thorax and arm, regardless if it is in the abduction plane, flexion plane, or in between.

2. Evaluation of movement—Range of motion of the injured shoulder should be compared with the opposite shoulder, along with the strength during abduction and rotation. This should be done both passively and actively. The shoulder should be inspected for any changes in synchrony, such as scapular winging, elevation of the scapula, muscle fasciculations indicating abnormal function, and any other irregular or asymmetric movements of the scapula. Information may be gained on loss of flexibility and instability resulting from muscle imbalance, fibrosis, and tendon, capsular, or ligament contractures. Loss of flexibility usually occurs in the capsular tissues of the glenohumeral joint. Sudden pain or clicking may indicate an intraarticular problem. Loss of motion in either internal or external rotation is suggestive of a chronic anterior or posterior dislocation, respectively.

3. Provocative tests—Specific tests are then performed that aid in making the correct diagnosis. The specific tests for instability, impingement syndrome, bicipital tendonitis, and superior capsulolabral/biceps anchor lesions are discussed as follows.

▶ Imaging and Other Studies

Many varieties of radiologic views and projections are available to examine shoulder injuries. An initial radiographic evaluation of the shoulder should consist of an

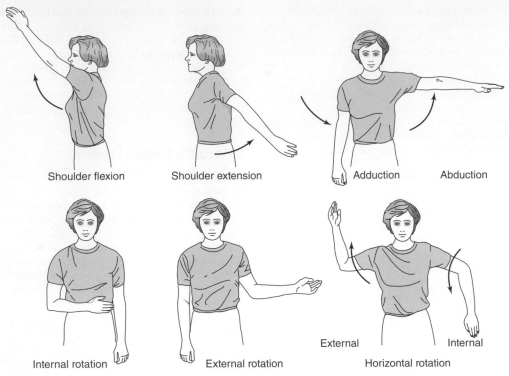

▲ **Figure 3–23.** Descriptions of shoulder motion.

anteroposterior view of the glenohumeral joint in both internal and external rotation and an axillary lateral view. Additional plain radiographic views depend on the underlying pathology. MRI may be indicated in evaluation of rotator cuff disorders recalcitrant to conservative treatment. A magnetic resonance arthrogram may be useful in detecting labral pathology. Ultrasonography is also useful in diagnosis of rotator cuff tendon injury, but it is operator dependent. Electromyographic examination can be useful in identifying shoulder pain of cervical origin.

▶ **Arthroscopic Evaluation**

A. Indications for Arthroscopic Evaluation of Shoulder Injuries

Indications for arthroscopic examination of the shoulder include the following:

1. Impingement syndrome, including subacromial bursitis, rotator cuff tendonitis, and rotator cuff tears

2. Acromioclavicular joint osteoarthritis

3. Loose bodies

4. Chronic synovitis

5. Glenohumeral instability

6. Superior capsulolabral/biceps anchor (ie, SLAP) lesions

7. Adhesive capsulitis (frozen shoulder)

B. Technique

With the patient either in the lateral decubitus or the beach chair position, the arthroscope is inserted into the posterior shoulder. With visualization of the glenohumeral joint, an anterior portal immediately lateral to the coracoid allows additional inflow and entrance of additional instruments. Additional portals may be used; for example, an additional anterior portal inferior to the first may be used for instability repair. The arthroscope is then removed from the joint and placed into the subacromial bursa. A portal lateral to the acromion allows subacromial decompression and rotator cuff repair.

C. Steps in Evaluation

Examination of shoulder range of motion and stability with the patient under anesthesia is helpful in the diagnosis and treatment of shoulder injuries. This should be performed in the operating room prior to arthroscopy. The steps in arthroscopic examination should then include the following:

1. Glenohumeral articular surfaces

2. Rotator cuff from inside the joint

3. Labrum including the biceps anchor

4. Anterior capsule

5. Rotator cuff from the subacromial bursal space

6. Coracoacromial ligament

7. Acromion

8. Acromioclavicular joint

Ludewig PM, Phadke V, Braman JP, Hassett DR, Cieminski CJ, LaPrade RF: Motion of the shoulder complex during multi-planar humeral elevation. *J Bone Joint Surg Am* 2009;91:378. [PMID: 19181982]

Saupe N, Zanetti M, Pfirrmann CW, Wels T, Schwenke C, Hodler J: Pain and other side effects after MR arthrography: prospective evaluation in 1085 patients. *Radiology* 2009;250:830. [PMID: 19164115]

Vlychou M, Dailiana Z, Fotiadou A, Papanagiotou M, Fezoulidis IV, Malizos K: Symptomatic partial rotator cuff tears: diagnostic performance of ultrasound and magnetic resonance imaging with surgical correlation. *Acta Radiol* 2009;50:101. [PMID: 19052931]

SHOULDER TENDON AND MUSCLE INJURY

▶ Rotator Cuff Tendon Injuries

Injury to the rotator cuff is the most common cause of shoulder pain and disability. Although shoulder weakness and decreased range of motion are associated with a rotator cuff tendon tear, pain from subacromial bursitis or rotator cuff tendinosis may also be the cause. Symptoms are often worsened by activity, especially with overhead activity. Night pain is also common, and many patients complain of awakening after rolling onto the affected shoulder.

Any prolonged repetitive activity involving overhead motion such as tennis, pitching, golf, or swimming may cause rotator cuff injury. Injury, whether repetitive or acute, can produce a continuous vicious cycle (Figure 3–24). Blood supply to this tendon is precarious, thus decreasing its capacity for healing.

1. Subacromial Bursitis and Rotator Cuff Tendinosis

▶ Essentials of Diagnosis

- *Mild or moderate pain with overhead shoulder motion.*
- *Occasional night pain.*
- *History of repetitive overhead activity.*
- *No muscle atrophy.*
- *No weakness or mild weakness from the shoulder pain.*
- *Pain is relieved with a subacromial lidocaine injection.*

▶ Prevention

Limiting repetitive overhead activities and maintenance of good rotator cuff strength are keys to prevention. Additionally, overall conditioning and stretching and strengthening with careful attention paid to technique can be helpful in minimizing many injuries resulting from overuse.

▶ Clinical Findings

Bursitis of the shoulder refers to an inflammation of the subacromial bursa. It may or may not be present along with rotator cuff tendinosis, and the two entities are similar. Pain is present with activity involving overhead motion, and there is usually no pain or only mild pain with the arm at the side.

Of the four rotator cuff muscles, the supraspinatus tendon is most often initially involved. Rotator cuff tendinosis also results from impingement syndrome and is characterized by pain with activity involving overhead motion. The patient may occasionally be awakened by pain at night.

Active range of shoulder motion may be limited by pain. No atrophy of the shoulder muscles is present, and manual muscle testing demonstrates mild weakness. Passively, when the internally rotated shoulder is moved into forward flexion, the patient will experience discomfort. This is called the Neer impingement sign (Figure 3–25). This pain then

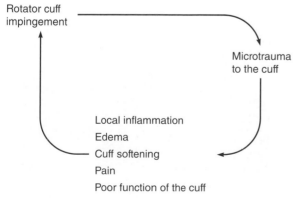

Rotator cuff
impingement

Microtrauma
to the cuff

Local inflammation
Edema
Cuff softening
Pain
Poor function of the cuff

▲ **Figure 3–24.** The cycle of injury and reinjury resulting from rotator cuff impingement.

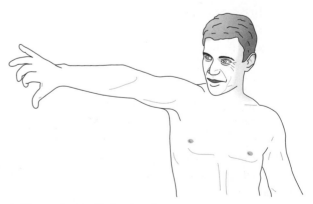

▲ **Figure 3–25.** Evaluating for impingement of the supraspinatus tendon with the "empty can" test.

resolves, and there is a dramatic increase in strength and range of motion with the Neer impingement test (10 mL of lidocaine is injected into the subacromial space).

Radiographic views of the subacromial space such as the supraspinatus outlet view may show a spur on the undersurface of the acromion, causing narrowing of the subacromial space. In recent years, advances in imaging methods such as ultrasonography and MRI have aided in the diagnosis of subacromial bursitis, rotator cuff tendinosis, and rotator cuff tendon tear (Figure 3–26).

▶ Treatment

Treatment starts with conservative measures such as activity modification, physical therapy, and oral nonsteroidal anti-inflammatory drugs (NSAIDs). Only with normal function of the rotator cuff tendons will glenohumeral mechanics be improved and the impingement syndrome cease. If this treatment fails, a subacromial injection of corticosteroids may be helpful. Most patients respond well to these nonoperative treatments.

Surgical intervention is indicated if symptoms do not resolve after a few months of such treatment. Then, acromioplasty, also called subacromial decompression, which is shaving the undersurface of the acromion, usually results in relief of symptoms. An exception is the young athlete with glenohumeral instability and secondary tendinosis. In this case, the instability should be treated first, and the rotator cuff tendinosis will then resolve. This procedure can be done arthroscopically to decrease postoperative discomfort and minimize the complication of deltoid muscle rupture from the acromion. Those who require surgical treatment are usually able to return to pain-free activities.

2. Rotator Cuff Tendon Tear

▶ Essentials of Diagnosis

- *Moderate or severe pain with activity involving overhead motion.*
- *Persistent night pain.*
- *History of repetitive overhead activity.*
- *Weakness with moderate and severe tears.*
- *Atrophy of rotator cuff muscles with severe tears.*
- *Pain is relieved with a subacromial lidocaine injection.*

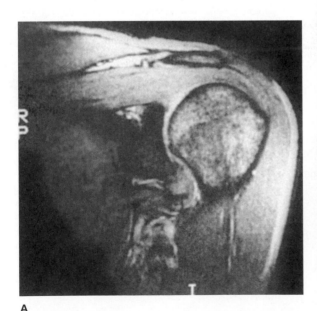

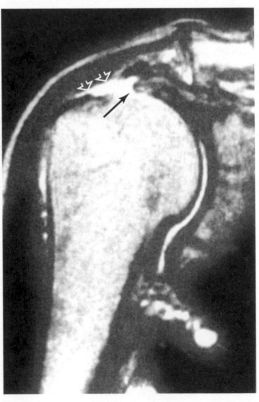

A   **B**

▲ **Figure 3–26.** MRI demonstrating (**A**) normal shoulder anatomy and (**B**) cystic changes at the greater tuberosity with rotator cuff tear (*arrow*).

▶ Prevention

Maintenance of overall body conditioning with regular stretching and strengthening of the rotator cuff and scapular stabilizing muscles can help prevent rotator cuff injuries.

▶ Clinical Findings

A rotator cuff tendon tear is characterized by pain with activity involving overhead motion. However, the patient is often awakened at night with pain as well. The athlete with a chronic rotator cuff tear may experience a gradual loss of strength. Pain may be persistent, occurring even when the arm is at the side. Active range of shoulder motion is limited, and if the tear is severe, there will be atrophy of the shoulder muscles. Manual muscle testing demonstrates weakness. The Neer impingement sign is positive, and the pain resolves with a subacromial injection of lidocaine. Radiographic evaluation is similar to that for subacromial bursitis and rotator cuff tendinosis.

▶ Treatment

Radiographic evaluation and treatment are similar to subacromial bursitis management. Unlike acute tears, chronic rotator cuff tears often present insidiously, with slow progression from subacromial bursitis to rotator cuff tendinosis and eventual tendon tear. Differentiating severe rotator cuff tendinosis from partial or small full-thickness chronic rotator cuff tears may be difficult.

There are two important considerations in treating an individual with a rotator cuff tear—the current symptoms and the risk of the tear progressing. Although the lesion location and size are helpful in describing a rotator cuff tear, symptoms do not correlate with these factors alone. Some individuals are able to cope with the symptoms of a rotator cuff tear, and some may be completely asymptomatic. The severity of symptoms is influenced by a number of other factors including pain tolerance, the acute or chronic nature of the injury, the age and activity level of the individual, humeral head superior migration, shoulder muscle strength, muscle atrophy, fatty changes in the muscle, arthritis, and workman's compensation status.

Rest, rehabilitation, and taking NSAIDs, sometimes for as long as 4–9 months, may relieve symptoms. Range-of-motion and strengthening exercises are recommended, unless they cause significant discomfort. Strengthening the other shoulder muscles may increase the individual's ability to cope with the rotator cuff tear. Avoidance of activities that exacerbate the symptoms, such as activities involving overhead motion, is also recommended. Symptoms of pain, weakness, or decreased range of motion that persist after a nonoperative treatment program has been tried indicate the need for surgical intervention.

Because rotator cuff tears may progress in size over time, immediate repair may be warranted in some at-risk individuals. Both epidemiologic and imaging studies of the general population indicate a high incidence of partial-thickness rotator cuff tears at younger ages and full-thickness rotator cuff tears at older ages. The increasing prevalence of rotator cuff injuries in older individuals may be the best evidence that rotator cuff tears progress in severity. Specifically, about 25% of individuals over 60 years of age have a tear, and in those over 80 years of age, there is a full-thickness rotator cuff tear in about 50% of individuals. The risk of a rotator cuff tear progressing to a more severe tear cannot currently be predicted, but it is thought to be higher in young, active individuals, partly because they have many more years to sustain an injury.

The thin degenerated tissue of a chronic rotator cuff tear makes surgical repair more difficult than repair of an acute tear. The repair can be accomplished with either an arthroscopic or an open technique. For years, surgical decompression has been routine with rotator cuff repair, but recently some have questioned whether it needs to be done. The arthroscopic technique yields results comparable to the open technique. There have been many recent changes to the arthroscopic technique such as using a double row of fixation rather than a single row and using novel methods of securing the sutures.

Some severe tears may be impossible to repair. This includes many of the tears that are large to massive in size or that involve two or more rotator cuff tendons; when the humeral head is positioned superior, against the acromion; and when there is meaningful atrophy of the rotator cuff muscles or fatty changes. Debridement of the rotator cuff and the subacromial spurs may diminish pain in such instances.

Rehabilitation after a repair lasts from 3 months to 1 year with gradual exercise progression needed to restore normal, or near-normal, function and strength. This varies with the size of the tear that was repaired and the type of surgery performed. Typically, immediately after the procedure, passive motion and isometric strengthening exercises start, along with elbow-, hand-, and grip-strengthening exercises. At 6 weeks, the athlete may be able to begin low-intensity active strengthening exercises against gravity. The goals are to bring the athlete to normal strength with a functional, pain-free range of motion.

▶ Prognosis

The prognosis following a rotator cuff tear depends on many factors, as described earlier. There are few specific criteria governing return to sports following rotator cuff injuries. Determining factors must be individualized to the athlete, considering the nature and treatment of the rotator cuff injury as well as the desired sport. Patients must be pain free and have attained full range of motion with near full strength prior to returning to their sport to minimize reinjury.

3. Partial-Thickness Rotator Cuff Tendon Tear

A partial articular-sided tendon avulsion is much more common than a bursal side tear of the rotator cuff. As with other rotator cuff injuries, symptoms may resolve with appropriate physical therapy and analgesics. Yet, some individuals with a partial-thickness tear have persistent or recurrent symptoms. If a conservative program of exercises and gradual return to activity do not lead to steady improvement, then further diagnostic evaluation with ultrasonography, MRI, or arthroscopy may be helpful. Whereas repair of the partial-thickness rotator cuff tear may be best in some, debridement of the abnormal cuff may diminish or relieve symptoms in others. Some clinicians use involvement of greater than 50% of the tendon thickness as an indication for repair. Repair necessitates a rehabilitation program similar to that described earlier for full-thickness rotator cuff tears. Following debridement, immediate resumption of range-of-motion and muscle-strengthening exercises begins. Typically, it requires 6–12 months for an athlete whose sport involves throwing to return to athletics following arthroscopic debridement of a partial-thickness rotator cuff tear.

4. Cuff "Arthropathy"

Severe rotator cuff tears may lead to the humeral head being positioned superior against the undersurface of the acromion. Because of the tear of the rotator cuff, the humeral head no longer stays centered on the glenoid and the pull of the deltoid is unopposed. Over time, the humeral head and the glenoid wear from the abnormal contact. Most individuals have severe shoulder dysfunction, sometimes described as pseudoparalysis. They are able to move their shoulder only the smallest amounts. Interestingly, others are able to lift their arms and complain only of pain and weakness. This is a difficulty in caring for rotator cuff injuries. Symptoms may not correlate with the severity; some are able to cope with the injury, while others cannot. Nonoperative treatment including rehabilitation, NSAIDs, and steroid injection is usually effective in diminishing symptoms. In the elderly, shoulder hemiarthroplasty diminishes pain but improves function mildly. More pain relief and improvement in function is possible with a shoulder replacement with reverse ball-and-socket prosthesis. But complications such as loosening are more prevalent, so it is reserved for the elderly.

Feeley BT, Gallo RA, Craig EV: Cuff tear arthropathy: current trends in diagnosis and surgical management. *J Shoulder Elbow Surg* 2009;18:484. [PMID: 19208484]

Levy O, Venkateswaran B, Even T, Ravenscroft M, Copeland S: Mid-term clinical and sonographic outcome of arthroscopic repair of the rotator cuff. *J Bone Joint Surg Br* 2008;90:1341. [PMID: 18827245]

Mall NA, Kim HM, Keener JD, et al: Symptomatic progression of asymptomatic rotator cuff tears: a prospective study of clinical and sonographic variables. *J Bone Joint Surg Am* 2010;92:2623. [PMID: 21084574]

Matsen FA 3rd: Open rotator cuff repair without acromioplasty. *J Bone Joint Surg Am* 2009;91:487. [PMID: 19182000]

Pennington WT, Gibbons DJ, Bartz BA, et al: Comparative analysis of single-row versus double-row repair of rotator cuff tears. *Arthroscopy* 2010;26:1419. [PMID: 20875720]

Zumstein MA, Jost B, Hempel J, Hodler J, Gerber C: The clinical and structural long-term results of open repair of massive tears of the rotator cuff. *J Bone Joint Surg Am* 2008;90:2423. [PMID: 18978411]

▶ CPT Codes for Rotator Cuff Injuries

23130 Acromioplasty or acromionectomy, partial, with or without coracoacromial ligament release

23410 Repair of ruptured musculotendinous cuff (eg, rotator cuff) open; acute

23412 Reconstruction of complete shoulder (rotator) cuff avulsion, chronic (includes acromioplasty)

23415 Coracoacromial ligament release, with or without acromioplasty

23420 Reconstruction of complete shoulder (rotator) cuff avulsion, chronic (includes acromioplasty)

28926 Arthroscopy, shoulder, surgical; decompression of subacromial space with partial acromioplasty, with or without coracoacromial release

29827 Arthroscopy, shoulder, surgical; with rotator cuff repair

GLENOHUMERAL JOINT INSTABILITY

Distinguishing between shoulder laxity and instability is difficult, both because of the wide variability of normal joint laxity and the absence of biomechanical studies defining laxity and instability. In contrast, other joints such as the knee have precise definitions of instability. A Lachman test revealing greater than 5 mm of translation compared to the contralateral side is widely accepted as being associated with an ACL rupture and resulting knee instability. At the shoulder, instability is often defined as translations that result in symptoms. This poor definition of shoulder instability hampers proper diagnosis and intra- and interobserver classification and makes comparison of research studies difficult. Future study of normal and abnormal joint kinematics is needed to aid clinicians in diagnosis and classification of shoulder instability.

To make the correct diagnosis, the glenohumeral joint must be tested for anterior, posterior, and inferior instability. Different classifications of glenohumeral joint instability have been proposed, based on various characteristics. TUBS and AMBRI have been used to distinguish the two main types of instability. TUBS is an acronym describing instability caused by a *t*raumatic event, which is *u*nidirectional, is associated with a *B*ankart lesion, and often requires *s*urgical treatment. AMBRI refers to *a*traumatic, *m*ultidirectional instability that may be *b*ilateral and is best treated by *r*ehabilitation. In this classification, the etiology of multidirectional instability is thought to be enlargement of the capsule from either a genetic or microtraumatic origin. TUBS and AMBRI are of historic interest as clinicians have recognized more types of instability.

FEDS is an acronym describing the four most important characteristics of shoulder instability (*frequency*, *etiology*, *direction*, and *severity*) and can be obtained by history and physical examination. Frequency is classified as solitary, occasional (two to five episodes) or frequent (more than five episodes). Etiology is classified as traumatic or atraumatic. Direction is classified as anterior, inferior, or posterior. Lastly, severity is classified as subluxation or dislocation. Easy to remember, a weakness of the FEDS classification is that it does not distinguish unidirectional from multidirectional instability.

The positive sulcus sign has been used as the diagnostic hallmark for multidirectional instability, but we now know that the sulcus sign is sometimes found in shoulders of asymptomatic individuals with increased laxity. Laxity or joint play is a trait of body constitution that differs from one individual to another. Individuals may be loose or tight jointed. A shoulder is hyperlax if the examiner can easily subluxate the humeral head out of the glenoid in the anterior, posterior, and inferior directions without eliciting symptoms. Unfortunately, this makes classification of instability based on etiology, or direction alone, extremely difficult. Instead, classification is best based on the direction of instability that elicits symptoms and the presence or absence of hyperlaxity (Table 3–2). Multidirectional instability is defined as instability in both the anterior and posterior directions, which is most often subluxation rather than dislocation.

Often there is a tear of the glenoid labrum, the fibrocartilaginous rim around the glenoid fossa that deepens the socket and provides stability for the humeral head. It also is a connection for the surrounding capsuloligamentous structures. Glenoid labrum tears may occur from repetitive shoulder motion or acute trauma. In the athlete with repeated anterior subluxation of the shoulder, tears of the anteroinferior labrum may occur and lead to progressive instability. Patients with glenoid labrum injuries may describe their pain as interrupting smooth functioning of the shoulder during their specific activity. A labrum tear may be felt as a "pop" or "click" with motion of the shoulder. MRI arthrogram is useful for detection of these lesions.

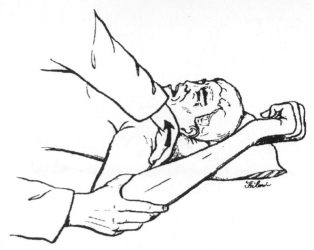

▲ **Figure 3–27.** The apprehension test for anterior instability.

Kuhn JE: A new classification system for shoulder instability. *Br J Sports Med* 2010;44:341. [PMID: 20371559]

▶ Glenohumeral Joint Instability Evaluation

A. Anterior Instability

The apprehension test is performed to assess anterior instability. The test applies an anterior-directed force to the humeral head from the back with the arm in abduction and external rotation (Figure 3–27). A positive test results from the patient's apprehension that the joint will dislocate. This maneuver mimics the position of subluxation, or dislocation, and causes reflex guarding. Conversely, the relocation test is positive if relief is obtained by applying a posterior-directed force to the humeral head (Figure 3–28).

B. Posterior Instability

No single test has high sensitivity and specificity for posterior instability. There is no posterior apprehension test, similar as that for anterior instability, that is helpful. The Jahnke test, sometimes called the jerk test, is performed by applying a posteriorly directed force to the forward flexed and internally rotated shoulder. The shoulder is then moved in horizontal abduction, into the coronal plane, as an anterior-directed force is applied to the humeral head. A clunk occurs as the humeral head reduces from the subluxed position (Figure 3–29). To perform the circumduction test, the patient is instructed to actively move the shoulder in a large circle starting from a flexed, internally rotated, and cross-body position, then to forward flexion, then to an abducted and externally rotated position, and lastly to the arm at the side. The examiner stands behind the patient and palpates the posterior shoulder. If positive, the joint subluxes in the flexed, internally

Table 3–2. Classification of glenohumeral instability based on the direction of instability and the presence or absence of hyperlaxity.

Direction / Laxity	UDI (Unidirectional Instability)	MDI (Multidirectional Instability)
Normal laxity	Very common 60%	Very rare 3%
Increased laxity	Common 30%	Rare 7%

Adapted, with permission, from Gerber C: Observations of the classification of instability. In: Warner JJP, Iannotti JP, Flatow EL, eds: *Complex and Revision Problems in Shoulder Surgery.* Philadelphia: Lippincott-Raven; 1997:9–18.

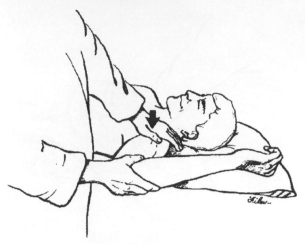

▲ **Figure 3–28.** The relocation test is positive if relief is obtained by applying a posterior-directed force to the humeral head.

rotated, and cross-body position and reduces as the shoulder is moved. In the Kim test, with the patient in a sitting position and the arm at 90 degrees of abduction, the examiner holds the elbow and lateral aspect of the proximal arm, and a strong axial loading force is applied. Then, while the arm is further elevated 45 degrees diagonally upward, downward and backward force is applied to the proximal arm. A sudden onset of posterior shoulder pain indicates a positive test result, regardless of accompanying posterior clunk of the humeral head.

C. Inferior Instability

The sulcus sign is used to evaluate laxity and inferior instability. The test is performed with the athlete in a sitting position with the arm at the side. A distraction force is applied longitudinally along the humerus. If positive, discomfort or apprehension of instability is experienced as the skin just distal to the lateral acromion hollows out (Figure 3–30).

GLENOHUMERAL DISLOCATION

When the shoulder is forced beyond the limit of its normal range of motion, the articular surface of the humeral head may be displaced from the glenoid to varying degrees. The majority of glenohumeral dislocations, or subluxations, are in the anteroinferior direction.

1. Anterior Dislocation

▶ Essentials of Diagnosis

- *The arm is typically held supported at the side.*
- *A visible dimple may be seen under the acromion due to the absence of the humeral head.*
- *The humeral head may be palpable under the coracoid or in the axilla.*
- *Range of motion will be extremely painful and limited.*
- *Appropriate radiographs will confirm the direction of dislocation and possible associated injuries.*

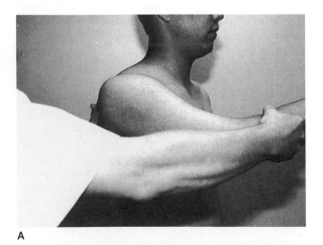

A

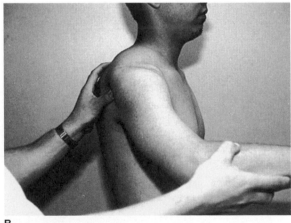

B

▲ **Figure 3–29.** The Jahnke test for posterior instability. **A:** A posterior-directed force applied to the forward flexed shoulder (in the upper left column). **B:** The shoulder is then moved into the coronal plane as an anterior-directed force is applied to the humeral head (in the lower left column). A clunk occurs as the humeral head reduces from the subluxed position. (Reprinted, with permission, from Hawkins RJ, Bokor DJ: Clinical evaluation of shoulder problems. In: Rockwood CA, Matsen F III, eds: *The Shoulder*. New York: WB Saunders; 1998, p. 186.)

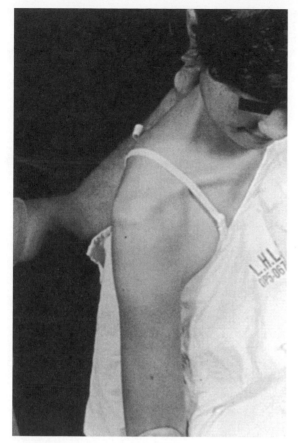

▲ **Figure 3–30.** The sulcus test for inferior instability. (Reprinted, with permission, from Hawkins RJ, Bokor DJ: Clinical evaluation of shoulder problems. In: Rockwood CA, Matsen F III, eds: *The Shoulder*. New York: WB Saunders; 1998, p. 189.)

▶ **Prevention**

Shoulder dislocations are typically the result of an acute traumatic injury. Therefore, although avoiding injury to the shoulder is the best form of prevention, minimizing the risk of dislocation following a blow can be achieved with regular stretching and strengthening of the rotator cuff musculature.

▶ **Clinical Findings**

Anterior glenohumeral dislocation occurs from either exceeding the normal range of motion in external rotation and/or abduction or a direct posterior or posterolateral blow on the shoulder strong enough to displace the humeral head. The anterior capsule is either stretched or torn within its attachment to the anterior glenoid. The head may be displaced into a sub-coracoid, subglenoid, or rarely subclavicular or intrathoracic

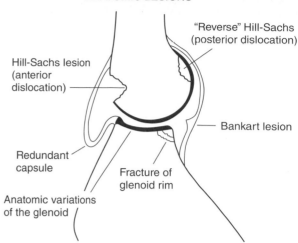

ANATOMIC LESIONS

"Reverse" Hill-Sachs (posterior dislocation)

Hill-Sachs lesion (anterior dislocation)

Bankart lesion

Redundant capsule

Fracture of glenoid rim

Anatomic variations of the glenoid

▲ **Figure 3–31.** Anatomic lesions producing shoulder instability.

position. Two major lesions are typically seen in patients with recurrent anterior dislocations (Figure 3–31). First is the Bankart lesion, an anterior capsular injury associated with a tear of the glenoid labrum off the anterior glenoid rim. The Bankart lesion may occur with fractures of the glenoid rim. Such fractures are often minimally displaced, and treatment is usually dictated by the joint instability. The second major lesion associated with recurrent anterior dislocations is the Hill-Sachs lesion, a compression fracture of the posterolateral articular surface of the humeral head. It is created by the sharp edge of the anterior glenoid as the humeral head dislocates over it. When large, both the Bankart and the Hill-Sachs lesions predispose to recurrent dislocations when the arm is placed in abduction and external rotation. If the glenoid rim fracture involves more than 20% of the glenoid diameter, then the joint becomes prone to instability, and treatment with open reduction and internal fixation is best. If the fracture is old, or the glenoid rim is worn to a similar level, then cortico-cancellous bone grafting of the glenoid rim is indicated.

Other injuries associated with anterior dislocation may occur. These include avulsion of the greater tuberosity from the humerus, caused by traction from the rotator cuff, and injury to the axillary nerve, which may be stretched or torn. Loss of axillary nerve function results in denervation of the deltoid and teres minor muscles and loss of sensation over the proximal lateral aspect of the arm. Axillary nerve palsy may also occur during reduction of the dislocation and therefore should be tested both before and after reduction. The deltoid extension lag sign, described in the section on axillary nerve injury, may be the best way to assess function of this nerve. Lastly, the dead arm syndrome may occur after anterior joint instability. For example, a pitcher may report a sudden inability to throw, with the arm going numb and becoming extremely weak after ball release. The symptoms are transient, resolving within a few seconds to minutes.

Athletes who sustain a shoulder dislocation will try to hold the injured extremity at their side, gripping the forearm with the opposite hand. Most athletes know their shoulder is dislocated and will immediately seek help. On physical examination of an anterior dislocation, the examiner will note a space underneath the acromion where the humeral head should lie and a palpable anterior mass representing the humeral head in the anterior axilla.

▶ Treatment

Acute and recurrent anterior glenohumeral dislocations must be distinguished, as an acute dislocation sustains severe trauma with the increased probability of associated injuries. The recurrent dislocation may occur with minimal trauma, and reduction may be accomplished with much less effort. Anterior dislocations may be reduced by one of several techniques. Longitudinal traction may be exerted on the affected arm with external rotation, followed by internal rotation of the arm. Care must be taken to avoid direct pressure on the neurovascular structures. Another method is to have the patient lie face down on the table and tie or tape a bucket to the injured arm and slowly fill it with water. This allows the musculature around the shoulder to relax from the force of the weight and effect a spontaneous reduction.

Following reduction of an initial dislocation, the shoulder should be immobilized in internal rotation for 2–6 weeks. Healing will generally take at least 6 weeks. Before returning to athletics, the patient should have normal range of motion without pain and normal strength in the shoulder. Emphasis must be placed on strengthening the rotator cuff muscles to compensate for the laxity of the ligamentous support. When weight training is begun, military press, fly exercises, a narrow grip while bench pressing, and deep shoulder dips must be excluded until considerable time has elapsed and healing is complete.

Recurrent dislocations should be treated with minimal immobilization until the pain subsides, followed by range-of-motion and muscle-strengthening exercises. Many restraining devices are available to help prevent recurrent dislocations during sporting activities, focusing on keeping the arm from going into abduction and external rotation. These orthotics may be effective, but because they limit the athlete's range of shoulder motion, their use is limited for certain competitive activities.

If an athlete has sustained multiple dislocations and is unresponsive to conservative treatment, surgical reconstruction of the shoulder joint may be indicated. There is a wide variety of repair procedures with either open or arthroscopic techniques. Repair of the labral lesion (ie, Bankart repair) and tightening of the anteroinferior capsule are integral to all of these procedures (Table 3–3), and success is frequent. When present, large Hill-Sachs and bony Bankart lesions should be treated as well.

Table 3–3. Repair of capsule and labrum back to the glenoid rim.

Bankart procedure
    duToit procedure
    Viek procedure
    Eyre-Brook procedure
    Moseley procedure
Muscle and capsule plication
    Putti-Platt procedure
    Symeonides procedure
Muscle and tendon sling procedures
    Magnuson-Stack procedure
    Bristow-Helfet-Latarjet procedure modifications
    Boytchev procedure
    Nicola procedure
    Gallie-LeMesurier procedure
    Boyd transfer of long head of biceps (for posterior dislocation)
Bone block
    Eden-Hybbinette procedure
    DeAnquin procedure (through a superior approach to the shoulder)
Osteotomies
    Weber (humeral neck)
    Saha (humeral shaft)

For most surgical procedures, aggressive range-of-motion exercises do not start until at least 3 weeks postoperatively. The goal is to have full abduction and 90 degrees of external rotation. By 12 weeks, patients have often progressed well into their initial programs and may begin a variety of weight-training exercises, avoiding exercises that strain the anterior capsule.

▶ Prognosis

Young patients are at a high risk for redislocation after a primary traumatic anterior shoulder dislocation if treated conservatively with rehabilitation. Surgical stabilization should be considered in these cases. In general, despite surgical stabilization, patients have up to a 10% chance of redislocation if returning to play in contact sports.

2. Posterior Dislocation

▶ Essentials of Diagnosis

- *Posterior dislocations are more difficult to diagnose than anterior dislocations.*
- *The arm is typically held in internal rotation and is not able to be externally rotated.*
- *Appropriate radiographs will confirm the direction of dislocation and possible associated injuries.*

Prevention

Shoulder dislocations are typically the result of an acute traumatic injury. Therefore, while avoiding injury to the shoulder is the best form of prevention, the risk of dislocation following a blow can be minimized with regular stretching and strengthening of the rotator cuff musculature.

Clinical Findings

Posterior glenohumeral dislocations result from the posterior capsule being torn, stretched, or disrupted from the posterior glenoid. A reverse Hill-Sachs lesion (see Figure 3–31) may appear on the anterior articular surface of the humerus. With a posterior dislocation, the subscapularis, or its insertion on the lesser tuberosity, may be injured. Posterior dislocations are often difficult to diagnose, as the patient may have a normal contour to the shoulder or the deltoid of a well-developed athlete may mask signs of a displaced humeral head. The patient holds the injured shoulder in internal rotation and the examiner cannot externally rotate it. Anteroposterior and axillary radiographs must be obtained to diagnose a posterior dislocation.

Treatment

Applying traction in the line of the adducted humerus, with an anterior directed force to the humeral head, reduces a posterior dislocation. Anesthesia often helps decrease the trauma of reduction. Following reduction, the shoulder is immobilized for 2–6 weeks in external rotation and a small amount of abduction. Surgical treatment should be considered if these measures fail to provide the desired results.

Prognosis

Patients with an acute posterior dislocation are often able to return to their sport following a course of rehabilitation emphasizing range-of-motion and rotator cuff strengthening.

3. Multidirectional Instability

Essentials of Diagnosis

- *Multidirectional instability is often difficult to diagnose.*
- *Shoulder pain is not specific to overhead activities or associated with other shoulder injuries.*
- *Fatigue or paresthesias may be present.*
- *Evidence of both anterior and posterior instability with the history and physical examination.*
- *Positive sulcus sign.*
- *Must be evaluated for hyperlaxity that must then be distinguished from instability.*

Clinical Findings

Some patients will have instability in both the anterior and posterior directions, which is most often subluxation rather than dislocation. This may result in a painful shoulder, especially if rotator cuff strength decreases. The pain is often primarily a result of rotator cuff inflammation, likely from attempts to stabilize the humeral head during activity. Patients may complain of vague symptoms, including upper extremity fatigue, discomfort, pain, apprehension, and paresthesias. They may describe frank episodes of instability. Physical examination should include evaluation for signs of generalized hyperlaxity, which include hyperextension of the metacarpophalangeal joints, elbows, and knees and the ability to adduct the thumb to the ipsilateral wrist. Generalized hyperlaxity does not necessarily indicate symptomatic instability of the shoulder. The shoulder examination should include tests for anterior, posterior, and inferior instability as described earlier. MRI can be a useful adjunct to plain radiographs and may reveal an enlarged axillary pouch and labral or rotator cuff pathology.

Treatment and Prognosis

Initial treatment for multidirectional instability is nonoperative and leads to successful results in the vast majority of cases. This includes patient education, modification of activity, and a strengthening program for the rotator cuff and scapular stabilizing muscles. When this fails, surgery is often effective in relieving symptoms. Because of differences in classifying multidirectional instability, results of treatment vary as well. For those with multidirectional instability classified as instability in both the anterior and posterior directions, about two thirds of patients, less than that with unidirectional anterior instability, will have relief after surgery.

Bahu MJ, Trentacosta N, Vorys GC, Covey AS, Ahmad CS: Multidirectional instability: evaluation and treatment options. *Clin Sports Med* 2008;27:671. [PMID: 19064150]

Barchilon VS, Kotz E, Barchilon Ben-Av M, Glazer E, Nyska M: A simple method for quantitative evaluation of the missing area of the anterior glenoid in anterior instability of the glenohumeral joint. *Skeletal Radiol* 2008;37:731. [PMID: 18523766]

Bartl C, Schumann K, Vogt S, Paul J, Imhoff AB: Arthroscopic capsulolabral revision repair for recurrent anterior shoulder instability. *Am J Sports Med.* 2011;39:511. [PMID: 21212311]

Bradley JP, Forsythe B, Mascarenhas R: Arthroscopic management of posterior shoulder instability: diagnosis, indications, and technique. *Clin Sports Med* 2008;27:649. [PMID: 19064149]

DiPaola MJ, Jazrawi LM, Rokito AS, et al: Management of humeral and glenoid bone loss—associated with glenohumeral instability. *Bull NYU Hosp Jt Dis* 2010;68:245. [PMID: 21162700]

Hovelius L, Olofsson A, Sandström B, et al: Nonoperative treatment of primary anterior shoulder dislocation in patients forty years of age and younger. A prospective twenty-five-year follow up. *J Bone Joint Surg Am* 2008;90:945. [PMID: 18451384]

Purchase RJ, Wolf EM, Hobgood ER, Pollock ME, Smalley CC: Hill-Sachs "remplissage": an arthroscopic solution for the engaging Hill-Sachs lesion. *Arthroscopy* 2008;24:723. [PMID: 18514117]

CPT Codes for Shoulder Instability

23650 Closed treatment of shoulder dislocation, with manipulation; without anesthesia

23655 Closed treatment of shoulder dislocation, with manipulation; requiring anesthesia

23600 Open treatment of acute shoulder dislocation

23450 Capsulorrhaphy, anterior; Putti-Platt procedure or Magnuson type operation

23455 Capsulorrhaphy, anterior; with labral repair (eg, Bankart procedure)

23460 Capsulorrhaphy, anterior, any type; with bone block

23462 Capsulorrhaphy, anterior, any type; with coracoid process transfer

23465 Capsulorrhaphy, glenohumeral joint, posterior, with or without bone block

23466 Capsulorrhaphy, glenohumeral joint, any type multidirectional instability

29806 Arthroscopy, shoulder, surgical; capsulorrhaphy

SLAP LESIONS

SLAP lesions involve the origin of the long head of the biceps brachii (biceps anchor) and the superior capsulolabral structures. The acronym SLAP is for *superior labrum anterior and posterior*. A type I lesion is fraying of the labrum. Type II lesions are most common, accounting for over 50% of patients with a SLAP lesion, and are detachment of the superior labrum from the glenoid. A type III lesion is a bucket-handle tear of the superior labrum with firm attachment of the remainder of the labrum. In a type IV lesion, there is a tear of the labrum that extends into the biceps tendon (Figure 3–32).

Types V to VII SLAP lesions were later added to this initial four-part classification. A type V lesion is an anterior-inferior Bankart lesion that continues superiorly to include separation of the biceps tendon. A type VI lesion includes a biceps separation with an unstable flap tear of the labrum. Finally, a type VII lesion involves a superior labrum-biceps tendon separation that extends anteriorly beneath the middle glenohumeral ligament.

Proposed mechanisms of injury include a fall onto an outstretched arm, with the shoulder positioned in abduction and slight forward flexion at the time of the impact, and in overhead athletes, posteroinferior capsular tightness that results in diminished internal rotation of the abducted shoulder, diagnosed with comparison to the contralateral side. With overhead throwing, this results in posterosuperior translation of the humeral head, accompanied by pain in the cocking phase of throwing and demonstrated on clinical examination by pain in the posterior shoulder when placed in the apprehension position of abduction and external rotation. A peel-back mechanism is proposed as being responsible for the SLAP lesion. Mild anterior shoulder instability also occurs due to these alterations in the glenohumeral joint and aberrations

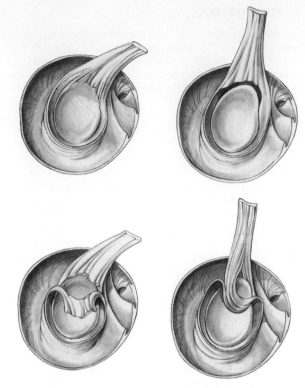

▲ **Figure 3–32.** The five types of the SLAP lesion include fraying of the superior capsulolabrum (type I), detachment of the superior capsulolabrum and the biceps anchor (type II), bucket-handle tearing of the superior capsulolabrum (type III), detachment of the superior capsulolabrum and tearing into the biceps anchor (type IV), and combinations of these (type V).

of scapulothoracic motion. However, SLAP lesions may most commonly be found incidentally in elderly individuals undergoing surgical treatment of a rotator cuff tear.

▶ Essentials of Diagnosis

- *Common clinical complaints are shoulder pain greater with activities involving overhead motion and a painful "catching" or "popping."*

- *Pain with resisted forward flexion with the arm in the internally rotated and slightly adducted position, relieved by externally rotating the arm.*

- *Magnetic resonance arthrography can aid in the diagnosis.*

▶ Prevention

Because labral injuries can result from repetitive activity or an acute traumatic event, it is important to maintain good strength and flexibility of the shoulder to minimize these injuries.

Clinical Findings

SLAP lesions cause shoulder pain both from mechanical symptoms and mild shoulder instability. Yet, they remain difficult to diagnose despite efforts to develop specific tests. No single test is both sensitive and specific for the diagnosis of SLAP lesions. Magnetic resonance arthrography can be helpful. However, diagnostic arthroscopy remains the best means to definitively diagnose SLAP lesions. The active compression test may prove to be the most useful single provocative maneuver. The internally rotated shoulder is forward flexed to 90 degrees and is then brought across the body in horizontal abduction about 10 degrees. The test is positive if the patient has pain with resisted forward flexion that is relieved by external rotation of the shoulder.

A complicating factor in making the diagnosis is that the majority of SLAP lesions are associated with other shoulder pathology such as rotator cuff tears, acromioclavicular joint pathology, and instability. Less than 28% of SLAP lesions are isolated.

Treatment

Although the history, physical examination, and imaging, specifically magnetic resonance arthrography, are helpful, definitive diagnosis of SLAP lesions is best made with diagnostic arthroscopy. Treatment can be simplified by noting whether the lesion would contribute to detachment of either the biceps anchor or the anterosuperior capsulolabrum. Lesions producing meaningful detachment of the anterior capsuloligamentous structures generally require repair of these structures back to the bony glenoid rim. Lesions extending into the biceps tendon may require debridement, biceps tenotomy, or tenodesis.

Alpert JM, Wuerz TH, O'Donnell TF, Carroll KM, Brucker NN, Gill TJ: The effect of age on the outcomes of arthroscopic repair of type II superior labral anterior and posterior lesions. *Am J Sports Med* 2010;38:2299. [PMID: 20739578]

Barber FA, Field LD, Ryu RK: Biceps tendon and superior labrum injuries: decision making. *Instr Course Lect* 2008;57:527. [PMID: 18399607]

Boileau P, Parratte S, Chuinard C, Roussanne Y, Shia D, Bicknell R: Arthroscopic treatment of isolated type II SLAP lesions: biceps tenodesis as an alternative to reinsertion. *Am J Sports Med* 2009;37:929. [PMID: 19229046]

Franceschi F, Longo UG, Ruzzini L, Rizzello G, Maffulli N, Denaro V: No advantages in repairing a type II superior labrum anterior and posterior (SLAP) lesion when associated with rotator cuff repair in patients over age 50: a randomized controlled trial. *Am J Sports Med* 2008;36:247. [PMID: 17940144]

Kanatli U, Ozturk BY, Bolukbasi S: Anatomical variations of the anterosuperior labrum: prevalence and association with type II superior labrum anterior-posterior (SLAP) lesions. *J Shoulder Elbow Surg* 2010;19:1199. [PMID: 21070956]

Meserve BB, Cleland JA, Boucher TR: A meta-analysis examining clinical test utility for assessing superior labral anterior posterior lesions. *Am J Sports Med* 2009;37:2252. [PMID: 19095895]

CPT Code for SLAP Lesions

29807 Arthroscopy, shoulder, surgical; repair of SLAP lesion

SHOULDER STIFFNESS

Essentials of Diagnosis

- *Very painful and/or limited range of motion of the shoulder.*
- *May be idiopathic or posttraumatic.*
- *Loss of active and passive range of motion, most notably internal rotation.*
- *Arthrography can aid in the diagnosis.*

Prevention

Most patients have some sort of antecedent trauma to their shoulder, be it minimal or severe. Initiating gentle range-of-motion and strengthening exercises immediately after the traumatic event are essential to minimizing the likelihood of developing shoulder stiffness.

Clinical Findings

Often called adhesive capsulitis or frozen shoulder, shoulder stiffness is a painful condition characterized by significant restriction in both active and passive range of motion. With shoulder stiffness, the articular surfaces are normal and the joint is stable, yet there is a restriction in range of motion. Stiffness usually results from soft-tissue contracture but can also occur from malaligned articular surfaces, bursal adhesions, or a shortened muscle-tendon unit. Often of uncertain etiology, the restrictions of shoulder motion are global. That is, none of the shoulder planes of motion is spared.

Shoulder stiffness may be separated into idiopathic and posttraumatic etiologies. Idiopathic shoulder stiffness is most common in older individuals, especially women between 40 and 60 years of age. Other factors that predispose to idiopathic shoulder stiffness include cervical, cardiac, pulmonary, neoplastic, neurologic, and personality disorders. Patients with diabetes mellitus are also at a high risk of developing shoulder stiffness, with 10–35% of diabetics having restriction of shoulder motion. Diabetics who have been insulin dependent for many years have the greatest incidence and bilateral involvement. Because of this close association, clinicians should ask their patients with shoulder stiffness about symptoms of diabetes; 70% of individuals with shoulder stiffness may have diabetes or a prediabetes condition. The pathophysiology of idiopathic shoulder stiffness remains uncertain, but the pathoanatomy is commonly limited to contracture of the glenohumeral capsule (Figure 3–33). Most prominently involved is the rotator interval, which includes the superior glenohumeral ligament and coracohumeral ligament.

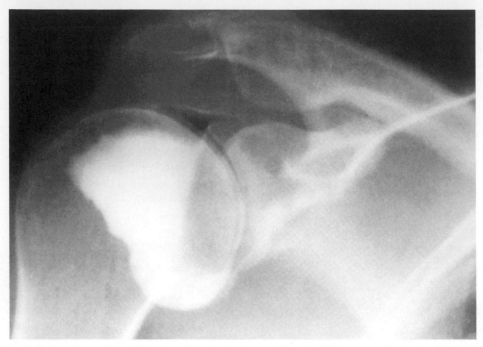

▲ **Figure 3–33.** Adhesive capsulitis of the shoulder. Note the small irregular joint capsule with addition of contrast material.

Although all patients can recall some traumatic event that preceded their shoulder stiffness, those with distinct trauma such as a prior fracture, rotator cuff tear, or surgical procedure have a posttraumatic etiology. Stiffness after shoulder surgery is typical and usually resolves with time and appropriate rehabilitation. The shoulder should not be neglected after any surgery about the shoulder girdle. This includes axillary or cervical lymph node dissections, especially when combined with radiation therapy, cardiac catheterization in the axilla, and coronary artery bypass grafting with sternotomy and thoracotomy. All surgeons should be aware that these procedures may result in restricted shoulder motion.

The clinical presentation of idiopathic shoulder stiffness is classically described as having three phases. The first phase is the painful, freezing phase. The pain is typically achy in nature, and sudden jolts or attempts at rapid motion exacerbate the chronic discomfort. The pain may begin at night, and shoulder motion becomes progressively limited. Patients often hold their arm at their side and in internal rotation with the forearm across the belly. They may also be treated for nonspecific shoulder pain with a sling in this position. This inflammatory phase often lasts between 2 and 9 months.

The second phase of progressive stiffness lasts between 3 and 12 months. Stiffness progresses to a point at which shoulder motion is restricted in all planes. Essentially, the shoulder has undergone fibrous arthrodesis. Fortunately, pain progressively decreases from the initial inflammatory phase. With time, patients are able to use the shoulder with little or no pain, within the restricted range of motion, but attempts to exceed this range are accompanied by pain. The patient's symptoms then plateau. Unfortunately, this phase may be persistent, with symptoms lasting for extended periods. In the resolution, or thawing phase, the shoulder slowly and progressively becomes more supple. It can be as short as a month, but typically lasts 1–3 years.

On clinical examination, there is loss of both active and passive range of shoulder motion. Often the first motion to be affected is internal rotation, demonstrated by an inability to bring the arm up the back to the same level as the normal shoulder. MRI reveals decreased rotator interval size, and arthrography demonstrates marked reduction in joint capacity; often the affected shoulder will not take more than a few milliliters of dye, whereas the normal capacity is 20–30 mL.

▶ Treatment

Treatment varies, but conservative modalities and progressive range-of-motion exercises seem effective. Range-of-motion exercises for external rotation and abduction will help minimize the length of restriction in motion and dysfunction. Nonoperative treatments are successful for most.

When operative treatments are chosen, manipulation under anesthesia and capsular distension, along the mainstays of intervention, are replaced by selective arthroscopic capsular release.

Prognosis

Whether treated nonoperatively or operatively, a return of about 80% shoulder range of motion is usual.

Blanchard V, Barr S, Cerisola FL: The effectiveness of corticosteroid injections compared with physiotherapeutic interventions for adhesive capsulitis: a systematic review. *Physiotherapy* 2010;96:95. [PMID: 20420956]

Hand C, Clipsham K, Rees JL, Carr AJ: Long-term outcome of frozen shoulder. *J Shoulder Elbow Surg* 2008;17:231. [PMID: 17993282]

Hand GC, Athanasou NA, Matthews T, Carr AJ: The pathology of frozen shoulder. *J Bone Joint Surg Br* 2007;89:928. [PMID: 17673588]

Milgrom C, Novack V, Weil Y, Jaber S, Radeva-Petrova DR, Finestone A: Risk factors for idiopathic frozen shoulder. *Isr Med Assoc J* 2008;10:361. [PMID: 18605360]

Rill BK, Fleckenstein CM, Levy MS, Nagesh V, Hasan SS: Predictors of outcome after nonoperative and operative treatment of adhesive capsulitis. *Am J Sports Med* 2011;39:567. [PMID: 21160014]

Saccommanni B: Inflammation and shoulder pain: a perspective on rotator cuff disease, adhesive capsulitis, and osteoarthritis: conservative treatment. *Clin Rheumatol* 2009;28:495. [PMID: 19224130]

Tauro JC, Paulson M: Shoulder stiffness. *Arthroscopy* 2008;24:949. [PMID: 18657745]

Thomas SJ, McDougall C, Brown ID, et al: Prevalence of symptoms and signs of shoulder problems in people with diabetes mellitus. *J Shoulder Elbow Surg* 2007;16:748. [PMID: 18061115]

CPT Codes for Shoulder Stiffness

23020 Capsular contracture release (eg, Sever-type procedure)

23700 Manipulation under anesthesia, shoulder joint, including application of fixation apparatus (dislocation excluded)

29825 Arthroscopy, shoulder, surgical; with lysis and resection of adhesions, with or without manipulation

FRACTURES ABOUT THE SHOULDER

1. Clavicular Fracture

The clavicle is one of the most commonly fractured bones in the body, with direct trauma being the usual cause in athletic events (Figure 3–34). Football, wrestling, and ice hockey are the sports most commonly involved in clavicular fractures, which is not surprising as all three are associated with high-speed contact between players.

Essentials of Diagnosis

- *History of injury to the shoulder.*
- *Swelling and ecchymosis overlying the injured clavicle.*
- *Pain and crepitation upon palpation of the fracture site.*
- *Pain and limited range of motion of the arm, specifically in forward flexion and abduction.*
- *Appropriate radiographs will define the location and severity of the fracture.*

Clinical Findings

Despite the proximity of vital structures, clavicular fractures that occur during athletic activities are rarely associated with

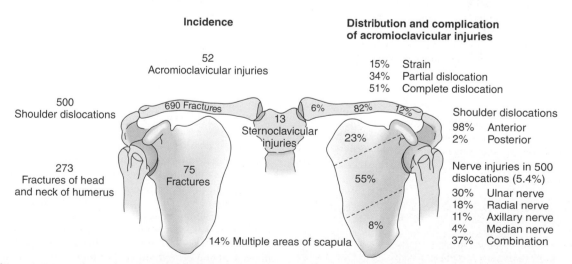

▲ **Figure 3–34.** Analysis of 1603 shoulder girdle injuries, showing the frequency and location of fractures and dislocations.

neurovascular damage, and accompanying soft-tissue disorders are uncommon. The patient will usually give a history of falling in the area of the shoulder or receiving a blow to the clavicle, experiencing immediate pain and an inability to raise the arm. Radiography will usually confirm the clinical impression and must show the entire clavicle, including the shoulder girdle, upper third of the humerus, and sternal end of the clavicle.

Of clavicular fractures, midclavicular fractures account for 80%, distal fractures for 15%, and proximal fractures for 5%. Most fractures of the shaft of the clavicle heal well. However, some neurovascular complications, such as a tear of the subclavian artery or a brachial plexus injury, are serious, although rare. Therefore, when evaluating and treating clavicular fractures, an initial neurovascular examination is very important. Pulses in the distal part of the upper extremity, strength, and sensation must be carefully evaluated.

Because the clavicle is the only bone structure that fixes the shoulder girdle to the thorax, a fracture through the clavicle causes the shoulder to sag forward and downward. The pull of the sternocleidomastoid muscle may displace the proximal fragment superiorly. These forces tend to hinder the initial reduction and maintenance of reduction. In addition, distal fractures, which are more common in older age groups, may involve tears in the coracoclavicular ligament, which allows the proximal clavicle to ride up superiorly, mimicking an acromioclavicular dislocation. Delayed union is much more common in this type of fracture than in other clavicular fractures.

Treatment

Mid and proximal clavicular fractures are usually treated with a short period of rest, with a sling on the affected side to support the extremity. Immobilization is usually discontinued at 3–4 weeks, and once the clavicular fracture has healed, range-of-motion and strengthening exercises should begin. Comminuted mid and proximal clavicular fractures with meaningful displacement and especially when it is shortening may be best treated with open reduction and internal fixation. Distal fractures with tears in the coracoclavicular ligament, mimicking an acromioclavicular dislocation, are best treated with open reduction and internal fixation.

Prognosis

Onset of exercises prior to healing may contribute to nonunion. Athletes should not be allowed to return to play until shoulder strength and range of motion return to preinjury levels. Generally, no special braces or pads are required when the athlete returns to play.

Khan LA, Bradnock TJ, Scott C, Robinson CM: Fractures of the clavicle. *J Bone Joint Surg Am* 2009;91:447. [PMID: 19181992]

Kulshrestha V, Roy T, Audige L: Operative versus nonoperative management of displaced midshaft clavicle fractures: a prospective cohort study. *J Orthop Trauma* 2011;25:31. [PMID: 21164305]

Robinson CM, Court-Brown CM, McQueen MM, et al: Estimating the risk of nonunion following nonoperative treatment of a clavicular fracture. *J Bone Joint Surg Am* 2004;86-A:1359. [PMID: 15252081]

▶ CPT Codes for Clavicle Fractures

23500 Closed treatment of clavicular fracture; without manipulation

23505 Closed treatment of clavicular fracture; with manipulation

23515 Open treatment of clavicular fracture, includes internal fixation, when performed

2. Proximal Humerus Fracture

▶ Essentials of Diagnosis

- *History of trauma to the shoulder.*
- *Swelling and ecchymosis overlying the shoulder that may extend down to the elbow.*
- *Tenderness and crepitation over the fracture site.*
- *Pain with attempted range of motion of the shoulder.*
- *Appropriate radiographs will define the location and severity of the fracture.*

Fractures of the proximal humerus, which represent approximately 4–5% of all fractures, are a relatively uncommon sports injury. They most often present in young adolescents with open growth plates or in elderly osteoporotic patients. When they do occur in the athlete, they are typically the result of a high-energy impact injury or are secondary to an underlying pathologic bone condition.

▶ Clinical Findings

The proximal humerus consists of four major bony components: the humeral head, the greater tuberosity, the lesser tuberosity, and the humeral shaft. Fractures, which can occur between any or all of these regions, are traditionally defined by the location and displacement of the fracture fragments (Figure 3–35). The patient with a proximal humerus fracture will usually be able to report the mechanism of injury and will complain of pain, swelling, and an inability to use the shoulder. A physical examination will often reveal loss of the normal contour of the shoulder, tenderness about the shoulder, ecchymosis that may extend down to the elbow, and crepitus on attempted range of motion. A thorough neurovascular examination is essential, as brachial plexus and axillary nerve injuries have been reported in association with proximal humerus fractures. Because the axillary nerve is the nerve most commonly injured in these cases, sensation to light touch and pin-prick over the lateral aspect of the upper arm and deltoid muscle function must be tested. An accurate radiographic evaluation is necessary to confirm the

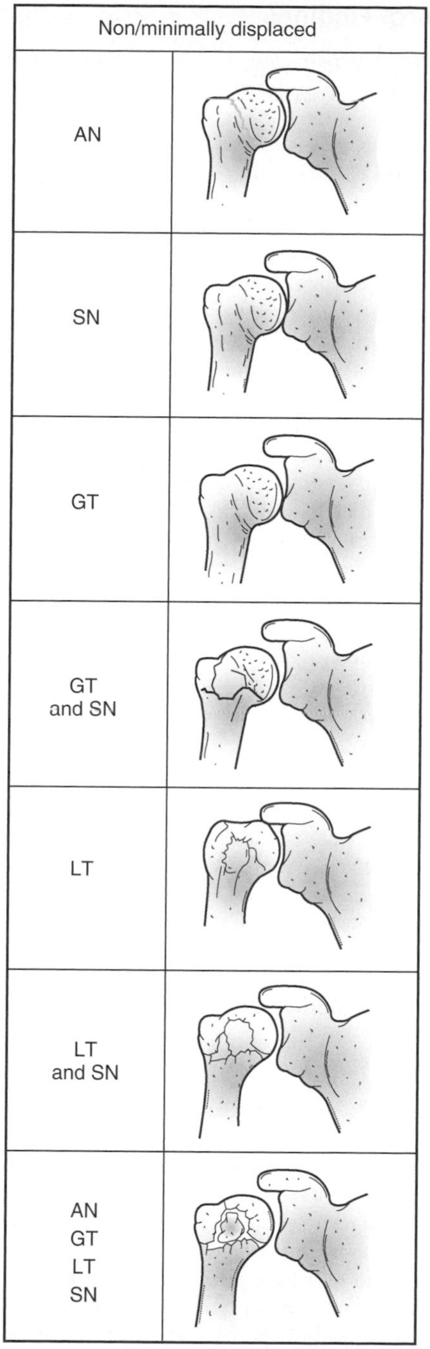

▲ **Figure 3–35.** Four-part classification for fractures of the proximal humerus. AN, anatomic neck; GT, greater tuberosity; LT, lesser tuberosity; SN, surgical neck. [Reprinted with permission from Norris TR, Green A: Proximal humerus fractures and fracture-dislocations. In: Browner BD, et al, eds: *Skeletal Trauma: Fractures, Dislocation and Ligamentous Injuries.* Elsevier; 1998.]

type and severity of the fracture and is essential in determining the treatment plan. Anteroposterior and lateral views in the plane of the scapula, as well as an axillary view to rule out an associated glenohumeral dislocation, are necessary.

▶ **Treatment**

Most proximal humerus fractures are minimally displaced and can be treated nonoperatively with sling immobilization and early passive range of motion. However, about 20% need to be treated operatively. Many factors contribute to this decision-making process, including fracture type and degree of displacement, bone quality, activity level, and associated injuries. Surgical options range from closed reduction and percutaneous pinning to open reduction with internal fixation to humeral head replacement.

▶ **Prognosis**

For minimally displaced fractures, the prognosis is generally good. Loss of motion is the most common complication. It can take 12–18 months to attain the maximal result, so range-of-motion exercises should be continued for an extended period of time.

Cannon CP, Paraliticci GU, Lin PP, Lewis VO, Yasko AW: Functional outcome following endoprosthetic reconstruction of the proximal humerus. *J Shoulder Elbow Surg* 2009;18:705. [PMID: 19186077]

Zhu Y, Lu Y, Shen J, Zhang J, Jiang C: Locking intramedullary nails and locking plates in the treatment of two-part proximal humeral surgical neck fractures: a prospective randomized trial with a minimum of three years of follow-up. *J Bone Joint Surg Am* 2011;93:159. [PMID: 21248213]

PROXIMAL HUMERAL EPIPHYSEAL FRACTURE

In young athletes, epiphyseal fractures of the proximal humerus may occur. The separate growth centers of the articular surface, greater tuberosity, and lesser tuberosity coalesce at approximately age 7 years, with the remaining growth plates closing at 20–22 years of age. Therefore, fracture separations may occur at any age until the growth plates have closed. Fortunately, fractures in this area usually do not arrest growth.

▶ **Essentials of Diagnosis**

- *Proximal humerus pain.*
- *Widening of the proximal humeral physis on radiographs.*

▶ **Clinical Findings**

Injury can occur to the shoulder in the growing musculoskeletal system of young athletes engaged in sports that involve overhead throwing. Proximal humerus pain associated with widening of the proximal humerus epiphysis, especially while throwing, has been termed "little league shoulder."

Although widening of the proximal humerus epiphysis can be an adaptive change to throwing, when painful, it may represent a fracture resulting from overuse.

Treatment

Cessation of throwing is the first step in treatment. Once pain has resolved, range-of-motion and strengthening exercises can be initiated. Ultimately, throwing can be resumed as long as the patient is pain free.

Bahrs C, Zipplies S, Ochs BG, et al: Proximal humeral fractures in children and adolescents. *J Pediatr Orthop* 2009;29:238. [PMID: 19305272]

CPT Codes for Proximal Humerus Fractures

23600 Closed treatment of proximal humeral (surgical or anatomic neck) fracture; without manipulation

23605 Closed treatment of proximal humeral (surgical or anatomic neck) fracture; with manipulation, with or without skeletal traction

23615 Open treatment of proximal humeral (surgical or anatomic neck) fracture, includes internal fixation, when performed, includes repair of tuberosity(s), when performed

23616 Open treatment of proximal humeral (surgical or anatomic neck) fracture, includes internal fixation, when performed, includes repair of tuberosity(s), when performed; with proximal humeral prosthetic replacement

23620 Closed treatment of greater humeral tuberosity fracture; without manipulation

23525 Closed treatment of greater humeral tuberosity fracture; with manipulation

23630 Open treatment of greater humeral tuberosity fracture, includes internal fixation, when performed

GLENOHUMERAL JOINT OSTEOARTHRITIS

Essentials of Diagnosis

- *Constant achy pain in all shoulder positions, even with the arm at the side.*
- *Pain worsened with activity.*
- *Crepitus with motion.*
- *Pain is relieved with lidocaine injection into glenohumeral joint.*

Prevention

It is best to curtail activity once the articular surfaces of the glenohumeral joint have been injured to minimize progression of osteoarthritis. Even rigorous activity in the uninjured shoulder is unlikely to result in osteoarthritis.

Clinical Findings

Achy, persistent pain and limitation of motion are often initial symptoms of osteoarthritis of the glenohumeral joint. Most common after the sixth decade, osteoarthritis can present at earlier ages in those having suffered injury earlier in life. Pain is exacerbated by activity and often persists for hours after the activity ceases. In mild to moderate cases, the pain diminishes with NSAIDs. Shoulder motion is associated with crepitus, and active and passive range of motion are the same, similar to adhesive capsulitis. Shoulder weakness and muscle atrophy are secondary to the pain and disuse of the shoulder that occur when the osteoarthritis is severe.

Radiographs of the shoulder reveal decreased joint space, osteophytes, subchondral sclerosis, and subchondral cysts of the glenohumeral joint. The prominence of these findings is associated with the severity of the disease but is only loosely associated with complaints of pain. Like the hip, knee, and other joints, some have severe pain with mild radiographic findings, whereas others cope well with severe findings. MRI may be useful to evaluate the shoulder for other injuries such as a rotator cuff tear.

Treatment

Rest, rehabilitation, and taking NSAIDs may diminish symptoms in those with mild to moderate osteoarthritis. Range-of-motion and strengthening exercises are recommended, unless they cause significant discomfort. Activities that exacerbate the symptoms should be avoided, and strengthening of the shoulder muscles should be done as long as they do not exacerbate symptoms. Injection of corticosteroids may relieve symptoms for a period of time, and repeated injections at intervals of a few months are sometimes effective. Individuals with pain, weakness, or decreased range of motion that persist after nonoperative treatment may elect surgical intervention with glenohumeral joint arthroplasty.

Prognosis

Glenohumeral joint arthroplasty is effective in diminishing shoulder pain when both the humeral head and the glenoid are resurfaced (total joint arthroplasty). Another option is hemiarthroplasty of the humeral head only, which decreases pain, on average, by about two thirds. The latter may yield a more durable arthroplasty as the glenoid component loosens more often over long periods of time than the humeral component. About 90% of total joint arthroplasties will last 10 years, and nearly 75% will last 20 years. Neither procedure yields normal joint function; patients have only partial improvement in strength and range of motion.

Hambright D, Henderson RA, Cook C, Worrell T, Moorman CT, Bolognesi MP: A comparison of perioperative outcomes in patients with and without rheumatoid arthritis after receiving a total shoulder replacement arthroplasty. *J Shoulder Elbow Surg* 2011;20:77. [PMID: 20655764]

Millett PJ, Gobezie R, Boykin RE: Shoulder osteoarthritis: diagnosis and management. *Am Fam Physician* 2008;78:605. [PMID: 18788237]

Saltzman MD, Mercer DM, Warme WJ, Bertelsen AL, Matsen FA 3rd: Comparison of patients undergoing primary shoulder arthroplasty before and after the age of fifty. *J Bone Joint Surg Am* 2010;92:42. [PMID: 20048094]

Singh JA, Sperling J, Buchbinder R, McMaken K: Surgery for shoulder osteoarthritis: a Cochrane systematic review. *J Rheumatol* 2011;38:598. [PMID: 21239751]

▶ CPT Codes for Glenohumeral Joint Osteoarthritis

23470 Arthroplasty, glenohumeral joint; hemiarthroplasty

23472 Arthroplasty, glenohumeral joint; total shoulder (glenoid and proximal humeral replacement [eg, total shoulder])

29822 Arthroscopy, shoulder, surgical; debridement, limited

29823 Arthroscopy, shoulder, surgical; debridement, extensive

ACROMIOCLAVICULAR JOINT INJURY

▶ Essentials of Diagnosis

- *Pain and swelling over the acromioclavicular joint.*
- *May have visible elevation or displacement of the clavicle relative to the acromion (asymmetric to the contralateral shoulder).*
- *Pain with forward elevation of the arm.*
- *Appropriate radiographs can be confirmatory.*

▶ Prevention

Avoiding activities that may result in a downward blow to the tip of the shoulder is the best way to prevent these injuries.

▶ Clinical Findings

Acromioclavicular dislocations or subluxations, commonly referred to as separations, vary in severity depending on the extent of injury to the stabilizing ligaments and capsule. The typical mechanism of injury is a direct downward blow to the tip of the shoulder. Clinically, pain at the top of the shoulder over the acromioclavicular joint is the predominant symptom, with varying decreases in motion depending on the severity of the injury. The athlete who has sustained this type of injury will typically leave the field holding the arm close to the side.

When checking for instability of the acromioclavicular joint, the examiner should manipulate the midshaft of the clavicle, rather than the acromioclavicular joint to rule out pain from contusion to the acromioclavicular area. For milder acromioclavicular injuries, the patient should put the hand of the affected arm on the opposite shoulder, and the

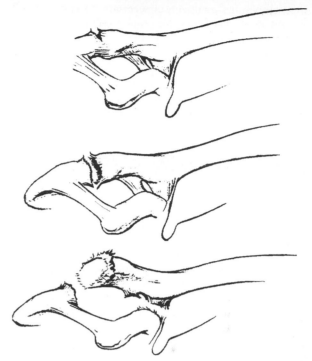

▲ **Figure 3–36.** Grades of acromioclavicular joint separations.

examiner may then gently apply downward pressure at the patient's affected elbow, noting if this maneuver causes pain at the acromioclavicular joint.

Acromioclavicular joint injuries were initially divided into grades I to III (Figure 3–36). Grade I injuries are typically produced by a mild blow causing a partial tear of the acromioclavicular ligament. When the acromioclavicular ligament is completely torn, but the coracoclavicular ligament remains intact, a grade II injury that involves subluxation or partial displacement results. When the force of injury is severe enough to tear the coracoclavicular and acromioclavicular ligaments in addition to the capsule, a grade III injury occurs.

Three additional injuries were later added to the classification. In grade IV injuries, the clavicle is displaced posterior and buttonholed through the fascia of the trapezius muscle. Grade V injuries demonstrate severe inferior displacement of the glenohumeral joint, with the clavicle often 300% superior to the acromion. Lastly, in grade VI injuries, the distal end of the clavicle is locked inferior to the coracoid.

Acromioclavicular joint displacement is often obvious on physical examination, but it is best classified by radiography. An anteroposterior radiograph that is aimed 10 degrees cephalad allows visualization of the acromioclavicular joint. A radiograph of the entire upper thorax allows the vertical distance between the coracoid and the clavicle on both the involved and uninvolved sides to be compared. Anteroposterior radiographs with weights applied to the upper extremities are usually unnecessary. An axillary lateral radiograph is also essential for proper classification.

Treatment

Management of acromioclavicular joint injuries depends on their severity. Grade I and II injuries may be treated with a sling until discomfort dissipates, usually within 2–4 weeks. Next a rehabilitation program starts, and normal range of motion and strength to the upper extremity begin to be restored. Treatment of acute grade III injuries or complete dislocations in athletes is controversial; most believe grade III injuries are best managed nonoperatively, but others advocate operative treatment. Grade IV to VI injuries are best treated with open reduction and internal fixation along with reconstruction of the coracoclavicular ligament.

Nonsurgical treatment usually includes a sling for comfort. Ice and other modalities are used for an acute acromioclavicular injury to reduce soreness and swelling. Pain is the limiting factor in beginning range-of-motion and isometric muscle-strengthening exercises. It should be used as a guide for initiation and progress through rehabilitation. Range-of-motion exercises can be begun rather quickly and strengthening added when pain permits.

Before resuming athletic activities, the patient should have full, painless range of motion, no tenderness on palpation, and sufficient strength.

Prognosis

Athletes who do not need to elevate their arms, such as soccer or football players, tend to return to sports earlier than players engaged in sports that require overhead arm activity, such as tennis, baseball, and swimming.

Johansen JA, Grutter PW, McFarland EG, Petersen SA: Acromioclavicular joint injuries: indications for treatment and treatment options. *J Shoulder Elbow Surg* 2011;20(2 Suppl):S70. [PMID: 21195634]

Rios CG, Mazzocca AD: Acromioclavicular joint problems in athletes and new methods of management. *Clin Sports Med* 2008;27:763. [PMID: 19064155]

CORACOID FRACTURE

Fractures of the coracoid process are rare; they are usually seen in professional riflemen and skeet shooters, although they have also been reported in baseball and tennis players. They are identified on radiographs, and conservative treatment, including cessation of activity, usually results in uncomplicated healing after 6–8 weeks.

STERNOCLAVICULAR JOINT INJURY

In the skeletally mature adult athlete, injury to the sternoclavicular joint usually involves the surrounding soft tissue and capsule tearing, leading to subluxation or dislocation.

The mechanism of injury is either a blow to the point of the shoulder, which predisposes the athlete to anterior dislocation, or a direct blow to the clavicle or chest with the shoulder in extension, which predisposes the athlete to posterior dislocation. The injury may range from a symptomatic sprain to a complete sternoclavicular dislocation with disruption of the capsule and its restraining ligaments.

1. Anterior Dislocation

Essentials of Diagnosis

- *History of trauma to the upper chest wall.*
- *Painful prominence overlying the proximal end of the clavicle.*
- *Appropriate radiographs or computed tomography (CT) scan can be diagnostic.*

Clinical Findings

The most common type of sternoclavicular dislocation is anterior dislocation. This is recognized clinically by an anterior prominence of the proximal clavicle on the involved side. Radiographic documentation of an anterior sternoclavicular dislocation is difficult because the rib, sternum, and clavicle overlap at the joint, but may be confirmed by oblique views. A CT scan is very sensitive and should be done if the radiograph appears normal but a dislocation is suspected.

Treatment

Although dislocation of the anterior sternoclavicular joint may cause considerable distress initially, the symptoms usually subside rapidly, with no loss of shoulder function. A variety of surgical and nonsurgical approaches have been advocated, but surgery for anterior dislocations often results in significant complications. Closed treatment modalities vary from using a sling to attempted closed reduction, which may be successful initially but is difficult to maintain.

2. Posterior Dislocation

Essentials of Diagnosis

- *History of trauma to the upper chest wall.*
- *Pain in the region of the proximal end of the clavicle.*
- *Patient may present with hoarseness, dysphagia, or severe respiratory distress.*
- *Appropriate radiographs or CT scan can be diagnostic.*

Clinical Findings

Posterior sternoclavicular dislocation is much less common but is associated with more complications because of the potential for injury to the esophagus, great vessels, and trachea. Presenting symptoms range from mild to moderate

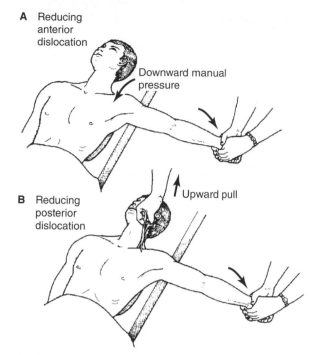

A Reducing anterior dislocation

Downward manual pressure

B Reducing posterior dislocation

↑ Upward pull

▲ **Figure 3–37.** Method for reducing (**A**) anterior sternoclavicular dislocation and (**B**) posterior sternoclavicular dislocation.

pain in the sternoclavicular region to hoarseness, dysphagia, severe respiratory distress, and subcutaneous emphysema from tracheal injury.

▶ **Treatment**

In most instances, closed reduction of posterior dislocations, if performed early, is successful and stable. To effect reduction, a pillow is placed under the upper back of the supine patient, and gentle traction is applied with the shoulder held in 90 degrees of abduction and at maximum extension (Figure 3–37). Rarely, closed reduction under general anesthesia or open reduction is required.

After reduction, the patient is put in an immobilization splint and is instructed to use ice and oral NSAIDs. Once the joint has healed sufficiently, usually within 2–3 weeks, range-of-motion exercises may begin. Elevation of the arm should not be attempted until 3 weeks after injury.

3. Medial Clavicular Epiphyseal Fracture

In athletes younger than 25 years of age, sternoclavicular injuries may not result in true dislocations, but rather in fractures through the growth plate of the proximal clavicle. These clavicular epiphyseal fractures may appear clinically as dislocations, particularly if some displacement is present, and may be treated conservatively. Typically, these are not

associated with growth deformities, and reduction of the fracture is not needed unless there is severe displacement. Symptomatic treatment for pain will usually suffice. Sometimes an adolescent presents with an enlarging mass at the sternoclavicular joint, accompanied by parents with worries of cancer. A careful history reveals trauma several weeks earlier, and the mass represents the callus of a healing clavicular epiphyseal fracture that can be demonstrated radiographically.

Jaggard MK, Gupte CM, Gulati V, Reilly P: A comprehensive review of trauma and disruption to the sternoclavicular joint with the proposal of a new classification system. *J Trauma* 2009;66:576. [PMID: 19204537]

▶ **CPT Codes for Acromioclavicular and Sternoclavicular Joint Injuries**

23101 Arthrotomy, acromioclavicular joint or sternoclavicular joint, including biopsy and/or excision of torn cartilage

23120 Claviculectomy; partial

23520 Closed treatment of sternoclavicular dislocation; without manipulation

23525 Closed treatment of sternoclavicular dislocation; with manipulation

23530 Open treatment of sternoclavicular dislocation, acute or chronic

23532 Open treatment of sternoclavicular dislocation, acute or chronic; with fascial graft (includes obtaining graft)

23540 Closed treatment of acromioclavicular dislocation; without manipulation

23545 Closed treatment of acromioclavicular dislocation; with manipulation

24550 Open treatment of acromioclavicular dislocation, acute or chronic

23552 Open treatment of acromioclavicular dislocation, acute or chronic; with fascial graft (includes obtaining graft)

▼ **OTHER SHOULDER TENDON AND MUSCLE**

BICEPS TENDON INJURIES

1. Bicipital Tendinosis

▶ **Essentials of Diagnosis**

- *Pain localized to the anterior proximal humerus and shoulder joint.*
- *Pain with resisted forward flexion and supination.*
- *Pain may be relieved by a steroid injection into the sheath of the biceps tendon.*

Prevention

Similar to the prevention of rotator cuff injuries, general conditioning and stretching and strengthening before activities can help minimize injury to the biceps tendon.

Clinical Findings

The long head of the biceps muscle is an intraarticular structure deep in the rotator cuff tendon as it passes under the acromion to its insertion at the top of the glenoid. The same mechanism that initiates symptoms of impingement syndrome in rotator cuff injuries may inflame the tendon of the biceps in its subacromial position, causing bicipital tendinosis. Tendinosis may also result from subluxation of the tendon out of its groove in the proximal humerus and can occur under, into, or on top of the subscapular tendon. Subluxation of the biceps tendon is almost always associated with a subscapularis tendon tear. The symptoms of bicipital tendinosis, whether the result of impingement or tendon subluxation, are essentially the same. Pain is localized to the proximal humerus and shoulder joint, with resisted supination of the forearm aggravating the pain. Pain may also occur on manual testing of the elbow flexors and on palpation of the tendon itself. The Yergason test is used to determine instability of the long head of the biceps in its groove.

Treatment

If the biceps tendinosis is associated with shoulder impingement, then therapy aimed at treating the impingement syndrome will relieve the bicipital tendinosis. If subluxation of the tendon within its groove is the cause of the irritation, conservative therapy includes NSAIDs and restriction of activities, followed by a slow resumption of activities after a period of rest. Strengthening of the muscles that assist the biceps in elbow flexion and forearm supination is also beneficial. Steroid injections into the sheath of the biceps tendon are helpful, but they may be hazardous if placed into the substance of the tendon because they will promote tendon degeneration. Persistent symptoms may warrant tenodesis of the biceps tendon directly into the humerus.

Prognosis

Recovery from biceps tenodesis is difficult, and it is doubtful if a competitive athlete could return to peak performance after treatment.

2. Biceps Tendon Tears at the Shoulder

Essentials of Diagnosis

- *"Popeye" appearance of the upper arm from distal retraction of the biceps muscle.*
- *May or may not be painful and ecchymotic depending on the chronicity of the injury.*

Prevention

Similar to the prevention of rotator cuff injuries, general conditioning and stretching and strengthening before activities can help minimize injury to the biceps tendon.

Clinical Findings

The long head of the biceps tendon may rupture proximally, either from the supraglenoid tubercle of the scapula at the entrance of the bicipital groove proximally or at the exit of the tunnel at the musculotendinous junction. The muscle mass moves distally, producing a bulging or "Popeye" appearance to the arm, but the short head remains intact; rupture of the biceps tendon distally involves both heads, and the muscle mass moves proximally. Rupture of the long head of the biceps may be predictive of a rotator cuff tear. The mechanism is usually a forceful flexion of the arm and is more common in older athletes or following direct trauma. Microtears probably serve to render the tendon vulnerable to an acute tearing event. The degree of ecchymosis is dependent on the location of the tear, with avascular areas having less ecchymosis and the musculotendinous junction producing quite a noticeable amount of ecchymosis. Diagnosis is usually easily accomplished, as the deformity is obvious.

Treatment

Surgical treatment of proximal ruptures, if indicated, is usually reserved for younger patients. The proximal end of the tendon is usually found beneath the attachment of the pectoralis major. Proximal biceps tendon rupture usually occurs with rotator cuff tears in middle-aged and older athletes.

Prognosis

Athletes are permitted to return to full contact play once they have achieved maximal functional strength and range of elbow motion, which typically occurs 4–6 months following a proximal biceps repair.

Nho SJ, Strauss EJ, Lenart BA, et al: Long head of the biceps tendinopathy: diagnosis and management. *J Am Acad Orthop Surg* 2010;18:645. [PMID: 21041799]

CPT Codes for Biceps Tendon Injuries at the Shoulder

23430 Tenodesis of long tendon of biceps

23440 Resection or transplantation of long tendon of biceps

29828 Arthroscopy, shoulder, surgical; biceps tenodesis

PECTORALIS MAJOR RUPTURE

Essentials of Diagnosis

- *Sudden pain.*
- *Ecchymosis and swelling along the pectoralis major muscle.*

Prevention

Similar to the prevention of rotator cuff injuries, general conditioning and stretching and strengthening before activities can help minimize injury to the pectoralis major.

Clinical Findings

Rupture of the pectoralis major tendon is an uncommon injury, usually occurring during bench press exercises in weight lifting and caused by sudden unexpected muscle contraction during pulling or lifting. The athlete usually experiences sudden pain and develops local ecchymosis and swelling. As the swelling subsides, a sulcus and deformity may be visible, and the patient notices weakness of the arm in adduction and internal rotation.

Treatment

The rupture may be partial or complete, and nonoperative treatment usually results in satisfactory function for the activities of daily life. Surgery may be considered if the athlete wishes to return to heavy weight lifting.

Prognosis

Athletes are permitted to return to contact sports once they have achieved full strength and range of motion, which typically occurs 6 months following a pectoralis major repair.

Antosh IJ, Grassbaugh JA, Parada SA, Arrington ED: Pectoralis major tendon repairs in the active-duty population. *Am J Orthop* 2009;38:26. [PMID: 19238264]

Provencher MT, Handfield K, Boniquit NT, Reiff SN, Sekiya JK, Romeo AA: Injuries to the pectoralis major muscle: diagnosis and management. *Am J Sports Med* 2010;38:1693. [PMID: 20675652]

SHOULDER NEUROVASCULAR INJURY

1. Brachial Plexus Injury

Essentials of Diagnosis

- *Often preceded by a fall onto the shoulder.*
- *Paresthesias and/or motor loss in the affected extremity that can be transient or permanent.*
- *EMG can help localize the lesion and aid in prognosis.*

Clinical Findings, Treatment, and Prognosis

Brachial plexus injuries are typically caused by a fall on the shoulder as seen in acromioclavicular joint injuries. Most brachial plexus injuries do not involve motor loss and exhibit paresthesias, which resolve in a period of minutes to weeks, although some cases may persist for months or years. Early in the course of the injury, a transient slowing of conduction across the plexus or a mild prolongation of nerve latency may be seen. The "burner" or "stinger" is one of the most common brachial plexus injuries encountered in athletes. The key to diagnosis is a short duration of upper extremity paresthesias and shoulder weakness, with pain-free range of motion of the cervical spine. Players may return to competition after shoulder strength and full, pain-free range of motion have returned.

Rarely, a severe injury will occur (eg, from motorcycle racing). Chronic injuries result in instability of the shoulder that may be treated with trapezius transfer. Arthrodesis is an alternative, initially or after failed muscle transfer.

Safran MR: Nerve injury about the shoulder in athletes. Part 2: long thoracic nerve, spinal accessory nerve, burners/stingers, thoracic outlet syndrome. *Am J Sports Med* 2004;32:1063. [PMID: 15150060]

2. Long Thoracic Nerve Injury

Essentials of Diagnosis

- *Palsy of the serratus anterior results in medial winging of the scapula.*
- *May be painless, but often there is medial scapula pain.*

Clinical Findings, Treatment, and Prognosis

Traction incidents may cause a long thoracic nerve palsy, with subsequent serratus anterior paralysis and winging of the scapula. Traction and blunt trauma may also cause injury to the spinal accessory nerve, another cause of winging of the scapula. These can be differentiated on physical examination by the position of the scapula. With serratus anterior palsy, the inferior portion of the scapula tends to go medially, whereas the opposite occurs with spinal accessory nerve palsy. Treatment is usually conservative, with return of function in weeks if the nerve has not been divided.

3. Suprascapular Nerve Injury

Essentials of Diagnosis

- *Poorly localized pain and weakness in the posterolateral shoulder.*
- *Weakness and atrophy of the supraspinatus and/or infraspinatus muscles.*
- *MRI may reveal the presence of a cyst in the suprascapular or spinoglenoid notch.*
- *Electromyography/nerve conduction velocity (EMG/NCV) can aid in the diagnosis.*

Clinical Findings, Treatment, and Prognosis

Entrapment of the suprascapular nerve is often associated with activities such as weight lifting, baseball pitching, volleyball, and backpacking. Traction and repetitive shoulder use are the mechanisms of injury. Compression of the nerve may occur from entrapment at the anterior suprascapular notch of the scapula or at the level of the spinoglenoid notch. The latter occurs in volleyball players and baseball players and is likely caused by rapid overhead acceleration of the arm. Compression is associated with poorly localized pain and weakness in the posterolateral aspect of the shoulder girdle. This may be followed by atrophy of the supraspinatus or infraspinatus muscles. Eventually, there is weakness of forward flexion and external rotation of the shoulder. The diagnosis is confirmed by EMG and nerve conduction studies.

Conservative therapy consists of rest, NSAIDs, and physical therapy designed to increase muscular tone and strength. If this is unsuccessful, then surgical exploration is indicated, which may reveal hypertrophy of the transverse scapular ligament, anomalies of the suprascapular notch, and ganglion cysts. Results of surgery vary with the lesion discovered, but many patients return to full function postoperatively.

4. Musculocutaneous Nerve Injury

Essentials of Diagnosis

- *Weak or absent biceps muscle function with sensory loss in the lateral forearm.*
- *EMG/NCV may aid in the diagnosis and prognosis.*

Clinical Findings, Treatment, and Prognosis

This nerve is susceptible to direct frontal blows or surgical procedures. Injury is associated with numbness in the lateral forearm to the base of the thumb and weak to absent biceps muscle function. Most injuries seen in sports are transient and respond to conservative treatment in a matter of days to weeks.

5. Axillary Nerve Injury

Essentials of Diagnosis

- *Present following a shoulder dislocation or proximal humerus fracture.*
- *Weakness or absence of deltoid muscle function.*
- *Positive deltoid extension lag sign.*
- *EMG/NCV can aid in diagnosis and prognosis.*

Clinical Findings, Treatment, and Prognosis

The mechanism of injury may be trauma by direct blow to the posterior aspect of the shoulder, following dislocation or fracture of the proximal humerus, and following surgery. The axillary nerve can be injured especially during arthroscopic capsular release procedures and is most prone to be injured with release of the anteroinferior capsule. The axillary nerve passes caudal to the glenohumeral joint capsule, and its position relative to the capsule varies with shoulder position; its distance from the capsule diminishes with abduction of the shoulder. With the arm at the side, it courses 1–1.5 cm lateral to the anteroinferior glenoid rim at the 5 o'clock position (right shoulder). As the nerve courses posterior, it is located increasing more lateral to the glenoid rim. It is 2–2.5 cm from the posteroinferior glenoid rim at the 7 o'clock position (right shoulder). The degree of injury to the nerve varies because the initial presentation may be mild weakness during elevation and abduction of the arm with or without numbness of the lateral arm. The deltoid extension lag sign is indicative of axillary nerve injury. To perform this test, the examiner elevates the arm into a position of near full extension, asks the patient to hold the arm in this position, and then releases the arm. If there is complete deltoid paralysis, the arm will drop. For partial nerve injuries, the magnitude of the angular drop, or lag, is an indicator of deltoid strength. Approximately 25% of all dislocated shoulder injuries are associated with axillary nerve traction injuries, which respond well to rest, physical therapy, and time. If recovery is not complete within 3–6 months, surgical intervention is recommended with exploration, using neurolysis or grafting, or both, as necessary. Results of surgery are usually favorable, with sensory recovery occurring before motor recovery.

Zarkadas PC, Throckmorton TW, Steinmann SP: Neurovascular injuries in shoulder trauma. *Orthop Clin North Am* 2008;39:483. [PMID: 18803978]

THORACIC OUTLET SYNDROME

Essentials of Diagnosis

- *Symptoms are often nonspecific; may be neurologic, venous, or arterial; and may include edema, pallor, or coolness as well as paresthesias.*
- *Doppler examination and EMG/NVC studies can assist in the diagnosis.*

Clinical Findings, Treatment, and Prognosis

The symptoms resulting from thoracic outlet compression may be neurologic, venous, or arterial in nature. Obstruction of the subclavian vein may lead to stiffness, edema, and even thrombosis of the limb. Arterial obstruction may be the result of direct compression and manifests with pallor, coolness, and forearm claudication. Doppler examination reveals changes in arterial and venous flow. EMG and nerve conduction studies are also helpful in diagnosis.

Nonoperative treatment is recommended for less severe forms of this syndrome, and once the pain subsides, an exercise program to strengthen the pectoral girdle muscles is beneficial. Special exercises to strengthen the upper and lower trapezius, along with the erector spinae and serratus anterior muscles, yield good results. Correcting poor posture and an ongoing maintenance program are mandatory once improvement is reached. Progression of symptoms or failure of nonoperative treatment is an indication for surgical exploration and correction of the pathologic factors encountered.

Laulan J, Fouquet B, Rodaix C, Jauffret P, Roquelaure Y, Descatha A: Thoracic outlet syndrome: definition, aetiological factors, diagnosis, management and occupational impact. *J Occup Rehabil.* 2011;21:366. [Epub ahead of print][PMID: 21193950]

▼ ELBOW INJURIES

EPICONDYLITIS (TENNIS ELBOW)

Tennis elbow is an eponym given to many painful conditions about the elbow. An anatomic location may usually be found and specific diagnosis made.

1. LATERAL EPICONDYLITIS

▶ Essentials of Diagnosis

- *A history of repetitive activity or overuse.*
- *Pain localized to the lateral elbow that may radiate to the forearm.*
- *Tenderness at the extensor carpi radialis brevis origin, just anterior and distal to the center of the lateral epicondyle.*
- *Normal elbow range of motion.*
- *Usually normal radiographs and rarely (<10%) calcification adjacent to the lateral epicondyle.*

Lateral epicondylitis is commonly known as tennis elbow and involves the tendons of the extensor muscles of the wrist and hand. Patients who perform repetitive wrist extension against resistance (such as the backhand stroke in tennis) are at risk. The pain they have is usually chronic in nature and more bothersome than disabling. Tenderness is located over the lateral humeral epicondyle, and pain is produced by extending the wrist against resistance. This is most marked when done with the elbow extended. The tendon of the extensor carpi radialis brevis is the most common site of the lesion. Other causes for lateral elbow pain should be considered, including radiocapitellar arthritis and posterior interosseous nerve compression. Radiographs only rarely reveal soft-tissue calcification near the lateral humeral epicondyle, and MRI is of questionable aid in making the diagnosis.

Treatment includes decreasing specific activities and using a counterforce brace that theoretically distributes the tension of the muscular pull over a larger area. A lighter racquet, proper grip size on the racquet, and proper technique are also helpful. Stretching the extensor and supinator muscles is done by flexing the wrist of the upper extremity with the elbow extended. It is often helpful to pronate the forearm. Exercises to strengthen the wrist extensor muscles should be included. If this approach fails, an injection of local anesthetic and cortisone into the most tender region is often curative. Surgical treatment yields satisfactory outcomes in recalcitrant cases, and multiple procedures, including arthroscopic techniques, have been described. Commonplace in all procedures is release of the common extensor origin. Histologic studies of the afflicted tendon show degenerative changes with angiofibroblastic proliferation. These are thought to be similar to the pathologic changes of the torn rotator cuff, with diminished vascularity, an altered nutritional state, and tearing of the susceptible tendon.

2. MEDIAL EPICONDYLITIS

▶ Essentials of Diagnosis

- *A history of repetitive activity or overuse, often from activities that result in valgus elbow forces, such as occurs with baseball throwing.*
- *Pain localized to the medial elbow that may radiate to the forearm*
- *Tenderness at the flexor-pronator origin, most commonly of the pronator teres and the flexor carpi ulnaris.*
- *Normal elbow range of motion.*
- *Usually normal radiographs and rarely (<10%) calcification adjacent to the medial epicondyle.*

Medial epicondylitis involves the common flexor pronator origin and is commonly known as golfer's elbow. Treatment is similar to the management of lateral epicondylitis, although with emphasis on the wrist flexors and the forearm pronators. Ulnar nerve compression at the elbow may occur in conjunction with medial tennis elbow. In about 60% of the cases treated surgically, ulnar nerve compression was present. The common flexor origin is an important medial stabilizer of the elbow, so if surgical treatment is indicated, the debrided tendon should be reattached rather than released from the medial epicondyle.

Baker CL Jr, Baker CL 3rd: Long-term follow-up of arthroscopic treatment of lateral epicondylitis. *Am J Sports Med* 2008;36:254. [PMID: 18202296]

Calfee RP, Patel A, DaSilva MF, Akelman E: Management of lateral epicondylitis: current concepts. *J Am Acad Orthop Surg* 2008;16:19. [PMID: 18180389]

Coombes BK, Bisset L, Vicenzino B: Efficacy and safety of corticosteroid injections and other injections for management of tendinopathy: a systematic review of randomised controlled trials. *Lancet* 2010;376:1751. [PMID: 20970844]

▶ CPT Codes for Lateral and Medial Epicondylitis

24357 Tenotomy, elbow, lateral or medial (eg, epicondylitis, tennis elbow, golfer's elbow); percutaneous

24358 Tenotomy, elbow, lateral or medial (eg, epicondylitis, tennis elbow, golfer's elbow); debridement, soft tissue and/or bone, open

24359 Tenotomy, elbow, lateral or medial (eg, epicondylitis, tennis elbow, golfer's elbow); debridement, soft tissue and/or bone, open with tendon repair or reattachment

ELBOW INSTABILITY

Rupture of the collateral ligaments of the elbow occurs most commonly from elbow dislocation. This can result from excessive valgus force, and initially, the ulnar collateral ligament ruptures. Excessive posterolateral rotatory force may also result in rupture of the lateral ulnar collateral ligament. In either case, the elbow may dislocate, and typically the direction is posterior. Treatment after relocation and brief immobilization consists of active range of motion exercises. Recurrent instability is rare; instead, a small loss of elbow extension, usually less than 10 degrees, commonly results.

1. Valgus Instability

▶ Essential of Diagnosis

- *Sudden or gradual onset of medial elbow pain after throwing.*
- *Pain greatest at late cocking and acceleration phase of throwing.*

- *Maximum tenderness about 1 cm distal to the medial epicondyle.*
- *Provocative maneuvers that place valgus stress on elbow reproduce symptoms.*
- *There may also be ulnar neuropathy and posteromedial elbow impingement, medial epicondylitis, and cubital tunnel syndrome.*

Valgus instability may result from overuse in overhead throwing sports such as baseball, football, and javelin throwing. With acute MCL rupture, a pop may be felt during a throw. Tenderness is present on the medial side of the elbow, usually just distal to the medial epicondyle. Instability can then be appreciated when a valgus force is applied to the elbow. This must be done with the elbow flexed 20 degrees, as failure to unlock the olecranon from within the olecranon fossa in full extension creates a false sense of stability. Comparison to the contralateral side aids in making the correct diagnosis. If the ulnar collateral ligament has been injured but remains intact, then the valgus stress test may elicit pain, but no instability. Then the "milking maneuver" (Figure 3–38) will also elicit pain along the medial side of the elbow. Eliciting pain while moving the elbow in flexion and extension with valgus stress during the milking maneuver may be the best test for diagnosing MCL injuries in the elbow.

A stress radiograph may aid in making the diagnosis. An anteroposterior radiograph can be taken while the examiner performs the valgus stress test. Alternatively, gravity can be used to apply the valgus stress. For this, an anteroposterior radiograph of the elbow is taken with the shoulder externally rotated at 90 degrees with the elbow flexed at approximately 20 degrees. When instability is present, there will be a wider medial opening than on the contralateral normal side. MRI may also be useful, especially if an arthrogram is performed concurrently, as dye leaking through the ulnar collateral ligament is diagnostic of a rupture.

Surgical repair may be indicated in overhead throwing athletes who suffer an acute rupture of their ulnar collateral ligament and still want to continue to participate in their

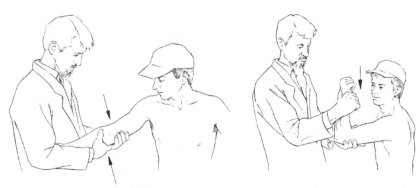

▲ **Figure 3–38.** The valgus stress and milking maneuver tests for medial ulnar collateral ligament injury. (Reprinted, with permission, from Chen FS, Rokito AS, Jobe FW: Medial elbow problems in the overhead-throwing athlete. *J Am Acad Orthop Surg* 2001;9:102.)

sport. Soccer, basketball players, and other athletes participating in nonoverhead throwing sports may be treated with a program of early active range-of-motion exercises with expectation of full return to their sport. Chronic ulnar collateral ligament injuries resulting from overuse are best treated with rehabilitation, NSAIDs, and avoidance of throwing for as long as 3 months. Only those with residual pain and instability after participation in such a program should undergo reconstruction of the anterior band of the ulnar collateral ligament. In this surgery pioneered by Dr Frank Jobe, a tendon graft, usually the palmaris longus, is used to reconstruct the ligament from the anterior and distal aspect of the medial humeral epicondyle to the sublime tubercle of the ulna. Up to 85% of athletes are able to return to highly competitive throwing after such surgery.

Cain EL Jr, Andrews JR, Dugas JR, et al: Outcome of ulnar collateral ligament reconstruction of the elbow in 1281 athletes: results in 743 athletes with minimum 2-year follow-up. *Am J Sports Med* 2010;38:2426. [PMID: 20929932]

Murthi AM, Keener JD, Armstrong AD, Getz CL: The recurrent unstable elbow: diagnosis and treatment. *J Bone Joint Surg Am* 2010;92:1794. [PMID: 20660245]

2. Posterolateral Rotatory Instability

▶ Essentials of Diagnosis

- *Sudden or gradual onset of lateral elbow pain.*
- *There may be snapping, catching, locking, or a sensation of elbow instability.*
- *A history of tennis elbow surgery.*
- *The provocative maneuver of the posterolateral rotator instability test reproduces symptoms.*

Posterolateral rotatory instability of the elbow may result from a fall on the outstretched upper extremity, surgery of the lateral side of the elbow, or chronic varus stress as may occur in long-term crutch walkers. The instability covers a spectrum of severity from mild subluxation to recurrent dislocation. Those with mild forms complain of intermittent symptoms on the lateral side of the elbow associated with supination of the forearm such as pain, snapping, or catching. More severe symptoms include locking or sensations of elbow instability. To perform the posterolateral rotatory instability test, a valgus stress is applied to the supinated elbow with the patient supine and the upper extremity over the head (Figure 3–39). Subluxation of the radial head occurs with the elbow in extension and resolves when the elbow is flexed. This maneuver also reproduces the patient's symptoms. A lateral stress radiograph, done with the elbow in extension as described for the posterolateral rotatory instability test, may also demonstrate the instability (see Figure 3–39). Treatment for acute cases consists of an elbow brace to hold the forearm in pronation and restrict terminal elbow extension for a 6-week period of time. Chronic cases are best treated with reconstruction of the lateral ulnar collateral ligament. Postoperatively, the patient is put in the same brace as used for acute posterolateral rotatory instability for 6–12 weeks.

Charalambous CP, Stanley JK: Posterolateral rotatory instability of the elbow. *J Bone Joint Surg Br* 2008;90:272. [PMID: 18310745]

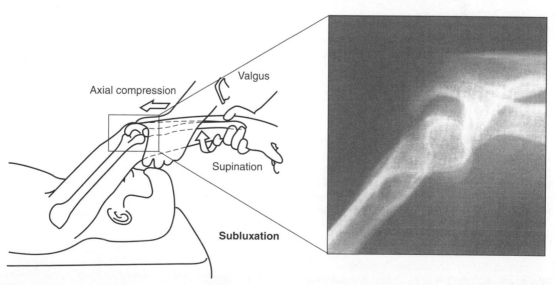

▲ **Figure 3–39.** The posterolateral rotatory instability test reproduces the patient's symptoms. At right is a lateral stress radiograph.

CPT Codes for Elbow Instability

24343 Repair lateral collateral ligament, elbow, with local tissue

24344 Reconstruction lateral collateral ligament, elbow, with tendon graft (includes harvesting of graft)

24345 Repair medial collateral ligament, elbow, with local tissue

24346 Reconstruction medial collateral ligament, elbow, with tendon graft (includes harvesting of graft)

CUBITAL TUNNEL SYNDROME

Essentials of Diagnosis

- *Medial elbow pain exacerbated by throwing and paresthesias in ring and little fingers.*
- *Positive Tinel sign over cubital tunnel and positive elbow flexion test.*
- *Associated with both medial epicondylitis and MCL injury.*

Prevention relies on sound throwing techniques, which minimize valgus load on elbow. Correction of known causes of nerve irritation including valgus instability of the elbow may also prevent the syndrome. The cubital tunnel is formed by the medial epicondyle, the elbow joint, and the two heads of the flexor carpi ulnaris. Structures proximal to, within, and distal to the tunnel can cause compression, entrapment, traction, subluxation, or irritation of the ulnar nerve. Proximally, these structures include the arcade of Struthers (not to be confused with the *ligament* of Struthers, which is associated with median neuropathy) and medial head of the triceps. Within the groove, they include the medial epicondyle, the epicondylar groove, anconeus epitrochlearis, the two heads of the flexi carpi ulnaris, and their interconnecting ligament of Osborne. Distally, an offending structure may be the deep flexor-pronator fascia. Regardless of cause or site, the final common pathway of cubital tunnel syndrome is the onset of nerve ischemia and fibrosis.

Initial symptoms may be medial elbow pain with occasional radiation to the medial forearm. Paresthesias may occur in the ulnar two fingers. Athletes will often present before onset of weakness. Mechanical complaints such as snapping may occur with nerve subluxation. Diagnosis is chiefly clinical and relies on two provocative tests: a positive Tinel sign over the nerve and a positive elbow flexion test. This test is performed by placing the elbow in full flexion and the wrist in maximal extension. A test is positive if pain or paresthesias are elicited within 1 minute. Sensory changes can be detected with Semmes-Weinstein monofilament testing and, in more advanced cases, with two-point discrimination tests. Motor deficits often occur late, and athletes usually complain before asymmetric hypothenar atrophy, decreased pinch and grip strength, abducted small finger or Wartenberg sign, Froment sign, and clawing of the ulnar two

fingers occur. Motor deficits may not be present, even in late cases, if the intrinsic muscles of the hand receive innervation from the median nerve—the result of an anatomic variant known as the Martin-Gruber anastomosis.

A thorough exam of the neck and proximal upper extremity is performed to eliminate neuropathic etiologies with similar manifestations such as cervical radiculopathy, brachial plexopathy (of the medial cord), and thoracic outlet syndrome.

Plain radiographs including special views such as cubital tunnel view may reveal bony abnormalities causing ulnar nerve compression. Similarly, MRI may identify soft-tissue abnormalities having the same effect. EMG and NCV studies will be negative in more than 50% of patients with the syndrome. Slowing of conduction velocities to less than 50 m/s when the elbow is flexed is indicative of disease. Reduction in sensory nerve action potential also confirms early neuropathy.

Treatment of ulnar neuropathy at the cubital tunnel is initially nonoperative: rest, ice, anti-inflammatory medication, and padded splinting at 30–45 degrees of elbow flexion. Nighttime extension splinting is often quite helpful in reducing symptoms early in the disease process. Corticosteroid injections are not recommended due to the superficial position of the nerve. Conservative management will often fail in athletes due to the high demands, especially if there is a subluxing ulnar nerve. Surgical indications include failed nonoperative management and ulnar nerve subluxation. Several techniques have been used, including simple decompression, medial epicondylectomy, subcutaneous transposition, and submuscular transposition. With each technique, the ulnar nerve should be released at all possible sites of compression, from the ligament of Struthers proximally, through the cubital tunnel, and past the two heads of the flexor carpi ulnaris. Each technique has potential complications and approximately an 85% success rate. After brief postoperative immobilization, passive and then active range of motion is begun (by 4 weeks). Strengthening and throwing exercises are started by the eighth postoperative week. Complications are uncommon but include injury to the medial antebrachial cutaneous nerve, injury to the MCL complex, and perineural scarring. Unrecognized medial elbow pathology will also limit success.

Conservative therapy has excellent results except in high-demand athletes. Results of surgical intervention vary inversely with degree of preoperative nerve involvement. Many patients with good to excellent results return to unrestricted play by 6 months postoperatively. This can be a career-ending insult to a throwing athlete if the pathology has been present for a prolonged time prior to treatment.

Gellman H: Compression of the ulnar nerve at the elbow: cubital tunnel syndrome. *Instr Course Lect* 2008;57:187. [PMID: 18399580]

CPT Codes for Cubital Tunnel Syndrome

64718 Neuroplasty and/or transposition; ulnar nerve at elbow

BICEPS TENDON TEARS AT THE ELBOW

Essentials of Diagnosis

- *"Popeye" appearance of the upper arm from proximal retraction of the biceps muscle.*
- *May or may not be painful and ecchymotic depending on the chronicity of the injury.*
- *Weakness of elbow flexion and forearm supination.*

Prevention

General conditioning and stretching and strengthening before activities can help minimize injury to the biceps tendon.

Clinical Findings

The long head of the biceps tendon may rupture distally at the insertion into the radial tuberosity, at the myotendinous junction, or within the muscle itself. The muscle mass moves proximally, producing a bulging or "Popeye" appearance to the arm. Rupture of the biceps tendon distally involves both heads. The mechanism is usually a forceful flexion of the arm and is more common in older athletes or following direct trauma. Microtears probably serve to render the tendon vulnerable to an acute tearing event. The degree of ecchymosis is dependent on the location of the tear, with avascular areas having less ecchymosis and the musculotendinous junction producing quite a noticeable amount of ecchymosis. Diagnosis is usually easily accomplished, as the deformity is obvious.

Treatment

In older individuals, nonoperative treatment is an option, although elbow flexion and forearm supination remain weak. In others, rupture of the distal biceps tendon often warrants surgical repair and is effective in restoring strength of elbow flexion and forearm supination. The tendon is easily found after acute injury, about 6 cm above the elbow joint, and care must be taken to avoid damage to the lateral antebrachial cutaneous nerve. After approximately 3 months, the tendon may be coiled up and scarred, and restoration of normal muscle may be very difficult. Surgical repair has traditionally been done with a two-incision technique, and the tendon that avulsed from bone is sewed back though drill holes. Newer, one-incision techniques using suture anchors are equally effective.

Prognosis

Athletes are permitted to return to full-contact play once healing is sufficient and they have achieved maximal functional strength and range of elbow motion, which typically occurs 4–6 months following a distal biceps repair.

Complications include loss of elbow range of motion, heterotopic bone, rerupture, nerve injuries (particularly the posterior interosseous portion of the radial nerve), and synostosis of the radius and ulna.

Frazier MS, Boardman MJ, Westland M, Imbriglia JE: Surgical treatment of partial distal biceps tendon ruptures. *J Hand Surg Am* 2010;35:1111. [PMID: 20610056]

Vidal AF, Drakos MC, Allen AA: Biceps tendon and triceps tendon injuries. *Clin Sports Med* 2004;23:707. [PMID: 15474231]

CPT Codes for Biceps Tendon Tears at the Elbow

24340 Tenodesis of biceps tendon at elbow (separate procedure)

24342 Reinsertion of ruptured biceps or triceps tendon, distal, with or without tendon graft

OTHER ELBOW OVERUSE INJURIES

1. Posterior and Posteromedial Elbow Impingement

Essentials of Diagnosis

- *Posterior elbow pain during terminal extension of the throwing arm or posteromedial elbow pain during the acceleration phase of throwing.*
- *Loss of elbow extension and tenderness along posterior or posteromedial olecranon.*
- *Pain elicited with forced rapid elbow extension in presence of valgus load.*
- *Posterior and posteromedial olecranon osteophyte sometimes visible on plain films.*
- *Associated with valgus extension overload and valgus instability.*

Impingement may result from mechanical abutment of bone and soft tissues in the posterior elbow. This may or may not be associated with injury of the ulnar collateral ligament.

Hyperextension injuries with an intact ulnar collateral ligament occur in gymnasts, football lineman, weightlifters, and others. The lesion is usually located in the center of the posterior elbow, and the pain is reproduced by forcible extension of the elbow. If there is insufficiency of the ulnar collateral ligament, as is often the case when there is posterior elbow impingement in overhead athletes, the lesion is posteromedial. In this case, the impingement is between the medial aspect of the olecranon and the lateral side of the medial wall of the olecranon fossa (Figure 3–40). Pain may be reproduced with the valgus stress test, as described earlier for valgus instability, but the pain is posteromedial and medial. Radiographs may demonstrate osteophytes of the olecranon fossa.

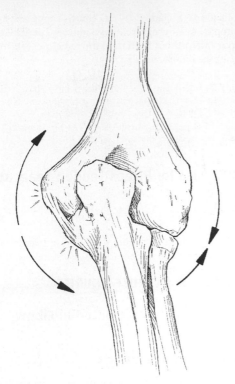

▲ Figure 3–40. Mechanism of posteromedial impingement between the medial aspect of the olecranon and the lateral side of the medial wall of the olecranon fossa. (Reprinted, with permission, from Chen FS, Rokito AS, Jobe FW: Medial elbow problems in the overhead-throwing athlete. *J Am Acad Orthop Surg* 2001;9:105.)

As with most injuries caused by repetitive trauma, treatment begins with prevention. The number of innings pitched is probably the most important factor relating to injury. If symptoms persist, removal of osteophytes is successful treatment, provided that no ulnar collateral ligament injury is present. Treatment of the valgus instability is also required for successful outcome.

Moskal MJ, Savoie III FH, Field LD: Arthroscopic treatment of posterior elbow impingement. *Instr Course Lect* 1999;48:399. [PMID: 10098066]

Sellards R, Kuebrich C: The elbow: diagnosis and treatment of common injuries. *Prim Care* 2005;32:1. [PMID: 15831310]

2. Fatigue Fracture of the Medial Epicondyle

▶ Essentials of Diagnosis

- *Sudden onset of medial epicondyle pain and swelling from throwing.*

In children, fatigue fractures of the medial epicondyle cause pain and swelling. This has been blamed on throwing curve balls, but some studies have shown that a properly thrown curve ball causes no more injuries than the traditional fastball. Prevention or minimization of damage involves several steps. First, it is important to maintain proper conditioning by continuing pitching practice in the off season or beginning the baseball season in a slow progressive fashion. Second, pain and inflammation should be avoided, and if the elbow becomes painful, the athlete should stop throwing immediately. An accurate pitching count should be kept during a game, and a stopping point should be planned in advance. If the pitcher begins having pain or shows loss of control, pitching should be temporarily terminated, and treatment to decrease the swelling and inflammation should begin. No competitive throwing is allowed until full range of motion returns and no pain or tenderness is associated with throwing.

3. Osteochondritis Dissecans of the Capitellum

▶ Essentials of Diagnosis

- *Gradual onset of lateral elbow pain in overhead athletes and gymnasts.*
- *Catching or locking of the elbow.*
- *Grinding of the lateral elbow.*
- *There may be loss of range of motion, especially if there is an effusion or there are associated loose bodies.*

Osteochondritis dissecans of the capitellum affects pitchers over 10 years of age (Figure 3–41) and gymnasts sometimes at an earlier age. Changes in the radiocapitellar joint are very worrisome because of possible permanent loss of function. Many surgical procedures have been described, but if fragmentation occurs, loose bodies may require excision. Recently, some have tried using osteochondral transplants to "repair" the lesion.

Rahusen FT, Brinkman JM, Eygendaal D: Arthroscopic treatment of posterior impingement of the elbow in athletes: a medium-term follow-up in sixteen cases. *J Shoulder Elbow Surg* 2009;18:279. [PMID: 19218052]

Ruchelsman DE, Hall MP, Youm T: Osteochondritis dissecans of the capitellum: current concepts. *J Am Acad Orthop Surg* 2010;18:557. [PMID: 20810937]

▶ CPT Codes for Posterior and Posteromedial Elbow Impingement and Osteochondritis Dissecans of the Capitellum

29834 Arthroscopy, elbow, surgical; with removal of loose body or foreign body

29837 Arthroscopy, elbow, surgical; debridement, limited

29838 Arthroscopy, elbow, surgical; debridement, extensive

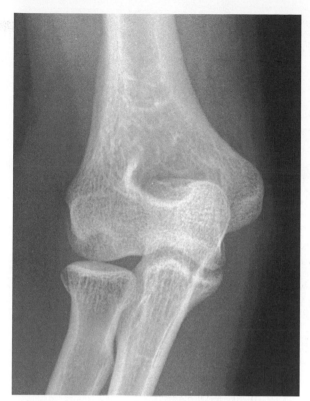

▲ **Figure 3-41.** Anteroposterior view of an elbow with osteochondritis dissecans of the capitellum.

CERVICAL SPINE INJURY

Cervical spine injuries in athletes are relatively infrequent, but the potential for serious injury to the nervous system exists. If spine injury is suspected, it is wise to be extremely cautious until a proper diagnosis can be made. This is the best way to prevent a repairable injury from becoming a catastrophe. Most often, a spine injury results from a collision and sometimes includes associated head injuries. The head and neck must be immobilized immediately, and ease of breathing and level of consciousness ascertained immediately.

1. Brachial Plexus Neuropraxia

The most common cervical injury is pinching or stretching neuropraxia of the nerve root and brachial plexus. The injury is of short duration, and the patient has a full pain-free range of motion of the neck. These injuries are commonly called "stinger" or "burner" injuries. They result from lateral impact of the head and neck with simultaneous depression of the shoulder. This may cause stretching and pinching of the nerves of the brachial plexus, with burning pain, numbness, and tingling extending from the shoulder down into the hand and arms. Symptoms frequently involve the C5 and C6 root levels. Usually, recovery is spontaneous within a few minutes after the acute episode.

Patients who demonstrate full muscle strength of the intrinsic muscles of the shoulder and upper extremity and have full pain-free range of motion of the cervical spine may return to their activities. If they have residual weakness or numbness, they should not be allowed to reenter the game. Absence of neck pain should alert one to the possibility of a cervical spine injury, as neck pain is not part of the syndrome.

Persistence of paresthesia or weakness requires further evaluation before returning to play. This includes neurologic, electromyographic, and radiographic evaluation. The athlete should not participate in contact sports until full muscle strength has been achieved and a repeat electromyogram shows evidence of axonal regeneration, usually at least 4–6 weeks.

Prevention of "stinger" injuries is chiefly through correct head and neck techniques and strengthening of the neck musculature. Additionally, the use of cervical rolls may eliminate extremes of motion during impact.

2. Cervical Strain

Acute strains of the muscles of the neck are probably the most frequent cervical injuries in athletes. The word *strain* implies injury to a muscle, whereas a sprain is a ligamentous injury. A strain happens when a muscle tendon unit is overloaded or stretched. The clinical picture is common to all musculotendinous injuries. Motion of the neck becomes painful, reaching a peak after several hours or the next day. Anti-inflammatory medication, heat, massage, and other modalities are beneficial.

3. Cervical Sprain

With cervical sprain, there has been damage to the ligamentous and capsular structure connecting the facet joints and vertebra. It is often difficult to differentiate from a strain. There is limited motion and pain in the area of the injury and along the muscle groups overlying the area of the injury. Ligamentous disruption may be extensive enough to result in instability with associated neurologic involvement. Routine cervical spine radiographs are indicated. In athletes with diminished motion as well as pain, stability of the cervical spine should be documented. This may be done with flexion and extension radiographs.

Treatment of a cervical sprain consists of immobilization, rest, support, and anti-inflammatory therapy. Return to participation is permitted when motion and muscle strength normalize.

4. Cervical Spinal Cord Neuropraxia With Transient Tetraplegia

The phenomenon of cervical spinal cord neuropraxia with transient tetraplegia is a distinct clinical entity. Sensory changes include a burning pain, numbness, tingling, or loss of sensation. Motor changes include weakness or complete paralysis, which is usually transient, with complete recovery occurring in 10–15 minutes, although in some cases, gradual resolution occurs over 36–48 hours. Complete motor function and full pain-free cervical motion return. Routine radiographs of the cervical spine are negative for fractures or dislocations. Some radiographic findings include spinal stenosis, congenital fusions, cervical instability, and intervertebral disk disease.

The risks of permanent neurologic injury from cervical stenosis are thought to be significant. The Torg ratio was previously used for diagnosis of cervical stenosis. It is defined as ratio of the anteroposterior diameter of the spinal canal divided by the anteroposterior diameter of the vertebral body (Figure 3–42) being less than 0.80. But this ratio has recently been thought to be of low predictive value. Current methods for diagnosis of cervical spinal stenosis rely on MRI and CT. A cervical canal diameter of less than 13 mm is considered stenotic and less than 10 mm is considered absolute stenosis. Patients who have had neurologic symptoms and are found to have cervical stenosis should not be cleared for contact sports. Those found to have spinal stenosis who have not had symptoms should be treated on an individual basis.

Athletes who have suffered transient tetraplegia are not known to be at any greater risk for permanent tetraplegia. Patients who have this syndrome and associated instability of the cervical spine or cervical disk disease should be precluded from further participation in contact sports.

More severe injuries, including fractures and dislocation of the cervical spine, may occur. Treatment of these begins on the playing field, with immobilization of the spine. A face mask, if worn, may be cut off with bolt cutters. After thoroughly stabilizing the spine, the patient is moved to a spine board. Sandbags are used to immobilize the head and neck. The patient may then be transported to a local emergency room for further evaluation and treatment. Fractures and dislocations with or without permanent neurologic injury are treated like other spine injuries.

Crowl AC, Kong JF: Cervical spine. In: Johnson DL, Mair SD, eds: *Clinical Sports Medicine*. Philadelphia: Mosby Elsevier; 2006:143-149.

Dailey A, Harrop JS, France JC: High-energy contact sports and cervical spine neuropraxia injuries: what are the criteria for return to participation? *Spine (Phila Pa 1976)* 2010;35(21 Suppl): S193. [PMID: 20881462]

Torg JS, Corcoran TA, Thibault LE, et al: Cervical cord neurapraxia: classification, pathomechanics, morbidity, and management guidelines. *J Neurosurg* 1997;87:843. [PMID: 9384393]

LUMBAR SPINE INJURY

▶ Clinical Findings

Spondylolysis is a disruption of the pars interarticularis, while spondylolisthesis involves anterior slippage of one vertebral body over the next. Spondylolysis is most often found at L5 and L4, but may occasionally be seen at L3 and L2. It is believed to result from repeated stress around the pars interarticularis during hyperextension of the lumbar spine. If continued hyperextension activity occurs, spondylolysis may become spondylolisthesis. Sports in which spondylolisthesis is commonly found include gymnastics, football, and weight lifting. Female teenage gymnasts, for example, often have back pain but normal early radiographs. Approximately 3–6 weeks later, a stress response may be seen around the pars interarticularis, with increased density developing. At this time, the bone scan will be positive, indicating an impending stress fracture that will show up on plain radiographs in 2–4 weeks. A physician who is aware of which sports put stress on the pars interarticularis should consider a bone scan to rule out spondylolisthesis.

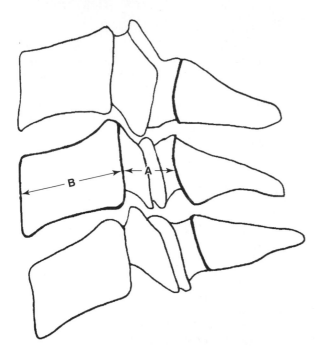

▲ **Figure 3–42.** The ratio of the spinal canal to the vertebral body is the distance from the midpoint of the posterior aspect of the vertebral body to the nearest point on the corresponding spinolaminar line (**A**) divided by the anteroposterior width of the vertebral body (**B**). (Reproduced, with permission, from Torg JS, Pavlov H, Genuario SE, et al: Neurapraxia of the cervical spinal cord with transient quadriplegia. *J Bone Joint Surg Am* 1986;68:1354.)

▶ Treatment and Prognosis

The treatment of spondylolisthesis involves cessation of all aggravating sports and other actions producing spinal hyperextension. A certain percentage of these fractures will heal spontaneously. Healing time for spondylolysis of the lumbar spine is usually about 6 months. If after that period of time no significant signs of healing are apparent, it is unlikely that spontaneous healing will take place. At this point, spinal fusion should be considered, or the patient should be willing to confine his activities to less stressful, pain-free sports.

Many patients with spondylolisthesis engage in high-level sporting activities without significant pain or neurologic deficit.

Only a small percentage actually present for evaluation and care. Complete evaluation and treatment recommendations for spondylolisthesis and spondylolysis are found in the section on the spine.

Leone A, Cianfoni A, Cerase A, Magarelli N, Bonomo L: Lumbar spondylolysis: a review. *Skeletal Radiol* 2011;40:683. [PMID: 20440613]

Milanese S, Grimmer-Somers K: What is adolescent low back pain? Current definitions used to define the adolescent with low back pain. *J Pain Res* 2010;3:57. [PMID: 21197310]

Purcell L: Causes and prevention of low back pain in young athletes. *Paediatr Child Health* 2009;14:533. [PMID: 20885805]

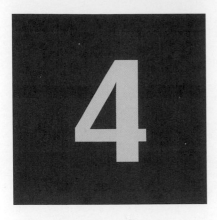

Disorders, Diseases, and Injuries of the Spine

Bobby K.B. Tay, MD
Brett A. Freedman, MD
John M. Rhee, MD
Scott D. Boden, MD
Harry B. Skinner, MD, PhD

▼ INFLAMMATORY DISEASES OF THE SPINE

Bobby K.B. Tay, MD

RHEUMATOID ARTHRITIS (ICD-9 720.0)

▶ Essentials of Diagnosis

- Up to 71% of patients with rheumatoid arthritis have C-spine involvement.
- C1-C2 instability, basilar invagination, and subaxial subluxation are common disease patterns.
- Inflammatory pannus causes synovial joint destruction.
- Eighty percent of patients are rheumatoid factor positive.

▶ General Considerations

Rheumatoid arthritis is the most common form of inflammatory arthritis. It affects 3% of women and 1% of men. The disease frequently affects the spine. Up to 71% of patients with rheumatoid arthritis show involvement of the cervical spine. The most common patterns of involvement are C1-C2 instability, basilar invagination, and subaxial subluxation (ICD-9 738.4). Of these patterns, both C1-C2 instability and basilar invagination have become less frequently encountered as a result of improvements in pharmacologic therapy. Sudden death associated with rheumatoid arthritis, most probably secondary to brainstem compression or vertebrobasilar insufficiency, is reported.

▶ Pathogenesis

The same inflammatory cells that destroy peripheral joints affect the synovium of apophyseal and uncovertebral joints of the spine, causing painful instability with or without neurologic compromise. The pannus, a conglomeration of hypertrophic synovium and inflammatory cells, often causes facet joint and transverse ligament destruction, leading to painful instability. The hypertrophic tissue can also cause

direct compression of the spinal cord and nerve roots at the affected levels.

▶ Prevention

Prevention of rheumatoid instability centers around control of the inflammatory component of the disease. The standard pharmacotherapeutic strategy initially involves the use of anti-inflammatory medication and ends the application of DMARDs.

▶ Clinical Findings

A. Symptoms and Signs

From 7 to 34% of patients present with neurologic problems. Documentation of neurologic function can be difficult because loss of joint mobility leads to general muscle weakness. Although many patients complain of nonspecific neck pain, atlantoaxial subluxation is the most common cause of pain in the upper neck, occiput, and forehead in patients with rheumatoid arthritis. Symptoms are aggravated by motion. Increasing compression of the spinal cord results in severe myelopathy with gait abnormalities, weakness, paresthesias, and loss of dexterity. Findings may also include Lhermitte sign (a tingling or electrical feeling that occurs in the arms, legs, or trunk when the neck is flexed), increased muscle tonus of the upper and lower extremities, and pathologic reflexes.

B. Imaging Studies

Instability of the upper cervical spine is determined on lateral flexion-extension radiographs. An atlantodens interval (ADI) that exceeds 3.5 mm is abnormal. Subluxation with an ADI of 10–12 mm indicates disruption of all supporting ligaments of the atlantoaxial complex (transverse and alar ligaments). The spinal cord in this position is compressed between the dens and the posterior arch of C1. Although the ADI is an important measurement for traumatic instability of the C1-C2 complex, the posterior atlantodens interval

(PADI) is more prognostic to assess neurologic compromise. The PADI is a direct measure of the space available for the spinal cord at the C1-C2 level. The PADI is measured from the posterior aspect of the odontoid process to the nearest posterior structure (the foramen magnum or the posterior ring of the atlas). If the space available for the spinal cord is less than 13 mm, the likelihood that the patient will develop myelopathy is extremely high.

Cranial settling is present in 5–32% of patients. The odontoid process should not project more than 3 mm above the Chamberlain line, which is a line between the hard palate and the posterior rim of the foramen magnum. The tip of the dens should not project more than 4.5 mm above the McGregor line, which is a line connecting the posterior margin of the hard palate to the occiput. The Clark classification divides the axis into thirds in the sagittal plane. In severe cases of cranial settling, the anterior arch of C1 moves from station 1 (the upper third of C2) to station 3 (the lower third of C2). Neurologic compromise occurs as a result of impingement of the dens into the brainstem and the upper cervical spinal cord. The vertebral arteries can also become occluded as they course between the dens and the foramen magnum to enter the skull.

Lateral subluxation and posterior atlantoaxial instability are less frequent. From 10 to 20% of patients with rheumatoid arthritis present with subaxial subluxation. Erosion of the facet joints and narrowing of the disks leads to subtle anterior subluxations often found on several levels. This results in the characteristic so-called stepladder deformity that occurs most commonly at the C2-C3 and C3-C4 levels.

C. Laboratory Studies

Rheumatoid factor is positive in up to 80% of patients. The erythrocyte sedimentation rate (ESR) rate is elevated and the hemoglobin is decreased in the active phase of the disease. After plain radiographs, which should include lateral flexion-extension views, magnetic resonance imaging (MRI) is the study of choice to evaluate the degree of neural compression and deformity.

▶ Differential Diagnosis

- Osteoarthritis
- Other inflammatory arthritides

▶ Complications

Untreated instability can lead to loss of neurologic function, paralysis, and sudden death. Medical treatment using disease-modifying antirheumatoid drugs (DMARDs) can cause immunosuppression and lead to a higher risk of contracting infections. Complications of surgical treatment include a higher rate of infection, poor wound healing, lower fusion rate, and potentially a higher rate of instrumentation failure due to poor bone quality.

▶ Treatment

Indications for surgery are severe neck pain and increasing loss of neurologic function. Most commonly, a posterior arthrodesis between C1 and C2 is performed (CPT 22590). A Gallie type or Brooks type of fusion can be done, or posterior transarticular screw fixation (CPT 22840) can be used (Figure 4–1). The latter obviates the need for postoperative halo immobilization. In cases of basilar invagination (cranial settling), extension of the fusion to the occiput (CPT 22590) is necessary. Preoperative halo traction (CPT 20661) is often required to reduce the subluxation or pull the odontoid process out of the foramen magnum. Often a suboccipital craniectomy (CPT 61343) is necessary to decompress the brainstem adequately. Good fixation can be obtained through the use of plate-screw and rod-screw constructs (CPT 22842). Subaxial subluxation with spinal cord compression should be treated with decompression and stabilization with spinal fusion. This can be done most easily via a posterior approach with laminectomy and posterior instrumented fusion or a combined anterior and posterior decompression and fusion for patients with poor bone stock or significant sagittal plane deformity (Figure 4–2).

Borenstein D: Inflammatory arthritides of the spine: surgical versus nonsurgical treatment. *Clin Orthop Relat Res* 2006;443:208. [PMID: 16462444]

Caird J, Bolger C: Preoperative cervical traction in cases of cranial settling with halo ring and Mayfield skull clamp. *Br J Neurosurg* 2005;19:488. [PMID: 16574561]

Gluf WM, Schmidt MH, Apfelbaum RI: Atlantoaxial transarticular screw fixation: a review of surgical indications, fusion rate, complications, and lessons learned in 191 adult patients. *J Neurosurg Spine* 2005;2:155. [PMID: 15739527]

Higashino K, Sairyo K, Katoh S, Nakano S, Enishi T, Yasui N: The effect of rheumatoid arthritis on the anatomy of the female cervical spine: a radiological study. *J Bone Joint Surg Br* 2009;91:1058. [PMID: 19651834]

Kauppi MJ, Neva MH, Laiho K, et al: Rheumatoid atlantoaxial subluxation can be prevented by intensive use of traditional disease modifying antirheumatic drugs. *J Rheumatol* 2009;36:273. [PMID: 19132793]

Kim DH, Hilibrand AS: Rheumatoid arthritis in the cervical spine. *J Am Acad Orthop Surg* 2005;13:463. [PMID: 16272271]

Paus AC, Steen H, Rislien J, Mowinckel P, Teigland J: High mortality rate in rheumatoid arthritis with subluxation of the cervical spine: a cohort study of operated and nonoperated patients. *Spine (Phila Pa 1976)* 2008;33:2278. [PMID: 18784629]

Ronkainen A, Niskanen M, Auvinen A, Aalto J, Luosujrvi R: Cervical spine surgery in patients with rheumatoid arthritis: long-term mortality and its determinants. *J Rheumatol* 2006;33:517. [PMID: 16511921]

Wolfs JF, Kloppenburg M, Fehlings MG, van Tulder MW, Boers M, Peul WC: Neurologic outcome of surgical and conservative treatment of rheumatoid cervical spine subluxation: a systematic review. *Arthritis Rheum* 2009;61:1743. [PMID: 19950322]

Wollowick AL, Casden AM, Kuflik PL, Neuwirth MJ: Rheumatoid arthritis in the cervical spine: what you need to know. *Am J Orthop (Belle Mead NJ)* 2007;36:400. [PMID: 17849024]

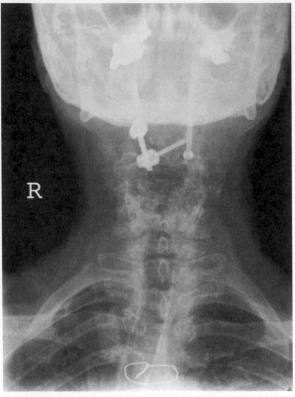

A

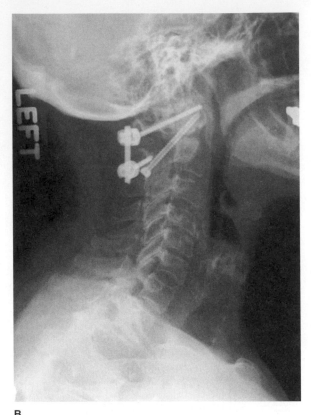

B

▲ **Figure 4–1.** (**A and B**) Anteroposterior and lateral radiographic images of a 50-year-old woman with rheumatoid arthritis who suffered a fracture of the odontoid treated with posterior C1-C2 fusion with a transarticular screw construct on the right and a C1 lateral mass/C2 translaminar screw construct on the left.

ANKYLOSING SPONDYLITIS (ICD-9 720.0)

▶ Essentials of Diagnosis

- *Seronegative spondyloarthropathy.*
- *Juvenile ankylosing spondylitis has a predisposition to hip involvement.*
- *Unlike rheumatoid arthritis, males are more often affected than females.*
- *Eighty-eight percent to 96% of patients with ankylosing spondylitis are HLA-B27 positive.*

▶ General Considerations

Ankylosing spondylitis is a chronic seronegative inflammatory disease that affects the axial skeleton, especially the sacroiliac joints, hip joints, and spine. Extraskeletal involvement is found in the aorta, lung, and uvea. The incidence of ankylosing spondylitis is 0.5–1 per 1000 people. Although males are affected more frequently than females, mild courses of ankylosing spondylitis are more common in the latter. The disease usually has its onset during early adulthood. However, juvenile ankylosing spondylitis affects adolescents (younger than 16 years) and has a predisposition to hip involvement.

▶ Pathogenesis

The human leukocyte antigen (HLA)-B27 surface antigen is found in 88–96% of patients, and investigators postulate that an endogenic component (ie, HLA-B27) and an exogenic component (eg, *Klebsiella* or *Chlamydia*) are responsible for triggering of the disease process. The ESR is elevated in up to 80% of the cases but does not accurately reflect disease activity. The serum creatine phosphokinase (CPK), however, is a good indicator of the severity of the disease process.

▶ Prevention

No preventive measures are available to avoid developing the disease. DMARDs may be useful in treating the pain that is associated with the inflammatory stage of the disease process. These include tumor necrosis factor-alpha (TNF-α) antagonists. Appropriate bracing prior to the onset of spinal ankylosis can minimize or prevent the development of spinal deformity.

▶ Clinical Findings

A. Symptoms and Signs

The onset is insidious, with early symptoms including pain in the buttocks, heels, and lower back. Patients complain typically of morning stiffness, the improvement of symptoms with activity during the day, and the return of symptoms in the evening. The earliest changes involve the sacroiliac joints and then extend upward into the spine. Spinal disease results in loss of motion and subsequent loss of lordosis in the cervical and lumbar spine. Synovitis in the early stages leads to progressive fibrosis and ankylosis of the joints during the reparative phase. Enthesitis occurs at the insertion of the annulus fibrosus on the vertebral body with eventual calcification that results in the characteristic "bamboo spine." The pain from

the inflammatory process subsides after full ankylosis of the affected joints occurs. Approximately 30% of patients develop uveitis, and 30% have chest tightness. Limited chest expansion indicates thoracic involvement. Fewer than 5% of patients have involvement of the aorta, characterized by dilation and possible conduction defects. In addition, patients may suffer from renal amyloidosis and pulmonary fibrosis.

B. Imaging Studies

The earliest radiographic changes are visible in the sacroiliac joints. Symmetric bilateral widening of the joint space is followed by subchondral erosions and ankylosis. Bony changes in the spine affect the vertebral body. Changes include loss of the anterior concavity of the vertebral body, squaring of the vertebra, and marginal syndesmophyte formation, which give the spine the appearance of bamboo. Ankylosis of the apophyseal joints also develops. The disease generally starts in the lumbar spine and migrates cephalad to the cervical spine. Atlantoaxial instability is seen occasionally.

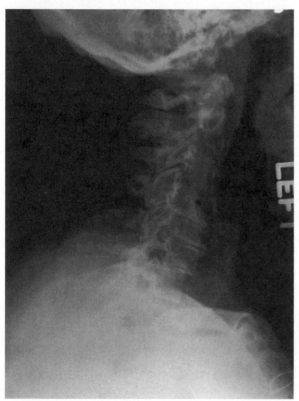

A

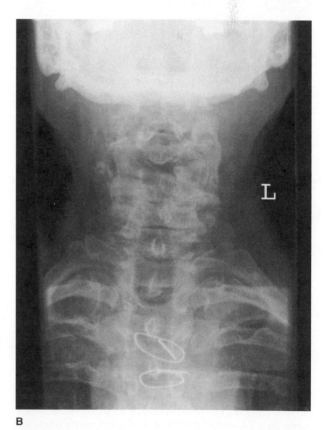

B

▲ **Figure 4–2.** (**A and B**) Preoperative anteroposterior (AP) and lateral images of a 58-year-old man with inflammatory arthritis demonstrating severe joint damage and subaxial subluxation. (**C and D**) Postoperative AP and lateral radiographic images after treatment with anterior and posterior decompression and reconstruction with fusion.

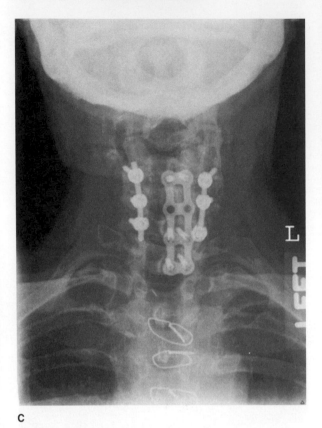

C

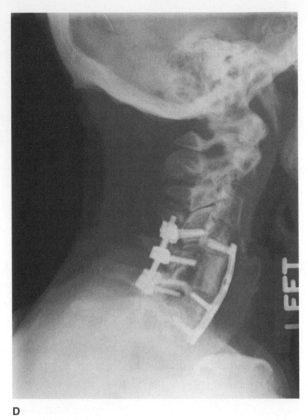

D

▲ **Figure 4–2.** (Continued)

▶ Differential Diagnosis

Early stages of the disease can appear to be similar to other inflammatory spondyloarthropathies.

▶ Complications

The main complications of untreated cervical spinal deformity include significant loss of functionality from inability to look forward (loss of horizontal gaze). Complications of surgical treatment include infection, paralysis, and C7 or T1 root injury leading to loss of triceps and intrinsic hand function, respectively. Because of medical treatments, these patients are at a higher risk for wound complications and post-surgical infections. TNF-α antagonists should be stopped for at least 2 weeks prior to surgical treatment to minimize the risk for infection. Prolonged use of a halo vest in the post-operative period (up to 6 months) can lead to halo-related complications, including pin site infection and intracranial perforation of the halo pins over time. The patient's osteoporotic bone (especially in the cervical spine lateral masses) increases the risk of hardware pullout.

▶ Treatment

The natural history of ankylosing spondylitis, with its slow progression over several decades, has to be considered in planning treatment. Initially, treatment consists of exercises and indomethacin. Approximately 10% of patients develop severe bony changes that eventually require surgical intervention. These changes characteristically include a fixed bony flexion deformity that limits their ambulatory potential. Hip disease should be addressed before correction of spinal deformities because correction of hip flexion deformities may allow significant compensation of the spinal kyphosis (ICD-9 737.9) to allow adequate horizontal gaze. When planning surgical treatment, it is important to stop treatment with TNF-α inhibitors for at least 2 weeks prior to surgery to minimize the risk for wound infection.

Loss of lumbar lordosis can be treated by multilevel V-shaped osteotomies posteriorly (the Smith-Petersen procedure; CPT 22214), by a decancellation procedure (the Heinig procedure; CPT 22207) of L3 or L4, or by pedicle subtraction osteotomy based at L3 or L4 (Thomassen osteotomy; CPT 22207) (Figure 4–3). The L3-L4 level is used

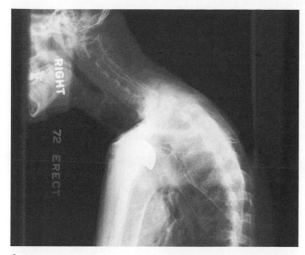

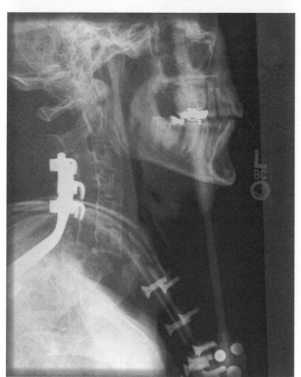

▲ **Figure 4–3.** Preoperative (**A**) and postoperative (**B**) lateral radiographs of a 38-year-old man with cervicothoracic kyphosis and loss of horizontal gaze who was treated with a posterior cervicothoracic osteotomy and instrumented fusion.

because this correlates with the apex of the normal lumbar lordosis and allows for adequate distal fixation to hold the osteotomy in a stable configuration.

The spine is then fused in the corrected position. Utilization of modern fixation systems such as a pedicle screw system allows for early mobilization of the patient. Thorough preoperative assessment of the deformity and measuring of the chin-eyebrow-to-floor angle are helpful for the exact planning of the corrective osteotomy. Relative contraindications to surgery are poor general health and significant scarring of the major vessels, which may be injured when the spine is extended.

The cervical osteotomy (CPT 22210) is performed between C7 and T1. This approach avoids injury to the vertebral artery that usually enters the transverse foramen at the C6 level. Historically the procedure was usually performed under local anesthesia in the semisitting position with facet wiring and halo application (CPT 20661) as the only forms of fixation. However, the evolution of somatosensory and transcranial motor evoked potential monitoring of the spinal cord permits the use of general anesthesia. After removal of the posterior elements and neural decompression, the kyphotic deformity is corrected with gentle extension of the head. The ossified disk space fractures under the extension force and hinges on the posterior longitudinal ligament. The head is held in the corrected position using internal fixation with rod-screw constructs or hook-rod constructs with adjunctive halo vest immobilization (see Figure 4–3). Long constructs with multiple levels of fixation often to C2 or C3 are necessary to obtain sufficient purchase in the ossified but osteoporotic bone to allow for adequate biomechanical stability. Other procedures, such as a decancellation wedge osteotomy of C7 (CPT 22206), have also been described. However, great care must be taken in these cases to avoid inadvertent spinal translation at the osteotomy site that can cause injury to the nerves or the spinal cord. More recently, the adoption of circumferential fusion and fixation techniques has allowed the potential to avoid halo vest immobilization.

Baraliakos X, Listing J, von der Recke A, Braun J: The natural course of radiographic progression in ankylosing spondylitis—evidence for major individual variations in a large proportion of patients. *J Rheumatol* 2009;36:997. [PMID: 19332632]

Einsiedel T, Schmelz A, Arand M, et al: Injuries of the cervical spine in patients with ankylosing spondylitis: experience at two trauma centers. *J Neurosurg Spine* 2006;5:33. [PMID: 16850954]

Etame AB, Than KD, Wang AC, La Marca F, Park P: Surgical management of symptomatic cervical or cervicothoracic kyphosis due to ankylosing spondylitis. *Spine (Phila Pa 1976)* 2008;33:E559. [PMID: 18628698]

Gill JB, Levin A, Burd T, Longley M: Corrective osteotomies in spine surgery. *J Bone Joint Surg Am* 2008;90:2509. [PMID: 18978421]

Hoh DJ, Khoueir P, Wang MY: Management of cervical deformity in ankylosing spondylitis. *Neurosurg Focus* 2008;24:E9. [PMID: 18290747]

Kanter AS, Wang MY, Mummaneni PV: A treatment algorithm for the management of cervical spine fractures and deformity in patients with ankylosing spondylitis. *Neurosurg Focus* 2008;24:E11. [PMID: 18290737]

Kelleher MO, Tan G, Sarjeant R, Fehlings MG: Predictive value of intraoperative neurophysiological monitoring during cervical spine surgery: a prospective analysis of 1055 consecutive patients. *J Neurosurg Spine* 2008;8:215. [PMID: 18312072]

Kubiak EN, Moskovich R, Errico TJ, Di Cesare PE: Orthopaedic management of ankylosing spondylitis. *J Am Acad Orthop Surg* 2005;13:267. [PMID: 16112983]

Maksymowych WP: Disease modification in ankylosing spondylitis. *Nat Rev Rheumatol* 2010;6:75. [PMID: 20125174]

Simmons ED, DiStefano RJ, Zheng Y, Simmons EH: Thirty-six years experience of cervical extension osteotomy in ankylosing spondylitis: techniques and outcomes. *Spine (Phila Pa 1976)* 2006;31:3006. [PMID: 17172997]

Smith MD, Scott JM, Murali R, Sander HW: Minor neck trauma in chronic ankylosing spondylitis: a potentially fatal combination. *J Clin Rheumatol* 2007;13:81. [PMID: 17414535]

Thumbikat P, Hariharan RP, Ravichandran G, McClelland MR, Mathew KM: Spinal cord injury in patients with ankylosing spondylitis: a 10-year review. *Spine (Phila Pa 1976)* 2007;32:2989. [PMID: 18091492]

Tokala DP, Lam KS, Freeman BJ, Webb JK: C7 decancellisation closing wedge osteotomy for the correction of fixed cervicothoracic kyphosis. *Eur Spine J* 2007;16:1471. [PMID: 17334795]

van der Heijde D, Landew R, Einstein S, et al: Radiographic progression of ankylosing spondylitis after up to two years of treatment with etanercept. *Arthritis Rheum* 2008;58:1324. [PMID: 18438853]

Vosse D, van der Heijde D, Landew R, et al: Determinants of hyperkyphosis in patients with ankylosing spondylitis. *Ann Rheum Dis* 2006;65:770. [PMID: 16219704]

Whang PG, Goldberg G, Lawrence JP, et al: The management of spinal injuries in patients with ankylosing spondylitis or diffuse idiopathic skeletal hyperostosis: a comparison of treatment methods and clinical outcomes. *J Spinal Disord Tech* 2009;22:77. [PMID: 19342927]

Woodward LJ, Kam PC: Ankylosing spondylitis: recent developments and anaesthetic implications. *Anaesthesia* 2009;64:540. [PMID: 19413825]

DISEASES AND DISORDERS OF THE CERVICAL SPINE

▶ Essentials of Diagnosis

- *Adequate imaging is essential to diagnosis.*
- *Imaging must include the entire cervical spine and the occiptocervical and cervicothoracic junctions.*
- *Lateral cervical spine view is the most important view in radiographic imaging of the cervical spine.*
- *Inadequate imaging will miss over 20% of cervical injuries.*

▶ General Considerations

In evaluating the cervical spine, the use of appropriate imaging studies is critical to a timely and precise diagnosis. Available imaging techniques include plain radiography, tomography, myelography, computed tomography (CT), CT with myelography, three-dimensional reconstruction CT, MRI, and scintigraphy. An understanding of the advantages and disadvantages of each technique is necessary for the proper selection of imaging studies and interpretation of results.

A. Plain Radiography

In evaluating the patient with neck pain, cervical spine radiographs are important in the initial search for a possible lesion. In the trauma setting, when a head or neck injury is suspected, radiographic studies must be carried out appropriately, or a life-threatening lesion may be overlooked. The trauma series includes anteroposterior (AP), right oblique, left oblique, and open-mouth (odontoid) views in addition to an initial cross-table lateral view. When all five views are taken, sensitivity is 92%. Cervical spine precautions must be implemented throughout the radiographic evaluation (see the section on injuries of the cervical spine later in the chapter). In the absence of a history of trauma, the oblique and odontoid views are not always required.

The lateral view reveals the majority of traumatic lesions if performed correctly. Inadequate views can miss more than 20% of cervical spine injuries, however. All seven vertebrae should be clearly visible. Gentle traction on the upper extremities may be necessary to view C7. If this is unsuccessful, a swimmer's view may be necessary. Careful scrutiny of the prevertebral soft tissue, the anterior border of the vertebral bodies, the vertebral bodies themselves, the posterior border of the bodies, the spinal canal proper, and the posterior elements must be done.

The prevertebral region may reveal swelling consistent with a hematoma, and this may serve as the only clue to a traumatic lesion. The upper limits for the prevertebral space are 10 mm at C1; 5 mm at C2; 7 mm at C3 and C4; and 20 mm at C5, C6, and C7. The contours of the cervical bony structures are regular, and subtle incongruities may indicate significant instability. Variations in normal cervical anatomy do exist, however, and a familiarity with them may prevent an overzealous workup. The ADI normally measures less than 3 mm in adults and less than 4 mm in children.

In reviewing the AP radiograph, careful assessment of the interspinous distance must be undertaken. Vertical widening at a given level greater than 1.5 times the level above and below indicates a hyperflexion injury with posterior instability or interlocking of the posterior facets. Traumatic tilting may also be noted in the AP plane while not appreciated on the lateral view.

Oblique views taken at 45 degrees allow visualization of the articulations of the facet joints. The open-mouth view permits evaluation of the odontoid process, the lateral masses, and the articulations of the lateral masses, and it also permits assessment of the distance between each lateral mass and the odontoid process. In atlantoaxial rotatory subluxation, the lateral mass of the atlas that is rotated forward is closer to the midline (medial offset); the opposite mass is farther away from the midline (lateral offset). Burst fractures of the C1 ring cause overhang of the C1 lateral masses on C2. A combined overhang exceeding 6.9 mm is highly correlated with insufficiency of the transverse ligament and C1-C2 sagittal instability.

This radiographic series is equally important in evaluating infants and children with suspected congenital or developmental defects and adults with insidious neck pain. Arthritic changes may be subtle or readily apparent with osteophytes, disk space narrowing, and facet sclerosis. Bone quality can also be assessed on plain radiographs.

B. Computed Tomography

CT scans allow excellent visualization of the bony architecture and the paravertebral soft tissues of the cervical spine. The pedicles, laminae, spinous processes, and bony spinal canal can be examined with significantly better resolution when CT is used than when conventional radiographs are taken (Figure 4–4). CT with myelography or intrathecal contrast enhancement permits visualization of the spinal canal contents.

CT is an appropriate modality for evaluating congenital variations and malformations, including spinal canal stenosis and spina bifida. Pars defects, atlantoaxial joint diseases, inflammatory changes, primary tumors, and metastatic carcinoma are well appreciated with CT. Although cervical disk disease is detectable when thin cuts and contrast enhancement are used with CT, it is better visualized with MRI.

In the trauma patient with questionable findings on plain radiographs, CT is integral in evaluating possible fractures or instability. Atrophy, deformity, and displacement of the spinal cord from acute or chronic injury are all appreciable with the use of intrathecal contrast. With the advent of MRI, however, CT is now reserved for the assessment of the bony architecture, which it does better than MRI.

Three-dimensional reconstruction of CT images gained wide clinical acceptance with the advancement of computer graphics. The reconstructions can be rotated in space to evaluate the anatomy from almost any perspective. This technique is valuable in the understanding of atlantoaxial rotatory subluxations or complex fractures of the spinal column.

C. Magnetic Resonance Imaging

MRI permits axial, sagittal, coronal, or oblique plane analysis of the anatomy. It is routinely noninvasive, requiring contrast material in only selected cases.

MRI is the standard for assessing cervical spinal cord damage. Spinal cord tumors and trauma, as well as central disk herniation, can be easily visualized. In the preoperative evaluation of patients with spondylosis or disk herniation, MRI is the neuroimaging test of choice (see Figure 4–4).

Intravenous paramagnetic agent gadolinium is commonly used to differentiate tissues receiving higher blood flow. This is helpful in the diagnosis of infection, tumor, and postsurgical scar.

High-resolution dynamic (flexion/extension/upright) MRIs have allowed the diagnosis of more subtle patterns of spinal impingement that may not be apparent in a supine (nonloaded) MRI study with the neck in a neutral position. These can allow imaging to be done in a neck position that reproduces the patient's symptoms.

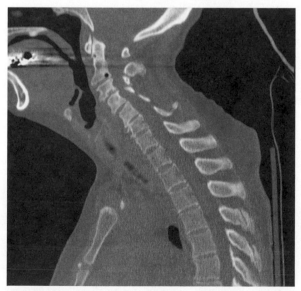

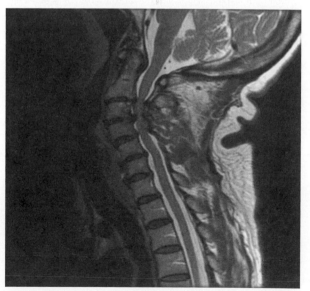

A   B

▲ **Figure 4–4.** Sagittal CT (**A**) and MRI (**B**) images of a patient with cervical spondylotic myelopathy and spinal stenosis. CT demonstrates excellent bony detail, and the MRI allows assessment of the spinal cord and disks.

D. Scintigraphy

Bone scans that employ technetium-99m phosphate permit assessment of physiologic processes within the musculoskeletal system. Metabolic, metastatic, and inflammatory abnormalities can be detected. Technetium-99m phosphate is a bisphosphonate. Its chemical similarity to pyrophosphate promotes its incorporation into bone hydroxyapatite and accumulates in areas of increased osteogenesis. Early-phase imaging with technetium-99m gives blood flow information. Accordingly, subtle fractures, avascular necrosis, and osteomyelitis can be detected. Other radioisotopes used in scintigraphy include gallium-67 citrate, which labels serum proteins, and indium-111, which labels white blood cells. These labeling techniques are helpful in discerning areas of neoplasia or acute infection.

Currently, positron emission scintigraphy combined with high-resolution CT provides a more precise image of the affected areas.

Anderson PA, Muchow RD, Munoz A, Tontz WL, Resnick DK: Clearance of the asymptomatic cervical spine: a meta-analysis. *J Orthop Trauma* 2010;24:100. [PMID: 20101134]

Bailitz J, Starr F, Beecroft M, et al: CT should replace three-view radiographs as the initial screening test in patients at high, moderate, and low risk for blunt cervical spine injury: a prospective comparison. *J Trauma* 2009;66:1605. [PMID: 19509621]

Barrett TW, Schierling M, Zhou C, et al: Prevalence of incidental findings in trauma patients detected by computed tomography imaging. *Am J Emerg Med* 2009;27:428. [PMID: 19555613]

Brandenstein D, Molinari RW, Rubery PT, Rechtine GR 2nd. Unstable subaxial cervical spine injury with normal computed tomography and magnetic resonance initial imaging studies: a report of four cases and review of the literature. *Spine (Phila Pa 1976)* 2009;34:E743. [PMID: 19752695]

Como JJ, Diaz JJ, Dunham CM, et al: Practice management guidelines for identification of cervical spine injuries following trauma: update from the Eastern Association for the Surgery of Trauma Practice Management Guidelines Committee. *J Trauma* 2009;67:651. [PMID: 19741415]

Gonzalez RP, Cummings GR, Phelan HA, Bosarge PL, Rodning CB: Clinical examination in complement with computed tomography scan: an effective method for identification of cervical spine injury. *J Trauma* 2009;67:1297. [PMID: 20009681]

Gore PA, Chang S, Theodore N: Cervical spine injuries in children: attention to radiographic differences and stability compared to those in the adult patient. *Semin Pediatr Neurol* 2009;16:42. [PMID: 19410157]

Grauer JN, Vaccaro AR, Lee JY, et al: The timing and influence of MRI on the management of patients with cervical facet dislocations remains highly variable: a survey of members of the Spine Trauma Study Group. *J Spinal Disord Tech* 2009;22:96. [PMID: 19342930]

Hashem R, Evans CC, Farrokhyar F, Kahnamoui K: Plain radiography does not add any clinically significant advantage to multidetector row computed tomography in diagnosing cervical spine injuries in blunt trauma patients. *J Trauma* 2009;66:423. [PMID: 19204517]

Lehman RA Jr, Helgeson MD, Keeler KA, Bunmaprasert T, Riew KD: Comparison of magnetic resonance imaging and computed tomography in predicting facet arthrosis in the cervical spine. *Spine (Phila Pa 1976)* 2009;34:65. [PMID: 19127162]

Manchikanti L, Dunbar EE, Wargo BW, Shah RV, Derby R, Cohen SP: Systematic review of cervical discography as a diagnostic test for chronic spinal pain. *Pain Physician* 2009;12:305. [PMID: 19305482]

Mummaneni PV, Kaiser MG, Matz PG, et al: Preoperative patient selection with magnetic resonance imaging, computed tomography, and electroencephalography: does the test predict outcome after cervical surgery? *J Neurosurg Spine* 2009;11:119. [PMID: 19769491]

Pieretti-Vanmarcke R, Velmahos GC, Nance ML, et al: Clinical clearance of the cervical spine in blunt trauma patients younger than 3 years: a multi-center study of the American Association for the Surgery of Trauma. *J Trauma* 2009;67:543. [PMID: 19741398]

Richards PJ, George J, Metelko M, Brown M: Spine computed tomography doses and cancer induction. *Spine (Phila Pa 1976)* 2010;35:430. [PMID: 20081559]

Saltzherr TP, Beenen LF, Reitsma JB, Luitse JS, Vandertop WP, Goslings JC: Frequent computed tomography scanning due to incomplete three-view x-ray imaging of the cervical spine. *J Trauma* 2009;68:1213. [PMID: 20016389]

Schoenfeld AJ, Bono CM, McGuire KJ, Warholic N, Harris MB: Computed tomography alone versus computed tomography and magnetic resonance imaging in the identification of occult injuries to the cervical spine: a meta-analysis. *J Trauma* 2010;68:109. [PMID: 20065765]

Simon JB, Schoenfeld AJ, Katz JN, et al: Are "normal" multidetector computed tomographic scans sufficient to allow collar removal in the trauma patient? *J Trauma* 2010;68:103. [PMID: 20065764]

Song KJ, Choi BW, Kim GH, Kim JR: Clinical usefulness of CT-myelogram comparing with the MRI in degenerative cervical spinal disorders: is CTM still useful for primary diagnostic tool? *J Spinal Disord Tech* 2009;22:353. [PMID: 19525791]

Xu-hui Z, Jia-hu F, Lian-shun J, et al: Clinical significance of cervical vertebral flexion and extension spatial alignment changes. *Spine (Phila Pa 1976)* 2009;34:E21. [PMID: 19127144]

CONGENITAL MALFORMATIONS (ICD-9 756.10)

▶ Essentials of Diagnosis

- *Os odontoideum (ICD-9 756.10) is a congenital nonunion of the dens that can lead to significant C1-C2 instability.*

- *Injuries can occur after minimal trauma.*

- *Klippel-Feil syndrome (ICD-9 756.16) exhibits a triad of clinical features: a short "web" neck, a low posterior hairline, and limited cervical neck motion.*

- *Syndromic conditions such as VATER (vertebrae, anus, trachea, esophagus, and renal abnormalities) must be ruled out in the presence of congenital failure of formation or segmentation in the cervical spine.*

▶ General Considerations

The atlanto-occipital region is a frequent location for abnormalities. Various combinations involving bone and nervous structures are possible. During embryologic development, 42 somites are formed from the paraxial mesoderm. The somites divide into sclerotomes, which form the vertebral bodies after separation into a caudal and cephalad portion. The middle portion builds the intervertebral disk. The second, third, and fourth somites fuse and become the occiput and posterior part of the foramen magnum. The fate of the first somite is unclear. The development of the neural tube progresses simultaneously with that of the cartilaginous skeleton.

Disturbances of embryologic development can result in incomplete development or absence of a tissue or part, as found in dysraphism, aplasia of the odontoid process, incomplete closure of the atlas, or absence of the atlas facet. Lack of segmentation results in atlanto-occipital fusion, block vertebrae, and possible instability at adjacent cervical levels. A disturbance of neurologic development, alone or in combination with bony defects, can lead to basilar impression, Arnold-Chiari malformation, and syringomyelia, all of which manifest in various states of spinal cord dysfunction (myelopathy).

1. Os Odontoideum

▶ Pathogenesis

Os odontoideum is an uncommon type of pseudarthrosis between the odontoid process and the body of the axis (Figure 4–5). It can cause significant atlantoaxial instability and myelopathy and can result in sudden death. Gross instability at the C1-C2 level can lead to spinal cord impingement or injury as it is compressed against the anterior portion of the axis or the posterior ring of the atlas. In some cases, extrinsic compression of the vertebral arteries results in ischemic insult to the brain.

▶ Prevention

There is no preventive measure to avoid this congenital anomaly. However, a stable os odontoideum (no motion on flexion and extension) may be treated without surgical stabilization. In this case, the patient should be counseled

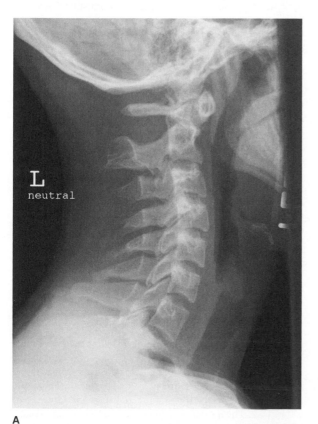

A

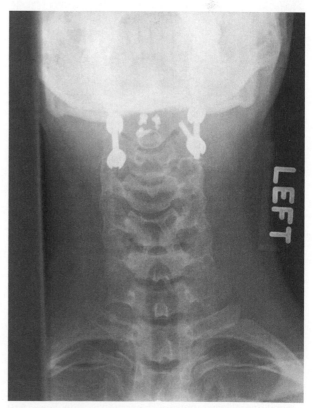

B

▲ **Figure 4–5. (A)** Lateral radiograph of a 24-year-old man with a symptomatic os odontoideum. **(B and C)** Anteroposterior and lateral radiographs after stabilization and fusion of C1-C2 to stabilize the os odontoideum.

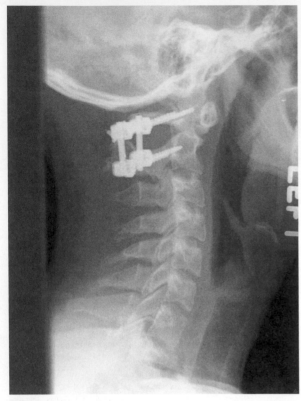

C

▲ **Figure 4–5.** (Continued)

about the risks of neurologic injury with potentially minor trauma.

▶ Clinical Findings

A. Symptoms and Signs

Patients with os odontoideum may be asymptomatic or may present with symptoms and signs that relate to atlantoaxial instability, such as ill-defined neck complaints or focal or diffuse neurologic deficits. A careful history may be needed to rule out trauma, although congenital os odontoideum may come to the attention of the surgeon secondary to a reported but inconsequential neck injury.

B. Imaging Studies

The radiographic findings may be extremely subtle and difficult to distinguish. In the mature skeleton, os odontoideum appears as a radiographic lucency. In children younger than 5 years, however, an anomalous gap may be confused with a normal neural synchondrosis. Flexion-extension views must therefore be obtained to demonstrate motion between the odontoid process and the body of the axis. The ossicle in os odontoideum is either round or ovoid, with a smooth surface and uniform cortical thickness. It is usually approximately

half the size of the normal odontoid process. In traumatic nonunion, the edge is irregular with a narrow gap. The fracture line may involve the body of C2 as well. An additional radiologic finding in os odontoideum is hypertrophy of the anterior ring of the atlas with a corresponding hypoplastic posterior ring. In flexion-extension views, the ossicle travels with the anterior ring of the atlas (see Figure 4–5). In cases that are difficult to diagnose, further studies include open-mouth views, tomograms, and CT reconstructions.

▶ Differential Diagnosis

Dens fractures (ICD-9 805.02) may appear similar to an os odontoideum. However, these fractures are often associated with more significant trauma (ie, motor vehicle accident).

▶ Complications

Complications of nonsurgical treatment include neurologic injury, chronic neck pain, and sudden death. Complications of surgical treatment include paralysis, infection, stroke, or death from vertebral artery injury.

▶ Treatment

Patients diagnosed with os odontoideum must be warned of the gravity of the situation because minimal trauma can be fatal. Patients with cervical myelopathy can be treated with traction, immobilization, or both, but they often require subsequent posterior fusion. Direct osteosynthesis of the os odontoideum fragment is often not possible due to its small size. Sometimes symptoms are reversible with or without intervention. Management of asymptomatic patients with instability is controversial. The benefits of surgical stabilization in an attempt to avoid potentially lethal injury from relatively minor trauma are counterbalanced by the possible complications of surgery. Improvements in image-guided surgery using systems such as STEALTH or BrainLAB have improved the accuracy and safety of placing internal fixation devices in this anatomically unique area. Alternative fixation techniques such as C1 lateral mass fixation combined with C2 translaminar or pars/pedicle fixation have minimized but not eliminated the potential for vertebral artery injury.

If fusion is indicated, usually a posterior fusion of C1-C2 (CPT 22595) is adequate. Different fusion techniques are available. Most surgeons use internal fixation with transarticular screws or C1 lateral mass/C2 screw fixation with rods (CPT 22840) combined with the Gallie or Brooks technique of structural bone grafting (CPT 20931, 20938). The Gallie technique involves the use of a single block-shaped bone graft between the posterior ring of C1 and the spinous process of C2. A single sublaminar wire holds the graft in place. The Brooks technique uses from two to four sublaminar wires, and two bone grafts are wedged between the laminae of C1 and C2. The loss of motion between atlas and axis results in an overall decrease of 50% of cervical rotation. Use of transarticular screws or screw-rod constructs that purchase into the lateral masses of C1 and the pedicle of C2 are rigid enough to allow the patient to mobilize without a soft cervical collar.

2. Klippel-Feil Syndrome (ICD-9 756.16)

▶ Essentials of Diagnosis

- *Syndrome associated with congenital fusion of cervical vertebrae.*
- *"Classic triad."*
- *Look for associated anomalies including scoliosis, renal disorders, deafness, and Sprengel deformity.*

▶ Pathogenesis

Klippel-Feil syndrome refers to an array of clinical disorders associated with congenital fusion of one or more cervical vertebrae. The fusion, which may be multilevel, results from a failure of the normal division of the cervical somites during the third through eighth weeks of embryogenesis. The cause of this failure is unknown. The syndrome was first described in 1912 by M. Klippel and A. Feil as a triad of clinical features: a short "web" neck, a low posterior hairline, and limited cervical neck motion. Interestingly, only 50% of patients with the syndrome that now bears the names of Klippel and Feil present with this classic triad.

Various conditions were subsequently seen in association with congenitally fused cervical vertebrae. These include scoliosis (seen in approximately 60% of cases), renal abnormalities (in 35%), deafness (in 30%), Sprengel deformity (in 30%), synkinesis or mirror movement (in 20%), congenital heart defects (in 14%), brainstem anomalies, congenital cervical stenosis, adrenal aplasia, ptosis, Duane contracture, lateral rectus palsy, facial nerve palsy, syndactyly, and upper extremity diffuse or focal hypoplasia.

▶ Prevention

There is no preventive measure to avoid this congenital anomaly. Children with mild involvement can be expected to grow up to lead healthy, normal lives. Patients with more severe involvement can do comparably well if the associated conditions are successfully treated at an early age.

▶ Clinical Findings

A. Symptoms and Signs

Decreased range of motion is the most frequent finding in patients with cervical spine involvement. Involvement of only the lower cervical spine or fusion of fewer than three vertebrae results in minimal loss of motion, however. Patients may also be able to compensate at other cervical interspaces, masking any loss of motion.

Neck shortening is difficult to detect unless extreme. Webbing of the neck (pterygium colli), facial asymmetry, or torticollis is seen in fewer than 20% of patients. Webbing of the neck can nevertheless be dramatic, with underlying muscle involvement extending from the mastoid to the acromion. Sprengel deformity, which results from a failure of either or both scapulae to descend from their embryologic origin at C4, is seen in approximately 30% of patients. Sometimes an omovertebral bone bridges the cervical spine to the scapulae and limits the neck and shoulder motion.

Cervical spine symptoms in Klippel-Feil syndrome are related to the secondary hypermobility of the unfused vertebrae. Except for atlantoaxial joint involvement, resulting in a significant decrease in occipital rotation, the fused joints at a given level are asymptomatic. Because of the increased mechanical demands placed on the uninvolved joints, secondary osteoarthritis, disk degeneration, spinal stenosis, and instability may result at these levels. Neurologic sequelae, usually confined to the head, neck, and upper extremities, result from impingement of the cervical nerve roots. With progressive cervical instability, the spinal cord may become involved, leading to spasticity, weakness, hyperreflexia, and even quadriplegia or sudden death from minor trauma.

B. Imaging Studies

Radiographic findings of congenital cervical vertebral fusion are diagnostic of Klippel-Feil syndrome (Figure 4–6). This may present as synostosis of two vertebral bodies or as a multilevel fusion, as originally described in 1912. Other noteworthy findings are flattening of the involved vertebral bodies and the absence of disk spaces. Hypoplastic cervical disks in a child are often hard to appreciate radiographically. If suspected, flexion-extension views can be taken. CT scanning and MRI have improved the assessment of bony and nerve root involvement.

Spinal canal stenosis is not usually seen until adulthood. Although anterior spina bifida is infrequent, the posterior form is not. Enlargement of the foramen magnum with fixed hyperextension often accompanies the cervical spina bifida. Hemivertebrae can also occur in this syndrome.

Involvement of the upper thoracic spine may be the first sign of an undiagnosed cervical synostosis. Because of the potential for multiorgan involvement in patients with Klippel-Feil syndrome, an electrocardiogram and renal ultrasound are also recommended.

▶ Differential Diagnosis

In the presence of associated congenital abnormalities such as hemivertebra, other syndromic conditions such as VATER should be ruled out.

▶ Complications

Complications are directly related to the treatment of the specific symptomatic conditions. The complications of surgical treatment include nerve injury and paralysis. Nonfusion-type procedures can lead to kyphosis because the levels adjacent to the congenitally fused levels are often degenerated at the time of presentation. Anterior fusion surgery can often span more than one motion segment and can lead to loss of range of motion (from fusion) and can potentially accelerate the rate of wear of the segments adjacent to the surgical fusion. Extensile anterior approaches

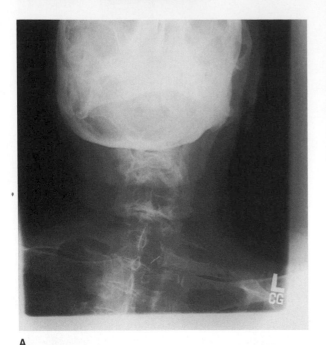

A

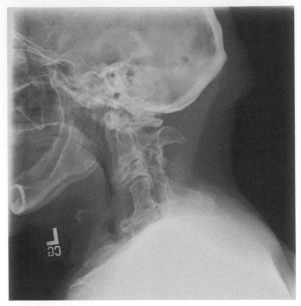

B

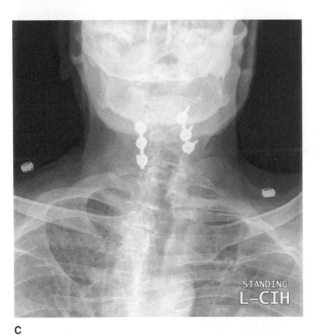

C

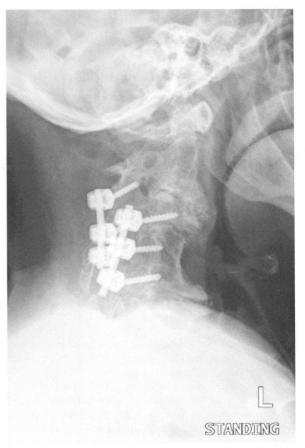

D

▲ **Figure 4–6.** (**A and B**) Anteroposterior (AP) and lateral radiographs of a 60-year-old man with Klippel-Feil demonstrating the congenitally fused cervical vertebrae that have led to deterioration of the adjacent disk segments, leading to severe spinal stenosis. (**C and D**) AP and lateral radiographs after posterior laminectomy and fusion with instrumentation.

can be complicated by postoperative swallowing disorders or unilateral vocal cord paralysis.

▶ Treatment

Treatment of cervical spine abnormalities is limited. Multilevel involvement leads to hypermobility at uninvolved joints, so affected patients should be cautious in their activities. Prophylactic surgical stabilization is not routinely performed in asymptomatic patients because the risk-benefit ratio has not been well defined. In some cases, however, surgical fusion is performed.

Secondary osteoarthritis may be treated in the usual manner, including use of a cervical collar, traction, and anti-inflammatory agents. Nerve root impingement requires careful evaluation before surgical decompression because more than one level may be involved and there may also be central abnormalities.

Surgical correction of the aesthetic deformities is only moderately successful. Carefully selected candidates may benefit from soft-tissue Z-plasty or tenotomies. This may improve the appearance of the patient but does not affect cervical motion.

Campbell RM Jr: Spine deformities in rare congenital syndromes: clinical issues. *Spine (Phila Pa 1976)* 2009;34:1815. [PMID: 19644333]

Grob D: Fusion in craniocervical malformation. *Eur Spine J* 2009; 18:1241. [PMID: 19693545]

Klimo P Jr, Kan P, Rao G, Apfelbaum R, Brockmeyer D: Os odontoideum: presentation, diagnosis, and treatment in a series of 78 patients. *J Neurosurg Spine* 2008;9:332. [PMID: 18939918]

Menezes AH: Pathogenesis, dynamics, and management of os odontoideum. *Neurosurg Focus* 1999;6:e2. [PMID: 16972748]

Samartzis D, Kalluri P, Herman J, Lubicky JP, Shen FH: The extent of fusion within the congenital Klippel-Feil segment. *Spine (Phila Pa 1976)* 2008;33:1637. [PMID: 18594455]

Samartzis D, Lubicky JP, Herman J, Shen FH: Faces of spine care: from the clinic and imaging suite. Klippel-Feil syndrome and associated abnormalities: the necessity for a multidisciplinary approach in patient management. *Spine J* 2007;7:135. [PMID: 17269206]

Sankar WN, Wills BP, Dormans JP, Drummond DS: Os odontoideum revisited: the case for a multifactorial etiology. *Spine (Phila Pa 1976)* 2006;31:979. [PMID: 16641773]

Shen FH, Samartzis D, Herman J, Lubicky JP: Radiographic assessment of segmental motion at the atlantoaxial junction in the Klippel-Feil patient. *Spine (Phila Pa 1976)* 2006;31:171. [PMID: 16418636]

Tracy MR, Dormans JP, Kusumi K: Klippel-Feil syndrome: clinical features and current understanding of etiology. *Clin Orthop Relat Res* 2004;424:183. [PMID: 15241163]

CERVICAL SPONDYLOSIS

▶ Essentials of Diagnosis

- *Cervical spondylosis is directly associated with disk degeneration.*

- *The most frequently involved levels are the more mobile segments: C5-C6, C6-C7, and C4-C5.*

- *Spinal canal stenosis is present when the canal diameter becomes less than 13 mm.*

- *Extension of the cervical spine often exacerbates the symptoms of spinal cord and nerve root compression.*

▶ General Considerations

Cervical spondylosis (ICD-9 721.0, 721.1) is defined as a generalized disease process affecting the entire cervical spine and related to chronic disk degeneration. In approximately 90% of men older than 50 years and 90% of women older than 60 years, degeneration of the cervical spine can be demonstrated by radiographs. Initial disk changes are followed by facet arthropathy, osteophyte formation, and ligamentous instability. Myelopathy, radiculopathy, or both may be seen secondarily. Cervical myelopathy is the most common form of spinal cord dysfunction in people older than 55 years. People older than 60 years are more likely to have multisegmental disease. The incidence of cervical myelopathy (ICD-9 721.1) is twice as great in men as in women.

▶ Pathogenesis

The relationship between the spinal cord and its bony arcade has been studied extensively. The first publication on the subject was written in the early 1800s and gave the first account of a "spondylotic bar," which was actually a thickened posterior longitudinal ligament protruding into the canal secondary to disk degeneration. Subsequent work revealed that disk degeneration and osteoarthritis could lead to spinal cord and nerve root impingement.

Acute traumatic disk herniation (ICD-9 722.0) was distinguished from the chronic spondylotic process in the mid-1950s. Concurrently, anterior spinal artery impingement by the disk or osteophyte was proposed as part of the pathogenesis. As indicated in these studies, disk degeneration starts with tears in the posterolateral region of the annulus. The subsequent loss of water content and proteoglycans in the nucleus then leads to a decrease of disk height. The longitudinal ligaments degenerate and form bony spurs at their insertion into the vertebral body. These so-called hard disks have to be distinguished from soft disks, which represent acute herniation of disk material into the spinal canal or into the neural foramen. The most frequently involved levels are the more mobile segments: C5-C6, C6-C7, and C4-C5. The converging of the cervical disk space may result in buckling of the ligamentum flavum, with further narrowing of the spinal canal. Segmental instability results in hypertrophic formation of osteophytes by the uncovertebral joint of Luschka and by the facet joints. These prominent spurs result in compression of both the exiting nerve roots and the spinal cord (ICD-9 722.71).

Further work revealed that the sagittal cervical canal diameter was appreciably smaller (3 mm on average) in the myelopathic spondylotic spine than in the normal spine.

The anterior-posterior dimensions of the cervical spinal canal measure between 17 and 18 mm in normal individuals. Spinal canal stenosis is present when the canal diameter becomes less than 13 mm. With extension of the neck, both the spinal canal diameter and the neuroforaminal diameter decrease.

► Prevention

Cervical spondylosis (ICD-9 721.0, 721.1, 721.90) is generally a progressive, chronic disease process (Figure 4–7). In a study of 205 patients with neck pain, Gore et al (2009) found that many patients had decreased pain at the 10-year follow-up, but those with the most severe involvement did not improve. Conservative measures may retard the disease process in its early stages. Maintaining overall aerobic conditioning and fitness and awareness, early diagnosis, and appropriate treatment of spinal cord compression can reduce or prevent functional losses.

► Clinical Findings

A. Symptoms and Signs

Headache (ICD-9 784.0) may be the presenting symptom of cervical spondylosis. Usually, the headache is worse in the morning and improves throughout the day. It is commonly located in the occipital region and radiates toward the frontal area. Infrequently, patients complain of a painful, stiff neck. Signs include decreased range of motion, crepitus, or both. With more advanced cases, radicular or myelopathic symptoms may be present.

1. Cervical spondylotic radiculopathy (ICD-9 722.0)— Cervical radiculopathy in spondylosis can be quite complex, with nerve root involvement seen at one or more levels and occurring either unilaterally or bilaterally. The onset may be acute, subacute, or chronic, and impingement on the nerve roots may be from either osteophytes or disk herniation. With radiculopathy, sensory involvement in the form of paresthesias or hyperesthesia is more common than motor or reflex changes. Several dermatomal levels may be involved, with radiation into the anterior chest and back. The chief complaint is radiation of pain into the interscapular area and into the arm. Typically, patients have proximal arm pain and distal paresthesias. Extension of the neck with rotation toward the side of neural impingement (Spurling sign) can reproduce the patient's pain pattern.

2. Cervical spondylotic myelopathy (ICD-9 722.1)— Cervical myelopathy has a variable clinical presentation, given the complex pathogenic mechanisms involved. These

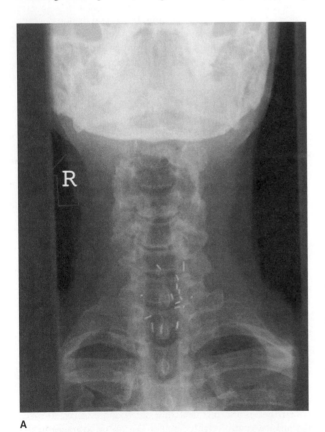

A

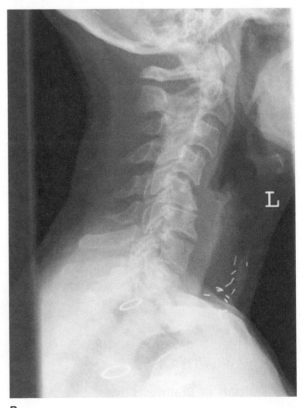

B

▲ **Figure 4–7.** (**A and B**) Anteroposterior and lateral radiographs of a 53-year-old woman with multilevel cervical spondylosis.

include static or dynamic canal impingement, facet arthropathy, vascular ischemia, and the presence of spondylotic transverse bars. In addition, given its neuronal topography, the cord may be affected in dramatically different ways by relatively minor differences in anatomic regions of compression. The clinical course of myelopathy is usually progressive, leading to complete disability over a period of months to years with stepwise deteriorations in function.

Patients often present with paresthesias, dyskinesias, or weakness of the hand, the entire upper extremity, or the lower extremity. Deep aching pain of the extremity, broad-based gait, loss of balance, loss of hand dexterity, and general muscle wasting are found in patients with advanced myelopathy. Impotence is not uncommon in these patients. Patients with severe myelopathy may exhibit a positive Lhermitte sign. In this situation, dropping the head rapidly into flexion elicits a "lightning/electrical" sensation that radiates into the arms and down the thoracic spine. Lhermitte sign is also positive in patients suffering from multiple sclerosis. Appropriate imaging studies, including a brain MRI, are necessary to rule this diagnosis out.

Hyperextension injuries of the spondylotic cervical spine can precipitate a central cord syndrome in which motor and sensory involvement is typically greater in the upper extremities than the lower extremities. Recovery from this injury is usually incomplete. Complete quadriplegia can also occur if the preexisting stenosis is severe. In this setting, the 1-year mortality approaches 80%.

Deep tendon reflexes can be either hyporeflexic or hyperreflexic, with the former seen in anterior horn cell (upper extremity) involvement and the latter seen in corticospinal tract (lower extremity) involvement. Hyporeflexia is found at the level of compression; hyperreflexia occurs on the level below. Long-tract signs, such as the presence of the Hoffmann reflex or Babinski reflex, indicate an upper motor neuron lesion. Clonus is often present although asymmetric. Upper extremity involvement is often unilateral, whereas lower extremities are affected bilaterally. High cervical spondylosis (C3-C5) leads to complaints of numb and clumsy hands; myelopathy of the lower cervical spine (C5-C8) presents with spasticity and loss of proprioception in the legs.

Abdominal reflexes are usually intact, enabling the clinician to differentiate spondylosis from amyotrophic lateral sclerosis, in which reflexes are often absent. Multiple compressions of the spinal cord cause more severe deterioration functionally and electrophysiologically than does a single-level compression.

B. Imaging Studies

Although spondylosis results from cervical spine degeneration, not every patient with radiographic evidence of cervical disk degeneration has symptoms. Furthermore, patients with all the radiographic stigmas of cervical spondylosis may be asymptomatic, and others with clinical evidence of myelopathy may show only modest radiographic changes.

This paradox is explainable by canal size differences, with the smaller-diameter canal having less space to buffer the degenerative lesion.

The average AP diameter of the spinal canal measures 17 mm from C3 to C7. The space required by the spinal cord averages 10 mm. The dural diameter increases by 2–3 mm in extension. The smallest sagittal AP diameter is measured between an osteophyte on the inferior aspect of the vertebral body to the base of the spinous process of the next vertebra below. An absolute spinal canal stenosis exists with a sagittal diameter of less than 10 mm. The stenosis is relative if the diameter measures 10–13 mm.

Plain film findings also vary according to the stage of spondylosis at which they were taken. Radiographs may appear normal in early disk disease. Alternatively, they may show single or multilevel disk space narrowing with or without osteophytes. C5-C6 and C6-C7 are the two most commonly involved segments. Vertebral body sclerosis at the adjacent base plates may also be seen. Cortical erosion is uncommon and indicates an inflammatory process such as rheumatoid arthritis.

Oblique views permit evaluation of the facet joints and detection of osteophytosis and sclerosis. The superior facets undergo degeneration more frequently than their inferior counterparts. The superior joints may then subluxate posteriorly and erode into the lamina below. Inferior osteophytes, however, may prevent significant slippage. If instability seen on flexion-extension views is significant (>3.5 mm when measured at the posteroinferior corner of the vertebral body), foraminal stenosis and vertebral artery impingement may result.

MRI permits visualization of the entire cervical canal and spinal cord by showing the spinal cord and nerve roots in two planes (Figure 4–8). The use of a contrast-enhanced CT scan is occasionally required in elderly (more than 60 years) patients with advanced degenerative bony changes of the cervical spine. Accurate identification of the location and extent of pathologic changes is necessary to determine the optimal approach for decompression. Selective nerve root blocks and electromyography may be useful to identify the level of involvement.

▶ Differential Diagnosis

Inflammatory, neoplastic, and infectious conditions can mimic cervical spondylotic radiculopathy and myelopathy.

The cervical spine is affected in most rheumatoid arthritis patients. Atlantoaxial subluxation or subaxial instability can cause symptoms similar to those seen in degenerative cervical myelopathy. A primary tumor or metastatic disease can present with unremitting neck pain, often more intense at night. MRI can distinguish neoplastic conditions from degenerative disorders. Infections of the cervical spine occur in children and in elderly (more than 60 years) or immunocompromised individuals. Multiple sclerosis should be considered in the differential diagnosis. It occurs in younger patients but can present with similar motor signs. Pancoast tumors may invade the brachial plexus, resulting in upper extremity symptoms. Syringomyelia presents with tingling

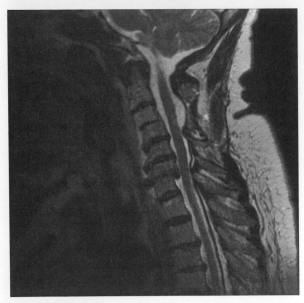

▲ Figure 4–8. Sagittal T2-weighted MRI image of a patient with cervical spondylotic myelopathy demonstrating severe multisegmental spinal stenosis.

sensations plus motor weakness. A low protein concentration in the cerebrospinal fluid and characteristic changes on MRI are found. Disorders of the shoulder, especially rotator cuff tendinitis, can imitate cervical radiculopathy. Compressive peripheral neuropathies, such as thoracic outlet syndrome, also have to be ruled out.

▶ Treatment

Patients should be divided into three groups, according to the predominance of their symptoms: neck pain alone, radiculopathy, and myelopathy. The duration and progression of symptoms need to be considered in the planning of treatment. Several studies suggest that patients with cervical radiculopathy or myelopathy have better long-term results from surgery if symptoms are of short duration.

▶ Prevention

Initial management of patients with cervical spondylosis may involve a soft collar, anti-inflammatory agents, and physical therapy consisting of mild traction and the use of isometric strengthening and range-of-motion exercises. The soft cervical collar should be worn only briefly, until the acute symptoms subside. Analgesics are important in the acute phase, and muscle relaxants are helpful in breaking the cycle of muscle spasm and pain. Diazepam should be avoided because of its side effects as a clinical depressant. Epidural corticosteroid injections may be efficacious in patients with radicular pain. Trigger point injections are an empirical form of therapy that seems to work well in patients with chronic neck pain.

The value of cervical traction remains unclear. It is contraindicated in patients with cord compression, rheumatoid arthritis, infection, or osteoporosis. A careful screening of roentgenograms before treatment is mandatory. No evidence indicates that home traction is more effective than manual traction. Isometric strengthening exercises of the paravertebral musculature should be started after the acute symptoms resolve. The patient should be instructed to start a home exercise program early to avoid long-term dependency on passive therapy modalities. Although ice, moist heat, ultrasound, transcutaneous electrical nerve stimulation (TENS), and interferential stimulation are safe to use, there is no scientific proof of their efficacy.

▶ Complications

Complications of surgical treatment include nerve injury (ICD-9 953.0), paralysis (ICD-9 952.00, 952.05), and infection (ICD-9 998.59). If anterior approaches are employed, dysphagia and vocal cord paralysis can occur. Postsurgical kyphotic deformity (ICD-9 737.10) can develop after multilevel laminectomy. If fusions are performed, failure of fusion (nonunions) that will require surgical augmentation/repair can occur.

▶ Surgical Treatment

Surgical intervention should be considered if the patient does not respond to a conservative treatment protocol or shows evidence of deteriorating myelopathy or radiculopathy. The spinal cord can be effectively decompressed by anterior, posterior, or combined approaches.

The anterior approach allows for multilevel diskectomy (CPT 63075, 63076), vertebrectomy (CPT 63081, 63082), foraminotomy, preparation of the interspaces (CPT 22554) and fusion with structural autograft (CPT 20938) taken from the iliac crest bone, structural allografts (CPT 20931), or synthetic fusion cages supplemented with autograft, allograft, or synthetic matrices. Cervical plating improves fusion rate, decreases the potential for bone graft dislodgement, and helps to maintain cervical alignment during the healing process. However, supplemental posterior fixation and fusion should be considered after two-level vertebrectomy and should be definitely performed after a three-level corpectomy. Posterior fixation minimizes the risk of anterior dislodgement of the graft even in the presence of solid anterior fixation. Alternatively, short (one-level) corpectomy combined with diskectomy for long fusions (three or more levels) improves fixation and thus decreases the potential for graft dislodgement (Figure 4–9). Anterior interbody fusion (CPT 22554) after decompression for a herniated cervical disk has a high success rate. However, fusion does lead to increased biomechanical stresses and intradiskal pressures at the adjacent unfused disk spaces. This may lead to premature degeneration of those adjacent levels.

Cervical disk replacement prostheses were also developed to provide a motion-sparing alternative to anterior cervical diskectomy and fusion (Figure 4–10). By maintaining existing motion or restoring motion to a diseased motion segment,

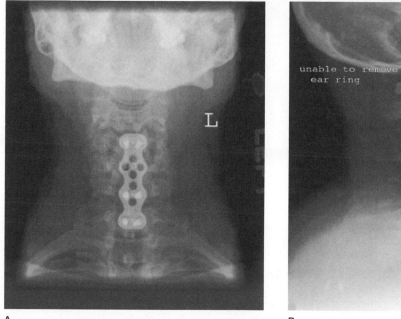
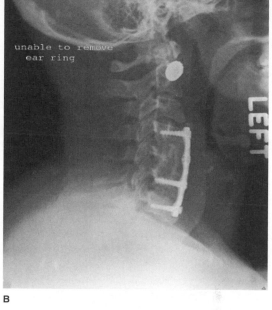

A **B**

▲ **Figure 4–9. (A and B)** Anteroposterior and lateral radiographs of a patient treated with an anterior decompression and fusion with a corpectomy of C5 and diskectomy of C6-C7 and anterior plating.

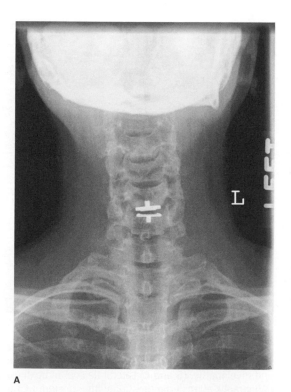
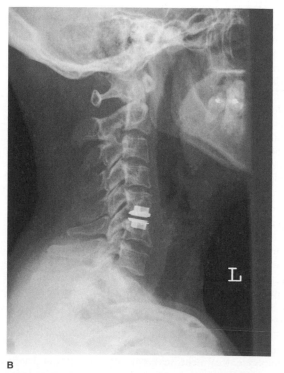

A **B**

▲ **Figure 4–10. (A and B)** Anteroposterior and lateral radiographs of a 45-year-old woman with a C5-C6 herniated disk treated with a diskectomy and reconstruction with a cervical disk replacement.

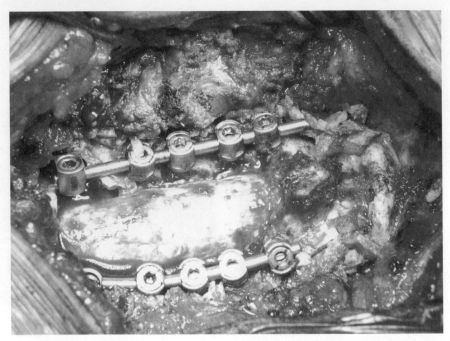

▲ **Figure 4–11.** Intraoperative image of the decompressed dura and stabilized spine after a posterior C3 to C7 laminectomy and fusion with instrumentation.

these prostheses have the potential to decrease the rate of symptomatic adjacent segment degeneration. Currently, 5-year data from clinical trials approved by the Food and Drug Administration (FDA) provide evidence that the disk prosthesis for one-level cervical disk disease achieves neurologic and neck pain relief comparable to anterior cervical diskectomy and fusion while maintaining near physiologic motion at the treated level. Function and segmental motion are also maintained at 5-year follow-up.

The number of involved levels may be important in deciding which of the surgical approaches to use. Patients with cervical myelopathy and involvement of more than three vertebral body levels may be best managed by a posterior approach. Multilevel laminectomy (CPT 63015) or laminoplasty (CPT 63050, 63051) shows excellent results. If laminectomies are performed, the facet joints and capsules should be preserved to minimize the chance of postlaminectomy deformity. Late swan-neck deformities after laminectomy can be avoided with simultaneous posterior fusion using lateral mass fixation (Figure 4–11). Laminoplasty is advantageous in that the cervical spinal cord can be decompressed while minimizing the development of late deformity (Figure 4–12). In addition, the morbidity associated with instrumentation and fusion can be avoided and some cervical motion can be preserved.

Operative treatment in cases of cervical spondylotic radiculopathy and myelopathy must be individualized for every patient.

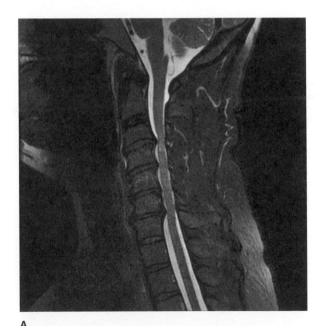

A

▲ **Figure 4–12.** (**A**) Preoperative sagittal T2-weighted MRI image of a patient with multilevel cervical spinal stenosis and myelopathy. (**B and C**) Lateral flexion and extension radiographs after decompression with a posterior C3 to C7 laminoplasty demonstrating excellent cervical motion.

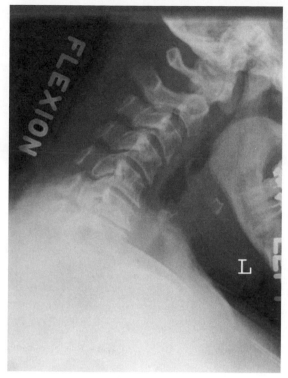

B

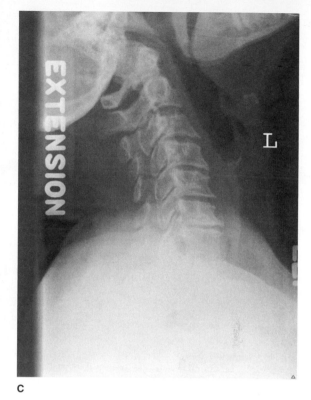

C

▲ **Figure 4–12.** (Continued)

Anderson PA, Matz PG, Groff MW, et al: Laminectomy and fusion for the treatment of cervical degenerative myelopathy. *J Neurosurg Spine* 2009;11:150. [PMID: 19769494]

Boakye M, Patil CG, Santarelli J, Ho C, Tian W, Lad SP: Cervical spondylotic myelopathy: complications and outcomes after spinal fusion. *Neurosurgery* 2008;62:455. [PMID: 18382324]

Buchowski JM, Anderson PA, Sekhon L, Riew KD: Cervical disc arthroplasty compared with arthrodesis for the treatment of myelopathy. Surgical technique. *J Bone Joint Surg Am* 2009;91(Suppl 2):223. [PMID: 19805586]

Dimar JR 2nd, Bratcher KR, Brock DC, Glassman SD, Campbell MJ, Carreon LY: Instrumented open-door laminoplasty as treatment for cervical myelopathy in 104 patients. *Am J Orthop (Belle Mead NJ)* 2009;38:E123. [PMID: 19714281]

Fehlings MG, Arvin B: Surgical management of cervical degenerative disease: the evidence related to indications, impact, and outcome. *J Neurosurg Spine* 2009;11:97. [PMID: 19769487]

Fehlings MG, Gray R: Importance of sagittal balance in determining the outcome of anterior versus posterior surgery for cervical spondylotic myelopathy. *J Neurosurg Spine* 2009;11:518. [PMID: 19929352]

Gwinn DE, Iannotti CA, Benzel EC, Steinmetz MP: Effective lordosis: analysis of sagittal spinal canal alignment in cervical spondylotic myelopathy. *J Neurosurg Spine* 2009;11:667. [PMID: 19951018]

Harrop JS, Naroji S, Maltenfort M, et al: Cervical myelopathy: a clinical and radiographic evaluation and correlation to cervical spondylotic myelopathy. *Spine (Phila Pa 1976)* 2010 Feb 10. [Epub ahead of print] [PMID: 20150835]

Holly LT, Matz PG, Anderson PA, et al: Clinical prognostic indicators of surgical outcome in cervical spondylotic myelopathy. *J Neurosurg Spine* 2009;11:112. [PMID: 19769490]

Holly LT, Matz PG, Anderson PA, et al: Functional outcomes assessment for cervical degenerative disease. *J Neurosurg Spine* 2009;11:238. [PMID: 19769503]

Holly LT, Moftakhar P, Khoo LT, Shamie AN, Wang JC: Surgical outcomes of elderly patients with cervical spondylotic myelopathy. *Surg Neurol* 2008;69:233. [PMID: 18325426]

Hyun SJ, Rhim SC, Roh SW, Kang SH, Riew KD: The time course of range of motion loss after cervical laminoplasty: a prospective study with minimum two-year follow-up. *Spine (Phila Pa 1976)* 2009;34:1134. [PMID: 19444059]

Matz PG, Anderson PA, Holly LT, et al: The natural history of cervical spondylotic myelopathy. *J Neurosurg Spine* 2009;11:104. [PMID: 19769489]

Matz PG, Anderson PA, Groff MW, et al: Cervical laminoplasty for the treatment of cervical degenerative myelopathy. *J Neurosurg Spine* 2009;11:157. [PMID: 19769495]

Matz PG, Holly LT, Mummaneni PV, et al: Anterior cervical surgery for the treatment of cervical degenerative myelopathy. *J Neurosurg Spine* 2009;11:170. [PMID: 19769496]

Mummaneni PV, Kaiser MG, Matz PG, et al: Cervical surgical techniques for the treatment of cervical spondylotic myelopathy. *J Neurosurg Spine* 2009;11:130. [PMID: 19769492]

Nikolaidis I, Fouyas IP, Sandercock PA, Statham PF: Surgery for cervical radiculopathy or myelopathy. *Cochrane Database Syst Rev* 2010;1:CD001466. [PMID: 20091520]

O'Shaughnessy BA, Liu JC, Hsieh PC, Koski TR, Ganju A, Ondra SL: Surgical treatment of fixed cervical kyphosis with myelopathy. *Spine (Phila Pa 1976)* 2008;33:771. [PMID: 18379404]

Pimenta L, McAfee PC, Cappuccino A, Cunningham BW, Diaz R, Coutinho E: Superiority of multilevel cervical arthroplasty outcomes versus single-level outcomes. *Spine (Phila Pa 1976)* 2007;32:1337. [PMID: 17515823]

Rao RD, Currier BL, Albert TJ, et al: Degenerative cervical spondylosis: clinical syndromes, pathogenesis, and management. *J Bone Joint Surg Am* 2007;89:1360. [PMID: 17575617]

Rao RD, Currier BL, Albert TJ, et al: Degenerative cervical spondylosis: clinical syndromes, pathogenesis, and management. *Instr Course Lect* 2008;57:447. [PMID: 18399602]

Riew KD, Buchowski JM, Sasso R, Zdeblick T, Metcalf NH, Anderson PA: Cervical disc arthroplasty compared with arthrodesis for the treatment of myelopathy. *J Bone Joint Surg Am* 2008;90:2354. [PMID: 18978404]

Rihn JA, Lawrence J, Gates C, Harris E, Hilibrand AS: Adjacent segment disease after cervical spine fusion. *Instr Course Lect* 2009;58:747. [PMID: 19385583]

Ryken TC, Heary RF, Matz PG, et al: Cervical laminectomy for the treatment of cervical degenerative myelopathy. *J Neurosurg Spine* 2009;11:142. [PMID: 19769493]

Ryu JS, Chae JW, Cho WJ, Chang H, Moon MS, Kim SS: Cervical myelopathy due to single level prolapsed disc and spondylosis: a comparative study on outcome between two groups. *Int Orthop* 2010 Jan 29. [Epub ahead of print] [PMID: 20108087]

Suk KS, Kim KT, Lee JH, Lee SH, Lim YJ, Kim JS: Sagittal alignment of the cervical spine after the laminoplasty. *Spine (Phila Pa 1976)* 2007;32:E656. [PMID: 17978640]

Wang X, Chen Y, Chen D, et al: Removal of posterior longitudinal ligament in anterior decompression for cervical spondylotic myelopathy. *J Spinal Disord Tech* 2009;22:404. [PMID: 19652565]

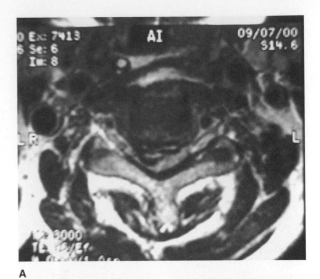

A

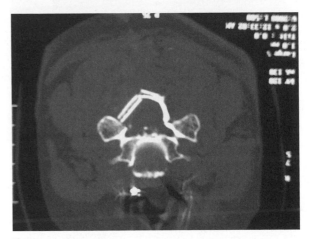

B

▲ **Figure 4–13.** (**A**) Preoperative axial T2-weighted MRI image showing severe cervical stenosis from ossification of the posterior longitudinal ligament (OPLL). (**B**) Postoperative axial CT image demonstrating the OPLL lesion after decompression.

OSSIFICATION OF THE POSTERIOR LONGITUDINAL LIGAMENT (ICD-9 723.7)

▶ Essentials of Diagnosis

- *Common cause of myelopathy in Asian population.*
- *Peak age of onset in the sixth decade of life.*
- *Disorder associated with other rheumatologic conditions.*
- *Males are more affected than females.*

▶ General Considerations

Ossification of the posterior longitudinal ligament (OPLL) is a relatively common cause of spinal canal stenosis and myelopathy in the Asian population (Figure 4–13). Its overall incidence is 2–3% in Japan, compared with 0.6% in Hawaii and 1.7% in Italy. Males are affected more often than females, and the peak age at onset of symptoms is the sixth decade.

▶ Pathogenesis

Although the cause of the disorder is unknown, it may be controlled by autosomal dominant inheritance because it is found in 26% of the parents and 29% of the siblings of affected patients. The disorder is associated with several rheumatic conditions, including diffuse idiopathic skeletal hyperostosis (ICD-9 728.89), spondylosis (ICD-9 721.0), and ankylosing spondylitis (ICD-9 720.0).

▶ Prevention

Currently, there are no preventive measures that affect the development of OPLL. Once symptomatic, fusion of the affected area halts the growth of the ossification.

▶ Clinical Findings

Almost all patients have only mild subjective complaints at the onset, although 10–15% of them complain of clumsiness and spastic gait. Nevertheless, minor trauma can lead to acute deterioration of symptoms and can result in quadriplegia. Spastic quadriparesis is the most common neurologic presentation.

OPLL can easily be diagnosed on plain lateral radiographs. The levels most frequently involved are C4, C5, and C6. A segmental type of disorder is distinguished from the continuous, local, and mixed type based on the distribution of lesions behind the vertebral bodies. CT scanning is helpful in assessing the thickness, lateral extension, and AP diameter of the ossified ligament. More than 95% of the ossification is localized in the cervical spine, although extension into the thoracic spine is reported to be a cause of persistent myelopathy following cervical decompression.

Endochondral ossification is mainly responsible for the formation of the ossified mass, which connects to the upper and lower margins of the vertebral bodies. In many cases, the ossified material is closely adherent to the underlying dura and makes excision quite hazardous. Compression of the spinal cord results in atrophy and necrosis in the gray matter and demyelinization of the white substance.

▶ Differential Diagnosis

OPLL must be considered in every case of cervical spondylotic myelopathy (ICD-9 721.1). OPLL must also be distinguished from idiopathic disk space calcification (ICD-9 722.91).

▶ Complications

Complications of surgical treatment include nerve injury (especially C5 root neurapraxia), paralysis, and infection. Removal of the ossification through an anterior approach has a high incidence of durotomy and subsequent spinal fluid leakage.

▶ Treatment

Neurologic improvement with either conservative or surgical treatment is achieved in a significant proportion of patients. Patients with severe myelopathy require neural decompression by an anterior, posterior, or combined approach. Sophisticated posterior decompression techniques, such as the open-door laminoplasty (CPT 63050, 63051), have yielded excellent long-term results for OPLL lesions that do not comprise more than 50% of the spinal canal cross-sectional area and in cases where the overall alignment of the cervical spine is neutral or lordotic.

Andres RH, Binggeli R: Ossification of the posterior longitudinal ligament. *J Rheumatol* 2008;35:528. [PMID: 18322975]

Chen Y, Chen D, Wang X, Guo Y, He Z: C5 palsy after laminectomy and posterior cervical fixation for ossification of posterior longitudinal ligament. *J Spinal Disord Tech* 2007;20:533. [PMID: 17912131]

Chen Y, Guo Y, Chen D, et al: Diagnosis and surgery of ossification of posterior longitudinal ligament associated with dural ossification in the cervical spine. *Eur Spine J* 2009;18:1541. [PMID: 19452175]

Dalbayrak S, Yilmaz M, Naderi S: "Skip" corpectomy in the treatment of multilevel cervical spondylotic myelopathy and ossified posterior longitudinal ligament. *J Neurosurg Spine* 2010;12:33. [PMID: 20043761]

Hida K, Yano S, Iwasaki Y: Considerations in the treatment of cervical ossification of the posterior longitudinal ligament. *Clin Neurosurg* 2008;55:126. [PMID: 19248677]

Inamasu J, Guiot BH: Factors predictive of surgical outcome for ossification of the posterior longitudinal ligament of the cervical spine. *J Neurosurg Sci* 2009;53:93. [PMID: 20075820]

Kim TJ, Bae KW, Uhm WS, Kim TH, Joo KB, Jun JB: Prevalence of ossification of the posterior longitudinal ligament of the cervical spine. *Joint Bone Spine* 2008;75:471. [PMID: 18448378]

Miyazawa N, Akiyama I: Ossification of the ligamentum flavum of the cervical spine. *J Neurosurg Sci* 2007;51:139. [PMID: 17641578]

Mochizuki M, Aiba A, Hashimoto M, Fujiyoshi T, Yamazaki M: Cervical myelopathy in patients with ossification of the posterior longitudinal ligament. *J Neurosurg Spine* 2009;10:122. [PMID: 19278325]

▼ DISEASES AND DISORDERS OF THE LUMBAR SPINE

Brett A. Freedman, MD; John M. Rhee, MD; Scott D. Boden, MD

OVERVIEW

Symptomatic degenerative conditions of the lumbar spine are among the most common reasons for referral to a spine surgeon. The differential diagnosis of back and radiating lower extremity pain is extensive (Table 4–1). Five of the most common forms of symptomatic degenerative lumbar spinal conditions, as well as spinal infections, tumors, and scoliosis, will be addressed.

DISK HERNIATION

▶ General Considerations

A disk herniation occurs when a piece of the nucleus pulposus (central gelatinous portion of the disk) pushes through a tear in the tougher annulus fibrosis, a dense collagenous ring encircling the nucleus pulposus. This can occur in the central (Figure 4–14A), posterolateral (Figure 4–14B), foraminal (Figure 4–14C), and extraforaminal zones (Figure 4–14D).

Table 4–1. Differential diagnoses for degenerative lumbar spinal conditions.

- Myofascial pain, "lumbar strain"; myofascial low back pain (second most common pain generator after disk) tends to respond more to muscle relaxers; possible role for Botox (botulinum toxin)
- Medical neuropathy (eg, vitamin B_{12} deficiency, thyroid disease)
- Central nervous system disease (eg, cerebrovascular accident, multiple sclerosis)
- Referred pain (eg, chronic pancreatitis, splenomegaly)
- Spondylodiskitis, epidural abscess, infected facet cyst
- Malignancy (metastatic disease most common neoplasm; night pain, atypical, nonpostural/mechanical, constitutional symptoms)
- Peripheral vascular disease, vascular claudication (VC); riding a bike makes VC worse and not neurogenic claudication (NC), standing makes NC worse and not VC; VC is typically associated with a specific distance tolerance and weak pulses
- Diabetes mellitus
- Degenerative joint disease of the hip
- Piriformis syndrome; about 20% of the time the sciatic nerve goes through the piriformis; with contraction of this muscle, sciatica occurs; steroids for inflammation and Botox have been used

The more central the herniation, the more likely it is to compress the traversing nerve root (ie, S1 at the L5/S1 disk), whereas the more lateral the herniation, the more likely it is to compress the exiting nerve root (ie, L5 at L5/S1 disk). Thus, a disk herniation at one spinal level can have different clinical presentations.

Herniated nucleus pulposus (HNP) can cause nerve root symptoms by two mechanisms. First, the herniation can cause a mechanical deformation of the nerve root. Second, the release of various inflammatory mediators by the herniated disk elicits a robust inflammatory response and irritates

the nerve root. It is thought that most cases of symptomatic radiculopathy from disk herniations have both a mechanical and inflammatory basis, which helps to explain in part why the size of the herniation does not necessarily correlate with the severity of symptoms.

Annually, about 5–20 per 1000 adults sustain disk herniations, resulting in a 13–40% lifetime incidence, occurring most commonly in the fifth decade. The L4/5 and L5/S1 levels are most commonly affected (80%); however, with age, proximal levels (such as L2/3 and L3/4) become increasingly involved. Recently, studies have identified genetic inheritance as the most important risk factor for developing lumbar disk herniations. Occupational and recreational exposures, obesity, and smoking are also important potentially modifiable risk factors.

▶ Clinical Findings

A. Signs and Symptoms

Disk herniations classically present with prodromal low back pain that acutely changes to a radiating leg pain. When this occurs, the low back pain may resolve or remain, but the leg symptoms most commonly predominate. More than 50% of the time, there is no inciting event noted. Along with pain, the patient can have numbness and/or weakness in the pattern of the compressed nerve. Diskogenic problems typically are worse in forward flexion and better in extension. Because sitting increases intradiskal pressure, many with symptomatic disk herniations feel more pain sitting than in other positions, such as lying down or even standing. Additionally, positions that put tension on the nerve root (ie, fully extending the knee) tend to reproduce or exacerbate the radiating pain.

All patients presenting with painful lumbar degenerative conditions need a thorough neurologic and physical examination (Tables 4–2 to 4–4). Representative dermatomes of the L1-S1 nerve roots should be assessed for light touch and pinprick sensation and should be compared to the contralateral side. The patient should be asked to stand and ambulate.

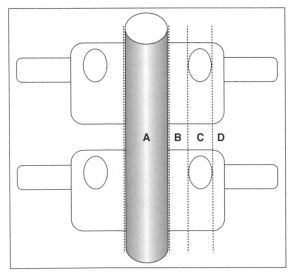

▲ **Figure 4–14.** Diagram depicting the four locations/zones for a disk herniation.

Table 4–2. Lumbar spine physical exam.

- Inspection: skin, signs of previous surgery, palpation, spasm
- Posture: alignment (scoliosis), sagittal balance, coronal balance, stance
- Range of motion: amount and motion that elicits pain
- Motor strength (5-point manual muscle testing scale; 0 = flaccid, 5 = normal)
- Sensation: by dermatome (L1-S1) + low sacral (anal sensation)
- Tension signs
  - ○ Supine and sitting straight leg raise test (L5-S1 radiculopathy)
  - ○ Femoral stretch test (L2-L4 radiculopathy)
- Sacroiliac joint testing: palpation, lateral compression, FABER (flexion, abduction, external rotation)
- Gait: heel walk, toe walk, in-line walk, standing squat, balance
- Mental status (mood/affect, orientation) and Waddell sign
- Targeted extremity exam: pulses, hip/knee range of motion

Table 4–3. Motor strength grades.

0–No motion, no twitch, complete paralysis
1–Muscle twitch/contraction or fasciculation, no motion
2–Full AROM[a] with gravity eliminated
3–Full AROM against gravity, but not against resistance
4–Able to overcome gravity and some degree of resistance
5–Normal muscle strength (ie, symmetric to contralateral side)

[a]AROM, active range of motion. "+" and "−" can be added to provided further degrees of description; this is helpful in more subtle degrees of motor loss (the more common clinical scenario), since the motor grading scale is skewed toward more profound deficit.

Gait should be assessed for independence, stability, and antalgia. Frequently patients will not bear full weight on the leg ipsilateral to a large disk herniation and may list to the contralateral side. To further test motor strength and coordination, patients should be asked to walk on their heels and toes. If possible, spine range of motion should be assessed, specifically seeking out whether spinal flexion or extension is more provocative. Last, tension signs should be assessed. In the supine position, each lower extremity should be elevated between 20 and 70 degrees. Reproduction of pain down the leg below the knee constitutes a positive straight leg raise (SLR) test. A crossed SLR occurs when elevation of the contralateral extremity reproduces pain in the symptomatic extremity. Prone SLR (femoral stretch test) can be performed to test for tension in the upper lumbar roots (L2, L3, and L4), indicated by anterior thigh pain. The SLR can be repeated in the sitting position, during motor strength testing of the quadriceps as the patient fully extends the knee.

B. Imaging

MRI is the gold standard for detecting and defining lumbar disk herniations but can be overly sensitive, because high proportions of asymptomatic volunteers may have abnormal-appearing disks on MRI. Thus, it is paramount

Table 4–4. Major motor groups and their innervation.

Nerve Root	Muscle	Action
L1,2	Iliopsoas	Hip flexion
L3,4	Quadriceps Adductors	Knee extension Hip adduction
L4,5	Tibialis anterior	Ankle dorsiflexion
L5	Extensor hallucis longus	Great toe extension
L5,S1	Peroneal longus/brevis	Ankle eversion
S1	Gastrosoleus	Ankle plantarflexion

to correlate MRI findings with clinical signs and symptoms when diagnosing and treating HNPs. Disk herniations typically have three distinct morphologies on MRI—protrusion (often called a "disk bulge"), extrusion, and sequestration. A protrusion is a general bulge of the posterior disk that is seen both in conjunction with disk degeneration and the normal aging process. It is the most common form of HNP, seen in 20–30% of asymptomatic adults under the age of 40, 60% between age 40 and 60, and 80–100% over the age of 60. Protrusions have the most variable outcomes following diskectomy, with a 7–13% reherniation rate and up to 38% with persistent sciatica complaints. Protrusions are a relatively poor prognosticator for either operative or nonoperative outcomes with treatment, which makes sense because a protrusion tends to indicate global disk failure, which is less likely to respond to focal interventions like injections or microdiskectomy. Disk extrusion is an HNP in which nuclear material pushes through and beyond the annulus, yielding a mushroom-like appearance with a cap and a stalk. Extrusions represent the HNP morphology most commonly treated with diskectomy (approximately two thirds of cases) (Figure 4–15). Sequestration is a progression of extrusion, in which the herniated nuclear fragment is no longer in continuity with the disk of origin. Extrusions and sequestrations typically have better outcomes than protrusion. Unlike protrusions or bulges, extrusions and sequestrations are seen in fewer than 1–10% of asymptomatic volunteers. Thus, the clinical relevance of extrusion and sequestration is generally more certain than that of a protrusion or disk bulge.

▶ Treatment

The first-line treatment for most degenerative, symptomatic conditions of the lumbar spine is nonoperative. Despite the multiple nonoperative therapies advocated, overall, they have had surprisingly limited evidential support; however, researchers in the last decade have made a concerted effort to overcome this prior limitation. Nonoperative treatment is initially attempted because of the overall favorable natural history of the disorder. Symptoms in 60–90% of HNPs will resolve spontaneously in the first 6–12 weeks. Table 4–5 lists some of the more common nonoperative treatment options. Treatments are added in a stepwise fashion, beginning with medications such as nonsteroidal anti-inflammatory drugs (NSAIDs). A short course of oral steroids often provides significant symptom relief as well. Muscle relaxants may help diminish spasms and pain. Narcotics should generally be used sparingly for a short period of time due to their addictive potential. Physical therapy may be helpful in those whose symptom level allows them to participate. Epidural steroid injections (ESIs) are a common nonoperative treatment option. These are best performed under fluoroscopic guidance, with the medication placed transforaminally at the level and side of the herniation to provide the maximal dose at the needed area. The results of clinical studies on ESIs have been variable, but there is level 1 evidence indicating that

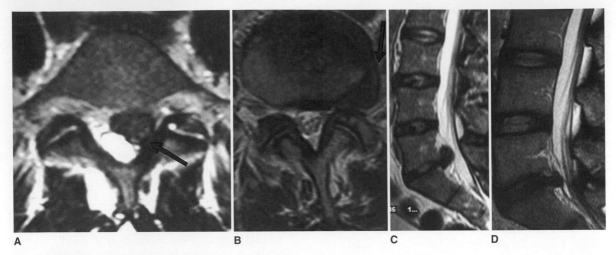

▲ **Figure 4–15.** Different types of disk herniations. (**A**) Axial T2 MRI of a large, extruded, posterolateral disk hernia-tion at L5-S1 compressing the S1 root (*purple arrow*). (**B**) Axial T2 MRI of an extraforaminal disk herniation at L4-L5 (*purple arrow*). This herniation compresses the exiting L4 root. (**C**) Sagittal MRI demonstrates disk herniation (extrusion type) that has migrated cephalad from the disk space of origin (L5-S1). (**D**) Sagittal MRI demonstrates disk herniation that has stayed at the level of the disk space (L5-S1).

they may be superior to placebo at least in the acute phase. It is unclear, however, whether ESIs change the natural history of disk herniations. Regardless, the immediate response to these injections can be diagnostic and prognostic. Patients with good to excellent initial response, regardless of whether it diminishes with time, have better outcomes following diskectomy than those with little to no response at any point following injection.

Indications for operative treatment include: (1) persistent symptoms despite a reasonable course of nonoperative treat-ment, (2) profound or progressive motor deficit, (3) cauda equina syndrome, (4) intractable pain, and (5) patient preference. Level 1 studies have consistently shown that

Table 4–5. Nonoperative treatment options.

Physical therapy/exercise
Counseling/education
Activity modification
NSAIDs/celecoxib
Narcotics pain medications
Muscle relaxers
Nerve-modulating agents (ie, gabapentin)
Oral steroids
Epidural or nerve root injection of steroids
Chiropractor/manipulation/traction
Massage/heat/cold/transcutaneous electrical nerve stimulation/ acupuncture
Psychology/biofeedback/psychiatry

NSAIDs, nonsteroidal anti-inflammatory drugs.

surgical decompression of the nerve root by removal of the offending disk fragment is significantly more efficacious than nonoperative care at time points up to 1–4+ years. These advantages exist for all outcomes commonly assessed, including pain reduction, functional improvement, and even improvement in mental health. Without question, the single most consistent finding is that the time to achieve maximal clinical outcome is substantially reduced with surgery compared with nonoperative care. The most impactful of these studies is the Spine Patient Outcomes Research Trial (SPORT), a National Institutes of Health–funded, 13-site multicenter study with observational and randomized clinical trial arms that evaluated the outcomes of surgical treatment versus conservative care for three of the most common degenerative spinal conditions—disk herniation (n = 289 randomized, n = 365 observational), spinal stenosis, and spondylolisthesis. The ample data collected from this land-mark 5-year prospective study have been subanalyzed to evaluate the impact of multiple factors, including cost and complications. The more proximal the herniated level (ie, L3/4 or L4/5 and above), the more likely surgical decompres-sion is superior to nonoperative care.

For all comers, the major advantage of surgery over non-operative care is quicker time to resolution of symptoms, especially radicular pain. This faster symptom resolution leads to a cost-benefit advantage over nonoperative care. Most patients who undergo microdiskectomy notice sub-stantial improvement in radicular leg pain in the immedi-ate postoperative period. Not infrequently, preoperative weakness and less commonly numbness may also improve quickly, although usually not as quickly or as completely as pain does, particularly if the numbness and weakness were long-standing and constant rather than intermittent. Diabetic patients may also have less recovery of nerve root function.

Conversely, nonoperatively treated patients have an overall slower time to improvement, with maximal outcomes not achieved until 1–2 years following symptom onset; however, at the 1- to 2-year mark, some studies have shown that the significant clinical advantage of surgery over nonoperative care may lessen or no longer exist. On the other hand, the results of the SPORT study show that patients who presented for treatment after 6 or more months of symptom duration had significantly less improvement than those who received treatment more acutely, which is consistent with prior prospective studies. Thus, there appears to be an optimal time window for maximal benefit from surgery that is somewhere between 6 weeks and 6 months. In the end, it is patient preference that should most direct treatment following symptomatic HNPs that do not resolve spontaneously or fail to respond to initial attempts at nonoperative care. Those with the most significant symptoms tend to select surgery, and those with more mild or intermittent symptoms may be best treated in a nonoperative fashion. There is little evidence that the method of surgery (eg, microdiskectomy, minimally invasive diskectomy, traditional "open" diskectomy) has a significant effect on outcomes as long as the nerve root is appropriately decompressed.

While the decision to treat an HNP with surgery or nonoperative therapy is largely one of patient and surgeon preference, there are rare exceptions in which acute operative treatment is absolutely indicated. The most agreed upon urgent surgical indication following HNP is cauda equina syndrome. Patients with cauda equina syndrome may demonstrate acute, profound bilateral lower extremity neurologic deficits, with saddle anesthesia and bowel/bladder incontinence (usually bowel incontinence and urinary retention). Cauda equina syndrome represents one of the true emergent/urgent conditions of the lumbar spine. Thus, all patients with suspected cauda equina syndrome should be immediately referred to a spine surgeon and undergo emergent MRI. Neurologic outcomes are traditionally thought to be best when decompression occurs within the first 48 hours, although recently, it has been shown that the severity (regardless of duration) of incontinence is the most important preoperative predictor of bowel/bladder functional recovery. Even when treated quickly, about 25–50% of patients will have continued bowel/bladder dysfunction. In addition to cauda equina syndrome, patients with any form of progressive neurologic deficit or those in whom pain is not well controlled in an outpatient setting are also candidates for early surgery.

Careful patient selection is mandatory when considering surgery. In addition to the disk pathology, psychosocial factors weigh heavily on outcomes. The presence of three or more of the five Waddell signs is associated with poor outcomes following surgical treatment due to underlying psychosocial issues. These signs include (1) a discrepancy between the seated and the supine SLR; (2) superficial and widespread tenderness that is nonanatomic; (3) pain with axial loading of the head or twisting the pelvis; (4) nondermatomal sensory deficits ("my whole leg is numb"); and (5) overreaction on exam.

▶ Complications

The most common complications of lumbar diskectomy include infection (1–3%), dural tears (3–10%), nerve root injury (<1%), and recurrent herniations (4–27%). Persistent low back pain is a not uncommon complaint despite excellent relief of radicular pain. It must be understood by the patient preoperatively that the primary goal of surgery is to relieve radicular nerve root pain and that midline axial low back pain may or may not improve even with an otherwise successful surgery.

Ahn UM, Ahn NU, Buchowski JM, Garrett ES, Sieber AN, Kostuik JP: Cauda equina syndrome secondary to lumbar disc herniation: a meta-analysis of surgical outcomes. *Spine (Phila Pa 1976)* 2000;25:1515. [PMID: 10851100]

Buttermann GR: Treatment of lumbar disc herniation: epidural steroid injection compared with discectomy. A prospective, randomized study. *J Bone Joint Surg Am* 2004;86-A:670. [PMID: 15069129]

Carragee EJ, Han MY, Suen PW, Kim D: Clinical outcomes after lumbar discectomy for sciatica: the effects of fragment type and annular competence. *J Bone Joint Surg Am* 2003;85-A:102. [PMID: 12533579]

Casal-Moro R, Castro-Menéndez M, Hernández-Blanco M, et al: Long-term outcome after microendoscopic diskectomy for lumbar disk herniation: a prospective clinical study with a 5-year follow-up. *Neurosurgery* 2011;68:1568. [PMID: 21311384]

Katayama Y, Matsuyama Y, Yoshihara H, et al: Comparison of surgical outcomes between macro discectomy and micro discectomy for lumbar disc herniation: a prospective randomized study with surgery performed by the same spine surgeon. *J Spinal Disord Tech* 2006;19:344. [PMID: 16826006]

Lebow R, Parker SL, Adogwa O, et al: Microdiscectomy improves pain-associated depression, somatic anxiety, and mental well-being in patients with herniated lumbar disc. *Neurosurgery* 2012;70:306. [PMID: 22251975]

Lurie JD, Berven SH, Gibson-Chambers J, et al: Patient preferences and expectations for care: determinants in patients with lumbar intervertebral disc herniation. *Spine (Phila Pa 1976)* 2008;33:2663. [PMID: 18981962]

Lurie JD, Faucett SC, Hanscom B, et al: Lumbar discectomy outcomes vary by herniation level in the Spine Patient Outcomes Research Trial. *J Bone Joint Surg Am* 2008;90:1811. [PMID: 18762639]

Manchikanti L, Buenaventura RM, Manchikanti KN, et al: Effectiveness of therapeutic lumbar transforaminal epidural steroid injections in managing lumbar spinal pain. *Pain Physician* 2012;15:E199. [PMID: 22622912]

McCarthy MJ, Aylott CE, Grevitt MP, Hegarty J: Cauda equina syndrome: factors affecting long-term functional and sphincteric outcome. *Spine (Phila Pa 1976)* 2007;32:207. [PMID: 17224816]

Osterman H, Seitsalo S, Karppinen J, Malmivaara A: Effectiveness of microdiscectomy for lumbar disc herniation: a randomized controlled trial with 2 years of follow-up. *Spine* 2006;31:2409. [PMID: 17023847]

Peul WC, van den Hout WB, Brand R, et al: Prolonged conservative care versus early surgery in patients with sciatica caused by lumbar disc herniation: two year results of a randomised controlled trial. *BMJ* 2008;336:1355. [PMID: 18502911]

Qureshi A, Sell P: Cauda equina syndrome treated by surgical decompression: the influence of timing on surgical outcome. *Eur Spine J* 2007;16:2143. [PMID: 17828560]

Rhee JM, Schaufele M, Abdu WA: Radiculopathy and the herniated lumbar disk: controversies regarding pathophysiology and management. *Instr Course Lect* 2007;56:287. [PMID: 17472314]

Rihn JA, Hilibrand AS, Radcliff K, et al: Duration of symptoms resulting from lumbar disc herniation: effect on treatment outcomes: analysis of the Spine Patient Outcomes Research Trial (SPORT). *J Bone Joint Surg Am* 2011;93:1906. [PMID: 22012528]

Ryang YM, Oertel MF, Mayfrank L, Gilsbach JM, Rohde V: Standard open microdiscectomy versus minimal access trocar microdiscectomy: results of a prospective randomized study. *Neurosurgery* 2008;62:174. [PMID: 18300905]

Stafford MA, Peng P, Hill DA: Sciatica: a review of history, epidemiology, pathogenesis, and the role of epidural steroid injection in management. *Br J Anaesth* 2007;99:461. [PMID: 17704089]

Weinstein JN, Tosteson TD, Lurie JD, et al: Surgical versus nonoperative treatment for lumbar spinal stenosis four-year results of the Spine Patient Outcomes Research Trial. *Spine (Phila Pa 1976)* 2010;35:1329. [PMID: 20453723]

Weinstein JN, Tosteson TD, Lurie JD, et al: Surgical vs. nonoperative treatment for lumbar disk herniation: the Spine Patient Outcomes Research Trial (SPORT): a randomized trial. *JAMA* 2006;296:2441. [PMID: 17119140]

Weinstein JN, Tosteson TD, Lurie JD, et al: Surgical vs. nonoperative treatment for lumbar disk herniation: the Spine Patient Outcomes Research Trial (SPORT) observational cohort. *JAMA* 2006;296:2451. [PMID: 17119141]

SPINAL STENOSIS

▶ Essentials of Diagnosis

- *Often due to degenerative conditions of the spine but can also occur from congenitally narrowed spinal canal or inflammatory and traumatic conditions.*

- *Symptoms are exacerbated by extension of the spine and improved by flexion of the spine.*

- *Need to assess for vascular insufficiency and osteoarthritis of the hips and knees.*

▶ General Considerations

Spinal stenosis refers to a narrowing of the spinal canal, most commonly due to the accumulation of space-occupying, degenerative material such as hypertrophic ligamentum flavum, osteophytes, and disk herniations or bulges (Figure 4–16). In rare instances, accumulation of epidural fat can also lead to spinal stenosis. Stenosis can occur in the central portion of the canal, the lateral recess (ie, the area underneath the facet joints), or the foramen. In most cases, stenosis occurs at the level of the facet joints. It is at that level that pathologic changes in the disk, facets, and ligamentum flavum hypertrophy converge to produce the greatest amount of narrowing. In contrast, stenosis is relatively uncommon at the level of the pedicles, and when it occurs at this level, it often indicates an underlying congenital or developmental stenosis of the bony canal.

Spinal stenosis is often seen in patients with a developmentally narrow spinal canal. Such patients may have had sufficient room for their nerve roots in youth, but possess little reserve capacity for the accumulation of degenerative lesions, which occur in all humans with age. Concomitant spinal instability (lateral listhesis or spondylolisthesis) and/or deformity (eg, scoliosis) may accentuate spinal stenosis: as one vertebra translates on the other, the portion of the spinal canal in between the two segments becomes narrowed in a manner similar to the closing of a cigar cutter. When foraminal stenosis occurs, it is usually due to the hypertrophy and/or proximal migration of the superior articular facet from the level below (ie, the S1 superior facet in L5-S1 foraminal stenosis), along with associated encroachment of the ligamentum flavum into the foramen. A decrease in disk height or disk herniation or bulging into the foramen can also lead to foraminal stenosis. The L4/5 level is the most commonly involved segment in spinal stenosis. Symptomatic patients can present at any adult age, with congenitally stenotic patients presenting as early as their late teen years, but most degenerative stenosis patients present in their 50s and beyond.

▶ Clinical Findings

A. Signs and Symptoms

Classically, patients complain of the insidious onset of radiating buttock and leg pain that is worse as the compromised spinal canal is further narrowed in extension (eg, standing upright or walking [downhill especially]) and improved as the canal is relatively enlarged in flexion (eg, sitting, lying down in a "fetal" position, or walking while bent over a shopping cart). Associated numbness, weakness, or a feeling of "heaviness" or easy fatigue in the legs with walking may be present. Patients may also complain of concomitant low back pain. Not all patients, however, present with these classic symptoms. Many will have significant radicular leg pain even at rest. Not infrequently, the leg symptoms may not radiate all the way down the leg but rather localize only to the buttock or posterior thigh area.

A thorough physical examination is necessary but is commonly nonfocal. Severe motor and sensory deficits are relatively uncommon. The hips and knee joints of all patients should be assessed, as osteoarthritis of those joints may often mimic spinal stenosis symptoms. Greater trochanteric bursitis can also masquerade as radiating leg pain. Sacroiliac joint

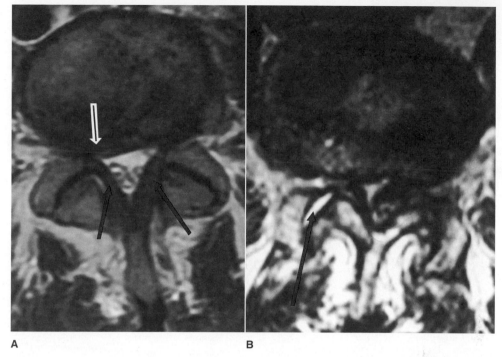

A   B

▲ **Figure 4-16.** (**A**) Axial MRI demonstrating lateral recess (subarticular) stenosis due to thickening of the ligamentum flavum (*purple arrows*). There is also an associated right posterolateral disk bulge (*white arrow*). (**B**) Severe central stenosis causing a pinhole-size spinal canal. Note associated facet joint synovitis and arthropathy (*purple arrow*).

pain, which can be very difficult to definitively diagnose, can also mimic stenotic pain localized only to the buttocks. In addition, a vascular examination should be performed in all patients to rule out vascular claudication.

B. Imaging

A noncontrast MRI scan is the most useful diagnostic tool for identifying spinal stenosis. In those who cannot have MRI scans (eg, those with pacemakers), a CT myelogram is necessary. There is little role for a plain CT scan in evaluating spinal stenosis, although it may be useful in identifying associated bony abnormalities or for surgical planning. Standing plain AP, lateral, and flexion-extension x-rays should be taken to rule out associated spinal instability or deformity.

▶ Treatment

Nonoperative treatment modalities include the same ones used to treat lumbar disk herniations. Because stenosis rarely leads to progressive neurologic injury, nonoperative modalities are generally attempted first. However, whereas disk herniations may spontaneously resolve over time with resorption of fragments, spinal stenosis due to bony or ligamentous hypertrophy does not spontaneously regress with either time or nonoperative treatment. Similar to lumbar disk herniations, nonoperative

treatment in lumbar spinal stenosis is purely symptomatic, meaning that it may help to improve pain symptoms but does not modify the underlying stenosis or make it "go away." As such, it is debatable whether nonoperative therapies alter the natural history of spinal stenosis, and the literature shows little evidence of such. A recent meta-analysis demonstrated that the evidence in support of various nonoperative treatments is low grade at best. ESIs are a common nonoperative treatment; however, unlike for disk herniation, there does not appear to be a clinical advantage between intralaminar and transforaminal techniques. In milder cases of lumbar spinal stenosis, nonoperative treatment may lead to long-term improvement in symptoms. More commonly, however, especially in those with severe stenosis, the symptoms tend to recur and progress with time.

In those with persistent symptoms or progressive neurologic deficits, surgical treatment affords excellent outcomes. In the majority of cases of central and lateral recess stenosis, the procedure of choice is a decompressive laminectomy of the stenotic areas (Figure 4–17). A fusion is not generally indicated for spinal stenosis in the absence of instability. In those with symptomatic foraminal stenosis, a foraminotomy is additionally performed. If there is symptomatic foraminal stenosis with a tilting of the segment in the coronal plane that further narrows the foramen, then a fusion may be necessary

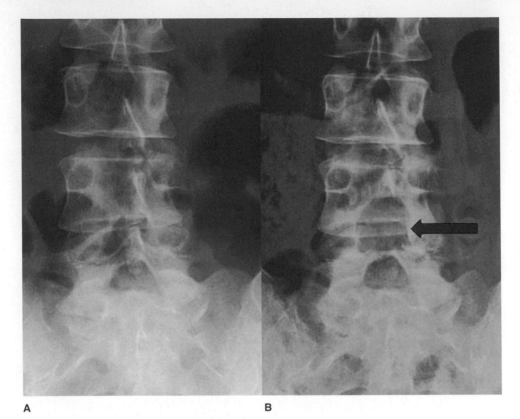

▲ **Figure 4–17.** Anteroposterior radiographs before (**A**) and after (**B**) L4-L5 laminectomy for spinal stenosis. In most cases, central and lateral recess stenoses occur at the level of the disk space, where the facets, ligamentum flavum, and disk can converge to compress the neural elements. Thus, adequate decompression is generally achieved when the area spanning the rostral to the caudal portion of the facet joints has been relieved of neurologic compression (*purple arrow*).

to keep the foraminal height sufficient to relieve root compression postoperatively, even if a foraminotomy has been performed. In certain instances, particularly in the upper lumbar spine where the pars tends to be narrower, a satisfactory foraminotomy may require enough resection of the pars such that a fusion should be added because of the iatrogenic instability created in the process of decompressing the root.

In the properly chosen patient, laminectomy provides excellent improvement in spinal stenosis symptoms. Reduction or elimination of radicular/claudicatory pain and improvement in physical function can be expected in 70–90% of cases. Again, patients should be counseled that the primary goal of treatment is relief of neurogenic rather than axial back pain, although a reduction in the latter may occur in up to 75% of cases.

Ammendolia C, Stuber K, de Bruin LK, et al: Nonoperative treatment of lumbar spinal stenosis with neurogenic claudication: a systematic review. *Spine (Phila Pa 1976)* 2012;37:E609. [PMID: 22158059]

Athiviraham A, Yen D: Is spinal stenosis better treated surgically or nonsurgically? *Clin Orthop Relat Res* 2007;458:90. [PMID: 17308483]

Atlas SJ, Keller RB, Wu YA, Deyo RA, Singer DE: Long-term outcomes of surgical and nonsurgical management of lumbar spinal stenosis: 8 to 10 year results from the Maine lumbar spine study. *Spine (Phila Pa 1976)* 2005;30:936. [PMID: 15834339]

Koc Z, Ozcakir S, Sivrioglu K, Gurbet A, Kucukoglu S: Effectiveness of physical therapy and epidural steroid injections in lumbar spinal stenosis. *Spine (Phila Pa 1976)* 2009;34:985. [PMID: 19404172]

Malmivaara A: Surgical or nonoperative treatment for lumbar spinal stenosis? A randomized controlled trial. *Spine (Phila Pa 1976)* 2007;32:1. [PMID: 17202885]

Ruetten S, Komp M, Merk H, Godolias G: Surgical treatment for lumbar lateral recess stenosis with the full-endoscopic interlaminar approach versus conventional microsurgical technique: a prospective, randomized, controlled study. *J Neurosurg Spine* 2009;10:476. [PMID: 19442011]

Smith CC, Booker T, Schaufele MK, et al: Interlaminar versus transforaminal epidural steroid injections for the treatment of symptomatic lumbar spinal stenosis. *Pain Med* 2010;11:1511. [PMID: 20735751]

Weinstein JN, Tosteson TD, Lurie JD, et al: Surgical versus nonsurgical therapy for lumbar spinal stenosis. *N Engl J Med* 2008;358:794. [PMID: 18287602]

Zouboulis P: Functional outcome of surgical treatment for multi-level lumbar spinal stenosis. *Acta Orthop* 2006;77:670. [PMID: 16929447]

DEGENERATIVE DISK DISEASE

▶ Essentials of Diagnosis

- *Aging of the disk leads to dehydration and internal disk disruption.*
- *Most degenerative disks are asymptomatic.*
- *It is not possible to diagnose a painful disk by imaging studies alone.*

▶ General Considerations

Aging of the intervertebral disk leads to a loss of water content, decrease in height, and an alteration in its normal mechanical properties. As a result, motion segment hypermobility, along with tears in the annulus, may occur. Although this degenerative cascade occurs ubiquitously in all spines with aging, it becomes symptomatic in only a small minority. It is currently unclear why some degenerative disks cause pain, whereas the vast majority do not, and there are no MRI or other imaging criteria that reliably differentiate symptomatic from nonsymptomatic degenerative disks. Thus, it is not possible to diagnose a painful degenerative disk on the basis of imaging studies alone.

We differentiate the term "degenerative disk," which is a radiographic and anatomic description, from "degenerative disk disease" (DDD), which refers to the clinical syndrome of pain in the presence of a degenerative disk (Figure 4–18). Because the diagnosis of DDD is difficult to make, surgically treating diskogenic low back pain has relatively low success rates compared to other types of spinal surgery. Thus, surgical treatment of DDD is reserved for patients with severe symptoms that fail to respond to extensive nonoperative measures and in whom a clear disk pain generator has been identified (see Table 4–5). Heritability and genetics have been shown to be important risk factors for developing DDD. Potentially modifiable risk factors include smoking, obesity, and occupational exposures.

▶ Clinical Findings

A. Signs and Symptoms

Diskogenic low back pain classically is worse in flexion and better in extension. As with disk herniations, sitting is often the most aggravating position because it leads to the highest intradiskal pressures. Axial back pain may radiate to the buttock, thigh, or groin, but usually not past the knee in the absence of neurologic compression. Radiation past

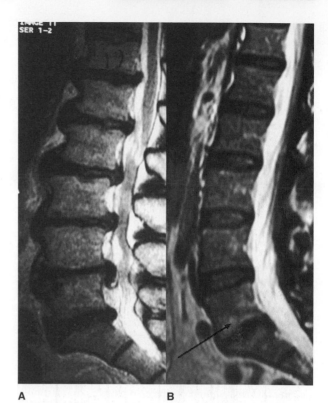

▲ **Figure 4–18.** (**A**) A 75-year-old man with symptoms of spinal stenosis and multilevel disk degeneration, but no low back pain. For reasons that are unclear, the majority of degenerative disks do not cause axial low back pain. Thus, one must not presume that degenerative changes found on imaging studies are necessarily responsible for symptoms, although they certainly can be. (**B**) A 37-year-old woman with single-level symptomatic degenerative disk disease at L5–S1. Note the relative loss of hydration (the central portion of the disk is darker, essentially black, compared to the more proximal disks) and disk height, along with Modic endplate changes (*purple arrow*).

the knee in a dermatomal distribution typically indicates concomitant nerve root compression/irritation. It is important to determine the degree of relief afforded by rest. Pain that never improves, even at rest, suggests that mechanically based procedures such as spinal fusion may be unlikely to improve the pain.

B. Imaging

Radiographs typically show disk space narrowing, vertebral body osteophytes, or endplate and facet sclerosis. Radiographs should be taken upright to evaluate for potential deformities or instabilities that may not be apparent in the recumbent position. Flexion-extension films may rule out spondylolisthesis and instability. CT scans may rule out occult spondylolysis or tumors. MRI without contrast is the study of choice and demonstrates decrease in disk height and water content (dark on T2 imaging) with disk degeneration. High-intensity zones (HIZs) are focal areas of increased signal on T2-weighted images in the normally dark posterior/outer annulus indicative of annular tears or fissures. Associated endplate changes ("Modic" changes) indicative of endplate edema, fatty degeneration, or sclerosis may occur with disk degeneration as well. Patients with HIZs and Modic changes who undergo surgery for DDD tend to have better outcomes than those without such MRI findings. However, the presence of these findings is not diagnostic of symptomatic DDD.

Diskography is a useful but imperfect diagnostic modality. Because it is impossible to determine whether a disk is painful simply by its radiographic appearance, the concept behind provocative diskography is to identify the symptomatic disk by injecting it with contrast material under pressure. If the injection reproduces the patient's typical low back pain (ie, demonstrates "concordant" pain), then that disk may be symptomatic. A CT scan can be obtained immediately following diskography to evaluate the morphology of the disk and its competence. Typically, a control level (an adjacent normal-appearing disk) is tested as well. Testing this level should produce no pain or a modest pressure sensation. If the patient reports severe pain at multiple levels, even those that are morphologically normal on MRI and postdiskography CT scan, he/she may be too sensitive to pain and less likely to benefit from a surgical procedure. The limited information to be gained from this test must be balanced against the risk of the procedure. A matched cohort study of patients who underwent diskography 7–10 years prior demonstrated significantly more disk degeneration and herniation at the side and levels of disks that had undergone diskography. This finding was consistent with those of previous animal studies.

▶ Treatment

DDD is a challenging problem to manage, and there are no excellent treatment options. Because surgery is appropriate for only a select few, treatment always starts in a nonoperative fashion. Nonoperative options include those listed in Table 4–5. Lifestyle modifications, behavioral therapies, and management of associated psychosocial stressors may help DDD patients better cope with and manage their pain. Level 1 evidence demonstrates that patients with symptomatic DDD that is refractory to at least 6 months of nonoperative therapy may benefit from surgical treatment.

The most common surgical treatment of symptomatic DDD is spinal fusion. Surgery can be performed either anteriorly or posteriorly. Anterior surgery has the benefits of high fusion rates and avoiding the morbidity related to disruption of lumbar extensor muscles, but carries risks

intrinsic to the anterior approach, such as vascular injury, retrograde ejaculation in men, and injury to the abdominal contents (Figure 4–19). Posterior fusion (either posterolateral and/or posterior interbody) generally involves pedicle screw instrumentation and provides rigid fixation, but it requires extensive posterior muscle dissection, which may exacerbate low back pain, and it also has higher infection rates and overall lower fusion rates than anterior surgery. All fusion techniques have been shown to demonstrate significantly better outcomes over nonoperative treatment in well-selected patients with single-level disk disease. Overall, about two thirds to three fourths of patients obtain significant and lasting relief from spinal fusion surgery directed at treating DDD.

Nonfusion approaches include posterior dynamic stabilization and anterior lumbar disk arthroplasty. There is little evidence to support the use of posterior dynamic stabilization. On the other hand, recent 2-year FDA Investigational Device Exemption clinical trials comparing anterior arthroplasty to single- and two-level fusion in well-selected patients have shown significant improvements from baseline for both surgical treatments. In these studies, arthroplasty had an equivalent or superior clinical effect over fusion. However, it must be stressed that these are short-term results; the long-term functionality and survival characteristics for lumbar

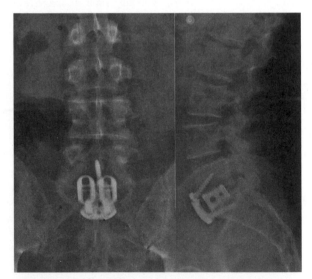

▲ **Figure 4–19.** Anteroposterior and lateral radiographs of a 43-year-old man status post anterior lumbar interbody fusion with cage and plate construct. Although this particular threaded, lumbar-tapered interbody cage can be used quite successfully (>95% fusion rate) as a stand-alone device, when the vascular anatomy permits and cage fixation is suboptimal, a plate can be added to further secure the construct. Excellent relief of symptoms was obtained.

arthroplasties are unknown. Potential catastrophic implant failures, including potentially life-threatening expulsion of implants into the iliac vessels, have been reported, tempering enthusiasm for this approach.

▶ Complications

Commonly reported complications of instrumented posterior fusions include infection, nonunions, and implant-related issues such as malposition, loosening of screws, or backout of cages. Anterior complications include vascular injury (up to 3%), retrograde ejaculation due to hypogastric plexus injury (up to 5%), and cage migration. Fusion rates of anterior lumbar interbody fusions using rhBMP-2 and a threaded cage approach 100%. However, it has recently been reported that the rate of retrograde ejaculation may be higher when rhBMP-2 is used versus autograft. Fusion rates for posterior one- and two-level arthrodesis are 80–95%.

▶ Prognosis

DDD displays relatively poor outcomes compared to other lumbar spinal diagnoses regardless of either surgical or nonoperative management. About one third of patients fail to respond to all forms of treatment. Careful patient selection is the key to successful surgical outcomes. Patients with refractory low back pain and untreated underlying psychosocial conditions that exacerbate pain perception consistently have poorer surgical outcomes. Other poor prognostic factors include worker's compensation status, pending litigation, obesity, and smoking. Proper counseling as to realistic expectations for pain reduction following surgery is paramount.

Berg S, Tullberg T, Branth B, Olerud C, Tropp H: Total disc replacement compared to lumbar fusion: a randomised controlled trial with 2-year follow-up. *Eur Spine J* 2009;18:1512. [PMID: 19506919]

Burkus JK: Six-year outcomes of anterior lumbar interbody arthrodesis with use of interbody fusion cages and recombinant human bone morphogenetic protein-2. *J Bone Joint Surg Am* 2009;91:1181. [PMID: 19411467]

Carragee EJ: Retrograde ejaculation after anterior lumbar interbody fusion using rh-BMP-2: a cohort controlled study. *Spine J* 2011;11:511. [PMID: 21612985]

Carragee EJ, Don AS, Hurwitz EL, et al: 2009 ISSLS Prize Winner: does discography cause accelerated progression of degeneration changes in the lumbar disc: a ten-year matched cohort study. *Spine (Phila Pa 1976)* 2009;34:2338. [PMID: 19755936]

Carragee EJ, Lincoln T, Parmar VS, Alamin T: A gold standard evaluation of the "discogenic pain" diagnosis as determined by provocative discography. *Spine (Phila Pa 1976)* 2006;31:2115. [PMID: 16915099]

Carreon LY, Glassman SD, Howard J: Fusion and nonsurgical treatment for symptomatic lumbar degenerative disease: a systematic review of Oswestry Disability Index and MOS Short Form-36 outcomes. *Spine J* 2008;8:747. [PMID: 18037354]

Cheh G: Adjacent segment disease following lumbar/thoracolumbar fusion with pedicle screw instrumentation: a minimum 5-year follow-up. *Spine (Phila Pa 1976)* 2007;32:2253. [PMID: 17873819]

Delamarter R, Zigler JE, Balderston RA, et al: Prospective, randomized, multicenter FDA IDE study of the ProDisc-L total disc replacement compared to circumferential arthrodesis for the treatment of two-level degenerative disc disease: results at twenty-four months. *J Bone Joint Surg Am* 2011;93:705. [PMID: 21398574]

Dimar JR: Clinical and radiographic analysis of an optimized rhBMP-2 formulation as an autograft replacement in posterolateral lumbar spine arthrodesis. *J Bone Joint Surg Am* 2009;91:1377. [PMID: 19487515]

Glassman SD, Polly DW, Bono CM, Burkus K, Dimar JR: Outcome of lumbar arthrodesis in patients sixty-five years of age or older. *J Bone Joint Surg Am* 2009;91:783. [PMID: 19339561]

Gornet MF, Burkus JK, Dryer RF, et al: Lumbar disc arthroplasty with MAVERICK disc versus stand-alone interbody fusion: a prospective randomized controlled multicenter IDE trial. *Spine (Phila Pa 1976)* 2011;36:E1600. [PMID: 21415812]

Guyer RD: Prospective, randomized, multicenter Food and Drug Administration investigational device exemption study of lumbar total disc replacement with the CHARITE artificial disc versus lumbar fusion: five-year follow-up. *Spine J* 2009;9:374. [PMID: 18805066]

Hsieh PC, Koski TR, O'Shaughnessy BA, et al: Anterior lumbar interbody fusion in comparison with transforaminal lumbar interbody fusion: implications for the restoration of foraminal height, local disc angle, lumbar lordosis, and sagittal balance. *J Neurosurg Spine* 2007;7:379. [PMID: 17933310]

Manchikanti L, Glaser SE, Wolfer L, Derby R, Cohen SP: Systematic review of lumbar discography as a diagnostic test for chronic low back pain. *Pain Physician* 2009;12:541. [PMID: 19461822]

Mirza SK, Deyo RA: Systematic review of randomized trials comparing lumbar fusion surgery to nonoperative care for treatment of chronic back pain. *Spine (Phila Pa 1976)* 2007;32:816. [PMID: 17414918]

Putzier M, Hoff E, Tohtz S, et al: Dynamic stabilization adjacent to single-level fusion: part II. No clinical benefit for asymptomatic, initially degenerated adjacent segments after 6 year follow-up. *Eur Spine J* 2010;19:2181. [PMID: 20632044]

Soegaard R, Bünger CE, Christiansen T, Høy K, Eiskjaer SP, Christensen FB: Circumferential fusion is dominant over posterolateral fusion in a long-term perspective: cost-utility evaluation of a randomized controlled trial in severe, chronic low back pain. *Spine (Phila Pa 1976)* 2007;32:2405. [PMID: 18090078]

Videbaek TS: Circumferential fusion improves outcome in comparison with instrumented posterolateral fusion: long-term results of a randomized clinical trial. *Spine (Phila Pa 1976)* 2006;31:2875. [PMID: 17139217]

FACET SYNDROME

▶ General Considerations

Facet arthropathy and facet syndrome are relatively common but often underappreciated pain generators in patients with degenerative lumbar conditions. Unlike disk degeneration,

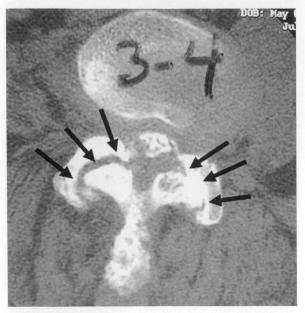

▲ **Figure 4–20.** CT myelogram demonstrates severe spinal stenosis at L3-L4 along with bilateral facet arthropathy (black arrows).

which is ubiquitous in symptomatic and asymptomatic people, 15–90% of patients with chronic low back have obvious arthritic changes to their lumbar facet joints, whereas fewer than 15% of asymptomatic volunteers have arthritic changes on advanced imaging. Upward of 10% of patients following diskectomy may develop clinically symptomatic lumbar facet joint syndrome, which can be responsive to facet blocks. Revision or radical diskectomies significantly increase this risk.

Facet joints appear to be an independent generator of back pain. Although facet arthrosis may follow disk degeneration, facet syndrome and diskogenic back pain syndrome usually do not occur concurrently, as facet anesthetic blocks and diskogram are positive at the same level in fewer than 3–10% of cases. L5/S1 is the most commonly involved level, followed by L4/5 and L3/4. Facet degeneration is characterized by changes similar to those seen at other synovial joints—osteophytes, subchondral cysts, cartilage wear, joint space narrowing, and deformation (Figure 4–20).

The facet capsule is richly innervated by the medial branch of the posterior ramus. Each posterior ramus divides to innervate two to three facet joints, including the joints associated with its neuroforamen and the ones above and below.

▶ Clinical Findings

A. Signs and Symptoms

One of the challenges with diagnosing facet syndrome (the cluster of chronic low back pain worse in extension, in the setting of facet arthritic changes that respond to facet local anesthetic blocks) is that it has no reliable signs or symptoms. Often there is referred pain that radiates into the buttock and posterior thigh (not below the knee) and sometimes into the groin as well. Lumbar extension, especially with the addition of truncal rotation, is often limited and painful. Controlled, comparative local anesthetic blocks are the diagnostic modality of choice. This requires two injections on two separate occasions of two types of local anesthetic—short acting (lidocaine) and long acting (bupivacaine). To confirm the diagnosis, the patient should have a positive response (pain relief and/or ability to perform previously painful maneuvers) after both injections and the response should be longer following the longer-acting anesthetic. Response to one and not the other is considered a false-positive result, which occurs in up to 50% of the cases. Unfortunately, multiple studies have demonstrated poor or no correlation between response to facet injections and response to nonoperative treatment or subsequent spinal fusion. Thus, while many spine surgeons believe facet degeneration is a pain generator in chronic low back pain, defining it as a unique entity or determining its contribution to a multifactorial etiology for low back pain remains unclear.

B. Imaging

It is thought in most instances that disk degeneration and height loss precede facet arthrosis. Facet orientation, which is best measured on CT scan, tends to become progressively more sagittal as arthrosis progresses. Patients with more sagittally oriented facet joints are more prone to develop spondylolisthesis. MRI and CT scans often demonstrate lateral recess and foraminal stenosis from hypertrophy of the superior articulating process in advanced facet arthropathy. Like other synovial joints, arthrosis can lead to the formation of synovial cysts. Facet cysts most commonly form on the posterior aspect of the joint, but those on the ventral or medial surface can compress nerve roots, causing radiculopathy.

▶ Treatment

Facet syndrome is primarily treated nonoperatively with the modalities listed in Table 4–5. After clinical examination, facet local anesthetic blocks are a potential next step for the diagnosis and treatment of facet syndrome. Patients who have a positive response to facet blocks (>50–80% pain reduction) are candidates for intraarticular steroid injections or radiofrequency ablations (RFAs). Steroid injections provide long-term back pain relief in 16–63% of patients. RFA involves placing a radiofrequency probe under radiographic guidance and thermocoagulating the medial branch of the posterior ramus as it enters the facet capsule. Using strict selection criteria (positive controlled comparative blocks), it is thought that RFA provides up to 1 year of 80–90% pain relief in 60% of patients, with 87% of patients getting at least 60% pain relief. Randomized controlled trials have shown that RFA is superior to placebo. Other studies have found no significant treatment effect following facet steroid injections or RFA compared to saline placebo. RFA and intraarticular steroid injections, like many nonoperative interventions, tend to produce diminishing returns with repeated application. Last, posterior fusion may be a final treatment option for facet syndrome, with limited and contradictory evidential support. In general, facet syndrome should not be viewed as a surgical disease; further, favorable results from facet injections may not predict good outcomes from fusion surgery.

Cohen SP: Lumbar zygapophysial (facet) joint radiofrequency denervation success as a function of pain relief during diagnostic medial branch blocks: a multicenter analysis. *Spine J* 2008;8:498. [PMID: 17662665]

Cohen SP, Hurley RW: The ability of diagnostic spinal injections to predict surgical outcomes. *Anesth Analg* 2007;105:1756. [PMID: 18042881]

Cohen SP, Raja SN: Pathogenesis, diagnosis, and treatment of lumbar zygapophysial (facet) joint pain. *Anesthesiology* 2007;106:591. [PMID: 17325518]

Dreyfuss P, Halbrook B, Pauza K, Joshi A, McLarty J, Bogduk N: Efficacy and validity of radiofrequency neurotomy for chronic lumbar zygapophysial joint pain. *Spine (Phila Pa 1976)* 2000;25:1270. [PMID: 10806505]

Esses SI, Moro JK: The value of facet joint blocks in patient selection for lumbar fusion. *Spine (Phila Pa 1976)* 1993;18:185. [PMID: 8441932]

Jackson RP, Jacobs RR, Montesano PX: 1988 Volvo award in clinical sciences. Facet joint injection in low-back pain. A prospective statistical study. *Spine (Phila Pa 1976)* 1988;13:966. [PMID: 2974632]

Nath S, Nath CA, Pettersson K: Percutaneous lumbar zygapophysial (facet) joint neurotomy using radiofrequency current, in the management of chronic low back pain: a randomized double-blind trial. *Spine (Phila Pa 1976)* 2008;33:1291. [PMID: 18496338]

Steib K, Proescholdt M, Brawanski A, et al: Predictors of facet joint syndrome after lumbar disc surgery. *J Clin Neurosci* 2012;19:418. [PMID: 22277562].

Stojanovic MP, Sethee J, Mohiuddin M, et al: MRI analysis of the lumbar spine: can it predict response to diagnostic and therapeutic facet procedures? *Clin J Pain* 2010;26:110. [PMID: 20090436]

van Wijk RM, Geurts JW, Wynne HJ, et al: Radiofrequency denervation of lumbar facet joints in the treatment of chronic low back pain: a randomized, double-blind, sham lesion-controlled trial. *Clin J Pain* 2005;21:335. [PMID: 15951652]

Wong DA, Annesser B, Birney T, et al: Incidence of contraindications to total disc arthroplasty: a retrospective review of 100 consecutive fusion patients with a specific analysis of facet arthrosis. *Spine J* 2007;7:5. [PMID: 17197326]

SPONDYLOLISTHESIS

▶ Essentials of Diagnosis

- *There are six distinct types of spondylolisthesis.*
- *Signs and symptoms are dependent on type but often include a combination of low back pain and leg pain.*

- *Degree of slippage and slip angle and overall sagittal balance are important considerations in choosing the optimal treatment.*

▶ General Considerations

Spondylolisthesis is derived from the Greek *spondylo* (meaning spine) and *olisthesis* (meaning slip) and refers to an abnormal slippage of one vertebra over the next. There are six types of spondylolisthesis (Table 4–6). The overall lifetime incidence of spondylolisthesis is 9–10%, with isthmic and degenerative being the most common types.

▶ Clinical Findings

A. Signs and Symptoms

1. Degenerative spondylolisthesis—Patients are typically older (50s and up) and complain of varying amounts of low back and/or leg pain. The radicular leg symptoms are similar

Table 4–6. Wiltse Classification of spondylolisthesis.

I **Dysplastic/congenital:** marked by dome-shaped sacrum, abnormal L5/S1 facet joints, elongated, thin L5 pars with a trapezoidal shape of the L5 vertebral body; prone to high-grade slip (ie, >50%).
II **Isthmic** (most common in adolescents/adults): due to a defect or acute fracture in the bilateral L5 pars interarticularis; allows L5 to slip forward up to 50%. Spondylolysis typically occurs spontaneously by age 5-6. It occurs in about 5–6% of Caucasians (higher rate in other races), but only about one third go on to develop listhesis. There is a familial predilection. If the lysis occurs from a traumatic cause, it can be treated nonoperative with a good outcome. Lytic spondylolisthesis does not predict low back pain (LBP); therefore when a low-grade slip is incidentally found, it does not require spine surgical consultation. When LBP and/or radiating lower extremity symptoms are present and fail to respond to nonoperative measures, spinal fusion with or without decompression and reduction provides favorable results for most.
III **Degenerative** (most common in older adults): the final outcome of progressive disk degeneration, height loss, instability, and facet arthropathy, most commonly at L4/5 level (>85% of cases) and often associated with neurogenic claudication. Strong female predilection (4-6:1). Decompression and fusion are indicated following failure of nonoperative treatment for symptomatic patients, typically in their fifties to sixties, with good to excellent outcomes in >75%.
IV **Traumatic:** spondylolisthesis following a destabilizing fracture of the lumbar spine other than a pars fracture. This injury requires spinal stabilization surgery.
V **Pathologic:** spondylolisthesis occurring secondary to primary or metastatic lesions weakening the supportive structures of the spinal unit. This condition requires spinal stabilization surgery with or without tumor resection and adjuvant therapies. This is a rare condition.
VI **Iatrogenic:** typically used to describe spondylolisthesis that occurs following lumbar decompression surgery without fusion, where the pars is thinned too much, resulting in acute or insufficiency pars fracture. Fusion is indicated in these cases.

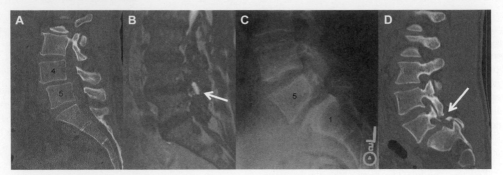

▲ **Figure 4–21.** (**A**) Degenerative spondylolisthesis at L4-L5, the most common level at which they occur. (**B**) MRI of same patient showing fluid (*white arrow*) in the severely degenerative L4/5 facet. (**C**) Isthmic spondylolisthesis at L5-S1 (grade 1) (0–25% slippage). Although isthmic defects occur most commonly at L5-S1, they can occur elsewhere. (**D**) Note the pars defect (*white arrow*).

to those of spinal stenosis, as central and lateral recess stenosis is exacerbated by the slip. Foraminal stenosis can also occur. Thus, the radicular symptoms may be associated with both the exiting and traversing roots at the level of stenosis. The L4/5 level is by far the most common level affected by degenerative spondylolisthesis, although it can occur at other lumbar levels. Associated axial low back pain from instability should typically be better with rest and worse with standing or walking.

2. Isthmic spondylolisthesis—Patients may present in their preteen to teen years or be relatively asymptomatic until their adulthood (30s to 50s). L5-S1 is by far the most common level involved, although isthmic defects can be seen at other levels (Figure 4–21). Central stenosis is relatively uncommon with isthmic defects, as the pars defect actually enlarges the spinal canal with slippage of the associated vertebrae. Instead, foraminal narrowing and resulting exiting root compression are typical, with the L5 root being most commonly involved with an L5-S1 isthmic slip. Low back pain when present tends to be mechanical (worse with activity) and may be acutely associated with a "clunking" sensation in flexion and extension.

B. Imaging

The degree of spondylolisthesis is commonly classified according to the Meyerding grade (Table 4–7). Degenerative slips tend to be low grade, with the majority being grade I or, less frequently, grade II or III. Standing lateral x-rays are paramount to diagnosis, as the slip may not be visible on recumbent films such as supine x-rays or CT/MRI scans. Flexion-extension films may demonstrate dynamic worsening of instability (>2–4 mm motion). Lateral listhesis (slippage in the coronal plane) can also occur alone or in combination with spondylolisthesis. MRI scans are obtained to evaluate associated neural impingement. CT scans with sagittal reformatting can be helpful in identifying pars

defects that may not be evident on x-ray or MRI. Bone scans are occasionally useful in identifying occult pars defects.

▶ Treatment

Slips in adults with isthmic or degenerative spondylolisthesis rarely progress. However, growing children with isthmic defects may progress. In addition, children with dysplastic slips and adults with iatrogenic slips (typically resulting from a pars insufficiency fracture after previous diskectomy/decompression procedure) are much more likely to progress and thus should be fused or at least followed carefully. The standard nonoperative treatment options (see Table 4–5) apply to the initial treatment of spondylolisthesis. Decompression alone is rarely appropriate for patients with any form of spondylolisthesis as it can further destabilize the segment or leave persistent symptoms (back and/or leg pain) related to instability. The most common treatment for either degenerative or isthmic spondylolisthesis is a posterior lumbar decompression and fusion. Recent randomized control trials have shown that surgery in the form of one- to two-level posterior decompression and fusion for degenerative

Table 4–7. Meyerding slippage grade.

Percent slippage is measured as the distance from the inferior posterior corner of L5 to the superior posterior corner of S1, divided by the length of the S1 superior endplate. Spondylolisthesis is often classified as low grade (0–50%) versus high grade (>50%) because this distinction impacts surgical treatment.

  I 0–25%
 II 26–50%
III 51–75%
IV 76–100%
 V Spondyloptosis: the condition in which the L5 (and the entire spinal column above) has slipped completely anterior to the S1 vertebra

spondylolisthesis with stenosis reliably and significantly outperforms nonoperative care at all times points out to 5 years. Fusion for degenerative and isthmic spondylolisthesis tends to be a very successful operation with 75% or more of patients reporting major improvement in their condition that lasts 2–4 years or longer. To put this in generic terms, the improvement in overall measures of general health and well-being (eg, Short Form-36) following fusion for spondylolisthesis is equivalent to that for hip/knee arthroplasty.

Ha KY, Na KH, Shin JH, Kim KW: Comparison of posterolateral fusion with and without additional posterior lumbar interbody fusion for degenerative lumbar spondylolisthesis. *J Spinal Disord Tech* 2008;21:229. [PMID: 18525481]

Hu SS, Tribus CB, Diab M, Ghanayem AJ: Spondylolisthesis and spondylolysis. *J Bone Joint Surg Am* 2008;90:656. [PMID: 18326106]

Kalichman L, Hunter DJ: Diagnosis and conservative management of degenerative lumbar spondylolisthesis. *Eur Spine J* 2008;17:327. [PMID: 18026865]

Kim JS, Kang BU, Lee SH, et al: Mini-transforaminal lumbar interbody fusion versus anterior lumbar interbody fusion augmented by percutaneous pedicle screw fixation: a comparison of surgical outcomes in adult low-grade isthmic spondylolisthesis. *J Spinal Disord Tech* 2009;22:114. [PMID: 19342933]

Müslüman AM, Yilmaz A, Cansever T, et al: Posterior lumbar interbody fusion versus posterolateral fusion with instrumentation in the treatment of low-grade isthmic spondylolisthesis: midterm clinical outcomes. *J Neurosurg Spine* 2011;14:488. [PMID: 21314280]

Rampersaud YR, Wai EK, Fisher CG, et al: Postoperative improvement in health-related quality of life: a national comparison of surgical treatment for (one- or two-level) lumbar spinal stenosis compared with total joint arthroplasty for osteoarthritis. *Spine J* 2011;11:1033.

Remes V, Lamberg T, Tervahartiala P, et al: Long-term outcome after posterolateral, anterior, and circumferential fusion for high-grade isthmic spondylolisthesis in children and adolescents: magnetic resonance imaging findings after average of 17-year follow-up. *Spine (Phila Pa 1976)* 2006;31:2491. [PMID: 17023860]

Resnick DK, Choudhri TF, Dailey AT, et al: Guidelines for the performance of fusion procedures for degenerative disease of the lumbar spine. Part 9: fusion in patients with stenosis and spondylolisthesis. *J Neurosurg Spine* 2005;2:679. [PMID: 16028737]

Swan J: Surgical treatment for unstable low-grade isthmic spondylolisthesis in adults: a prospective controlled study of posterior instrumented fusion compared with combined anterior-posterior fusion. *Spine J* 2006;6:606. [PMID: 17088191]

Weinstein JN: Surgical compared with nonoperative treatment for lumbar degenerative spondylolisthesis. Four-year results in the Spine Patient Outcomes Research Trial (SPORT) randomized and observational cohorts. *J Bone Joint Surg Am* 2009;91:1295. [PMID: 19487505]

Weinstein JN, Lurie JD, Tosteson TD, et al: Surgical versus nonsurgical treatment for lumbar degenerative spondylolisthesis. *N Engl J Med* 2007;356:2257. [PMID: 17538085]

SPINAL INFECTIONS

▶ Essentials of Diagnosis

- *Most common forms of spinal infections include diskitis, osteomyelitis, epidural abscess, and postoperative infections.*
- *Lumbar spine is most commonly involved followed by the thoracic spine in bacterial infections.*
- *Thoracic spine most commonly involved in fungal infections.*
- *Pathophysiology of infection differs between children and adults.*
- *Back pain is the most common symptom and is severe and unremitting.*

▶ General Considerations

Spinal infections represent fewer than 5% of orthopedic infections. The lumbar spine is the most common region involved (50%), followed by the thoracic spine (35%). The most common forms of spinal infection include (1) diskitis, (2) osteomyelitis, (3) epidural abscess, and (4) postoperative (infection complicates 0–5% of spinal surgeries). *Staphylococcus aureus* is the most common (40–60%) organism for all types of spinal infection, followed by coagulase-negative *Staphylococcus* and gram-negative enteric organisms, and a culture-specific diagnosis remains paramount to treatment. *Propionibacterium acne* and *Staphylococcus epidermidis* are common pathogens in late-onset spinal infections following instrumented spinal fusion. These low-virulence pathogens are cultured from the skin in over 80% of subjects prior to skin preparation for surgery.

The pathoanatomy of pyogenic diskitis and osteomyelitis is different in children versus adults. In children, the disk can become primarily infected via blood vessels that cross the endplate and connect the vertebrae to the nucleus. In adults, the disk is avascular and becomes secondarily infected from a primary focus of infection in the vertebral body (ie, osteomyelitis). Hematogenous osteomyelitis typically starts in the anterior-inferior corner of the vertebral body. In this portion of the vertebral body, the end-arterioles loop and create sluggish blood flow. Additionally, the venous drainage of the vertebral body is valveless (Batson plexus) and communicates with the pelvic venous system. These two anatomic features may facilitate bacterial sludging and extravasation. As the infection progresses, the endplates erode, allowing spread of infection into the adjacent avascular disk (Figure 4–22). It is the involvement of adjacent vertebral levels and the intervening disk that most reliably differentiates pyogenic diskitis from neoplasm, as tumors rarely cross the disk space. From the disk space, infection can spread to adjacent vertebral bodies and/or paravertebral structures. In some advanced cases (5–18%), infection can spread posteriorly into the spinal canal as an epidural abscess. Epidural abscess can also form hematogenously into the posterior epidural space without associated diskitis/osteomyelitis. An epidural abscess is

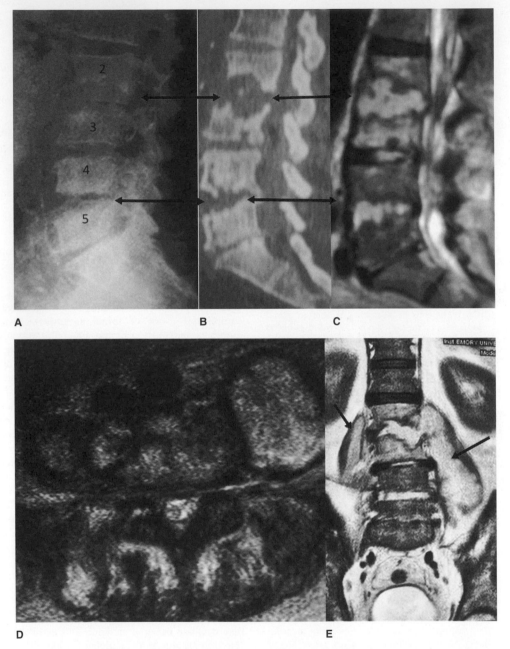

▲ **Figure 4–22.** (**A**) Lateral radiograph of a morbidly obese brittle diabetic man with osteomyelitis-diskitis involving L2-L3 and L4-L5. (**B**) CT reconstruction demonstrates erosion of the endplates at the bottom of L2, top of L3, bottom of L4, and top of L5 due to infection. (**C, D, and E**) Sagittal, axial, and coronal MRIs show extensive infection at L2-L3 and L4-L5 with bilateral psoas abscesses (*black arrows*).

the most urgent of spinal infections due to the potential for progressive neurologic deficit.

Nonbacterial infections are less common. Fungal infections are often indolent but can lead to multilevel involvement and significant deformity. Tuberculous spinal infection (Pott disease) is also an indolent infection, which has a predilection for the thoracic spine, but only affects about 1–5% of patients with tuberculosis (TB). Like fungal infections, kyphotic deformity is often the most clinically significant adverse effect. TB may mimic tumor because it tends to spare the disk space, presumably because TB is an obligate aerobic organism and the oxygen tension in the disk space is low. A purified protein derivative test will be positive in >95% of immune-competent patients, but may be anergic in immune-compromised patients. Traditional TB cultures took 21 days or longer for results, but recently polymerase chain reaction has become the test of choice to confirm TB infection.

▶ Clinical Findings

A. Signs and Symptoms

Symptoms of spinal infection are widely variable. Back pain localized to the area of infection is the most common symptom. Back pain associated with infections is classically more severe and unremitting (often worse at night) compared to that seen with degenerative disorders, although many patients do have mechanical symptoms that modulate with level of activity. Constitutional symptoms such as fever are not sensitive and may be present in only about 33–50% of spinal infections. Furthermore, fever is a common (>40%, >75% following major fusion surgery) phenomenon in the immediate postoperative period for uncomplicated spinal surgeries. Neurologic symptoms, such as radiating pain, numbness, or weakness, may occur and are associated with epidural extension of infection or pathologic fracture of infected vertebrae causing kyphosis and compression of the neural elements. Those at risk for infection include the elderly, diabetics, and those on chronic steroids.

Hemodynamically unstable septic shock is rare but can occur with spinal infections. The physical exam may be normal or demonstrate limited range of motion of the affected spine. Neurologic deficits are relatively uncommon at presentation (10–17%).

B. Laboratory Studies

Baseline laboratories for patients presenting with suspected spinal infection include complete blood count (CBC) with differential, C-reactive protein (CRP), ESR, and blood cultures from two separate sites. Leukocytosis and a left shift will be present in less than 50%, but CRP and ESR will be elevated in more than 90% at presentation. The CRP starts to elevate within 24–48 hours of infection onset, whereas ESR can take up to 1 week to elevate. In addition to being first to elevate, CRP is the first to normalize following initiation of successful treatment. As such, it is

an important tool in monitoring treatment response. Blood cultures are positive in only 30–50% of patients. Antibiotics should be withheld until blood cultures and preferably tissue cultures can be obtained. CT-guided needle biopsy of the most accessible site of presumed infection is the culture method of choice and yields positive results in 50–80% of patients, but it is imperative to obtain large enough samples to culture. If an organism cannot be identified or in patients with obvious infections requiring surgical debridement and reconstruction, open biopsy is performed with 80–90% positive yield in patients without recent antibiotic exposure.

C. Imaging

Plain radiographs in osteomyelitis may demonstrate radiolucency from osteolysis or sclerosis in chronic infections. However, plain films may be negative early in the disease process, as radiolucency is not seen until 30–50% of the trabeculae have been lost, which may take up to 3–4 weeks to develop. Disk space narrowing is an early radiographic finding of diskitis. As the infection progresses, spinal deformities such as focal kyphosis may be seen.

MRI with gadolinium contrast is the study of choice for diagnosing all forms of spinal infections. Its sensitivity and specificity are more than 95%. MRI changes occur within 24–48 hours of infection onset. MRI additionally allows for evaluation of neurologic compression. However, the true extent of bony destruction is better evaluated on CT scans. Typically, both an MRI and CT scan are needed to fully evaluate spinal infections. Nuclear medicine studies (technetium-99 or gallium studies) reliably (90% accuracy) show uptake in areas of infection within 3–7 days of onset but are less commonly used now that MRI is widely available and provides better anatomic detail.

▶ Treatment

The goals of treating pyogenic infections are fourfold: (1) to eradicate the infection; (2) relieve pain; (3) preserve or improve neurologic function; and (4) maintain or restore spinal alignment and stability. Indications for surgical treatment include the following: (1) to obtain a microbiologic diagnosis; (2) presence of abscess (intradiskal, bony, soft tissue, or epidural); (3) presence of neurologic deficit; (4) spinal instability; (5) progressive or severe spinal deformity; and (6) failure of nonoperative treatment, including refractory pain. The major goal of surgery is thorough debridement of all infected, nonviable tissue. Spinal reconstruction with instrumentation is often used to stabilize the spine after debridement. Although somewhat counterintuitive, the use of spinal implants, particularly those made of titanium, to fuse and stabilize the infected spine helps to successfully eradicate the infection, provided there has been adequate debridement and institution of culture-specific antibiotics. In the absence of the above indications, a term of nonoperative treatment may be considered. Failure of nonoperative treatment is indicated by lack of improvement in pain, fever, and/or laboratory parameters despite 2–3 weeks of appropriate antibiotic coverage.

In most cases, an anterior approach is necessary to radically debride the infection. Supplemental posterior instrumentation and fusion are usually needed to provide additional stability in the majority of cases, as the spine is rendered unstable either by the infection or the debridement needed to remove the infection. Anterior bone quality is generally poor in patients with infection and should not routinely be relied upon alone for fixation. Epidural abscesses are most commonly drained through a dorsal approach and are most common in the thoracolumbar spine. Classically, autograft has been used to graft anterior column deficits. More recently, allograft or titanium mesh cages combined with rhBMP-2 have been used with success to avoid the morbidity of autograft harvest. A prolonged course of postoperative antibiotics, typically parenteral for a minimum of 6 weeks, is needed. Nutritional supplementation plays a crucial role in healing of these patients, who are or become malnourished by the chronic infection.

▶ Prognosis

Spinal infection is a serious disease, which historically was fatal in 50–70% of cases and even today has an overall mortality rate of 5–20%. Debridement and instrumented fusion can be successfully performed in a single stage with 90–100% initial response and less than 10% recurrence. When postoperative infections are identified and adequately treated in the acute phase (<4–6 weeks after surgery), originally placed implants can generally be left.

Allen RT, Lee YP, Stimson E, Garfin SR: Bone morphogenetic protein-2 (BMP-2) in the treatment of pyogenic vertebral osteomyelitis. *Spine (Phila Pa 1976)* 2007;32:2996. [PMID: 18091493]

Grane P, Josephsson A, Seferlis A, Tullberg T: Septic and aseptic post-operative discitis in the lumbar spine—evaluation by MR imaging. *Acta Radiol* 1998;39:108. [PMID: 9529438]

Hahn F, Zbinden R, Min K: Late implant infections caused by *Propionibacterium acnes* in scoliosis surgery. *Eur Spine J* 2005;14:783. [PMID: 15841406]

Kuklo TR, Potter BK, Bell RS, Moquin RR, Rosner MK: Single-stage treatment of pyogenic spinal infection with titanium mesh cages. *J Spinal Disord Tech* 2006;19:376. [PMID: 16826013]

Mok JM, Pekmezci M, Piper SL, et al: Use of C-reactive protein after spinal surgery: comparison with erythrocyte sedimentation rate as predictor of early postoperative infectious complications. *Spine (Phila Pa 1976)* 2008;33:415. [PMID: 18277874]

Ogden AT, Kaiser MG: Single-stage debridement and instrumentation for pyogenic spinal infections. *Neurosurg Focus* 2004;17:E5. [PMID: 15636575]

O'Shaughnessy BA, Kuklo TR, Ondra SL: Surgical treatment of vertebral osteomyelitis with recombinant human bone morphogenetic protein-2. *Spine (Phila Pa 1976)* 2008;33:E132. [PMID: 18317180]

Petignat C, Francioli P, Harbarth S, et al: Cefuroxime prophylaxis is effective in noninstrumented spine surgery: a double-blind, placebo-controlled study. *Spine (Phila Pa 1976)* 2008;33:1919. [PMID: 18708923]

Savage JW, Weatherford BM, Sugrue PA, et al: Efficacy of surgical preparation solutions in lumbar spine surgery. *J Bone Joint Surg Am* 2012;94:490. [PMID: 22437997]

Schimmel JJ, Horsting PP, de Kleuver M, et al: Risk factors for deep surgical site infections after spinal fusion. *Eur Spine J* 2010;19:1711. [PMID: 20445999]

SPINAL TUMORS

▶ Essentials of Diagnosis

- *Metastatic tumors are the most common tumors of the spine.*
- *Eighty percent of metastases to the spine come from cancer of the prostate, breast, or lung.*
- *Most common benign primary tumor of the spine is hemangioma.*
- *Back pain is the most common presenting symptom.*

▶ General Considerations

Metastases represent the most common tumors of the spine. The spine is the most common location for skeletal metastasis, with the thoracic spine being the most commonly involved region. Typical spinal metastases include tumors of the prostate, breast, lung, thyroid, and kidney. Not unexpectedly, since they are the most prevalent cancers, 80% of spinal metastases originate from prostate, breast, or lung primary malignancies. In contrast, primary malignant bone tumors are comparatively rare and include chondrosarcoma, osteosarcoma, and chordoma. Lymphomas, solitary plasmacytomas, and multiple myelomas are also seen in the spine. Most (70%) malignant tumors arise in patients older than 21 years and typically occur in the anterior spine (vertebral body and pedicles). Chondrosarcoma is a notable exception that typically arises from the posterior elements.

The most common benign tumor of the spine is hemangioma, present in 10–12% of people. Most patients present with asymptomatic, incidental findings on MRI scans for other reasons (eg, back pain or sciatica), but in rare cases, hemangiomas can become large and symptomatic. Other than hemangiomas, which are frequently seen in older patients, benign bone tumors are much more common in younger patients. Osteoid osteomas and osteoblastomas are benign primary bone tumors that tend to involve the posterior elements. They are classically associated with nonmechanical back pain that tends to be worse at night and that improves with NSAIDs. Other benign bone tumors of the spine include aneurysmal bone cyst, fibrous dysplasia, and giant cell tumors. Giant cell tumors, although histologically benign, may be locally aggressive and even metastasize.

Another tumorlike finding that is a relatively common incidental finding on routine MRI for evaluation of back pain or sciatica is syrinx (a fluid-filled space within the spinal cord) or persistence of the central canal of the spinal cord. When seen, pathologic reasons, such as intramedullary tumor, Chiari malformation, spinal canal anomaly, tethered cord, or severe spinal stenosis, can be excluded with a screening MRI of the whole spine, preferably with contrast. However, about 90% of syringes are stable incidental findings not correlated with the clinical symptoms that elicited the MRI. In such cases, in the absence of progressive neurologic deficits or planned surgical intervention, expectant observation is a reasonable option as well.

▶ Clinical Findings

A. Signs and Symptoms

The presentation of spinal tumors is often similar to that of spinal infections. Axial back pain is the most common complaint, present in about 90% of cases. Associated neurologic symptoms may be present if the tumor impinges neural elements or is associated with pathologic fracture and neural compression (ie, metastatic spinal cord compression). The presence of constitutional symptoms such as fevers, night sweats, or weight loss should be elicited. Back pain is often constant and unremitting, classically worse at night time, but may also have a component made worse by mechanical loading. Patients with new-onset back pain and a history of cancer need to be ruled out for metastatic disease to the spine. Physical findings include local tenderness over the tumor, limited range of motion, and, in advanced cases, deformity from vertebral body collapse and kyphosis.

B. Imaging and Laboratory Data

The radiologic workup of spinal tumors is similar to that of spinal infections. MRI remains the mainstay of diagnosis, with CT scans also obtained to assess the degree of bony destruction, the pattern of bone response to the lesion, and the presence of matrix, and weight-bearing plain films to assess overall alignment and deformity. Plain films are poorly sensitive for tumors: approximately 40% trabecular bone loss must be present before being detectable on plain film as a lucent area. Thus advanced imaging is critical to making a prompt diagnosis. Because of its ability to provide fine bony detail, CT scans are helpful in determining the aggressiveness of lytic lesions. Slow-growing benign tumors usually display a sharp transition zone with reactive, sclerotic bone surrounding the tumor as the bone has had time to respond. This is called a geographic 1A lesion. Aggressive, fast-growing tumors usually demonstrate a moth-eaten appearance with little reactive bone and a wide transition zone. Biopsy should be considered for spinal tumors that cannot be diagnosed based on imaging alone. Most commonly, needle biopsy under CT guidance is sufficient, but several large-bore specimens should be obtained to ensure a tissue diagnosis. In the case of widely metastatic disease, biopsy of a more superficial tumor may be considered if it is easier to access. If a needle biopsy is inconclusive, then open biopsy may be needed. In cases in which a curative resection is contemplated, the biopsy must be planned appropriately to allow for excision of the biopsy tract during the definitive operation.

A metastatic workup should be considered in all patients with spinal tumors, which includes a CT scan of the chest, abdomen, and pelvis. Whole-body bone scan can also be helpful in detecting malignant or metastatic foci. Unfortunately, only about 50% of multiple myelomas display increased uptake on bone scans. Bone scans detect tumors based on increased regional blood flow to the tumor and by radiolabeling (with technetium-99) phosphates, which are deposited in areas of active bone formation. Routine laboratory data include CBC with differential, calcium, Mg, Po_4, and liver function tests. Serum and urine electrophoresis can be helpful in diagnosing multiple myeloma.

Preoperative embolization of tumors may be helpful in decreasing intraoperative bleeding, making surgery safer, easier, and more effective. Likewise, selective embolization is a treatment option for large, symptomatic hemangiomas. In addition, with tumors involving the lower thoracic spine, angiography may be helpful in identifying the major feeding vessel to the spinal cord (the artery of Adamkiewicz) so that it can be spared surgically and avoid potential vascular infarction of the spinal cord.

▶ Treatment

Treatment is dictated by a number of factors, including age (<65 or >65 years), tumor type and stage, symptom severity, presence of neurologic compression or neurologic symptoms (most importantly, ambulatory status), expected life span (<3 or >3 months), and mechanical stability. Most benign asymptomatic lesions require no treatment, but depending on the certainty of the diagnosis, periodic follow-up with CT scans is prudent. Timely repeat imaging is also indicated if symptoms worsen during clinical observation. Indications for surgery include absence of viable nonsurgical treatment modalities, intractable pain despite nonsurgical treatment, mechanical instability, neurologic preservation or need for decompression, and, rarely, in certain primary tumors of the spine, curative resection. Percutaneous cement augmentation is a minimally invasive intervention with an expanding role in the treatment of painful spinal neoplastic lesions. The treatment of hemangiomas was the initial indication for this technique, which is now most commonly used to treat osteoporotic vertebral compression fractures.

Steroids are often used in the setting of tumors causing myelopathy from spinal cord compression. Bisphosphonates are also commonly used by oncologists to manage bone loss associated with neoplastic disease of the spine. They have been shown to significantly reduce the incidence of skeletally related (adverse) events (pathologic fracture, need for radiation or surgery to bone, or spinal cord compression) in patients with multiple myeloma and osteolytic metastases.

A. Metastatic Tumors

Most metastatic tumors without neurologic compression are treated nonsurgically with radiation and/or chemotherapy, depending on the tumor type and its responsiveness to those modalities. However, in the presence of symptomatic spinal cord compression, recent level 1 evidence, which has since been corroborated in other studies, concludes that surgery prior to radiation therapy is superior to radiation therapy alone or radiation prior to surgery in terms of neurologic outcomes. An exception arises if neurologic compression is due solely to a highly radiosensitive tumor, with no significant spinal instability or bony compressive component, in which case radiation may be considered first. Unless the tumor is highly radiosensitive or the patient is a poor surgical candidate, we generally advocate performing surgery first in patients with symptomatic neurologic compression in order to avoid progressive neurologic deterioration and complications associated with surgery through a previously irradiated field.

Surgery may also be considered in those without actual but impending neurologic compromise due to spinal instability. In general, those with more than 50% vertebral body involvement or destruction of the facet joints, pars, and pedicles are at risk for instability and resultant neurologic compromise. Unfortunately, in clinical practice, the assessment of spinal stability is often not straightforward, typically requiring a nuanced interpretation of biomechanical criteria based on the "personality" or pattern of tumor involvement seen on a combination of plain film, CT, and MRI.

The choice of surgical approach depends on a number of factors. In the vast majority of metastatic cases, the goal is palliation of pain and prevention or reversal of neurologic impairment. Thus the operation should be designed to achieve those goals while minimizing morbidity. Depending on the location and pattern of compression, the decompression and reconstruction can be performed anteriorly, posteriorly, or combined.

Postoperative radiation may be helpful in removing residual tumor left behind in order to decrease recurrence. However, acute postoperative radiation therapy may increase the rate of nonunions and wound infection. Thus, it is generally preferable to wait anywhere from 3 to 6 weeks after surgery to institute radiation. The choice of spinal reconstruction will depend on the patient's overall prognosis. Those with a reasonable life expectancy beyond 1–2 years may benefit from achieving solid bony union, but this must be balanced against the potentially higher bleeding and infection risks associated with bone grafting and fusion. Those with poor prognoses for survival may be best managed with decompression and instrumentation only. In these circumstances, cement can be used to augment vertebral corpectomies and provide immediate mechanical stability of vertebral body defects. Pain related to impending or actual pathologic fractures may be managed in certain instances with percutaneous cement procedures, such as vertebroplasty or kyphoplasty, which have the advantage of being less invasive.

B. Benign Primary Bone Tumors

Osteoid osteomas are typically seen in the posterior elements of teenagers (10–20 years old) and may be associated with acute scoliosis. CT scans demonstrate a central (lucent) nidus of tumor (sometimes with a small focus of bone at its center) surrounded by a sclerotic rim of reactive bone. Spontaneous regression can occur. If the symptoms are severe or persist despite time and NSAIDs, thorough curettage of the lesion yields good outcomes. If the nidus is removed, recurrence is relatively unlikely. Good results have also been reported with RFA. Most cases of osteoid osteoma or osteoblastoma-related scoliosis are not structural and spontaneously improve after tumor resection.

Osteoblastomas represent osteoid osteomas that are larger than 2 cm. They typically occur in patients younger than 30 years and can also be associated with scoliosis. When they occur in the spine, they tend to be in the posterior arch. Marginal excision provides excellent outcomes with relatively low recurrence rates. Depending on the extent of the excision, a fusion may be necessary.

Aneurysmal bone cysts cause hyperemic lytic lesions, most commonly in the posterior elements but not infrequently extending into the anterior column of the lumbar spine as well (Figure 4–23). As with most benign primary bone tumors, patients tend to be younger, typically younger than 20 years. Expansion may cause neural compression and radiculopathy or myelopathy. MRI demonstrates characteristic fluid-fluid levels due to the layering of blood within the lesion. Curettage and resection of aneurysmal bone cysts with bone grafting is the treatment of choice. Again, fusion may be needed depending on the extent of the lesion. Preoperative embolization should strongly be considered to limit intraoperative bleeding.

Giant cell tumors are seen in slightly older individuals (20s to 40s) and arise most commonly in the anterior spine. Curettage and bone grafting may be performed but have a high recurrence rate of up to 45%. Thus, en bloc resection should be considered when feasible to prevent long-term recurrences. Radiation treatment may be associated with sarcomatous transformation in up to 15% of patients and thus is not routinely recommended.

C. Malignant Primary Bone Tumors

Multiple myeloma is the most common primary malignant bone tumor of the spine and is usually seen in patients in their 50s to 60s. It and its unifocal counterpart, solitary plasmacytoma, are B-cell lymphoproliferative cancers. In the absence of instability, myeloma can be treated with radiation, chemotherapy, and stem-cell transplants. However, surgery may be the option of choice in the face of neurologic compression associated with spinal instability, pathologic fractures, or impending fractures. Typically, patients will receive an antiresorptive medicine (like bisphosphonates) to reduce the incidence of skeletally related adverse events.

Chordomas are tumors arising from notochordal cells within the vertebral body, typically during the fifth and sixth decades and beyond. The sacrum accounts for over half of cases involving the spine, with the occipitocervical region accounting for another third. Because the local recurrence

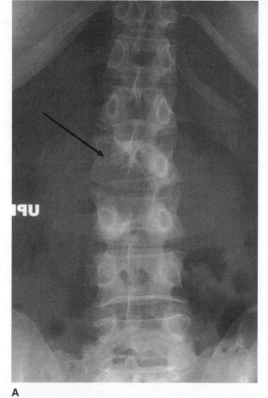

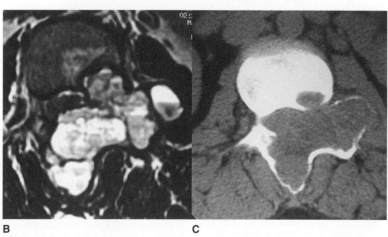

▲ **Figure 4–23.** Aneurysmal bone cyst of the spine in a 27-year-old woman with severe low back pain and leg weakness. (**A**) Anteroposterior radiograph demonstrates destruction of the L2 pedicle along with lytic changes in the L2 vertebra (*black arrow*). (**B**) Axial MRI shows an expansile, cystic lesion with fluid-fluid level causing compression of the spinal canal. (**C**) CT scan shows expansile cortical margin with lytic erosion.

rate of chordoma is extremely high, care must be taken to obtain wide margins and avoid tumor contamination into the surgical field. Adjuvant radiation therapy may be helpful, particularly if complete resection is not possible or tumor contamination occurs during resection. Most patients with

chordoma eventually die from complications related to local recurrence.

Chondrosarcomas are cartilaginous tumors typically arising in the posterior elements of the spine in patients in their 40s to 60s. Radiographs and CT scans demonstrate calcification within the tumor. Because they are radio-resistant, wide surgical excision is the mainstay of treatment. It is important to try to obtain clean surgical margins in order to avoid local recurrences, because local recurrence and progression are the most common causes of death from chondrosarcoma.

▶ Prognosis

The prognosis will vary widely depending on the tumor. In the case of acute myelopathy associated with metastatic disease, it has been shown in a randomized controlled trial that immediate surgical decompression followed by radiation therapy is superior to radiation therapy alone. In general, surgical counseling must include specific discussion of quality of remaining life weighed against the degree of pain and/or actual versus impending neurologic deficit. Patients with less than 3 months of expected survival are typically provided nonoperative care. Surgery becomes a more reasonable option in those with better prognoses, and it should at least be considered in all patients with actual or impending neurologic deficits, especially spinal cord level compression. Even in those with relatively poor prognoses, surgery may provide substantial benefit in terms of neurologic preservation and pain relief during a patient's remaining life.

Acosta FL Jr, Dowd CF, Chin C, Tihan T, Ames CP, Weinstein PR: Current treatment strategies and outcomes in the management of symptomatic vertebral hemangiomas. *Neurosurgery* 2006;58:287. [PMID: 16462482]

Barr JD, Barr MS, Lemley TJ, McCann RM: Percutaneous vertebroplasty for pain relief and spinal stabilization. *Spine (Phila Pa 1976)* 2000;25:923. [PMID: 10767803]

Berenson J, Pflugmacher R, Jarzem P, et al: Balloon kyphoplasty versus non-surgical fracture management for treatment of painful vertebral body compression fractures in patients with cancer: a multicentre, randomised controlled trial. *Lancet Oncol* 2011;12:225. [PMID: 21333519]

Chaichana KL, Woodworth GF, Sciubba DM, et al: Predictors of ambulatory function after decompressive surgery for metastatic epidural spinal cord compression. *Neurosurgery* 2008;62:683. [PMID: 18425015]

Chi JH, Gokaslan Z, McCormick P, Tibbs PA, Kryscio RJ, Patchell RA: Selecting treatment for patients with malignant epidural spinal cord compression-does age matter? Results from a randomized clinical trial. *Spine (Phila Pa 1976)* 2009;34:431. [PMID: 19212272]

Gerszten PC, Monaco EA 3rd: Complete percutaneous treatment of vertebral body tumors causing spinal canal compromise using a transpedicular cavitation, cement augmentation, and radiosurgical technique. *Neurosurg Focus* 2009;27:E9. [PMID: 19951062]

Henry DH, Costa L, Goldwasser F, et al: Randomized, double-blind study of denosumab versus zoledronic acid in the treatment of bone metastases in patients with advanced cancer (excluding breast and prostate cancer) or multiple myeloma. *J Clin Oncol* 2011;29:1125. [PMID: 21343556]

Kondo T, Hozumi T, Goto T, Seichi A, Nakamura K: Intraoperative radiotherapy combined with posterior decompression and stabilization for non-ambulant paralytic patients due to spinal metastasis. *Spine (Phila Pa 1976)* 2008;33:1898. [PMID: 18670344]

Magge SN, Smyth MD, Governale LS, et al: Idiopathic syrinx in the pediatric population: a combined center experience. *J Neurosurg Pediatr* 2011;7:30. [PMID: 21194284]

Patchell RA, Tibbs PA, Regine WF, et al: Direct decompressive surgical resection in the treatment of spinal cord compression caused by metastatic cancer: a randomised trial. *Lancet* 2005;366:643. [PMID: 16112300]

Singh K, Samartzis D, Vaccaro AR, Andersson GB, An HS, Heller JG: Current concepts in the management of metastatic spinal disease. The role of minimally-invasive approaches. *J Bone Joint Surg Br* 2006;88:434. [PMID: 16567775]

▼ DEFORMITIES OF THE SPINE

Bobby K.B. Tay, MD; Harry B. Skinner, MD, PhD

SCOLIOSIS

▶ Essentials of Diagnosis

- *Scoliosis is deviation of the spine from the vertical axis greater than 10 degrees.*
- *Ninety percent of cases do not progress.*
- *Curve magnitude greater than 45 degrees is likely to progress into adulthood.*
- *Most cases in young people are asymptomatic; adults are more likely to have symptoms of back pain and sciatica.*

▶ General Considerations

Scoliosis as defined by the Scoliosis Research Society is any lateral deviation of the spine from the normal vertical line of 10 degrees or greater. Minor "wiggles" less than 10 degrees are termed spinal asymmetry and do not require follow-up. Using the 10-degree standard, about 2–4% of the U.S. population has scoliosis with an equal distribution between the sexes. At this low threshold for diagnosis, over 90% of cases will not progress to the point of warranting further intervention. Thus, referral to a spine surgeon is typically reserved for curves that are more than 15–20 degrees, for curves that demonstrate progression on serial assessment by the primary care provider, or for patients with worrisome history or physical exam findings. When coronal curvature is greater than 20–30 degrees, a strong female predominance (8–10:1) is noted. Idiopathic scoliosis is a disease that is driven by skeletal growth until a significant magnitude of curvature is obtained (>30–50 degrees). As such, there are essentially three stages of treatment for scoliosis—observation alone (the most common), bracing (only appropriate in the skeletally immature), and surgical correction.

If by skeletal maturity the coronal curve has not exceeded 30 degrees, then this mild spinal deformity is not likely to progress in adulthood, and it is unlikely to have future clinical impact on the patient. On the other hand, when the magnitude of curvature exceeds 45–50 degrees, progression in adulthood is predicted, typically at a pace of 1 degree per year. With continued progression, clinical manifestations are likely, which include back pain and radiculopathy/sciatica (especially when the major curve involves the lumbar spine), and in the most severe cases (>75–90 degrees), pulmonary and gastrointestinal (GI) compromise can occur. As such, surgery, in the form of instrumented spinal fusion, is typically indicated when coronal curvature exceeds 45–50 degrees. The goals of surgical correction are to arrest curve progression and provide sufficient curve correction to produce a stable, well-balanced spine centered over the pelvis by fusing as few segments as possible. In addition to this primary structural goal, additional benefits may include improved cosmesis and reduced back pain and neurologic dysfunction. Traditionally, scoliosis clinical research has focused on the primary goal, which has been deformity correction. Recent clinical studies have focused on the overall well-being of scoliosis patients as assessed by validated outcome tools.

Scoliosis is most commonly divided into subsets, based on the age at diagnosis. When scoliosis is present at birth, it is termed congenital scoliosis, which occurs by one of two structural anomalies. Either there is a failure of formation of part of the spine (for instance, a hemi-vertebra, which is the most common anomaly producing congenital scoliosis), or there is failure of segmentation (ie, a block vertebra). The crucial period for formation and segmentation of the spine occurs in the fourth to sixth week of gestation, which is also a critical time for spinal cord, renal, and cardiac development. As a result, when congenital scoliosis is diagnosed, the health of these additional structures should be screened as well. When scoliosis presents within the first 3 years of life, it is termed infantile scoliosis. Infantile scoliosis is a rare (<1% of all cases) form of scoliosis, which has strong genetic associations, and it too requires further screening (ie, screening MRI of the spine). It commonly produces a left thoracic curve, and the vast majority (~90%) resolves spontaneously. When it presents between 3 and 10 years of age, it is called juvenile scoliosis. This type behaves and is treated like adolescent scoliosis, although the greater growth potential predisposes to a greater risk of progression to the point of surgical indication. Adolescent idiopathic scoliosis, the most common type of scoliosis, is diagnosed when scoliosis presents after 10 years of age and prior to skeletal maturity (typically 2 years after menarche in females). Adult scoliosis refers to scoliosis detected after skeletal maturity. It typically has two primary distinctions—de novo (meaning it developed in adulthood, often as an advanced form of spinal degeneration, typified by low-degree lumbar curves with significant rotatory subluxation[s]) and progressive (meaning it was the progression of a curve that started earlier in life). Aside from congenital and infantile forms of scoliosis, which have unique anatomic considerations, the distinctions between juvenile, adolescent, and adult are not as significant.

Last, the aforementioned classifications describe idiopathic scoliosis, which is the etiology of 85% of cases;

however, scoliosis can be associated with skeletal syndromes (eg, Marfan syndrome or neurofibromatosis), termed syndromic scoliosis, or neuromuscular conditions (cerebral palsy being most common). These two rarer causes of scoliosis tend to produce more significant degrees of curvature and more commonly require surgical intervention. Neuromuscular scoliosis is often treated with fusion of the entire thoracic and lumbar spine to the pelvis. An important consideration for these two rare forms of scoliosis is that they are part of a syndrome. When diagnosed, comprehensive evaluation for other known associated manifestations (eg, aortic dilation in Marfan syndrome) of the syndrome should be undertaken.

▶ Clinical Findings

A. Signs and Symptoms

Scoliosis is most commonly detected incidentally on screening examinations or during routine pediatric appointments in the preteen years. Uneven ribs, shoulders, or pelvis may be noted by the patient or parents and should be assessed on examination. While the vast majority of patients are asymptomatic at presentation, about one third of patients will complain of back pain, which is often in the interscapular area. When it is in the low lumbar area, radiographs should be inspected for evidence of spondylolisthesis, which can coexist in scoliotic patients. Since reports of back pain can be elicited in a similar percentage of young adults with straight spines, the clinical significance of this complaint and the direct association with the underlying spinal deformity may not be clear. That being said, reports of severe back pain may prompt further evaluation, to include screening whole-spine MRI to ensure that no intraspinal anomalies (eg, syrinx, tumor, or diastematomyelia) are present. The yield from these additional studies is exceedingly low and likely does not offset the cost and difficulty (eg, some level of sedation is often needed to obtain the MRI). Since indications for MRI in the setting of scoliosis are not universally accepted, this determination is probably best left to the consultant. When patients present with positive findings on neurologic examination (eg, weakness, sensory deficits, altered gait, bowel or bladder problems), then screening MRI should be ordered.

The Adams forward bend test is the classic screening assessment for scoliosis. It is carried out in most states on an annual basis in school for adolescent females (and commonly males as well). This test requires the examiner to stand posterior to the patient, while the child bends over at the waist until their trunk is level with the ground. Scoliosis is not simply a lateral deviation, but a rotation of the spine. The rotation at the thoracic level causes the ribs to rise up on the side of the curve apex, which is most commonly the right side (90% of cases). It is so common for the main thoracic curve to be apexed to the right that many experts feel screening MRI is indicated whenever the main thoracic curve points to the left. This truncal rotation can simply be viewed or palpated, but a scoliometer is a device, which looks like a carpenter's level, used to directly measure the degree of rotation in the chest cavity. Screening thresholds for radiograph and/or spine surgical consultation vary between 5- and 7-degree tilt, as measured by the scoliometer. The lower threshold is more sensitive (minimal to no false negatives), whereas the upper limit is more specific (less false positives).

B. Imaging

The gold standard for diagnosing scoliosis is an upright posterior-anterior long cassette (36") frontal and lateral radiograph of the entire thoracic and lumbar spine. This is often called a scoliosis survey. This should be obtained at a radiology suite that is versed in the proper protocol for obtaining high-quality scoliosis films. The radiologist or spine surgeon then views the spine and looks for the three common curves that occur in scoliosis—proximal thoracic, main thoracic, and lumbar. The magnitude of the curvature is measured using the Cobb method, which subtends the angle between lines drawn at the upper endplate of the upper vertebra in the measured curve (termed the upper end vertebrae) to the lower endplate of the lower vertebrae (lower end vertebra). The apex is the direction that the convex side of the curve points (often reported using the Latin prefixes *dextro*, meaning right, or *levo*, meaning left); specifically, it is the lateral-most deviated point in the curve, which can be a vertebral body or disk space. The largest of the curves is called the major curve. Any additional curves are called minor curves. The major curve, in addition to having the greatest degree of coronal curvature, also has the greatest degree of rotation. Rotation is graded based on the degree to which the apical vertebral pedicles are rotated from their normal owl's eyes appearance. Minor curves are frequently compensatory. Compensatory curves typically do not have a rotatory component, as they are simple lateral deviations in the spine that naturally occur to compensate for the major curve, thereby keeping the head centered over the pelvis.

The most common method in current use for classifying adolescent idiopathic scoliosis curves is the Lenke classification system. It replaces the King classification system, because it is more reliable, better predicts surgical plan, and takes into account the three-dimensional nature of scoliosis. In addition to standing scoliosis films, supine bending films are also needed to assess the flexibility and structural nature of each curve. The Lenke classification system has three components. First, there are six curve types. Then there is a lumbar modifier, which demonstrates the degree to which the lumbar curve deviates from the vertical midline. Last, there is a sagittal modifier, which assesses the degree of thoracic (T5-T12) kyphosis.

Many patients with main thoracic scoliosis (Lenke type 1, most common type) have flat (hypokyphotic) thoracic spines, as the normal thoracic kyphosis has rotated into the coronal plane. Kyphosis (abnormal forward curvature of the spine; normal = 10–50 degrees) can occur in the setting of scoliosis or as an independent deformity.

When global thoracic kyphosis of more than 50 degrees occurs in the setting of three or more consecutive thoracic vertebral bodies having a wedging of 5 degrees or more, typically with Schmorl nodes present, it is termed Scheuermann kyphosis. Most cases of Scheuermann kyphosis require no specific treatment, although bracing can be attempted during growth. Corrective surgical fusion may be considered in severe cases (>75–90 degrees).

▶ Treatment

As stated earlier, there are three stages of treatment for scoliosis. The first and commonly the only stage needed is serial observation. Because scoliosis is a disease of progression, it takes at least two points in time to fully assess the significance of the deformity, unless the deformity is severe at presentation. Three factors most affect the likelihood of progression: (1) female gender, (2) growth remaining, and (3) current curve magnitude. To minimize repeated radiation exposure, serial follow-up typically occurs at 4-month intervals during periods of peak growth and 6-month intervals during periods of less expected growth, especially in lower magnitude curves (<20 degrees). Curves that are less than 30 degrees in adulthood do not require routine follow-up. While there is some variation, a consensus of the reported methods for predicting progression to more than 40–45 degrees shows that major curves that are less than 20–30 degrees at or in the year prior to menarche or the start of the skeletal growth spurt in males have less than 5–20% risk of progression to the point of requiring surgical intervention. Asymptomatic curves of less than 30 degrees detected as incidental findings in females more than 2 years out from menarche and skeletally mature males do not require spine surgical consultation solely for evaluation of scoliosis. Since curve progression in adulthood occurs at a much slower pace than in adolescence, serial images, when indicated, should be separated by 1–3+ years in adults. The measurement error for coronal curve measurement on scoliosis films is 3–5 degrees. Thus, with an expected progression of 1 degree per year in adulthood, it would take at least 3 years to demonstrate a real progression exceeding measurement error. Indications for scoliosis surgery in adults are largely based on clinical complaints, as opposed to curve magnitude and deformity.

If the major curve progresses to 20–25 degrees (up to 35 degrees) in a skeletally immature patient, then bracing is the next stage of treatment offered. There are several types of braces, with two major subsets—thoracolumbar orthoses and nighttime braces. Thoracolumbar orthoses (eg, Boston brace) are the most common type of brace and are intended to be worn 20–22 hours a day. They are typically made of thin plastic, so they can be worn under clothes to reduce the stigma of wearing a brace. Compliance significantly affects the ability of braces to prevent progression, which is the goal of bracing. Bracing is not intended to permanently correct scoliosis, but rather to arrest curve progression at a magnitude below which it is unlikely to produce lifelong impact (ie, <30 degrees). With compliant wear, bracing can arrest/slow scoliosis progression and prevent need for surgical intervention in up to 75% of those treated. Bracing is a challenging treatment for image-conscious adolescents to tolerate, because when it is started, it must be maintained through the remainder of skeletal growth and then some time after (often 2–3 years of total wear time). To avoid brace wear during school, nighttime braces were introduced, which hold the spine in an overcorrected position during nighttime only. This technique is more painful and may be less effective. Physical therapy and activity modification do not influence the natural history of scoliosis. There is no reason to restrict activity in patients diagnosed with scoliosis. That being said, reducing the weight of book bags, encouraging the wear of both shoulder straps (versus using just one shoulder), and best yet, rolling book-bags with two sets of books (one for school and one for home) can help reduce back pain complaints and do demonstrate short-term measureable difference in curvature.

Last, when the degree of curvature exceeds 45–50 degrees, surgical intervention in the form of instrumented spinal fusion is indicated. This can occur via posterior, anterior, or combined posterior-anterior spinal fusion. Clear clinical superiority between the approaches is uncertain. Each has its own specific risk-benefit profile. Multiple techniques exist for correcting the curvature seen in scoliosis. All methods include rigid fixation of the spine, some degree of destabilization of the instrumented spinal segment (ie, facetectomies and ligament releases), correction of the deformity via forces applied through the implants, and securing the correction by locking the screws (or fixation devices) to rods and then placement of bone graft to encourage solid fusion across the instrumented segment. The most common means for instrumenting the spine is a pedicle screw and rod construct. Pedicle screws provide strong three-column fixation capable of delivering three-dimensional corrective forces to the spine.

Outside the scope of this chapter is the complex decision process that goes into level selection and whether to fuse all curves or only the major curve, expecting the minor/compensatory curves to spontaneously correct. Current surgical techniques, especially in young healthy patients, produce solid fusions with excellent correction in the vast majority of patients with very low rates of complications. The most dreaded complication is spinal cord injury (<1%). This can occur through implant malposition, but more commonly is related to the acute correction of the deformity, especially in the setting of significant kyphosis. Intraoperative neuromonitoring allows for real-time or near real-time assessment of spinal cord function during scoliosis surgery to reduce the risk of this severe complication. Comorbidities, such as osteoporosis, obesity, cardiac disease, and diabetes, increase the rate of complication associated with adult scoliosis surgery. Further, younger patients have significantly more flexible curves, which can be more effectively corrected with simpler

techniques, than the rigid curves seen in adult scoliosis. When the primary presenting symptom is pain or neurologic deficit, deformity correction in the setting of low-magnitude curves (30–50 degrees) in patients with neutral sagittal balance (ie, the spine is maintained in a rather vertical stature, without fixed forward tipping of the spine) is not always a goal of surgery in adult scoliosis. When sagittal imbalance is present through scoliosis or kyphoscoliosis, long-segment thoracolumbar fusions are often indicated to secure the spine and restore the sagittal balance in adults. This is crucial, because sagittal balance is the structural parameter most predictive of successful clinical outcome following adult scoliosis surgery. More recently, it has been shown that in addition to achieving these technical goals, scoliosis surgery significantly improves cosmesis, pain, and overall well-being.

Belmont PJ Jr, Kuklo TR, Taylor KF, Freedman BA, Prahinski JR, Kruse RW: Intraspinal anomalies associated with isolated congenital hemivertebra: the role of routine magnetic resonance imaging. *J Bone Joint Surg Am* 2004 Aug;86-A(8):1704-1710. [PMID: 15292418]

Bridwell KH, Baldus C, Berven S, et al: Changes in radiographic and clinical outcomes with primary treatment adult spinal deformity surgeries from two years to three- to five-years followup. *Spine (Phila Pa 1976)* 2010;35:1849. [PMID: 20802383]

Carreon LY, Sanders JO, Diab M, Sturm PF, Sucato DJ; Spinal Deformity Study Group: Patient satisfaction after surgical correction of adolescent idiopathic scoliosis. *Spine (Phila Pa 1976)* 2011;36:965. [PMID: 21224771]

Charles YP, Daures JP, de Rosa V, Diméglio A: Progression risk of idiopathic juvenile scoliosis during pubertal growth. *Spine (Phila Pa 1976)* 2006 Aug 1;31(17):1933-1942. [PMID: 16924210]

Clements DH, Marks M, Newton PO, Betz RR, Lenke L, Shufflebarger H; Harms Study Group: Did the Lenke classification change scoliosis treatment? *Spine (Phila Pa 1976)* 2011 Jun 15;36(14):1142-1145. [PMID: 21358471]

Diab M, Landman Z, Lubicky J, et al: Use and outcome of MRI in the surgical treatment of adolescent idiopathic scoliosis. *Spine (Phila Pa 1976)* 2011;36:667. [PMID: 21178850]

Fu KM, Smith JS, Polly DW Jr, et al: Correlation of higher preoperative American Society of Anesthesiology grade and increased morbidity and mortality rates in patients undergoing spine surgery. *J Neurosurg Spine* 2011;14:470. [PMID: 21294615]

Hamilton DK, Smith JS, Sansur CA, et al: Rates of new neurological deficit associated with spine surgery based on 108,419 procedures: a report of the scoliosis research society morbidity and mortality committee. *Spine (Phila Pa 1976)* 2011;36:1218. [PMID: 21217448]

Howard A, Wright JG, Hedden D: A comparative study of TLSO, Charleston, and Milwaukee braces for idiopathic scoliosis. *Spine (Phila Pa 1976)* 1998 Nov 15;23(22):2404-2411. [PMID: 9836354]

Isaacs RE, Hyde J, Goodrich JA, Rodgers WB, Phillips FM: A prospective, nonrandomized, multicenter evaluation of extreme lateral interbody fusion for the treatment of adult degenerative scoliosis: perioperative outcomes and complications. *Spine (Phila Pa 1976)* 2010;35(26 Suppl):S322. [PMID: 21160396]

Lange JE, Steen H, Gunderson R, Brox JI: Long-term results after Boston brace treatment in late-onset juvenile and adolescent idiopathic scoliosis. *Scoliosis* 2011;6:18. [PMID: 21880123]

Lehman RA Jr, Lenke LG, Keeler KA, et al: Operative treatment of adolescent idiopathic scoliosis with posterior pedicle screw-only constructs: minimum three-year follow-up of one hundred fourteen cases. *Spine (Phila Pa 1976)* 2008;33:1598. [PMID: 18552676]

Lenke LG: Lenke classification system of adolescent idiopathic scoliosis: treatment recommendations. *Instr Course Lect* 2005;54:537. [PMID: 15948478]

Little DG, Song KM, Katz D, Herring JA: Relationship of peak height velocity to other maturity indicators in idiopathic scoliosis in girls. *J Bone Joint Surg Am* 2000;82:685. [PMID: 10819279]

Lowe TG, Line BG: Evidence based medicine: analysis of Scheuermann kyphosis. *Spine (Phila Pa 1976)* 2007;32(19 Suppl): S115. [PMID: 17728677]

Newton PO, Faro FD, Lenke LG, et al: Factors involved in the decision to perform a selective versus nonselective fusion of Lenke 1B and 1C (King-Moe II) curves in adolescent idiopathic scoliosis. *Spine (Phila Pa 1976)* 2003;28:S217. [PMID: 14560195]

Potter BK, Kuklo TR, Lenke LG: Radiographic outcomes of anterior spinal fusion versus posterior spinal fusion with thoracic pedicle screws for treatment of Lenke Type I adolescent idiopathic scoliosis curves. *Spine (Phila Pa 1976)* 2005;30:1859. [PMID: 16103856]

Ramirez N, Johnston CE, Browne RH: The prevalence of back pain in children who have idiopathic scoliosis. *J Bone Joint Surg Am* 1997;79:364. [PMID: 9070524]

Reames DL, Smith JS, Fu KM, et al: Complications in the surgical treatment of 19,360 cases of pediatric scoliosis: a review of the Scoliosis Research Society Morbidity and Mortality database. *Spine (Phila Pa 1976)* 2011;36:1484. [PMID: 21037528]

Smucny M, Lubicky JP, Sanders JO, Carreon LY, Diab M: Patient self-assessment of appearance is improved more by all pedicle screw than by hybrid constructs in surgical treatment of adolescent idiopathic scoliosis. *Spine (Phila Pa 1976)* 2011;36:248. [PMID: 21248593]

Thuet ED, Winscher JC, Padberg AM, et al: Validity and reliability of intraoperative monitoring in pediatric spinal deformity surgery: a 23-year experience of 3436 surgical cases. *Spine (Phila Pa 1976)* 2010;35:1880. [PMID: 20802388]

NEUROFIBROMATOSIS

Spinal deformity associated with neurofibromatosis poses some special considerations. Curvatures seen in affected patients may be of the idiopathic type or the dysplastic type. Curvatures of the first type exhibit the same curve patterns as seen in patients with idiopathic scoliosis and are most commonly right thoracic curves and may be managed in a similar manner. Curvatures of the second type can be much more malignant in behavior.

Dysplastic curves can be identified by evidence of dysplastic bone: penciling of the ribs or transverse processes, enlargement of the foramina, erosion of the vertebrae, and evidence of a shorter, more abrupt curve than that seen in idiopathic scoliosis. Dysplastic curves usually are associated with kyphosis, which also exists through a fairly short sharp segment. They may occur in the thoracic, thoracolumbar, or lumbar spine.

Dysplastic curves in patients with neurofibromatosis can progress rapidly and lead to severe deformity. Bony erosion can occur secondary to neurofibromas or dural ectasia (expansions of the dural sac, which can account for enlargement of the foramina or erosion of the vertebrae). The short kyphotic curves and erosion of bone can, in severe cases, result in neurologic impairment, including paraplegia.

Surgery in patients with dysplastic curves is associated with a high incidence of pseudarthrosis. If surgery is indicated, it is usually recommended to perform both an anterior and a posterior fusion. This combined approach results in a satisfactory fusion rate of up to 80%. Because of the dysplastic bone stock, it may be necessary to use a combination of sublaminar wires, hooks, and screws. Preoperative MRI may be useful in assessing the extent of dural ectasia. Fusion levels are selected according to the end vertebra of the curvature. The end fusion level must lie centered over the middle of the sacrum (the Harrington stable zone), much like the selection for idiopathic scoliosis. Clearly, however, the fusion should not end above or below a dysplastic vertebra, although it would be rare for such a level not to be within the curve.

Funasaki H, Winter RB, Lonstein JB, et al: Pathophysiology of spinal deformities in neurofibromatosis: an analysis of 71 patients who had curves associated with dystrophic changes. *J Bone Joint Surg Am* 1994;76:692. [PMID: 8175817]

Greggi T, Martikos K: Surgical treatment of early onset scoliosis in neurofibromatosis. *Stud Health Technol Inform* 2012;176:330. [PMID 22744522]

Vitale MG, Guha A, Skaggs DL: Orthopaedic manifestations of neurofibromatosis in children: an update. *Clin Orthop Relat Res* 2002;401:107. [PMID: 12151887]

CONGENITAL SCOLIOSIS

Congenital scoliosis is caused by one of the two types of structural bony abnormality (Figure 4–24). Type I is a failure of formation, such as that seen with hemivertebrae. Type II is a failure of segmentation, such as that seen with block vertebrae and that seen with unsegmented bars, where there is a tether to growth on one side of the spine. Mixed abnormalities are also found in patients with congenital scoliosis. Unilateral unsegmented bars with contralateral hemivertebrae have the greatest tendency for rapid progression and should be surgically fused as soon as the bony abnormality is evident. Unilateral unsegmented bars also tend to progress.

With respect to progression, hemivertebrae have a variable prognosis, depending on whether a contralateral hemivertebra is present that results in overall balance of the spine, whether multiple hemivertebrae are on one side of the spine, and how much growth potential is predicted for

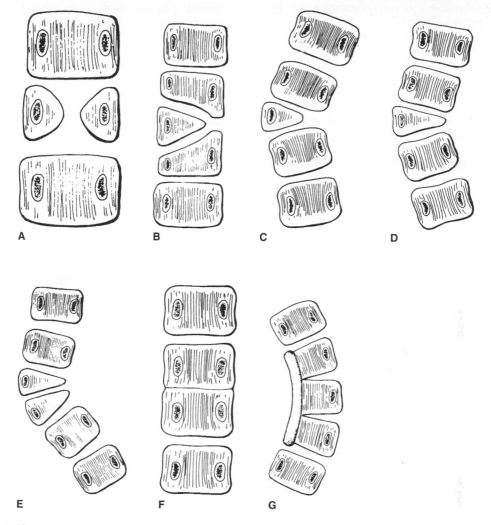

▲ **Figure 4–24.** The major types of congenital scoliosis are failure of formation, as shown in diagrams **A** through **E**, and failure of segmentation, as shown in diagrams **F** and **G**. (Reproduced, with permission, from Hall JE: Congenital scoliosis. In Bradford DS, Hensinger RN, eds: *The Pediatric Spine*. New York: Thieme; 1985.)

each endplate of the hemivertebra. Hemivertebrae at the cervicothoracic junction and the lumbosacral junction have a relatively poor prognosis because the spine above or below the abnormality cannot compensate. Hemivertebrae should be observed so as to delineate their growth potential and progression.

Bracing is ineffective in treating congenital scoliosis because the curves are inflexible. Bracing is sometimes used to prevent progression of the compensatory curve, however.

In patients with congenital scoliosis, the incidence of cardiac abnormalities is increased, as is the incidence of renal abnormalities (20–30%) and intracanal abnormalities (10–50%).

Abdominal ultrasound or other imaging tests should be used to rule out absent or abnormal kidneys. Intracanal abnormalities may include a syrinx (cyst within the cord), diastematomyelia or diplomyelia (division or reduplication of the cord, respectively), and tethered cord (presence of a tight filum terminale that does not permit the conus medullaris to migrate upward normally with growth).

If surgical intervention in patients with congenital scoliosis is indicated, several options are available. "Growth-friendly" surgical management is preferred in early-onset scoliosis so that the curve can be controlled while the spine and thorax continue to grow. Various distraction/compression systems are available for such surgery without fusion. Fusion in situ is the simplest procedure. For very young (<10 years) patients, however, a posterior fusion alone results in tethering of the posterior elements while the anterior elements continue to grow. This situation may lead to the crankshaft phenomenon, whereby the anterior growth in the spine results in a twisting deformity around the fused posterior elements. For this reason, combined anterior and posterior fusion is usually recommended for very young patients, halting growth circumferentially about the spine. (The crankshaft phenomenon can also occur in very young patients with noncongenital forms of scoliosis who were treated by posterior fusion. Age younger than 10 years, Risser stage 0 or 1, and the presence of an open triradiate cartilage are indicators of skeletal maturity at risk for development of crankshaft.)

In some cases of hemivertebra, hemiepiphysiodesis may be performed, arresting growth on the curve convexity but permitting continued growth on the curve concavity, with resultant gradual curve correction. This procedure has good results in selected patients but can be unpredictable with respect to the amount of actual correction that can be achieved.

In cases in which a hemivertebra is accompanied by significant coronal decompensation and compensatory growth would not be adequate to result in spinal balance, consideration can be given to hemivertebra excision via a combined anterior and posterior approach. Although this procedure is technically more demanding and has greater potential risks, it allows for better overall curve correction and improvement of coronal balance. Newer surgical techniques may allow for a single-stage posterior hemivertebral decancellation and excision. This approach may obviate the need for a separate anterior approach to the spine. Hemivertebra excision may be the preferred option in the lumbar spine or lumbosacral junction, where the neurologic risk is to the cauda equina rather than the spinal cord and where oblique takeoff of the vertebra above the hemivertebra can result in significant truncal decompensation.

Bradford DS: Partial epiphyseal arrest and supplemental fixation for progressive correction of congenital spinal deformity. *J Bone Joint Surg Am* 1982;64:610. [PMID: 7068703]

Gomez JA, Lee JK, Kim PD, et al: "Growth friendly" spine surgery: management options for the young child with scoliosis. *J Am Acad Orthop Surg* 2011;19:722. [PMID: 22134204]

Lenke LG, Newton PO, Sucato DJ, et al: Complications following 147 consecutive vertebral column resections for severe pediatric spinal deformity: a multicenter analysis. *Spine (Phila Pa 1976)* 2013;38:119. [PMID: 22825478]

Thompson AG, Marks DS, Sayampanathan SR, et al: Long term results of combined anterior and posterior convex epiphysiodesis for congenital scoliosis due to hemivertebrae. *Spine (Phila Pa 1976)* 1995;20:1380. [PMID: 7676336]

Wang S, Zhang J, Qiu G, et al: Dual growing rods technique for congenital scoliosis: More than 2 years outcomes: the preliminary results of a single centre. *Spine (Phila Pa 1976)* 2012;37:E1639. [PMID: 22990366]

Yaszay B, O'Brien M, Shufflebarger HL, et al: Efficacy of hemivertebra resection for congenital scoliosis: a multicenter retrospective comparison of three surgical techniques. *Spine (Phila Pa 1976)* 2011;36:2052. [PMID: 22048650]

KYPHOSIS

The normal sagittal contour of the spine includes cervical lordosis, thoracic kyphosis, and lumbar lordosis (Figure 4–25). Increases or decreases in any of these can be seen. If they are

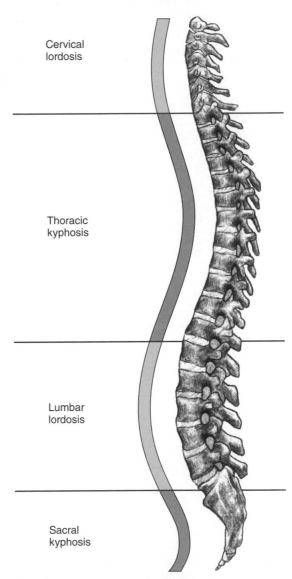

Cervical lordosis

Thoracic kyphosis

Lumbar lordosis

Sacral kyphosis

▲ **Figure 4–25.** The normal sagittal contour of the spine. (Reproduced, with permission, from Bullough PG, Boachie-Adjei O: *Atlas of Spinal Diseases*. London: Gower; 1988.)

severe enough, they can cause disability, as discussed later in the cases of congenital kyphosis and Scheuermann kyphosis.

1. Congenital Kyphosis

As in congenital scoliosis (see previous discussion), congenital kyphosis can result from a failure of formation or a failure of segmentation. In congenital kyphosis, however, failures of formation have a much more dangerous clinical prognosis. These can lead to congenital or progressive "dislocation" of the spinal column (Figure 4–26) and paralysis if not treated appropriately. If performed early enough, posterior fusion may be sufficient to prevent neurologic problems. Severe deficiencies, however, may require anterior and posterior fusion to achieve stability.

2. Scheuermann Kyphosis

Normal thoracic kyphosis ranges from 25 to 45 degrees. Postural kyphosis can increase this curvature, but if no abnormalities are present, the curve is flexible and the posture can be easily corrected by the child. If endplate abnormalities are present and three or more vertebral bodies are wedged as seen on the lateral radiograph, the diagnosis of Scheuermann kyphosis can be made. Schmorl nodules, characterized by herniation of the disk material at the vertebral endplates, and increased thoracic kyphosis are also seen. Clinically, patients with this type of kyphosis have a curvature that is more abrupt than that observed in people with postural roundback, and this type is only partly correctable by forced extension. It can be demonstrated either by having the patient hyperextend or by taking a lateral radiograph with the patient lying over a bolster at the apex of the kyphosis so the Cobb angle can be measured. Thoracic curves may cause pain and discomfort, although some report that pain is more commonly seen in thoracolumbar curves.

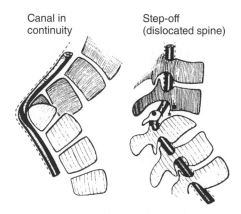

▲ Figure 4–26. Congenital kyphosis and congenital "dislocation" of the spinal column. (Reproduced, with permission, from Dubousset J: Congenital kyphosis. In Bradford DS, Hensinger RN, eds: *The Pediatric Spine.* New York: Thieme; 1985.)

Bracing can be instituted if the kyphosis measures more than 45 or 55 degrees in a skeletally immature patient, particularly if the curvature is progressive or accompanied by pain. If lesser degrees of deformity are symptomatic, they can be treated with physical therapy exercises and observed for progression. Brace treatment requires the use of the Milwaukee brace, with two paraspinal pads placed over the apical ribs posteriorly. Radiographs should be taken with the patient in the brace to confirm that adequate correction is being effected. The brace can be removed for sports and bathing but should otherwise be worn 23 hours a day. Repeat lateral radiographs should be taken at intervals of 4–6 months. If bracing is successful at controlling the curve, it should be continued until the patient nears skeletal maturity. Weaning should be performed slowly, so as to maintain correction. Although some correction may be lost, proper use of the Milwaukee brace can result in long-lasting improvement in many patients with kyphosis (which is not the case with brace treatment of adolescent idiopathic scoliosis).

Surgical treatment of kyphosis may be indicated if the curve magnitude increases despite bracing, if the patient has significant associated symptoms, or if the patient who is nearing skeletal maturity has a severe curvature. Posterior spinal fusion with multilevel posterior Smith-Peterson osteotomies is the treatment of choice in these cases. Segmental instrumentation using pedicle screws with a compression-type construct is used to correct the deformity and hold the correction until fusion occurs. If the curve flexibility does not permit adequate correction as demonstrated on a hyperextension lateral radiograph, an anterior release and fusion prior to the posterior spinal fusion is indicated. Care should be taken to extend the fusion to the upper thoracic spine, sometimes to T1, to minimize the risk of developing junctional problems at the cervicothoracic junction.

Reports describe the natural history of Scheuermann kyphosis, suggesting some functional limitations but little actual interference with lifestyle. The deformity can worsen over time. It appears clear, however, that many patients have their symptoms of back pain and deformity improved by surgery. Proper patient education and selection are essential for appropriate treatment of these patients.

Arlet V, Schlenzka D: Scheuermann's kyphosis: surgical management. *Eur Spine J* 2005;14:817. [PMID: 15830215]

Noordeen MH, Garrido E, Tucker SK, et al: The surgical treatment of congenital kyphosis. *Spine (Phila Pa 1976)* 2009;34:1808. [PMID: 19644332]

Tsirikos AI, McMaster MJ: Infantile developmental thoracolumbar kyphosis with segmental subluxation of the spine. *J Bone Joint Surg Br* 2010;92:430. [PMID: 20190317]

MYELODYSPLASIA

Neural tube defects can result in complex spinal deformities secondary both to the neuromuscular collapsing nature of the spine and to the vertebral anomalies that can give rise to congenital kyphosis or congenital scoliosis. Myelomeningocele or meningocele is present at birth in a patient whose neural tube failed to close in utero. Sac closure is usually performed shortly after birth. In many cases, the affected infant also requires placement of a ventriculoperitoneal shunt because of hydrocephalus. The level of neurologic function usually corresponds to the level of the defect. For example, a low thoracic myelomeningocele patient has no lumbar nerve roots functioning and therefore no lower extremity function. An L4 myelomeningocele patient has a functioning tibialis anterior but no extensor hallucis and no gastrocnemius and usually no voluntary bowel and bladder control.

Neurologic function in patients with myelodysplasia is static and should not deteriorate with growth. Neurologic changes, especially during growth spurts, require evaluation for tethered cord, a common occurrence in affected children, which results in traction on the spinal cord.

Orthopedic management includes maximizing the function of patients through the use of braces, ambulatory aids, wheelchairs, or surgery. The degree of spinal deformity is related to the neurologic level, with spinal collapse more likely in those with a higher neurologic level of involvement than in those with a lower level. The presence of bony abnormalities can affect this prognosis, of course.

As with many neuromuscular spinal deformities, curvatures may present early in life. If the clinician elects to treat a patient with bracing, it is important to remember that bracing in the presence of insensate skin can result in pressure sores if the brace is not adequately padded and the parents are not instructed regarding skin care.

In many cases, the curvature eventually requires surgical stabilization. Because of the magnitude and stiffness of the curvature as well as the absence of posterior elements, the preferred treatment is anterior and posterior fusion. Anterior instrumentation may improve rigidity of the surgical construct. In patients with myelodysplasia, fusion to the sacrum is invariably required because of pelvic obliquity or lack of sitting balance. Instrumentation from the pelvis (iliac fixation) to the proximal thoracic spine is preferred, as with many neuromuscular deformities.

The lack of posterior elements in the myelodysplastic spine can lead to congenital kyphosis. Although kyphosis in these patients does not compromise neurologic function, it can lead to pressure sores over the prominent area. The treatment of choice for this problem is posterior kyphectomy and fusion. The neural elements can be cut and tied off at the site of the kyphotic deformity since the patient usually has no neurologic function below the kyphus.

Banit DM, Iwinski HJ Jr, Talwalkar V, et al: Posterior spinal fusion in paralytic scoliosis and myelomeningocele. *J Pediatr Orthop* 2001;21:117. [PMID: 11176365]

Hwang SW, Thomas JG, Blumberg TJ, et al: Kyphectomy in patients with myelomeningocele treated with pedicle screw-only constructs: case reports and review. *J Neurosurg Pediatr* 2011;8:63. [PMID: 21721891]

THORACIC DISK DISEASE

Disk herniation is found much less commonly in the thoracic spine than in the cervical and lumbar spine, presumably because of the decreased mobility seen in this region with the rib cage and sternum. Herniated thoracic disks account for 1–2% of operative disks, although the reported incidence in autopsy series is 7–15%.

Patients with thoracic disk disease may present with radicular symptoms at the level of involvement and complain of back or lower extremity pain, extremity weakness, numbness corresponding to the level of the disk herniation or below, and bowel or bladder dysfunction. They may demonstrate a spastic gait, with long-tract signs, if the disk is more central. Diagnosis is made by myelography, sometimes in conjunction with CT scanning or MRI.

In the absence of long-tract signs and paraparesis, conservative measures may include rest, anti-inflammatory medications, and physical therapy, with a 70–80% success rate.

Surgical treatment is recommended for patients with signs of myelopathy, including paraparesis or hyperreflexia. Decompression is most safely performed via an anterior approach. The anterior extrapleural approach is advocated and yields good results.

When an anterior approach is used, 58–86% of patients show neurologic improvement and 72–87% experience pain relief. Neurologic deterioration is reported in up to 7% of patients who undergo surgery via an anterior or anterolateral approach and in 28–100% of patients who undergo posterior decompression. A major complication rate of 6.7% and a reoperation rate of 5% were reported for a minimally invasive lateral approach. Posterior laminectomies are associated with a high rate of complications, including worsening neurologic function from manipulation of the cord and incomplete decompression of an inadequately visualized disk.

Brown CW, Deffer PA Jr, Akmakjian J, et al: The natural history of thoracic disc herniation. *Spine (Phila Pa 1976)* 1992;17:97. [PMID: 1631725]

Russo A, Balamurali G, Nowicki R, et al: Anterior thoracic foraminotomy through mini-thoracotomy for the treatment of giant thoracic disc herniations. *Eur Spine J* 2012;21(Suppl 2):S212. [PMID: 22430542]

Uribe JS, Smith WD, Pimenta L, et al: Minimally invasive lateral approach for symptomatic thoracic disc herniation: initial multicenter clinical experience. *J Neurosurg Spine* 2012;16:264. [PMID: 22176427]

Vanichkachorn JS, Vaccaro AR: Thoracic disk disease: diagnosis and treatment. *J Am Acad Orthop Surg* 2000;8:159. [PMID: 10874223]

OSTEOPOROSIS AND VERTEBRAL COMPRESSION FRACTURES

Osteoporosis is characterized by a decline in overall bone mass in the axial and appendicular skeleton. The disease affects between 15 and 20 million people in the United States. Peak bone mass, attained between 16 and 25 years of age, slowly declines with age as the rate of bone resorption exceeds that of bone formation. This phenomenon occurs in both men and women and is known as senile osteoporosis. Women are also susceptible to postmenopausal osteoporosis that occurs during the 15–20 years after the onset of menopause and is directly linked to estrogen deficiency. Environmental factors also play a role in accelerating the rate of skeletal bone loss. These include chronic calcium deficiency, smoking, excessive alcohol intake, hyperparathyroidism, and inactivity. Genetic influences may also play a role.

Vertebral compression fractures are one of the most frequent manifestations of osteoporosis in the elderly (>60 years). Over 700,000 vertebral compression fractures occur each year. Fortunately, the overwhelming majority of patients are asymptomatic or become asymptomatic after a period of conservative care.

Clinical Findings

Patients with symptomatic vertebral compression fractures typically complain of axial pain localized to the fractured level. Occasionally, the patient's family notices that the patient's back is becoming increasingly rounded, and significant loss of height has occurred. This spinal deformity is known as the "dowager's hump." In general, there is no neurologic dysfunction and no radiation of the pain in any dermatomal distribution. There is often no history of significant trauma or an inciting event.

Imaging

Plain radiographs and densitometric scans are the major imaging modalities in the assessment of osteoporotic bone and their pathologic counterparts (insufficiency fractures). Dual-energy x-ray absorptiometry (DXA or DEXA) is the most useful of the densitometric imaging techniques because it carries a high degree of precision (0.5–2%) and subjects the patient to minimal amounts of radiation. It is also quite accurate for assessment of osteoporosis in both the axial and appendicular skeleton. It is important to note, however, that hypertrophic osteophytes in the spine that are radiodense can cause an inaccurate reading on the DXA and should not be used as the sole site of assessment for osteoporosis. Other imaging modalities include single-energy x-ray absorptiometry (SXA), quantitative computed tomography (QCT), and radiographic absorptiometry.

Posterior/anterior and lateral radiographs of the affected area of the spine are likely to reveal the location and severity of the osteoporotic fracture(s). In the thoracic spine, wedge compression fractures are most commonly encountered. In the lumbar spine, both compression and burst fractures can occur. Other imaging modalities include technetium bone scans and MRI scans. These studies should be reserved for the evaluation of fractures that remain symptomatic or progress after a course of conservative treatment. MRI is extremely useful in differentiating nonunited fractures from

those that have healed and in differentiating osteoporotic fractures from those caused by malignancy.

Bone biopsy is indicated if a metabolic bone disease or a malignancy is suspected as the cause of the osteoporosis. The sample, typically retrieved from the anterior iliac crest or from the vertebral body at the time of vertebral augmentation, is examined using bone histomorphometry.

Treatment

Prevention still remains the best treatment for osteoporosis. Maximizing bone mineral density prior to the onset of bone loss and minimizing the bone loss that occurs is the optimal regimen to prevent the painful sequelae of the disease. In women, estrogen replacement therapy can be initiated if there is no history of breast cancer, thromboembolic disease, or endometrial disease. Routine gynecologic examination is necessary once therapy is initiated. Calcitonin therapy can be used if estrogen therapy is contraindicated. Parathyroid hormone is currently under clinical trials for the treatment of osteoporosis. Early evidence suggests that it may help to increase skeletal bone mass significantly and may be useful as a first-line treatment for severe osteoporosis.

The bisphosphonates, etidronate and alendronate, prevent osteoclastic resorption of bone. They are the only FDA-approved compounds in widespread use that increase bone mineral density. However, the increase is relatively small. The use of chronic continuous bisphosphonate therapy has been linked to insufficiency fractures of the proximal femur.

The initial treatment of symptomatic vertebral compression fractures involves a trial of analgesic therapy and bracing for comfort. Evaluation and treatment for osteoporosis can be initiated if not done already. Conservative therapy should be attempted for at least 6–12 weeks or longer if the patient is improving.

Surgical Treatment

Patients who have fractures that cause neurologic deficits or significant spinal cord compression should be treated with anterior decompression and fusion followed by posterior segmental instrumentation and fusion. The poor bone quality makes correction of deformity and maintenance of posterior only constructs a challenging task (Figure 4-27).

Patients who have recalcitrant back pain from a nonunited vertebral compression fracture and have failed a course of conservative management can obtain excellent symptomatic relief from fracture stabilization through injection of PMMA bone cement into the fracture through a percutaneous technique. The two most popular procedures, vertebroplasty and kyphoplasty, are both safe and efficacious. In both techniques, a cannula is inserted intrapedicularly or extrapedicularly (lateral to the pedicle) into the anterior portion of the affected vertebral body, and acrylic cement is instilled into the fractured bone under fluoroscopic control. Once the cement cures, the fracture is immediately stabilized.

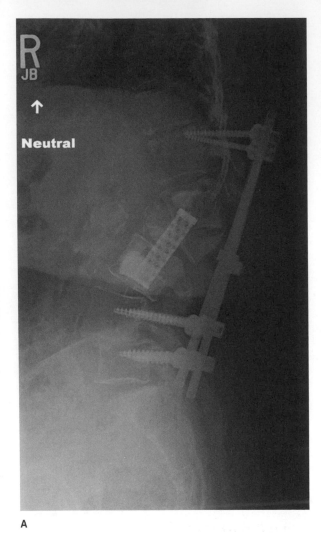

A

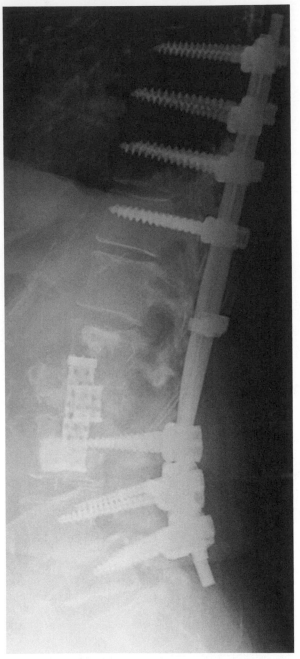

B

▲ **Figure 4–27.** Complex revision osteotomy surgery. A 65-year-old woman with incapacitating back and leg pain after two failed prior operations done at an outside hospital for an osteoporotic burst fracture. (**A**) Preoperative lateral x-ray demonstrates pullout of the screw construct, multiple nonunions, sagittal imbalance, and inability to walk due to pain. She underwent third-time revision decompression, complete removal of the L2 vertebral body (vertebral column resection [VCR]), and revision instrumentation and fusion, all done through a posterior approach. This procedure allows for shortening of the spinal column and correction of kyphotic deformity. (**B**) Postoperative lateral x-ray demonstrates markedly improved alignment. Patient was able to walk with minimal pain.

In the kyphoplasty technique, a balloon is inflated in the vertebral body in an attempt to compress the existing bone, create a void for instillation of more viscous cement under lower pressure, and correct the wedge deformity. This technique has the theoretical advantage of allowing some deformity correction and preventing high-pressure-related extrusion of PMMA into the spinal canal.

The mechanism of pain relief achieved through vertebroplasty and kyphoplasty is unclear. Multiple mechanisms may play a role, including fracture stabilization, denervation of pain fibers by the heat generated during the cement curing process, and neurotoxicity of the PMMA monomer. In addition, longer follow-up has raised concerns over predisposing the adjacent segment to fracture by overstiffening the affected level. These concerns are currently under active investigation.

Asenjo JF, Rossel F: Vertebroplasty and kyphoplasty: new evidence adds heat to the debate. *Curr Opin Anaesthesiol* 2012;25:577. [PMID: 22914353]

Coumans JV, Reinhardt MK, Lieberman IH: Kyphoplasty for vertebral compression fractures: 1-year clinical outcomes from a prospective study. *J Neurosurg* 2003;99(Suppl 1):44. [PMID: 12859058]

Do HM, Kim BS, Marcellus ML, et al: Prospective analysis of clinical outcomes after percutaneous vertebroplasty for painful osteoporotic vertebral body fractures. *AJNR Am J Neuroradiol* 2005;26:1623. [PMID: 16091504]

Garnier L, Tonetti J, Bodin A, et al: Kyphoplasty versus vertebroplasty in osteoporotic thoracolumbar spine fractures. Short-term retrospective review of a multicentre cohort of 127 consecutive patients. *Orthop Traumatol Surg Res* 2012;98:S112. [PMID: 22939104]

Grohs JG, Matzner M, Trieb K, et al: Minimal invasive stabilization of osteoporotic vertebral fractures: a prospective nonrandomized comparison of vertebroplasty and balloon kyphoplasty. *J Spinal Disord Tech* 2005;18:238. [PMID: 15905767]

Steinmann J, Tingey CT, Cruz G, et al: Biomechanical comparison of unipedicular versus bipedicular kyphoplasty. *Spine (Phila Pa 1976)* 2005;30:201. [PMID: 15644756]

Svedbom A, Alvares L, Cooper C, et al: Balloon kyphoplasty compared to vertebroplasty and nonsurgical management in patients hospitalised with acute osteoporotic vertebral compression fracture: a UK cost-effectiveness analysis. *Osteoporos Int* 2013;24:355. [PMID: 22890362]

▼ INJURIES OF THE CERVICAL SPINE

The cervical spine is the most mobile area of the spine, and as such, it is prone to the greatest number of injuries. Injuries to the cervical spine and spinal cord are also potentially the most devastating and life altering of all injuries compatible with life. In the United States, approximately 10,000 spinal cord injuries occur each year (about 39 per million). An estimated 80% of the victims are younger than 40 years, with the highest proportion of injuries reported in those between 15 and 35 years of age. Approximately 80% of all people who suffer from spinal column injuries are male. Falls account for 60% of injuries to the vertebral column in patients older than 75 years. In younger patients, 45% of injuries result from motor vehicle accidents, 20% from falls, 15% from sports injuries, 15% from acts of violence, and the remainder from other causes.

With the use of seat belts and air bags in motor vehicles and the advent of trauma centers and improved emergency service awareness of potential cervical injuries, fewer patients with cervical spine injuries are dying secondary to respiratory complications. The approach in treating these patients is early recognition of cervical spine injuries with rapid immobilization to prevent neurologic deterioration while the evaluation and treatment of associated injuries are carried out. After the patient is stabilized, the goals are restoration and maintenance of spinal alignment to provide stable weight bearing and facilitate rehabilitation.

▶ Identification and Stabilization of Life-Threatening Injuries

Eighty-five percent of all neck injuries requiring medical evaluation are a result of a motor vehicle accident. Many of the affected patients are multiple-trauma victims and therefore may have more urgent life-threatening conditions. The ABCs of trauma are followed in order of priority, with *a*irway, *b*reathing (ventilation), and *c*irculation secured before further evaluation proceeds. Throughout the evaluation of other body systems, the cervical spine should be presumed injured and thus immobilized. Approximately 20% of patients with cervical trauma are hypotensive upon presentation. The hypotension is neurogenic in origin in approximately 70% of cases and related to hypovolemia in 30%. Concomitant bradycardia is suggestive of a neurogenic component. Another finding suggestive of cervical spine injury is an altered sensorium secondary to head trauma or lacerations and facial fractures. Appropriate diagnosis and fluid management are critical in the early hours of postinjury management. After all life-threatening injuries are identified and stabilized, the secondary evaluation, including an extremity examination and neurologic examination, can be safely carried out.

▶ History and General Physical Examination

Details of the history of the injury should be obtained. If the patient is conscious, much of the information can be obtained directly. If not, family members or witnesses of the injury should be questioned. In the case of a motor vehicle accident, for example, pertinent questions include the following: Which part of the patient's body was the point of impact? Was the patient thrown from the car? Was there head trauma or a loss of consciousness? Were there any transient signs of paresis? Was the patient able to move any of his or her extremities at any time following the accident and before loss of function? What were the speeds of the involved motor vehicles? Was the patient restrained with a seat belt? Did an air bag deploy?

The history taken from the patient or family members should also include information about preexisting conditions such as epilepsy or seizures and about preexisting injuries. If the patient had any previous radiographic examinations, the radiographs might be useful for comparison.

It is helpful to question patients about what they are experiencing at the time of the examination. Are there areas of numbness, paresthesia, or pain? Can they move their extremities? The examiner should then proceed with the physical evaluation, beginning by observing the face and head of the patient for any areas of potential injury and attempting to determine the potential mechanism of injury. For instance, any lacerations or contusions to the forehead might indicate a hyperextension-type injury because as the head hits the windshield and stops, the body continues to move forward from the momentum of the impact. Observation should next include watching the extremities for any signs of motion. A genital examination should be performed because a sustained penile erection may be indicative of severe spinal cord injury. Then without moving the patient, palpation can be performed. Although palpation can be helpful in identifying potential levels of injury of the spine, it should not be used as the sole screening examination because false-negative results are possible.

▶ Neurologic Evaluation

A meticulous neurologic examination should be performed following the history and general physical examination.

A. Neurologic Tests

The neurologic evaluation should start with documentation of the function of the cranial nerves, working proximally to distally. Observation is particularly important in the unconscious patient. Spontaneous motion in an extremity may be a sole source of information regarding spinal cord function. Respiratory efforts made with intrathoracic musculature versus abdominal musculature are also significant. In the conscious patient who is able to follow commands, a motor

examination should be fairly straightforward. Rectal and perianal sensations should be documented because these may be the sole signs of intact distal spinal cord function.

An extensive sensory examination should also be performed with careful attention to dermatomal innervation. In the acute setting, it is useful to document sharp and dull sensations as well as proprioception. Sharp and dull sensations are carried via the lateral spinothalamic tract, whereas proprioception is carried through the posterior columns. Sharp and dull sensations are effectively tested with the sharp and blunt ends of a pen, and proprioception is tested by having the patient verify the position of the large toe and other joints as the examiner places them in dorsiflexion and plantarflexion. It proves helpful to make ink markings directly on the patient's skin to show the level of the dermatomal deficit, which decreases the chance for intraobserver or interobserver error over sequential examinations.

Reflexes should be checked bilaterally. In the upper extremity, the biceps reflex at the flexor side of the elbow evaluates the C5 nerve root, and the brachioradialis stretch reflex at the radial aspect of the forearm just proximal to the wrist checks the C6 nerve root. The triceps reflex is innervated by C7. In the lower extremity, the knee jerk reflex is innervated by L4, and the ankle jerk is innervated by S1.

The presence or absence of the four reflexes listed in Table 4–8 should be checked. The Babinski reflex (plantar reflex) is evaluated by firmly stroking the lateral plantar aspect of the foot distally and then medially over the metatarsal heads and then observing the toes. If the toes flex, the response is considered negative (normal). If the toes extend and spread, the response is considered positive (abnormal) and indicative of an upper motor neuron lesion. The bulbocavernosus reflex has its root in the S3 and S4 nerves and is evaluated by squeezing on the glans in a male patient or applying pressure to the clitoris in a female patient. This action should elicit a contraction of the anal sphincter. If a Foley catheter is in place, simply pulling on the Foley catheter can stimulate the anal sphincter contraction. The cremasteric reflex is evaluated by stroking the inner thigh and observing the scrotal sac, which should retract upward secondary to contraction of the cremasteric muscle. This function is innervated by T12 and L1. Finally, the anal wink, innervated by S2, S3, and S4, is elicited by stimulating the skin about the anal sphincter and eliciting a contraction.

Table 4–8. Evaluation of reflexes in patients with injuries of the cervical spine.

Reflex	Root	Positive Response	Significance
Babinski	Upper motor neurons	Extension and spread of toes	Upper motor neuron lesion is present
Bulbocavernosus	S3 and S4	Contraction of anal sphincter	Spinal shock is over
Cremasteric	T12 and L1	Retraction of scrotal sac	Spinal shock is over
Anal wink	S2, S3, and S4	Contraction of anal sphincter	Spinal shock is over

The presence of spinal shock causes the absence of all reflexes below the level of injury and typically lasts up to 24 hours after the injury. The bulbocavernosus reflex is the reflex that returns first (see Table 4–8), thus marking the end of spinal shock. This point has prognostic importance because recovery from a complete neurologic deficit that is still present at the end of spinal shock is extremely unlikely. A complete neurologic examination should be repeated over time as the patient is manipulated and treated.

B. Anatomic Considerations

The ability to interpret the results of a patient's neurologic examination appropriately depends on a thorough knowledge of the anatomy of the spinal cord and peripheral nerves.

Peripheral nerves are a combination of afferent fibers, which carry information from the periphery to the central nervous system, and efferent fibers, which carry information away from the central nervous system. As the peripheral nerve approaches the spinal cord, it becomes known as the spinal nerve. Prior to entering the spinal cord, the fiber splits, with the afferent fibers becoming the dorsal root or sensory root and the efferent fibers becoming the ventral root. The afferent fibers are often regrouped in various plexuses that are located between the spinal cord and the periphery. This regrouping takes place before the fibers enter the dorsal root, therefore leading to significant overlap between the dorsal root and the respective dermatomes. The implications of this anatomic fact should be kept in mind by the clinician when performing a sensory examination. For example, a sectioned peripheral nerve is demonstrated by a highly specific sensory loss in that particular area served by that nerve, whereas the clinical findings are more variable for a sectioned dorsal root.

The spinal cord is a caudal continuation of the brain, extending in an organized fashion from the foramen magnum at the base of the skull down to the proximal lumbar spine. The spinal cord has three primary functions: It provides a relay point for sensory information; it serves as a conduit for ascending sensory information and descending motor information; and it mediates body and limb movements because it contains both interneurons and motor neurons. Headed from caudal to rostral, the spinal cord is highly organized with a central butterfly-shaped area of gray matter and surrounding white matter.

The overall diameter of the spinal cord varies as a relative percentage of the spinal canal. The cord fills approximately 35% of the canal at the level of the atlas but increases to approximately 50% of the canal in the lower cervical spine. This variation results from the relative increasing and decreasing size of the spinal gray matter and spinal white matter. As the spinal roots become larger, as occurs at the base of the cervical spine, the size of the gray matter increases relative to the white matter, whereas the size of the white matter decreases linearly from cephalad to caudal.

The gray matter, so called because it appears gray on unstained cross sections, is divided into three zones: the dorsal horn, the intermediate zone, and the ventral horn. Made up predominantly of lower motor neurons, it is prominent in the cervical swellings and lumbar swellings, where axons concentrate before exiting to innervate the upper extremities and lower extremities, respectively.

The white matter derives its name from the fact that the axons in this area are myelinated, casting a white hue on unstained sections. White matter is functionally and anatomically divided into three bilaterally paired columns: the ventral columns, the lateral columns, and the dorsal columns.

The two major ascending systems that relay somatic sensory information are the dorsal columns and the anterolateral system. The ascending axon has its cell body located in the dorsal root ganglion before proceeding without synapsing through the dorsal horn at that level and then ascending along the dorsal column before synapsing at the approximate level of the medulla and crossing over to the contralateral side before proceeding to the cerebral cortex. The topography of the dorsal column is such that the sacrum and lower extremities are medial, with the trunk and cervical region being lateral. The anterolateral system carries pain and temperature sensorium. The afferent fibers have a cell body in the dorsal root ganglion and then synapse at that given level in the dorsal horn before crossing directly to the contralateral side and traveling up the spinothalamic tract.

Motor pathways originate in the cerebral cortex and travel distally to the contralateral side approximately at the level of the medulla and travel down the lateral corticospinal tract before synapsing with the lower motor neuron in the ventral horn of the gray matter. The topography of the corticospinal tract is such that the sacrum and legs lie lateral to the trunk and cervical axons. Thus, at the level of the cervical spine, the spinal cord contains both lower motor neurons traversing to the upper extremities and upper motor neurons being transmitted to the lower extremities. Therefore, injury in this area can give both upper and lower motor findings.

The anatomy of the reflex arc and especially its relationship to spinal shock should be kept in mind. The basic reflex circuitry is an afferent nerve coming from a stretch receptor through the dorsal horn of gray matter before synapsing with the lower motor neuron in the ventral horn of the gray matter, which sends a positive signal to the same muscle via an alpha motor neuron. This simple arc, however, is modulated by input from higher centers. If all descending influence is interrupted, such as would occur in a traumatic transection of the spinal cord, all reflexes are lost. This is also seen during spinal shock. If the local circuitry of the reflex arc is not disturbed, reflexes return at the end of spinal shock. The earliest reflex to return is the bulbocavernosus reflex, which typically returns within 24 hours of injury. Peripheral reflexes may take several months before they return.

C. Risk of Neurologic Damage

As mentioned earlier, the spinal cord varies in its diameter from cephalad to caudad. In the upper cervical spine, it occupies approximately a third of the spinal canal. In the lower cervical spine, it occupies approximately half of the canal. As inferred from this anatomy, the risk of neurologic damage from injury is greater in the lower cervical spine.

Cord compromise extends from two causes: mechanical destruction resulting directly from the trauma and vascular insufficiency. With vascular insufficiency, hypoxia and edema follow and result in further tissue damage. By approximately 6 hours after the trauma, axonal transport ends, and by 24 hours, cord necrosis begins.

D. Classification of Neurologic Status

1. Intact—Approximately 60% of injuries to the cervical spine result in no neurologic sequelae. In most of these cases, the injuries are in the upper cervical spine, where the ratio of the spinal cord to the spinal canal is smaller. It is obviously critical to identify unstable injuries of the cervical spine in the intact patient because the evolution of neurologic deficits is both potentially catastrophic and preventable.

2. Nerve root injuries—Eight cervical nerve roots correspond to the seven cervical vertebral bodies. Each of the first seven nerve roots exits above its respective body (the C1 nerve exiting above the C1 vertebral body, the C2 nerve exiting above the C2 body, and so forth), whereas the C8 nerve root exits through the foramen between the C7 and T1 vertebral bodies. Nerve root injuries can happen either in isolation or in conjunction with more severe spinal cord injuries. Injury to the nerve root alone may result from a compression or fracture of the lateral bone mass and thus impingement on the neural foramen. The clinical findings of a root injury would be those of a lower motor neuron lesion. If the nerve root is still intact and the ongoing pressure to the root is removed, the prognosis for recovery of nerve root function is good.

3. Incomplete versus complete neurologic injury—In the acute setting, any evidence of neurologic function distal to the level of injury is significant and defines the lesion as being incomplete rather than complete. As Lucas and Ducker reported in a prospective study published in 1979, "The less the injury, the greater the recovery," and "partial lesions partially recover, whereas complete lesions do not."

The motor and sensory examination outlined by the American Spinal Injury Association (ASIA) is the most widely accepted and utilized system to assess the impact of spinal cord injury on the patient. It involves the use of a grading system to evaluate the remaining sensory and motor function. The system allows the patients to be assessed through scales of impairment and functional independence.

The sensory level is determined by the patient's ability to perceive pinprick (using a disposable needle or safety pin) and light touch (using a cotton ball). Testing of a key point in each of the 28 dermatomes on the right and the left sides of the body and evaluation of perianal sensation are required.

The variability in sensation for each individual stimulus is graded on a three-point scale:

0 = absent

1 = impaired

2 = normal

NT = not testable

In the cervical spine, the C3 and C4 nerve roots supply sensation to the entire upper neck and chest in a cape-like distribution from the tip of the acromion to just above the nipple line. The next adjacent sensory level is the T2 dermatome. The brachial plexus, C5-T1, supplies the upper extremities.

ASIA also recommends testing of pain and deep pressure sensation in the same dermatomes as well as an evaluation of proprioception by testing the position sense of the index fingers and great toes on each side.

The motor level is determined by manual testing of a key muscle in the 10 paired myotomes from rostral to caudal. The strength of each muscle is graded on a six-point scale:

0 = total paralysis

1 = palpable or visible contraction

2 = full range of motion of the joint powered by the muscle with gravity eliminated

3 = full range of motion of the joint powered by the muscle against gravity

4 = active movement with full range of motion against moderate resistance

5 = normal strength

NT = not testable

For myotomes that are not clinically testable by manual muscle evaluation, the motor level is presumed to be the same as the sensory level (C1-C4, T2-L1, S2-S5).

ASIA also recommends evaluation of diaphragmatic function (via fluoroscopy, C4 level) and the abdominal musculature (via the Beevor sign, which is the upward migration of the umbilicus from upper abdominal contraction in the absence of lower abdominal contraction due to paralysis at the T10 level). Evaluation of medial hamstring and hip adductor strength is also recommended but not required.

E. Clinical Features of Spinal Cord Syndromes

Combining the findings on examination with knowledge of the cross-sectional anatomy of the spinal cord allows the examiner to identify specific injury patterns (Figure 4–28).

1. Central cord syndrome—The most common of the incomplete cord syndromes is the central cord syndrome, which occurs most frequently in elderly (>65 years) people with underlying degenerative spondylosis but can also be found in younger people who have had a severe hyperextension

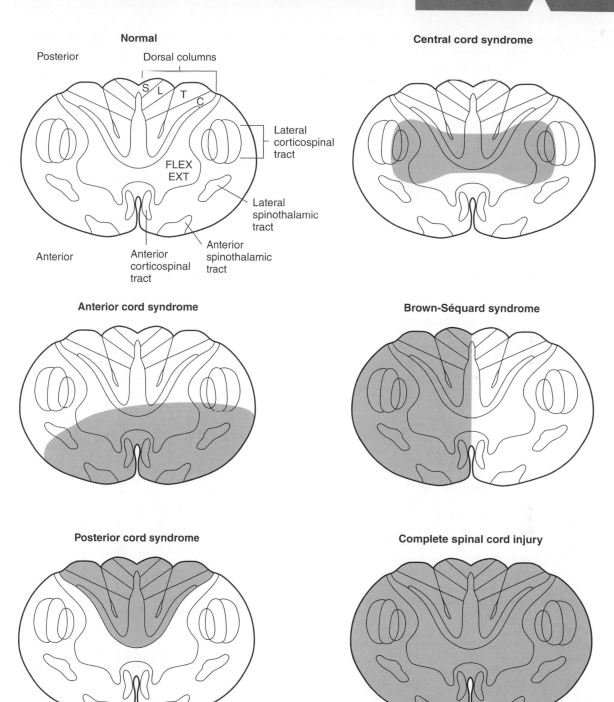

▲ **Figure 4–28.** Diagrams illustrating cross-sectional views of the normal and injured spinal cord. The diagram of the normal spinal column shows the segmental arrangement (C, cervical; L, lumbar; S, sacral; T, thoracic) and the area of flexors and extensors (FLEX and EXT). Central cord syndrome, anterior cord syndrome, Brown-Séquard syndrome, and posterior cord syndrome are incomplete injuries, with affected areas shaded. In complete spinal cord injury, all areas are affected.

injury with or without evidence of a fracture, known as spinal cord injury without radiographic abnormality (SCIWORA). Central cord syndrome is defined by ASIA as a clinical presentation characterized by "dissociation in degree of motor weakness with lower limbs stronger than upper limbs and sacral sensory sparing." The syndrome typically occurs following a hyperextension injury and is thought to be caused by an expanding hematoma or edema forming in the central aspect of the spinal cord. Central cord syndrome can be quite variable in presentation and in recovery. A mild presentation may consist of a slight burning sensation in the upper extremities, whereas a severe central cord syndrome includes motor impairment in both the upper and lower extremities, bladder dysfunction, and a variable sensory deficit below the level of injury. The pattern of clinical presentation is directly related to the cross-sectional anatomy of the spinal cord. Because the lower extremity and sacral tracts of the spinothalamic and corticospinal tracts are lateral, these areas are often spared in central cord syndrome. In cases in which they are involved, they are the areas whose function returns first. The upper extremity deficit is caused by a lesion in the gray matter, and the damage here is largely irreversible.

From 50 to 75% of patients with central cord lesions show some neurologic improvement, but the amount of improvement varies considerably among patients. The usual order in which motor function recovery occurs is as follows: return of lower extremity strength, return of bladder function, return of upper extremity strength, and return of intrinsic function of the hand.

2. Anterior cord syndrome—The patient with an anterior cord syndrome typically presents with immediate paralysis and loss of pain and temperature sensation. Both the spinothalamic and corticospinal tracts are located in the anterior aspect of the spinal cord and are therefore involved. With the dorsal columns preserved, the patient still has intact proprioception and vibratory sense as well as intact sensation to deep pressure. This clinical presentation is the most common in the younger (<35 years) trauma victim. The mechanism of injury is typically a flexion injury to the cervical spine. It is usually associated with an identifiable lesion of the cervical spine, most commonly a vertebral body burst fracture or a herniated disk. Return of useful motor function is reported in only 10–16% of patients with anterior cord syndrome. The prognosis is slightly improved, however, if evidence of spinothalamic tract function is present early.

3. Brown-Séquard syndrome—Patients with this syndrome have a motor weakness on the ipsilateral side of the lesion and a sensory deficit on the contralateral side caused by a functional hemisection of the spinal cord. For example, a cervical lesion on the right side of the spinal cord disrupts the ipsilateral corticospinal tract, which is the tract that carries motor function to the right side of the body distal to the level of the lesion. The right spinothalamic tract is also disrupted. This tract carries pain and temperature fibers from the contralateral side of the body distal to the level of injury. Position sense and vibratory sense, which are carried in the posterior column, have not yet crossed the midline; therefore, these sensory functions are disrupted on the ipsilateral side of the injury.

Brown-Séquard syndrome may result from a closed rotational injury such as a fracture-dislocation or may result from a penetrating trauma such as a stab wound or from iatrogenic injury while placing surgical instruments within the spinal canal. The prognosis in cases resulting from a closed injury is quite favorable, with 90% of patients regaining function of the bowel and bladder as well as the ability to walk.

4. Posterior cord syndrome—The posterior cord syndrome is the least common of the incomplete syndromes and typically a result of an extension-type injury. Its clinical presentation is one of loss of position and vibratory sense below the level of injury secondary to disruption of the dorsal columns. With these deficits as isolated findings, the prognosis for recovery of ambulation and function of the bowel and bladder is excellent.

5. Complete spinal cord injury—A complete neurologic deficit is characterized by a total absence of sensation and voluntary motor function caudal to the level of spinal cord injury in the absence of spinal shock. Initial evaluation must rule out any evidence of sacral sparing and the presence of a bulbocavernosus reflex. In the absence of sacral sparing and with the return of the bulbocavernosus reflex, which typically occurs within 24 hours, the spinal cord injury is termed complete and there is virtually no likelihood of functional spinal cord recovery. Affected patients may gain some root function about the level of the injury—a phenomenon called root escape because this damage to nerve roots is a peripheral nerve injury. Although the presence of root escape should not be taken as a potential return of spinal cord function, it can significantly improve the patient's rehabilitation efforts because vital function of the upper extremities may be regained.

▶ Imaging Studies

A. Radiography

1. Screening radiograph—A lateral radiograph of the cervical spine may be the only screening tool obtained upon initial radiographic evaluation of the multiple-trauma patient. This radiograph must be carefully reviewed. Should a patient present with a complete neurologic injury or a densely affected incomplete neurologic injury indicating a traumatically malaligned cervical spine, closed reduction of the cervical spine should be urgently attempted with axial traction through Gardner-Wells tongs. Once the patient is fully evaluated and life-threatening injuries are stabilized, secondary diagnostic studies can then be undertaken. If the patient is fully alert, has full pain-free rotational range of motion, no palpable tenderness, and no other injuries, the cervical spine can be cleared on clinical grounds.

2. Subsequent plain radiographs—Full radiographic evaluation of the cervical spine with plain radiographs includes lateral, AP, open-mouth (odontoid), right oblique, and left oblique views. The lateral radiograph, if adequate, visualizes approximately 85% of significant cervical spine injuries. It must display the base of the skull with all seven cervical vertebrae, as well as the proximal half of the T1 vertebral body. If the C7-T1 junction is not visualized, a repeat radiograph should be done with axial traction on the upper extremities caudally to attempt to visualize the C7-T1 junction. If this is unsuccessful, a swimmer's view, which is a transthoracic lateral with the patient's arm fully abducted, should be taken. If this plain radiograph is not satisfactory and if suspicion of injury is still high, a CT scan must be obtained.

When evaluating a lateral cervical spine radiograph, the clinician should first evaluate the bony anatomy. Four lines or curves should be kept in mind (Figure 4–29). The anterior spinal line and the posterior spinal line are imaginary lines drawn from the anterior cortex and posterior cortex, respectively, of the cervical vertebral body from C2 all the way down to T1. The spinal laminar curve is an imaginary line drawn from the posterior aspect of the foramen magnum connecting the anterior cortex of each successive spinous process. These three lines (labeled A, B, and C in Figure 4–29) should have a gentle, continuous lordotic curve with no areas of acute angulation. The fourth line (labeled D in Figure 4–29) is known as the basilar line of Wackenheim, and it is drawn along the posterior surface of the clivus and should thus be tangent to the posterior cortex of the tip of the odontoid process. After the clinician examines the radiograph in terms of these four lines or curves, he or she should look at the individual vertebral bodies to see if there is loss of height of any of them or if a rotational deformity is present with alterations in the alignment of the facets.

The evaluation of soft tissues can also prove valuable diagnostically. Prevertebral soft tissues have an upper limit of normal width beyond which a prevertebral hematoma indicative of vertebral injury can be suspected. The upper limits of normal are 11 mm at C1, 6 mm at C2, 7 mm at C3, and 8 mm at C4. The measurements below C4 become more variable and therefore less reliable clinically.

The AP view of the cervical spine is at first a confusing projection to those who are unfamiliar with cervical anatomy, yet careful attention to bony detail in the AP view can be of significant diagnostic aid in picking up subtle injuries. The bony and soft-tissue anatomy seen on the AP projection should be symmetric. The spinous processes should be equally spaced because a single level of increased intraspinous process distance suggests posterior instability. Abrupt malalignment of the spinous processes suggests a rotatory injury such as a unilateral facet dislocation. After checking for these problems, the clinician should inspect the lateral

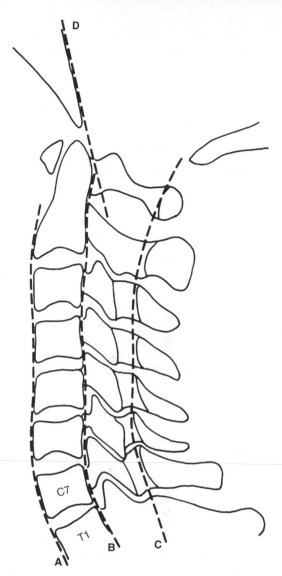

▲ **Figure 4–29.** Diagram illustrating normal lines and curves in the bony anatomy of the cervical spine. The anterior spinal line (line A), the posterior spinal line (line B), and the spinal laminar curve (line C) should have a gentle, continuous lordotic curve. The basilar line of Wackenheim (line D) is drawn along the posterior surface of the clivus and should thus be tangent to the posterior cortex of the tip of the odontoid process. (Reproduced, with permission, from El-Khoury GY, Kathol MH: Radiographic evaluation of cervical spine trauma. *Semin Spine Surg* 1991;3:3.)

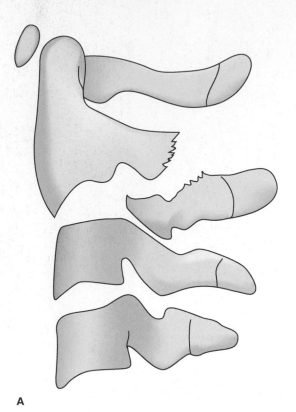

A

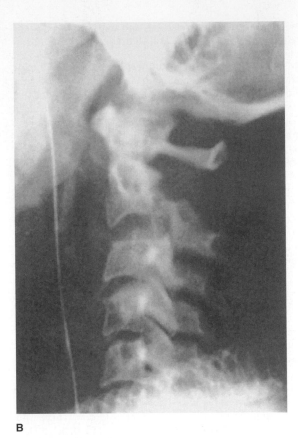

B

▲ **Figure 4–30.** **(A)** Diagram illustrating an increase of the C2-C3 interdisk space in a patient with type IIA traumatic spondylolisthesis. **(B)** Radiograph demonstrating an increased space. (Reproduced, with permission, from Levine AM, Rhyne AL: Traumatic spondylolisthesis of the axis. *Semin Spine Surg* 1991;3:47.)

masses. The facet joints are typically angled away from the vertical and therefore not clearly seen on the AP projection. If, however, the facet joint can be seen at a particular level, this is indicative of a fracture through the lateral masses and a rotational malalignment of the facet.

The open-mouth (odontoid) view is the projection most useful for looking at C1-C2 anatomy. It permits visualization of both the dens in the AP plane and the lateral masses of C1 on C2.

The right and left oblique views can be taken of the cervical spine with the patient in the supine position. These views are useful as confirmatory studies in ruling in or out lateral mass injuries.

3. Stress radiographs—Two techniques are used in obtaining cervical stress radiographs. The first is to apply axial distraction to the cervical spine through a halo or traction device and obtain a lateral radiograph. This technique should be carefully performed in the presence of a physician and only after gross instabilities of the cervical spine are ruled out. Serial lateral radiographs are taken as weight

is sequentially added, reaching an amount equivalent to approximately a third of body weight or 30 kg, depending on the level of suspected injury. Occult instability can be inferred by noting an interspace angulation of at least 11 degrees or an interspace separation of at least 1.7 mm (Figure 4–30).

The second technique, which should only be performed in a fully alert and cooperative patient, is used to obtain flexion-extension lateral radiographs that are helpful in the diagnosis of late instability. The technique is to have the patient flex the head forward as far as possible while a lateral radiograph is taken and then to have the patient put the head in full extension while another radiograph is taken. Findings presumptive of instability are facet subluxation, forward subluxation of 3.5 cm of one vertebral body on the next, and interbody angulation of greater than 11 degrees.

B. Computed Tomography

CT scanning is the most useful means for definitive delineation of bony fracture anatomy. Its advantages are its ready availability and its ability to be performed with a minimal amount of patient manipulation. CT scans provide excellent axial detail, and if thin enough sections are taken, the computer can reconstruct images in sagittal, coronal, or oblique planes. CT scans can now even be reformatted into a three-dimensional construct for excellent visualization of the bony anatomy.

C. Magnetic Resonance Imaging

MRI is the most effective way to evaluate the soft-tissue component of cervical trauma. The major advantage of MRI is that it can visualize occult disk herniation, hematoma, or edema about the spinal cord, as well as ligamentous injury. Current disadvantages are that MRI is disrupted by metallic objects, so these should be removed from the area of examination, and it also requires a prolonged amount of time to perform, therefore making close monitoring of the acutely ill patient difficult.

▶ Diagnostic Checklist of Spinal Instability

The concept of spinal stability is central to the understanding and treatment of cervical spine injuries. In a broad sense, patients with injuries that are deemed unstable require surgical intervention, whereas those deemed to have stable injury patterns can be treated nonoperatively. Spinal injuries, however, are not readily divided into unstable and stable injuries, and in actuality, they fall along a spectrum of spinal instability.

White and Panjabi's diagnostic checklist of spinal instability (Table 4–9) has nine categories, each of which is assigned a point value. If a total of 5 points is present in a given patient, the injury is deemed unstable.

Holdsworth's two-column theory of spine stability, as well as Denis's three-column theory, proposed for application to the thoracolumbar spine, are also applied to the cervical spine in an attempt to better predict stability in the neck.

▶ General Principles of Managing Acute Injuries of the Cervical Spine

Management of acute cervical spine injury is predicated on two principles: protection of the uninjured spinal cord and prevention of further damage to the injured spinal cord. This is accomplished by following spine precaution principles from the very onset of medical care, starting at the accident scene. The cervical spine should be considered injured until proven otherwise and securely immobilized before the patient is transported to a medical center. The equipment for initial immobilization should not be removed until the definitive means of immobilization can be put in place or the cervical spine is cleared of injury. Use of a spinal board, with the patient's head taped to the board and held between two sandbags, is the most secure form of immobilization readily available in the field. This technique can be

Table 4–9. White and Panjabi's diagnostic checklist of spinal instability.

Checklist Category	Description	Point Value[a]
1	Disruption of the anterior elements, with >25% loss of height	2
2	Disruption of the posterior elements	2
3	Sagittal plane translation of >3.5 mm or >20% of the anteroposterior diameter of the vertebral body	2
4	Intervertebral sagittal rotation of >11 degrees	2
5	Intervertebral distance of >1.7 mm on a stretch test	2
6	Evidence of cord damage	2
7	Evidence of root damage	1
8	Acute intervertebral disk space narrowing	1
9	Anticipated abnormally large stress	1

[a]If a total of 5 points is present in a given patient, the injury is deemed unstable.
Modified and reproduced, with permission, from White AA III, Panjabi MM: Update on the evaluation of instability of the lower cervical spine. *Instr Course Lect* 1987;36:513.

supplemented by a Philadelphia collar. When the medical center is reached, if a definitive cervical spine injury is identified and deemed unstable, skeletal traction for immobilization, reduction, or both may be applied. Gardner-Wells traction is easily applied and adequate for axial traction. Halo traction affords the added advantage of four-point fixation and thus controlled traction in three planes. Prior to application of traction, it is important to make sure that the patient does not have an occipitocervical dislocation. In these cases, application of traction can lead to worsening of the dislocation and neurologic injury. These specific cases should be treated with immediate application of a halo vest. Halo traction can also be easily converted at a later time to halo-vest immobilization.

Among the various agents that show potential benefits in laboratory studies of models of spinal cord injury are corticosteroids, opiate receptor antagonists (such as naloxone or thyrotropin-releasing hormone), and diuretics (such as mannitol). The National Acute Spinal Cord Injury Studies (NASCIS) II and III reported neurologic improvement with steroid treatment given within 8 hours of injury. Those treated within 3 hours did best; those treated between hours 3 and 8 only did better by extending to 48 hours of treatment. Criticism of the NASCIS studies called to question the validity of the conclusions, and many professional organizations downgraded their enthusiasm for the use of methylprednisolone in the patient with the acutely injured spinal cord. However, many hospitals still use the protocol in blunt trauma cord injuries if the medicine can be administered within 3 hours of the injury. The recommended dosage of methylprednisolone in an acute setting is 30 mg/kg given as a bolus and followed by 5.4 mg/kg/h for 24 hours. However, some thought should be given to its use because, for example, the Congress of Neurological Surgeons stated that steroid therapy "should only be undertaken with the knowledge that the evidence suggesting harmful side effects is more consistent than any suggestion of clinical benefit."

Cripps RA, Lee BB, Wing P, et al: A global map for traumatic spinal cord injury epidemiology: towards a living data repository for injury prevention. *Spinal Cord* 2011;49:493. [PMID: 21102572]

Denis F: The three-column spine and its significance in the classification of acute thoracolumbar spinal injuries. *Spine (Phila Pa 1976)* 1983;8:817. [PMID: 6670016]

Ito Y, Sugimoto Y, Tomioka M, et al: Does high dose methylprednisolone sodium succinate really improve neurological status in patient with acute cervical cord injury? A prospective study about neurological recovery and early complications. *Spine (Phila Pa 1976)* 2009;34:2121. [PMID: 19713878]

White AA III, Panjabi MM: Update on the evaluation of instability of the lower cervical spine. *Instr Course Lect* 1987;36:513. [PMID: 3437146]

INJURIES OF THE UPPER CERVICAL SPINE

With the exception of occipitoatlantal dissociation, traumatic injuries to the upper cervical spine are less frequently associated with significant neurologic injury than are traumatic injuries to the lower cervical spine. This is secondary to the fact that the spinal cord occupies only a third of the upper spinal canal versus a half of the lower spinal canal.

▶ Occipitoatlantal Dissociation

Occipitoatlantal dissociation is a disruption of the cranial vertebral junction, and it implies a subluxation or complete dislocation of the occipitoatlantal facets. This injury is typically fatal, yet the clinician must be aware of it because unrecognized occipitoatlantal dissociation may have catastrophic results. The mechanism of dissociation is poorly understood, but it most likely results from either a severe flexion or distraction type of injury. Anterior translation of the skull on the vertebral column is a common presentation and most likely a hyperflexion injury. Bucholz, however, presented the pathologic anatomic findings of fatal occipitoatlantal dissociation and proposed a mechanism of hyperextension with resultant distractive force applied across the craniovertebral junction.

When the dissociation is a frank dislocation, the findings are clear on a lateral radiograph. When the dissociation is a subluxation, however, findings may be more subtle. In normal individuals, the distance between the tip of the dens and the basion (the anterior aspect of the foramen magnum) should be no greater than 1.0 cm, and the previously described Wackenheim line should run from the base of the basion tangentially to the tip of the dens. If the dens penetrates this line, anterior translation of the cranium is implied.

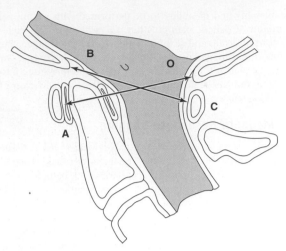

▲ **Figure 4–31.** Diagram showing lines used in the calculation of the Powers ratio, which is helpful in diagnosing occipitoatlantal dissociation. The distance between the basion (point B) and the posterior arch (point C) is divided by the distance between the anterior arch of C1 (point A) and the opisthion (point O). The normal ratio of BC to AO is 1:1. A ratio of greater than 1 suggests the head is dislocated anteriorly on the spine.

Calculation of the Powers ratio can also be helpful in securing the diagnosis. Powers and his colleagues described a ratio of two lines (Figure 4–31), the first of which runs from the tip of the basion to the midpoint of the posterior lamina of the atlas (line BC) and the second of which runs from the anterior arch of C1 to the opisthion (line AO). When the ratio of BC to AO is greater than 1:1, anterior occipitoatlantal dissociation is present. Other radiographic signs include marked soft-tissue swelling and the presence of avulsion fractures at the occipitovertebral junction.

Early recognition and surgical stabilization are the mainstays of treatment in cases of occipitoatlantal dissociation.

▶ Fractures of Vertebra C1 (Atlas Fractures)

The mechanism of injury in the fracture of the atlas is most typically axial compression with or without extension force, and the anatomic findings of the fracture are indicative of the specifics of the force and the position of the head at the time of impact. In 1920, Jefferson presented his classic description of the four-part fracture of the atlas following an axial injury. This fracture is a burst type that occurs secondary to the occipital condyles being driven into the interior portions of the ring of the atlas and driving the lateral masses outward, resulting in a two-part fracture of the anterior ring of the atlas as well as a two-part fracture of the posterior ring. More common than the classic four-part atlas fracture, however, are the two-part and three-part fractures. Isolated anterior arch fractures are the least common, and they are

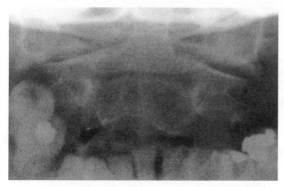

▲ **Figure 4–32.** Open-mouth (odontoid) radiographic view demonstrating asymmetry of the lateral masses of C1 on C2 with overhang in a patient with a Jefferson fracture. (Reproduced, with permission, from El-Khoury GY, Kathol MH: Radiographic evaluation of cervical spine trauma. *Semin Spine Surg* 1991:3:3.)

typically associated with fractures of the dens, whereas the more common posterior arch fracture is typically the result of a hyperextension injury.

A fracture of the atlas is typically diagnosed on plain radiographs. Findings may be subtle on the lateral cervical spine radiograph. The open-mouth (odontoid) view may show asymmetry of the lateral masses of C1 on C2 with overhang (Figure 4–32). A bilateral overhang totaling more than 6.9 mm is presumptive evidence of a disruption to the transverse ligament and suggests potential late instability. Presumptive evidence for transverse ligament disruption can also be seen on the lateral radiograph if the ADI is greater than 4 mm.

The treatment for fractures of the atlas as isolated injuries is typically nonoperative (Figure 4–33). If there are signs of transverse ligament disruption, halo traction is indicated with later transfer to halo-vest immobilization for a total of 3–4 months. Immediate halo-vest application is indicated in cases involving a moderately displaced fracture with lateral mass overhang up to 5 mm, although collar immobilization is preferred in cases involving a minimally displaced fracture of the atlas. At completion of bony union, flexion-extension views should be obtained to rule out any evidence of late instability. If late instability is present and the bony elements were allowed to heal, a limited C1-C2 fusion can address the instability. If a nonunion is present or if the posterior arch remains disrupted, an occiput to C2 fusion is necessary to control the late instability.

▶ Dislocations and Subluxations of Vertebrae C1 and C2

A. Atlantoaxial Rotatory Subluxation

Atlantoaxial rotatory subluxation is most common in children and may be associated with minimal trauma or even

occur spontaneously. Although some patients are asymptomatic, others present with neck pain or torticollis (a position in which the head is tilted toward one side and rotated toward the other). Inasmuch as the mechanism of injury is often unclear, the propensity for the C1-C2 location is based on anatomic factors. In approximately 50% of cases, cervical spine rotation occurs at the C1-C2 junction, where the facet joints are more horizontal and less inherently stable in rotation.

The diagnosis of atlantoaxial rotatory subluxation is typically suspected on the basis of radiographs taken in several views. The odontoid view may show displacement of the lateral masses with respect to the dens; a lateral view may show an increased ADI; and the AP view may show a lateral shift of the spinous process of C1 on C2. CT scanning can be used to confirm the diagnosis, and a dynamic CT scan with full attempted right and left rotation can demonstrate a fixed deformity.

There are four types of atlantoaxial rotatory subluxations. In type I, the ADI is less than 3 mm, which suggests the transverse ligament is still intact. In type II, the interval is 3–5 mm, which suggests the transverse ligament is not structurally intact. In type III, the interval exceeds 5 mm, which is indicative of disruption of the transverse ligament as well as secondary stabilization of the alar ligament. In type IV, there is a complete posterior dislocation of the atlas on the axis, a finding typically associated with a hypoplastic odontoid process such as that seen in several forms of mucopolysaccharidosis (eg, the Morquio syndrome).

Treatment of atlantoaxial subluxation is typically conservative, consisting of traction followed by immobilization. Approximately 90% of patients respond to this treatment regimen. There is a high incidence of recurrence, however. For patients who do not respond to conservative measures and for patients with recurrent problems, C1-C2 arthrodesis may be required to control the deformity.

B. Disruption of the Transverse Ligament

The transverse ligament and secondarily the alar ligament are the main constraints to anterior displacement of C1 on C2. It was previously presumed that because anterior subluxation of C1 on C2 typically involves a fracture through the dens, the transverse ligament is in fact stronger than the bony elements of the dens. Fielding and his colleagues, however, showed that experimentally this was not the case, yet clinically the higher association of anterior dislocation of dens fractures still holds true.

The mechanism of disruption is typically a flexion injury, and the diagnosis is made on lateral radiographs. The ADI should not exceed 3 mm in the adult. If the interval is 4 mm or larger and the dens is intact, a rupture of the transverse ligament is presumed.

High-resolution CT scan can be used to categorize this injury into two types. Type 1 is a disruption in the substance of the transverse ligament, whereas type 2 involves

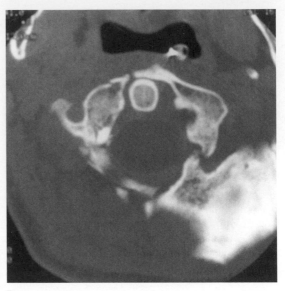

B

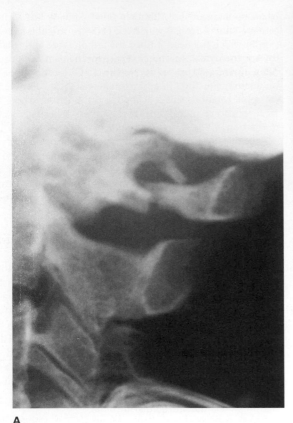

A

▲ **Figure 4–33.** Imaging studies in a patient who was in a motor vehicle accident and sustained a distractive extension injury to his cervical spine and a three-part fracture of his atlas (a Jefferson fracture). (**A**) Lateral radiographic view showing a fracture of the posterior arch. (**B**) Axial section of a CT scan further delineating the fracture anatomy. This injury was deemed stable and treated nonoperatively in a halo vest.

an avulsion fracture of the insertion of the transverse ligament on the lateral mass of C1. Type 1 injuries predictably fail conservative treatment and should be managed with a C1-C2 arthrodesis. A trial of nonoperative care in type 2 injuries using a rigid cervical orthosis may be a reasonable alternative. A 74% success rate can be anticipated, with surgery reserved for patients who fail nonoperative care, showing persistent instability after 12 weeks in mobilization.

C. Fracture of the Odontoid Process

Fracture of the odontoid process is typically associated with high-velocity trauma, and the mechanism of injury is flexion in most cases. Depending on the fracture pattern, extension may be the predominant force in a smaller subset of cases. Associated injuries, particularly fractures of the ring of the atlas, should be ruled out. Neurologic involvement is relatively rare with odontoid fractures. In a study of 60 patients

with acute fractures of the odontoid process, Anderson and D'Alonzo reported that 15 had some neurologic deficit on presentation, but only five of the 15 had major neurologic involvement, and only two of this group of five remained quadriparetic at follow-up.

Odontoid fractures may be suspected on the basis of clinical presentation and confirmed on plain radiographs, although spasm and overlying shadows can obscure the diagnosis. CT scan with sagittal and coronal reconstruction is the most sensitive study to diagnose these injuries. CT scan with axial sectioning alone may miss the horizontal fracture line typical of these injuries; thus, the reconstructions are necessary.

Both the risk of nonunion with delayed instability and the method of treating odontoid fracture depend on the classification of the fracture. Reported rates of nonunion range from 20 to 63%. According to the classification system proposed in 1974 by Anderson and D'Alonzo,

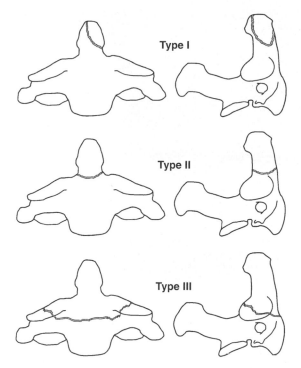

▲ Figure 4–34. Diagram showing the three types of fractures of the odontoid process.

there are three types of fracture of the odontoid process (Figure 4–34).

Type I is a fracture through the tip of the odontoid process. In this configuration, the blood supply is maintained through the base of the odontoid process and through the attachment of the alar transverse ligaments. The mechanical stability of this fracture pattern is left intact. Symptomatic care and immobilization are the treatment of choice.

Type II, the most common type, is a fracture through the base of the odontoid process at its junction with the body of the axis. In this configuration, soft-tissue attachments to the fracture fragment cause distraction at the fracture site. Because the amount of cancellous bone available for opposition is limited, a high nonunion rate is expected, particularly if displacement is significant or the patient is older (>60 years). In this case, primary surgical treatment may be indicated. Anterior screw fixation of the odontoid process is now the treatment of choice for most type II odontoid fractures. Although it is technically demanding, it does allow for the maintenance of motion at C1-C2 (Figure 4–35).

Type III is a fracture through the body of the axis. The blood supply is maintained through soft-tissue attachments, and abundant cancellous bone opposition at the fracture site facilitates a high rate of union. The treatment, therefore, is conservative, consisting of halo traction or halo-vest immobilization until bony union occurs. Although the rate

of union is acceptable, there is a relatively high rate of malunion that may limit the patient's cervical rotation.

D. Hangman's Fracture (Traumatic Spondylolisthesis of Vertebra C2)

Hangman's fracture occurs when a fracture line passes through the neural arch of the axis. The anatomy of the axis is such that the superior facets are anterior and the inferior facets are posterior, thus concentrating stress through the neural arch. Because of the high ratio of spinal canal size to spinal cord size at this level, neurologic damage associated with hangman's fracture should be unusual. However, in his postmortem studies, Bucholz reported that traumatic spondylolisthesis was second only to occipitoatlantal dislocations in cervical injuries leading to fatalities.

According to the scheme proposed by Levine and Rhyne, hangman's fractures can be classified on the basis of anatomic factors and the presumed mechanism of injury. Treatment depends on the type of fracture. Imaging studies in a patient with hangman's fracture are shown in Figure 4–36.

Type I is typically caused by hyperextension with or without additional axial load. There is no angulation of the deformity, and the fracture fragments are separated by less than 3 mm. Treatment should consist of immobilization in a cervical collar or halo vest until union occurs, which is typically 12 weeks.

Type II is thought to be caused by hyperextension and axial load with a secondary flexion component leading to displacement of the fracture. Reduction of the anterior angulation in this type of fracture is necessary and typically obtained by traction therapy and then followed by placement of a halo vest until union occurs. An atypical type II hangman's fracture is described. This fracture occurs through the posterior aspect of the vertebral body, potentially resulting in cord compromise as the anterior aspect of the vertebral body flexes forward. A higher likelihood of neurologic injury with this atypical pattern is seen, and halo-vest immobilization is recommended.

Type IIA has the same fracture pattern as type II but with a component of distraction that also occurred at the time of injury and led to disruption of the C2-C3 disk space, rendering this injury inherently unstable. Traction should be avoided in cases of type IIA fracture because it exacerbates the injury. Treatment should consist of immediate halo-vest application, with the patient's head positioned in slight extension to afford a reduction.

Type III includes a fracture through the neural arch, a facet dislocation, and a disruption of the C2-C3 disk space that renders the injury highly unstable. Treatment generally consists of early closed reduction of the facet dislocation and application of a halo vest to maintain the reduction. If the reduction cannot be obtained in a closed fashion or cannot be maintained conservatively, treatment with open reduction of the dislocation and anterior or posterior fusion is indicated.

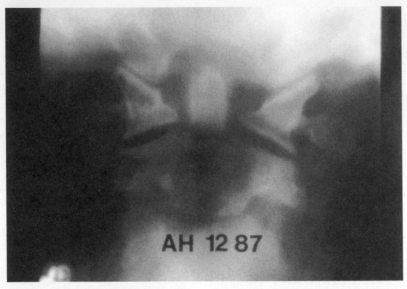

A

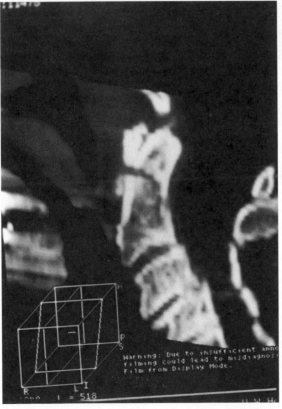

B

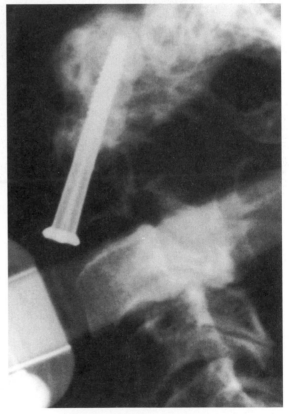

C

▲ **Figure 4–35.** Imaging studies in a patient with a type II odontoid fracture nonunion. (**A**) Open-mouth radiographic view showing the fracture line at the base of the odontoid process. (**B**) Sagittal reconstruction using CT scanning to better delineate the fracture anatomy. (**C**) Radiograph taken after the patient underwent anterior placement of two odontoid screws under fluoroscopic control using a cannulated screw system.

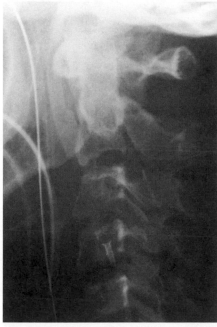

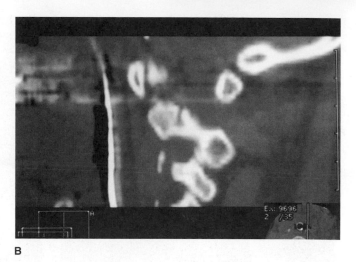

B

A

▲ **Figure 4–36.** Imaging studies in a patient who was in a motor vehicle accident and sustained a hangman's fracture, or traumatic spondylolisthesis of C2. (**A**) Lateral radiographic view, which is largely unremarkable. (**B**) Sagittal reconstruction using CT scanning to better delineate the fracture site at the base of the posterior elements. The patient was treated nonoperatively.

Anderson LD, D'Alonzo RT: Fractures of the odontoid process of the axis. *J Bone Joint Surg Am* 1974;56:1663. [PMID: 4434035]

Hsu WK, Anderson PA: Odontoid fractures: update on management. *J Am Acad Orthop Surg* 2010;18:383. [PMID: 20595131]

Huybregts JG, Jacobs WC, Vleggeert-Lankamp CL: The optimal treatment of type II and III odontoid fractures in the elderly: a systematic review. *Eur Spine J* 2013;22:1. [PMID: 22941218]

Ramieri A, Domenicucci M, Landi A, et al: Conservative treatment of neural arch fractures of the axis: computed tomography scan and x-ray study on consolidation time. *World Neurosurg* 2011;75:314. [PMID: 21492736]

INJURIES OF THE LOWER CERVICAL SPINE

As stated earlier, fractures and dislocations of the lower cervical spine have a greater frequency of catastrophic neurologic involvement because of the decreased ratio of spinal canal to spinal cord in the lower levels. Treatment of affected patients again relies on early recognition of the injury, recognition of inherent stability or instability of the injury pattern, and institution of appropriate definitive care.

In 1982, Allen and colleagues developed a classification system for closed indirect fractures and dislocations of the lower cervical spine. After reviewing numerous cases previously described by other authors as well as 165 of their own cases, they grouped the injuries into six categories, based on the position of the cervical spine at the time of impact and on the dominant mode of failure. The six categories were compressive flexion, vertical compression, distractive flexion, compressive extension, distractive extension, and lateral flexion. Of these, the distractive flexion injuries were the most common, followed by the compressive extension injuries and the compressive flexion injuries. Some of the categories were further divided into stages, as described next.

▶ Compressive Flexion Injury

There are five stages of compressive flexion injuries, which are labeled compression flexion stage (CFS) I through V (Figure 4–37). CFS I shows a slight blunting and rounding to the anterior superior vertebral margin, without any evidence of posterior ligamentous damage. CFS II shows some additional loss of height of the anterior vertebral body, again sparing the posterior elements. CFS III has an additional fracture line passing from the anterior surface of the vertebral body through to the inferior subchondral plate, with minimal displacement. CFS IV has less than 3 mm of displacement of the inferior posterior vertebral fragment into the neural canal. CFS V has severe displacement of the inferior posterior fragment

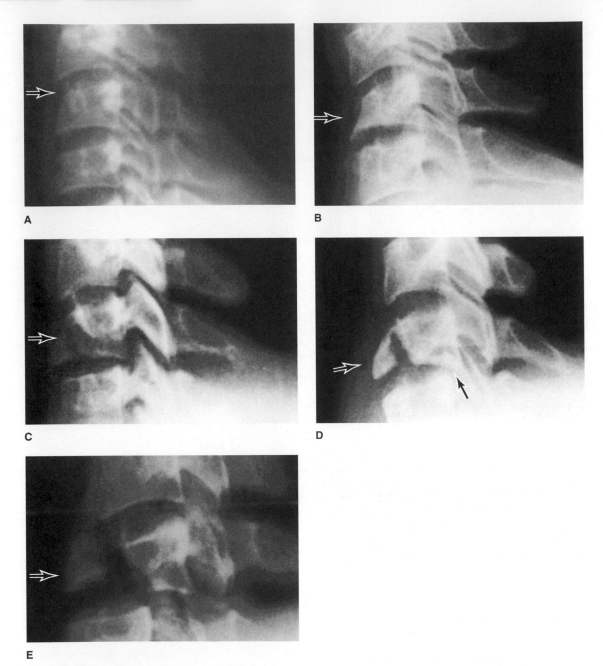

▲ **Figure 4–37.** Radiographs showing the five stages of compressive flexion injury. **A** shows compression flexion stage (CFS) I. **B** shows CFS II. **C** shows CFS III. **D** shows CFS IV. **E** shows CFS V. (Reproduced, with permission, from Allen BL, Ferguson RL, Lehmann TR, et al: A mechanistic classification of closed, indirect fractures and dislocations of the lower cervical spine. *Spine (Phila Pa 1976)* 1982;7:1.)

into the canal, with widening of the spinous processes posteriorly, indicative of three-column disruption.

Within the compressive flexion category are two types of fractures, more commonly referred to as the **compression fracture** and the **teardrop fracture.** Most compression fractures without disruption of the posterior elements are thought to be stable, so no surgical intervention is required. The more severe compression fracture injuries, however, can result in displacement of bone into the spinal canal, and if a neurologic injury is present, these require anterior decompression and stabilization. All patients should be carefully checked with flexion-extension views at the completion of their treatment to rule out any evidence of late instability.

▶ Vertical Compression Injury

Vertical compression spinal (VCS) injuries occur secondary to axial loading and are divided into three stages. VCS I consists of an endplate central fracture with no evidence of ligamentous failure. VCS II is a fracture of both vertebral endplates, again with only minimal displacement. VCS III is the more commonly termed **burst fracture** with a spectrum of fragmentation of the vertebral body, with or without posterior element disruption.

The treatment for VCS injuries is typically nonoperative. Traction is applied to obtain and maintain alignment, and bony union is generally complete after 3 months of halo-vest immobilization. Flexion-extension views should be obtained at the completion of healing because a posterior ligamentous injury can result in late instability.

▶ Distractive Flexion Injury

The category of distractive flexion spinal (DFS) injury was the most common injury category reported by Allen and colleagues, and it includes both unilateral and bilateral facet subluxation and dislocation. There are four stages of DFS injury. DFS I, termed a **flexion sprain,** is characterized by subluxation of the facet joint, with possible interspinous process widening. This injury has subtle radiographic findings and may easily be missed during initial evaluation and therefore result in late symptomatic instability (Figure 4–38).

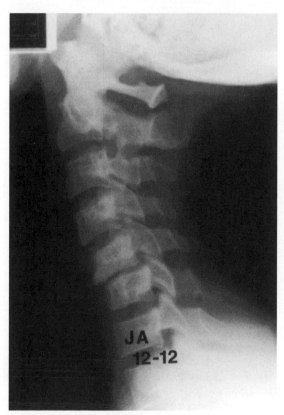

A

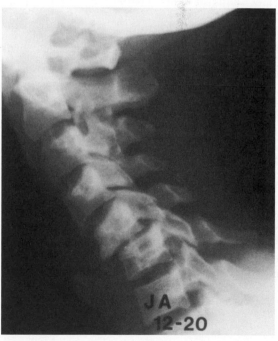

B

▲ **Figure 4–38.** Imaging studies in a patient with a distractive flexion injury of the cervical spine. **(A)** This lateral radiographic view demonstrates anterior subluxation of C5 on C6. **(B)** The follow-up radiograph shows progression of the subluxation. The patient was treated with a posterior spinal fusion of C5-C6.

DFS II is a unilateral facet dislocation, the diagnosis of which can be confirmed on plain radiographs. The lateral radiograph would reveal an anterior subluxation of one vertebra of approximately 25% of vertebral body width at the affected level. The facet itself may be perched or fully dislocated. DFS III is a bilateral facet dislocation with approximately 50% anterior dislocation at the affected level. DFS IV, which is also termed a **floating vertebra,** is a bilateral facet dislocation with displacement of a full vertebral width.

Treatment of DFS injuries depends on the severity of the injury. Achievement of anatomic alignment and spinal stability yields the best results. Patients with unilateral facet dislocation should be treated with closed reduction in the acute phase, followed by immobilization. If closed reduction is not possible, open reduction and fusion are indicated (Figure 4–39). Bilateral facet dislocations are associated with a higher incidence of both neurologic injury and instability. Treatment consisting of closed reduction and immobilization

is feasible, but because it results in a high percentage of late instability, which eventually requires posterior fusion, the use of early posterior fusion is indicated.

Another fracture pattern that should be included in the discussion on flexion injuries is the clay shoveler's fracture, which is a fracture of the spinous process, typically at level C6, C7, or T1. This is an avulsion injury that generally occurs in flexion by the counteractive forces of the muscular attachments. As an isolated injury, it is considered stable and usually treated nonoperatively.

▶ Compressive Extension Injury

The category of compressive extension (CES) injury was the second most common injury category reported by Allen and colleagues. It is divided into five stages. CES I is a fracture of the vertebral arch unilaterally, with or without displacement, and CES II is a bilateral fracture. CES III and CES IV

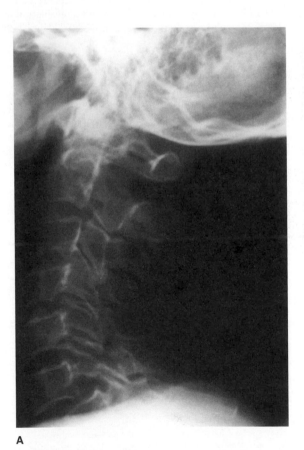

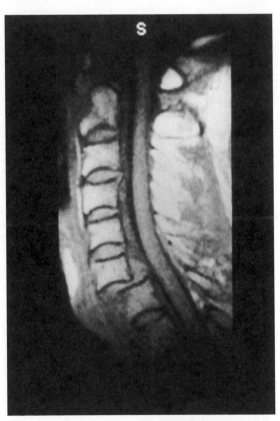

A

B

▲ **Figure 4–39.** Imaging studies in a man who fell from a height and suffered a C6-C7 fracture-dislocation with a perched facet but remained neurologically intact. (**A**) Lateral radiographic view demonstrating the fracture-dislocation at C6-C7. (**B**) MRI demonstrating the anterior subluxation of C6 on C7, with the intervertebral disk retropulsed behind the C6 vertebral body. The patient was treated with an anterior diskectomy, reduction, and fusion.

were not encountered in the series reported by Allen and colleagues but are theoretic interpolations between CES II and CES V. CES III is a bilateral fracture of the vertebral arch articular processes, lamina, or pedicle without vertebral displacement, whereas CES IV is the same fracture pattern but with moderate vertebral body displacement. Three patients in the Allen series had CES V injuries, which were bilateral vertebral arch fractures with 100% anterior displacement.

Treatment of CES injuries is related to the three-column theory. Stabilization with a posterior, anterior, or combined approach is indicated if there is significant disruption of the middle column or of two of the three columns.

▶ Distractive Extension Injury

Distractive extension (DES) injuries are typically soft-tissue lesions and divided into two stages. DES I is a disruption of the anterior ligamentous complex or, rarely, a nondisplaced fracture of the vertebral body. Radiographs may appear entirely normal. One clue to the diagnosis is widening of the disk space, which is sometimes present. DES II is a disruption of the posterior soft-tissue complex, which can allow posterior displacement of the upper vertebral body into the spinal canal. This lesion is often reduced at the time of lateral radiographs and may show only subtle or no changes on routine radiographs. When neurologic involvement is present, it is most commonly a central cord syndrome, and provided that no coexisting compression lesions are present, some neurologic recovery is expected.

The DES injury is usually stable and does not require surgical intervention. Late flexion-extension views, however, are indicated to rule out any evidence of late instability.

▶ Lateral Flexion Injury

Allen and colleagues included the injuries of five patients in the category of lateral flexion (LFS) injury. This category is further divided into two stages. LFS I is an asymmetric compression fracture of the vertebral body and ipsilateral posterior arch, with no displacement in the coronal plane. LFS II has a similar fracture pattern but with displacement in the coronal plane, which suggests ligamentous disruption on the tension side of the injury. This mechanism can lead to brachial plexus injuries of varying degrees on the distracted side.

Because of the rarity of LFS injuries, treatment protocols are not well established. Surgical stabilization should be considered if late instability is expected or if there is a neurologic deficit.

▶ Treatment Decisions

Ultimately the treating physician must decide on a treatment plan. The Allen classification, although quite useful to describe an injury, is a mechanistic system that is challenging to apply to the individual patient to assess operative indications. The decision whether to operate is based on a spectrum of spinal stability and neurologic compromise. A patient with a three-column injury, continued neurologic compression, and neurologic symptoms has a clear operative indication either through an anterior, posterior, or combined approach. A fully neurologically intact patient with a one-column injury generally does fine in a brace. Patients with injury patterns in between must be treated on a case-by-case basis.

CERVICAL STRAINS AND SPRAINS (WHIPLASH INJURY)

Cervical strains and sprains, which are commonly referred to as a whiplash injury when associated with motor vehicle accidents, can produce a protracted and confusing clinical picture. Pain is typically the one unifying feature, yet there may be numerous other complaints, including local tenderness, decreased range of motion, headaches that are typically occipital, blurred or double vision, dysphagia, hoarseness, jaw pain, difficulty with balance, and even vertigo. It is often difficult for the physician to correlate radiographic findings, diagnostic test results, and other objective findings with the subjective complaints of the patient. The constellation of symptoms is fairly uniform, however, and should certainly not be discounted, and many investigators propose an anatomic basis for the clinical complaints. McNabb proposed that paresthesias in the ulnar distribution may be secondary to spasm of the scalenus muscle, and certainly symptoms such as hoarseness and dysphagia can be related to retropharyngeal hematoma. The cervical zygapophysial joint and facet capsule are implicated as a source for chronic pain after whiplash injury.

Figure 4–40 presents an algorithm for management of cervical strain. Radiographs should be taken because the amount of neck trauma that the patient has sustained may be significant. Radiographic findings, however, may be subtle or entirely negative. Cervical lordosis may be reversed, indicating spasm. Subtle signs of instability may also be present, and these can be further delineated on flexion-extension views if symptoms persist. The prevertebral soft-tissue window should be within normal limits to rule out any prevertebral hematoma. MRI is not helpful in the acute setting to definitively diagnose whiplash injury.

Once the stability of the spine is ensured, the care of the cervical sprain or whiplash injury should be symptomatic. Initial rest, bed rest if necessary, and soft collar immobilization are indicated, along with the use of anti-inflammatory medications. Early mobilization with progressive range of motion and weaning from external supports should be encouraged, however. Frequent reassurance is often necessary because the symptoms may be long lasting. Some patients with chronic unrelenting symptoms despite maximal conservative management may benefit from facet injections and rhizotomies.

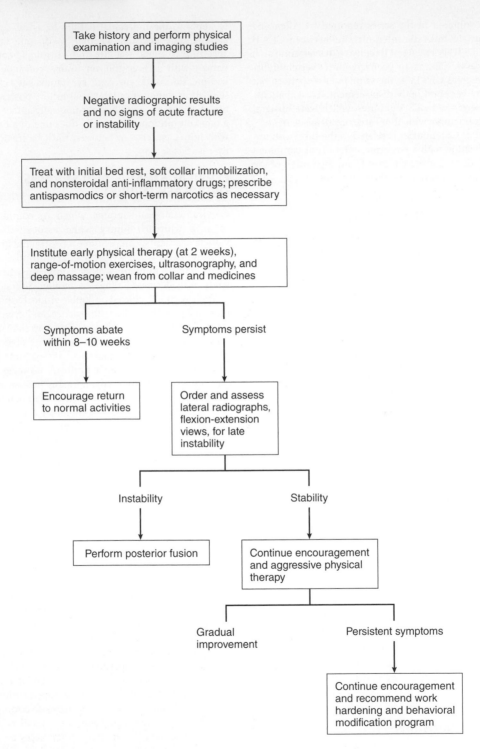

▲ **Figure 4–40.** Algorithm for management of patients with cervical strain.

Approximately 42% of patients have persistent symptoms beyond 1 year, with approximately a third having persistent symptoms beyond 2 years. Most patients who do improve do so within the first 2 months. Factors associated with a poor prognosis include the presence of occipital headaches, interscapular pain, or reversal of cervical lordosis. Women have a worse prognosis than men, and hyperextension injuries are thought to have a worse prognosis than hyperflexion injuries.

Anderson SE, Boesch C, Zimmermann H, et al: Are there cervical spine findings at MR imaging that are specific to acute symptomatic whiplash injury? A prospective controlled study with four experienced blinded readers. *Radiology* 2012;262:567. [PMID: 22187629]

McNabb I: The "whiplash syndrome." *Orthop Clin North Am* 1971;2:389. [PMID: 5150390]

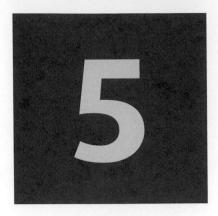

Musculoskeletal Oncology

R. Lor Randall, MD, FACS

Russell Ward, MD

Bang H. Hoang, MD

Musculoskeletal oncology is a field of medicine that involves the diagnosis and management of neoplastic conditions affecting the musculoskeletal system. This not only entails neoplasia of mesenchymal origin (derived from embryonic mesoderm), but also metastatic carcinoma and a variety of pseudotumorous conditions. Mesenchymal tumors are an extremely heterogeneous group of neoplasms including over 200 benign conditions and 90 types of sarcoma, and so the majority of this chapter is dedicated to them. The relative incidence of benign to malignant disease is 200:1. These tumors are classified histomorphologically based on features of differentiation, but there is considerable overlap. It is favorable to consider these separate conditions as points on a continuum, rather than entirely distinct entities. Classification, nevertheless, is important because it may yield insight to the behavior, treatment response, and overall prognosis. Benign disease, by definition, behaves in a nonaggressive fashion and exhibits little tendency to locally recur or metastasize. Sarcomas (malignant tumors of mesenchymal origin), however, can be rapidly destructive, have metastatic potential, and have a tendency to locally recur.

Neoplastic processes arise in tissues of mesenchymal origin far less frequently than those of ectodermal or endodermal origin. In 2004, soft-tissue and bone sarcomas had an annual incidence in the United States of just more than 8600 and 2400 new cases, respectively. When compared with the overall cancer mortality of 563,000 cases per year in 2004, sarcomas are a small fraction of the problem. However, although they are a relatively uncommon form of cancer, these tumors behave in an aggressive fashion, with currently reported mortality rates in some series of greater than 50%. According to the National Cancer Institute's Surveillance, Epidemiology, and End Results (SEER) program, approximately 8600 new soft-tissue sarcomas developed in the United States in 2004 with over 3600 sarcoma-related deaths. The associated morbidity is much higher. These tumors inflict a tremendous emotional and financial toll on individuals and society alike. Furthermore, sarcomas preferentially affect older patients, with only 15% occurring in patients younger than 15 years and 40% in patients older than 55 years. Accordingly, as the population ages, the incidence of these conditions will increase.

ETIOLOGY OF MUSCULOSKELETAL TUMORS

Tumorigenesis is a multifactorial process, which, despite considerable fiscal and intellectual interest, is still poorly understood. There is commonality in genetic mutation that confers to cells the ability to replicate in an unregulated fashion. The development of a colony of abnormally proliferating cells out of normal tissue is referred to as transformation. This process involves acquired mutations in oncogenes, tumor suppressor genes, and other genes that directly or indirectly control proliferation, cell motility, and properties of invasiveness. Such a process may progress beyond the state of benign disease to an aggressive, dedifferentiated state with considerable genomic instability.

To appreciate how bone or soft-tissue tumors develop, one must have a basic understanding of the cell cycle and the regulation thereof. The cell cycle is divided into four distinct phases: G1 (gap 1), S (DNA synthesis), G2 (gap 2), and M (mitosis). After a copy of the entire cellular genome has been synthesized, these duplicate chromosomes are separated, and the cell divides during mitosis. The majority of cell growth occurs during G1. The mature state for mesenchymal cells is normally in a resting, nonproliferative phase designated G0.

Control of the cell cycle is a function of numerous regulatory proteins and checkpoints. These checkpoints allow for the monitoring and repair of the genetic sequence. These proteins are encoded by two basic gene types: oncogenes (stimulatory) and tumor suppressor genes (inhibitory). Oncogenes are genes encoding proteins, which have the inherent ability to transform the host cell to a neoplastic phenotype. Protooncogenes (eg, *RAS*, *WNT*, *MYC*) are wild-type genes that can become oncogenes upon mutation

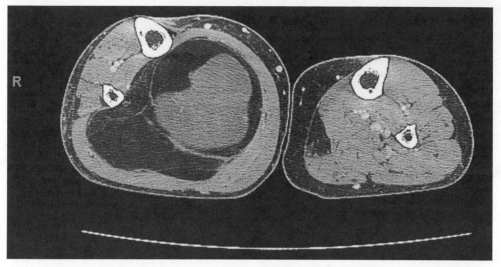

▲ **Figure 5–1.** CT scan of a myxoid liposarcoma within the substance of a long-standing intramuscular lipoma.

or dysregulation of expression. Tumor suppressor genes (eg, *p53*, *Rb*, *p21*) typically require loss-of-function mutations or mutations in other regulatory genes to impart the neoplastic phenotype. These genes are primarily involved with cell-cycle checkpoints.

Inherited mutations in these genes result in neoplastic predisposition syndromes. In syndromes such as hereditary retinoblastoma and Li-Fraumeni syndrome, one mutated copy of a tumor suppressor gene (*Rb* and *p53*, respectively) is inherited. Through a variety of causes including deletion, translocation, point mutation, promoter silencing, or other means of loss of heterozygosity, the remaining function of that gene product is lost, and from that cell a tumor is born. Once checkpoint machinery has been disrupted, additional mutations may be accumulated at an increasing rate, allowing genomic instability to spiral out of control. At the extreme, as seen commonly in osteosarcoma, cells contain up to four times the normal number of chromosomes with multiple chromosomal aberrations.

In addition to hereditary factors that predispose one to the development of neoplasia, many well-described environmental factors exist, such as radiation exposure, chemical carcinogens, and certain oncogenic viral infections. More of these factors may surface as meticulous investigation continues in the field of cancer research.

The neoplastic process may arrest in the so-called benign state, with further genomic instability curtailed, or it may progress to a sarcomatous state. For example, if a cell type of origin is a lipoblast, then a lipoma or a liposarcoma may develop. Furthermore, a liposarcoma may progress in its differentiation such that its phenotype, as a high-grade lesion, minimally reflects its lipoblastic origin. This principle is

illustrated in Figure 5–1, which shows a myxoid liposarcoma within the substance of a typical intramuscular lipoma. This possibility does not imply, however, that all benign lesions are necessarily at risk for malignant degeneration. It is not a surgical indication to resect a lipoma because of concern for secondary liposarcoma.

Although a plethora of molecular pathways are being studied, understanding of the details of genomic instability and subsequent tumor formation is lacking. There is no single pathway by which all neoplasms arise; instead, multiple genetic targets are altered in a variety of sequences and combinations with the common result of cellular proliferation that is tumorigenesis.

▼ EVALUATION AND STAGING OF TUMORS

▶ History and Physical Examination

When evaluating a new patient with a possible tumor, the workup must commence with a thorough history and physical examination. Prior to ordering any diagnostic studies, particular questions must be answered, and the physical characteristics of the mass in question must be assessed. This procedure prevents unnecessary tests and better enables the physician to determine which tests will be most helpful in diagnosing the condition as well as facilitating therapeutic interventions if needed.

The clinical history is of paramount importance (Table 5–1). The age of the patient permits the development of a list of potential diagnoses (Table 5–2), which, when combined with the history, physical examination, and a few additional studies, should permit establishing a diagnosis.

Table 5–1. Questions that must be asked in the workup of a possible tumor.

1. **The patient's age.** Certain tumors are relatively specific to particular age groups.
2. **Duration of complaint.** Benign lesions generally have been present for an extended period (years). Malignant tumors usually have been noticed for only weeks to months.
3. **Rate of growth.** A rapidly growing mass, as in weeks to months, is more likely to be malignant. Growth may be difficult to assess by the patient if it is deep seated, as can be the case with bone. Deep lesions may be much larger than the patient thought ("tip-of-the-iceberg" phenomenon).
4. **Pain associated with the mass.** Benign processes are usually asymptomatic. Osteochondromas (see text) may cause secondary symptoms because of encroachment on surrounding structures. Malignant lesions may cause pain.
5. **History of trauma.** With a history of penetrating trauma, one must rule out osteomyelitis. With a history of blunt trauma, healing fracture must be entertained.
6. **Personal or family history of cancer.** Adults with a history of prostate, renal, lung, breast, or thyroid tumors are at risk for developing metastatic bone disease. Children with neuroblastoma are prone to bony metastases. Patients with retinoblastoma are at an increased risk for osteosarcoma. Secondary osteosarcomas and other malignancies can result from treatment of other childhood cancers. Family history of conditions such as Li-Fraumeni syndrome must raise suspicion of any bone lesion. Furthermore, certain benign bone tumors can run in families (eg, hereditary multiple exostoses; see text).
7. **Systemic signs or symptoms.** Generally there should be no significant findings on the review of systems with benign tumors. Fevers, chills, night sweats, malaise, change in appetite, weight loss, and so on should alert the physician that an infectious or neoplastic process may be involved.

The duration and timing of symptoms, rate of growth, presence of pain, and a history of trauma can help elucidate the diagnosis. Specifically, pain or other symptoms occurring at rest or during the night are of particular concern. Additionally, a careful past medical history, family history, and review of systems must not be overlooked.

A thorough physical examination is also critical (Table 5–3). The clinician must assess the location and size of the mass, the quality of the overlying skin, the presence of warmth, any associated swelling, the presence of tenderness, and the firmness of the lesion. For superficial lesions, transillumination and auscultation may also be beneficial. Range of motion of all joints in proximity to the tumor must be recorded, and a complete neurovascular exam must be performed. An assessment of the related lymph node chains and an examination for an enlarged liver or spleen should also be performed.

The clinician must also consider pseudotumors in addition to true neoplastic conditions. A history of trauma suggests possible stress fracture of myositis ossificans as a diagnosis. The association of symptoms with physical activity and variations of symptoms with the passage of time are important considerations in establishing a differential diagnosis.

▶ Imaging Studies

A. Radiography

Initial evaluation should begin with plain radiography. In every patient with a suspected tumor, orthogonal antero-posterior (AP) and lateral views of the affected area should be obtained. This includes soft-tissue masses as well. Furthermore, in the case of a bone lesion, the entire bone should be imaged. In many cases, radiographic examination is diagnostic, and no further imaging studies are indicated. Although in the case of a more aggressive process the diagnosis may be determined on plain radiographs, further evaluation with advanced studies is usually indicated to determine the extent of disease involvement, as well as the degree of systemic involvement (staging).

The initial radiographic images must be scrutinized. For bone lesions, the location within the bone (eg, diaphyseal, metaphyseal, or epiphyseal; eccentric or central; medullary or surface) facilitates the diagnosis. Epiphyseal tumors are usually benign. Primary sarcomas of bone are usually metaphyseal; however, round cell tumors, such as Ewing sarcoma, multiple myeloma, and lymphoma, are usually medullary diaphyseal lesions. A tumor arising from the surface of a bone may be benign, such as an osteochondroma, or may be malignant, such as a parosteal osteosarcoma.

Terms such as *geographic*, *well-circumscribed*, and *permeative* are useful in describing radiographic abnormalities. Geographic or well-circumscribed implies that the lesion has a distinct, sharply marginated boundary, and suggests benignity (Figure 5–2). Lesions with this feature may exhibit sclerotic borders if the bone itself has reacted to contain the process. A poorly defined, infiltrative process is described as permeative or moth-eaten and reflects a more aggressive process such as malignancy (Figure 5–3), although benign, aggressive processes can exhibit this radiographic feature as well (Figure 5–4). An exception to this rule is multiple myeloma, which frequently demonstrates a punched-out, well-demarcated appearance but in multiple locations.

Matrix quality is another radiographic feature that aids in diagnosis. Lesions may be entirely radiolucent, sparsely mineralized, or predominantly mineralized, and mineralization may be spiculated, stippled, or composed of rings and arcs. Most osteosarcomas, for example, have a spiculated pattern of mineralization expanding out from the host bone in a sunburst appearance. In contrast, chondroid matrix characteristically forms rings and arcs of mineralization. In soft-tissue lesions, matrix mineralization can be very helpful in diagnosis, as in hemangiomas showing smooth, round mineralized phleboliths, as opposed to synovial sarcoma frequently showing irregular mineralization.

With a careful history, physical examination, and appropriate radiographs, the physician can usually reach a working

Table 5–2. Distribution of bone tumors by age (years).

Type of Tumor	0	10	20	30	40	50	60	70	80
Benign bone tumors									
Osteoid osteoma									
Osteoblastoma									
Osteofibrous dysplasia									
Enchondroma									
Periosteal chondroma									
Osteochondroma									
Chondroblastoma									
Chondromyxoid fibroma									
Fibrous cortical defect									
Nonossifying fibroma									
Fibrous dysplasia									
Solitary bone cyst									
Aneurysmal bone cyst									
Epidermoid cyst									
Giant cell tumor									
Hemangioma									
Malignant bone tumors									
Classic osteosarcoma									
Hemorrhagic osteosarcoma									
Parosteal osteosarcoma									
Periosteal osteosarcoma									
Secondary osteosarcoma									
Low-grade intramedullary osteosarcoma									
Irradiation-induced osteosarcoma									
Multicentric osteosarcoma									
Primary chondrosarcoma									
Secondary chondrosarcoma									
Clear cell chondrosarcoma									
Dedifferentiated chondrosarcoma									
Mesenchymal chondrosarcoma									
Ewing sarcoma									
Lymphoma									
Multiple myeloma									
Solitary plasmacytoma									
Fibrosarcoma									
Malignant fibrous histiocytoma									
Adamantinoma									
Vascular sarcoma									
Chordoma									
Metastatic carcinoma									

Table 5–3. Aspects of physical examination that should be documented when evaluating a patient with a mass.

1. **Skin color**
2. **Warmth**
3. **Location**
4. **Swelling.** Swelling, in addition to the primary mass effect, may reflect a more aggressive process.
5. **Neurovascular exam.** Changes may reflect a more aggressive process.
6. **Joint range of motion** of all joints in proximity to the region in question, above and below.
7. **Size.** A mass greater than 5 cm should raise the suspicion of malignancy.
8. **Tenderness.** Tenderness may reflect a more rapidly growing process.
9. **Firmness.** Malignant tumors tend to be firmer on examination than benign processes. This applies more to softtissue tumors than osseous ones.
10. **Lymph nodes.** Certain sarcomas (eg, rhabdomyosarcoma, synovial sarcoma, epithelioid, and clear cell sarcomas) all have increased rates of lymph node involvement.

diagnosis of the lesion. Although some benign and malignant tumors mimic each other, many diagnoses can be ruled out based on information gained without advanced imaging. Factors such as patient age and location as well as radiographic features such as boundary, matrix quality, and

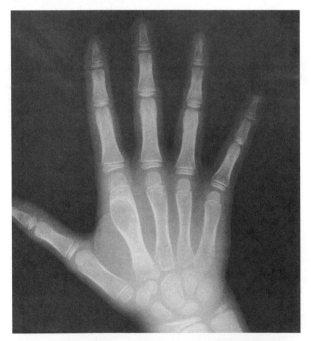

▲ **Figure 5–2.** Radiograph of an enchondroma of the second metacarpal. Notice its geographic appearance.

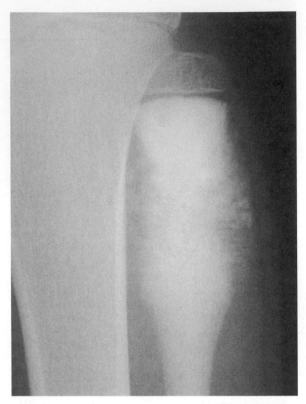

▲ **Figure 5–3.** Radiograph of a proximal fibular osteosarcoma demonstrating the destructive, permeative nature of malignant bone tumors.

reaction of the bone to the lesion can be used to narrow the differential diagnosis. It should be noted that infection can have an extremely variable radiographic appearance, and frequently remains on the differential until ruled out by laboratory studies or biopsy. Tables 5–1 through 5–6 can be used in a step-wise fashion to illustrate the process of focusing the differential diagnosis prior to any advanced imaging and can assist in obtaining the most appropriate studies.

B. Isotope Bone Scanning

Technetium-99 radioisotope scans are used to assess the degree of osteoblastic activity of a given lesion (Figure 5–5). In general, they are quite sensitive, with a few exceptions, for active lesions of bone. Accordingly, technetium-99 scans are excellent screening studies for remote lesions (staging). The best indication for a bone scan is suspected multiple bony lesions, such as in metastatic carcinomas and lymphomas of bone. Isotope bone scanning is far simpler to perform, less expensive, and requires less total-body irradiation than skeletal surveys. It is common practice to use serial isotope scans to follow patients with suspected metastatic disease and, at the same time, evaluate the effectiveness of their systemic therapy.

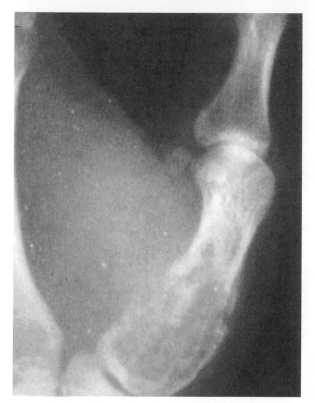

▲ Figure 5–4. Radiograph of a giant cell tumor of the thumb. This is a typical moth-eaten appearance.

Isotope scanning is also used in the staging process of a primary sarcoma of bone such as osteosarcoma to rule out an asymptomatic remote skeletal lesion. Technetium-99 scans are also useful in distinguishing blastic lesions of bone. Given that the study reflects osseous metabolic activity, dormant lesions such as enostoses (bone islands) would not demonstrate significantly increased tracer uptake compared with a blastic prostate metastasis. Inflammatory and traumatic lesions also demonstrate increased activity. It is important to note, however, that multiple myeloma and some metastatic carcinomas (eg, renal cell carcinoma) may not demonstrate increased uptake (ie, false-negative result). Skeletal surveys are preferable for screening for distant involvement in such cases.

C. Computed Tomography and Magnetic Resonance Imaging

Computed tomography (CT) remains a standard imaging procedure for use in well-selected clinical situations. Perhaps the best indication for CT is for smaller lesions that involve cortical structures of bone or spine (Figure 5–6). In such cases, CT is superior to magnetic resonance imaging (MRI) because the resolution of cortical bone using MRI is inferior.

CT scan of the chest is the modality of choice for evaluating patients for pulmonary metastasis. Abdominal CT is invaluable in surveying for primary tumor in patients who present with skeletal metastases. For tumors involving the pelvis and sacrum, CT can help elucidate the extent of bone involvement (Figure 5–7). In cases involving a soft-tissue lesion, MRI is far superior to CT unless there is a heavily mineralized process.

MRI is the imaging modality of choice for evaluating bone marrow involvement and noncalcific soft-tissue lesions. The two most common sequences are the T1-weighted and T2-weighted spin echo (Figure 5–8). Short tau inversion recovery (STIR) sequences have been shown to further elucidate the conspicuity of tumors and bone marrow edema against a nonpathologic background. MRI can also demonstrate the normal anatomy of soft structures, including nerves and vessels, thereby eliminating the need for arteriography and myelograms. Dynamic-enhanced MRI, with its ability to estimate tumor blood flow by examining the rate of contrast uptake and clearance, may serve as a predictor of clinical outcome or tumor response to chemotherapy.

▶ Laboratory Studies

A. Biopsy

The biopsy is usually the last staging procedure. It is preferred to obtain advanced imaging prior to biopsy to avoid postsurgical artifact on these studies, which may aid in determining a definitive diagnosis. There are three types of biopsy for musculoskeletal neoplasia: excisional, incisional, and needle biopsies. Excisional biopsy is discouraged unless the lesion is particularly small (2–3 cm) or in a location where a cuff of healthy tissue can be resected as a margin without significantly increased morbidity.

Complications relating to biopsy are very common. Accordingly, careful preoperative planning is imperative. Imaging studies aid the surgeon in planning biopsy approach and technique. The highest-quality diagnostic tissue is usually found at the periphery of the lesion, where it interfaces with the normal surrounding tissue. In the case of extracompartmental primary bone lesions, the periphery of the soft-tissue extension can be sampled without further compromising the structural integrity of the bone. In the case of intramedullary lesions, a round or ovular window should be developed to decrease the risk of fracture, and the defect should be filled with bone wax or cement to avoid unnecessary contamination of the uninvolved soft tissue. There is also evidence that biopsies performed by the treating oncologic surgeon enjoy a lower complication rate than those performed by inexperienced practitioners prior to referral.

The placement of the biopsy site is a major consideration, since resection of the biopsy tract is necessary for many malignant diagnoses. Serious contamination of vital structures such as the popliteal artery or sciatic nerve may result in amputation rather than limb-sparing surgery.

Table 5–4. Skeletal distribution of bone tumors, ranked from most common (1) to least common (5) sites.

Type of Tumor	Femur	Tibia	Foot or Ankle	Humerus	Radius	Ulna	Hand or Wrist	Scapula	Clavicle	Rib	Vertebra	Sacrum	Pelvis	Skull	Face
Benign bone tumors															
Osteoid osteoma	1	2		4			5				3				
Osteoblastoma	3	4		5							1				2
Osteofibrous dysplasia		1													
Chondroma	2		4	3			1								
Osteochondroma	1	3		2				5					4		
Chondroblastoma	1	3		2				5					4		
Chondromyxoid fibroma	3	1	2		5								4		
Fibrous cortical defect	2	1		3	4				5						
Nonossifying fibroma	2	1		3	4				5						
Solitary bone cyst	2	3		1		5							4		
Aneurysmal bone cyst	1	2		4							3		5		
Giant cell tumor	1	2		5	3							4			
Hemangioma	3	4		5							2			1	
Malignant bone tumors															
Classic osteosarcoma	1	2		3									4		
Hemorrhagic osteosarcoma	1	2		3							5		4		
Parosteal osteosarcoma	1	2		3		4									
Periosteal osteosarcoma	1	2	5	3		4									
Secondary osteosarcoma	2	5		3									1	4	
Low-grade intramedullary osteosarcoma	1	2		2											
Irradiation-induced osteosarcoma	1			2							3	5			
Primary chondrosarcoma	1			4						3	5		2		
Secondary chondrosarcoma	2			3				4			5		1		4

	C1	C2	C3	C4	C5	C6	C7	C8	C9	C10	C11	C12	C13	C14
Dedifferentiated chondrosarcoma	1			3			4		5			2		4
Mesenchymal chondrosarcoma	5								3	2		1		
Ewing sarcoma	1			3			5		4			2		
Lymphoma	1			4					5	3		2		
Myeloma	4			5					2	1		3		
Fibrosarcoma	1	2		4								3		
Malignant fibrous histiocytoma	1	3		5								2		5
Adamantinoma	3	1			4								4	
Vascular sarcoma		4		3					5	1		2		
Chordoma										3	1		3	
Metastatic carcinoma	2			5					4	1		3		

Table 5-5. Bone tumors: imaging characteristics, location in a long bone, and beneficial studies, ranked from most common or most beneficial (1) to least common or least beneficial (3).

Type of Tumor	Imaging Characteristics			Location in a Long Bone					Beneficial Studies				
	Geographic	Moth Eaten	Permeative	Epiphyseal	Metaphyseal	Metadiaphyseal	Diaphyseal	Surface	Plain Radiograph	CT Scan	MRI	Isotope Bone Scan	Blood Studies
Benign bone tumors													
Osteoid osteoma	1				1	2	3		1	2		3	
Osteoblastoma	2	1			2	1	3		1	2		3	
Osteofibrous dysplasia	1	1				2	1		1	2		3	
Chondroma	1				3	1	2		1	2		3	
Osteochondroma	1				2			1	1	2			
Chondroblastoma	1	2		1	2				1	2			
Chondromyxoid fibroma	1	2			1	2			1	2		3	
Fibrous cortical defect	1				1	2			1				
Nonossifying fibroma	1	2			1	2			1	2			
Solitary bone cyst	1				1	2	3		1				
Aneurysmal bone cyst	3	2	1		1	2		3	1	2	3		
Giant cell tumor	3	1	2	1	2				1	2			3
Hemangioma	2	1			3	1	2		1	2			
Malignant bone tumors													
Classic osteosarcoma	3	1	2		1	2	3		1		2	3	
Hemorrhagic osteosarcoma		1	2		1	2			1		2		3
Parosteal osteosarcoma	2	1			2	3		1	2	1			

	1	2	3	4	5	6	7	8	9	10	11	12	13
Periosteal osteosarcoma				1	2	1		2	3			1	2
Secondary osteosarcoma			3	1	2			2	1		2	1	1
Low-grade intramedullary osteosarcoma		3		2	1		3	2	1			1	1
Irradiation-induced osteosarcoma		3	2		1	1	3	2	1		2	1	1
Primary chondrosarcoma			3	1	2			2	1	3		1	2
Secondary chondrosarcoma				1	2		3	3	2			1	1
Dedifferentiated chondrosarcoma			1	3	2			2	1		2	1	
Mesenchymal chondrosarcoma			1	3	2			2	1		2	1	
Ewing sarcoma		3	1		2		3	2	1		1	2	
Lymphoma		2	1		3		2	1	3		1	2	
Myeloma	2	3			1		2	3	1			2	1
Fibrosarcoma			1		2		3	2	1		2	1	
Malignant fibrous histiocytoma			1		2		3	2	1		2	1	
Adamantinoma			3	2	1		1	2	3			1	2
Vascular sarcoma		3	2		1		3	2	1		3	1	2
Chordoma			1	2	3		2	1				1	2
Metastatic carcinoma		1		3	2		3	2	1		2	1	3

Table 5–6. Distribution of soft-tissue tumors by age.

Type of Tumor	0	10	20	30	40	50	60	70	80
Benign soft-tissue tumors									
Desmoid tumor		▓	▓	▓	▓				
Intramuscular lipoma			▓	▓	▓	▓	▓		
Spindle-cell lipoma					▓	▓	▓		
Angiolipoma		▓	▓	▓					
Diffuse lipomatosis		▓							
Benign lipoblastoma	▓	▓	▓						
Hibernoma			▓	▓					
Capillary hemangioma	▓								
Cavernous hemangioma		▓	▓	▓					
Arteriovenous hemangioma	▓	▓	▓						
Epithelioid hemangioma			▓	▓					
Pyogenic granuloma		▓	▓						
Lymphangioma		▓	▓						
Glomus tumor			▓	▓					
Benign hemangiopericytoma			▓	▓					
Neurilemoma					▓				
Solitary neurofibroma			▓	▓					
Neurofibromatosis		▓	▓	▓					
Intramuscular myxoma					▓	▓	▓	▓	
Malignant soft-tissue tumors									
Pleomorphic MFH						▓	▓		
Myxoid MFH						▓	▓		
Giant cell MFH						▓	▓		
Angiomatoid MFH			▓	▓					
Dermatofibrosarcoma protuberans			▓	▓	▓				
Fibrosarcoma						▓			
Leiomyosarcoma					▓	▓			
Well-differentiated liposarcoma					▓	▓			
Myxoid liposarcoma				▓	▓				
Round cell and pleomorphic liposarcoma					▓	▓	▓		
Embryonal rhabdomyosarcoma	▓	▓							
Alveolar rhabdomyosarcoma		▓	▓						
Pleomorphic rhabdomyosarcoma					▓	▓	▓	▓	
Synovial sarcoma		▓	▓	▓					
Solitary malignant schwannoma					▓	▓	▓		
Multiple malignant schwannoma				▓	▓	▓	▓		
Angiosarcoma					▓	▓	▓	▓	
Alveolar soft part sarcoma		▓	▓						
Epithelioid sarcoma			▓	▓					
Clear cell sarcoma			▓	▓					

MFH, malignant fibrous histiocytoma.

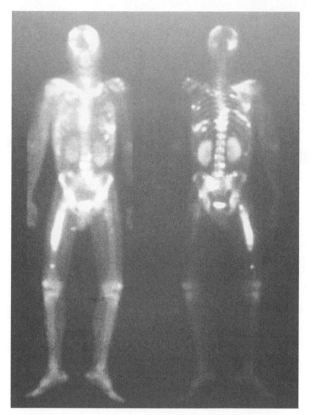

▲ **Figure 5–5.** Technetium-99 scan demonstrating extensive osteoblastic activity in a patient with metastatic adenocarcinoma.

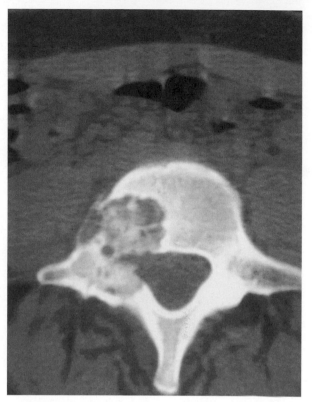

▲ **Figure 5–6.** CT scan of an osteoblastoma arising from the right pedicle of a lumbar vertebra.

Furthermore, transverse incisions should be avoided due to the swath of uninvolved tissue that would need to be resected to incorporate such a biopsy tract into a surgical approach. In many cases, this mandates the use of free or rotational flap coverage that otherwise would not be necessary. Meticulous hemostasis is also mandatory to avoid the formation of a contaminating hematoma. In rare instances, a drain may be helpful, but should exit the skin in line with the biopsy incision.

Obtaining an adequate specimen is critical. A frozen section determines, if viable, diagnostic tissue has been obtained. Definitive diagnosis is rarely possible based on frozen section. In most circumstances, definitive resection should be delayed until final histopathologic diagnosis has been rendered. For the diagnosis of some histologies, special studies may be required such as immunohistochemistry, flow cytometry, fluorescence in situ hybridization, or other cytogenetic studies. Adequate material, handled appropriately, is required for the completion of many of these studies.

Needle biopsies, either core or fine needle, are increasingly being used at experienced tumor centers, especially for presumed lesions that are easily diagnosed, such as round

cell tumors or metastatic carcinoma. Because the subtype of tumor frequently determines treatment, architecture of the tumor is generally needed, which requires core rather than fine-needle biopsy. For spine or deep pelvic lesions image-directed needle biopsy is ideal because it avoids

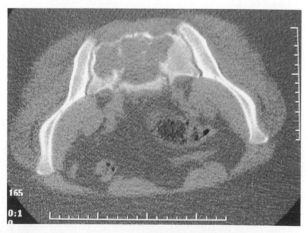

▲ **Figure 5–7.** Pelvic CT demonstrating the bony destruction of the sacrum caused by a giant cell tumor.

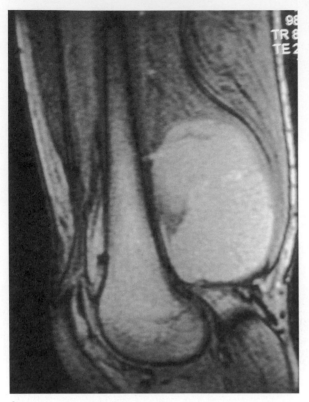

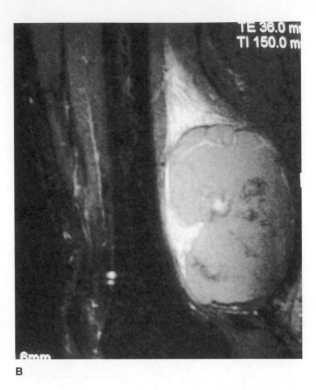

A

B

▲ **Figure 5–8.** Synovial sarcoma involving the popliteal fossa. (**A**) T1-weighted. (**B**) T2-weighted.

excessive multicompartmental contamination. Fine-needle biopsy should be reserved for use in consultation with an experienced cytopathologist. Most current studies show a diagnostic accuracy of 75–85% for needle biopsy compared with more than 95% accuracy for incisional biopsy.

B. Cultures and Special Studies

The damage of biopsy specimens after retrieval can make it impossible to perform special studies such as immuno-histochemistry, cytogenetics, flow cytometry, and electron microscopy. For this reason, the surgeon should consult with the pathologist prior to biopsy. For example, formalin pres-ervation of the specimen will preclude many of the above studies. Not only is it important for the operating room personnel to be aware of this, but it is also important for the pathologist to be aware of the clinical history and differential diagnoses, so that the specimen is handled appropriately. It is also wise to culture for bacteria, fungus, and acid-fast bacilli when clinical suspicion warrants.

Molecular diagnostics continue to revolutionize sarcoma diagnostics. This is particularly evident in the decreasing inci-dence of undifferentiated pleomorphic sarcoma as technologic advances allow better determination of the cell lineage of origin. Specific genomic rearrangements and mutations have been identified in a variety of tumors (Table 5–7). This is not only improving diagnostics, but also treatment. Gastrointestinal stromal tumor (GIST), a malignant mesenchymal neoplasm of the gastrointestinal tract, omentum, and mesentery, expresses a mutant form of *c-kit*. The *KIT* gene encodes a tyrosine kinase receptor for which targeted therapy has been developed and has shown significant efficacy. Targeted therapy has also been developed for some subtypes of lymphoma based on the expression pattern of cell surface markers. The status of these cell surface proteins is most often established using flow cytometry.

▶ Staging Systems

Staging refers to a critical assessment of the grade and size of a tumor and the extent to which the disease has spread. There are two dominant staging systems for both soft-tissue sarcoma and primary bone sarcoma, which are described in the following sections. The goals of cancer staging include treatment guidance, prognostic stratification, and investiga-tion continuity.

Table 5–7. Common translocations seen in sarcomas.

Ewing/primitive neuroectodermal tumor: t(11; 22) (q24; q12), (t21; 22) (q22; q12), (t7; 22) (p22; q12)
Myxoid chondrosarcoma: t(9; 22) (q22; q12)
Myxoid and round cell liposarcoma: t(12; 16) (q12; p11)
Synovial sarcoma: t(X; 18) (p11; q11)
Alveolar rhabdomyosarcoma: t(2; 13) (q35; q14), t(1; 13) (p36; q14)
Alveolar soft parts sarcoma: t(X; 17) (p11.2; q25)
Desmoplastic small round cell tumor: t(11; 22) (p13; q12)
Congenital fibrosarcoma: t(12; 15)

A. System of the American Joint Committee on Cancer

The American Joint Committee on Cancer (AJCC) system (6th edition) is used by most surgical oncologists. This is the four-stage tumor, node, metastasis (TNM) classification system that provides staging criteria for both soft-tissue sarcoma and primary bone sarcoma, as well as all other major malignancies. The distinct staging systems for both soft-tissue sarcoma and primary bone sarcoma entail the size and grade of the primary tumor as well as presence of nodal or distant metastases.

For soft-tissue sarcoma, stage I represents any grade 1 or 2 (out of 4) tumor without nodal or distant metastases. Stage II and III tumors are grade 3 or 4 tumors without metastases. The distinction is in size and depth, where stage III is a tumor of more than 5 cm and deep to fascia (T2b), and stage II is any superficial tumor (T1a and T2a) or less than 5 cm and deep (T1b). Stage IV is any grade, size, or depth tumor with nodal or distant metastases.

For primary bone sarcoma, stage I represents any grade 1 or 2 (out of 4) tumor without noncontiguous or metastatic disease. This is further subdivided by size, with stage IA including tumors of less than 8 cm in largest dimension and stage IB including tumors of 8 cm or greater. It should be noted that this has changed since the AJCC fifth edition, where the distinction was based on intra- versus extracompartmental designation. Stage II represents any grade 3 or 4 tumor without noncontiguous or metastatic disease. This group also is divided into stage IIA and IIB based on 8-cm size. Stage III is any grade or size tumor with noncontiguous disease in the same bone and no distant metastases. Stage IV is any grade or size tumor with distant metastatic disease and is divided into stage IVA and IVB based on isolated pulmonary metastases versus extrapulmonary disease including lymph nodes, respectively.

B. Musculoskeletal Tumor Society System (Surgical Staging System or Enneking System)

Many orthopedic oncologists prefer the Enneking system, which addresses both primary bone and soft-tissue sarcoma, and specifically addresses unique problems associated with

sarcoma affecting the extremities. It is a three-stage system with stage I representing low-grade tumors without metastases. Stage II represents high-grade tumors without metastases. The first two groupings are further subdivided into type A and B based on intra- or extracompartmental designation, respectively. Stage III is any tumor with metastatic disease. Although compartmentalization is an important surgical concept, to date, it has not been shown to be a statistically significant prognostic factor.

▶ Essentials of Diagnosis

- *Meticulous history and physical examination are critical in the diagnosis of bone and soft-tissue tumors.*

- *Plain radiography should be the initial imaging modality in the evaluation of bone and soft-tissue tumors. Frequently, it is diagnostic, obviating the need for advanced imaging and, at times, biopsy.*

- *When biopsy is necessary, it should be performed with careful planning by the surgeon prepared to definitively treat all possible diagnoses.*

Heck RK, Peabody TD, Simon MA: Staging of primary malignancies of bone. *CA Cancer J Clin* 2006;56:366. [PMID: 17135693]

Jaffe CC: Response assessment in clinical trials: implications for sarcoma clinical trial design. *Oncologist* 2008;13:14. [PMID: 18434633]

Kotilingam D, Lev DC, Lazar AJ, et al: Staging soft tissue sarcoma: evolution and change. *CA Cancer J Clin* 2006;56:282. [PMID: 17005597]

Mankin HJ, Mankin CJ, Simon MA: The hazards of the biopsy, revisited. *J Bone Joint Surg Am* 1996;78:656. [PMID: 8642021]

Mitsuyoshi G, Naito N, Kawai A, et al: Accurate diagnosis of musculoskeletal lesions by core needle biopsy. *J Surg Oncol* 2006;94:1. [PMID: 16788939]

Moley JF, Eberlein TJ: Soft-tissue sarcomas. *Surg Clin North Am* 2000;80:687. [PMID: 10836012]

Oliviera AM, Nascimento AG: Grading in soft tissue tumors: principles and problems. *Skeletal Radiol* 2001;30:543. [PMID: 11685477]

Ordonez JL, Martins AS, Osuna D, et al: Targeting sarcomas: therapeutic targets and their rational. *Semin Diagn Pathol* 2008;25:304. [PMID: 19013896]

Simon MA, Finn HA: Diagnostic strategy for bone and soft tissue tumors. *J Bone Joint Surg Am* 1993;75:622. [PMID: 8478392]

Zahm SH, Fraumeni JF Jr: The epidemiology of soft tissue sarcoma. *Semin Oncol* 1997;24:504. [PMID: 9344316]

▼ DIAGNOSIS AND TREATMENT OF TUMORS

BENIGN BONE TUMORS

Benign bone tumors have certain characteristics that favor their diagnosis over malignant conditions. Benign lesions are frequently asymptomatic and, many times, are detected incidentally during workup of an unrelated condition such as minor trauma. The diagnosis can often be made with plain radiography alone. Benign bone tumors are usually well circumscribed, and there is evidence of the host bone successfully reacting to contain the lesion, characterized radiographically by sclerotic margins or a dense osteoblastic reactive zone. In contrast, if the condition is malignant, the patient usually complains of pain, and the radiograph commonly shows a more permeative lesion with lytic destruction and poorly defined margins that suggest rapid progression. Further studies such as MRI or bone scintigraphy are unnecessary for typical benign lesions, such as fibrous dysplasia, enchondroma, or nonossifying fibroma. There is far less cytogenetic information available for benign bone tumors, likely because there is less implication in the treatment. A system of staging exists for benign bone tumors. Stage 1 lesions are considered latent. They are generally asymptomatic, but not always. Although they can progress, they usually resolve. Initially, these lesions should be observed. Stage 2 lesions are considered active. They tend not to resolve spontaneously and are less well demarcated than stage 1 lesions. They frequently require surgical intervention with meticulous attention to complete extirpation because of their propensity for recurrence. Stage 3, or aggressive, lesions demonstrate extensive destruction. Treatment often requires wide en bloc resection.

The more common types of benign bone tumors seen by the practicing orthopedic surgeon are discussed in this section.

▶ Benign Osteoid-Forming Tumors

A. Osteoid Osteoma: ICD-9-CM 213.x

The most common benign osteoid-forming tumor is the osteoid osteoma, accounting for 10% of all benign bone tumors. It is more common in males than in females with a peak incidence in the second decade of life. Although it may be present in almost any bone, the proximal femur is the most common location. Dull, aching, nocturnal pain is characteristic, and it is commonly relieved entirely by nonsteroidal anti-inflammatory drugs (NSAIDs) secondary to a high concentration of prostaglandins in the nidus. Osteoid osteoma may have a unique pathogenic nerve supply as well, a unique finding among the bone tumors.

The characteristic radiographic feature of the osteoid osteoma is a central, lytic nidus usually 1 cm or less in diameter. The more common cortically based lesion (Figure 5–9) exhibits extensive reactive sclerosis, creating a fusiform bulge on the bone surface. However, if the nidus is more centrally located in metaphyseal bone, less sclerosis is seen and the radiographic appearance is less diagnostic. If the nidus is close to, or actually in, a joint, as in a femoral neck lesion, the resulting reactive synovitis may mimic a pyarthrosis or rheumatoid arthritis. Technetium bone scans are invariably positive. A CT scan is recommended to better anatomically locate the nidus and confirm the diagnosis.

In the spine, the typical location for an osteoid osteoma is in the posterior elements. The lumbar spine is most commonly involved followed by the thoracic spine. A secondary scoliosis is usually associated with this presentation with the lesion located at the apex of the concavity. Furthermore, if the nidus is in proximity to a nerve root, radicular pain may develop, which may obscure timely diagnosis.

Histologically, the nidus is seldom larger than 1 cm, and for lesions greater than 2 cm, the term osteoblastoma is reserved, suggesting somewhat more aggressive proliferative features. The nidus is composed of loose, vascular connective tissue and immature, lacy osteoid lined by plump osteoblasts. At the periphery of the nidus, there is bone organized into a tiny trabecular network with centripetally increasing maturity. There is a paucity of cytogenetic data for this entity, which is unlikely to increase rapidly, secondary to the fact that diagnostic tissue is rarely procured in the course of the diagnosis or treatment.

Many cases of osteoid osteoma are stage 1 lesions and can be treated symptomatically with aspirin or NSAIDs until they spontaneously resolve. If the patient fails such treatment, surgical intervention is warranted. If surgery is undertaken, the entire nidus must be eradicated. Resection of surrounding sclerotic bone should not be excessive, because it can severely compromise the structural integrity of the host bone. The so-called burr-down technique is preferred over en bloc resection. The nidus is recognized by the hyperemic, pink hue and is removed by curettage. The burr is then used to advance the margin another 2–3 mm. CT-guided radiofrequency ablation is emerging as an accepted treatment modality. This method employs probes with high-frequency alternating current to induce ionic agitation and frictional heat to induce tumor necrosis. Radiofrequency ablation is used extensively as a less invasive treatment modality with similar success rate as surgical excision.

B. Osteoblastoma: ICD-9-CM 213.x

Osteoblastoma is a large osteoid osteoma that demonstrates a propensity for the posterior elements of the spine. Osteoblastomas are found more commonly in males than in females and occur in the same age group as osteoid osteomas. Osteoblastomas are less common than osteoid osteomas, accounting for 1% of all benign bone tumors. They can occur in the metaphyses of long bones, raising concern of osteosarcoma, and a few are seen in the ankle and wrist. These are usually stage 1–2 lesions.

Radiographically, the osteoblastoma has a more lytic and destructive appearance than the osteoid osteoma. Its nidus, which is greater than 1–2 cm, has a less sclerotic boundary and may take on the appearance of an aneurismal bone cyst. Histologically, however, the nidus is identical to that of an osteoid osteoma. There is rich vascularity in a bed of

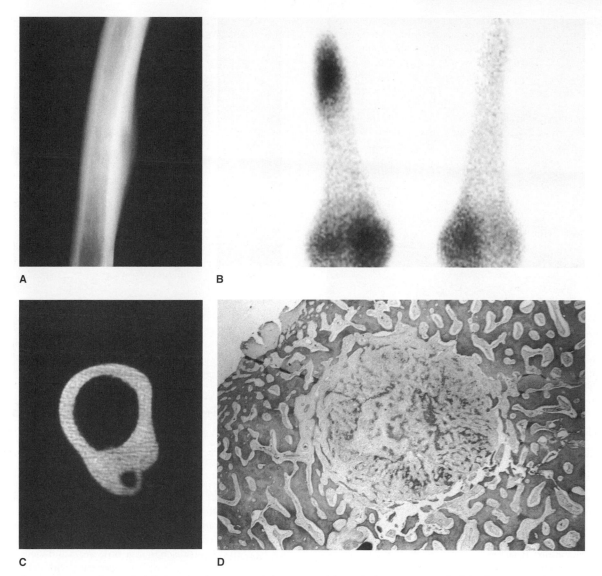

A

B

C

D

▲ **Figure 5–9.** Radiograph (**A**), isotope bone scan (**B**), CT scan (**C**), and photomicrograph (**D**) of an osteoid osteoma in the femur of a 19-year-old man.

disorganized, immature osteoid and microtrabeculae lined with a single layer of plump osteoblasts. Multinucleated, osteoclast-like giant cells may be present. Although little cytogenetic data are available, preliminary evidence suggests moderately increased genetic instability over that of osteoid osteoma.

In the spine, the effects of osteoblastoma are similar to osteoid osteoma, although at times more pronounced, including radiating pain and other effects of nerve root or spinal cord impingement (Figure 5–10).

In patients with osteoblastoma, treatment usually consists of vigorous curettage of the lesion, which may require structural bone grafting if instability results. Radiofrequency ablation may also prove useful in the management of this lesion in certain circumstances.

C. Osteofibrous Dysplasia: ICD-9-CM 213.7

Osteofibrous dysplasia is a rare condition, usually presenting as a stage 1–2 lesion, that is seen almost exclusively in the

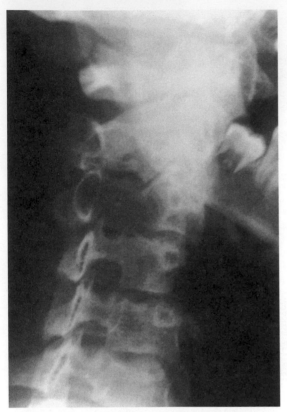

▲ **Figure 5–10.** Radiograph of an osteoblastoma in the pedicle area of the C3 vertebra of a 14-year-old boy.

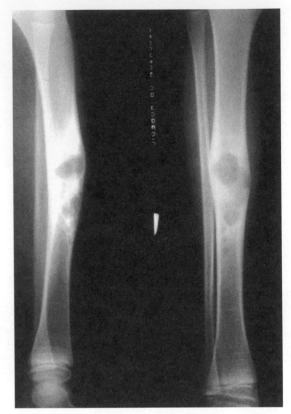

▲ **Figure 5–11.** Radiograph of osteofibrous dysplasia in the tibia of an 8-year-old boy.

tibia of children during the first two decades of life. There is a strong male predilection. It commonly affects the anterior cortex resulting in an anterior tibial bow. Osteofibrous dysplasia can be seen in the fibula, and even more rarely, can be seen bilaterally. It is most likely a hamartomatous process and tends to involute spontaneously with skeletal maturity.

In osteofibrous dysplasia (Figure 5–11), lytic changes are seen in the anterior tibial cortex surrounded by sclerotic margins creating a soap-bubble appearance similar to the radiographic picture of fibrous dysplasia and adamantinoma. Histologically, the lytic lesion shows a benign trabecular alphabet soup pattern in a fibrous stroma. Notably, there is prominent osteoblastic rimming of the trabeculae, in contrast with fibrous dysplasia.

As previously eluded to, there is a significant diagnostic dilemma in distinguishing between osteofibrous dysplasia and adamantinoma. If progression is documented or there are other alarming features, diagnostic biopsy is warranted. Osteofibrous dysplasia is vimentin positive but keratin negative, whereas adamantinoma exhibits prominent nests of keratin-positive epithelial cells. When a few scattered keratin-positive cells are seen, it is termed osteofibrous dysplasia–like adamantinoma.

In a report of experience with 35 cases of osteofibrous dysplasia, investigators indicated that early attempts at curettage and grafting of the lesions resulted in a high failure rate because of recurrence. For this reason, they suggested waiting until patients reach the age of 15 years and their disease spontaneously arrests before proceeding with debridement and grafting.

▶ Essentials of Diagnosis

- *Benign osteoid-forming lesions of bone are typically painful and, especially in the case of osteoid osteoma, may be relieved by aspirin or NSAIDs.*

- *Osteoblastoma is very similar to osteoid osteoma, but larger, and both show a predilection to the posterior elements of the spine. If there is an associated painful scoliosis, the convexity will point away from the side of the lesion.*

- *Osteofibrous dysplasia is characterized histologically by the presence of osteoblastic rimming of the immature trabeculae, in contrast to fibrous dysplasia, which has absent osteoblastic rimming.*

▶ Benign Chondroid-Forming Tumors

A. Enchondroma and the Multiple Enchondromatoses: ICD-9-CM 213.x

Enchondroma refers to a centrally located chondroma of bone. These tumors are relatively common, accounting for greater than 10% of benign bone tumors. In 50% of cases, the tumor is found in the small tubular bones of the hands and feet. It arises in growing bones as a hamartomatous process, but is frequently asymptomatic and may avoid detection until the patient reaches adulthood, at which time it may be discovered in association with a pathologic fracture or as an incidental finding.

Radiographs of enchondromas show geographic lysis with sharp margination and central calcification (Figure 5–12). In the case of an enchondroma of the hand, the cortex is frequently thinned out with slight expansion. In contrast, with involvement of the large long bones, the lesion is centrally located with minimal cortical erosion. Enchondromas are either stage 1 or 2 lesions.

Multiple enchondromatosis, or Ollier disease (Figure 5–13), is a rare nonfamilial dysplasia typically seen on half of the body and appears similar to fibrous dysplasia. This condition can be quite extensive with significant involvement of the metaphyses resulting in bowing and shortening of the long bones. Such dramatic changes are not seen in solitary enchondroma. In patients with Maffucci syndrome, multiple enchondromatosis is seen in association with multiple soft-tissue hemangiomas.

A large solitary enchondroma converts to low-grade chondrosarcoma in fewer than 5% of cases, and the conversion takes place during adulthood. A solitary enchondroma in the hand rarely converts to chondrosarcoma, although histologically these appear more biologically active. A secondary

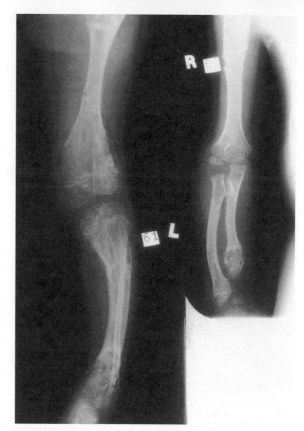

▲ **Figure 5–13.** Radiograph of Ollier disease of the upper and lower extremities.

chondrosarcoma can occur in enchondromatosis up to 20% of the time and may be related to acquired inactivation of certain tumor suppressor genes.

There is no need to treat an asymptomatic patient with a solitary enchondroma, but the patient should be followed radiographically for changes suggesting dedifferentiation. In cases of impending fracture or persistently symptomatic lesions, curettage with margin extension and bone grafting may be performed with a low risk of recurrence. Patients with multiple enchondromatosis must be followed closely because of the increased risk of secondary chondrosarcoma. Patients with Maffucci syndrome are at additional risk for the development of other mesenchymal neoplasia, including hemangiosarcoma and lymphangiosarcoma.

B. Periosteal Chondroma: ICD-9-CM 213.x

A benign chondroma seen on the surface of a bone is called a periosteal chondroma. Patients frequently have more than one lesion, and the most common location is on the proximal humeral metaphysis. Radiographically, the lesions appear to saucerize the underlying cortex (Figure 5–14).

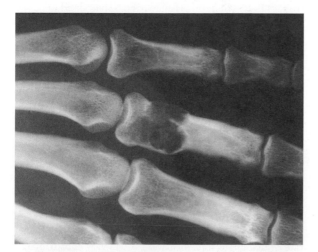

▲ **Figure 5–12.** Radiograph of an enchondroma of the proximal phalanx of the ring finger.

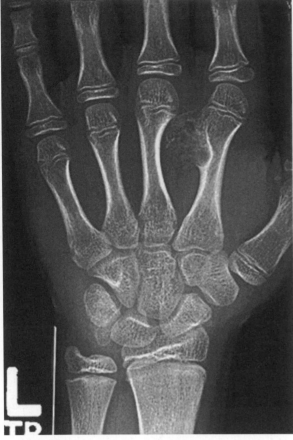

▲ **Figure 5–14.** Radiograph of a periosteal chondroma on the index metacarpal of a 12-year-old boy. Notice the buttress of bone proximally and the characteristic matrix mineralization.

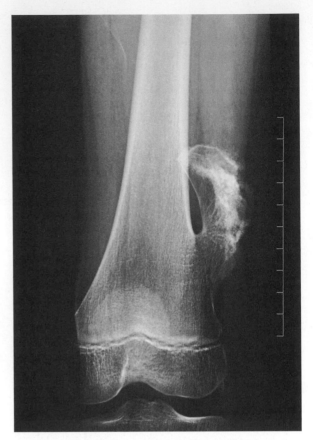

▲ **Figure 5–15.** Radiograph of a solitary osteochondroma on the distal femur of a skeletally immature individual.

These stage 1–2 lesions may grow to a sizable mass, but those larger than 4 cm suggest peripheral chondrosarcoma. Management usually consists of serial imaging to ensure it does not continue growing into adulthood. In concerning cases, simple excision results in low recurrence rates.

C. Osteochondroma: ICD-9-CM 213.x

The nonossifying fibroma is the most common benign bone tumor, and the osteochondroma is the second most common. Like the enchondroma, the osteochondroma is a developmental, or hamartomatous, process that arises from a defect in the outer edge of the metaphyseal side of a growth plate, resulting in an exostosis that points away from the joint and moves away from the physis with growth.

Macroscopically, there is a bony base, sharing a medullary communication with the host bone, and a cartilaginous cap

(Figures 5–15 and 5–16). They may be pedunculated or sessile. The cartilage cap has a similar columnar organization as a growth plate and synchronously stops growth at skeletal maturity.

A familial form of osteochondromata, called hereditary multiple exostosis (HME), is an autosomal dominant disorder that is one tenth as common as solitary osteochondroma. Three genetic loci are associated with HME involving the tumor suppressor *EXT* genes (*EXT1, EXT2,* and *EXT3*). This condition exhibits variable penetrance, with the severest forms resulting in severe angular deformities and limb shortening from hundreds of osteochondromata. Forearm involvement can be quite deforming. The metaphyseal portions of the long bones are deformed and widened (Figures 5–17 and 5–18). The histologic findings in the lesions of HME are similar to those in solitary osteochondroma.

Conversion to chondrosarcoma is exceedingly rare in solitary osteochondroma and occurs in adulthood. The rate of malignant transformation in HME is approximately 1%, occurring in the cartilaginous cap, usually in the larger proximal lesions.

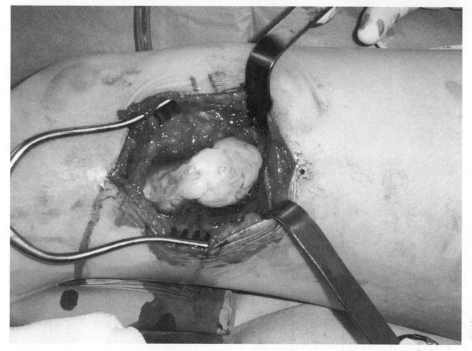

▲ **Figure 5–16.** Typical glistening white appearance of the cartilage cap seen on the same osteochondroma in Figure 5–15.

Osteochondromas are stage 1 lesions. Most children with a solitary osteochondroma are asymptomatic and therefore do not require surgical treatment. In some cases, the lesion may be palpable and irritating. Surgical resection is appropriate in these cases to address the symptoms only and not as a prophylaxis for chondrosarcomatous degeneration. In HME, symptomatic lesions are addressed surgically as needed. Corrective osteotomy is occasionally required for angular deformity.

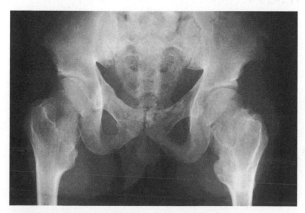

▲ **Figure 5–17.** Radiograph of multiple exostoses involving both hips.

If a previously quiescent lesion begins to enlarge in an adult, it should be removed. The surgical margin should be wide enough to include the entire cartilaginous cap.

D. Chondroblastoma: ICD-9-CM 213.x

The chondroblastoma is a benign cartilage-forming tumor that occurs in the epiphyses or apophyses. When it is diagnosed near or at skeletal maturity, it may expand across the physis or physeal scar. The peak incidence is during the second decade of life with a slight male predominance. The long bones are most often affected, but the patella, talus, and calcaneus are also commonly reported locations. There may be joint involvement presenting with an effusion.

Radiographically, there is sharp demarcation of a radiolucent lesion in the epiphysis with stippled or flocculent calcification. There may be erosion of the subchondral bone with collapse or pathologic fracture (Figure 5–19). There may also be a recognizable aneurismal component. Histologically, there is a background of uniform polyhedral cells with grooved nuclei producing sparse, amorphous chondroid. The cells may be separated by a fine lace of mineralization producing a "chicken wire" appearance. Osteoclast-like giant cells and macrophages are present, especially near areas of hemorrhage or aneurismal conversion.

Although chondroblastoma presents in a younger age group than giant cell tumor, the two are comparable.

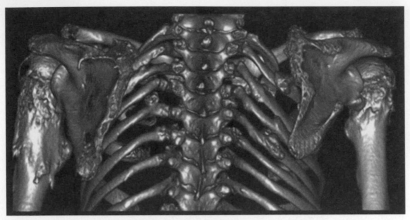

▲ **Figure 5–18.** Three-dimensional reconstructed CT scan of the bilateral shoulders and upper thorax of a skeletally immature female with hereditary multiple exostoses.

Similarities include the location, radiographic appearance, and strikingly similar histologic features. They both typically present as stage 2 or 3 lesions. Also in common is the rare incidence of pulmonary metastasis. When pulmonary metastasis develops, the histology is the same, and they respond well to resection, carrying an excellent prognosis.

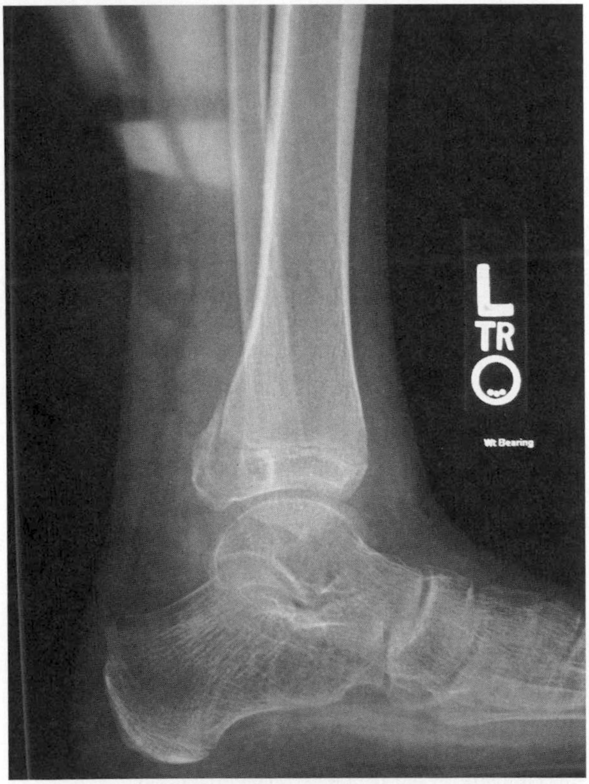

Treatment of chondroblastoma usually consists of intralesional curettage with margin extension and bone grafting or structural supplementation with polymethyl methacrylate. The recurrence rate is less that 10% with this form of treatment. When the subchondral bone has been destroyed or the lesion is otherwise more locally aggressive, wide resection with osteoarticular allograft reconstruction has been used with success. Transformation to secondary chondrosarcoma is extremely rare but occurs with increased frequency following radiation therapy.

E. Chondromyxoid Fibroma: ICD-9-CM 213.x

The chondromyxoid fibroma, a very rare tumor, generally affects males in the second or third decade of life. The most common location is the proximal tibial metaphysis, followed by the distal femur and the metatarsals. The tumor is slow growing and accompanied by mild pain and symptoms.

Radiographs of chondromyxoid fibroma show a lytic tumor with sharp sclerotic margins and a pseudoloculated pattern resembling that of a bone cyst. They are eccentric in metaphyseal bone with thinning of the involved cortex (Figure 5–20). Histologic findings include a strange but specific mixture of fibrous, myxomatous, and chondroid tissues, which could mistakenly suggest the diagnosis of chondrosarcoma. There are also frequent osteoclast-like giant cells. The expression pattern of collagens seems to be unique to this entity with predominantly type II, but also types I, III, and VI.

Chondromyxoid fibroma usually presents as a stage 2 lesion and has a markedly high propensity for local recurrence. With recurrence rates approaching 25% following simple curettage and bone grafting, aggressive margin extension should be performed. The conversion of chondromyxoid fibroma to secondary chondrosarcoma is extremely rare.

▲ **Figure 5–19.** Radiograph of a chondroblastoma in the distal tibia of a 15-year-old boy.

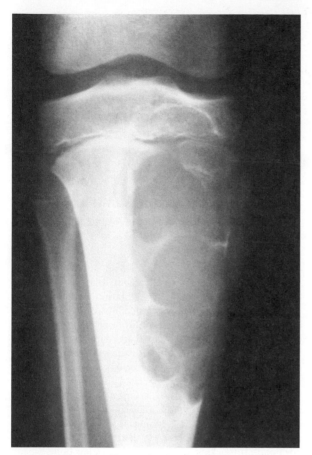

▲ **Figure 5–20.** Radiograph of a chondromyxoid fibroma in the proximal tibia of an 11-year-old boy.

▶ **Essentials of Diagnosis**

- *The matrix of chondroid tumors is characterized by stippled calcification or the presence of rings and arcs of calcification.*
- *The hallmark of osteochondroma is continuity of the medullary portion of the lesion with the host bone in contrast to the periosteal chondroma, where the host cortex separates the medullary canal of the host bone from the lesion itself.*
- *Chondromyxoid fibroma is a rare lesion but may be aggressive and have a very high rate of local recurrence.*

▶ **Benign Fibrous Tumors of Bone**

A. Fibrous Cortical Defect: ICD-9-CM 213.x

Fibrous cortical defects, or cortical desmoids, are small, hamartomatous fibromas seen almost exclusively in the metaphyseal areas of the lower extremities of growing children. They can be multiple, and as many as 25% of normal children demonstrate these asymptomatic lesions

at 5 years of age. The lesions tend to disappear as a result of bone remodeling before skeletal maturity. They may show increased uptake on isotope bone scans.

In the case of fibrous cortical defects, microscopic studies show benign-appearing fibroblasts in a whorled pattern with occasional histiocytes, foam cells, and benign giant cells. The radiographic appearance is so characteristic of this entity (Figure 5–21) that a biopsy is usually not necessary. These are stage 1 lesions and can generally be observed.

B. Nonossifying Fibroma: ICD-9-CM 213.x

Just as the osteoblastoma is considered a larger or more extensive form of osteoid osteoma, the nonossifying fibroma is considered a larger form of the fibrous cortical defect. It is typically seen in the lower extremity of children. Because of its size, it may not entirely resolve by skeletal maturity and can persist into adult life. If the lesion is quite large, approaching 50% of the diameter of the bone, pathologic fracture may ensue. The fracture healing process may facilitate resolution of the lesion. Careful consideration to fracture prophylaxis should be reserved for large lesions in children older than 10 years. Nonossifying fibromas are stage 1 lesions, and neither they nor fibrous cortical defects require biopsy because their radiographic appearance is so characteristic.

With nonossifying fibroma, multiple lesions may take on the appearance of fibrous dysplasia and can be associated with café-au-lait skin defects. Large defects in the tibia can assume the appearance of chondromyxoid fibroma (Figure 5–22). The lesions have a well-defined sclerotic margin with a pseudoloculated lytic center that gives them a soap-bubble radiographic appearance. Histologically, they appear identical to fibrous cortical defects and are characterized by abundant benign fibrous tissue speckled with areas of histiocytes, foam cells, and giant cells. As the lesion involves in adulthood and the number of giant cells and histiocytes diminishes, large areas of cholesterol deposits become evident, which

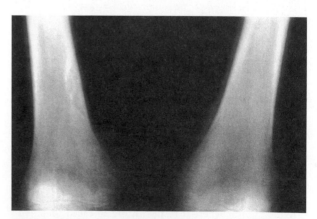

▲ **Figure 5–21.** Radiograph of a metaphyseal fibrous cortical defect in a 15-year-old boy.

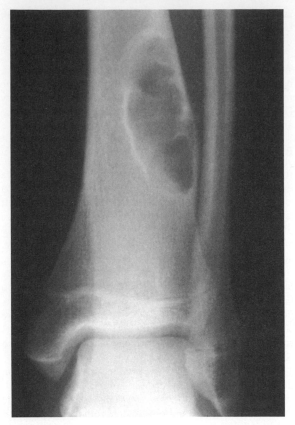

▲ **Figure 5–22.** Radiograph of a nonossifying fibroma of the distal tibia.

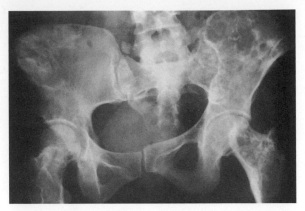

▲ **Figure 5–23.** Radiograph of polyostotic fibrous dysplasia of the pelvis.

may suggest the diagnosis of xanthofibroma or xanthoma of bone. Nonossifying fibromas are clearly separated from fibrous dysplasia by the absence of metaplastic osteoid formation in the fibrous stroma.

C. Fibrous Dysplasia: ICD-9-CM 756.54

Fibrous dysplasia can present in a variety of ways: monostotic, polyostotic, and with or without associated syndromes (Figure 5–23). Most cases are diagnosed in the first three decades and have a distinct female predilection. The monostotic presentation is more common than the polyostotic. This condition is a dysplastic anomaly of bone forming mesenchymal tissue with an inability to produce mature lamellar bone. Accordingly, the bone is arrested in an immature woven state with a resultant proliferation of spindled fibroblasts. In the polyostotic form, it tends to be unilateral rather than bilateral. Nevertheless, it can involve any bone in the body. The most common location is the proximal femur where it results in the so-called shepherd's crook deformity. Other areas frequently involved include the tibia, pelvis, humerus, radius, and ribs.

In addition to bony involvement, patients can demonstrate café-au-lait skin pigmentation. These patches usually have a rough border, in contrast to the smooth border of those seen in neurofibromatosis. Patients with fibrous dysplasia may have associated endocrine problems. For example, 5% of patients with the polyostotic form of fibrous dysplasia also exhibit precocious puberty (McCune-Albright syndrome). Other associated endocrine abnormalities include hyperthyroidism, acromegaly, Cushing disease, and hypophosphatemic osteomalacia. Polyostotic fibrous dysplasia with soft-tissue myxomas is known as Mazabraud syndrome. Fibrous dysplasia can also involve the skull and jaw bones, mimicking ossifying fibroma of jaw bone.

Radiographically, fibrous dysplasia has a ground-glass appearance due to the fine mineralization pattern of the immature woven trabeculae. There is surrounding remodeling of the host bone, which is often expansile. In fibrous dysplasia, microscopic findings include an alphabet soup pattern of metaplastic woven bone scattered through a benign fibrous tissue stroma. The woven trabeculae have a characteristic absence of osteoblastic rimming. Foam cells, giant cells, and cholesterol deposits can be seen. Large cystic areas and even areas of cartilage formation are commonly present.

The molecular basis for fibrous dysplasia is associated with mutations affecting the alpha subunit of G protein. Cells of the osteoblastic lineage are affected, resulting in decreased differentiation and increased proliferation. These mutations cause constitutive elevation of cyclic adenosine monophosphate (cAMP) in fibrous dysplasia and thus alter cAMP target genes such as *c-fos, c-jun, IL-6,* and *IL-11.*

Fibrous dysplasia tends to be active during the growing years and then burns out in adult life. Fewer than 1% of lesions convert to osteosarcoma, fibrosarcoma, or even chondrosarcoma. If conversion does occur, it almost always happens during adulthood. Generally, this disease is either stage 1 or 2.

In pediatric patients with active disease, curettage and grafting should be avoided because of high recurrence rates.

The goals in treating pediatric patients should be the prevention and treatment of deformity, especially in the lower extremity. Most cases should become quiescent with skeletal maturity. If not, the best surgical treatment in adults consists of rigid fixation with an intramedullary implant with strut grafting as needed. Medical management with bisphosphonates is of benefit in some cases. Irradiation is contraindicated because it may lead to irradiation-induced sarcoma at a later date.

▶ Essentials of Diagnosis

- *Nonossifying fibromas/fibrous cortical defects may be present in up to one third of the population and are usually detected incidentally.*

- *If fibrous dysplasia is suspected, a careful examination of the skin should be performed for café-au-lait spots, which are seen in McCune-Albright syndrome.*

▶ Cystic Lesions of Bone

A. Simple Bone Cyst: ICD-9-CM 733.21

Simple bone cysts are a common pseudotumor of bone and the most frequent cause of pathologic fractures in children. Bone cysts usually affect patients between 5 and 15 years of age and occur more often in boys than in girls (2:1) with an incidence of 1 per 10,000 children per year. They are found in the proximal humerus in 50% of cases and in the upper femur in 25%. The calcaneus and pelvis are also uniquely common locations. Patients are asymptomatic until a pathologic fracture occurs. The cystic process continues to grow away from the physis. When it remains in contact with the physis, it is termed "active." When it separates, it is termed "inactive."

Radiographs typically show a solitary cyst that is centrally located in the metaphyseal area and has marked thinning of the adjacent cortical bone and a pseudoloculated appearance (Figure 5–24). The bone cyst is filled with a clear serous fluid, and there is increased pressure during the active phase. The fact that this pressure gradually decreases as the cyst becomes inactive suggests a hydrodynamic mechanism. If there is associated fracture, radiographs may show the characteristic "fallen leaf" sign (Figure 5–25).

The cyst cavity, lined with a fibrinous membrane that contains giant cells, foam cells, and a slight osteoid formation, is similar to the fibrous tissues seen in other fibrous bone lesions, including fibrous dysplasia. The periosteal covering in the area of a cyst is normal, and thus the pathologic fractures heal normally and in most cases do not require surgery. Unfortunately, the cyst usually persists after fracture union and requires further treatment. Bone-resorbing factors, such as matrix metalloproteinases, prostaglandins, interleukin (IL)-1, IL-6, tumor necrosis factor-alpha (TNF-α), and oxygen-free radicals, are demonstrated in the cyst fluid. Nitrate and nitrite levels are also noted to be higher than in serum.

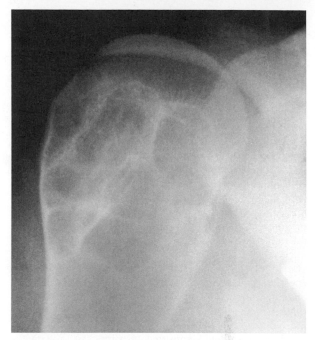

▲ **Figure 5–24.** Radiograph of a solitary bone cyst on the proximal humerus of a 13-year-old boy.

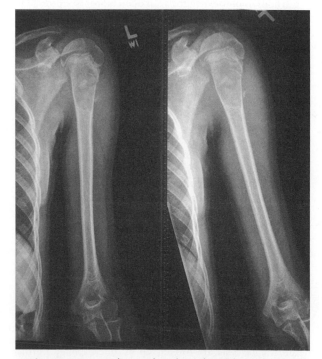

▲ **Figure 5–25.** Radiographs of a solitary bone cyst with associated pathologic fracture and a "fallen leaf" sign in a 12-year-old girl.

Before the mid-1970s, the standard treatment for a solitary bone cyst was aggressive curettage or even resection followed by bone grafting. In patients with active disease, the recurrence rate was 30–50%, and repeated grafting was frequently necessary. In patients with inactive disease, particularly those older than 15 years, the surgical results were much better and the recurrence rate was lower. Unicameral bone cysts are generally considered stage 1 lesions, but occasionally they may be stage 2. Currently, treatment is a function of location. In weight-bearing bones, such as the proximal femur, lesions should be treated aggressively. Initial management usually involves aspiration/injection with either bone marrow or corticosteroid. The injections are carried out with bone biopsy needles and are repeated three to five times at intervals of 2–3 months, depending on the radiographic response. The best results are when the patient is between 5 and 15 years of age, at which time the disease is active and macrophage activity is greatest in the cyst lining. Curettage and bone grafting may also be an effective modality. Demineralized bone matrix injected in combination with autogenous bone marrow shows encouraging results, with a relatively low recurrence rate and low morbidity.

Physicians should note that sarcomas can take on the radiographic appearance of a solitary bone cyst. For this reason, if needle aspiration does not reveal cystic fluid or if it is impossible to inject contrast material and obtain radiologic confirmation of the diagnosis, an open biopsy is indicated to rule out a sarcoma.

B. Aneurysmal Bone Cyst: ICD-9-CM 733.22

Aneurysmal bone cyst is a hemorrhagic lesion with many characteristics of a giant cell tumor but occurs only half as frequently. Although 75% of the cases of aneurysmal bone cyst occur in patients aged 10–20 years old, giant cell tumor is rare in patients younger than 20 years of age. Both aneurysmal bone cyst and giant cell tumor are more common in females than in males. The femur is the most frequently affected site, followed by the tibia, pelvis, and spine. In the spine, two thirds of aneurysmal bone cysts arise from the posterior elements, and one third arise from the vertebral body.

Initially, the aneurysmal bone cyst appears on radiograph as an aggressive osteolytic lesion with extensive permeative cortical destruction that gives the impression of a malignant process such as Ewing sarcoma or hemorrhagic osteosarcoma. Next, a large aneurysmal bulge occurs outside the bone, with a thin reactive shell of bone forming at the outer edge. Less soap-bubbly pseudoseptation is seen in an aneurysmal bone cyst than in a solitary bone cyst (Figure 5–26).

At the time of biopsy, the aneurysmal bone lesion demonstrates large hemorrhagic cysts, but bleeding is modest. The hemorrhagic cysts are broken up by thick spongy fibrous septae that histologically contain great numbers of large giant cells and have thin osteoid seams. Even if a few mitotic figures are seen, the diagnosis of a benign lesion can remain.

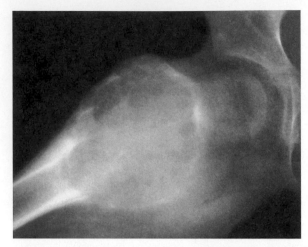

▲ **Figure 5–26.** Radiograph of an aneurysmal bone cyst on the proximal femur of a 5-year-old boy.

A carefully placed biopsy with multiple samples is needed to rule out other well-known skeletal tumors that may demonstrate an aneurysmal component. These include giant cell tumor, chondromyxoid fibroma, and malignant hemorrhagic osteosarcoma. Some authors believe there is no such entity as the aneurysmal bone cyst and that it is merely a morphologic variant of some other underlying neoplastic process. Like the solitary bone cyst, this cyst may have a hydraulic pressure origin that is secondary to hemorrhage and could be traumatically induced. However, abnormal cytogenetic findings were noted in aneurysmal bone cysts, which may suggest a distinct cellular pathogenetic etiology. Specifically, a t(16,17) translocation resulting in a *CDH11-USP6* fusion gene product is frequently observed in aneurismal bone cyst. Aneurysmal bone cyst is either a stage 2 or 3 lesion and frequently symptomatic.

If an aneurysmal bone cyst is left untreated, it may involute spontaneously, during which time it develops a heavy shell of reactive bone at the periphery. This involutional process can be hastened by surgical curettage and bone grafting. Radiation is no longer recommended. Another option for treating extremely large lesions is repeated embolization to reduce the rate of hemorrhagic expansion.

C. Epidermoid Cyst: ICD-9-CM 213.x

The least common bone cyst is the epidermoid bone cyst. This lesion is found either in the distal phalanx or in the skull. No other bone is affected. In the case of the phalanx, the cyst is usually the result of nail bed epithelium being driven into the distal phalanx by a crushing blow. The ectopic squamous epithelium produces a keratinized cavity that is filled with clear fluid and creates a surface erosion with a sclerotic reactive base (Figure 5–27). The bulbous cyst seen at the fingertip transilluminates with flashlight examination. Other conditions that might have a similar appearance are the glomus tumor and the

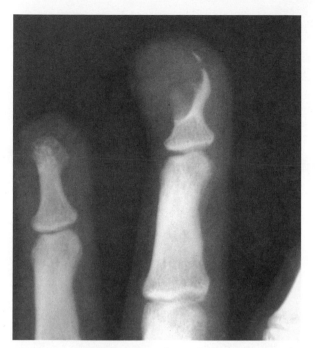

▲ **Figure 5–27.** Radiograph of an epidermoid cyst in the distal phalanx.

enchondroma. The epidermoid cyst is treated with a simple curettage and, in some cases, a bone graft.

▶ Essentials of Diagnosis

- *In the treatment of solitary bone cysts, there is a significant rate of recurrence, but the cysts will usually resolve with skeletal maturity.*

- *If an aneurysmal bone cyst is suspected in the differential diagnosis prior to biopsy, then a telangiectatic osteosarcoma should also be considered.*

▶ Giant Cell Tumor of Bone: ICD-9-CM 213.x

Numerous types of tumors contain giant cells but are not true benign giant cell tumors of bone. Most of the variants are seen in children and include aneurysmal bone cyst, chondroblastoma, simple bone cyst, osteoid osteoma, and osteoblastoma. The giant cell–rich osteosarcoma is the most malignant of the variants, and it is sometimes difficult to distinguish from an aggressive benign giant cell tumor. The giant cell reparative granuloma is a benign variant seen in jaw bones or hand bones and has more spindle cells than a classic giant cell tumor. The brown tumor of hyperparathyroidism is a nonneoplastic variant seen in both primary and secondary hyperparathyroidism. Only after all of the variant conditions are excluded can the diagnosis of benign giant cell tumor be made. Giant cell tumor of bone is now associated with an imbalance in the receptor activator of nuclear factor kappa B/receptor activator of nuclear factor kappa B ligand (RANK/RANKL) system, which is normally associated with osteoclastogenesis.

Between 5 and 10% of all benign bone tumors are true giant cell tumors, occurring most frequently in the third decade of life. They are more frequently found in females than in males. In approximately half of the cases, the tumor is found about the knee. The next most common locations are the distal radius and the sacrum. The tumor is usually painful for several months prior to diagnosis and can cause a pathologic fracture. It can also cause a painful effusion because of its juxtaposition to a major joint. Giant cell tumors may present as either stage 2 or stage 3 disease and less frequently as stage 1. On radiograph, the lesion appears lytic in nature and is located in the epiphyseal-metaphyseal end of a long bone (Figure 5–28). The lesion grows toward the joint surface and frequently comes into contact with articular cartilage but rarely breaks into the joint.

Like the chondroblastoma, the benign giant cell tumor has a 1–2% chance of metastasizing to the lung. Recurrent tumors have up to a 10% chance. Accordingly, pulmonary staging is an important component in the initial evaluation and follow-up of giant cell tumor of bone. The prognosis

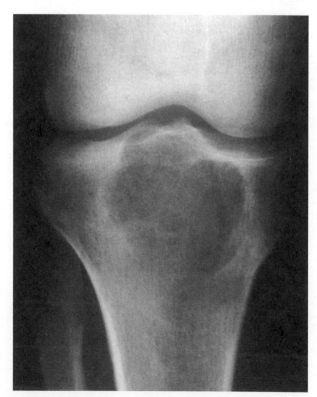

▲ **Figure 5–28.** Radiograph of a giant cell tumor on the proximal tibia of a 22-year-old woman.

for survival with this complication is favorable, and the tumors may resolve spontaneously. The benign giant cell tumor can later convert to a malignant condition such as an osteosarcoma or malignant fibrous histiocytoma. It is generally believed that this is secondary to treatment. A conversion rate of 15–20% is reported in patients who were treated previously with more than 3000 cGy of radiation, with conversion occurring 3 or more years after treatment. The conversion rate in patients who do not receive radiation is less than 5%. This finding has come into question with newer radiation therapy modalities.

Until recent years, the standard treatment for giant cell tumor was curettage and bone grafting. The recurrence rate with this treatment was reported to be up to more than 50%. Follow-up treatment consisted of an aggressive resection of the lesion and reconstruction with a large osteoarticular allograft, endoprosthesis, or an excisional arthrodesis. Currently, most surgeons elect an aggressive curettage, followed by high-speed burring and adjuvant phenol, hydrogen peroxide, or liquid nitrogen and by subsequent packing of the defect with bone cement. With this new approach, the recurrence rate is between 10 and 25%. When giant cell tumor infrequently involves an expendable bone, such as the fibula or ilium, it should be primarily resected. En bloc resection continues to be used to treat multiple recurrent tumors, intensive soft-tissue involvement, or massively destructive cases. Embolization may also prove palliative or curative in unresectable cases. For advanced, multiply recurrent, or aggressive metastatic cases, investigators are developing and testing experimental medical protocols, but these remain to be proven. Close follow-up for locally recurrent disease and pulmonary involvement is critical. Surveillance should include a plain chest radiograph every 6–12 months for the first 2–3 years at least.

Hemangioma: ICD-9-CM 213.x

Hemangioma of bone is a hamartomatous process that occurs more frequently in females than in males. It is most commonly found in vertebral bodies. It is found only rarely in the diaphysis of a long bone (Figure 5–29). Hemangiomas of bone can be associated with hemangiomas of soft tissue. The spinal lesion is usually discovered as an incidental radiographic finding and demonstrates a characteristic vertically oriented honeycombed or moth-eaten appearance. On rare occasions, a lesion can cause cord compression that may require surgical resection. In such cases, preoperative angiography is critical in evaluating the blood supply to the spinal cord. Alternatively, an attempt at arterial embolization may prove successful and is less aggressive.

Gorham disease, characterized by massive osteolysis in children or young adults, is usually associated with the presence of benign cavernous hemangiomas or lymphangiomas of bone. This strange condition usually affects a particular area (such as the spine or the hip) but can involve multiple bones of the area and tends to resolve spontaneously (Figure 5–30).

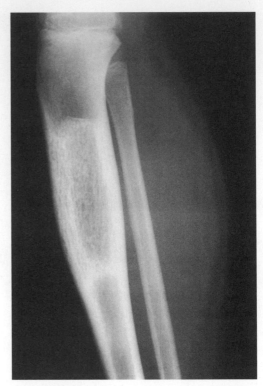

▲ **Figure 5–29.** Radiograph of a hemangioma of the tibia in a 14-year-old boy.

▶ Essentials of Diagnosis

- *Plain radiography is usually diagnostic, and advanced imaging is usually not required except for preoperative planning in benign bone lesions.*

- *Surgical treatment of most benign bone tumors is reserved for symptomatic lesions unresponsive to conservative measures, those at significant risk of fracture, or for documented enlargement over time.*

- *Giant cell tumor of bone and chondroblastoma both have an incidence of pulmonary seeding, and chest imaging should be included in the workup and surveillance of these entities.*

Balke M, Ahrens H, Streitbuerger A, et al: Treatment options for recurrent giant cell tumors of bone. *J Cancer Res Clin Oncol* 2009;135:149. [PMID: 18521629]

Balke M, Schremper L, Gebert C, et al: Giant cell tumor of bone: treatment and outcome of 214 cases. *J Cancer Res Clin Oncol* 2008;134:969. [PMID: 18322700]

Baruffi MR, Neto JB, Barbieri CH, et al: Aneurysmal bone cyst with chromosomal changes involving 7q and 16p. *Cancer Genet Cytogenet* 2001;129:177. [PMID: 11566352]

Bottner F, Roedl R, Wortler K, et al: Cyclooxygenase-2 inhibitor for pain management in osteoid osteoma. *Clin Orthop Relat Res* 2001;393:258. [PMID: 11764357]

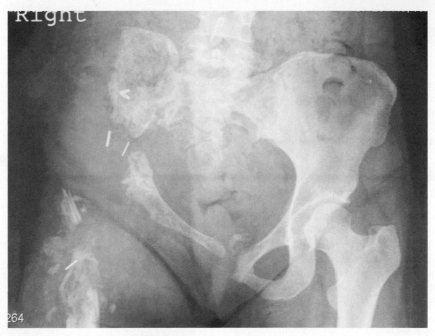

▲ **Figure 5–30.** Radiograph of a pelvis affected with Gorham disease in a 48-year-old woman.

Bovee JV, van Roggen JF, Cleton-Jansen AM, et al: Malignant progression in multiple enchondromatosis (Ollier's disease): an autopsy-based molecular genetic study. *Hum Pathol* 2000;31:1299. [PMID: 11070122]

Cantwell CP, Obyrne J, Eustace S: Current trends in treatment of osteoid osteoma with an emphasis on radiofrequency ablation. *Eur Radiol* 2004;14:607. [PMID: 14663625]

DiCaprio MR, Enneking WF: Fibrous dysplasia. *J Bone Joint Surg Am* 2005;87:1848. [PMID: 16085630]

Flemming DJ, Murphey MD, Carmichael BB, et al: Primary tumors of the spine. *Semin Musculoskelet Radiol* 2000;4:299. [PMID: 11371321]

Harish S, Saifuddin A: Imaging features of spinal osteoid osteoma with emphasis on MRI findings. *Eur Radiol* 2005;15:2396. [PMID: 15973540]

Kjar RA, Powell GJ, Schilcht SM, et al: Percutaneous radiofrequency ablation for osteoid osteoma: experience with a new treatment. *Med J Aust* 2006;184:563. [PMID: 16768663]

Knochentumoren A: Local recurrence of giant cell tumor of bone after intralesional treatment with and without adjuvant therapy. *J Bone Joint Surg Am* 2008;90:1060. [PMID: 18451399]

Oliveira AM, Hsi BL, Weremowicz S, et al: USP6 (Tre2) fusion oncogenes in aneurysmal bone cyst. *Cancer Res* 2004;64:1920. [PMID: 15026324]

Parekh SG, Donthineni-Rao R, Ricchetti E, et al: Fibrous dysplasia. *J Am Acad Orthop Surg* 2004;12:305. [PMID: 15469225]

Radhakrishnan K, Rockson SG: Gorham's disease: an osseous disease of lymphangiogenesis. *Ann N Y Acad Sci* 2008;1131:203. [PMID: 18519972]

Randall RL, Nork SE, James PJ: Aggressive aneurysmal bone cyst of the proximal humerus. *Clin Orthop Relat Res* 2000;370:212. [PMID: 10660716]

Robinson P, White LM, Sundaram M, et al: Periosteal chondroid tumors: radiologic evaluation with pathologic correlation. *Am J Roentgenol* 2001;177:1183. [PMID: 11641198]

Romeo S, Oosting J, Rozeman LB, et al: The role of noncartilage-specific molecules in differentiation of cartilaginous tumors: lessons from chondroblastoma and chondromyxoid fibroma. *Cancer* 2007;110:385. [PMID: 17559135]

Rougraff BT, Kling TJ: Treatment of active unicameral bone cysts with percutaneous injection of demineralized bone matrix and autogenous bone marrow. *J Bone Joint Surg Am* 2002;84-A:921. [PMID: 12063325]

Salerno M, Avnet S, Alberghini M, et al: Histogenic characterization of giant cell tumor. *Clin Orthop Relat Res* 2008;466:2081. [PMID: 18543051]

Staals EL, Bacchini P, Mercuri M, et al: Dedifferentiated chondrosarcomas arising in preexisting osteochondromas. *J Bone Joint Surg Am* 2007;89:987. [PMID: 17473135]

Suneja R, Grimer RJ, Belthur M, et al: Chondroblastoma of bone: long-term results and functional outcome after intralesional curettage. *J Bone Joint Surg Br* 2005;87:974. [PMID: 15972914]

Sung AD, Anderson ME, Zurakowski D, et al: Unicameral bone cyst: a retrospective study of three surgical treatments. *Clin Orthop Relat Res* 2008;466:2519. [PMID: 18679761]

MALIGNANT BONE TUMORS

Malignant bone tumors are primarily treated with wide resection followed by limb salvage surgery in current treatment regimens. Depending on the histology, this is augmented with the use of adjuvant chemotherapy or radiation therapy or both. Limb salvage surgery has been advanced significantly in the past two decades with improvements in megaprostheses and techniques associated with the use of allografts. Recent series report survival of megaprostheses about the knee of 80–90% and 60–80% at 5 and 10 years, respectively. Newer methods of fixation of megaprostheses are showing promising results for long-term survival and ease of revision surgery.

Allograft reconstruction continues to be useful but is used less frequently in the reconstruction of a major weight-bearing joint and is now primarily used in metadiaphyseal reconstructions.

▶ Osteoid-Forming Sarcomas

Aside from multiple myeloma, osteosarcoma of bone is the most common primary malignant tumor of bone, constituting 20% of all primary malignancies of bone. In the United States, between 500 and 1000 new cases are diagnosed each year. The global incidence is felt to be between 1 and 3 per million people annually. There are currently many subtypes of osteoid-forming sarcomas, ranging from the extremely low-grade variants, such as parosteal osteosarcoma, to the extremely high-grade variants, such as osteosarcoma secondary to Paget disease.

The molecular pathobiology is a subject of intense investigation. Several gene families were investigated as potential biomarkers of disease progression. Among these are genes involved with angiogenesis (eg, vascular endothelial growth factor [VEGF]), growth factors and their receptors (eg, transforming growth factor beta, Wnt receptor LRP5, HER2), cytoskeletal protein (eg, ezrin), and cellular senescent protein (ie, telomerase).

This discussion begins with the more common, central form of sarcoma that is seen in children and known as classic osteosarcoma.

A. Classic Osteosarcoma: ICD-9-CM 170.x

The classic form of osteosarcoma is typically seen in patients in their second or third decade, with a peak in the adolescent growth spurt. It occurs more frequently in males than in females and is found in the metaphyseal areas of long bones, with 50% of lesions about the knee joint (Figures 5–31 and 5–32). The distal femur is the most common site, followed by the proximal tibia and then the proximal humerus. It is rare to see osteosarcoma in the small bones of the feet or hands or in the spine. When seen in the foot, it occurs in the larger bones of the hindfoot. The prognosis is more favorable for a tumor in a small bone than for one in a large bone.

Most patients with classic osteosarcoma have symptoms of pain before a tumor is noticeable. A mass near a major joint may exist for several weeks or even months before a diagnosis is made. Dilated veins may be seen in the overlying skin. The radiographic findings include permeated lytic destruction of metaphyseal bone, with eventual cortical breakthrough into the subperiosteal space and subsequent

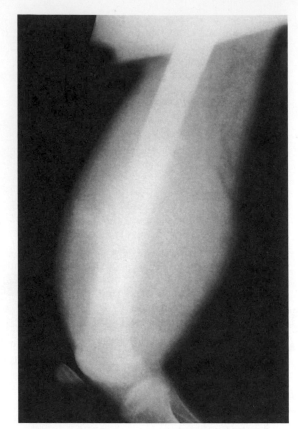

▲ **Figure 5–31.** Osteosarcoma of the distal femur of a 15-year-old female patient. Notice the sunburst appearance.

formation of a Codman triangle at the diaphyseal end of the tumor (Figure 5–33). As the tumor continues to push its way into the extracortical soft tissue, a typical sunburst pattern of neoplastic bone may be seen outside the involved bone.

In fewer than 2–25% of cases, an additional lesion may be found at a higher level in the femur. Such a so-called skip lesion may portend a worse probability of survival and should be considered a true metastatic focus (stage III [Enneking], stage III [AJCC]). Approximately 50% of osteosarcomas are of the more typical osteoblastic type, followed by chondroblastic, with a small percentage of them fibroblastic. Whether the subtype portends a better or worse prognosis is controversial. Confounding variables such as multidrug resistance (P-glycoprotein expression) may be differentially expressed in different subtypes. P-glycoprotein overexpression itself bears a substantial relationship to clinical outcome. More recently, higher serum VEGF levels, as a presumed surrogate marker for higher levels of tumor VEGF production, have been associated with poorer survival.

Staging of osteosarcoma must include an MRI of the entire involved bone (Figure 5–34). This technique offers

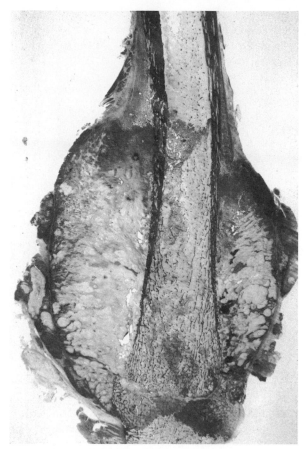

▲ **Figure 5–32.** Gross surgical specimen from Figure 5–31. Notice the sharp upper medullary margin located about the same level as the extracortical mass. The tumor has not invaded the growth plate.

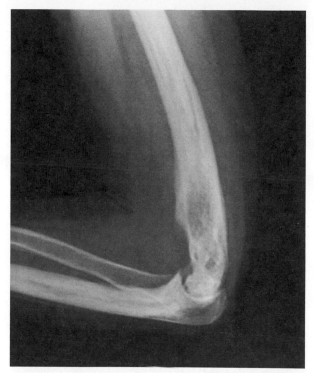

▲ **Figure 5–33.** Radiograph of the elbow of a 16-year-old patient who carries diagnoses of hereditary retinoblastoma and melorheostosis. Increasing elbow pain and the anterior diaphyseal Codman triangle were the presentation of an underlying osteosarcoma.

excellent contrast of the extracortical portion of the tumor and at the same time gives good intramedullary contrast of the high-signal tumor next to a low-signal fatty marrow. The periphery of the tumor can readily be appreciated and represents the most anaplastic and rapidly growing part of the tumor. This region is the best tissue for a biopsy because it is easy to reach, soft enough for a diagnostic frozen section, and representative of the most aggressive portion of the tumor. Furthermore, the MRI provides the necessary anatomic data to determine the level of transection through the host bone for a safe margin and to determine whether a limb-sparing procedure is feasible.

Before the advent of adjuvant multidrug chemotherapy, the treatment of osteosarcoma was radical amputation. Eighty percent of these patients proceeded to die from disseminated pulmonary disease. Today, with the combination of chemotherapy and surgical treatment, the prognosis for 5-year survival approaches 70%.

The drugs commonly used today include high-dose methotrexate, doxorubicin, cisplatin, and ifosfamide. The use of interferon in poor responders and patients suffering from disseminated disease is currently under investigation. They are administered intravenously in cyclic intervals of 3–4 weeks for approximately 11–15 weeks prior to surgery. Surveillance imaging studies are performed during this period to assess possible reduction in tumor volume. Tumor necrosis secondary to neoadjuvant chemotherapy, determined at the time of tumor resection, is an important prognostic factor. Patients with greater than 90% tumor necrosis have a significantly improved 5-year survival rate, approaching 85%. Approximately half of patients demonstrate this response to current chemotherapy regimens. Furthermore, the postoperative drug regimen can be adjusted based on this evaluation.

In extremity osteosarcoma, limb-sparing surgery, with wide resection of the tumor, is the standard approach. Amputation is reserved for the exceptional or recurrent case. In fewer than 10% of cases, amputation is performed at a level approximately 5 cm above the upper pole of the tumor. Limb salvage techniques continue to evolve with reconstruction

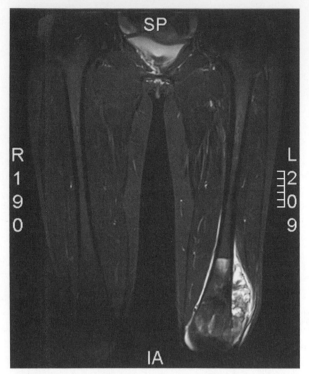

▲ **Figure 5–34.** Short tau inversion recovery sequence MRI of osteosarcoma of the femur of a 19-year-old woman.

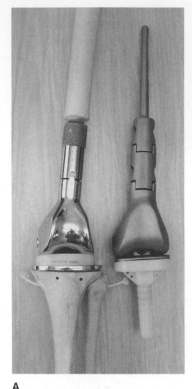
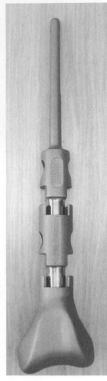

A

B

▲ **Figure 5–35.** (**A**) Two examples of distal femoral replacement systems. (**B**) Modularity of system allows different-size intercalary body segments.

options including large prostheses, structural allografts, and composite reconstructions. Endoprosthetics are composed of modular components in various lengths, linked together with taper fittings (Figures 5–35 and 5–36). The intramedullary stems are of various diameters and lengths and are usually cemented. The immediate functional results are excellent, with minimal early complications. However, subsequent loosening at 5–10 years occurs in as many as 15–30% of cases. Newer methods of fixation of megaendoprosthetics are showing promising results. Another limb-sparing procedure consists of the use of an osteoarticular allograft alone or in combination with a prosthesis. The major drawback with large bone allografts is a 10–15% chance of infection, nonunion, or stress fracture, especially in the immunosuppressed patient receiving chemotherapy. The use of an excisional arthrodesis was more popular in the past but is rarely elected today because patients have better function with a mobile joint.

Prior to the introduction of chemotherapy, the finding of pulmonary metastasis portended a very poor prognosis. Today, however, in larger tumor centers where aggressive surgical approaches with multiple thoracotomies and continued chemotherapy are used, the 5-year survival rate is approximately 30%. Patients with skeletal metastases, or so-called metachronous osteosarcoma, however, have a significantly worse prognosis, unless it is a solitary, resectable metastasis.

Molecular oncologic evaluation of osteosarcoma specimens is beginning to elucidate factors involved in its pathogenesis. The *p53* suppressor genes have an increased mutation rate in osteosarcoma. Osteosarcomas with a mutation in the *p53* gene have a significantly higher rate of genomic instability, including multiple duplicate chromosomes and frequent hyperdiploid state. However, wild-type *TP53* and *MDM2* in and of themselves are not of prognostic value. Loss of heterozygosity of the *Rb* gene is a predictive feature of osteosarcoma. The *F33* isoform also demonstrates a strong correlation with osteosarcoma disease progression. *ErbB-2* (*HER-2/neu*), a protooncogene, and transforming growth factor-beta, isoform 3 expression is also correlated with a worse prognosis in osteosarcoma patients. Controversy surrounds the significance of cytoplasmic versus membranous staining in *HER-2/neu* expression as it relates to prognosis in osteosarcoma.

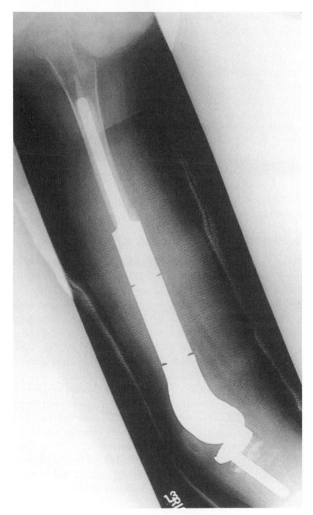

▲ **Figure 5–36.** Lateral radiograph of distal femoral replacement system in skeletally immature patient. Expansion with larger intercalary body segment is possible.

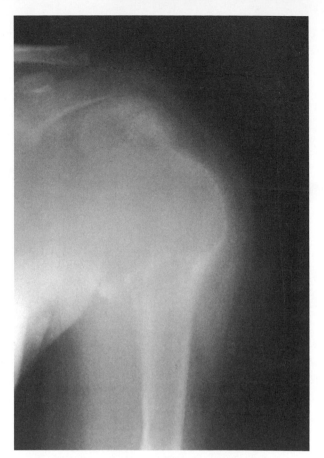

▲ **Figure 5–37.** Radiograph of hemorrhagic osteosarcoma in a 6-year-old girl.

B. Hemorrhagic or Telangiectatic Osteosarcoma: ICD-9-CM 170.x

Telangiectatic osteosarcoma, an extremely lytic and destructive variant of classic osteosarcoma, is seen in the same age group and location. Its radiographic appearance is similar to that of an aneurysmal bone cyst, thereby making the diagnosis difficult (Figure 5–37). The pathologic specimen is hemorrhagic, with microscopic evaluation demonstrating the presence of malignant-appearing stromal cells with giant cells.

Because hemorrhagic osteosarcoma is a high-grade, purely lytic tumor, the incidence of pathologic fracture in the early course of the disease is high. If significant contamination of the adjacent neurovascular structures results, a pathologic fracture may necessitate amputation rather than limb salvage (Figure 5–38). This situation must be carefully evaluated with a preoperative MRI. Accordingly, in cases with significant risk for fracture during the preoperative treatment regimen, it may be appropriate to immobilize the involved extremity or proceed with limb-sparing surgery earlier than usual. Prior to the advent of aggressive multidrug chemotherapy, the prognosis for patients with hemorrhagic osteosarcoma was extremely poor. At present, however, it is the same as the prognosis for patients who have classic osteosarcoma and is treated with similar protocols.

C. Parosteal Osteosarcoma: ICD-9-CM 170.x

Parosteal osteosarcoma is a low-grade variant arising in an exophytic pattern from the cortical surface of bone. There is no medullary involvement. It is low grade, with a 5-year survival rate in excess of 90% and a 10-year survival rate of 80%. It accounts for 3–4% of all osteosarcomas.

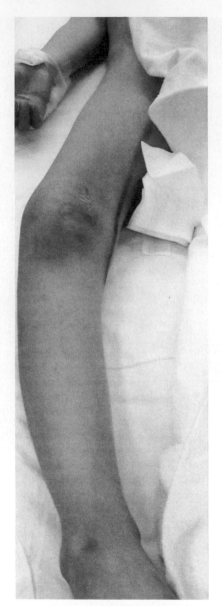

▲ **Figure 5–38.** Clinical photograph of patient who sustained pathologic fracture through a distal femoral osteosarcoma contaminating the neurovascular structures precluding limb salvage.

The tumor is composed of a spindle cell fibroblastic component with well-developed bone trabeculae. There also may be areas of cartilage present. Osteoblasts are well differentiated, and few mitotic figures are present.

Parosteal osteosarcoma is more common in females than in males and affects a slightly older age group than classic osteosarcoma (see Table 5–2). It is a slow-growing tumor with minimal symptoms initially. It is metaphyseal in origin, with the vast majority of cases involving the posterior aspect of the distal femur (Figure 5–39).

Because the parosteal osteosarcoma is low grade, it does not respond well to either chemotherapy or radiation therapy. Therefore, the only treatment is wide surgical resection. This usually requires distal femur removal, but in smaller cases, side resection of the posterior cortex and tumor only may be feasible, sparing the knee joint. Nevertheless, a negative tumor margin is imperative. Otherwise, recurrence is likely. Recurrence may occur as late as 5–10 years because of the tumor's slow growth.

On occasion, low-grade parosteal osteosarcoma can dedifferentiate into a high-grade sarcoma. Such a lesion carries a similar prognosis to classic osteosarcoma.

D. Periosteal Osteosarcoma: ICD-9-CM 170.x

Periosteal osteosarcoma is another surface osteosarcoma of low to intermediate grade. This lesion represents less than 2% of all osteosarcomas. It arises beneath the periosteum, elevating it and inducing vigorous neoosteogenesis with a predominant chondroblastic differentiation. It is slightly more common in females, with a peak incidence in the second decade of life. It almost exclusively arises in the long bone. The lesion can mimic an aneurysmal bone cyst or periosteal chondroma radiographically (Figure 5–40).

Because of its low to intermediate grade, periosteal osteosarcoma is generally not treated with chemotherapy but may be in more advanced cases. Wide surgical resection is the modality of choice. It also carries a better prognosis than classic osteosarcoma. Approximately 25% of patients succumb to metastatic disease within 2–3 years. The surgical treatment is usually a limb-sparing procedure, and because the tumor is more diaphyseal in location, the adjacent joints may often be spared.

E. Secondary Osteosarcoma: ICD-9-CM 170.x

Osteosarcoma can arise from benign disease through a process that may involve a second mutation and usually occurs at a later age (see Table 5–2). Among the benign conditions that can result in secondary osteosarcoma are Paget disease, osteoblastoma, fibrous dysplasia, benign giant cell tumor, bone infarction, and chronic osteomyelitis.

The classic example of a secondary osteosarcoma is seen in a small percentage of patients with Paget disease. Pagetic osteosarcomas, which represent approximately 3% of all osteosarcomas, are the most common osteosarcomas in the older (>65 years) age group. The most frequent location for pagetic osteosarcoma is the humerus, followed next by the pelvis and femur. The typical patient has a long history (15–25 years) of dull, aching pain associated with the inflammation of Paget disease before a new acute pain arises in an area of recent lytic destruction and the diagnosis of pagetic osteosarcoma is established (Figure 5–41). The prognosis for

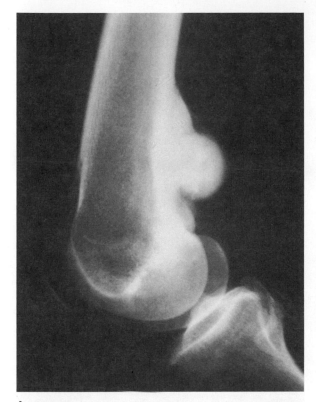

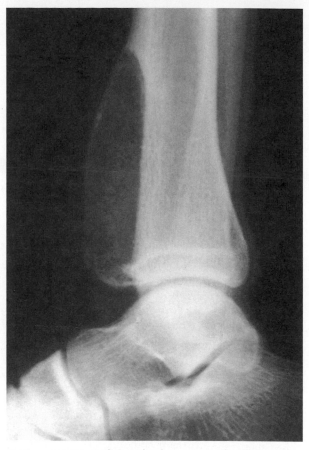

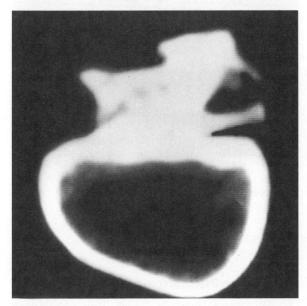

▲ **Figure 5–40.** Radiograph of a periosteal osteosarcoma of the distal tibia in a 15-year-old boy.

▲ **Figure 5–39.** Radiograph (**A**) and CT scan (**B**) of a parosteal osteosarcoma of the distal femur in a 21-year-old woman.

patients with pagetic osteosarcoma is extremely poor (5-year survival rate of approximately 8%). Because of the older age group involved, chemotherapy is usually not an option secondary to intolerance.

F. Low-Grade Intramedullary Osteosarcoma: ICD-9-CM 170.x

Another rare and low-grade osseofibrous variant of osteosarcoma is the central or intramedullary form. Although this variant has a microscopic appearance similar to that of parosteal osteosarcoma, it is usually located in metaphyseal bone about the knee joint in adults between 15 and 65 years of age. Males and females are equally affected. Radiographically, intramedullary osteosarcoma creates a sclerotic density in metaphyseal bone (Figure 5–42). Like the parosteal osteosarcoma, the low-grade intramedullary osteosarcoma carries an excellent prognosis and can be treated with local surgery alone.

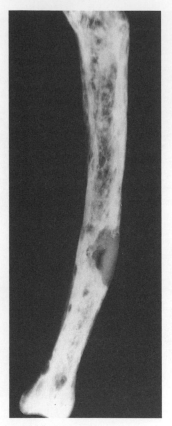

▲ **Figure 5–41.** Radiograph of a pagetic osteosarcoma of the tibia.

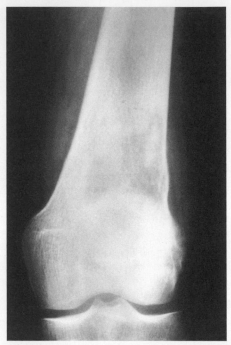

A

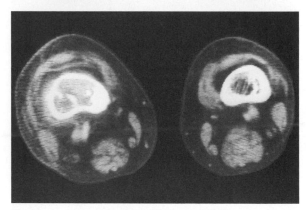

B

▲ **Figure 5–42.** Radiograph (**A**) and CT scan (**B**) of a low-grade intramedullary osteosarcoma in the distal femur of a 65-year-old man.

G. Irradiation-Induced Osteosarcoma: ICD-9-CM 170.x

Radiation-induced osteosarcoma may arise after any form of significant radiation exposure (in excess of 30 Gy) (Figure 5–43). Onset is usually delayed an average of 15 years (range, 3–55 years). Other irradiation-induced sarcomas, besides the osteosarcoma type, include irradiation-induced fibrosarcoma and malignant fibrous histiocytoma. All of these secondary sarcomas are invariably high grade and carry a poor prognosis for survival, with a very high rate of metastasis.

H. Multicentric Osteosarcoma: ICD-9-CM 170.x, or 199.0

Multicentric osteosarcoma has two clinical presentations: (1) synchronous, occurring in childhood and adolescence, and (2) metachronous, occurring in adults. The synchronous type is a high-grade sclerosing intramedullary type, which is lethal. The adult form is less aggressive, with a lower-grade histologic appearance, but prognosis remains grim (Figure 5–44).

I. Soft-Tissue Osteosarcoma: ICD-9-CM 171.x

Osteosarcoma can occur in muscle tissue outside bone and accounts for approximately 4% of all osteosarcomas (Figure 5–45). Soft-tissue osteosarcoma is rarely seen in patients younger than 40 years. The number of cases is equal in females and males, and the tumor is usually seen in large muscle groups of the pelvis and thigh areas.

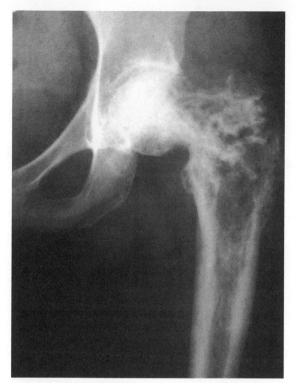

▲ **Figure 5–43.** Radiograph of irradiation-induced osteosarcoma of the peritrochanteric area in a 35-year-old woman.

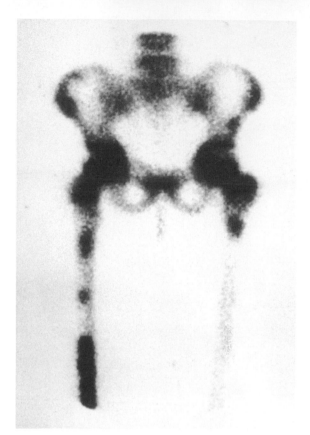

▲ **Figure 5–44.** Isotope bone scan of multicentric osteosarcoma in an 8-year-old girl.

Soft-tissue osteosarcoma must be differentiated from the more common myositis ossificans. Although soft-tissue osteosarcoma shows heavy mineralization in the central area (see Figure 5–45), myositis ossificans has a zonal pattern of ossification, with the mature, dense ossification concentrating at the periphery of the lesion.

The treatment of soft-tissue osteosarcoma is the same as for the high-grade osseous form and includes a wide resection and adjuvant chemotherapy. The prognosis is worse with the soft-tissue form of osteosarcoma, with a high rate of chemotherapy resistance.

▶ **Essentials of Diagnosis**

- *Osteosarcoma is best confirmed by biopsy of the leading edge of the soft-tissue component if possible.*
- *Parosteal osteosarcoma usually occurs on the posterior aspect of the distal femur, exhibiting a "stuck-on" appearance.*

▶ **Chondroid-Forming Sarcomas**

Chondroid-forming sarcomas are a heterogeneous group of neoplasms consisting of a cartilage-based histology. A cornerstone to the diagnosis of chondrosarcoma is the absence of osteoid formation. If any osteoid is present with a malignant stroma, the tumor is considered an osteosarcoma with chondroblastic features. It is important to make the distinction because chondrosarcomas behave differently from osteosarcomas. However, this can be a difficult task. The surgeon must consider the age of the patient and carefully assess the radiographic and histologic features to confirm the diagnosis.

A. Primary or Central Conventional Chondrosarcoma: ICD-9-CM 170.x

The typical primary chondrosarcoma is a low-grade tumor seen in adults between 30 and 60 years of age. The tumor is found more frequently in men than in women. Minimal symptoms of pain may occur over a period of several years before a radiograph is obtained. The pelvis and femur are the most common locations, followed by the rib cage, proximal humerus, scapula, and upper tibia. Primary chondrosarcoma is extremely rare in small bones, including the hand and foot. The metaphysis is the most common location in a long bone; however, a diaphyseal location is not unusual.

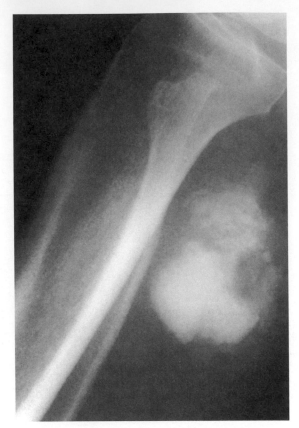

▲ **Figure 5–45.** Radiograph of a soft-tissue osteosarcoma in the calf area of a 67-year-old woman.

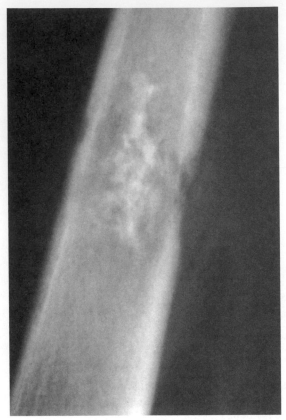

▲ **Figure 5–46.** Radiograph of a low-grade primary chondrosarcoma in the distal femur of an 83-year-old man.

Approximately 85% of central chondrosarcomas are low-grade lesions with a typical matrix calcification that can be described as flocculated with multiple rings and arcs. Radiographic criteria are more useful in distinguishing between enchondroma and low-grade chondrosarcoma than are histologic ones. Frequently cited radiographic criteria suggestive of more aggressive biologic potential include endosteal scalloping greater than 50% of the cortical width, change over time, and adjacent radiolucency near an area of typical chondroid matrix calcification (Figure 5–46). The high-grade lesions are rare, and radiographically, they lose their typical lobulated and calcific pattern and take on the appearance of a more permeative high-grade tumor, such as a malignant fibrous histiocytoma. At the same time, histologically, the high-grade chondrosarcomas lose their chondroid matrix pattern, which is replaced with that of a more aggressive spindle cell tumor.

Because of the weakened cortex, the patient usually complains of local pain not experienced with an enchondroma. Because most chondrosarcomas are low grade, they do not respond well to adjuvant irradiation or chemotherapy.

Therefore, aggressive surgical management is imperative. However, optimal surgical management is controversial. Although wide en bloc resection is ideal from a margin standpoint, it can often produce considerable morbidity. On the contrary, aggressive intralesional resection (curettage) and margin expansion with adjuvant therapy (eg, phenol or liquid nitrogen) can reduce morbidity and may provide equal local control. In fact, some authors found that for grade 1 chondrosarcoma the margin of resection is not significant in terms of local recurrence or disease progression.

In general, the prognosis for low-grade central chondrosarcoma is very good, with a low rate of pulmonary metastasis if the primary lesion is widely resected. Nevertheless, recurrences can occur late, even over 15 years later. For any intermediate- or high-grade chondrosarcomas, wide en bloc resection is mandatory (Figure 5–47).

B. Secondary Chondrosarcoma: ICD-9-CM 170.x

The vast majority of secondary chondrosarcomas arise from osteochondromas in patients afflicted with HME.

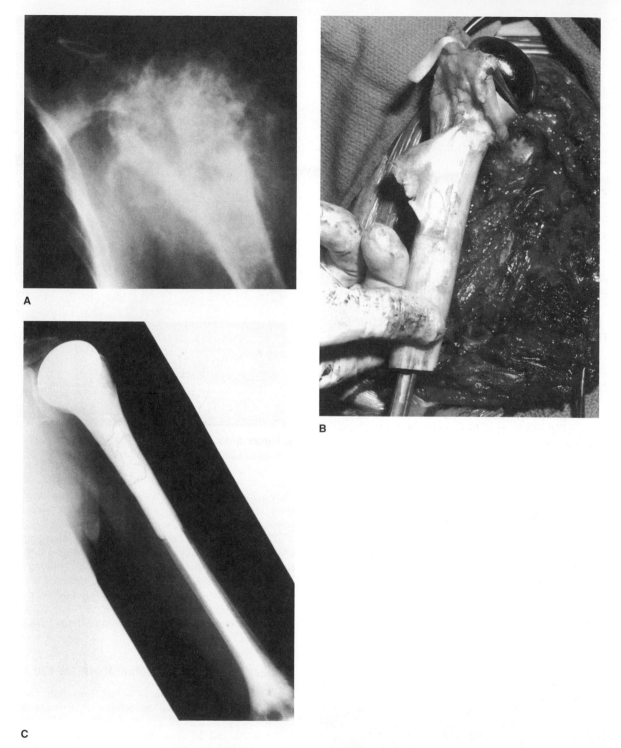

▲ **Figure 5–47.** Preoperative radiograph of a large central chondrosarcoma in the proximal humerus of a 52-year-old woman (**A**), placement of a Neer prosthesis (**B**), and postoperative radiograph (**C**).

Patients with solitary osteochondromas do not generally form secondary chondrosarcomas in their lesions, making prophylactic removal unnecessary and unwarranted unless the solitary lesion is otherwise symptomatic. Even in patients with HME, the rate of malignant degeneration is less than 1% and generally does not occur in patients prior to skeletal maturity. However, patients with secondary chondrosarcoma tend to be younger than those with primary chondrosarcomas (see Table 5–2). The lesions tend to be slow growing with minimal to mild symptoms. The most common site is the pelvis, followed by the proximal femur, proximal humerus, and ribs. Plain radiographs demonstrate a flocculated calcific pattern (Figure 5–48). An osteochondroma with a cartilage cap thicker than 1–2 cm should raise suspicion of a secondary chondrosarcoma. The overall prognosis for patients with secondary or peripheral chondrosarcoma is even better than that for patients with primary or central chondrosarcoma. Surgical removal, without violation of the cartilage cap, is the only effective treatment modality.

C. Dedifferentiated Chondrosarcoma: ICD-9-CM 170.x

Dedifferentiated chondrosarcoma is the most malignant variant of chondrosarcoma, accounting for between 5 and 10% of all chondrosarcomas. It is heralded by the transformation of areas of conventional chondrosarcoma into malignant fibrous histiocytoma or osteosarcoma. Histologically, it is characterized by two distinct but neighboring areas of low- to intermediate-grade malignant chondroid tumor and heterogeneous high-grade sarcoma. Dedifferentiated chondrosarcoma occurs in older patients, usually between 50 and 70 years of age. It is found in the same areas affected by central primary chondrosarcomas, including the pelvis,

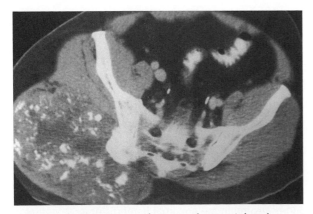

▲ **Figure 5–48.** CT scan of a secondary peripheral chondrosarcoma in the ilium of a 56-year-old man with hereditary multiple exostoses.

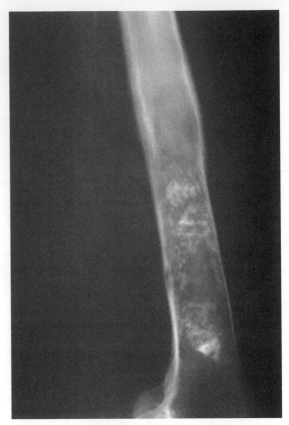

▲ **Figure 5–49.** Radiograph of dedifferentiated chondrosarcoma in the distal femur of a 73-year-old woman.

femur, and proximal humerus (Figure 5–49). Radiographs show areas of rarefaction within the tumor with cortical attenuation. Pathologic fracture is not uncommon.

The prognosis in dedifferentiated chondrosarcoma is bleak, with the majority of patients developing and dying of metastatic disease within 1 year (historically, 1-year survival rate approached 10%). Chemotherapy and radiation therapy are less effective than in malignant fibrous histiocytoma or osteosarcoma that arose de novo. Surgical resection remains the mainstay of treatment, with adjuvant modalities employed in younger patients.

D. Clear Cell Chondrosarcoma: ICD-9-CM 170.x

Clear cell chondrosarcoma is a rare low-grade variant of chondrosarcoma. Clear cell lesions occur more often in males than in females and are usually seen in patients between 20 and 50 years of age. The vast majority of lesions are found in the femoral head (Figure 5–50). The radiographic appearance is one of a lytic tumor with sharp margination and a central matrix calcification, creating the appearance of a chondroblastoma. Although microscopic

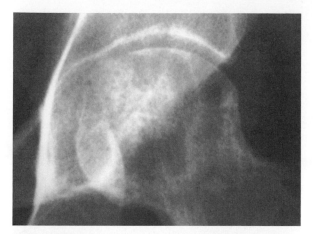

▲ **Figure 5–50.** Radiograph of clear cell chondrosarcoma of the femoral head in a 25-year-old man.

examination reveals the presence of some giant cells, as seen in chondroblastoma, areas of low-grade chondrosarcoma are also evident in which no giant cells are seen. Even on gross examination, the clear cell chondrosarcoma does not look like a chondrosarcoma, which explains why it is frequently mistaken for a chondroblastoma in younger adult patients. The tumor cells have abundant glycogen, giving them their characteristic clear cell phenotype. Although no significant genetic alteration is found in clear cell chondrosarcoma, newer findings show that alkaline phosphatase activity may correlate with prognosis.

The treatment for clear cell chondrosarcoma is a wide excision and reconstruction. The prognosis with this type of treatment is good. In contrast, when lesions are mistaken for chondroblastomas and treatment consists of simple curettage and bone grafting, the prognosis is poor and the recurrence rate is high.

E. Mesenchymal Chondrosarcoma: ICD-9-CM 170.x, or 171.x

Another rare variant of chondrosarcoma is the mesenchymal chondrosarcoma. It is a highly cellular tumor composed of primitive mesenchymal cells with foci of cartilage differentiation. This tumor involves the soft tissue in a third of cases, occurs more frequently in females than in males, and is seen in young adults (see Table 5–2). The jaw is the most common location, followed by the spine and ribs, with few cases noted in long bones.

Mesenchymal chondrosarcoma is a high-grade tumor with histologic features of low-grade chondrosarcoma. Heavily calcified areas, mixed with areas of malignant round cells, may give it the appearance of Ewing sarcoma or solitary fibrous tumor.

Treatment consists of resection, with a wide margin if possible, and adjuvant chemotherapy and radiation therapy. Despite aggressive treatment, the prognosis is very poor, with a high incidence of pulmonary metastasis.

▶ **Essentials of Diagnosis**

- *Typical chondroid-forming sarcomas are not sensitive to radiation therapy or chemotherapy and are treated with surgery alone.*
- *Pain, endosteal scalloping greater than 50% of the cortical width, or radiolucency adjacent to an otherwise typical-appearing enchondroma should alert the practitioner to the possibility of chondrosarcoma.*

▶ **Round Cell Tumors**

This so-called group of tumors is composed of distinct tumors that, other than their similar microscopic appearance using hematoxylin-eosin stain, are quite different. They behave and are treated in a variety of ways, given that each arises from a different cell type.

A. The Ewing Sarcoma Family of Tumors

1. Ewing sarcoma: ICD-9-CM 170.x—Ewing sarcoma is a well-known clinical entity originally described by James Ewing as a diffuse endothelioma of bone. Since the time of his description, many theories have evolved regarding the tumor's true histogenesis. Based on electron microscopic and immunohistochemical findings, experts currently believe the tumor represents an undifferentiated member of the family of neural tumors distinct from neuroblastoma. The Ewing sarcoma family of tumors (ESFT) also includes the less common primitive neuroectodermal tumor (PNET) and Askin tumors. ESFTs have been shown to express chimeric transcription factors that result from reciprocal translocations involving chromosome 22, containing the Ewing sarcoma gene (*EWS*). Ninety percent of the time t(11:22) is seen, resulting in a *EWS/FLI-1* chimera. Less frequently, t(21:22) and t(7:22) are seen. The resulting transcription factors are put under the control of the *EWS* promoter. Recently, investigations have elucidated a handful of downstream targets, including VEGF (encoding vascular endothelial growth factor) and CAV1 (encoding caveolin-1), which are thought to be necessary for tumorigenesis. Furthermore, they are being investigated as possible targets for directed therapy.

In 90% of cases, Ewing sarcoma is found in patients between 5 and 25 years of age. If the patient is younger than 5 years, the most likely diagnosis is metastatic neuroblastoma. Males are affected more frequently than females and carry a worse prognosis. The pelvis is the most common location, followed by the femur, tibia, humerus, and scapula. However, because Ewing sarcoma is a myelogenous tumor, it can be found in any bone in the body (Figure 5–51).

Ewing sarcoma appears radiographically as a central lytic tumor of the diaphyseal-metaphyseal bone. It creates extensive permeative destruction of cortical bone, and as it breaks through under the periosteum, it takes on a typical onion-skin, multilaminated appearance. Another radiographic feature is the reactive hair-on-end appearance created by

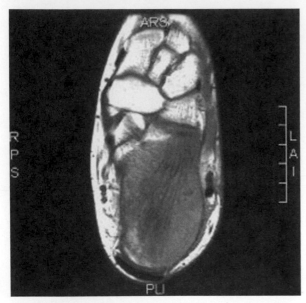

▲ **Figure 5–51.** MRI of the hindfoot of a 9-year-old girl with calcaneal Ewing sarcoma.

bone forming along the periosteal vessels that run perpendicularly between the cortex and the elevated periosteum (Figure 5–52).

Ewing sarcoma can frequently masquerade as osteomyelitis because it is a high-grade lesion with resultant areas of necrosis; liquefaction may occur that may be mistaken for pus. Furthermore, patients frequently present with systemic symptoms of low-grade intermittent fever and elevated white cell count and erythrocyte sedimentation rate (ESR). Microscopically, small roundlike cells predominate in densely packed sheets. Formation of pseudorosettes may also be seen (in <20%). The rosette-like patterns are more frequently seen in PNET.

Ewing sarcoma is an aggressive malignancy with high local recurrence and metastatic rates. Patients with locally resectable disease treated with multidrug chemotherapy have a 5-year survival rate of approximately 70% (Figure 5–53). Currently, most chemotherapy is driven by large cooperative trials including induction and adjuvant multidrug chemotherapy with drugs such as vincristine, doxorubicin, cyclophosphamide, dactinomycin, and ifosfamide. Unfortunately, 15–25% of patients present with nonlocalized disease. For the patient who presents with advanced metastatic disease, the 5-year survival rate is 30%. Resection of lung metastasis, if possible, does improve survival.

Ewing sarcoma is a radiosensitive tumor. Historically, this was a modality of choice, employing 45–50 Gy over 5 weeks to treat local disease. Because of the not insignificant risk of secondary sarcomas, surgery was investigated as the primary modality for local control. If the margins are contaminated, local irradiation must still be used postoperatively.

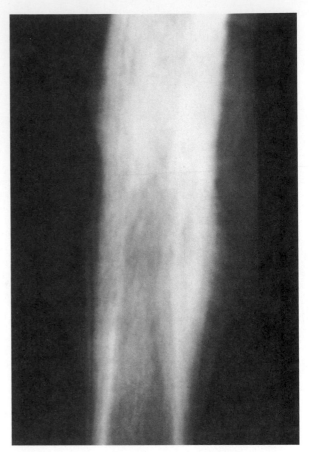

▲ **Figure 5–52.** Radiograph of periosteal response in Ewing sarcoma of the femur in a 15-year-old boy.

Postoperative radiotherapy is also generally accepted after complete resection of a tumor showing a poor response to neoadjuvant chemotherapy, with improved local control rates having been illustrated. Preoperative radiotherapy, although not generally used, may have a role in lesions that are on the border of resectability.

2. Primitive neuroectodermal tumor: ICD-9-CM 170.x, or 171.x—PNET is the less common relative to Ewing sarcoma. Like Ewing, this tumor demonstrates expression of neural markers by immunocytochemistry. PNET also exhibits the t(11:22) translocation with the resulting EWS/FLI-1 fusion protein. In fact, because of such similarities, it is generally agreed that PNET and Ewing sarcoma represent ends of a spectrum of disease.

By strict criteria, PNET is a rare tumor, representing approximately 10% of Ewing-like tumors. The demographics are identical to those of Ewing-like tumors. Treatment of PNET is similar to that of Ewing sarcoma; however, the survival rate is slightly less. Accordingly, some authors feel it should be distinguished from Ewing sarcoma.

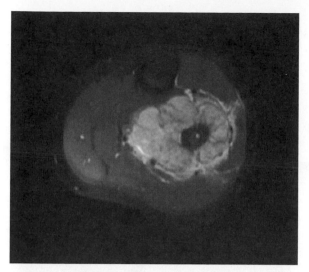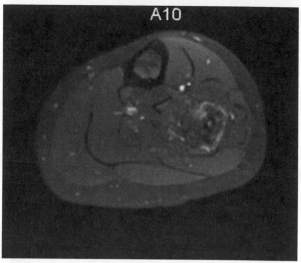

▲ **Figure 5–53.** Pretreatment MRI (**A**) and MRI following 10 weeks of neoadjuvant chemotherapy (**B**) of Ewing sarcoma of the fibula in a 14-year-old boy.

B. Lymphoma: ICD-9-CM 200.x

Lymphoblastic tumors are considered systemic neoplasms of the lymphatic organs, including the bone marrow, and they account for 7% of all malignant bone tumors. They can be roughly divided into Hodgkin lymphomas and non-Hodgkin lymphomas, both of which can affect bone. Of the two groups, the lymphomas associated with Hodgkin disease carry a much better prognosis. When they are found in bone, they tend to be localized and have a considerable blastic response, especially when involving the vertebra.

There are two main types of non-Hodgkin lymphomas. The type emphasized in this section is the primary lymphoma of bone, in which a localized lytic destruction occurs in a single bone, and the results of staging studies (including an isotope bone scan, a CT scan of the chest and abdomen, and marrow aspiration) all prove negative for other areas of involvement. The other type is the more generalized or systemic form of lymphoma, in which many lymphoid organs are involved, including the lymph nodes, liver, spleen, and bone. The prognosis is better for an isolated primary lymphoma of bone, but years later involvement may become generalized or systemic and carry a worse prognosis. This is similar to the case with plasma cell tumors, in which the findings in a patient can change from that of a solitary plasmacytoma with an excellent prognosis to that of the multiple myeloma form of the disease with a poor prognosis.

Primary lymphoma of bone, which was formerly called reticulum cell sarcoma of bone, accounts for approximately half of all lymphomas. To meet the criteria of being a primary bone lymphoma, there must be a 4- to 6-month interval from the onset of skeletal manifestations to the development of systemic disease. It occurs more frequently in males than in females, is usually found in patients older than 25 years, and affects the spine or pelvis in more than 50% of the cases. In the extremities, the femur is the most commonly involved area, followed next by the humerus and the tibia. Polyostotic involvement occurs in 10–40% of cases.

Radiographic findings in primary lymphoma include extensive lytic permeation of cortical bone, with minimal sclerotic response in diaphyseal, metaphyseal, and epiphyseal locations (Figure 5–54). MRI studies demonstrate that the actual marrow involvement is frequently more extensive than the cortical disruption seen on simple radiographs suggests.

The most common histologic types of lymphoma of bone are the large cell or mixed small and large cell types. The cells tend to demonstrate little cytoplasmic structure. However, the nuclear pattern shows indented and folded nuclear patterns and a prominent pink-staining nucleolus, which may help to distinguish it histologically from Ewing sarcoma. Immunohistochemical staining is often necessary to differentiate Ewing sarcoma from the B-cell and T-cell subtypes of lymphoma. In the case of lymphomas, the glycogen stain is usually negative, but the reticulum stain is often positive.

In primary lymphoma of bone, as in Ewing sarcoma, multidrug chemotherapy has greatly improved the 5-year survival rate, which now is approximately 70% for patients with either of these tumors. Like Ewing sarcoma, primary lymphoma of bone is highly sensitive to local irradiation. If the primary lymphoma is localized, a wide resection and limb-salvage reconstruction may be carried out, thereby avoiding the need for local irradiation, and possibly effect a cure. However, if the involvement is more extensive, as is commonly the case, it is necessary to use intralesional techniques such as cemented intramedullary nails or a long-stem

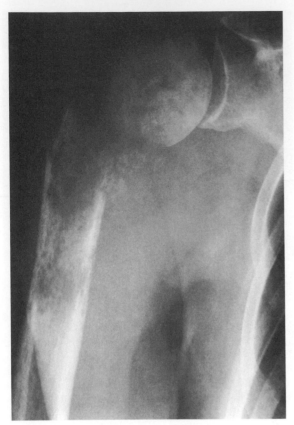

▲ **Figure 5–54.** Radiograph of a lymphoma in the proximal humerus of a 64-year-old woman.

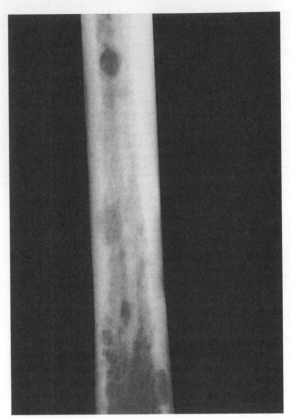

▲ **Figure 5–55.** Radiograph of multiple myeloma in the femoral shaft of a 72-year-old man.

prosthesis and subsequently use whole bone irradiation, similar to the management of metastatic carcinoma with pathologic fractures. In cases of extensive systemic involvement, bone marrow transplantation can be used.

C. Plasma Cell Tumor

A bone tumor composed of malignant monoclonal plasma cells is referred to as a myeloma or plasmacytoma. It is rare for a patient to have a solitary myeloma or plasmacytoma. Tumors are almost always found on multiple bony sites, in which case the term *multiple myeloma* is used.

1. Myeloma: ICD-9-CM 203.x—Multiple myeloma, which is the most common primary tumor of bone, accounts for 45% of all malignant bone tumors. It is the second most common hematopoietic malignancy. An estimated 90% of cases are in patients older than 40 years. It accounts for 1% of all malignancies in Caucasians and 2% in African Americans.

The disease is characterized by a triad of osteolytic punched-out lesions (multifocal) (Figure 5–55), neoplastic proliferation of atypical plasma cells, and a monoclonal gammopathy. Diagnostic criteria are established for myeloma. Major criteria include plasmacytosis on biopsy of a lesion, marrow plasmacytosis, and an abnormal serum protein electrophoresis and light (Bence Jones) proteinuria. It causes bony destruction similar to that caused by lymphomas, with most lesions occurring in the trunk, hip, and shoulder areas. Knowledge of the biology of multiple myeloma continues to increase at an astounding rate, and investigation toward targeted therapy grows proportionally. Targeted therapy trials have included inhibitors of cell surface receptors such as VEGF-R and IGF-1R, inhibitors of cell signaling pathways such as the MAPK pathway and the MTOR pathway, janus kinase inhibitors, histone deacetylase inhibitors, and many others.

Lesions are rarely found distal to the knee or elbow. Approximately 3% of patients with myeloma have a sclerotic form of the disease, which appears to carry a better prognosis and is associated with peripheral neuropathy. The serum protein electrophoresis shows an elevated monoclonal immunoglobulin on either the *a* or *y* spike. Bence Jones proteinuria is secondary to light-chain immunoglobulin spillover. Occasionally, electrophoresis of a urine sample yields positive results, whereas that of a serum sample yields negative results. In aggressive forms of myeloma, the extensive bone breakdown causes hypercalcemia, which can lead to a semicomatose state and, over a long period, results in nephrocalcinosis. Renal damage also results from protein plugging of the renal tubules, and renal failure may ensue.

A marrow aspirate usually demonstrates the abnormal plasma cells. These cells show an eccentrically placed nucleus in a well-structured eosinophilic cytoplasm. Although normal B-cell–derived plasma cells produce antibodies, the abnormal B-cell–derived plasma cells produce immunoglobulin that is ineffective, which helps explain the increased infection rate in patients with myelomas. Patients may also demonstrate extraosseous infiltrates, with the majority seen in the upper airway and oral cavity. Amyloidosis may be seen concurrently in 10–15% of cases. A quarter of these have extensive cardiac involvement. In such cases, the median survival is 4 months.

Plain radiographs show myeloma lesions to be sharply demarcated lytic lesions with minimal periostitis. Pathologic fixation is frequent. Bone scans have a high false-negative rate thought to be caused by almost exclusive osteoclast activity. For this reason, a skeletal survey instead of a bone scan is important in the staging of this disease.

Fewer than 2% of myeloma cases demonstrate the POEMS syndrome (*p*olyneuropathy, *o*rganomegaly, *e*ndocrinopathy, *M*-component spike, *s*kin changes, *s*cleroses of bone).

Although treatment and prognosis have improved, myeloma remains a fatal disease, with more than 90% of patients dying within 2–3 years. Chemotherapy such as melphalan and cortisone may induce a transient remission in 50–70% of cases. Bisphosphonates have been introduced to the treatment algorithm with results showing reduced skeletal-related events, pain, and increased time to progression.

Local treatment of myeloma is similar to that of metastatic disease, with cemented intramedullary nails and prosthetic devices used after an intralesional debridement. The amount of bleeding at the surgical site is usually extensive, similar to that encountered with surgery for metastatic renal cell carcinoma and certain thyroid metastases. After surgery, the entire bone should be irradiated with 5500 cGy. Spinal lesions should be handled just like metastatic tumors, as discussed in a later section.

2. Solitary myeloma: ICD-9-CM 203.8—Solitary lesions are rare (Figure 5–56). By definition, there must be no marrow involvement. Seventy-five percent of these cases have an entirely normal serum protein electrophoresis (SPEP) and urine protein electrophoresis (UPEP). The remaining 25% may have mild abnormalities. Vertebral involvement is the most common site. Patients also tend to be younger (<50 years old). Unfortunately, 70% of these solitary cases develop multiple myeloma within 3 years. Until this happens,

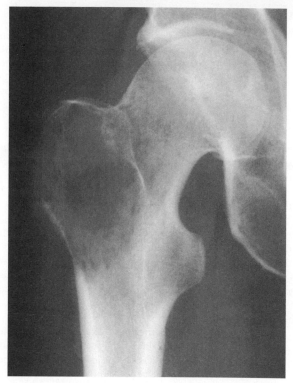

▲ **Figure 5–56.** Radiograph of a solitary plasmacytoma in the proximal femur of a 46-year-old man.

the treatment is only local, with a wide resection if possible or intralesional debridement and reconstruction followed by radiation therapy.

▶ Essentials of Diagnosis

- *Ewing sarcoma is characterized by a chimeric transcription factor that is a product, most often, of the t(11:22), resulting in an altered expression pattern in the neoplastic lineage.*

- *Because of the high level of sensitivity of lymphoma to chemotherapy and radiation therapy, wide resection is infrequently performed.*

- *Because of the propensity for myeloma to remain cold on isotope bone scanning, a skeletal survey is the study of choice for skeletal staging.*

▶ Fibrous Sarcomas of Bone

Malignant fibrous tumors of bone are clinically similar to osteosarcoma, but they affect an older (<20 years) age group of patients and show a complete absence of tumor osteoid formation. The two major tumors in this category are fibrosarcoma and malignant fibrous histiocytoma.

A. Fibrosarcoma of Bone: ICD-9-CM 170.x

Fibrosarcoma of bone is a malignant spindle cell tumor seen in an older patient population with a peak incidence in the fourth decade. It is 10 times less frequent than osteosarcoma but tends to involve similar locations. The most common site of fibrosarcoma is the distal femur, followed next in order by the proximal tibia, pelvis, proximal femur, and proximal humerus. It is rarely seen in the spine, hand, or foot.

On radiograph, fibrosarcomas appear to be almost purely osteolytic and permeative, similar to lymphomas. For this reason, they are painful and can lead to a pathologic fracture. Microscopically, myofibroblastic differentiation with osteoid formation or histiocytes permits distinction from fibroblastic osteosarcoma and malignant fibrous histiocytoma (MFH) of bone. The low-grade form is characterized by malignant-appearing fibroblasts that form a large amount of collagen fiber, giving the appearance of an aggressive desmoplastic fibroma. The high-grade form is characterized by a more anaplastic fibroblast with a higher index of mitotic activity and less collagen fiber formation. It is common to see a basket-woven or storiform pattern in the microscopic picture.

The prognosis and treatment are directly related to the histologic grade of the tumor. Low-grade fibrosarcoma has a better prognosis than osteosarcoma does, but it must be treated by means of an aggressive and wide resection to avoid local recurrence. Because the low-grade form has a low mitotic index, adjuvant chemotherapy and radiation therapy are of little help. High-grade fibrosarcoma has a prognosis and a rate of metastasis that are similar to those of osteosarcoma, and it is usually treated in a similar manner with a combination of surgery and, if the patient is young enough to tolerate the systemic toxicity, adjuvant chemotherapy.

B. Malignant Fibrous Histiocytoma of Bone: ICD-9-CM 170.x

Prior to 1970, MFH was rarely diagnosed in bone but was commonly found in soft tissue. Now MFH is more common in bone than fibrosarcoma, but the two types of tumor run a similar clinical course. MFH of bone is seen in middle-age and older adults (see Table 5–2), is more common in males than in females, and affects the same bony sites as fibrosarcoma and osteosarcoma.

MFH is a purely lytic tumor that shows aggressive permeation of metaphyseal-diaphyseal bone, similar to the findings in lymphoma (Figure 5–57). Lytic destruction is diffuse, with no evidence of a periosteal response of blastic repair. Microscopic analysis of MFH usually shows the tumor to be high grade and have highly anaplastic fibroblasts mixed with malignant histiocytes and a few giant cells in a typical storiform pattern.

Because MFH is closely related to the high-grade fibrosarcoma, it carries a poor prognosis, with high rates of local recurrence and metastasis. The treatment program is therefore similar to that for high-grade fibrosarcoma and osteosarcoma, and it includes an aggressive wide resection and the use of adjuvant chemotherapy.

▶ Adamantinoma of Bone: ICD-9-CM 170.x

Adamantinomas account for only 0.33% of all malignant bone tumors; occur with equal frequency in males and females, usually during the second and third decades of life; are found in the tibia in 90% of cases; and are usually diaphyseal in location, frequently starting in the anterior cortex. The cause of adamantinoma remains unknown, although angioblastic synovial cells and epithelial cells were considered in the past. Newer investigations, including immunohistochemistry and electron microscopic studies, lend support to the hypothesis of an epithelial origin, which goes along with the histologic appearance of a basal cell carcinoma and might explain the common site of origin subcutaneously in the anterior tibial cortex. The name *adamantinoma* was given to the tibial lesion because its histologic appearance is similar to that of the adamantinoma of jaw bone (ameloblastoma), but the two entities have no other relationship clinically.

In patients with adamantinoma, the radiograph shows a benign tumor with a lytic central core that is surrounded by reactive sclerotic bone that typically bulges the anterior cortex and thus takes on the appearance of either fibrous dysplasia or osteofibrous dysplasia (Figure 5–58). One consideration in the differential diagnosis is that osteofibrous dysplasia is painless, whereas pain is a frequent symptom in adamantinoma. Another is that benign fibrous lesions of bone stop growing at bone maturity, whereas the adamantinoma continues on into adult life, at which point a biopsy of the progressive lytic portion of the disease should be performed. There have been cases of osteofibrous dysplasia combined with small areas of adamantinoma scattered in the benign osseofibrous tissue. In fact, more recently, one variant has been termed osteofibrous dysplasia–like adamantinoma and appears to have less overall biologic potential. Adamantinoma is also occasionally found in both the tibia and fibula, so the physician should look for multiple sites.

Microscopic findings include nests or cords of epithelial or angioid tissue growing in a fibrous tissue stroma, which can give adamantinoma the appearance of a low-grade angiosarcoma or a metastatic carcinoma. Cytologically, chromosomal abnormalities are frequent, especially gains of chromosomes 7, 8, 12, and 19.

Adamantinoma grows extremely slowly, over many years, but on occasion metastasizes to regional lymph nodes and the lung. For this reason, it should be treated by a wide resection, which in most cases is a segmental diaphyseal resection followed by an allograft reconstruction over an intramedullary nail. Because of the low-grade nature of this tumor, adjuvant irradiation or chemotherapy is rarely indicated. Even if pulmonary metastases occur, they can be resected, and there is a fairly good prognosis for survival.

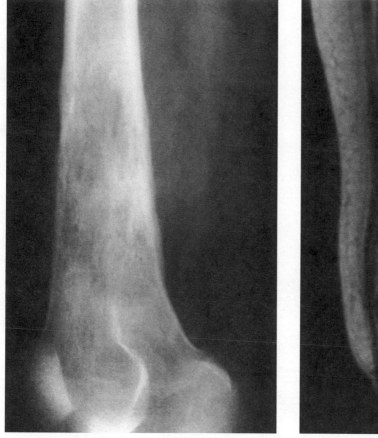 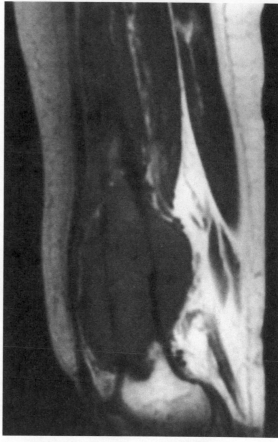

A   B

▲ **Figure 5–57.** Radiograph (**A**) and T1-weighted MRI (**B**) of malignant fibrous histiocytoma in the distal femur of a 50-year-old woman.

▶ Essentials of Diagnosis

- *Adamantinoma is on a continuum with osteofibrous dysplasia and should be distinguished by increasing pain and radiographic progression.*

▶ Vascular Sarcomas of Bone

Vascular sarcomas are relatively rare. They include the hemangioendothelioma, angiosarcoma, and hemangiopericytoma of bone. The terms *hemangioendothelioma* and *angiosarcoma* are frequently used synonymously; however, the first term refers to a low-grade tumor, and the second term usually suggests a higher grade lesion with a poorer prognosis.

A. Hemangioendothelioma: ICD-9-CM 170.x

The hemangioendothelioma, also known as angiosarcoma, which is more common in males than in females, is seen in a wide range of ages between the second and seventh decades. The femur, pelvis, spine, and ribs are the usual sites of origin, and the diaphyses and metaphyses of the long bones are also involved. One third of cases are multicentric, usually in the same bone or limb.

Radiographically, the lesion appears purely lytic. The more anaplastic the disease process is, the less reactive bone is. The clinical picture varies widely, depending on the histologic grade of the tumor. The low-grade lesions look like benign hemangiomas, are slow growing, and carry an excellent prognosis. The high-grade lesions are fast-growing lytic lesions with a poor prognosis.

Treatment depends on the histologic grade. The low-grade lesions do well with simple curettage and bone graft, but the high-grade lesions require a more aggressive wide resection and reconstruction. Adjuvant chemotherapy and radiation therapy can be considered for high-grade lesions, especially in patients with multifocal disease.

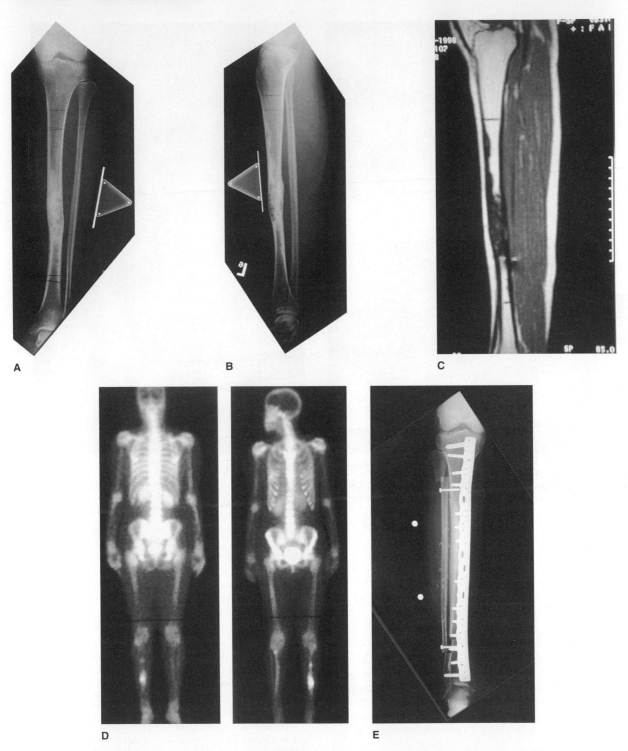

▲ **Figure 5–58.** Adamantinoma of the tibia. Initial anteroposterior radiograph (**A**), lateral radiograph (**B**), bone scan (**C**), and MRI (**D**). Immediate postoperative radiographs after resection with intercalary allograft reconstruction and vascularized fibula transport are shown in **E** and **F**. Anteroposterior and lateral radiographs from 3 years postoperatively are shown in **G** and **H**. Clinical photographs from 3 years postoperatively are shown in **I–K**.

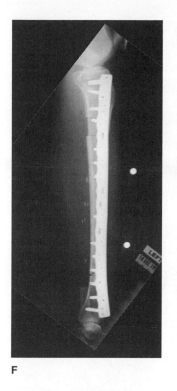

F

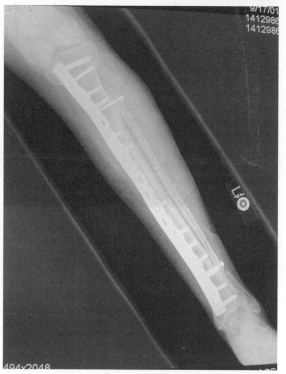

G

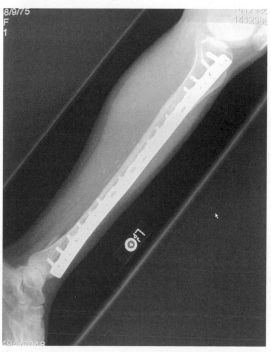

H

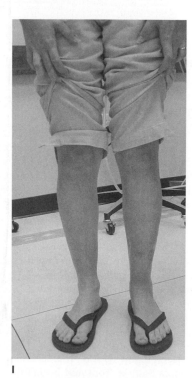

I

▲ **Figure 5–58.** (Continued)

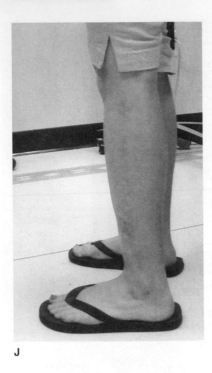

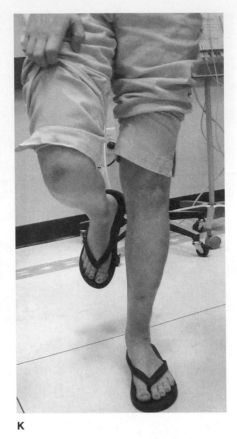

▲ **Figure 5–58.** (Continued)

▶ Chordomas: ICD-9-CM 170.x

Chordoma of bone is rare and accounts for 4% of malignant bone tumors. It takes its origin from the primitive notochord and has the clinical appearance of a chondrosarcoma. Chordomas affect males more frequently than females and are seen in patients between 30 and 80 years of age. Although 50% of the tumors are sacrococcygeal in origin, 37% arise in the sphenoccipital area, and the remainder of tumors arise from vertebral bodies of the cervical or lumbar spine. The cranial lesions are seen in a younger age group and carry a poor prognosis because of the dangerous location next to the brain, where surgical removal is difficult.

On radiograph, the chordoma appears as a centrally located lytic process that has minimal sclerotic response at the periphery and may show slight matrix calcification, as in a chondrosarcoma. By definition, chordoma is a midline lesion. If the sacrum is involved, the lesion is seen usually in the lower three sacral segments and presents as an extracortical lobulated mass both in front and behind the sacrum. Because of the slow tumor growth, pain may not occur early, but constipation can be an early symptom that results from pressure on the rectum. Because the true anatomic borders are not readily defined by routine radiography, it is best to image this tumor with CT or MRI (Figure 5–59).

Microscopically, nests or cords of cells, sprinkled in a sea of mucinous tissue, give an appearance similar to low-grade chondrosarcoma. In most cases, large vacuolated cells appear like a signet ring and are referred to as physaliferous cells.

Treatment for the sacral lesions is an aggressive wide resection, which can be difficult because of excessive bleeding. Significant neurogenic bowel and bladder deficits can result. At present, it is common to use adjuvant radiation therapy to help reduce the chance of postoperative recurrence. Newer studies recommend using up to 5000 cGy preoperatively, followed by a boost of 1500 cGy postoperatively. If the surgeon is successful in obtaining clean margins, the local recurrence rate is approximately 30%. With contaminated margins, the recurrence rate climbs to 65%. Recurrence 10–15 years following surgery is common. Because of the low-grade characteristics of the chordoma, it is rare to see a pulmonary metastasis, even after a local recurrence following an inadequate local surgical resection.

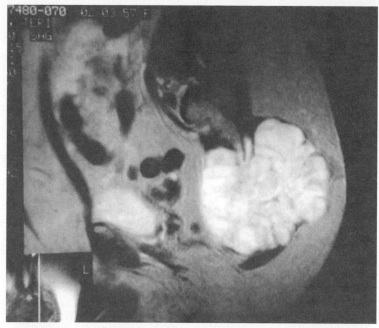

A

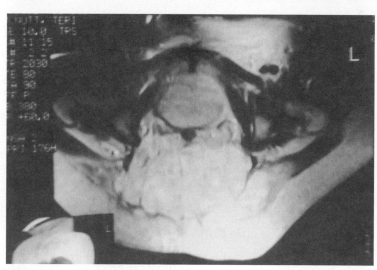

B

▲ **Figure 5–59.** Sacral chordoma in middle-aged woman: T2 sagittal image (**A**) and T2 transverse image (**B**).

▶ Essentials of Diagnosis

- *Information provided in the history and physical examination is critical in determining malignant versus benign characteristics of bone tumors.*

- *Survival in Ewing sarcoma and osteosarcoma has been dramatically improved with refined neoadjuvant*

chemotherapy, and the timing and duration of that treatment modality can affect outcome.

- *Biopsy of bone lesions with suspected malignant potential should include a portion of the periphery of the lesion, particularly when there is an associated soft-tissue component, as this is where the most diagnostic tissue is found.*

Anthouli-Anagnostopoulou FA, Hatziolou E, Papachristou G, et al: Juxtacortical osteosarcoma. A distinct malignant bone neoplasm. *Adv Clin Pathol* 2004;3:127. [PMID: 11080792]

Avnet S, Longhi A, Salerno M, et al: Increased osteoclast activity is associated with aggressiveness of osteosarcoma. *Int J Oncol* 2008;33:1231. [PMID: 19020756]

Bacci G, Balladelli A, Palmerini E, et al: Neoadjuvant chemotherapy for osteosarcoma of the extremities in preadolescent patients: the Rizzoli Institute experience. *J Pediatr Hematol Oncol* 2008;30:908. [PMID: 19131777]

Bacci G, Ferrari S, Bertoni F, et al: Histologic response of high-grade nonmetastatic osteosarcoma of the extremity to chemotherapy. *Clin Orthop Relat Res* 2001;386:186. [PMID: 11347833]

Bacci G, Forni C, Longhi A, et al: Local recurrence and local control of non-metastatic osteosarcoma of the extremities: a 27-year experience in a single institution. *J Surg Oncol* 2007;96:118. [PMID: 17577221]

Barrille-Nion S, Barlogie B, Bataille R, et al: Advances in biology and therapy of multiple myeloma. *Hematology (Am Soc Hematol Educ Program)* 2003;248. [PMID: 14633785]

Bruns J, Elbracht M, Niggemeyer O: Chondrosarcoma of bone: an oncological and functional follow-up study. *Ann Oncol* 2001;12:859. [PMID: 11484965]

Burger R, Le Gouill S, Tai YT, et al: Janus kinase inhibitor INCB20 has antiproliferative and apoptotic effects on human myeloma cells in vitro and in vivo. *Mol Cancer Ther* 2009;8:26. [PMID: 19139110]

Cesari M, Bertoni F, Bacchini P, et al: Mesenchymal chondrosarcoma. An analysis of patients treated at a single institution. *Tumori* 2007;93:423. [PMID: 18038872]

Crapanzano JP, Ali SZ, Ginsberg MS, et al: Chordoma: a cytologic study with histologic and radiologic correlation. *Cancer* 2001;93:40. [PMID: 11241265]

Desai SS, Jambhekar N, Agarwal M, et al: Adamantinoma of tibia: a study of 12 cases. *J Surg Oncol* 2006;93:429. [PMID: 16550582]

Donati D, Yin J, Di Bella C, et al: Local and distant control in non-metastatic pelvic Ewing's sarcoma patients. *J Surg Oncol* 2007;96:19. [PMID: 17345611]

Ewing J: Diffuse endothelioma of bone. *Proc NY Pathol Soc* 1921;21:17. [No PMID]

Gelderblom H, Hogendoorn PC, Dijkstra SD, et al: The clinical approach towards chondrosarcoma. *Oncologist* 2008;13:320. [PMID: 18378543]

Han I, Oh JH, Na YG, et al: Clinical outcome of parosteal osteosarcoma. *J Surg Oncol* 2008;97:146. [PMID: 18050289]

Hoang BH, Kubo T, Healey JH, et al: Expression of LDL receptor-related protein 5 (LRP5) as a novel marker for disease progression in high-grade osteosarcoma. *Int J Cancer* 2004;109:106. [PMID: 14735475]

Kanamori M, Antonescu CR, Scott M, et al: Extra copies of chromosomes 7, 8, 12, 19, and 21 are recurrent in adamantinoma. *J Mol Diagn* 2001;3:16. [PMID: 11227067]

Khanna C, Wan X, Bose S, et al: The membrane-cytoskeleton linker ezrin is necessary for osteosarcoma metastasis. *Nat Med* 2004;10:182. [PMID: 14704791]

Kilpatrick SE, Geisinger KR, King TS, et al: Clinicopathologic analysis of HER-2/neu immunoexpression among various histologic subtypes and grades of osteosarcoma. *Mod Pathol* 2001;14:1277. [PMID: 11743051]

Mandahl N, Gustafson P, Mertens F, et al: Cytogenetic aberrations and their prognostic impact in chondrosarcoma. *Genes Chromosomes Cancer* 2002;33:188. [PMID: 11793445]

Ocio EM, Mateos MV, Maiso P, et al: New drugs in multiple myeloma: mechanisms of action and phase I/II clinical findings. *Lancet Oncol* 2008;9:1157. [PMID: 19038762]

Ogose A, Hotta T, Kawashima H, et al: Elevation of serum alkaline phosphatase in clear cell chondrosarcoma of bone. *Anticancer Res* 2001;21:649. [PMID: 11299821]

Overholtzer M, Rao PH, Favis R, et al: The presence of p53 mutations in human osteosarcomas correlates with high levels of genomic instability. *Proc Natl Acad Sci USA* 2003;100:11547. [PMID: 12972634]

Pring ME, Weber KL, Unni KK, et al: Chondrosarcoma of the pelvis. A review of sixty-four cases. *J Bone Joint Surg Am* 2001;83-A:1630. [PMID: 11701784]

Rizzo M, Ghert MA, Harrelson JM, et al: Chondrosarcoma of bone: analysis of 108 cases and evaluation for predictors of outcome. *Clin Orthop Relat Res* 2001;391:224. [PMID: 11603673]

Roland Durr H, Wegener B, Krödel A, et al: Multiple myeloma: surgery of the spine: retrospective analysis of 27 patients. *Spine (Phila Pa 1976)* 2002;27:320. [PMID: 11805699]

Schwab JH, Antonescu CR, Athanasian EA, et al: A comparison of intramedullary and juxtacortical low-grade osteogenic sarcoma. *Clin Orthop Relat Res* 2008;466:1318. [PMID: 18425560]

Scully SP, Ghert MA, Zurakowski D, et al: Pathologic fracture in osteosarcoma: prognostic importance and treatment implications. *J Bone Joint Surg Am* 2002;84-A:49. [PMID: 11792779]

Streitburger A, Ahrens H, Balke M, et al: Grade I chondrosarcoma of bone: the Munster experience. *J Cancer Res Clin Oncol* 2009;135:543. [PMID: 18855011]

Tallini G, Dorfman H, Brys P, et al: Correlation between clinicopathological features and karyotype in 100 cartilaginous and chordoid tumours. A report from the Chromosomes and Morphology (CHAMP) Collaborative Study Group. *J Pathol* 2002;196:194. [PMID: 11793371]

Tian E, Zhan F, Walker R, et al: The role of the Wnt-signaling antagonist DKK1 in the development of osteolytic lesions in multiple myeloma. *N Engl J Med* 2003;349:2483. [PMID: 14695408]

Weiss A, Khoury JD, Hoffer FA, et al: Telangiectatic osteosarcoma: the St. Jude Children's Research Hospital's experience. *Cancer* 2007;109:1627. [PMID: 17351949]

BENIGN SOFT-TISSUE TUMORS

Soft tissue can be defined as nonepithelial, extraskeletal mesenchymal tissue exclusive of the reticuloendothelial system and glia. This definition would include fat, fibrous tissue, muscle, and the relating neurovascular structures.

Benign soft-tissue tumors, by definition, represent a differentiated neoplastic process with a limited capacity for autonomous growth. They generally demonstrate a marginal capacity to invade locally with infrequent local recurrence. Because of the extensive numbers of benign soft-tissue tumors, discussion is limited here to the more common entities.

▶ Lipomas

The lipoma is by far the most common soft-tissue tumor, accounting for approximately 50% of all soft-tissue tumors. Lipoma outnumbers liposarcoma by a ratio of 100:1. Cytogenetic abnormalities have been reported in 50–80% of lipomas. There are a large number of variants including the superficial subcutaneous lipoma; the intramuscular lipoma; the spindle cell lipoma; the angiolipoma; the benign lipoblastoma; and the lipomas of tendon sheaths, nerves, synovium, periosteum, and lumbosacral area.

A. Superficial Subcutaneous Lipoma: ICD-9-CM 214.x

The most frequently seen type of lipoma is the superficial subcutaneous type, which can be solitary or multiple. Subcutaneous lipomas occur with equal frequency in men and women and seem to arise spontaneously during the fifth and sixth decade of life. The most common locations are the back, shoulder, and neck.

On palpation, this tumor is soft and ballotable. Although it is found more commonly in obese patients, the size of the lipoma does not correlate with the weight of the patient. Lipomas do not reduce in volume with weight loss. They generally grow to a limited size, and sarcomatous degeneration does not occur. Surgical treatment is usually cosmetic in nature, and the recurrence rate is less than 5%.

B. Intramuscular Lipoma: ICD-9-CM 214.8

The deep intramuscular lipoma is seen in adults between 30 and 60 years of age, affects men more frequently than women, and is commonly found in the large muscles of the extremities. The lesions are slow growing and painless. The intramuscular lipoma has a characteristic radiolucency that contrasts with the surrounding muscle (Figure 5–60).

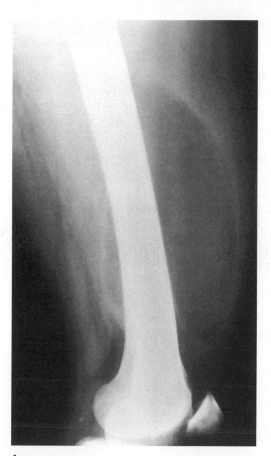
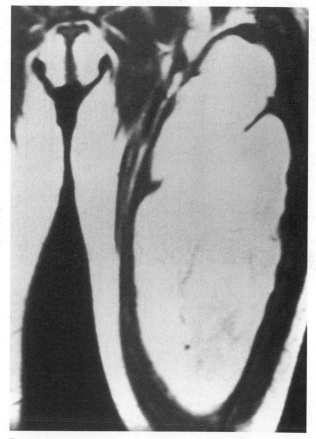

A   B

▲ **Figure 5–60.** Radiograph (**A**) and coronal view T1-weighted MRI (**B**) of an intramuscular lipoma in the quadriceps muscle of a 72-year-old man.

On MRI, this tumor demonstrates a uniform high-signal image on the T1-weighted spin-echo sequence. On gross examination, the tumor can appear quite infiltrative in surrounding muscle and has a faint yellow color on sectioning. Histologic studies show that the intramuscular lipoma, like the subcutaneous lipoma, is composed of benign lipocytes with small pyknotic nuclei that are difficult to see on the surface of the large fat-laden cell. When samples are taken for biopsy purposes, the pathologist must take care to rule out a low-grade, well-differentiated liposarcoma that can coexist with a benign lipoma. On rare occasions, a lipoma can have chondroid or osseous hamartomatous elements that have caused it to be classified as a mesenchymoma in the past. In other cases, evidence of hemorrhage or necrosis can be found in a lipoma and creates low-signal changes on the MRI that are similar to the changes seen in liposarcoma.

A marginal surgical excision is indicated for treatment of intramuscular lipoma. Local recurrence rates of 15–60% are reported.

C. Spindle Cell Lipoma: ICD-9-CM 214.x

The spindle cell lipoma is seen typically in the posterior neck and shoulder area in men between 45 and 64 years of age. On gross examination, the spindle cell lipoma has the appearance of an ordinary lipoma but with areas of gray-white gelatinous foci streaking through it. Microscopic examination of these areas reveals the presence of benign fibroblasts. Thus, with imaging studies, dense areas are scattered throughout the normal radiolucent areas of a lipoma. On MRI, findings generally consist of a low-signal streaking through the typical high-signal pattern of a benign lipoma.

The treatment for this lesion is a simple marginal resection. The chance for local recurrence is minimal.

D. Angiolipoma: ICD-9-CM 214.x

The angiolipoma (Figure 5–61) is a subcutaneous lesion seen in young adults (see Table 5–6), usually on the forearm. Multiple lesions are frequently present and usually painful because of their vascularity. Grossly, the lobular lipoma demonstrates vascular channels. Treatment of angiolipoma consists of marginal excision.

E. Diffuse Lipomatosis: ICD-9-CM 214.9

An extremely rare variant of the lipoma is diffuse lipomatosis, characterized by the presence of multiple superficial and deep lipomas that involve one entire extremity or the trunk and usually have their onset during the first 2 years of life. Histologically, an individual lesion in a patient with diffuse lipomatosis looks no different from a typical solitary lipoma. When lipomatosis of a nerve occurs, the involved limb or digit may become massive in size, sometimes making it impossible to remove the fatty tumors surgically. If this is the case, amputation may be indicated.

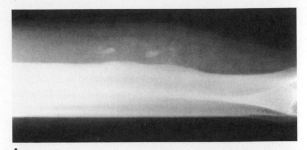

A

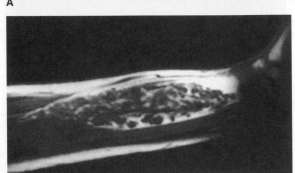

B

▲ **Figure 5–61.** Radiograph (**A**) and T1-weighted MRI (**B**) of a soft-tissue angiolipoma in the volar aspect of the forearm of a 27-year-old woman.

F. Lumbosacral Lipoma: ICD-9-CM 214.8

The lumbosacral lipoma occurs in the lumbosacral area posterior to a spina bifida defect. It is frequently associated with both intradural and extradural lipomas and thus can result in neurologic deficits. Although lumbosacral lipoma is generally considered a pediatric tumor, it can be seen in adults (Figure 5–62).

Surgical treatment consists of a marginal resection of the entire lipoma, including the portion arising from the vertebral canal and lumbosacral roots.

G. Benign Lipoblastoma and Diffuse Lipoblastomatosis: ICD-9-CM 215.x

The benign and diffuse types of lipoblastoma are seen in the extremities or trunk of infants. The lesions, solitary or multiple, can be superficial or deep in muscle tissue. They demonstrate cellular immaturity, with lipoblasts similar to the myxoid form of liposarcoma. Even with the cellular aggressiveness of the lesions, the prognosis is excellent following simple surgical resection.

H. Hibernoma: ICD-9-CM 215.x

Hibernoma, a rare lipoma usually seen in young adults (see Table 5–6), commonly occurs in the scapular and

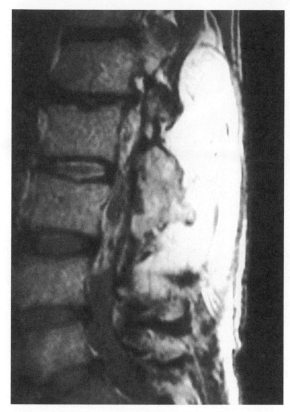

▲ **Figure 5–62.** T1-weighted MRI of a lumbosacral lipoma.

interscapular regions, is painless and slow growing, and ranges between 10 and 15 cm in diameter. The hibernoma is composed of finely granular or vacuolated cells characteristic of brown fat and contains a considerable amount of glycogen. The treatment is marginal surgical resection with a low potential for recurrence.

▶ **Essentials of Diagnosis**

- *In the histologic characterization of lipomatous lesions, biopsy is subject to considerable sampling error. Therefore, if incisional biopsy is indicated, the most suspicious portion of the lesion should be obtained.*
- *The differential diagnosis of macrodactyly should include lipomatosis of nerve.*
- *MRI findings of a lesion that shares the same signal intensity as subcutaneous fat on all sequences are diagnostic of a benign to low-grade lipomatous lesion.*

▶ **Benign Vascular Tumors**

Benign vascular proliferative tumors are the second most common benign tumor after lipomas. Three types of vascular tumors are discussed here: hemangiomas, lymphangiomas, and glomus tumors.

Like lipomas, angiomas occur in a wide variety of clinical conditions seen more often in females than in males. The most common type of angioma is the hemangioma, which can be a superficial cutaneous lesion or a deep, intramuscular one. The lymphatic counterpart of the hemangioma is known as the lymphangioma or hygroma. In most cases, the lesion is solitary or localized. If it is extensive and involves an entire limb, the term *angiomatosis* is used. Because most hemangiomas and lymphangiomas are congenital, the term *hamartomatous* or *arteriovenous malformation* is applied in their classification. Hemangiomas and lymphangiomas arise from developmental dysplasias of the endothelial tube, whereas glomus tumors arise from pericytes, which are cells that lie outside the endothelial tube. Most vascular anomalies arise sporadically, but some familial, autosomal dominant inheritance patterns are also described. Genetic analysis of these families identified specific gene mutations supporting the genomic role in the regulation of angiogenesis.

A. Hemangioma: ICD-9-CM 228.x

Hemangiomas are the most frequently seen tumors of childhood and account for 7% of all benign tumors.

1. Capillary hemangioma: ICD-9-CM 228.x—The most common type of hemangioma is the solitary capillary type, also referred to as the port-wine stain, which appears as an elevated red to purple cutaneous lesion on the head or neck. The lesion occurs during the first few weeks after birth, grows rapidly over a period of several months, and regresses over a 7-year period in 75–90% of cases.

Because of the spontaneous regression, no treatment is needed in most cases. In the past, treatment consisted of cryosurgery, sclerotherapy, or irradiation, but frequently this treatment was worse than the disease itself. Today, when treatment is required, the treatment of choice involves the use of selective laser coagulation.

2. Cavernous hemangioma: ICD-9-CM 228.x—The cavernous hemangioma is larger and less common than the capillary hemangioma. The enlarged vascular spaces of the cavernous lesion give it the appearance of a cluster of purple grapes. It lies deep in the extremity, with common involvement of muscles and even the synovial membrane of the joints (synovial hemangioma).

Imaging may be characteristic (Figure 5–63). In some patients with deep intramuscular forms of hemangioma, the skin shows no abnormalities and no phleboliths are apparent on radiograph. With MRI, deep intramuscular hemangiomas can be easily detected by the characteristic mixed-signal serpiginous pattern seen in the T1-weighted image.

The muscle lesions are usually asymptomatic until intralesional hemorrhage occurs either spontaneously or after a minor injury. The pain symptoms are usually short lived but

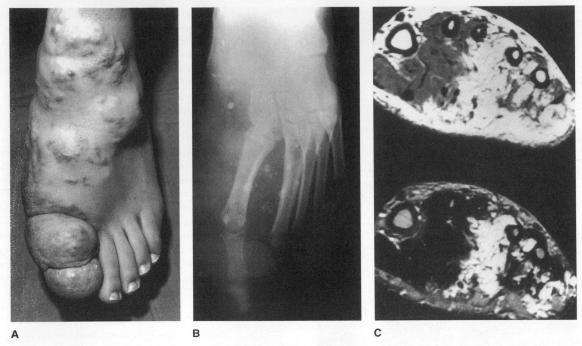

A   **B**   **C**

▲ **Figure 5–63.** Clinical appearance (**A**) and radiographic appearance (**B**) of a cavernous hemangioma in the foot of one patient, and T1-weighted and T2-weighted MRIs (**C**) of a cavernous hemangioma of another patient.

recur infrequently. In some patients, the pain is more severe and associated with muscle contracture and joint deformity. These patients may require surgical resection of the scarred-down lesion to allow for better joint function and to reduce the pain. In rare cases of multiple hemangiomas involving the entire limb, amputation may be indicated. Vascular embolization of the feeder vessels can be attempted but may lead to a significant compartment syndrome, with severe contractures or with loss of muscle strength and limitation of joint movement.

3. Arteriovenous hemangioma: ICD-9-CM 228.x—The arteriovenous hemangioma is seen in young patients (see Table 5–6), usually in the head, neck, or lower extremity. It is associated with significant arteriovenous shunting in the tumor, which creates increased perfusion. This results in increased local temperature, pain, and continuous thrill or bruit over the mass. In the extremity, it also results in an overgrowth of the limb (Klipel-Trenaunay syndrome).

If shunting is excessive, surgical removal of the hemangioma may be necessary to prevent consumptive coagulopathy and high-output cardiac failure (Kasabach-Merritt syndrome). Arteriograms are helpful in determining the degree of shunting prior to treatment. Embolization or surgical ligation of feeder vessels is frequently not a successful form of treatment.

4. Epithelioid hemangioma (Kimura disease): ICD-9-CM 228.x—This cutaneous hemangioma is found on the head or neck in women between 20 and 40 years old. It is associated with inflammatory changes and eosinophilia, and it sometime ulcerates. Its name is derived from the epithelial appearance of the endothelia-lined capillary structures.

5. Pyogenic granuloma: ICD-9-CM 228.x—The pyogenic granuloma is a polypoid capillary hemangioma that affects the skin or mucosal surfaces of males and females in all age groups. It may be associated with trauma and is found about the mouth, gingivae, or fingers. The lesions have a purple-red color, bleed easily, and ulcerate.

B. Lymphangioma: ICD-9-CM 228.x

The lymphangioma is nothing more than an angioma composed of lymphatic endothelial tubes filled with lymphatic fluid, rather than being filled with blood, as the hemangioma is. Lymphangiomas can be localized, which occurs with the cystic hygroma, and they are usually seen about the head, neck, or axilla of young boys and girls (see Table 5–6). As with hemangiomas, the larger lymphomas are cavernous lesions seen in older patients with deeper involvement. In both lymphangioma and hemangioma, because of increased regional perfusion, bony overgrowth can occur (Figure 5–64).

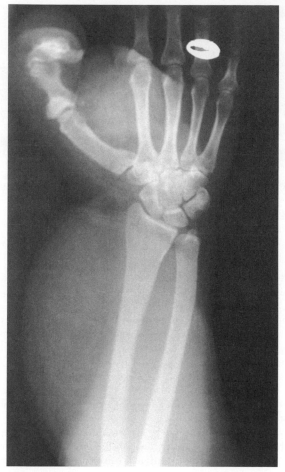

▲ **Figure 5–64.** Radiograph of a lymphangioma in the forearm and hand of a 23-year-old woman.

C. Glomus Tumor: ICD-9-CM 215.x

The glomus tumor arises from the hemangiopericyte, which is a cell seen at the periphery of the capillary vascular network and normally involved with the regulation of blood flow through the capillary system. Microscopic examination of the tumor reveals large vascular spaces surrounded by a homogeneous field of round epithelioid hemangiopericytes, with no evidence of mitotic activity.

The glomus tumor is a pink lesion that usually measures less than 1 cm in diameter. It represents 1.6% of all soft-tissue tumors and occurs with equal frequency in men and women, usually between 20 and 40 years of age. Although the tumor is found most commonly in the subungual area of a digit, where it is readily visible, it also occurs subcutaneously on the hand, wrist, forearm, or foot, where it may be invisible and thus difficult to diagnose until localized lancinating pain leads to a surgical exploration. Glomus tumors

have sporadically been reported in deep soft tissues, viscera, and intraosseous locations as well. After the lesion is surgically removed, the pain subsides and recurrence occurs in fewer than 10% of cases.

► Essentials of Diagnosis

- *Radiographic findings of phleboliths are diagnostic of hemangioma.*
- *Glomus tumors are usually diagnosed at a very small size due to characteristic location in the fingertip and extreme cold sensitivity.*

► Extraabdominal Desmoid Tumors (Aggressive Fibromatosis): ICD-9-CM 215.x

In comparison with the infantile fibrous lesions mentioned earlier, the desmoid tumor is seen in older children and young adults up through 40 years of age. Whereas abdominal desmoids are seen in the abdominal wall of women following pregnancy, the extraabdominal desmoids usually occur in men and are more common in proximal areas about the shoulder and buttock, followed next by the posterior thigh, popliteal area, arm, and forearm. In most cases, it presents as a solitary tumor. Multicentric involvement is seen at times, however, and can be associated with Gardner syndrome, which is characterized by polyposis of the large bowel and by craniofacial osteomas. In patients with familial adenomatous polyposis (FAP), an inherited disease caused by mutations in the *APC* gene, desmoids are a significant source of morbidity and mortality. The *APC* gene, located on chromosome 5, encodes for a 300-kDa protein, in which a germline mutation is an early event in tumor formation.

Desmoids are deep-seated tumors that arise from muscle fascial planes and infiltrate extensively into adjacent muscle tissue, tendons, joint capsules, and even bone. Compared with malignant fibrosarcomas, desmoids are poorly marginated and thus difficult to resect surgically. Desmoids can engulf surrounding vessels and nerves, whereas fibrosarcomas usually push these structures aside. A desmoid may cause local pain and grow quite rapidly, suggesting a malignant tumor. The desmoid tends to grow more longitudinally along muscle planes to a considerable size, frequently resulting in restricted joint motion about the shoulder, hip, or knee. Because the local aggressiveness of desmoids is so similar to that of malignant fibrosarcomas or MFHs, some experts believe the desmoid may be a low-grade fibrosarcoma that has lost its potential to metastasize; however, molecular analyses may suggest otherwise.

On gross examination, a desmoid tumor is firm and heavily collagenized. Microscopically, it has a low mitotic index, similar to that of a plantar or palmar fibromatosis. Radiographically, a desmoid is noncalcified and appears dense in comparison with normal muscle. It is easily seen in soft window CT scanning. More exact presurgical imaging can be obtained with MRI (Figure 5–65). As with an

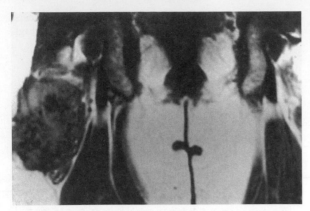

▲ **Figure 5–65.** T1-weighted MRI of a desmoid tumor in the gluteal area of a 45-year-old woman.

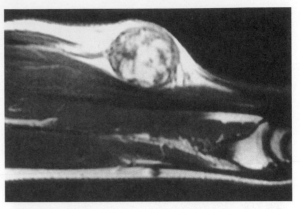

▲ **Figure 5–66.** T1-weighted MRI of a neurilemoma of the ulnar nerve in a 69-year-old man.

abdominal desmoid, an extraabdominal desmoid physical injury may play a role in the activation of a preexisting oncogene located in the damaged fibroblast.

Desmoids are usually treated surgically with an aggressive wide resection similar to that used in treating a primary sarcoma. Even following a margin-negative resection of the desmoid, the recurrence rate may approach 50%. For this reason, it is common to administer 50 Gy of radiation to the surgical site starting 2 weeks postoperatively. With radiation therapy, the recurrence rate decreases to 15%. In rare cases an amputation may be necessary after multiple recurrences. A few cases of spontaneous involution of desmoid tumors are reported after 40 years of age.

Based on clinical and experimental evidence, estrogen may play a role in the development of desmoid tumors. Accordingly, agents such as tamoxifen are being used in some centers because of their antiestrogen effects. NSAIDs were also implemented in attempts to treat aggressive cases. Cytotoxic chemotherapy has also been instituted in selected unresectable cases, especially associated with familial adenomatous polyposis, with some success.

▶ **Essentials of Diagnosis**

- *Desmoids are benign but may be extremely locally aggressive, with up to 50% recurring locally after margin-negative resection alone.*

▶ **Benign Tumors of Peripheral Nerves**

Benign tumors of peripheral nerve sheaths are common and take their origin from Schwann cells, which normally produce myelin and collagen fiber.

A. Neurilemoma: ICD-9-CM 215.x

The neurilemoma (neurinoma or benign schwannoma) is the least common of the benign tumors of peripheral nerve sheaths.

It usually affects individuals between 20 and 50 years of age and occurs with equal frequency in men and women. It has a predilection for spinal roots and for superficial nerves on the flexor surfaces of both upper and lower extremities. In most cases, the lesion is solitary, but multiple lesions are occasionally seen in von Recklinghausen disease. The neurilemmoma is slow growing and rarely causes pain or a neurologic deficit.

Unlike the neurofibroma, which has a fusiform appearance, the neurilemoma is round (Figure 5–66). Microscopic studies reveal the presence of a characteristic Verocay body, which consists of palisading Schwann cells and is found in the fibrotic Antoni A substance of the tumor. Other areas reveal a more mucinous Antoni B substance. Neurilemomas may occur in an axial fashion involving spinal roots, often presenting as a dumbbell-shaped extradural defect (Figure 5–67). In comparison with the less restricted peripheral lesions, the nerve root lesions are more apt to cause pain associated with neurologic deficiency because of their bony constriction.

In some cases, simple excision of the neurilemoma is clinically indicated, which often can be performed without serious damage to the nerve. If the patient is asymptomatic, observation is appropriate because there is little chance for malignant degeneration.

B. Solitary Neurofibroma: ICD-9-CM 215.x

The solitary neurofibroma is a fusiform fibrotic tumor arising centrally from a smaller peripheral nerve (Figure 5–68). The tumor is seen with equal frequency in men and women, usually between 20 and 30 years of age. It is 10 times more common than the multiple form seen in von Recklinghausen disease, is usually smaller, and carries less chance of malignant degeneration. Microscopic examination of the solitary neurofibroma shows interlacing bundles of elongated spindle cells with benign-appearing nuclei and

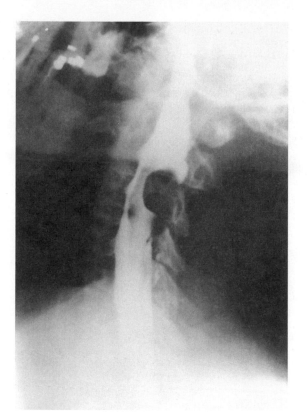

▲ **Figure 5–67.** Myelogram of a neurilemoma in the cervical spine.

occasionally with areas resembling the Antoni A tissue seen in the neurilemoma.

Treatment of the solitary neurofibroma consists of simple excision. Iatrogenic damage to the nerve fascicles is more likely than with resection of the neurilemoma, due to the intertwined growth of the neurofibroma.

C. Neurofibromatosis (von Recklinghausen Disease): ICD-9-CM 237.7

von Recklinghausen disease is a familial dysplasia, inherited as an autosomal dominant trait, with an incidence of approximately 1 in every 3000 live births. The disease usually begins during the first few years of life with the emergence of small café-au-lait spots. Over time, these lesions grow in number and size. Unlike the lesions seen in fibrous dysplasia, the lesions in von Recklinghausen disease do not have rough edges. If a patient has more than six lesions that have smooth edges and are greater than 1.5 cm in diameter, the diagnosis of von Recklinghausen disease is certain.

Later in life, the patient develops multiple neurofibromas, each of which appears as a soft cutaneous nodule (Figure 5–69). This pedunculated skin lesion, which is called fibroma molluscum, can be large and pendulous. More pathognomonic of the disease is the plexiform neurofibroma, occurring in 25% of patients, which appears in larger nerves and can involve an entire extremity (see Figure 5–69). When the overlying skin of an extremity is loose and hyperpigmented, the condition is called elephantiasis neuromatosa, or "elephant man syndrome." (It is now thought that John Merrick, the so-called elephant man, was actually affected by Proteus syndrome.) Among the bony

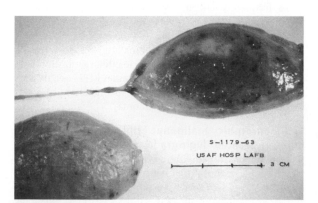

▲ **Figure 5–68.** Photographic appearance of a solitary neurofibroma.

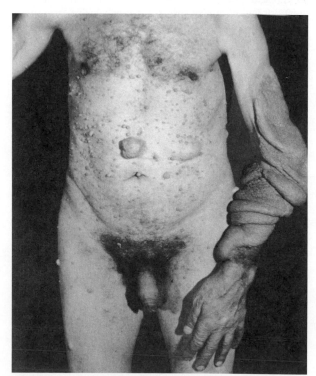

▲ **Figure 5–69.** Cutaneous manifestations of neurofibromatosis.

changes seen in von Recklinghausen disease are scoliosis in up to 20%, bowing and/or pseudarthrosis of the tibia in 5%, spinal meningocele, scalloping of the vertebra, and osteolytic lesions in bone.

A major threat to the patient's life is that a malignant sarcoma will develop from one of the large and deep neurofibromas. This occurs at a later age in 3–5% of patients.

▶ Essentials of Diagnosis

- *Neurilemomas are usually easily dissected off the associated nerve, whereas neurofibromas generally are far more intertwined in the nerve fascicles, making nerve-sparing resection more difficult.*

- *Patients with neurofibromatosis have a lifetime risk of secondary sarcoma of up to 5%.*

▶ Intramuscular Myxomas: ICD-9-CM 215.x

The intramuscular myxoma is a rare tumor seen in patients older than 40 years and affecting the large muscles about the thighs, shoulders, buttocks, and arms. It is a slow-growing, well-marginated tumor that has the gelatinous physical quality of a ganglion cyst or myxoid liposarcoma. The intramuscular myxoma causes no pain and can grow to greater than 15 cm in diameter. Although it appears radiolucent on CT scan, MRI demonstrates an intermediate signal on the T1-weighted image and an extremely high signal on the T2-weighted image. Multiple myxomas are associated with polyostotic fibrous dysplasia in Mazabraud syndrome.

The intramuscular myxoma can be resected marginally. After this procedure, the recurrence rate is extremely low.

▶ Essentials of Diagnosis

- *Many soft-tissue lesions have very characteristic findings on imaging studies, but those with nonspecific findings should be diagnosed with needle or incisional biopsy rather than excisional biopsy.*

Blei F: Basic science and clinical aspects of vascular anomalies. *Curr Opin Pediatr* 2005;17:501. [PMID: 16012263]

Blei F: Congenital lymphatic malformations. Ann N Y Acad Sci 2008;1131:185. [PMID: 18519970]

Crawford AH, Schorry EK: Neurofibromatosis update. *J Pediatr Orthop* 2006;26:413. [PMID: 16670560]

Faurschou A, Togsverd-Bo K, Zachariae C, et al: Pulsed dye laser vs. intense pulsed light for port-wine stains: a randomized side-by-side trial with blinded response evaluation. *Br J Dermatol* 2009;160:359. [PMID: 19120324]

Gega M, Yanagi H, Yoshikawa R, et al: Successful chemotherapeutic modality of doxorubicin plus dacarbazine for the treatment of desmoid tumors in association with familial adenomatous polyposis. *J Clin Oncol* 2006;24:102. [PMID:16382119]

Gombos Z, Zhang PJ: Glomus tumor. *Arch Pathol Lab Med* 2008;132:1448. [PMID: 18788860]

Kang HJ, Shin SJ, Kang ES: Schwannomas of the upper extremity. *J Hand Surg Br* 2000;25:604. [PMID: 11106529]

Lev D, Kotilingam D, Wei C, et al: Optimizing treatment of desmoid tumors. *J Clin Oncol* 2007;25:1785. [PMID: 17470870]

Marler JJ, Mulliken JB: Current management of hemangiomas and vascular malformations. *Clin Plast Surg* 2005;32:99. [PMID: 15636768]

Murphey MD, Carroll JF, Flemming DJ, et al: From the archives of the AFIP: benign musculoskeletal lipomatous lesions. *Radiographics* 2004;24:1433. [PMID: 15371618]

Nielsen GP, O'Connell JX, Rosenberg AE: Intramuscular myxoma: a clinicopathologic study of 51 cases with emphasis on hypercellular and hypervascular variants. *Am J Surg Pathol* 1998;22:1222. [PMID: 9777984]

Shields CJ, Winter DC, Kirwan WO, et al: Desmoid tumours. *Eur J Surg Oncol* 2001;27:701. [PMID: 11735163]

Signoroni S, Frattini M, Negri T, et al: Cyclooxygenase-2 and platelet-derived growth factor receptors as potential targets in treating aggressive fibromatosis. *Clin Cancer Res* 2007;13:5034. [PMID: 17785554]

Skapek SX, Frattini M, Negri T, et al: Vinblastine and methotrexate for desmoid fibromatosis in children: results of a Pediatric Oncology Group Phase II Trial. *J Clin Oncol* 2007;25:501. [PMID: 17290057]

Sorensen SA, Mulvihill JJ, Nielsen A: Long-term follow-up of von Recklinghausen neurofibromatosis: survival and malignant neoplasms. *N Engl J Med* 1986;314:1010. [PMID: 3083258]

MALIGNANT SOFT-TISSUE TUMORS

Sarcomas are capable of invasive, locally destructive growth with a tendency to recur and to metastasize. All sarcomas do not behave the same, however. Some sarcomas, such as dermatofibrosarcoma protuberans, rarely metastasize. Undifferentiated pleomorphic sarcoma, in contrast, does so with alacrity.

A. Fibrohistiocytic Tumors: ICD-9-CM 171.x

Until recently, MFH was the most common soft-tissue sarcoma seen in adults (Figure 5–70). Strangely, although more frequently encountered than other adult soft-tissue sarcomas, the cell type(s) of origin remain unclear. However, ongoing developments in molecular diagnostics have allowed the determination of the origin of an increasing number of cases. The latest World Health Organization classification for sarcomas no longer includes MFH as a distinct entity. The current nomenclature for the majority of MFH is undifferentiated pleomorphic sarcoma.

1. Pleomorphic malignant fibrous histiocytoma/ undifferentiated high-grade pleomorphic sarcoma: ICD-9-CM 171.x—Undifferentiated high-grade pleomorphic sarcoma occurs more frequently in men than in women by a ratio of 1.2:1, primarily affecting individuals between 50 and 70 years of age. Usually it is a deep lesion found in the large muscles about the thigh, hip, and retroperitoneal areas. The tumor may be asymptomatic.

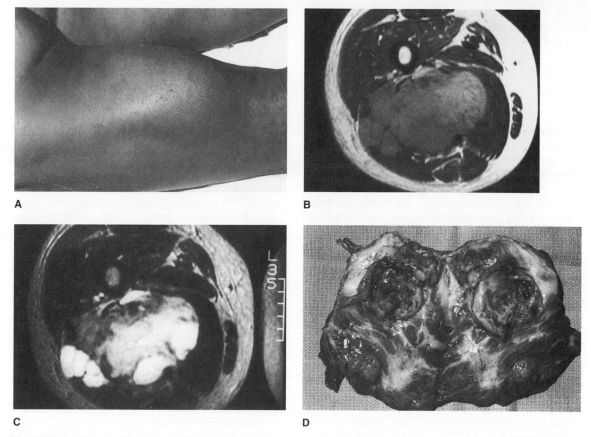

▲ Figure 5–70. Clinical appearance (**A**), T1-weighted MRI (**B**), T2-weighted MRI (**C**), and resected surgical specimen (**D**) of a large pleomorphic malignant fibrous histiocytoma in the posterior thigh of a 55-year-old man.

On gross examination, the tumor appears multinodular and may demonstrate several separate satellite lesions in the same muscle belly, especially at the superior and interior poles. It may be necrotic and ranges in color from dirty gray to a reddish tan. Microscopy demonstrates that it is composed of malignant fibroblasts mixed with anaplastic and pleomorphic histiocytes.

The prognosis and treatment vary, depending on the size and location of the tumor. The overall local recurrence potential is 45%, with a 40% incidence of metastasis to the lung and with a 10% incidence of regional lymph node involvement. Tumors smaller than 5 cm in diameter and found in a subcutaneous location in the distal body parts carry a good prognosis, with a 5-year survival rate of 80%, whereas tumors that are 5 cm or more in diameter and located deep in a more proximal muscle group carry a poor prognosis, with a 5-year survival rate of only 55%.

Although the treatment depends on the clinical situation, it generally consists of an aggressive wide resection after careful preoperative staging, including an MRI of the primary tumor and CT scan of the chest. Amputation is rare, with limb salvage possible in the majority of cases.

The use of adjuvant radiation therapy is important in reducing the local recurrence rate. Many clinicians administer 50–55 Gy to a wide area, followed by a boost of 60–66 Gy aimed at the surgical site. An attempt is made to leave a longitudinal strip of tissue out of the field of radiation to reduce the chance of postirradiation edema distal to the treatment site. Some centers advocate preoperative and postoperative radiation with 50 Gy given before resection and approximately 15 Gy given postoperatively. Some institutions employ preoperative radiation exclusively. Local recurrence rates are generally between 5 and 25%.

The use of adjuvant chemotherapy is more controversial. Because limited data suggest that chemotherapy results in a significant improvement in survival and because most patients are older individuals who cannot tolerate the high-dose protocols, medical oncologists are divided on whether to advocate the use of chemotherapeutic agents in the treatment of undifferentiated pleomorphic sarcoma.

2. Giant cell malignant fibrous histiocytoma/undifferentiated pleomorphic sarcoma with giant cells: ICD-9-CM 171.x

—The giant cell type of MFH also affects older patients and is seen in large muscle groups. Histologically, multiple osteoclastic giant cells are seen, and there may be areas of hemorrhage. It carries a similar prognosis for pulmonary metastasis, local recurrence, and overall survival.

3. Inflammatory malignant fibrous histiocytoma/undifferentiated pleomorphic sarcoma with prominent inflammation: ICD-9-CM 171.x

—The inflammatory type of MFH affects the older age groups and is more common in the retroperitoneal areas. Histologically, it has prominent benign-appearing xanthomatous cells and mixed inflammatory cells including neutrophils, eosinophils, and occasional lymphocytes and plasma cells. There is some evidence that this entity may be a form of dedifferentiated liposarcoma. Although it has a similar rate of pulmonary metastasis, review of the literature suggests less favorable overall survival with an increased rate of disease-related mortality. This is probably related to the more frequent retroperitoneal location.

B. Fibrosarcoma: ICD-9-CM 171.x

Fifty years ago, fibrosarcoma was considered the most common of the soft-tissue sarcomas, secondary to imprecise pathologic classification of MFH, certain liposarcomas, rhabdomyosarcoma, leiomyosarcomas, and malignant peripheral nerve sheath tumors. Currently, fibrosarcoma is considered one of the least common soft-tissue sarcomas. The diagnosis is reserved for those tumors in which the histology demonstrates a uniform fasciculated growth pattern of spindle cells (malignant fibroblasts). It is clinically similar to MFH, occurs with nearly equal frequency in men and women, is found in patients between 30 and 55 years of age, is sometimes slow growing and painless, and tends to affect deep fascial structures of muscle about the knee and thigh, followed next by the forearm and leg.

On gross examination, fibrosarcoma appears as a firm and lobulated lesion that has a yellowish white to tan color. The lesion may demonstrate a few calcific or osseous deposits on radiographic exam. Microscopy reveals spindle, uniformly shaped fibroblasts oriented in a herringbone pattern. Cells show varying degrees of mitotic activity. Fibrosarcomas contain no malignant histiocytes.

The treatment and prognosis depend on the grade of tumor in a particular patient. Low-grade fibrosarcoma is nearly the same tumor as a benign desmoid tumor and has an extremely low rate of metastasis. However, high-grade fibrosarcoma requires an aggressive wide surgical resection, along with radiation therapy, and has a pulmonary metastasis rate of 50–60%. Lymph node involvement is rare. The use of chemotherapy is considered controversial in patients with fibrosarcoma, as it is in patients with MFH.

C. Myxofibrosarcoma: ICD-9-CM 171.x

Also known as myxoid MFH, myxofibrosarcoma is a relatively common sarcoma in the elderly, seen in the 50- to 80-year age group. The thigh is the most common location followed by the arm and shoulder girdle. Most are large at presentation and may be low grade, with little metastatic potential, or high-grade, with metastases occurring in 20–35% of cases. Larger tumors with increased necrosis exhibit an increased rate of metastasis. Local recurrence is seen in approximately one half of cases after resection, and it is well described that lesions have the propensity to recur at a higher grade, having accumulated chromosomal aberrations. This property, combined with the fact that no specific cytogenetic abnormalities have been identified, highlights the role of genomic instability in the malignant degeneration of this entity. Largely because of the peak age group, chemotherapy is infrequently recommended; however, radiotherapy is routinely delivered either preoperatively or postoperatively.

D. Dermatofibrosarcoma Protuberans: ICD-9-CM 171.x

Dermatofibrosarcoma protuberans, a low- to intermediate-grade fibrohistiocytic tumor, is unique because of its nodular cutaneous location. It is seen more commonly in males than females and occurs in young or middle-age (20–40 years) adults. It is typically located about the trunk and proximal extremities. Antecedent trauma is recorded in 10–20% of cases. Dermatofibrosarcoma protuberans begins as a painless subcutaneous nodule or nodules and slowly develops into an elevated multinodular plaque (Figure 5–71). Microscopic examination of the lesion reveals the same storiform or basket-weave pattern of a benign or malignant fibrous histiocytoma but with a very low mitotic index. The pattern tends to infiltrate extensively into surrounding

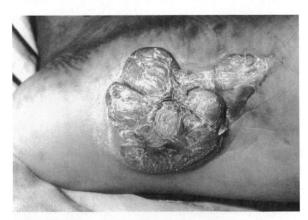

▲ **Figure 5–71.** Clinical appearance of dermatofibrosarcoma protuberans on the bottom of the heel of a 30-year-old man.

subcutaneous fat and skin, which accounts for the high local recurrence rate, sometimes reported to approach 50%.

Characteristic cytogenetic abnormalities are described with characteristic features such as reciprocal t(17;22) (q22;q13) or, more commonly, supernumerary ring chromosomes containing sequences from chromosomes 17 and 22. The specific cytogenetic rearrangement may not be as critical as the resulting fusion product of collagen 1 alpha 1 and platelet-derived growth factor (COL1A1-PDGFB), which is detected in the vast majority of cases.

Surgical treatment, consisting of an aggressive resection, is associated with a lower recurrence rate of 20%. Because of the low mitotic index, radiation therapy is not usually indicated, and the chance of pulmonary metastasis is only 1%.

▶ Essentials of Diagnosis

- *Malignant fibrous histiocytoma has recently been reclassified largely due to increased ability to determine cell lineage with modern molecular techniques.*

E. Liposarcomas: ICD-9-CM 171.x

Liposarcoma is the second most common soft-tissue sarcoma after undifferentiated pleomorphic sarcoma. Like MFH, liposarcoma is a tumor of older (40–60 years) patients and can be large and deep seated. Four types of liposarcoma are discussed in the following sections. The well-differentiated type and the myxoid type are associated with a low chance for lung metastasis, whereas the round cell and the pleomorphic types tend to behave more aggressively.

1. Well-differentiated liposarcoma: ICD-9-CM 171.x—

This very low-grade tumor affects individuals who are 40–60 years of age and occurs more frequently in men than in women. It grows extremely slowly and reaches a large size without causing pain. The deep-seated tumor is found in the retroperitoneum, buttock, or thigh. In some cases of well-differentiated liposarcoma, findings include inflammation and sclerosis.

On gross examination, this tumor has a fatty lobulated appearance similar to a benign lipoma. Even under the microscope, many large areas of the tumor appear benign. However, with proper sampling, the pathologist will find a few areas of lipoblast activity to suggest the diagnosis of a liposarcoma. MRI findings are sometimes difficult to distinguish from a large deep lipoma (Figure 5–72).

In cases of well-differentiated liposarcoma, a conservative wide resection is performed to avoid local recurrence. Adjuvant radiation therapy is not helpful, and chemotherapy is never used. The chance of metastatic disease is very low, and the prognosis for survival is excellent.

2. Myxoid liposarcoma: ICD-9-CM 171.x—

Myxoid liposarcoma is the most common fat sarcoma, accounting for 40–50% of all liposarcomas. The myxoid type is low to intermediate grade and seen in older patients (see Table 5–6).

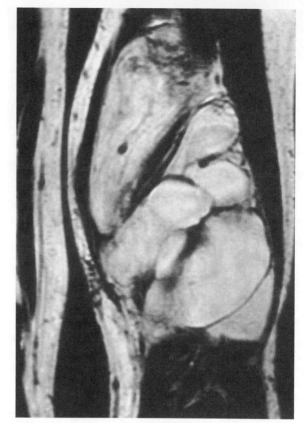

▲ **Figure 5–72.** T1-weighted MRI of a well-differentiated liposarcoma in the thigh of a 63-year-old man.

The clinical presentation is similar to the well-differentiated liposarcoma.

Gross examination of a myxoid liposarcoma reveals a lobulated pattern with some areas that appear similar to those of a lipoma but with other myxomatous areas. Microscopic examination shows myxoid tissue with areas of signet ring lipoblasts. It is common to find a delicate pattern of capillaries running through the myxoid areas. MRI frequently demonstrates a heterogeneous high- and low-signal pattern typical of myxoid liposarcoma but not present in cases of benign lipoma (Figure 5–73).

Characteristic translocations are also seen in myxoid liposarcoma. The predominant type is t(12;16)(q13;p11); however, t(12;22)(q13;q12) is also described. Multifocal myxoid liposarcoma is also described. Consideration for additional advanced axial imaging should be entertained with this histologic subtype. Although myxoid liposarcoma carries a very good prognosis, the tumor should be removed with wide margins. There is current debate over the use of neoadjuvant chemotherapy versus neoadjuvant radiotherapy, with this

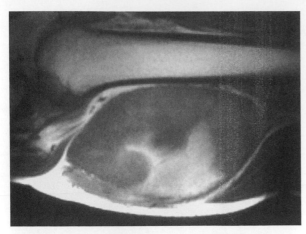

▲ Figure 5–73. Sagittal view T1-weighted MRI of a myxoid liposarcoma in the thigh of a 32-year-old man.

entity showing responsiveness to both. Adjuvant radiotherapy is still widely used today.

3. Round cell and pleomorphic liposarcoma: ICD-9-CM 171.x—These high-grade liposarcomas are seen in the same locations and age group as the well-differentiated and myxoid subtypes. But unlike the latter, the round cell and pleomorphic types are fast-growing tumors that may be painful.

In cases of round cell or pleomorphic liposarcoma, the lesion does not have a fatty appearance on gross examination but instead looks more like an MFH or a fibrosarcoma. Moreover, on MRI, the lesion appears more like an MFH, with a low-signal pattern in the T1-weighted image and a high-signal pattern in the T2-weighted image. Microscopically, the round cell type of liposarcoma shows areas of uniformly shaped round cells similar to those found in Ewing sarcoma or lymphoma and also shows areas of myxoid tissue. In the pleomorphic type of liposarcoma, large and bizarre giant cells occur similar to those found in undifferentiated pleomorphic sarcoma and rhabdomyosarcoma.

In round cell and pleomorphic liposarcoma, there is an early and high rate of pulmonary metastasis. Accordingly, the prognosis for survival is poor. Thus, the treatment should include aggressive resection, adjuvant radiation therapy as necessary, and chemotherapy in selected patients.

▶ Essentials of Diagnosis

- *CT scan of the abdomen and pelvis should be included in the staging and surveillance of liposarcomas due to the incidence of associated retroperitoneal tumors.*
- *Liposarcoma is particularly subject to sampling error with biopsy, so every effort should be made to sample the most aggressive-appearing portion of the tumor.*

F. Rhabdomyosarcomas: ICD-9-CM 171.x

Rhabdomyosarcomas account for 20% of all soft-tissue sarcomas. The embryonal and alveolar types of rhabdomyosarcoma affect pediatric patients, and the rarer pleomorphic type affects adults.

1. Embryonal rhabdomyosarcoma: ICD-9-CM 171.x— The embryonal type is seen in patients from birth to 15 years of age and encountered more frequently in boys than in girls. It is most common in the head and neck area. The so-called botryoid form is seen as a cluster of grapes under mucous membranes in the vagina, bladder, or retroperitoneal area. Histologically, it is a round cell tumor-like Ewing sarcoma, but some rhabdomyoblasts with cross striations are present in a few areas. The presence of anaplasia, or areas of cells containing enlarged, bizarre, hyperchromatic nuclei, is associated with a more aggressive phenotype.

Embryonal rhabdomyosarcoma is treated with local surgical resection plus preoperative and postoperative chemotherapy consisting of vincristine, dactinomycin, cyclophosphamide, and doxorubicin given in cyclic courses during a 2-year span. If the surgical margins are contaminated, local radiation therapy is used. With this program, the 5-year survival rate is 80%. Prior to the advent of chemotherapy, it was only 10%.

2. Alveolar rhabdomyosarcoma: ICD-9-CM 171.x—This type of rhabdomyosarcoma affects individuals between 10 and 25 years of age and is found more commonly in males than in females. Besides affecting the head and neck, it can be seen in the extremities, especially the thigh and calf. Microscopic examination of the lesion reveals a typical alveolar pattern of round cells, with fewer rhabdomyoblasts seen in this type of rhabdomyosarcoma than in the embryonal type. This type of rhabdomyosarcoma is associated with the fusion genes *PAX3-FKHR* or *PAX7-FKHR*. Although not definitive, the presence of the translocation t(2;13)/*PAX3-FKHR* may be an adverse prognostic factor, with molecular screening being implemented in the future. Currently, the treatment is the same as for the embryonal type, but the prognosis is a bit worse.

3. Pleomorphic rhabdomyosarcoma: ICD-9-CM 171.x— In the 1940s, pleomorphic rhabdomyosarcoma was a popular histologic diagnosis, and MFH was a rare one. Based on today's criteria, most of the old cases classified as pleomorphic rhabdomyosarcoma would now be classified as undifferentiated pleomorphic sarcoma. Currently, the pleomorphic type of rhabdomyosarcoma is the rarest type.

Pleomorphic rhabdomyosarcoma is a high-grade tumor that affects middle-age and older adults and is seen most commonly in the large muscle groups of the proximal extremities, usually the lower extremities. Microscopic examination of the tumor reveals large atypical giant cells, along with racket- or tadpole-shaped malignant rhabdomyoblasts that stain positive for glycogen, actin, and myosin. The tumor carries a poor prognosis and is associated with a high rate of metastasis to the lung. The treatment for pleomorphic rhabdomyosarcoma is similar to that for undifferentiated pleomorphic sarcoma and consists of a wide local resection and adjuvant radiation therapy. Chemotherapy is rarely indicated.

▶ Essentials of Diagnosis

- *Alveolar rhabdomyosarcoma is associated with characteristic translocations t(1;13) or t(2;13) resulting in the PAX7-FKHR or PAX3-FKHR fusion products, respectively. This affects prognosis and may ultimately affect treatment protocols as well.*

G. Leiomyosarcoma: ICD-9-CM 171.x

Leiomyosarcoma is a rare soft-tissue tumor whose cell type of origin is smooth muscle. It is seen in the middle-age adult (see Table 5–6) and is much more common in women than in men. Its usual locations, in order of frequency, are retroperitoneal, intraabdominal, cutaneous, and subcutaneous. In some cases, the lesion has a venous wall origin and is found in the vena cava or large vessels of the leg. On microscopic examination, leiomyosarcoma can demonstrate a palisading, orderly fascicular pattern similar to a malignant schwannoma. A specific immunohistochemical staining for actin may be helpful in the differential diagnosis.

The prognosis and treatment for leiomyosarcoma are similar to those for fibrosarcoma. However, leiomyosarcomas of venous wall origin have a worse prognosis because they are difficult to resect and have a high rate of pulmonary metastasis.

H. Synovial Sarcomas: ICD-9-CM 171.x

Synovial sarcoma (Figure 5–74) is the fourth most common soft-tissue sarcoma. It is seen in young adults between 15 and 35 years of age and affects males slightly more than females. The name of this tumor suggests a synovial cell origin, but only 10% of synovial sarcomas are found in a major joint. Nevertheless, they frequently arise from juxta-articular structures, especially around the knee, and they can also arise from tendon sheaths, bursal sacs, fascial planes, and deep muscles. Synovial sarcomas can be seen about the shoulder, arm, elbow, and wrist and are the most common soft-tissue sarcoma in the foot.

Synovial sarcomas initially grow slowly and cause pain in approximately half of affected patients. The tumors may appear after an injury, and because dystrophic calcification or even heterotopic bone formation is seen in half of the cases, the tumors are assumed to be a benign process for 2–4 years before a diagnostic biopsy is performed.

Microscopic examination of the tumor shows a typical biphasic pattern composed of epithelium-like cells that form nests, clefts, or tubular structures surrounded by malignant fibroblastic spindle cells. The epithelium-like cells produce a mucinous material that suggests a synovial cell origin, although this origin is unlikely. A monophasic form of synovial sarcoma is described and reported to consist of a dominant fibroblastic or epithelial cell pattern. If the lesion shows no biphasic component, however, it is difficult to confirm the diagnosis of synovial sarcoma.

Molecular characterization of this tumor reveals a particular translocation, t(X;18), representing the fusion of *SYT* (at 18q11) with either *SSX1* or *SSX2* (both at Xp11). Both *SYT* and *SSX* are transcription factors whose fusion product is seen in the majority of synovial sarcomas.

Despite the slow growth of synovial sarcoma, the 5- and 10-year survival rates are only 50 and 25%, respectively. In cases in which the tumors are heavily calcified, the 5-year survival rate is 80%. Because of the poor prognosis, the treatment plan should include aggressive wide resection, along with both radiation therapy and chemotherapy. Recent evidence shows

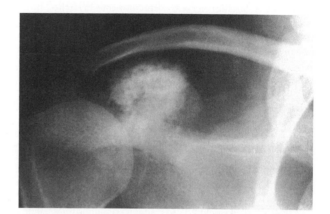

A

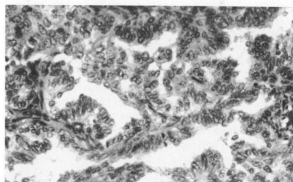

B

▲ **Figure 5–74.** Radiograph (**A**) and microscopic appearance (**B**) of a synovial sarcoma in the shoulder of a 20-year-old woman.

that ifosfamide-based regimens are associated with improved patient outcomes. Lymph node involvement is seen in 20% of affected patients and may require a surgical excision followed by local radiation therapy.

▶ Essentials of Diagnosis

- *Synovial sarcomas can present as small, calcified soft-tissue tumors in up to 50% of cases.*

I. Malignant Peripheral Nerve Sheath Tumor: ICD-9-CM 171.x

A malignant peripheral nerve sheath tumor can arise from a preexisting benign solitary neurofibroma but more frequently arises from the multiple lesions of neurofibromatosis type 1. In both cases, the tumor mass is usually larger than 5 cm in diameter and may arise from a large deep neurogenic structure such as the sciatic nerve (Figure 5–75) or one of the spinal roots. Smaller nerves, even cutaneous branches, however, can give rise to these sarcomas. Malignant degeneration from a solitary neurofibroma usually occurs after 40 years of age with a 5-year survival rate of 75%. In contrast, patients whose tumor arose from the lesions of neurofibromatosis type 1 are generally younger and have a 5-year survival rate of 30%. Surgical treatment consists of a wide resection if possible. Adjuvant radiation and chemotherapy are used in selected cases.

J. Malignant Vascular Tumors

1. Kaposi sarcoma: ICD-9-CM 176.x—Of the malignant vascular tumors, Kaposi sarcoma is the most common with four specific subtypes: (1) chronic, (2) lymphadenopathic, (3) transplant associated, (4) acquired immunodeficiency syndrome (AIDS) related. Its pathogenesis is related to infection with Kaposi sarcoma–associated herpesvirus while in the immunocompromised state. It is found directly beneath the skin, generally in the lower extremity of adults, is seen more often in men than in women, and is endemic in central Africa. The cutaneous lesions seen frequently in the foot and ankle area are purplish in color and are nodular (Figure 5–76). Microscopic examination of Kaposi sarcoma shows an aggressive vascular pattern with rare mitosis. However, over a period of many years, the tumor progresses into a full-blown angiosarcoma or fibrosarcoma. Cytotoxic chemotherapeutic alternatives are limited due to the immunocompromised status of the host. With continued investigation in the field, antiviral medications will likely become a mainstay in the treatment of this disease. Although the behavior of Kaposi sarcoma is a function of the immunologic status of the patient and other variables, the overall mortality rate is 10–20%.

2. Angiosarcoma: ICD-9-CM 171.x—Soft-tissue angiosarcoma is rare, accounting for less than 1% of all sarcomas. Although angiosarcomas are usually cutaneous lesions and

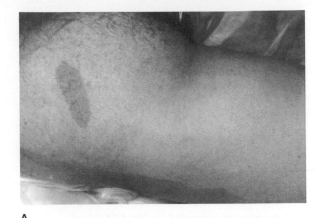

A

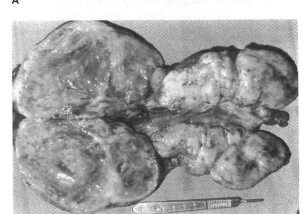

B

▲ **Figure 5–75.** Clinical appearance of a café-au-lait defect in the skin overlying a malignant schwannoma in the buttock area of a 42-year-old man (**A**), and gross appearance of the tumor in the resected sciatic nerve (**B**).

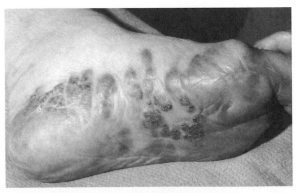

▲ **Figure 5–76.** Clinical appearance of Kaposi sarcoma of the foot.

tend to affect men more than women, they sometimes take the form of a deep tumor, and they are typically seen in the upper extremities of women who have chronic lymphedema following radical breast surgery and radiation therapy. Histologic examination of angiosarcoma shows anaplastic endothelial cells surrounded by reticulum fiber. Prognosis for the older patient is poor. Smaller lesions in younger (<50 years) patients have a distinctively better outcome. The treatment is wide resection, sometimes with radiation therapy.

3. Solitary fibrous tumor/hemangiopericytoma: ICD-9-CM 171.x—The diagnosis of solitary fibrous tumor versus hemangiopericytoma is a topic of debate. It is now thought that many lesions previously characterized as hemangiopericytomas are actually extrapleural solitary fibrous tumors. Both may range from very low-grade to high-grade sarcoma. These rare perivascular tumors are thought to arise from pericytes. Pericytes are highly arborized perivascular cells that line capillaries and venules. The lesion, which affects male and female adults with equal frequency, is usually found deep in muscle bellies and generally located in the thigh or retroperitoneal area of the pelvis. Microscopic examination of the malignant solitary fibrous tumor reveals tightly packed cells with round nuclei with moderate amounts of cytoplasm with poorly defined borders. Bifurcating sinusoidal vessels that have a typical staghorn appearance are characteristic of the classic hemangiopericytoma. Cytogenetic analysis reveals multiple chromosome translocations including $t(12:19)$ and $t(13:22)$. Treatment consists of a wide surgical resection, followed by local radiation therapy. Some authors recommend preoperative embolization or afferent vessel ligation (or both) intraoperatively.

MISCELLANEOUS SOFT-TISSUE SARCOMAS

The remaining soft-tissue sarcomas are rare and only a brief description of their clinical patterns is summarized.

A. Soft-Tissue Chondrosarcoma: ICD-9-CM 171.x

There are three types of soft-tissue chondrosarcomas.

1. Myxoid chondrosarcoma: ICD-9-CM 171.x—The myxoid chondrosarcoma is sometimes referred to as a chordoid sarcoma because it looks like a chordoma. It is a slow-growing tumor seen in adults, usually in deep structure of the leg. It has a myxoid appearance, does not calcify, and is low grade. Like the chordoma, the myxoid chondrosarcoma responds only to surgical removal.

2. Mesenchymal chondrosarcoma: ICD-9-CM 171.x—This tumor affects individuals between 15 and 40 years of age, is found deep in the lower extremity and neck areas, is fast growing, and carries a poor prognosis because of the high risk of pulmonary metastasis. Calcification may be seen on radiograph, and microscopic examination reveals round

cells scattered in a chondroid matrix. Treatment consists of a wide resection in conjunction with chemotherapy and radiation therapy.

3. Synovial chondrosarcoma: ICD-9-CM 171.x—The conversion of a synovial chondromatosis to a malignant synovial chondrosarcoma is an extremely rare phenomenon. It can occur with lesions of the hip or knee region in older (>60 years) adults.

B. Ewing Sarcoma: ICD-9-CM 171.x

Extraskeletal Ewing sarcoma can be found in individuals between 10 and 30 years of age and is usually located in the paravertebral area, thorax, or deep muscle area of the lower extremity. It is a fast-growing tumor with minimal pain symptoms. It carries the same prognosis as its counterpart in bone and is treated with the same combination of surgery, chemotherapy, and radiation therapy.

C. Alveolar Soft Part Sarcoma: ICD-9-CM 171.x

This round cell sarcoma affects more females than males, is usually found in patients between 15 and 35 years of age, and arises in the deep muscle tissue of the lower extremity, usually the thigh. Alveolar soft part sarcoma is a slow-growing tumor but carries a poor prognosis because of early pulmonary metastasis. The tumor has increased vascularity and is thought to originate from a neurogenic stem cell. It derives its name from its alveolar pattern, which is seen on microscopic examination and can cause this tumor to be mistaken for an alveolar form of rhabdomyosarcoma. A cytogenetic, unbalanced abnormality, $t(x;17)(p11.2;q25)$, is described. Treatment of alveolar soft part sarcoma consists of a wide surgical resection plus radiation therapy and chemotherapy.

D. Epithelioid Sarcoma: ICD-9-CM 171.x

Although this superficial skin lesion is seen most commonly in the palm of the hand, it can also be found on the dorsum of the forearm or on the plantar aspect of the foot. It is a slow-growing tumor that affects patients between 20 and 30 years of age, causes minimal pain symptoms, and is associated with ulceration.

Because epithelioid sarcoma has a whitish color that under the microscope demonstrates cords of epithelium-like cells, it can be mistaken for a synovial sarcoma. Moreover, because of its firm multilobulated presentation, the epithelioid sarcoma may be mistaken for a plantar of palmar fibromatosis (Figure 5–77).

Epithelioid sarcoma spreads as a lumpy nodularity along tendon sheaths or fascial planes and frequently involves local lymph nodes. Local surgical resection is followed by a high local recurrence rate, and a late pulmonary metastasis is common. For this reason, early treatment should consist of an aggressive wide surgical resection.

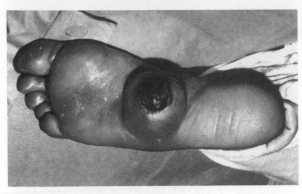

▲ **Figure 5–77.** Clinical appearance of epithelioid sarcoma on the plantar aspect of the foot of a 36-year-old man.

E. Clear Cell Sarcoma: ICD-9-CM 171.x

The clear cell sarcoma is thought to be a deep, noncutaneous variant of the well-known cutaneous melanoma. It is extremely rare, affects women more often than men, and commonly occurs between 20 and 40 years of age. It arises in tendon sheaths and fascial planes, most frequently in the foot and ankle but also in the knee and arm. Clear cell sarcoma starts slowly as a painless lump and has a high potential to spread to local lymph nodes. The lesion in many cases demonstrates evidence of melanin and melanosomes and may be of neural crest origin. The microscopic clear cell appearance can cause this sarcoma to be confused with epithelioid sarcoma and synovial sarcoma.

The prognosis is poor because of a high rate of pulmonary metastasis. This tumor may spread via lymphatics as well. Treatment consists of early aggressive wide resection and may include chemotherapy and local radiation therapy.

▶ Essentials of Diagnosis

- *Although most mesenchymal malignancies do not usually metastasize to lymph nodes, synovial sarcoma, epithelioid sarcoma, and rhabdomyosarcoma are exceptions.*
- *Soft-tissue sarcoma in the adult is generally more sensitive to radiation therapy than chemotherapy.*

Ahmad SA, Patel SR, Ballo MT, et al: Extraosseous osteosarcoma: response to treatment and long-term outcome. *J Clin Oncol* 2002;20:521. [PMID: 11786582]

Anderson J, Gordon T, McManus A, et al: Detection of the PAX3-FKHR fusion gene in paediatric rhabdomyosarcoma: a reproducible predictor of outcome? *Br J Cancer* 2001;85:831. [PMID: 11556833]

Canter RJ, Qin LX, Ferrone CR, et al: Why do patients with low-grade soft tissue sarcoma die? *Ann Surg Oncol* 2008;15:3550. [PMID: 18830667]

Canter RJ, Qin LX, Maki RG, et al: A synovial sarcoma-specific preoperative nomogram supports a survival benefit to ifosfamide-based chemotherapy and improves risk stratification for patients. *Clin Cancer Res* 2008;14:8191. [PMID: 19088035]

Casper C, Wald A: The use of antiviral drugs in the prevention and treatment of Kaposi sarcoma, multicentric Castleman disease and primary effusion lymphoma. *Curr Top Microbiol Immunol* 2007;312:289. [PMID:17089802]

Coindre JM, Hostein I, Maire G, et al: Inflammatory malignant fibrous histiocytomas and dedifferentiated liposarcomas: histological review, genomic profile, and MDM2 and CDK4 status favour a single entity. *J Pathol* 2004;203:822. [PMID: 15221942]

Davicioni E, Anderson MJ, Finckenstein FG, et al: Molecular classification of rhabdomyosarcoma: genotypic and phenotypic determinants of diagnosis. *Am J Pathol* 2009;174:550. [PMID: 19147825]

Eilber FC, Brennan MF, Eilber FR, et al: Chemotherapy is associated with improved survival in adult patients with primary extremity synovial sarcoma. *Ann Surg* 2007;246:105. [PMID: 17592298]

Eilber FC, Eilber FR, Eckardt J, et al: The impact of chemotherapy on the survival of patients with high-grade primary extremity liposarcoma. *Ann Surg* 2004;240:686. [PMID: 15383796]

Guadagnolo BA, Zagars GK, Ballo MT, et al: Long-term outcomes for synovial sarcoma treated with conservation surgery and radiotherapy. *Int J Radiat Oncol Biol Phys* 2007;69:1173. [PMID: 17689031].

Huang HY, Lal P, Qin J, et al: Low-grade myxofibrosarcoma: a clinicopathologic analysis of 49 cases treated at a single institution with simultaneous assessment of the efficacy of 3-tier and 4-tier grading systems. *Hum Pathol* 2004;35:612. [PMID: 15138937]

Jones RL, Fisher C, Al-Muderis O, et al: Differential Sensitivity of liposarcoma subtypes to chemotherapy. *Eur J Cancer* 2005;41:2853. [PMID: 16289617]

Koch M, Nielsen GP, Yoon SS: Malignant tumors of blood vessels: angiosarcomas, hemangioendotheliomas, and hemangiopericytomas. *J Surg Oncol* 2008;97:321. [PMID: 18286475]

Kuklo TR, Temple HT, Owens BD, et al: Preoperative versus postoperative radiation therapy for soft-tissue sarcomas. *Am J Orthop* 2005;34:75. [PMID: 15789525]

Ladanyi M: Fusions of the SYT and SSX genes in synovial sarcoma. *Oncogene* 2001;20:5755. [PMID: 11607825]

Lazar AJ, Das P, Tuvin D, et al: Angiogenesis-promoting gene patterns in alveolar soft part sarcoma. *Clin Cancer Res* 2007;13:7314. [PMID: 18094412]

Lehnhardt M, Daigeler A, Homann HH, et al: MFH revisited: outcome after surgical treatment of undifferentiated pleomorphic or not otherwise specified (NOS) sarcomas of the extremities—an analysis of 140 patients. *Langenbecks Arch Surg* 2009;394:313. [PMID: 18584203]

Nakayama R, Nemoto T, Takahashi H, et al: Gene expression analysis of soft tissue sarcomas: characterization and reclassification of malignant fibrous histiocytoma. *Mod Pathol* 2007;20:749. [PMID: 17464315]

Nascimento AF, Raut CP: Diagnosis and management of pleomorphic sarcomas (so-called "MFH") in adults. *J Surg Oncol* 2008;97:330. [PMID: 18286476]

Patel KU, Szabo SS, Hernandez VS, et al: Dermatofibrosarcoma protuberans COL1A1-PDGFB fusion is identified in virtually all dermatofibrosarcoma protuberans cases when investigated by newly developed multiplex reverse transcription polymerase chain reaction and fluorescence in situ hybridization assays. *Hum Pathol* 2008;39:184. [PMID: 17950782]

Pisters PW, O'Sullivan B, Maki RG: Evidence-based recommendations for local therapy for soft tissue sarcomas. *J Clin Oncol* 2007;25:1003. [PMID: 17350950]

Pitson G, Robinson P, Wilke D, et al: Radiation response: an additional unique signature of myxoid liposarcoma. *Int J Radiat Oncol Biol Phys* 2004;60:522. [PMID: 15380587]

Qualman S, Lynch J, Bridge J, et al: Prevalence and clinical impact of anaplasia in childhood rhabdomyosarcoma: a report from the Soft Tissue Sarcoma Committee of the Children's Oncology Group. *Cancer* 2008;113:3242. [PMID: 18985676]

Spunt SL, Skapek SX, Coffin CM: Pediatric nonrhabdomyosarcoma soft tissue sarcomas. *Oncologist* 2008;13:668. [PMID: 18586922]

West RB, Harvell J, Linn SC, et al: Apo D in soft tissue tumors: a novel marker for dermatofibrosarcoma protuberans. *Am J Surg Pathol* 2004;28:1063. [PMID: 15252314]

Willems SM, Debiec-Rychter M, Szuhai K, et al: Local recurrence of myxofibrosarcoma is associated with increase in tumor grade and cytogenetic aberrations, suggesting a multistep tumour progression model. *Mod Pathol* 2006;19:407. [PMID: 16415793]

MANAGEMENT OF CARCINOMA METASTASIZED TO BONE

▶ Incidence and Natural History of Metastases: ICD-9-CM 199

A. Common Metastatic Carcinomas and Areas of Skeletal Involvement

Metastatic involvement of the musculoskeletal system is one of the most significant clinical issues facing orthopedic oncologists. The number of patients with metastasis to the skeletal system from a carcinoma is 15 times greater than the number of patients with primary bone tumors of all types. Approximately a third of all diagnosed adenocarcinomas include skeletal metastases, resulting in approximately 300,000 cases per year. Furthermore, 70% of patients with advanced terminal carcinoma demonstrate bone metastases at autopsy. The carcinomas that commonly metastasize to bone are prostate, breast, kidney, thyroid, and lung carcinomas. One study showed that nearly 90% of patients with these types of carcinoma had bone metastases. Among the carcinomas that less commonly metastasize to bone are cancers of the skin, oral cavity, esophagus, cervix, stomach, and colon.

The spine is the most frequent area of bone metastasis. Other common skeletal sites include the pelvis, femur, rib, proximal humerus, and skull, in that order. Metastatic lesions are rarely found distal to the elbow or knee. If lesions are found in these areas, so-called acral metastases, the lung is the most common source. Solitary bone lesions comprise only approximately 10% of cases of bone metastasis.

B. Clinical Course of Metastases

The mechanism of metastases is accounted for in a modified "seed/soil" theorem. Fewer than 1 in 10,000 neoplastic cells that escape into the circulation from the primary site are able to set up a metastatic focus, a complex multistep process by which the cell must first break free. This is a function of *degradative* enzymes such as collagenases, hydrolases, cathepsin D, and proteases. Once the cell invades the vascular channel, it circulates through the body. It is theorized that the cell is protected by a fibrin platelet clot. However, clinical trials with heparin do not show a significant change in metastatic outcome. Local factors such as integrins are instrumental in attracting the circulating metastatic cell to a particular remote tissue site. Once within the new tissue, the metastatic cell releases factors such as tumor angiogenesis factor, inducing neovascularization, which in turn facilitates growth of the metastatic focus.

Patients with advanced metastatic disease frequently experience dysfunction of their hematopoietic and calcium homeostasis systems. Patients may develop a normochromic, normocytic anemia with leukocytosis. In response to the anemia, the increased production of immature cells is noted on the peripheral blood smear. This is termed the *leukoerythroblastic reaction.* Hypercalcemia may result in up to 30% of cases with extensive metastases. This is most frequently seen in myeloma, breast cancer, and non–small cell lung cancer.

Blastic metastases are frequently painless and associated with a lower incidence of pathologic fracture because the bone is not as severely weakened (Figures 5–78 and 5–79). Not all tumors that metastasize from the prostate to the bone are blastic. The lytic variants are painful and more likely to cause pathologic fractures.

Most tumors that metastasize from the breast to the bone are blastic, but some demonstrate mixtures of blastic and lytic areas in the same bone. By taking serial radiographs and noting the appearance of bone metastases, it is possible to follow the progress of treatment consisting of systemic therapy with hormones or chemotherapeutic agents plus local radiation therapy. A favorable response may show a gradual conversion from a lytic to a blastic appearance as the pain decreases.

Bone destruction in lytic lesions is a response by native osteoclasts to the tumor. Neovascularity is common. Among the tumors that are characteristic for this hemorrhagic response are thyroid carcinomas (Figure 5–80), renal cell carcinoma (Figure 5–81), and multiple myeloma. Before a surgical intervention, it is beneficial to perform a prophylactic embolization of the area to reduce perioperative bleeding. If a lesion is unexpectedly found to be aneurysmal at the time of surgical exploration, it is best to debulk the friable tumor mass rapidly down to normal bone and then pack the area until it can be stabilized with bone cement.

▶ Diagnosis

A. General Approach

A methodical approach is mandatory in the workup of a patient with presumed metastatic disease to bone to locate the primary tumor. A thorough history and physical examination

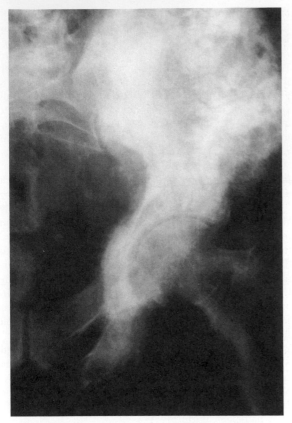

▲ **Figure 5–78.** Radiograph of a blastic carcinoma that metastasized from the prostate to the pelvis in an 85-year-old man.

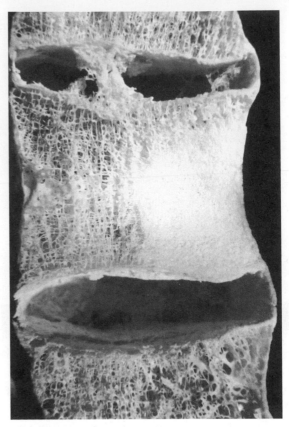

▲ **Figure 5–79.** Skeletal specimen of a blastic carcinoma that metastasized from the prostate to the lumbar spine.

must be completed prior to laboratory and radiographic analysis. Eight percent of patients may have their primary carcinoma detected on physical exam. Laboratory analysis should include complete blood count, ESR, renal and liver panels, alkaline phosphate, and serum protein electrophoresis.

Radiographic examination should follow with a plain chest radiograph and radiographs of known involved bones. Approximately 45% of primaries are detected in the lung on the chest radiograph. The workup should also include a staging bone scan. If this is negative, myeloma should be suspected. Furthermore, a lesion at a more convenient biopsy site may be found. Bone scan is also more sensitive than plain radiographs in detecting early lesions. CT scans of the chest, abdomen, and pelvis should be performed. Lung CT can detect up to 15% of primaries missed on the plain radiograph.

These studies in conjunction with a well-planned biopsy detect the majority of cases. Routine radiographic screening studies in search of early metastatic disease are not very helpful (Figure 5–82). Lytic changes become evident

on routine radiographs only when cortical destruction approaches 30–50% (Figure 5–83).

▶ Treatment and Prognosis

A. Nonsurgical Treatment

Nonsurgical management of metastatic carcinoma to bone includes observation, radiation treatment, and hormonal/ cytotoxic chemotherapy. Radiation is reserved for palliative management. Each patient must be carefully evaluated as a candidate for radiation therapy. The histologic type of disease, extent of disease, prognosis, marrow reserve, and overall constitution must be assessed.

After sustaining a pathologic fracture secondary to metastatic carcinoma, the average survival time is 19 months. Each histologic type has varying lengths of survival (prostate, 29 months; breast, 23 months; renal, 12 months; lung, 4 months). Furthermore, each type of carcinoma exhibits varying radiosensitivity. Prostate and lymphoreticular types

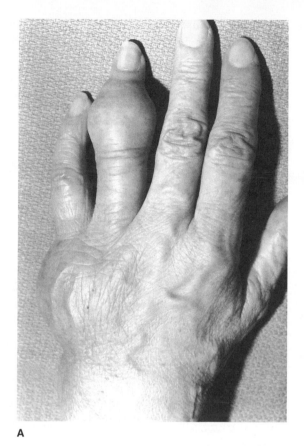

A

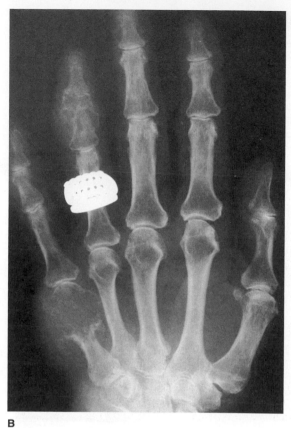

B

▲ **Figure 5–80.** Clinical appearance (**A**) and radiographic appearance (**B**) of aneurysmal lesions in a case of carcinoma that metastasized from the thyroid to the hand.

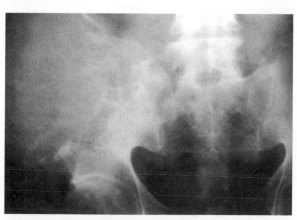

▲ **Figure 5–81.** Radiograph of a metastatic hyperne-phroma in the ilium.

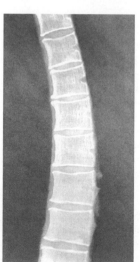

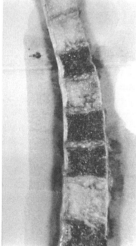

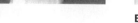

A B

▲ **Figure 5–82.** Radiograph (**A**) and gross appearance (**B**) of bone in a case of carcinoma that metastasized from the lung to the spine.

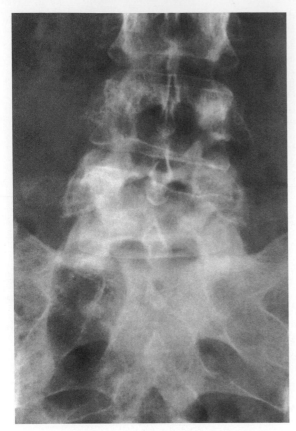

▲ **Figure 5–83.** Radiograph of the spine of a 45-year-old woman whose cancer had metastasized from the breast.

demonstrate excellent sensitivity. Breast is intermediate, and renal and gastrointestinal are poor. When used, appropriately 90% of patients gain at least minimal relief, with up to two thirds obtaining complete relief. Seventy percent of patients who are ambulatory retain this function after radiation therapy to the lower extremities. Systemic radioisotopes are also used in selected cases.

Hormonal therapy has an important role in the management of metastatic breast and prostate cancer. Fortunately, these agents are easy to administer and have few side effects.

For breast cancer, medical hormonal manipulation can be done by use of antiestrogens, progestins, luteinizing hormone–releasing hormone, or adrenal-suppressing agents. Tamoxifen is effective in 30% of all breast cancer cases but increases to 50–75% of cases when the tumor is known to be estrogen receptor, progesterone receptor positive. Surgical ablation (oophorectomy) may also have a role in certain cases.

For prostate cancer, reduction in testosterone levels via bilateral orchiectomy or administration of estrogens

or antiandrogens may produce dramatic results in certain cases. Estrogens are no longer used as a first agent because of the risk of cardiovascular complication.

The use of agents aimed at decreasing bone turnover, including bisphosphonates, osteoprotegerin, and nuclear factor kappa B inhibitor, has also been introduced to limit progression of bone metastases. Although the effect on overall tumor burden is unclear, there is evidence that bisphosphonates decrease skeletal-related events. Preclinical studies also suggest that when combined with cytotoxic agents, bisphosphonates may synergistically reduce the incidence of osseous metastases and prolong survival.

Cytotoxic chemotherapy is used in adenocarcinoma treatment quite extensively. In older (>60 years) patients with advanced disease, however, the side effects of the drugs may be too severe.

▶ **B. Surgical Treatment**

The goals for surgical intervention in the patient with metastatic carcinoma to bone are relief of pain; prevention of pathologic fractures; stabilization of realized pathologic fractures; enhancement of mobility, function, and quality of life; and perhaps improvement of survival. It is generally agreed that a patient must have a life expectancy of at least 6 weeks to warrant operative intervention. Special considerations to surgical management include noting that bone quality is attenuated and healing will be delayed if even possible. Cancer patients, irrespective of their age, may have increased difficulty protecting their fixation device/prosthesis secondary to systemic debilitation. Accordingly, rigid fixation, with polymethylmethacrylate (PMMA) augmentation as needed, is mandatory.

1. Hip—Seventy-five percent of all surgery for cancer that has metastasized to bone is performed in the hip area (Figure 5–84). Prior to 1970, surgeons attempted to stabilize these fractures with conventional hip nails or Austin Moore

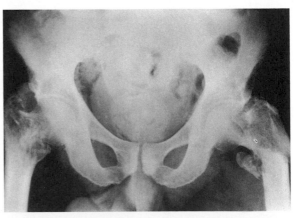

▲ **Figure 5–84.** Radiograph of the pathologic fractures of both hips in a 55-year-old man with lung carcinoma.

prostheses, but results were poor because of deficient local bone stock. After 1970, with the advent of bone cement as an adjuvant form of therapy, these same devices could be used, with improved results in most cases, along with local radiation therapy starting 2 weeks after the surgery. This technique allowed for early ambulation with less pain. However, as time passed and survival times increased, more failures were noted after 1–2 years with the hip nail and cement technique. For this reason, most surgeons currently use a cemented bipolar hemiarthroplasty for the femoral neck fractures and a longer stem calcar replacement hemiarthroplasty for the intertrochanteric fractures. Before these procedures are performed, it is wise to evaluate the entire shaft of the femur and the supraacetabular area for other lytic lesions that might require a longer stem femoral component for the shaft or a modified cemented acetabular component with a total hip replacement for acetabular lesions.

In many cases, the diagnosis of metastasis to the proximal femur is made before a fracture occurs. In these cases, it is the responsibility of the orthopedic surgeon to decide whether the patient should receive some form of internal stabilization prior to radiation therapy. A CT scan of the involved area helps make this decision. Criteria for the performance of a prophylactic stabilization procedure include the following: (1) 50% cortical lysis, (2) a femoral lesion greater than 2.5 cm in diameter, (3) an avulsion fracture of the lesser trochanter, and (4) persistent pain in the hip area 4 weeks following the completion of radiation therapy. These criteria are not perfect, however, and large errors arise in estimation of the load-bearing capacity of the bone.

2. Supraacetabular area—In the case of a small supraacetabular lesion with intact cortical bone, a cemented cup with a total hip system is generally most appropriate. Augmentation of the fully cemented reconstruction with threaded Steinmann pins or similar anchoring screws may be necessary in advanced cases (Figure 5–85). The principles of treatment are always the same, irrespective of the extent of disease: aggressive intralesional curettage of the area back to healthy bone, followed by the placement of large (4.76 mm) threaded Steinmann pins into the sacroiliac area. The pins are placed with an initial foundation batch of cement, leaving them exposed for a second batch of cement, on top of which the cup is placed. A routine femoral component is then cemented.

3. Femoral shaft—Diaphyseal lesions that affect the femur but spare the peritrochanteric area are best handled with some form of intramedullary nail (Figure 5–86). Fixation of the entire femur, including the peritrochanteric area, with a reconstruction-type nail is preferable in the event the disease progresses within the bone. Current intramedullary fixation devices often do not need cement augmentation. However, in cases of severe bone deficiency, PMMA introduction,

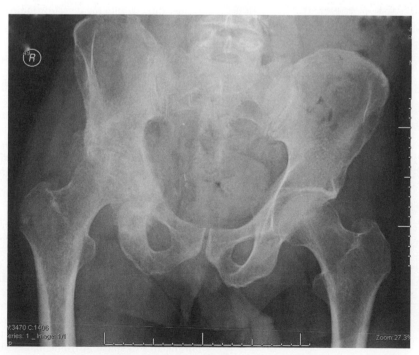

▲ **Figure 5–85.** Preoperative (**A**) and postoperative (**B**) radiographs of the pelvis of a 65-year-old man with metastatic transitional cell carcinoma to the right acetabular region.

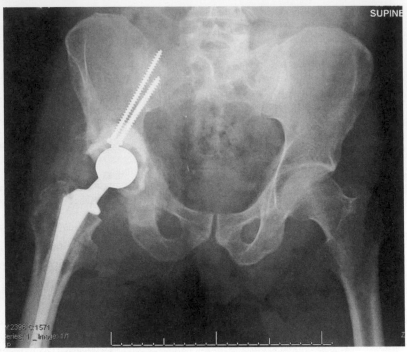

SUPINE

▲ **Figure 5–85.** (Continued)

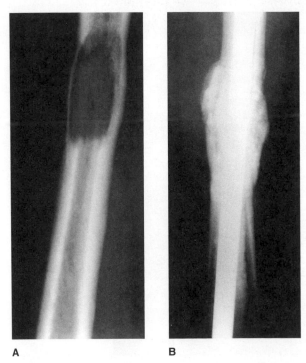

A
B

▲ **Figure 5–86.** Preoperative (**A**) and postoperative (**B**) radiographs of the midshaft of the femur of a patient whose treatment involved fixation with a cemented intramedullary nail.

either directly into the defect or indirectly at the nail insertion site, is preferable.

4. Humerus—The principle for the management of metastatic disease to the humerus is no different from that for the femur. In the case of diaphyseal lesions, surgeons either use a conventional intramedullary rod or they plate the lesion. PMMA may be used with either technique.

In the case of the proximal humerus involving a large amount of the humeral head and neck, it is frequently necessary to cement a long-stem prosthesis (Figure 5–87). Just as with the proximal femur, in the proximal humerus, there is no need to widely resect the tumor, and the rotator cuff is usually left intact.

5. Spine—In most cases of metastasis to the spine, the patient's pain can be managed adequately with local radiation therapy and medication. However, in cases of mechanical collapse associated with bony protrusion into the vertebral canal and cord compromise, surgical decompression and stabilization are frequently indicated. In the past, most of these problems were treated with posterior decompression by laminectomy alone. The results were poor because the spine was further destabilized, which resulted in increased kyphosis and anterior cord compression. With advances in the area of spinal instrumentation, the treatment shifted toward a more aggressive anterior decompression and stabilization if the patient's general condition allows. Even in cases in which the patient's general health does not tolerate

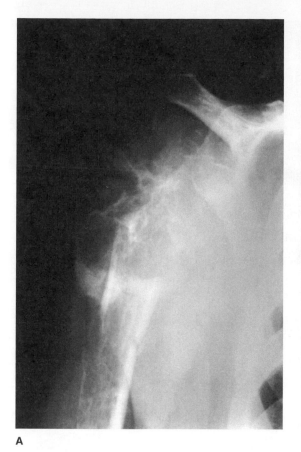 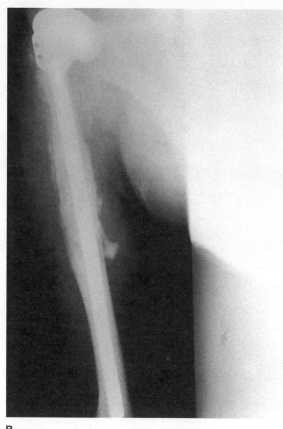

A   **B**

▲ **Figure 5–87.** Preoperative (**A**) and postoperative (**B**) radiographs of the proximal humerus of a patient whose treatment involved the use of a long-stem Neer prosthesis.

the larger anterior approach, a less aggressive alternative might include posterior decompression supplemented by posterior spinal fixation.

The midthoracic spine is the most common area for paraplegia secondary to metastasis because of the narrow vertebral canal at this level of the spine. The ideal surgical approach to the problem in a patient with a reasonable prognosis consists of an anterior thoracotomy and anterior decompression by vertebrectomy, followed by anterior stabilization. As an alternative approach in a patient with a worse prognosis and circumferential cord compression, a posterior decompression stabilization can be considered (Figure 5–88).

The second most common site for cord compression is the thoracolumbar region. The anterior reconstruction is the same in the thoracolumbar area as in the midthoracic area. A posterior stabilization may be advisable, especially in cases in which the prognosis is good.

The cervical spine is the least likely area for surgical treatment, mainly because the vertebral canal is wide at this level

and cord compromise is uncommon. If surgery is needed, an ideal reconstruction is an anterior decompression and stabilization.

Radiation therapy is required postoperatively with all of these reconstructions. The use of bone graft is therefore undesirable because of inhibited osteoblastic healing.

▶ **Essentials of Diagnosis**

- *Prostate, breast, kidney, thyroid, and lung carcinomas are the most common to metastasize to bone.*

- *Surgical treatment of metastatic bone disease should focus on early return to function and maximization of quality of life.*

- *Ionized calcium should routinely be checked in metastatic bone disease due to the morbidity and mortality of hypercalcemia of malignancy.*

- *Carcinoma of the lung is the most likely to cause distal, or so-called acral, metastases.*

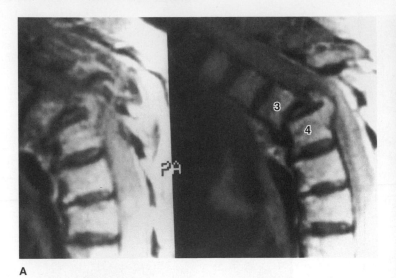

A

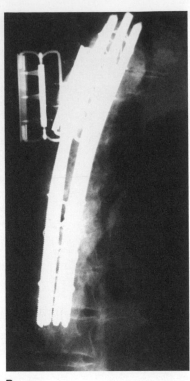

B

▲ **Figure 5–88.** Preoperative T1-weighted MRI (**A**) and postoperative radiograph (**B**) of the spine of a patient whose treatment involved use of posterior rods and sublaminar wires for stabilization.

Cappucio M, Gasbarrini A, Van Urk P, et al: Spinal metastasis: a retrospective study validating the treatment algorithm. *Eur Rev Med Pharmacol Sci* 2008;12:155. [PMID: 18700686]

Guise TA: Antitumor effects of bisphosphonates: promising preclinical evidence. *Cancer Treat Rev* 2008;34(Suppl 1):S19. [PMID: 18486348]

Hatoum HT, Lin SJ, Smith MR, et al: Zoledronic acid and skeletal complications in patients with solid tumors and bone metastases: analysis of a national medical claims database. *Cancer* 2008;113:1438. [PMID: 18720527]

Hipp JA, Springfield DS, Hayes WC: Predicting pathologic fracture risk in the management of metastatic bone defects. *Clin Orthop Relat Res* 1995;312:120. [PMID: 7634597]

Kohno N, Aogi K, Minami H, et al: Zoledronic acid significantly reduces skeletal complications compared with placebo in Japanese women with bone metastases from breast cancer: a randomized, placebo-controlled trial. *J Clin Oncol* 2005;23:3314. [PMID: 15738536]

Lu S, Zhang J, Zhou Z, et al: Synergistic inhibitory activity of zoledronate and paclitaxel on bone metastasis in nude mice. *Oncol Rep* 2008;20:581. [PMID: 18695909]

Manabe J, Kawaguchi N, Matsumoto S, et al: Surgical treatment of bone metastasis: indications and outcomes. *Int J Clin Oncol* 2005;10:103. [PMID: 15864695]

Mirels H: Metastatic disease in long bones. A proposed scoring system for diagnosing impending pathologic fractures. *Clin Orthop Relat Res* 1989;249:256. [PMID: 2684463]

Rougraff BT, Kneisl JS, Simon MA: Skeletal metastases of unknown origin: a prospective study of a diagnostic strategy. *J Bone Joint Surg Am* 1993;75:1276. [PMID: 8408149]

Wedin R, Bauer HC: Surgical treatment of skeletal metastatic lesions of the proximal femur: endoprosthesis or reconstruction nail? *J Bone Joint Surg Br* 2005;87:1653. [PMID: 16326880]

Wedin R, Bauer HC, Rutqvist LE: Surgical treatment for skeletal breast cancer metastases: a population-based study of 641 patients. *Cancer* 2001;92:257. [PMID: 11466677]

▼ DIFFERENTIAL DIAGNOSIS OF PSEUDOTUMOROUS CONDITIONS

In addition to benign, malignant, and metastatic neoplasms, a group of pseudotumors masquerade as bone and soft-tissue tumors. These lesions actually appear with greater frequency than either primary bone or soft-tissue tumors.

Stress-Reactive Lesions

The most common pseudotumors are those related to either bone or soft-tissue injury.

A. Stress Fracture of Bone: ICD-9-CM 733.9x

Stress fractures are common in young (<30 years) athletic individuals and can produce radiographic features that might suggest the diagnosis of a bone-forming sarcoma or Ewing sarcoma. It is important to obtain a careful history from patients regarding their physical activity both at work and at play. There will be no history of a single injury if the bone symptoms are caused by repetitive impact loading stress such as occurs with working out or cross-country running. The stress fracture usually occurs several weeks after a sudden increase in physical activity for which the patient is not properly conditioned. This is a common situation in the military, particularly during initial training.

Stress fractures are commonly located in the metaphyseal-diaphyseal areas of long weight-bearing bones. Early radiographs frequently appear normal before periosteal new bone begins to form. The most sensitive early diagnostic tool is a bone scan, which can appear hot or abnormal in the case of stress fractures, neoplasms, and infections. The MRI is sensitive to early fluid shifts in the periosteum overlying a stress fracture, but it is also sensitive to neoplastic and infectious conditions. One of the best methods to help rule out tumors and infection is to simply stop all physical stress to the injured bone for a period of 4 weeks. In patients with stress fracture, the pain should resolve spontaneously during this period, and a follow-up radiograph taken after this period reveals a typical fusiform circumferential periosteal callous formation. In patients with a tumor or infection, the pain persists, and the radiographic signs of permeative osteolysis predominate, in which case a biopsy and culture are indicated.

At times, the clinical picture of a stress fracture is confused by the preexistence of a benign stress raiser, such as a nonossifying fibroma or fibrous cortical defect (Figure 5–89).

In older patients, especially in postmenopausal women, stress fractures can occur with minimal physical activity. The circumstances under which the fracture occurred might not come out in a routine history. A common location of osteoporotic stress fractures is in the sacrum (Figure 5–90).

B. Myositis Ossificans: ICD-9-CM 728.12

Another common stress-reactive pseudotumor seen in the extremity is myositis ossificans, which occurs most frequently in the lower extremity in young men. The quadriceps muscle is commonly involved because of direct blows or tearing injury to this muscle. The pseudotumor mass may not arise for several months after the injury and may not be related to a specific injury. In older (>40 years), more sedentary patients, there may be no history of stress injury.

Early radiographs may not reveal soft-tissue calcification. With maturation, ossification occurs in the traumatized muscle fascial planes, which may suggest the diagnosis of a synovial sarcoma or other calcifying sarcoma. If the myositis pseudotumor is attached to the subjacent bone, it can mimic a parosteal osteosarcoma (Figure 5–91).

Infectious Diseases

Bacterial, viral, tuberculous, or fungal infections of the bone or soft tissue can frequently mimic a neoplastic process. This is particularly the case with infections that are

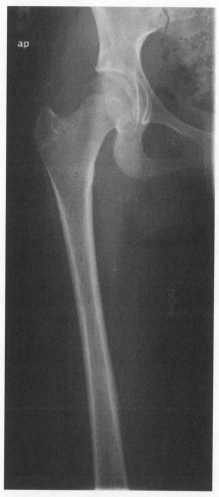

A

▲ **Figure 5–89.** Radiograph (**A**), isotope bone scan (**B**), and CT scan (**C**) of the femur of a 14-year-old girl with a stress fracture. Notice the subtle increased uptake in the contralateral femur in **B** and the absence of a nidus, which would be seen in osteoid osteoma, but rather a linear lucency in **C**.

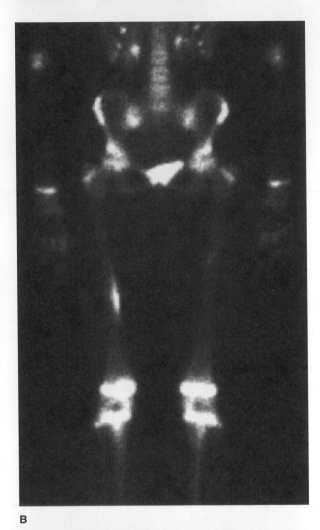

B

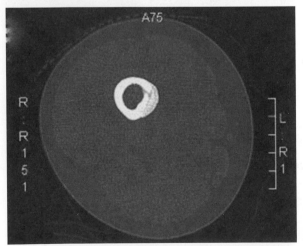

C

▲ **Figure 5–89.** (Continued)

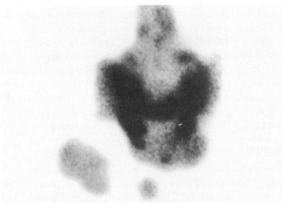

A

B

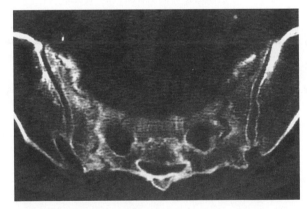

C

▲ **Figure 5–90.** T1-weighted MRI (**A**), isotope bone scan (**B**), and CT scan (**C**) of the sacrum in a 71-year-old woman with stress fracture.

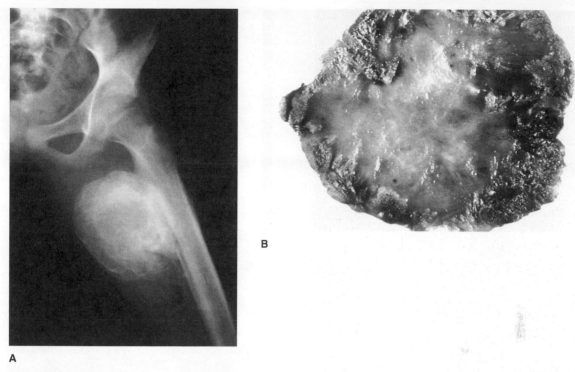

▲ **Figure 5–91.** Radiograph (**A**) and gross appearance of a resected specimen (**B**) of myositis ossificans in the adductor muscles of a 12-year-old girl.

not highly virulent, do not create systemic symptoms or a febrile response, and do not cause a large alteration in acute-phase reactant laboratory work. If a tender mass is present on examination and a bone or soft-tissue tumor is suggested by imaging studies, a biopsy may be indicated and should include a tissue culture to make the correct diagnosis. Inflammatory pseudotumors can be seen in any age group but are more common in children and frequently affect the lower extremity.

A. Bacterial Infection: ICD-9-CM 730.0-2x

Bacterial infections of bone can take on the appearance of a round cell tumor such as Ewing sarcoma in children or lymphoma in adults (Figure 5–92). In contrast, tuberculous and fungal infections are less inflammatory and thus have more localized, well-marginated lesions that take on the imaging appearance of a benign tumor.

B. Tuberculous or Fungal Infection: ICD-9-CM 015.x, or 730.2x

A tuberculous or fungal infection of the spine or extremity can present as a pseudotumor in children or young adults, especially in Asian or Mexican patients (Figure 5–93). The incidence of tuberculous and fungal infections, which are

low-grade infections that typically have an insidious onset, is also increased in patients with AIDS.

C. Caffey Disease: ICD-9-CM 730.3x

Caffey disease can mimic a neoplastic process. It is an idiopathic form of periostitis that is seen in infants younger than 6 months and affects the extremities, shoulder girdle, and mandible (Figure 5–94). It may have a viral origin and is currently much rarer than it was 30 years ago. The bony changes are osteoblastic and could suggest the diagnosis of an osteosarcoma, which is rare in infants. Caffey disease is self-limiting and usually clears spontaneously without disability.

▶ Metabolic Disorders

A. Brown Tumor of Primary Hyperparathyroidism: ICD-9-CM 733.90

Brown tumor is the most common metabolic disorder that mimics a neoplastic process in bone. The lytic giant cell lesions occur symmetrically in metaphyseal-epiphyseal bone as the result of increased parathyroid hormone production by a solitary parathyroid adenoma, by hyperplastic parathyroid glands, or by a solitary parathyroid carcinoma. Brown tumors occur three times more often in females than in

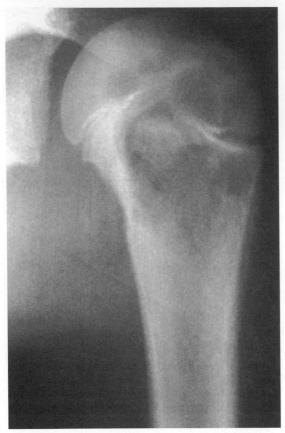

▲ **Figure 5–92.** Radiograph of acute osteomyelitis caused by *Staphylococcus aureus* in the proximal humerus of a 13-year-old boy.

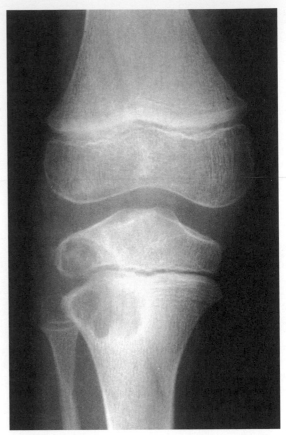

▲ **Figure 5–93.** Radiograph of tuberculous osteomyelitis in the proximal tibia of a 10-year-old girl.

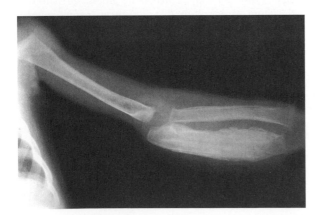

A

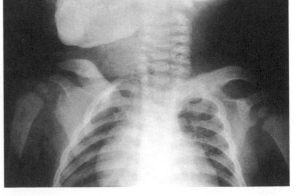

B

▲ **Figure 5–94.** Radiographs of the upper extremity (**A**) and the bilateral shoulders (**B**) of a 5-month-old infant with Caffey disease.

males and are usually seen between 15 and 70 years of age. They are most common in the ends of the long bone, followed next in frequency in the pelvis, long bone diaphysis, maxillary bone, cranium, rib, and hand. Brown tumors are rarely seen in the spine. Symptoms of pain are related to the local bone destruction, but widespread pain may result from generalized osteomalacia. The hyperparathyroid condition can lead to weight loss, psychological disorders, gastrointestinal disorders, renal stones, polyuria, and polydipsia.

The radiographic features of the brown tumor in bone include a round lytic area that may be multicentric and may suggest the diagnosis of metastatic carcinoma, multiple myeloma, or histiocytic lymphoma (Figure 5–95). In the case of a solitary lesion, it may suggest the diagnosis of a nonossifying fibroma, fibrous dysplasia, giant cell tumor, or aneurysmal bone cyst. At the time of biopsy, the brown tumor has the reddish brown appearance of a giant cell tumor. Microscopically, it looks like a giant cell tumor except that the background stromal cells are more fibroblastic and the bone trabeculae demonstrate abnormally thick and poorly mineralized osteoid seams. Because of the marked similarity between the brown tumor and the giant cell tumor, clinicians should routinely order an analysis of serum calcium,

phosphorus, and alkaline phosphatase levels in all patients with bone lesions that produce giant cells.

In patients with brown tumors, the treatment consists of removing the source of the excessive parathyroid hormone. After this, the bony defects usually heal spontaneously. Bone grafting is rarely required. Although the secondary hyperparathyroidism seen in renal failure patients does not usually develop into brown tumors, it does produce pseudotumorous calcification in soft tissue, a condition similar to tumoral calcinosis, which is discussed later in this section.

B. Paget Disease: ICD-9-CM 731.0

Paget disease is frequently included in discussions of metabolic bone disorders, although the demonstration of cytoplasmic and nuclear inclusion bodies in osteoclasts of pagetic bone similar to paramyxovirus infections may suggest a viral origin. Most clinicians are familiar with the late changes in Paget disease, which include the bowing of long bones and the finding of dense blastic changes on radiographic examination. However, many are unfamiliar with the early lytic phase of Paget disease when the radiographic findings are more suggestive of metastatic carcinoma, histiocytic

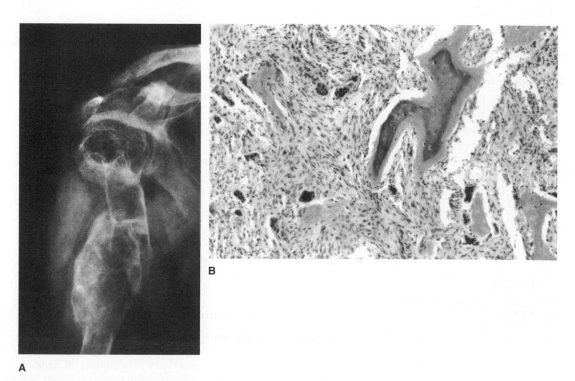

B

A

▲ **Figure 5–95.** Radiograph (**A**) and photomicrograph (**B**) of a brown tumor of hyperparathyroidism in the proximal humerus of a 40-year-old woman.

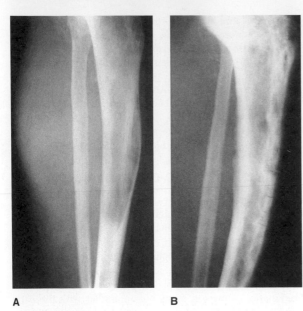

A   B

▲ **Figure 5–96.** Early and late radiographs of Paget disease of the tibia, taken when the patient was 45 years of age (**A**) and when he was 65 years of age (**B**).

lymphoma, primary sarcoma, or even primary hyperparathyroidism (Figure 5–96).

C. Gaucher Disease: ICD-9-CM 272.7

Gaucher disease is a rare familial disorder in which accumulation of glucocerebroside causes enlargement of the liver, spleen, and marrow tissues. The marrow infiltration in children and young adults causes a gradual loss of bone that can mimic a neoplastic condition. The most common areas involved include the distal femur, tibia, humerus, vertebral column, skull, and mandible. Isolated focal destructive changes with endosteal scalloping and moth-eaten patterns may suggest the diagnosis of metastatic disease, myelomatosis, primary sarcoma, or fibrous dysplasia (Figure 5–97).

▶ Hemorrhagic Conditions
A. Pseudotumor of Hemophilia: ICD-9-CM 733.90

A hematoma in the soft tissue or bone under the periosteum may be difficult to distinguish from a tumor. Hematoma formation is frequently precipitated by some form of trauma, and the bones most commonly involved are the femur, pelvis, tibia, and small bones of the hand. It is rare to see multiple lesions. The bony lesions can be

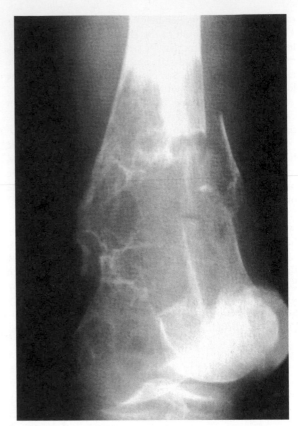

▲ **Figure 5–97.** Radiograph of a pathologic fracture secondary to Gaucher disease involving the distal femur in a 29-year-old man.

central or eccentric. The finding of lytic destruction followed by sclerotic reaction at the periphery may mimic the radiographic picture of an aneurysmal bone cyst or a giant cell tumor. In the hand bones, the osseous pseudotumors take on the appearance of a giant cell reparative granuloma or an osteoblastoma. The subperiosteal lesions bulge into the surrounding soft tissue and show reactive periosteal new bone formation and subjacent cortical erosion that may mimic Ewing sarcoma or hemorrhagic osteosarcoma (Figure 5–98).

B. Intramuscular Hematoma: ICD-9-CM 729.92

Another hemorrhagic disorder that can produce a pseudotumor of soft tissue is the intramuscular hematoma. It is similar to the soft-tissue pseudotumor of hemophilia but without a bleeding abnormality. Intramuscular hematomas are almost always related to blunt trauma, but they occasionally result from a traction injury that may subsequently

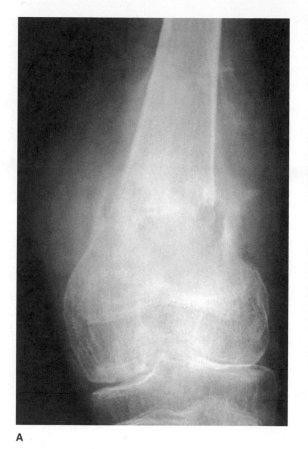

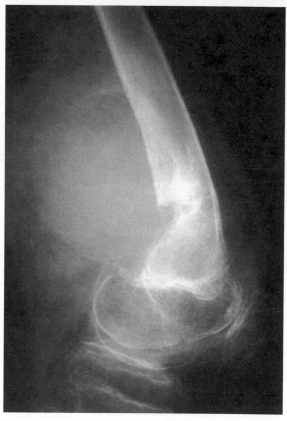

A

B

▲ **Figure 5–98.** Anteroposterior (**A**) and lateral (**B**) radiographs of a pseudotumor of hemophilia in the distal femur of a 14-year-old boy.

produce myositis ossificans. There may be no superficial signs of bruising in the overlying skin, and sometimes the hematoma grows in size at a later date, even as long as several years after the initial injury. The radiographic examination is of little help because no calcification or bony abnormality is evident. The MRI is the best imaging study, but unfortunately, the appearance of an intramuscular hematoma on MRI can mimic that of a deep soft-tissue sarcoma such as a malignant fibrous histiocytoma (Figure 5–99).

▶ Ectopic Calcification

Ectopic calcification in soft tissue has many causes, most of which are related to chronic degenerative disorders in collagenous structures such as tendons or ligaments about a joint. However, in cases in which the dystrophic calcification is associated with a soft-tissue mass, the clinician must rule out the diagnosis of a soft-tissue sarcoma such as synovial sarcoma.

A. Tumoral Calcinosis: ICD-9-CM 275.49

Tumoral calcinosis, seen about the hip, shoulder, and elbow, is characterized by extensive calcium phosphate deposition in a benign fibrous mass. There is a familial form associated with a loss-of-function mutation in the *FGF23* gene. A gain-of-function mutation in the same gene results in autosomal dominant hypophosphatemic rickets. Otherwise, it is an idiopathic condition that affects patients between 10 and 30 years of age and occurs more frequently in males than in females. Multiple lesions occur, and the lesions cause minimal pain and tenderness.

In cases of tumoral calcinosis, the extensive central fluffy calcification might suggest the diagnosis of a synovial sarcoma, soft-tissue chondrosarcoma, or tuberculosis (Figure 5–100). At biopsy, a chalky white paste exudes from a spongelike fibrous mass. Microscopic findings include extensive amorphous calcium phosphate deposits in a fibrous stroma speckled with macrophages and inflammatory cells.

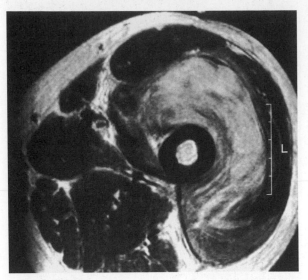

▲ **Figure 5–99.** Axial view T2-weighted MRI of a hematoma in the quadriceps muscles of a 46-year-old woman.

If the pseudotumor is not completely removed, a recurrence is very likely.

A similar condition is seen in patients with renal osteo-dystrophy with secondary hyperparathyroidism, and the mechanism for the deposition in this case is a high level of calcium phosphorus production.

▶ B. Compartment Syndrome: ICD-9-CM 728.12

The ischemic calcification and even ossification that occur in traumatic compartment syndromes in the lower extremity can often mimic a tumor. The initial injury is usually a crushing type that causes increased compartment pressure from muscle swelling. This pressure eventually leads to ischemic necrosis of the compartment muscle, which several years later becomes calcific or even ossified. Because the muscle appears firm and calcified on radiographic examination, the clinician may not relate the finding to an old injury and may suspect a calcifying sarcoma such as synovial sarcoma. The most common place for this pseudotumor is in one of the muscle compartments of the leg, and it causes stiffness and muscle weakness at the ankle and foot area (Figure 5–101). This process can mimic soft-tissue calcifications secondary to a neoplastic process (Figure 5–102).

▶ Dysplastic Disorders

Many developmental or dysplastic conditions can create bony abnormalities, which, on radiographic examination, can mimic a bone tumor. These are usually focal defects in enchondral bone formation that result from a failure to

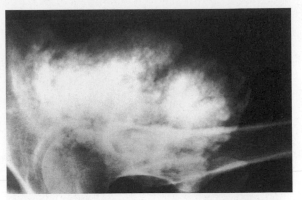

A

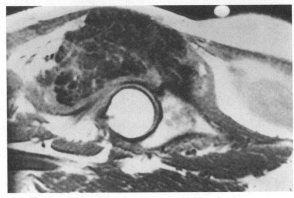

B

▲ **Figure 5–100.** Radiograph (**A**) and T1-weighted MRI (**B**) of tumoral calcinosis in the hip of a 54-year-old woman.

remodel primary woven bone forming at the metaphyseal end of the physis.

A. Osteoma: ICD-9-CM 213.x

Osteoma commonly occurs in the skull or maxilla and is composed of dense unorganized woven bone seen just beneath the cortex. There is no lytic component in or around the dense bone, and no symptoms are associated with the presence of osteomas. Because the lesions are commonly seen in the metaphyseal areas about the knee, the clinician may become concerned about the diagnosis of an early osteosarcoma. However, the lack of periosteal response and minimal uptake on an isotope bone scan help rule out sarcoma (Figure 5–103). In such cases, there should be no concern about future problems from the lesion, and usually no intervention is necessary.

B. Bone Island: ICD-9-CM 213.x

The bone island, or enostosis, is an even more sharply marginated dysplastic process than the osteoma. It is most

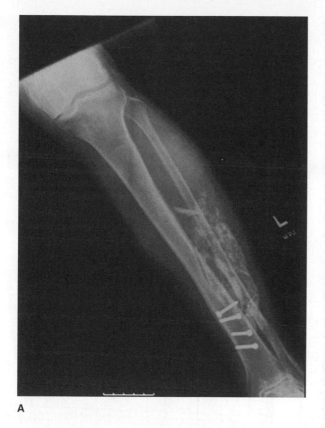

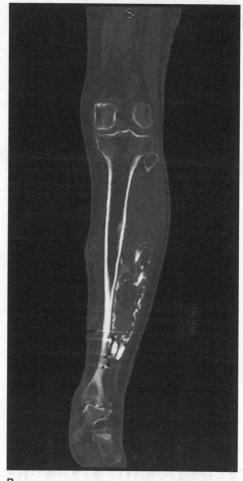

▲ **Figure 5–101.** Radiograph (**A**) and CT scan (**B**) of an old compartment syndrome of the anterior compartment of the leg of an 81-year-old woman who had a history of fracture treated with internal fixation 60 years prior.

commonly located in the pelvis. It can mimic a blastic metastatic lesion in patients with prostate cancer. However, with a bone island, as with an osteoma, the bone scan shows minimal and very focal activity, and the CT scan and MRI show no reaction in the surrounding marrow. Figure 5–104 shows the findings of a bone island through the pelvis of a 35-year-old man.

▶ Bone Infarcts

The two types of bone infarcts that can mimic bone tumors are the metaphyseal type and the epiphyseal type. They can be idiopathic in origin or secondary to increased alcohol consumption or corticosteroid use.

A. Metaphyseal Bone Infarct: ICD-9-CM 733.4x

The most common bone infarct is in the metaphyseal region, which is typically seen about the knee, hip, and shoulder in adults. Radiographically, the infarct can mimic a low-grade cartilaginous tumor such as an enchondroma. An infarct presents with a sclerotic honeycombed pattern (Figure 5–105), whereas a cartilaginous lesion presents with central flocculated calcification (Figure 5–106).

B. Epiphyseal Bone Infarct: ICD-9-CM 733.4x

Although epiphyseal bone infarcts have the same etiology as those in the metaphysis, these are most commonly found in the femoral condyles and the proximal femoral and

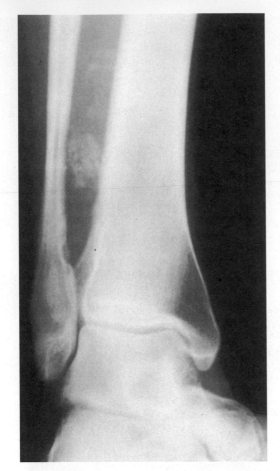

▲ **Figure 5–102.** Radiograph of calcification in synovial sarcoma of the leg.

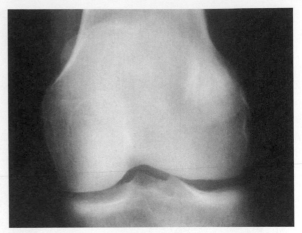

A

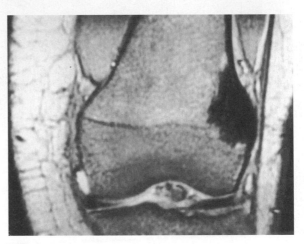

B

▲ **Figure 5–103.** Radiograph (**A**) and T2-weighted MRI (**B**) of a dysplastic process in the distal femur of a 64-year-old woman.

humeral epiphyses. In these locations, the lytic change seen in the epiphyseal bone can mimic a chondroblastoma. The differential diagnosis can be difficult before the appearance of a crescent sign or other radiographic signs of subchondral collapse that usually rule out the chondroblastoma (Figure 5–107).

▶ Histiocytic Disorders

A. Langerhans Cell Histiocytosis: ICD-9-CM 277.89

Sometimes inappropriately called histiocytosis X, Langerhans cell histiocytosis can present in a variety of ways. Previously considered distinct diseases, including eosinophilic granuloma, Hand-Schüller-Christian disease, and Letterer-Siwe disease, they are now considered part of

the same spectrum of histiocytosis presentation. Of these, the localized granulomatous form, which is called eosinophilic granuloma or Langerhans cell granulomatosis, is the one that mimics a tumor radiographically. Eosinophilic granuloma is seen twice as often in boys as in girls and commonly occurs between 5 and 15 years of age. It is usually monostotic but in 10% of cases involves two or three separate areas. It is a histiocytic process of unknown cause but may have a viral origin. It causes local inflammatory pain and may result in low-grade fever associated with an elevated sedimentation rate. Although the most common location of eosinophilic granuloma is the skull, it is also seen in the rib, pelvis, maxilla, vertebral body (vertebra plana)

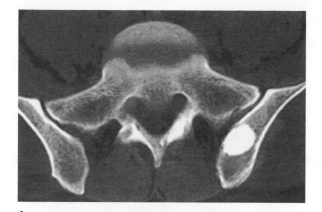

A

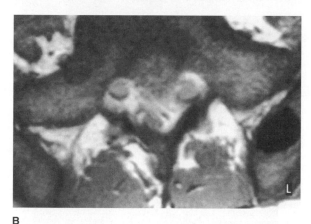

B

▲ **Figure 5–104.** CT scan (**A**) and T2-weighted MRI (**B**) of a bone island in the ilium of a 35-year-old man.

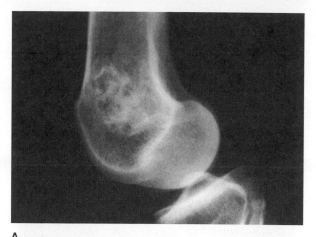

A

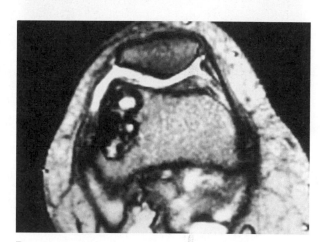

B

▲ **Figure 5–105.** Radiograph (**A**) and T1-weighted MRI (**B**) of a metaphyseal infarct in the distal femur of a 52-year-old woman.

(Figure 5–108), clavicle, and scapula, listed in the order of frequency. Besides affecting flat bones, it can arise in the diaphysis of long bones, followed next by the metaphysis, and it is least common in the epiphysis.

Eosinophilic granuloma can be extremely permeative and destructive, especially in long bones (Figure 5–109) and vertebrae (Figure 5–110), thereby mimicking a more aggressive process, such as Ewing sarcoma, metastatic neuroblastoma, or osteomyelitis. It can also produce a so-called onionskin periostitis of the type seen in Ewing sarcoma. The lesion has a more aggressive pattern in younger children and later becomes more focal and granulomatous. Microscopic findings include large pale-staining histiocytes speckled with small bright-staining eosinophils and an occasional giant cell.

Eosinophilic granulomas tend to involute spontaneously without treatment, and therefore, treatment should be conservative. Simple curettement and corticosteroid injections are beneficial. In difficult areas such as the spine or pelvis, low-dose radiation treatment (10 Gy) can be considered. In more disseminated cases that do not respond to simple treatment, low-dose chemotherapy is appropriate.

B. Pigmented Villonodular Synovitis: ICD-9-CM 716.9

Although this form of synovitis can mimic a histiocytic tumor, it is thought to be a nonneoplastic condition involving histiocytic proliferation. It occurs in the subsynovial tissue about major joints of the lower extremity in patients

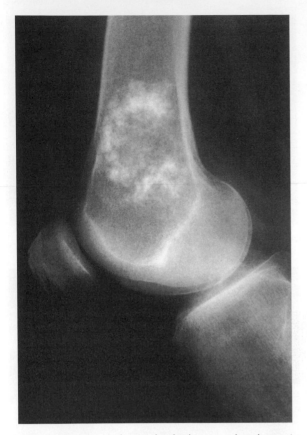

▲ **Figure 5–106.** Radiograph of a large enchondroma in the distal femur.

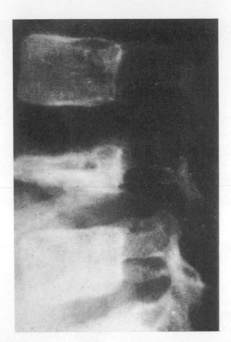

▲ **Figure 5–108.** Lateral radiograph of spine demonstrating characteristic vertebra plana of Langerhans cell histiocytoisis.

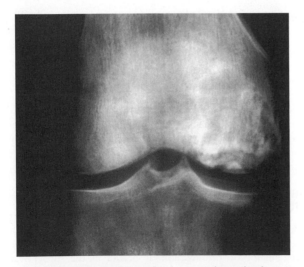

▲ **Figure 5–107.** Radiograph of an epiphyseal infarct in the femoral condyle of a 45-year-old woman.

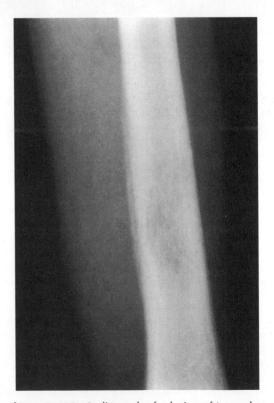

▲ **Figure 5–109.** Radiograph of a lesion of Langerhans cell histiocytosis of the humerus in a 12-year-old boy.

between 20 and 40 years of age. The knee joint is the most common site of involvement, followed next by the hip, ankle, and foot. Involvement of the upper extremity is rare.

The histopathology of pigmented villonodular synovitis is similar to that of a giant cell tumor of the tendon sheath, which presents with soft-tissue tumors about the ankle and on the fingers of the hand. The usual situation involves spontaneous swelling of one knee secondary to synovial hypertrophy. The swelling can grow gradually to a massive amount and be associated with intermittent hemarthroses. The inflamed synovium can cause juxtaarticular erosion into bone at the point of attachment of the joint capsule, as is seen in any chronic proliferative synovitis, including hemophilia and coccidioidomycosis.

In fewer than 10% of cases, pigmented villonodular synovitis is more localized and presents as a focal soft-tissue mass high in the suprapatellar pouch or in the popliteal space, and no generalized swelling of the knee occurs. In these cases, the mass can mimic a soft-tissue sarcoma such as a synovial sarcoma (Figure 5–111). Cortical erosion with secondary bony changes can also be appreciated frequently (Figure 5–112).

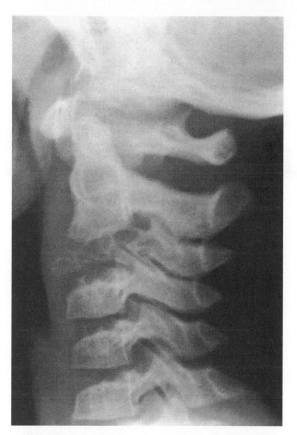

▲ **Figure 5–110.** Radiograph of a Langerhans cell histiocytosis in the body of the C3 vertebra in a 5-year-old girl.

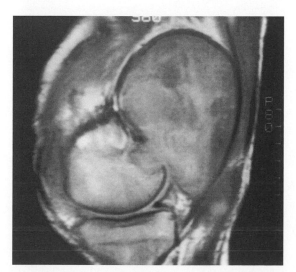

▲ **Figure 5–111.** T1-weighted MRI of pigmented villonodular synovitis in the popliteal space of a 50-year-old man.

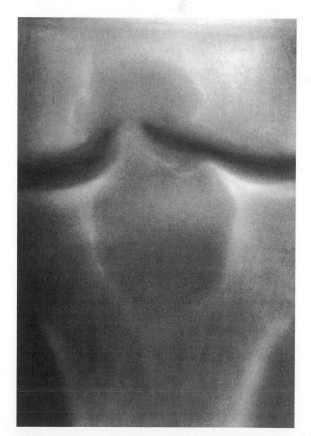

▲ **Figure 5–112.** Tomogram of pigmented villonodular synovitis in the proximal tibia of a young man.

► Essentials of Diagnosis

- *Myositis ossificans exhibits peripheral or centripetal calcification as opposed to calcifying soft-tissue malignancies.*
- *Infection of bone can take on many appearances, but clues to the diagnosis include violation of anatomic boundaries usually respected by tumors, such as the growth plate and the intervertebral disk.*

Garringer HJ, Malekpour M, Esteghamat F, et al: Molecular genetic and biochemical analyses of FGF23 mutations in familial tumoral calcinosis. *Am J Physiol Endocrinol Metab* 2008;295:E929. [PMID: 18682534]

Gasent Blesa JM, Alberola Candel V, Solano Vercet C, et al: Langerhans cell histiocytosis. *Clin Trans Oncol* 2008;10:688. [PMID: 19015065]

Mankin HJ, Rosenthal DI, Xavier R: Gaucher disease. New approaches to an ancient disease. *J Bone Joint Surg Am* 2001; 83-A:748. [PMID: 11379747]

Roodman GD: Studies in Paget's disease and their relevance to oncology. *Semin Oncol* 2001;28(4 Suppl 11):15. [PMID: 11544571]

Seton M: Paget's disease: epidemiology and pathophysiology. *Curr Osteoporos Rep* 2008;6:125. [PMID: 19032921]

Adult Reconstructive Surgery

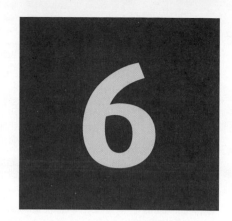

Harry B. Skinner, MD, PhD

Jon K. Sekiya, MD

Omar Jameel, MD

Patrick J. McMahon, MD

Adult reconstructive surgery in orthopedics has changed rapidly over the past several decades. Prior to the successful development of so-called low-friction arthroplasty of the hip in the late 1960s, treatment options for severe joint disease were limited. Reconstructive procedures with high success rates are now available for a variety of disorders, from marked degenerative hip and knee disease to rotator cuff tears of the shoulder. Research has increased the understanding of joint function and contributed to the success of almost all reconstructive procedures, and there is now tremendous demand for these procedures. In 2010, total knee arthroplasty and total hip arthroplasty procedures were estimated to number 770,000 and 280,000, respectively, in the United States and are increasing by approximately 65,000/year and 15,000/year, respectively. This is the result of their great success in returning patients to active lifestyles and the increasing numbers of older patients. Millions of Americans are now benefiting from these procedures for extended periods. Because the cumulative procedure failure rate is approximately 1% per year, 10 years after the operation, patients have approximately a 90% chance of still having a successful, well-functioning joint replacement.

Kurtz S, Ong K, Lau E, et al: Projections of primary and revision hip and knee arthroplasty in the United States from 2005 to 2030. *J Bone Joint Surg* 2007;89a:780. [PMID: 17403800]

▼ ARTHRITIS AND RELATED CONDITIONS

▶ Evaluation of Arthritis

To treat arthritic conditions of the joints appropriately, an understanding of the disease process is essential. This begins with accurate diagnosis and a history of the progression of the disease, so that the future progression can be predicted and appropriate decisions regarding treatment can be made. The physician must evaluate the possibility of traumatic, inflammatory, developmental, idiopathic, and metabolic causes of the arthritis (Table 6–1). Evaluation of the history, physical examination, and laboratory data is helpful in arriving at a diagnosis.

A. History

The history is very important in defining the disease process. The mechanism of injury and timing and duration of symptoms since onset are key factors. The mechanism of injury is most often insidious. The individual is often unable to recall a specific event that elicited the symptoms. However, when there was a sudden traumatic event in the past and especially when there was prior surgery, this information is important. The timing and severity of pain are valuable pieces of information. Most often, symptoms are initially mild and gradually worsen. Constant pain, night and day, implies infection, cancer, or a functional disorder. Perception of pain differs among individuals, but pain that awakens the patient is considered severe and requires evaluation. Symptoms frequently alternatively worsen and improve over time, and the patient's recollection of this and especially of whether there has been swelling is an important sign; also important is the distribution of joints if more than one is involved. The degree of interference with activities indicates the seriousness of the disorder. Pain only with activity such as walking, standing, or running suggests that joint loading is the cause.

Pain location helps distinguish referred pain from joint pain. Hip pain, for example, is felt typically in the groin or in the lateral aspect of the hip or anterior thigh but seldom in the buttock. Patients may complain of pain being in the "hip," but questioning by the physician may reveal it actually to be pain in the buttock, and this most often arises from the spine. Acetabular pain or femoral head pain is frequently felt in the groin. Proximal femur pain is usually appreciated in the anteroproximal thigh. As another example of the importance of pain location, knee pain may be localized as anterior (patellofemoral), medial (medial compartment), or lateral (lateral compartment). Or, it may also be poorly localized

Table 6–1. Causes of arthritic conditions.

Traumatic causes	Traumatic arthritis, osteonecrosis (posttraumatic)
Inflammatory causes	Infectious arthritis, gout, pseudogout, rheumatoid arthritis, systemic lupus erythematosus, ankylosing spondylitis, juvenile rheumatoid arthritis, Reiter syndrome
Developmental causes	Developmental dysplasia of the hip, hemophilic arthritis, following slipped capital femoral epiphysis, following Legg-Calvé-Perthes disease
Idiopathic causes	Osteoarthritis, osteonecrosis
Metabolic causes	Gout, calcium pyrophosphate deposition disease, ochronosis, Gaucher disease

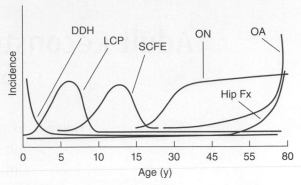

▲ **Figure 6–1.** The age distribution of hip disorders is given in a schematic representation. DDH, developmental dysplasia of the hip; Hip Fx, hip fracture; LCP, Legg-Calvé-Perthes disease; OA, osteoarthrosis; ON, osteonecrosis; SCFE, slipped capital femoral epiphysis.

by the patient. Pain in the back of the knee may result from a popliteal cyst (Baker cyst) or a torn meniscus. A swollen knee may be painful because of pressure, and this can be diffuse pain or may be posterior. Pain with any motion may indicate a septic joint or possibly a gouty joint. Arthritic pain in the elbow and shoulder is less clearly defined by patients, and in such cases, the physical examination is important. Shoulder pain may be caused by cervical, cardiac, or even diaphragmatic disorders.

Knowledge of the age distribution of the various arthritic disorders can be very helpful in diagnosing the disease. For example, a hip disorder in a patient under age 40 is unlikely to be osteoarthritis unless a predisposing condition is present, such as trauma. A more likely diagnosis is osteonecrosis. Similarly, a chronic condition of the knee in a 45-year-old man is likely to be a degenerative meniscus tear, unless the patient had a meniscectomy in his early 20s. This concept applies to all of the common disorders of the hip and knee (Figures 6–1 and 6–2). Further, a history of one of these disorders at an earlier age predisposes a patient to earlier osteoarthrosis.

B. Physical Examination

1. Hip—The physical examination of the hip is important to verify that the reported pain arises from the hip joint and to determine the severity of the arthritis. This begins with visual inspection and palpation of the muscles, bones, and joints. Many muscles surround the hip joint and large portions of the bone, limiting this portion of the examination. Other causes of the pain must be sought, such as pain referred from the lumbar spine. It is useful to document range of motion (ROM), gait, leg-length discrepancy, and muscle weakness. Pain arising from the hip is typically elicited at the extremes of ROM. Active straight leg raising or resisted straight leg raising may produce hip pain (Figure 6–3). Log rolling (internal and external rotation of

the hip in extension) usually elicits hip pain if pain is severe. Frequently, internal rotation of the hip in flexion is limited; this condition is one of the first signs of osteoarthritis of the hip. Abduction of the hip against gravity loads the hip and may produce hip pain of arthritis but does not do so if pain in the buttock or thigh is referred from the spine. Increased loading may be achieved by applying resistance to abduction. In the young (under age 40) patient with groin pain, provocative maneuvers can be used to diagnose labral tears. Flexion of the hip with external rotation (ER) and

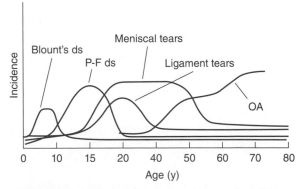

▲ **Figure 6–2.** The age distribution of knee disorders is given schematically as a function of age. Blount's ds, tibia vara; OA, osteoarthrosis; P-F ds, patellofemoral arthralgia. Meniscal tears can be either medial or lateral and are traumatic in the younger age group and degenerative in the older age group. Osteoarthrosis shows an earlier onset with the knee than with the hip because there is an incidence of medial gonarthrosis in the 40s and 50s caused by medial meniscectomy in the late teens and early 20s.

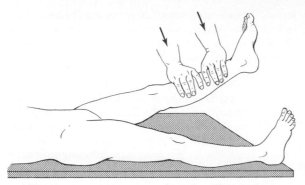

▲ **Figure 6–3.** Resisted straight leg raising test. The examiner asks the patient to actively raise the straight leg to approximately 30 degrees. This produces hip pain in severe arthritis. If no pain is produced, the examiner applies pressure to the thigh, which the patient resists. This increased joint loading uncovers mild to moderate hip pain.

abduction (ABD) is followed by extension, adduction (ADD), and internal rotation (IR). Clicking or catching is observed in patients with anterior labral tears. Posterior tears of the labrum are identified by moving the hip from extension, ABD, and ER to flexion, ADD, and IR.

The ROM in flexion, extension (flexion contracture), ABD, ADD, and IR and ER is measured. Decreased IR is an early finding in osteoarthritis.

2. Knee—The physical examination of the knee localizes the pain to the knee and to the specific involved compartment. As with the hip, this begins with visual inspection and palpation of the muscles, bones, and joints. Because knee pain can be referred from the hip, evaluation of the hip should be routine. Ligamentous evaluation of the knee is performed to discern knee stability (see Chapter 3). Instability is not common in osteoarthritis but is often seen in rheumatoid osteoarthritis and results from bone loss rather than ligament injury. Alignment of the knee while standing is measured to evaluate for varus or valgus deformities. Varus and valgus malalignment increase the odds of progression of osteoarthritis fourfold and fivefold, respectively, in 18 months. ROM of the knee is measured, and any flexion contracture or extensor lag is noted. Flexion contracture is an inability to come to full extension passively, whereas an extensor lag indicates an inability to extend the knee actively as far as it will extend passively. The contracture is common in advanced osteoarthritis, whereas the lag is generally a quadriceps muscle or tendon problem. The medial and lateral compartments are loaded during flexion and extension with varus and valgus stress, respectively, to elicit pain arising from each compartment. The patellofemoral joint may be assessed for pain and bone-on-bone crepitation by flexion and extension with pressure on the patella. The presence of fluid, synovitis, and erythema is also important.

3. Shoulder—Since shoulder pain can be referred from the cervical spine, evaluation of both is often necessary. Examination of the shoulder begins with visual inspection for asymmetry of bone and muscle contours in comparison to the other side. Palpation of the muscle to evaluate tone and of each of the three bones, including the humerus, clavicle, and scapula, follows. Not only the glenohumeral but also the acromioclavicular and sternoclavicular joints should be palpated. As with the hip, many muscles surround the portions of the shoulder, limiting this portion of the examination. However, tenderness over the anterolateral humeral head can often be found with rotator cuff disorders. Tendinitis of the long head of the biceps yields pain with palpation on the anteromedial humeral head. Active ROM is then assessed in flexion and abduction. External rotation is reproducibly measured by keeping the elbow on the waist and rotating the hand away from the body. Internal rotation is best evaluated by the patient positioning the hand behind the back and then measuring the highest vertebral level of the spine that the thumb can be positioned. Most individuals can position the thumb to the midthoracic area (eg, T6 or T7). When internal rotation is limited, the thumb can be elevated to lower levels, for example, L5. If active ROM is at all limited, passive ROM should be assessed. Strength of the upper extremity muscle is then evaluated along with sensation and deep tendon reflexes. Decreased strength in external rotation with the elbow at the side indicates significant rotator cuff weakness. Provocative tests can help evaluate the cause of symptoms including instability, biceps tendon injuries, and rotator cuff injuries (see Chapter 3).

4. Elbow—Inspection of the elbow includes measurement of the "carrying angle," the normal being a 5- to 7-degree angle of valgus alignment between the humerus and forearm. Visual inspection for scars and obvious deformities, as well as swelling, is performed. The joint and bony prominences are palpated, including the medial and lateral epicondyles, radial head, and olecranon. Active and passive motions are recorded for both flexion and extension and pronation and supination. Strength and provocative tests ensue (see Chapter 3). For example, the most common malady of the elbow is epicondylitis. Tenderness over the lateral epicondyle exacerbated by resisted wrist dorsiflexion is present with lateral epicondylitis (tennis elbow). Tenderness over the medial epicondyle with pain exacerbated by resisted wrist flexion is present with medial epicondylitis. As other examples, limitation of flexion and extension is seen not only with arthritis but also with posttraumatic stiffness.

C. Imaging Studies

The most fundamental data aiding in diagnosis of arthritis can be provided by plain radiographs with a minimum of two views. Views of the hip include a modified anteroposterior (AP) view of the pelvis (which clips the iliac wings to show the proximal femora) and a lateral view of the affected hip (either "frog," an AP view with the hip externally rotated and

Table 6–2. Radiographic findings in arthritis.

Disease State	Findings in Hip or Knee
Osteoarthritis	Joint space narrowing, subchondral sclerosis, osteophytes, subchondral cysts Hip: Superior or medial narrowing Knee: Early narrowing on Rosenberg views; flattening of femoral condyles
Rheumatoid arthritis or systemic lupus erythematosus	Uniform joint narrowing, erosion near joint capsule
Ankylosing spondylitis	Osteopenia, osteophytes, ankylosis of sacroiliac joints
Gout	Tophi, erosions
Calcium pyrophosphate deposition disease	Calcification of menisci and articular cartilage
Osteonecrosis	Crescent sign, spotty calcification
Gaucher disease	Erlenmeyer flask appearance, distal femora
Neuropathic joint	Four D's: destruction, debris, dislocation, densification (sclerosis, hypertrophy)
Hemophilic arthropathy	Epiphyseal widening, sclerosis, cysts, joint space narrowing

abducted, or a true lateral view). Views of the knee should include a 10-degree down-angled beam posteroanterior radiograph of the knee bent in 30–45 degrees of flexion taken while the patient is standing (the flexion weight-bearing view), a lateral view, and a tangential patellar view (Merchant view, 45 degrees of flexion) (Table 6–2). Osteoarthritis of the hip and knee can be quantitated using the Kellgren-Lawrence five-level scale where 0 is normal, 1 is doubtful, 2 is mild or minimal, 3 is moderate, and 4 is severe. Views of the shoulder should include AP, axillary, and lateral views of the scapula. Supraspinatus outlet views may be helpful in revealing acromial bone spurs, which produce impingement. The elbow usually can be visualized with AP and lateral radiographs.

D. Laboratory Findings

Basic blood testing should include a complete blood count and erythrocyte sedimentation rate (ESR). These are indicated in a suspected septic process or in the evaluation of a painful joint replacement. A normal white cell count may be helpful in the diagnosis of gout, especially if the inflamed joint is atypical (other than the first metatarsophalangeal joint).

Synovial fluid analysis is indicated in evaluation of infection, and it may also be quite helpful in the diagnosis of other arthritides. Aspiration of synovial fluid may reveal hemorrhagic fluid. If this is the result of a traumatic tap, it should be so noted and the fluid should be sent for analysis. If the fluid

is grossly hemorrhagic, several diagnoses must be entertained, including hemophilia, neuropathic arthropathy, pigmented villonodular synovitis, hemangioma, or trauma. A finding of fat floating on the bloody fluid in the setting of a traumatic injury suggests the presence of an intraarticular fracture.

The combined history, physical examination, radiographs, and appropriate laboratory studies should narrow the diagnoses to a relative few, if not the definitive one. It is helpful to consider diagnoses in categories, which, despite some overlap, provide a framework for further workup. Many of these arthritic conditions are described in the following sections.

Parvizi J, Della Valle CJ: AAOS Clinical Practice Guideline: diagnosis and treatment of periprosthetic joint infections of the hip and knee. *J Am Acad Orthop Surg* 2010;18:771. [PMID: 21119143]

Sharma L, Song J, Felson DT, et al: The role of knee alignment in disease progression and functional decline in knee osteoarthritis. *JAMA* 2001;286:188. [PMID: 11448282]

Solomon DH, Simel DL, Bates DW, et al: Does this patient have a torn meniscus or ligament of the knee? Value of physical exam of the knee. *JAMA* 2001;286:1610. [PMID: 11585485]

1. Noninflammatory Arthritis

The term **osteoarthritis** is a misnomer, because inflammation is not the primary pathologic process observed in this form of articular joint disruption. More accurately described as degenerative joint disease, the disease represents a final common pathway of injury to articular cartilage. Although the true nature and cause of osteoarthritis are unclear, radiographic findings and gross and microscopic pathologic features are fairly typical in most cases.

Categorization of primary and secondary forms of osteoarthritis, although still useful, is blurred. A designation of primary or idiopathic osteoarthritis was made when no identifiable predisposing conditions could be recognized. Osteoarthritis is considered secondary when an underlying cause such as trauma, previous deformity, or systemic disorder exists. Although many cases of hip osteoarthritis were considered idiopathic when the end-stage changes were observed, careful analysis indicated predisposing conditions such as slipped capital femoral epiphysis and mild forms of acetabular dysplasia in many cases.

The joints most commonly involved include the hip; knee; distal interphalangeal, proximal interphalangeal, and first carpometacarpal joints of the hand; and cervical, thoracic, and lumbar spine.

▶ Primary Osteoarthritis

A. Epidemiologic Features

Osteoarthritis is a widespread joint disorder in the United States, significantly affecting approximately 40 million people. Although autopsy studies show degenerative changes of weight-bearing joints in 90% of people older than 40 years, clinical symptoms are usually not present. The prevalence and severity of osteoarthritis increase with age.

When all ages are considered, men and women are equally affected. In those younger than 45 years, the disease is more prevalent in men; after age 55 years, women are more commonly afflicted. The pattern of joint involvement commonly includes the joints of the hands and knees in women and the hip joints in men. The risk of hip joint arthritis is significantly associated with increasing body mass index (BMI).

The incidence of hip osteoarthritis is higher in European and American white males than in Chinese, South African blacks, and East Indian persons. Primary hip osteoarthritis in Japanese persons is rare, but secondary osteoarthritis is common because of developmental dysplasia of the hip.

Evidence indicates that some distinct forms of osteoarthritis may be inherited as a dominant trait with a Mendelian pattern. A primary generalized osteoarthritis of the interphalangeal joints, particularly the distal interphalangeal joints of the hand, is a prominent feature, and symmetric and uniform loss of articular cartilage of the knee and hip joints is evident. Other types of inherited osteoarthritis include familial chondrocalcinosis (with deposition of calcium pyrophosphate dihydrate crystals in cartilage), Stickler syndrome (characterized by vitreoretinal degeneration), hydroxyapatite deposition disease, and multiple epiphyseal dysplasias. In summary, osteoarthritis has a genetic component that may be further elucidated by genome-wide association studies.

B. Pathologic Features

Early features of osteoarthritis include focal swelling and softening of the cartilage matrix. Mild loss of metachromatic staining ability represents loss of proteoglycans in the extracellular matrix. Surface irregularities in the form of fibrillation occur. Diffuse hypercellularity of the chondrocytes can be seen. The tidemark, an interface plane between articular cartilage and the zone of calcified cartilage, is thin and wavy early in osteoarthritis. During the second stage of articular cartilage degeneration with osteoarthritis, there is increased chondrocyte activity with proliferation and increased production of extracellular matrix. At the same time, there is an increase in catabolic activity with removal of damaged matrix to facilitate matrix remodeling. Chondrocyte repair response decreases with aging. Matrix degradation includes decreased proteoglycan production, less aggregation, and shorter glycosaminoglycan chains.

Later features of osteoarthritis include progressive loss of proteoglycans manifesting as reduction in safranin-O staining. Fibrillations in the surface deepen into fissures and later into deeper clefts. Chondrocyte cloning is seen and also reduplication of the tidemark, with discontinuous parallel lines indicating progression of calcification of the basal portion of the articular cartilage. Regions of eburnated bone represent complete loss of cartilage.

New bone formation occurs in a subchondral location as well as at margins of the articular cartilage. Areas of rarefaction of bone below eburnation are represented by "cysts" on radiographs and on gross inspection.

C. Laboratory Findings

Specific diagnostic tests for osteoarthritis are currently not available. Routine blood tests, urinalysis, and even synovial fluid analysis do not provide useful information, except for exclusion of inflammatory or infectious arthritis. Experimental work on identification of markers of cartilage degradation in osteoarthritis may provide diagnostic tests in the future. These include sensitive and specific assays for synovial fluid cytokines, proteinases and their inhibitors, matrix components and their fragments, serum antibodies to cartilage collagen, and identification of proteoglycan subpopulations.

D. Imaging Studies

Typical radiographic features indicate late pathologic changes in osteoarthritis, specifically narrowing of the joint space, subchondral sclerosis, subchondral bony cysts, and marginal osteophytes. End-stage disease is complicated by bony erosions, subluxation, loose bodies, and deformity.

Heberden nodes are commonly seen in primary osteoarthritis, represented by bony and cartilaginous enlargement of the distal interphalangeal joints of the fingers. Similar enlargements of the proximal interphalangeal joints of the fingers are called **Bouchard nodes**.

▶ Secondary Osteoarthritis

The term **secondary osteoarthritis** is applied when an underlying recognizable local or systemic factor exists. These include conditions leading to joint deformity or destruction of cartilage, followed by signs and symptoms typically seen with primary osteoarthritis. Examples of preexisting conditions leading to secondary osteoarthritic changes in joints include acute and chronic trauma, Legg-Calvé-Perthes disease, developmental dysplasia of the hip, rheumatoid arthritis, bleeding dyscrasias, achondroplasia, infection, crystal deposition disease, neuropathic disorders, overuse of intraarticular steroids, and multiple epiphyseal dysplasias. Radiographic features of secondary osteoarthritis reflect the underlying pathologic changes plus the changes resulting from the primary osteoarthritis.

Dai J, Ikegawa S: Recent advances in association studies of osteoarthritis susceptibility genes. *J Hum Genet* 2010;55:77. [PMID: 20075947]

Hoaglund FT, Steinbach LS: Primary osteoarthritis of the hip: etiology and epidemiology. *J Am Acad Orthop Surg* 2001;9:320. [PMID: 11575911]

Jiang L, Rong J, Wang Y, et al: The relationship between body mass index and hip arthritis: a systematic review and meta-analysis. *Joint Bone Spine* 2011;78:150. [PMID: 20580591]

Schiphof D, Boers M, Bierma-Zeinstra SMA: Differences in descriptions of Kellgren and Lawrence grades of knee osteoarthritis. *Ann Rheum Dis* 2008;67:1034. [PMID: 18198197]

2. Inflammatory Arthritis

▶ Rheumatoid Arthritis

A chronic systemic inflammatory disorder, rheumatoid arthritis is a crippling disease affecting approximately 0.5–1% of the population in the United States. Although similar synovial histopathologic and joint abnormalities are identifiable in all patients, the articular and systemic manifestations, outcomes, and differences in genetic makeup and serologic findings vary widely in individual patients. The cause is unknown, although the disease probably occurs in response to a pathogenic agent in a genetically predisposed host. Smoking has been identified as the main environmental risk. Possible other triggering factors include bacterial, mycoplasmal, or viral infections, as well as endogenous antigens in the form of rheumatoid factor, collagens, and mucopolysaccharides.

Joint involvement is typically symmetric, affecting the wrist, metacarpal phalangeal, proximal interphalangeal, elbow, shoulder, cervical spine, hip, knee, and ankle joints. The distal interphalangeal joints are typically spared. Extraarticular manifestations include vasculitis, pericarditis, skin nodules, pulmonary fibrosis, pneumonitis, and scleritis. The triad of arthritis, lymphadenopathy, and splenomegaly, known as Felty syndrome, is associated with anemia, thrombocytopenia, and neutropenia.

A. Epidemiologic Features

Rheumatoid arthritis occurs two to four times more often in women than men. The disease occurs in all age groups, but increases in incidence with advancing age, with a peak between the fourth and sixth decades.

Evidence for a genetic basis is provided by the association of rheumatoid arthritis with a certain haplotype of class II gene products of the major histocompatibility complex. Seventy-five percent of patients with rheumatoid arthritis carry circulating rheumatoid factors, which are autoantibodies against portions of the IgG antibody. In rheumatoid factor–positive patients, there is a high incidence of HLA-DR4, except in black patients. Only a minority of individuals with HLA-DR4 develop rheumatoid arthritis, however. (See Chapter 12, especially Tables 12–5 and 12–6.)

B. Pathologic Features

Early rheumatoid synovitis consists of a local inflammatory response with accumulation of mononuclear cells.

The antigen-presenting cell (macrophage) activates T lymphocytes, resulting in cytokine production, B-cell proliferation, and antibody formation. Chronic inflammation results in formation of a pannus, a thickened synovium filled with activated T and B lymphocytes and plasma cells, as well as fibroblastic and macrophagic types of synovial cells. Joint destruction begins with exposed bone at the margins of articular cartilage denuded of articular cartilage. Eventually, the cartilage itself is destroyed by inflammatory byproducts of the pannus. The synovial fluid, in contrast to the mononuclear cell infiltrate seen in the synovial membrane, has neutrophils forming 75–85% of the cells.

Rheumatoid factors are antibodies specific to antigens on the Fc fragment of IgG. The antibodies include IgM, IgG, IgA, and IgE classes, but the IgM rheumatoid factor is typically measured. Rheumatoid factor may be a triggering factor for rheumatoid arthritis and may contribute to the chronic nature of the disease, but it is not found in all patients with rheumatoid arthritis. Rheumatoid factor is also frequently found in patients with other inflammatory diseases, however, as well as in 1–5% of normal patients.

C. Laboratory Findings

No specific laboratory test exists for rheumatoid arthritis, but a series of test results help in the diagnosis. A high titer of rheumatoid factor (>1:160) is the most significant diagnostic finding. Anemia is moderate, and leukocyte counts are normal or mildly elevated. Acute-phase reactants are not specific yet reflect the degree of inflammation and are often elevated in rheumatoid arthritis. These include ESR and levels of C-reactive protein and serum immune complexes. Anticitrullinated peptide antibodies may add sensitivity and specificity to the diagnosis of rheumatoid arthritis. Antinuclear antibodies are often positive in patients with severe rheumatoid arthritis (up to 37% in one study) but are not specific for the disease.

D. Imaging Studies

Early radiographic changes in rheumatoid osteoarthritis include swelling of the small peripheral joints and marginal bony erosions. Joint space narrowing occurs later and is uniform, unlike the focal narrowing seen in osteoarthritis. Regional osteoporosis occurs, unlike the sclerosis seen in osteoarthritis. Advanced changes include bone resorption, deformity, dislocation, and fragmentation of affected joints. For example, protrusio acetabuli may be seen in the hips, and ulnar subluxation is common in the metacarpophalangeal joints.

Scott DL, Wolfe F, Huizinga TW: Rheumatoid arthritis: *Lancet* 2010;376:1094. [PMID: 20870100]

Whiting PF, Smidt N, Sterne JA, et al: Systematic review: accuracy of anti-citrullinated peptide antibodies for diagnosing rheumatoid arthritis. *Ann Intern Med* 2010;152:456. [PMID: 20368651]

▶ Ankylosing Spondylitis

A seronegative (negative rheumatoid factor) inflammatory arthritis, ankylosing spondylitis consists of bilateral sacroiliitis with or without associated spondylitis and uveitis. An insidious disease, the diagnosis is often delayed because of vagueness of the early symptom of low back pain and late x-ray changes of sacroiliitis. Diagnostic clinical criteria include low back pain, limited lumbar spine motion, decreased chest expansion, and sacroiliitis, which can now be diagnosed earlier with magnetic resonance imaging (MRI).

Joint involvement is primarily axial, including all portions of the spine, sacroiliac joint, and hip joints. Extraskeletal involvement includes dilation of the aorta, anterior uveitis, and restrictive lung disease secondary to restriction of thoracic cage mobility.

A. Epidemiologic Features

The association of HLA-B27 and ankylosing spondylitis is strong, with 90% of patients testing positive for this haplotype; however, only 2% of HLA-B27–positive patients develop ankylosing spondylitis. First-degree family members of a patient who has ankylosing spondylitis and is positive for HLA-B27 have a 20% risk of developing the disease.

B. Laboratory Findings

During the active phase of the disease, the ESR is increased. Testing for rheumatoid factor and antinuclear antibodies is negative.

C. Imaging Studies

Early in the course of ankylosing spondylitis, the sacroiliac joints may be widened, reflecting bony erosions of the iliac side of the joint. Later, the inflamed cartilage is replaced by ossification, resulting in ankylosis of the bilateral sacroiliac joints. Vertebrae of the thoracolumbar spine are squared off, with bridging syndesmophytes, forming a so-called bamboo spine. Ankylosis of peripheral joints may be seen. MRI may provide early, sensitive, and specific imaging evidence of sacroiliitis.

Marzo-ortega H, McGonagle D, Bennett AN: Magnetic resonance imaging in spondyloarthritis. *Curr Opin Rheumatol* 2010;22:381. [PMID: 20386452]

Rudwaleit M: New approaches to diagnosis and classification of axial and peripheral spondyloarthritis. *Curr Opin Rheumatol* 2010;22:375. [PMID: 20473175]

▶ Psoriatic Arthritis

A seronegative inflammatory arthritis associated with psoriasis, psoriatic arthritis was in the past considered a variant of rheumatoid arthritis. The discovery of rheumatoid factor

led to the division of inflammatory arthritides into seropositive and seronegative diseases, separating psoriatic arthritis from rheumatoid arthritis.

Although psoriatic arthritis is characterized by a relatively benign course in most patients, up to 20% develop severe joint involvement. The distal interphalangeal joints of the fingers are commonly affected, but several patterns of peripheral arthritis exist, including an asymmetric oligoarthritis, a symmetric polyarthritis (similar to rheumatoid osteoarthritis), arthritis mutilans (a destructive, deforming type of arthritis), and a spondyloarthropathy (similar to ankylosing spondylitis, with sacroiliac joint involvement).

In addition to the dry erythematous papular skin lesions, nail changes are found. These include pitting, grooves, subungual hyperkeratosis, and destruction.

A. Epidemiologic Features

In the United States, about 3.15% of the population is diagnosed with psoriasis. A third of patients with psoriasis have arthritis, with joint symptoms delayed as long as 20 years after onset of skin lesions. Both sexes are affected equally. The genes *IL12B* and *IL23R* are associated with psoriasis.

B. Laboratory Findings

There are no specific laboratory tests for psoriatic arthritis. Nonspecific inflammatory markers may be elevated, including ESR. Rheumatoid factor is usually negative but is present in up to 10% of patients.

C. Imaging Studies

Coexistence of erosive changes and bone formation is seen in peripheral joints, with absence of periarticular osteoporosis. Gross destruction of phalangeal joints (so-called pencil-in-cup appearance) and lysis of terminal phalanges are seen. Bilateral sacroiliac joint ankylosis and syndesmophytes of the spine are seen, as in ankylosing spondylitis.

Anandarajah AP, Ritchlin CT: The diagnosis and treatment of early psoriatic arthritis. *Nat Rev Rheumatol* 2009;5:634. [PMID: 19806150]

Chandran V, Raychaudhuri SP: Geoepidemiology and environmental factors of psoriasis and psoriatic arthritis. *J Autoimmun* 2010;34:J314. [PMID: 20034760]

▶ Juvenile Idiopathic Arthritis

Juvenile idiopathic arthritis (JIA) is an inflammatory arthritic syndrome with a variety of symptoms and is a diagnosis of exclusion in children with arthritis onset before age 16. It was previously called juvenile rheumatoid arthritis, but was renamed because it is not obviously related to adult rheumatoid arthritis. Early diagnosis is often difficult. Criteria for JIA include distinction of mode of onset as systemic, polyarticular, or pauciarticular. Systemic onset (also known as **Still disease**) occurs in 20% of patients and is characterized by high fever, rash, lymphadenopathy, splenomegaly, carditis, and varying degrees of arthritis. Polyarticular onset occurs in 30–40% of patients and is notable for fewer systemic symptoms, low-grade fever, and synovitis of four or more joints. Pauciarticular onset develops in 40–50% of patients and involves one to four joints; there are no systemic signs, but there is an increased incidence of iridocyclitis. Iridocyclitis is an insidious complication that requires early ophthalmologic slit-lamp evaluation, if JIA is suspected, to prevent blindness.

A. Epidemiologic Features

The two peak ages of onset are between 1 and 3 years and between 8 and 12 years. Females are affected twice as often as males.

B. Laboratory Findings

Leukocytosis up to 30,000/mL is seen with systemic-onset JIA, with mild elevations in polyarticular-onset disease and normal values in pauciarticular-onset disease. White blood cell counts in synovial fluid range from 150 to 50,000/mL. The ESR is elevated, as are other acute-phase reactants.

Rheumatoid factor is typically negative in JIA. As many as 50% of patients have positive antinuclear antibodies, a finding correlated with iridocyclitis and pauciarticular-onset disease.

C. Imaging Studies

Soft-tissue swelling and premature closure of physes may be seen early, as well as juxtaarticular osteopenia. Erosive changes are seen late and resemble those of rheumatoid osteoarthritis.

Dannecker GE, Quartier P: Juvenile rheumatoid arthritis: classification, clinical presentation and current treatments. *Horm Res* 2009;72(Suppl 1):4. [PMID: 19940489]

Martini A, Lovell DJ: Juvenile idiopathic arthritis: state of the art and future perspectives. *Ann Rheum Dis* 2010;69:1260. [PMID: 20525835]

▶ Systemic Lupus Erythematosus

Systemic lupus erythematosus (SLE) is a chronic inflammatory disease that may affect multiple organ systems. It is an autoimmune disorder in which autoantibodies are formed. The large variety of clinical appearances and laboratory findings may mimic many disorders. The diagnosis is based on the presence of four of the following 11 criteria: (1) malar rash; (2) discoid rash; (3) photosensitivity; (4) oral ulcers; (5) arthritis; (6) serositis; (7) renal disorders (proteinuria or casts); (8) neurologic disorders (seizures or psychosis);

(9) hematologic disorders (hemolytic anemia, leukopenia, lymphopenia, thrombocytopenia); (10) immunologic disorders (positive lupus erythematosus [LE] cell preparation, anti-DNA antibody, anti-Sm antibody, false-positive serologic test for syphilis); and (11) abnormal titer of antinuclear antibody.

A. Epidemiologic Features

Females are affected eight times as often as males. An increased risk for SLE is noted for Asians and Polynesians over whites in Hawaii. Black females are also associated with an increased risk over white females. Genetic susceptibility is demonstrated with increased frequency (5%) among relatives of patients with the disease. An inherited complement deficiency is inferred from the absence, or near absence, of individual complement components, the most common being C2. Evidence of a statistical association of SLE with tobacco smoke exposure has been found.

B. Laboratory Findings

Antinuclear antibody determination is the most helpful screening test for SLE. The LE cell preparation was the first immunologic test for SLE, but it is laborious, insensitive, and difficult to interpret. In patients with untreated active disease, 98% have positive antinuclear antibody tests. The higher the titer of antinuclear antibodies, the more likely is the diagnosis of SLE or related rheumatic syndrome. A low value for the antinuclear antibody test is 1:320; values greater than 1:5120 are considered high.

If antinuclear antibody levels are positive, more specific tests may be performed, including testing for anti-DNA antibodies, antibodies to extractable nuclear antigens, and complement levels. High titers of antibodies to double-stranded DNA are highly suggestive for SLE. Low complement levels (C3, C4, and total hemolytic complement levels) are found in the disease but are also seen in related illnesses.

Anemia, leukopenia, and thrombocytopenia are seen, as well as elevations in the ESR. Renal function tests and muscle and liver enzyme tests are often abnormal, reflecting multiple organ system involvement.

C. Imaging Studies

The radiographic features of arthritis in SLE are similar to those of rheumatoid osteoarthritis. Much of the joint pain may be related to osteonecrosis, particularly of the femoral and humeral heads.

Crispin JC, Liossis SN, Kis-Toth K, et al: Pathogenesis of human systemic lupus erythematosus: recent advances. *Trends Mol Med* 2010;16:47. [PMID: 20138006]

Kaiser R, Criswell LA: Genetics research in systemic lupus erythematosus for clinicians: methodology, progress, and controversies. *Curr Opin Rheumatol* 2010;22:119. [PMID: 20035223]

▶ Arthritis Associated With Inflammatory Bowel Disease

Peripheral arthritis and spondylitis are associated with ulcerative colitis and Crohn disease. Joint involvement is typically monoarticular or oligoarticular and often parallels the activity of the bowel disease. The arthritis, frequently migratory, is self-limiting in most cases, with only 10% of patients having chronic arthritis. The joints most commonly affected are the knees, hips, and ankles, in order of prevalence. Spondylitis associated with inflammatory bowel disease occurs in two forms. One is very similar to ankylosing spondylitis, including the increased incidence of the HLA-B27 haplotype. The other form has no identifiable genetic predisposition.

A. Epidemiologic Features

Up to 30% of patients with inflammatory bowel disease develop arthritis. There is no difference between the sexes in incidence.

B. Laboratory Findings

There is no specific diagnostic test. Synovial fluid analysis reveals an inflammatory process, with leukocyte counts of 4000–50,000/mL.

C. Imaging Studies

Peripheral arthritis is nonerosive, with juxtaarticular osteopenia and joint space narrowing. Spondylitis associated with inflammatory bowel disease resembles ankylosing spondylitis.

De Vos M: Joint involvement in inflammatory bowel disease: managing inflammation outside the digestive system. *Expert Rev Gastroenterol Hepatol* 2010;4:81. [PMID: 20136591]

Larsen S, Bendtzen K, Nielsen OH: Extraintestinal manifestations of inflammatory bowel disease: epidemiology, diagnosis, and management. *Ann Med* 2010;42:97. [PMID: 20166813]

▶ Reiter Syndrome

The classic triad of conjunctivitis, urethritis, and peripheral arthritis is known as **Reiter syndrome. Reactive arthritis** is becoming accepted as a more precise term because the initiating condition may be enteritis as well as a sexually transmitted disease. The peripheral arthritis is polyarticular and asymmetric, with knees, ankles, and foot joints most commonly affected.

A. Epidemiologic Features

Nongonococcal urethritis caused by *Chlamydia* accounts for the precipitating event in approximately 20% of cases. Patients who test positive for HLA-B27 are predisposed to developing arthritis after contracting nongonococcal urethritis. A reactive arthritis following enteric infection with *Salmonella*, *Shigella*, *Yersinia*, and *Campylobacter* is also noted. For enteric infections with *Shigella*, the risk of developing arthritis in individuals positive for HLA-B27 is close to 20%.

B. Laboratory Findings

There are no specific diagnostic tests for Reiter syndrome. Anemia, leukocytosis, and thrombocytosis occur, and the ESR is often elevated.

C. Imaging Studies

The radiographic features of Reiter syndrome are similar to those of ankylosing spondylitis, with calcifications of ligamentous insertions and ankylosing of joints. The sacroiliitis is unilateral, unlike in ankylosing spondylitis.

Bradshaw CS, Tabrizi SN, Read TR, et al: Etiologies of nongonococcal urethritis, bacteria, viruses, and the association with orogenital exposure. *J Infect Dis* 2006;193:366. [PMID: 16388480]

Carter JD, Hudson AP: The evolving story of *Chlamydia*-induced reactive arthritis. *Curr Opin Rheumatol* 2010;22:424. [PMID: 20445454]

3. Metabolic Arthropathy

▶ Gout

Deposition of monosodium urate crystals in the joints produces gout. Although most patients with gout have hyperuricemia, few patients with hyperuricemia develop gout. The causes of hyperuricemia include disorders resulting in overproduction or undersecretion of uric acid or a combination of these two abnormalities. Examples of uric acid overproduction include enzymatic mutations, leukemias, hemoglobinopathies, and excessive purine intake.

The first attack involves sudden onset of painful arthritis, most often in the first metatarsophalangeal joint, but also in the ankle, knee, wrist, finger, and elbow. The intensity of the pain is comparable to that from a septic joint, and differentiation is necessary because the treatment is different. Coexistence of a septic joint is unusual but possible. Rapid resolution with colchicine or indomethacin is seen. Chronic gouty arthritis is notable for tophaceous deposits, joint deformity, constant pain, and swelling.

A. Epidemiologic Features

Primary gout has hereditary features, with a familial incidence of 6–18%. It is likely that the serum urate concentration is controlled by multiple genes (most likely *SLC2A9* and *ABCG2*, which regulate urate excretion). Gout occurs in women, but at a later age, usually postmenopausal, and in association with hypertension and/or renal insufficiency, use of diuretics, and less alcohol consumption than men.

B. Laboratory Findings

The key diagnostic test is detection of monosodium urate crystals in white blood cells in synovial fluid. Negative birefringence of the needle-shaped crystals is seen by their yellow coloration on polarized light microscopy.

Hyperuricemia is usually seen, but up to a fourth of gout patients may have normal uric acid levels. Uric acid levels are elevated when they exceed 7 mg/dL. An elevated white blood cell count and ESR can be seen in acute gout, and thus these tests cannot be used to differentiate between the two processes. Aspirates should be sent for culture to rule out coexisting infection.

C. Imaging Studies

Tophi may be seen when they are calcified. Soft-tissue swelling is seen, as well as erosions. Chronic changes consist of extensive bone loss, joint narrowing, and joint deformity.

Agudelo CA, Wise CM: Gout: diagnosis, pathogenesis, and clinical manifestations. *Curr Opin Rheumatol* 2001;13:234. [PMID: 11333355]

Dirken-Heukensfeldt KJ, Teunissen TA, van de Lisdonk H, et al: Clinical features of women with gout arthritis. A systematic review. *Clin Rheumatol* 2010;29:575. [PMID: 20084441]

Vanitallie TB: Gout: epitome of painful arthritis. *Metabolism* 2010;59(Suppl 1):s32. [PMID: 20837191]

► Calcium Pyrophosphate Crystal Deposition Disease

Calcium pyrophosphate crystal deposition disease, a goutlike syndrome, is also known as pseudogout or chondrocalcinosis. Crystals of calcium pyrophosphate dihydrate are deposited in a joint, most commonly the knee and not the first metatarsophalangeal joint, as in gout. The diagnosis is made by demonstration of the crystals in tissue or synovial fluid and by the presence of characteristic radiographic findings.

Aging and trauma are associated with this disorder, as well as conditions such as hyperparathyroidism, gout, hemochromatosis, hypophosphatasia, and hypothyroidism. In patients over age 55, hyperparathyroidism should be considered as a cause.

A. Epidemiologic Features

Aging is the most common risk factor for chondrocalcinosis and the prevalence is 7–10% of people at age 60 with equal sex distribution. Hereditary forms of calcium pyrophosphate dihydrate deposition disease are reported, with mutations in the ankylosis (*ANKH*) gene as the cause.

B. Pathologic Features

Calcification of multiple joint structures occurs, including articular cartilage and capsules, with heaviest deposition in fibrocartilaginous structures such as the menisci. The crystals are more difficult to see than urate crystals and have negative birefringence on polarized light microscopy.

C. Imaging Studies

Calcification of menisci and articular cartilage is seen as punctate or linear radiodensities, which delineate these normally radiolucent structures. Bursas, ligaments, and tendons may have calcifications as well. Bony signs include subchondral cyst formation, signs of carpal instability, sacroiliac joint erosions with vacuum phenomenon, and crowning of the odontoid process.

Kohn NN, Hughes RE, McCarty DJ Jr, et al: The significance of calcium phosphate crystals in the synovial fluid of arthritis patients: the "pseudogout syndrome." II. Identification of crystals. *Ann Intern Med* 1962;56:738. [PMID: 14457846]

McCarty DJ, Kohn NN, Faires JS: The significance of calcium phosphate crystals in the synovial fluid of arthritis patients: the "pseudogout syndrome." I. Clinical aspects. *Ann Intern Med* 1962;56:711. [No PMID]

Richette P, Bardin T, Doherty M: An update on the epidemiology of calcium pyrophosphate dehydrate crystal deposition disease. *Rheumatology (Oxford)* 2009;48:711. [PMID: 19398486]

► Ochronosis

A hereditary deficiency in the enzyme homogentisic acid oxidase is present in the disease known as **alkaptonuria**. The presence of unmetabolized homogentisic acid results in a brownish black color of the urine (thus the name of the disease). The term **ochronosis** describes the clinical condition of homogentisic acid deposited in connective tissues, manifested by bluish black pigmentation of the skin, ear, and sclera, and in cartilage.

The diagnosis is made when the triad of dark urine, degenerative arthritis, and abnormal pigmentation is present. Freshly passed urine is normal in color but turns dark when oxidized. Spondylosis is common, with knee, shoulder, and hip joint involvement also seen.

A. Epidemiologic Features

Alkaptonuria is caused by a recessive autosomal gene encoding homogentisate 1,2-dioxygenase. Genetic testing is available.

B. Imaging Studies

Spondylosis is seen, with calcification of intervertebral disks with few osteophytes. Joint involvement is similar in appearance to that of osteoarthritis, except for protrusio acetabuli.

Introne WJ, Kayser MA, Gahl WA: Alkaptonuria. *Gene Reviews* (internet), May 9, 2003. [PMID: 20301627]

Zhao BH, Chen BC, Shao de C, et al: Osteoarthritis? Ochronotic arthritis! A case study and review of the literature. *Knee Surg Sports Traumatol Arthrosc* 2009;17:778. [PMID: 19381613]

4. Osteochondroses

▶ Osteonecrosis of the Femoral Head

A variety of conditions and diseases are associated with osteonecrosis, but the pathogenesis is unknown in most cases. Direct injury to the blood supply of the femoral head is implicated in traumatic causes of femoral head avascular necrosis such as subcapital femoral neck fracture and dislocation of the hip. The disorder is bilateral in more than 60% of cases and affects other bones in approximately 15% of cases. The leading nontraumatic causes of osteonecrosis include alcoholism, idiopathic causes, and systemic steroid treatment. The mechanism by which steroids cause osteonecrosis may be by adipogenesis because the effects may be reduced, at least in an animal model, by using lovastatin.

Other associated conditions include hemoglobinopathies, Gaucher disease, caisson disease, hyperlipidemia, tobacco use, hypercoagulable states, irradiation, and diseases of bone marrow infiltration such as leukemia and lymphoma.

A. Pathologic Features

Regardless of underlying causes, the early lesions in femoral head osteonecrosis include necrosis of marrow and trabecular bone, usually in a wedge-shaped area in the region of the anterolateral superior femoral head. The overlying articular cartilage is largely unaffected because it is normally avascular, obtaining nutrition from the synovial fluid. The deep calcified layer of cartilage, however, does derive nutrition from epiphyseal vessels and also undergoes necrosis. Histologically, necrotic marrow and absence of osteocytes in lacunae are seen.

Leukocytes and mononuclear cells collect around necrotic and fibrovascular tissue and eventually replace necrotic marrow. Osteoclasts resorb dead trabeculae, and osteoblasts then attempt to repair the damaged tissue; during attempted repair, the necrotic trabeculae are susceptible to fracture. Grossly, a subchondral fracture forms, with deformation of overlying articular cartilage. With time, fragmentation of articular cartilage ensues, resulting in degenerative arthritis.

B. Imaging Studies

Ficat created a classification based on the plain radiographic appearance of femoral head osteonecrosis in progressive stages. Stage I represents normal or minimal changes (mild osteopenia or sclerotic regions) in an asymptomatic hip. In stage II, subchondral sclerosis and osteopenia are evident, often in a well-demarcated wedge in the anterolateral femoral head seen best with radiographs taken with the patient in the frog-leg position from the lateral views. Stage III is heralded by collapse of subchondral bone, known as the crescent sign, and is pathognomonic for femoral head osteonecrosis. Femoral head flattening is often seen, but the joint space is preserved. Stage IV consists of advanced degenerative arthritic changes, with loss of joint space and bony changes in the acetabulum.

A newer classification system, devised by Steinberg, is popular and based on extent of head involvement as determined by MRI. This system, called the University of Pennsylvania system, has seven stages from normal (stage 0) to stage VI in which advanced degenerative changes are evident. Stages I–V are divided into three subcategories of mild, moderate, and severe. Stage III of the Steinberg system corresponds to stage III of the Ficat system.

Ficat RP: Idiopathic bone necrosis of the femoral head: early diagnosis and treatment. *J Bone Joint Surg Br* 1985;67:3. [PMID: 3155745]

Mont MA, Zywiel MG, Marker DR, et al: The natural history of untreated asymptomatic osteonecrosis of the femoral head: a systematic review. *J Bone Joint Surg Am* 2010;92:2165. [PMID: 20844158]

Steinberg ME, Steinberg ME, Garino JP, et al: A quantitative system for staging avascular necrosis. *J Bone Joint Surg Am* 1995;77B:34. [PMID: 17079364]

5. Other Disorders Associated With Arthritis

▶ Hemophilia

Hemophilia A is a heritable bleeding disorder produced by deficiency of factor VIII. Hemophilia B is a disease caused by lack of clotting factor IX. Both hemophilia A (classic hemophilia) and hemophilia B (Christmas disease) are sex-linked recessive disorders, although 30% of patients may have no family history of the disease. Hemophilic arthropathy primarily involves the knee joint, with the elbow and ankle joints affected less frequently.

A. Pathologic Features

Recurrent hemarthrosis produces deposits of hemosiderin and synovitis. In the acute phase, hypertrophy of synovium occurs, causing a higher risk of repeated bleeding. A pannus may form, as in rheumatoid osteoarthritis, with underlying cartilage destruction, possibly a result of the promotion of apoptosis of chondrocytes and cellular proliferation of the synovium by iron. With time, synovial fibrosis occurs, resulting in joint stiffness.

B. Imaging Studies

Soft-tissue swelling, seen early, is associated with hemarthroses. Later stages include widening of epiphyseal regions caused by overgrowth from increased vascularity. Skeletal changes are manifested as subchondral sclerosis and cyst formation early, with later loss of cartilage and secondary osteophyte formation. Squaring of the patella is seen, possibly resulting from overgrowth.

Lafeber FP, Miossec P, Valentino LA: Physiopathology of haemophilic arthropathy. *Haemophilia* 2008;14(Suppl 4):3. [PMID: 18494686]

Mann HA, Choudhury MZ, Allen DJ, et al: Current Approaches in haemophilic arthropathy of the hip. *Haemophilia* 2009;15:659. [PMID: 19298335]

Gaucher Disease

A rare familial disorder, Gaucher disease is an inborn error of metabolism caused by a deficiency of the lysosomal hydrolase enzyme β-glucocerebrosidase. Accumulation of glucosylceramidase in phagocytic cells of the reticuloendothelial tissues occurs, including the liver, spleen, lymph nodes, and bone marrow.

The femur is the most commonly affected bone, but the vertebrae, ribs, sternum, and flat bones of the pelvis may also be affected. The manifestations of skeletal disease are the result of mechanical effects of infiltration of the abnormal cells, leading to erosion of cortices and interference with the normal vascular supply. Expansion of bone and areas of osteolysis predispose affected bones to pathologic fracture, and vascular interruption leads to avascular necrosis of the femoral hip.

A. Epidemiologic Features

Inherited in an autosomal recessive manner, Gaucher disease is the most common inherited disorder of lipid metabolism. The disease is especially common in the Ashkenazi Jewish community.

B. Pathologic Features

Histologic examination of involved reticuloendothelial tissues demonstrates foam cells, which are large lipid-laden macrophages.

C. Imaging Studies

Early stages of skeletal involvement in Gaucher disease include diffuse osteoporosis and medullary expansion. The distal femur may expand to form a characteristic Erlenmeyer flask deformity. Localized erosions and sclerotic areas are seen. Osteonecrosis may be seen in the femoral head, humeral head, and distal femur. Secondary degenerative changes follow collapse of necrotic articular bone. Treatment is now possible with enzyme replacement therapy using imiglucerase, but bone response is usually slower than soft-tissue response.

Goldblatt J, Fletcher JM, McGill J, et al: Enzyme replacement therapy "drug holiday": results from an unexpected shortage of an orphan drug supply in Australia. *Blood Cells Mol Dis* 2011;46:107. [PMID 20684886]

Piran S, Amato D: Gaucher disease: a systematic review and meta-analysis of bone complications and their response to treatment. *J Inherit Metab Dis* 2010;33:271. [PMID: 20336376]

Trochanteric Bursitis

Trochanteric bursitis is a term applied to pain elicited to palpation of the lateral side of the hip in the side-lying position. The tenderness is attributed to friction between the greater trochanter and the iliotibial band during motion. Extended pressure to that area, such as with bedridden patients lying on their side, can be an inciting cause. Trochanteric bursitis is one of several disorders that falls under the term "greater trochanteric pain syndrome," which includes gluteus medius and minimus tears and "snapping hip." It affects about 1.8 patients per 100 per year. Risk factors include female gender, coexisting low back pain, iliotibial band tenderness, and obesity. It is diagnosed in the patient with a compatible history by point tenderness over the greater trochanter. A lack of tenderness suggests other sources of the pain, including referred lumbar pain.

Strauss EJ, Nho SJ, Kelly BT: Greater trochanteric pain syndrome. *Sports Med Arthrosc* 2010;18:113. [PMID: 20473130]

Williams BS, Cohen SP: Greater trochanteric pain syndrome: a review of anatomy, diagnosis and treatment. *Anesth Analg* 2009;108:1662. [PMID: 19372352]

Hip Labral Tears

The hip has a cartilaginous extension of the bony acetabulum called the labrum that deepens the acetabulum and stabilizes the hip. Labral tears were newly rediscovered as a source of pain and a cause of osteoarthrosis, partially because of the relative ease of evaluating their presence and subsequently treating them. Arthroscopy can be used to remove the torn labrum, similar to torn menisci.

A. Pathologic Features

The normal labrum is triangular in shape and variable in size from 1 to 10 mm in length. The pathologic labrum is classified into types A and B, depending on whether the labrum is traumatic (triangular: A) or degenerative (thick and rounded: B), and three stages: (1) intrasubstance degeneration, (2) partial tear, and (3) complete tear.

B. Imaging Studies

MRI arthrography is the test of choice for suspected labral tears. Contrast is seen going into the tear, which is frequently in the weight-bearing area of the acetabulum. Computed tomography (CT) arthrography and MRI are not as sensitive.

Safran MR: The acetabular labrum: anatomic and functional characteristics and rationale for surgical intervention. *J Am Acad Orthop Surg* 2010;18:338. [PMID: 20511439]

MEDICAL MANAGEMENT

▶ Nonsteroidal Anti-inflammatory Drugs

The use of nonsteroidal anti-inflammatory drugs (NSAIDs) in the management of osteoarthritis is widespread but controversial. Because only minimal inflammatory changes are present in joints with osteoarthritis, the use of acetaminophen is advocated as a first-line drug. In a short-term study of patients treated for osteoarthritis, acetaminophen (4000 mg/d) was found to be as effective as ibuprofen (2400 mg/d).

The therapeutic effect of NSAIDs can be dramatic in the osteoarthritic patient, even with severe disease. The main problems with routine NSAID therapy are the gastrointestinal (GI) and renal complications and the inhibition of normal platelet function. Thus, alternative therapies should be carefully considered, and therapy should be closely monitored. Current NSAIDs work by altering prostaglandin synthesis through nonspecific inhibition of both cyclooxygenase isoforms 1 (COX-1) and 2 (COX-2). COX-1 inhibition can have deleterious effects on hemostasis and the GI tract.

Patients treated with NSAIDs have a three times greater relative risk of developing GI complications than nonusers. In one study, NSAIDs were associated with acute hospital admissions of 30% of elderly patients. Patients at high risk for developing ulcers with use of NSAIDs are those with any of the following characteristics: age older than 65 years, history of prior ulcer disease, use of multiple-dose or high-dose NSAIDs, or use of concomitant corticosteroids. The antiprostaglandin effects of NSAIDs can reduce renal blood flow, leading to acute and chronic renal insufficiency. Patients at risk for acute renal insufficiency because of NSAIDs are elderly patients, those with atherosclerotic cardiovascular disease, and those with preexisting renal impairment. The platelet effects of these drugs are variable, depending on the NSAID half-life, on whether the NSAID inhibits thromboxane A, and on whether that inhibition is reversible. Aspirin, for example, is permanent for the life of the platelet. Many patients report increased bruising as a result of taking these drugs.

Table 6–3 compares the toxicities of currently available NSAIDs. Because the effects are not caused solely by the inhibitory effects on prostaglandin synthesis, the various chemical origins of these drugs may lead to slightly different clinical effects in different patients.

The chemical families of these drugs are noted in Table 6–4 with their half-lives and their dosing frequency. Dosing frequency is important because patient compliance with use of these drugs goes up with less frequent dosing, such as daily or twice daily.

COX-2–selective NSAIDs are now available. Most of the side effects attributable to NSAIDs are caused by inhibition of COX-1, an isoform that is normally present ("constitutive") in renal and GI tissues. COX-2–selective NSAIDs inhibit the isoenzyme that develops ("inducible") as a response to inflammation. By selectively inhibiting COX-2, the efficacy of NSAIDs is retained with much less side effects. Most NSAIDs have some effect on both enzymes, but in most cases, they largely affect either COX-1 or COX-2. Although COX-2–selective NSAIDs are purportedly safe, they are not without side effects. For example, celecoxib did not exhibit statistically significant decreased rates of complicated upper GI events in a randomized controlled trial.

The choice of an appropriate NSAID should be based on the following factors: clotting problems, compliance of the patient, GI symptom history, renal function, drug cost, and the effect on the patient with previously used NSAIDs. Patients taking warfarin would probably be better treated with a drug having no platelet effect that is COX-2 specific. Patients with a poor response to one type of NSAID may benefit from a trial with one from another chemical family. A patient with a history of poor drug compliance with other medications would benefit from once-daily dosing, whereas a patient already taking another drug three times daily would probably find three-times-daily dosing more convenient. Obviously, a patient with renal disease should be treated with a drug having not only low renal toxicity, but also a short half-life to minimize the accumulation of the drug in the body because of lack of renal excretion. The COX-2–selective NSAIDs will not eliminate the need for the other drugs. The vast majority of patients tolerate the side effects of the older drugs, and the risk-benefit ratio for these drugs is quite favorable, especially for short courses of treatment.

The advent of the COX-2–specific NSAIDs adds to their safety as analgesics for acute pain because the COX-2 inhibitors block the pain, fever, and inflammatory response while not affecting clotting. Thus, their use in the perioperative setting is significantly increased.

Surgical intervention is generally indicated for patients who have failed conservative therapy with NSAIDs. For patients who are not surgical candidates, a long-term regimen of narcotic medication may be considered.

Bingham S, Beswick PJ, Blum DE, et al: The role of the cyclooxygenase pathway in nociception and pain. *Semin Cell Dev Biol* 2006;17:544. [PMID: 17071117]

Gan TJ: Diclofenac: an update on its mechanism of action and safety profile. *Curr Med Res Opin* 2010;26:1715. [PMID: 20470236]

Hawkey C, Kahan A, Steinbrück K, et al: Gastrointestinal tolerability of meloxicam compared to diclofenac in osteoarthritis patients. International MELISSA Study Group. Meloxicam Large-scale International Study Safety Assessment. *Br J Rheumatol* 1998;37:937. [PMID: 9783757]

Table 6–3. Toxicity profiles of currently available NSAIDs.

Generic Name	Proprietary Name	Gastrointestinal Toxicity	Renal Toxicity	Platelet Effects (d)[a]	Other Toxicity[b]
Diclofenac	Voltaren	Moderate	Moderate	1	Hepatitis
Etodolac	Lodine	Low[c]	Moderate	NA	—
Indomethacin	Indocin	High	Moderate	1	Headache
Nabumetone	Relafen	Low[c]	Moderate	NA	Hepatitis
Sulindac	Clinoril	Moderate	Low	1	Dermatitis
Tolmetin	Tolectin	Moderate	Moderate	2	—
Meclofenamate	Meclomen	Moderate	Moderate	1	Diarrhea
Piroxicam	Feldene	Moderate	Moderate	14	—
Fenoprofen	Nalfon	Moderate	Moderate	1	—
Flurbiprofen	Ansaid	Moderate	Moderate	1	—
Ibuprofen	Motrin	Moderate	Moderate	1	—
Ketoprofen	Orudis	Moderate	Moderate	2	—
Naproxen	Naprosyn	Moderate	Moderate	4	—
Oxaprozin	Daypro	Moderate	Moderate	NA	—
Ketorolac	Toradol	High	Moderate	1	—
Salicylsalicylic acid[d]	Disalcid	None	None	None	—
Sodium salicylate[d]	—	None	None	None	—
Aspirin	—	High	Moderate	10	Tinnitus
Diflunisal[e]	Dolobid	Low	Low	None	—
Celecoxib	Celebrex	Low	Low	None	Sulfa allergies
Meloxicam	Mobic	Low	Moderate	None	—

[a]Average time to normal platelet function after discontinuation of drug.
[b]Other NSAIDs may have similar toxicity, but the effects are more prevalent with these agents.
[c]Simultaneous efficacy comparisons in inflammatory disease not available.
[d]No prostaglandin inhibition.
[e]Weak prostaglandin inhibitor.
NA, data not available.

Jones P, Lamdin R: Oral cyclooxygenase 2 inhibitors versus other oral analgesics for acute soft tissue injury: systematic review and meta-analysis. *Clin Drug Invest* 2010;30:419. [PMID: 20527999]

Lynch ME, Watson CPN: The pharmacology of chronic pain: a review. *Pain Res Manag* 2006;11:11. [PMID: 16511612]

Rainsford KD: Ibuprofen: pharmacology, efficacy and safety. *Inflammopharmacology* 2009;17:275. [PMID: 19949916]

Silverstein FE, Faich G, Goldstein JL, et al: Gastrointestinal toxicity with celecoxib vs nonsteroidal anti-inflammatory drugs for osteoarthritis and rheumatoid arthritis: the CLASS study: a randomized controlled trial. Celecoxib Long Term Arthritis Safety Study. *JAMA* 2000;284:1247. [PMID: 10979111]

Simon LS, Lanza FL, Lipsky PE, et al: Preliminary study of the safety and efficacy of SC-58635, a novel cyclooxygenase 2 inhibitor: efficacy and safety in two placebo-controlled trials in osteoarthritis and rheumatoid arthritis, and studies of gastrointestinal and platelet effects. *Arthritis Rheum* 1998;41:1591. [PMID: 9751091]

▶ Disease-Modifying Agents in Rheumatoid Arthritis

Several new disease-modifying antirheumatic drugs (DMARDs) are now available for the medical treatment of rheumatoid

Table 6–4. Dosage data of currently available NSAIDs.

Generic Name	Proprietary Name	Largest Unit Dose (mg)	Half-Life (h)	Dosing Frequency[a]	Family
Diclofenac	Voltaren	75	2	bid	Acetic acid
Etodolac	Lodine	300	6	qid	Acetic acid
Indomethacin	Indocin	50	4	tid	Acetic acid
Nabumetone	Relafen	500	20–30	2 qd	Acetic acid
Sulindac	Clinoril	200	8–14	bid	Acetic acid
Tolmetin	Tolectin	400	1–2	tid	Acetic acid
Meclofenamate	Meclomen	100	2	tid	Fenamates
Piroxicam	Feldene	20	30–86	qd	Oxicams
Meloxicam	Mobic	15	15–20	qd	Oxicams
Fenoprofen	Nalfon	600	2–3	qid	Propionates
Flurbiprofen	Ansaid	100	6	tid	Propionates
Ibuprofen	Motrin	800	2	qid	Propionates
Ketoprofen	Orudis	75	3	tid	Propionates
Naproxen	Naprosyn	500	14	bid	Propionates
Oxaprozin	Daypro	600	40–50	2 qd	Propionates
Ketorolac	Toradol	10	5	qid	Pyrrolo-pyrrole
Salicylsalicylic acid	Disalcid	750	1	qid	Salicylates
Sodium salicylate	—	650	0.5	q4h	Salicylates
Aspirin	—	325	0.25	2q4h	Salicylates
Diflunisal	Dolobid	500	10	bid	Salicylates
Celecoxib	Celebrex	200	11	bid	Sulfonamide

[a]Dosage required for treatment of inflammation.
bid = twice a day; qd = each day; q4h = every 4 hours; qid = four times a day; tid = three times a day.

arthritis, in addition to methotrexate and glucocorticoids. Although the experience of these new agents is limited, the mechanisms of their actions may guide orthopedic surgeons with respect to their potential effect on surgical procedures. Etanercept is an artificially bioengineered molecule that binds to the receptor of tumor necrosis factor (TNF), preventing activation of the inflammatory cascade. Infliximab is a chimeric antibody that also targets TNF. Both of these drugs probably have little effect on healing and most likely can be continued up to any surgical procedure. Rituximab targets the B cell, and tocilizumab inhibits interleukin-6, and both have shown significant improvements in rheumatoid arthritis. Leflunomide inhibits an enzyme, decreasing levels of pyrimidine nucleotides and inhibiting clonal expansion of T cells in rheumatoid arthritis. This DMARD should probably be discontinued 1 week prior to surgery, similar to methotrexate.

Cohen SB: Targeting the B cell in rheumatoid arthritis. *Best Pract Res Clin Rheumatol* 2010;24:553. [PMID: 20732652]

Scott DL, Wolfe F, Huizinga TW: Rheumatoid arthritis. *Lancet* 2010;375:1094. [PMID: 20870100]

Singh JA, Beg S, Lopez-Olivo MA: Tocilizumab for rheumatoid arthritis. *Cochrane Database Syst Rev* 2010;7:CD008331. [PMID: 20614469]

OTHER THERAPIES

▶ Nutritional Supplements

The nutritional supplements glucosamine sulfate and chondroitin sulfate are popular as nonprescription products for arthritis therapy. This popularity arises from the concept that these products may serve as substrate for the reparative processes in cartilage. Glucosamine sulfate is found as an intermediate product in mucopolysaccharide synthesis, and an elevated urinary excretion is seen in patients with osteoarthritis and rheumatoid osteoarthritis. Oral administration of glucosamine sulfate was compared with analgesic doses of ibuprofen in a 4-week trial in patients with osteoarthritis of the knee. Ibuprofen was found to provide pain relief more quickly, but the response rates were similar at 4 weeks.

Chondroitin sulfate is another glycosaminoglycan present in articular cartilage; its oral administration in one study resulted in no change in serum levels. In another study, patients with osteoarthritis of the hip and knee used fewer NSAIDs when given chondroitin sulfate compared with a placebo control group. Although glucosamine sulfate and chondroitin sulfate are unproven therapies at this time, their use may provide safe and effective symptomatic relief in some patients with osteoarthritis. Newer reports indicate improved symptoms of osteoarthritis with oral glucosamine and chondroitin sulfate, but the mechanisms of action are unknown. A recent meta-analysis showed no effect of these two supplements on joint pain or joint space narrowing when compared to placebo.

Brief AA, Maurer SG, Di Cesare PE: Use of glucosamine and chondroitin sulfate in the management of osteoarthritis. *J Am Acad Orthop Surg* 2001;9:71. [PMID: 11281631]

Reginster JY, Deroisy R, Rovati LC, et al: Long term effects of glucosamine sulphate on osteoarthritis progression: a randomized, placebo-controlled clinical trial. *Lancet* 2001;357:251. [PMID: 11214126]

Wandel S, Jüni P, Tendal B, et al: Effects of glucosamine, chondroitin, or placebo in patients with osteoarthritis of the hip or knee: network meta-analysis. *BMJ* 2010;341:c4675. [PMID: 20847017]

▶ Injections

One of the mainstays of the treatment of osteoarthrosis and rheumatoid osteoarthritis is the cortisone injection, which can be used for joints, bursae, and trigger points. Generally, injections of shoulders, elbows, wrists, finger joints, knees, ankles, and joints of the foot can be given in the office without radiographic or ultrasound control. While more accurate injection of corticosteroid was obtained under ultrasound guidance, no significant difference was noted in the clinical outcome. Hips and some joints of the foot and hand are best done with radiographic control to ensure location of the injection. The injections can be therapeutic with steroids or diagnostic with local anesthetic. For example, differentiation between the amount of a patient's pain coming from the back and the proportion coming from the hip can be ascertained with a lidocaine injection into the hip. This reliably informs the patient as to the realistic expectations of pain relief after a hip replacement.

Similarly, an ankle injection predicts pain relief after ankle fusion. Intraarticular administration of hyaluronic acid is now available for treatment of osteoarthritis of the knee with products of different molecular weight. The initial treatment protocols for these drugs called for weekly injections for 3–5 weeks to obtain a therapeutic effect. A single injection treatment is now available.

Hyaluronic acid is a long-chain polysaccharide responsible for the viscoelastic properties of synovial joint fluid. In pathologic states, such as osteoarthritis and rheumatoid osteoarthritis, both the concentration and the molecular size of hyaluronic acid are diminished. In animal experimental models, evidence indicates that hyaluronic injections may retard progression of osteoarthritis. Serial injections of hyaluronic acid in patients with osteoarthritic knees are reported to reduce pain for up to 10 months, but the mechanism of action is unknown. Because of the short half-life of hyaluronic acid, it is unlikely that the injections significantly boost lubrication of arthritic joints. Rather than being a disease-modifying therapy, the injectable hyaluronic acid products should be considered long-acting pain-relieving drugs. Questions about the efficacy of these products still remain, as studies and meta-analyses indicate a weak effect if any.

Cunnington J, Marshall N, Hide G, et al: A randomized, double-blind, controlled study of ultrasound-guided corticosteroid injection into the joints of patients with inflammatory arthritis. *Arthritis Rheum* 2010;62:1862. [PMID: 20222114]

Jergensen A, Stengaard-Pedersen K, Simonsen O, et al: Intra-articular hyaluronan without clinical effect in knee osteoarthritis: a multicentre, randomized, placebo-controlled, double-blind study of 337 patients followed for 1 year. *Ann Rheum Dis* 2010;69:1097. [PMID: 20447955]

Lo GH, LaValley M, McAlindon T, et al: Intra-articular hyaluronic acid in treatment of knee osteoarthritis: a meta-analysis. *JAMA* 2003;290:3115. [PMID: 14679274]

▶ Orthotic Treatment

The use of orthotics can ameliorate the symptoms of osteoarthrosis in the knee, the ankle, and possibly the elbow, but other joints are not really amenable to this treatment. The medial compartment of the knee is more commonly affected than the lateral, leading to, or resulting from, varus deformity. Thus, this disorder lends itself to orthotic treatment to remove the deformity. Heel wedges and valgus braces can be helpful in relieving the pain and improving the ambulatory function of patients with medial gonarthrosis. Similarly, orthotics to control varus and valgus forces at the ankle can be very helpful for ankle arthrosis.

Draper ER, Cable JM, Sanchez-Ballester J, et al: Improvement of function after valgus bracing of the knee. *J Bone Joint Surg Br* 2000;82:1001. [PMID: 11041589]

Pollo FE: Bracing and heel wedging for unicompartmental osteo-arthritis of the knee. *Am J Knee Surg* 1998;11:47. [PMID: 9606092]

Sgaglione NA, Chen E, Bert JM, et al: Current strategies for non surgical, arthroscopic, and minimally invasive surgical treatment of knee cartilage pathology. *Instr Course Lect* 2010;59:157. [PMID: 20415378]

▼ SURGICAL MANAGEMENT

PROCEDURES FOR RESTORATION OF FUNCTION/IMPROVEMENT OF PAIN

▶ Hip Arthroscopy

A. Femoroacetabular Impingement

Femoroacetabular impingement (FAI) is due to an incongruity of the hip joint. There are two types of FAI, cam and pincer impingement, although the two frequently coexist (Figure 6–4). Cam impingement results from abutment of an abnormally shaped femoral head into the acetabulum. The resultant shear forces are transmitted along the acetabular rim, causing injury to the labrum. Pincer impingement results from relative acetabular overcoverage. The labrum impinges on the femoral neck, which causes labral injury and subsequent ossification of the labrum, further deepening the socket and worsening the situation. Both cam and pincer types of impingement result in decreased clearance of the head–neck junction and labral injury.

Although in the past, FAI was treated with an open procedure (surgical dislocation of the hip), arthroscopic techniques for FAI have become very popular due to quicker recovery and less morbidity. For pincer lesions, anterior and anterolateral portals are established in the hip joint. A burr is inserted through the anterolateral portal, and the rim of the acetabulum is resected. The labrum can be preserved by placing the burr behind and underneath the labrum and subsequently refixing it after the rim of the acetabulum is adequately resected. For the treatment of cam lesions, a femoral osteochondroplasty is performed. A burr is inserted through the anterior portal, and the femoral head–neck junction is progressively resected until it no longer impinges on the acetabulum. Care must be taken not to damage the blood supply to the femoral head. The deep branch of the medial femoral circumflex courses along the posterior aspect of the greater trochanter, posterior to the tendon of obturator externus, and anterior to the tendons of superior gemellus, obturator internus, and inferior gemellus. It perforates the capsule above the superior gemellus and distal to the

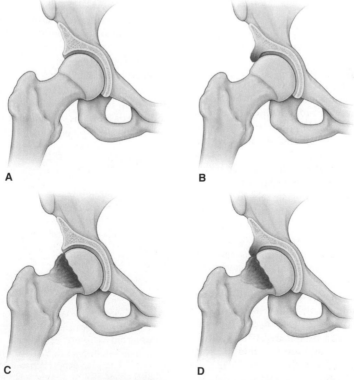

A   **B**

C   **D**

▲ **Figure 6–4.** **A:** Normal. **B:** Pincer. **C:** Cam. **D:** Combined.

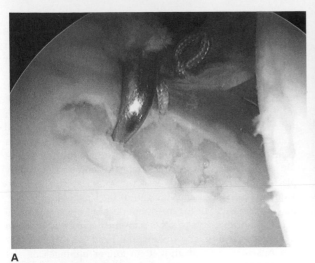

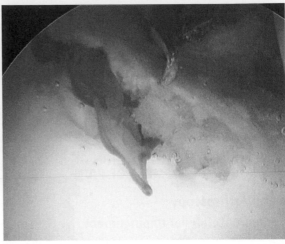

A   B

▲ **Figure 6–5.** Microfracture of an osteochondral defect in the hip joint.

tendon or piriformis, before dividing into two to four terminal retinacular branches. Maintaining the attachment of the external rotators maintains the blood supply to the femoral head. Additionally, the superior-lateral retinacular vessels must also be maintained during femoral neck osteoplasty.

Short-term outcomes of these arthroscopic techniques have been comparable to the open procedures for the treatment of FAI.

B. Labral Tears

The most common causes of acetabular labral tears are FAI and trauma. They are rarely an isolated event, with one study finding over 90% of patients undergoing hip arthroscopy for atraumatic labral tears having radiographic evidence of a bony abnormality such as dysplasia or FAI. Patients commonly complain of mechanical symptoms, such as clicking, catching, and/or a locking sensation.

Arthroscopic techniques for labral injury include debridement versus repair of the lesions. The goal of arthroscopic debridement of a torn hip labrum is to relieve pain by eliminating the unstable flap tear that causes the observed hip discomfort. Recently repair of the labrum, rather than debridement, has gained attention with the hope that it will improve functional outcomes and delay the onset of osteoarthritis. Type I tears occur when there is detachment of the labrum at the zone of transition to the articular cartilage. These tears can be repaired with reattachment of the labrum to the acetabular rim, usually with a suture anchor. Type II tears are intrasubstance splits with one or more cleavage planes. These tears can be repaired with a suture lasso technique and a bioabsorbable suture. Good to excellent short-term results have been achieved in 67–93% of cases of arthroscopic partial labrectomy. Outcome data on labrum repairs are still lacking; however, some investigators have demonstrated the healing capabilities of the labrum in an ovine model, whereas others have shown the superior biomechanical properties of a repaired labrum in a cadaver model.

▶ Microfracture

Microfracture is another arthroscopic technique that helps to restore function and decrease pain. It is used for the treatment of small- to medium-sized osteochondral defects. Through the use of an awl, the surgeon creates tiny fractures in the subchondral bone plate (Figure 6–5). This causes a clot to develop, which eventually forms fibrocartilage. Recovery is quick, and short-term results show 95–100% defect coverage. Functional outcome data for this procedure are lacking in the hip, but it is well established with good outcomes in the knee.

Bardakos NV, Vasconcelos JC, Villar RN: Early outcome of hip arthroscopy for femoroacetabular impingement: the role of femoral osteoplasty in symptomatic improvement. *J Bone Joint Surg Br* 2008;90:1570. [PMID: 19043126]

Byrd JW, Jones KS: Prospective analysis of hip arthroscopy with 2-year follow up. *Arthroscopy* 2000;16:578. [PMID: 10976117]

Crawford K, Philippon MJ, Sekiya JK, et al: Microfracture of the hip in athletes. *Clin Sports Med* 2006;25:327. [PMID: 16638495]

Larson CM, Giveans MR: Arthroscopic debridement versus refixation of the acetabular labrum associated with femoroacetabular impingement. *Arthroscopy* 2009;25:369. [PMID: 19341923]

Philippon MJ, Arnoczky SP, Torrie A: Arthroscopic repair of the acetabular labrum: a histologic assessment of healing in an ovine model. *Arthroscopy* 2007;23:376. [PMID: 17418329]

Philippon MJ, Briggs KK, Yen YM, et al: Outcomes following hip arthroscopy for femoroacetabular impingement with associated chondrolabral dysfunction: minimum two-year follow-up. *J Bone Joint Surg Br* 2009;91:16. [PMID: 19091999]

Philippon MJ, Schenker ML, Briggs KK, et al: Can microfracture produce repair tissue in acetabular chondral defects? *Arthroscopy* 2008;24:46. [PMID: 18182201]

Sampson T: Arthroscopic treatment of femoroacetabular impingement. *Am J Orthop* 2008;37:608. [PMID: 19212569]

PROCEDURES FOR JOINT PRESERVATION

A joint can potentially deteriorate for many reasons. The wear and tear of many years may be most common. In addition, infection can result in articular cartilage damage that then progresses over the years. Trauma may distort the joint, cause instability, or result in abnormal muscle forces, as occurs, for example, with a rotator cuff tear leading to cuff arthropathy. Other causes include (1) synovitis, as occurs, for example, with hemophilia, which forces the joint to dispose of blood on multiple occasions, and rheumatoid arthritis, which causes a proliferation of the synovium, which may destroy the articular cartilage; (2) osteonecrosis, which may result in fatigue fractures and collapse of the joint, with subsequent incongruity; and (3) abnormal distribution of load in the joint that results, for example, from malalignment. Certain procedures can slow progression of the deterioration resulting from these three causes and prolong the useful service of the joint. These procedures include synovectomy, core decompression, and osteotomy.

▶ Synovectomy

Synovectomy is a treatment that may prolong the life of the articular cartilage through removal of proliferative synovitis, which damages cartilage. Synovectomy is indicated for chronic but not acute synovitis. Chronic synovitis is a clinical entity characterized by proliferation of the synovium and may be monoarticular, as in pigmented villonodular synovitis, or polyarticular, as in rheumatoid arthritis or hemophilia. The term **synovitis** is relatively nonspecific, and the disorder is usually the result of a reaction to joint irritation.

A. Indications and Contraindications

The most common indication for synovectomy is rheumatoid arthritis, but the procedure may be beneficial in many other conditions, such as synovial osteochondromatosis, pigmented villonodular synovitis, and hemophilia, and occasionally following chronic or acute infection.

More specific indications for synovectomy include the following conditions:

1. Synovitis with disease limited to the synovial membrane with little or no involvement of the other structures of the joint
2. Recurrent hemarthroses in conditions such as pigmented villonodular synovitis or hemophilia
3. Infection when along with irrigation and debridement of the joint there is imminent destruction by lysosomal enzymes derived from white blood cells that may be liberated from the infection
4. Failure of conservative management

Contraindications include reduced ROM, significant degenerative arthrosis of the involved joint or other joint, or cartilage involvement.

B. Technique

Synovectomy is most commonly performed on the knee but also often on the elbow, ankle, and wrist. Three main techniques are available: open synovectomy, synovectomy with use of the arthroscope, and radiation synovectomy.

1. Open synovectomy—Open synovectomy is becoming less common because of pain that causes difficulty in obtaining full motion following surgery. Continuous passive motion may be beneficial in these cases. Open synovectomy may be necessary in cases of pigmented villonodular synovitis or synovial osteochondromatosis, although these diseases may also be treated by arthroscopy, which permits noninvasive complete removal of the synovium in many cases.

2. Synovectomy with use of arthroscope—Synovectomy with use of the arthroscope may be tedious, especially in large joints such as the knee, because complete treatment requires removal of the entire synovium in many cases.

A study of pigmented villonodular synovitis of the knee treated by total and partial arthroscopic synovectomy demonstrated that total synovectomy resulted in a low recurrence rate, whereas partial synovectomy resulted in symptomatic and functional improvement but a fairly high recurrence rate. Arthroscopic synovectomy was recommended only for localized lesions.

3. Radiation synovectomy—Radiation synovectomy is a technique that is becoming much more popular. It is used in knee joints affected by rheumatoid osteoarthritis. An injection of dysprosium-165-ferric hydroxide macroaggregates is given and leads to improvement in a significant percentage of patients. Proliferation of synovium decreases following this procedure, and there is less pain, blood loss, and expense than with more invasive procedures.

A similar technique is used in the knee joint in hemophiliacs. Phosphorus-32 chromic phosphate colloid is used and can be given on an outpatient basis. This is a safer technique for health care personnel, who have less contact with the blood of the hemophiliac patients, many of whom have become human immunodeficiency virus (HIV) positive through contaminated blood factor replacement.

Mendenhall WM, Mendenhall CM, Reith JD, et al: Pigmented villonodular synovitis. *Am J Clin Oncol* 2006;29:548. [PMID: 17148989]

► Cartilage Repair Techniques

Defects of articular cartilage were long considered permanent injuries, and the irrevocable sequela was gradual deterioration over time. The treatment of cartilaginous diseases and injuries was limited by the slow and poorly understood metabolism of articular chondrocytes. Current cartilage repair procedures pertain only to focal full-thickness cartilage defects. Such injuries are typically found in young (<40 years) patients injured during athletic activities or in patients with osteochondritis dissecans. Cartilage repair techniques are contraindicated in smokers and patients with high BMI (>35 kg/m^2), malalignment, meniscal deficiency, ligamentous laxity, or inflammatory conditions.

Because articular cartilage is avascular, prior surgical treatment consisted of chondroplasty, where underlying subchondral bone was either drilled, burred, or microfractured to produce bleeding and an inflammatory response. Although multiple growth factors may be released with bleeding, the ensuing repair tissue is essentially fibrous scar tissue with inferior load-bearing capabilities compared with articular cartilage. As a result, the repair tissue eventually degrades, leaving the defect little better than if left alone. Microfracture is still an option, primarily for smaller lesions.

Larger lesions (>4 cm^2) can be treated with autologous or allograft cartilage transplant. Much enthusiasm followed autologous cartilage transplant in which viable articular chondrocytes are harvested from a patient with a focal cartilaginous defect and cultured in a laboratory. The population of chondrocytes is expanded and placed back in the patient at the site of the cartilage injury. The cells are held in place with a flap of periosteum sutured to surrounding healthy cartilage. Although encouraging early clinical results were reported with this method, similar results are shown using only the flap of periosteum, and recent analyses suggest that the evidence for the efficacy of this technique is inconclusive. Mosaicplasty is another method of dealing with small- to medium-sized focal defects of cartilage and includes transplantation of small osteochondral plugs of mature cartilage and bone from another region of the patient's joint. Small cylinders of cartilage and bone are removed from non–weight-bearing portions of cartilage and transplanted into focal femoral defects. Although encouraging short-term results are reported, whether the reconstructed cartilage endures remains to be seen. Larger lesions, such as those comprising an entire compartment of the knee, may be treated with bulk osteochondral allografts.

In contrast to these focal lesions, osteoarthritis with involvement of significant portions of a joint is a more prevalent affliction, affecting more than 40 million individuals in the United States. The early pathologic observations of osteoarthritis indicate structural degradation of the superficial layers of the cartilage architecture. Meaningful spontaneous repair of injuries limited to cartilage are not observed clinically, but a variety of experimental evidence suggests a latent ability to affect some degree of healing after injury and possibly in osteoarthritis. These suppositions include observation of increased DNA synthesis and proteoglycan synthesis in chondrocytes during intermediate stages of osteoarthritis. The procedures just described for cartilage repair do not apply for osteoarthritics when there is involvement of significant portions of a joint.

Bedi A, Feeley BT, Williams RJ 3rd: Management of articular cartilage defects of the knee. *J Bone Joint Surg Am* 2010;92:992. [PMID: 20360528]

Brittberg M, Lindahl A, Nilsson A, et al: Treatment of deep cartilage defects in the knee with autologous chondrocyte implantation. *N Engl J Med* 1994;331:889. [PMID: 8078550]

Gomoll AH, Farr J, Gillogly SD, et al: Surgical management of articular cartilage defects of the knee. *J Bone Joint Surg* 2010;92:2470. [PMID: 20962200]

Vasiliadis HS, Wasiak J: Autologous chondrocyte implantation for full thickness articular cartilage defects of the knee. *Cochrane Database Syst Rev* 2010;10:CD003323. [PMID: 20927732]

► Core Decompression With or Without Structural Bone Grafting

A. Indications and Contraindications

Core decompression with or without bone grafting is a surgical treatment primarily used for the femoral head because the hip is the joint most commonly affected by osteonecrosis. The knee and the shoulder are affected less commonly. Osteonecrosis results from loss of blood supply to the bone and is associated with a variety of conditions. Under repetitive stress, microfractures occur, are not repaired, and eventually lead to collapse of the necrotic bone and disruption of the joint surface.

Several factors have been examined as potentially predictive of progression in the patient with an asymptomatic osteonecrotic lesion of the femoral head. While lesion location, lesion stage, age, gender, and BMI have all been suspected as important, the size of the lesion, particularly when over one third of the size of the femoral head, is probably the most significant risk factor for progression.

The treatment of osteonecrosis is controversial because the outcome is frequently unsatisfactory. Spontaneous repair of the osteonecrotic lesion may occur but is an exception to the usual natural history of osteonecrosis. Core decompression, core decompression with electrical stimulation and bone grafting, and core decompression with structural bone grafting are considered acceptable forms of treatment for this disorder. Another treatment involves use of a free vascularized fibula transplant after core decompression.

B. Technique

The goal of core decompression is to alleviate hypertension in the bone caused by obstructed venous egress from the affected area. The theory is that drilling a hole in an involved bony area diminishes pressure and permits the ingrowth of new blood vessels, which allow repair of the avascular bone and prevent joint destruction. Corticocancellous bone grafting is considered an alternative to simple core decompression because some evidence indicates this would place the femoral head at less risk of collapse in the postoperative period before new bone formation can occur. Core decompression or structural bone grafting is indicated in early osteonecrosis prior to collapse of the femoral head (Ficat stage I or II).

Core decompression is usually performed on the hip but may also be done on the knee or the shoulder. A lateral approach is used for the hip, and a pin is placed into the osteonecrotic area under fluoroscopic control. A reamer or core device is then passed over the pin to achieve decompression, and a sample of bone may be obtained for pathologic analysis. If structural bone grafting is to be performed, the graft may be placed over the pin (allograft or autograft fibula). Again, placement is performed under direct radiograph control.

The results of core decompression are mixed, possibly as a result of differences in technique, lack of standardization of staging, and different etiologies of the osteonecrosis. The major complication of the procedure in the hip is fracture from torsional failure that results from the stress concentration site in the lateral aspect of the cortex. Reports of structural bone grafting by some investigators are highly favorable, with a high percentage of asymptomatic hips showing no evidence of progression of necrosis or collapse. One series reported a relatively high rate of postoperative or intraoperative fracture (four of 31 cases).

▶ Osteotomy

Osteotomy should be considered part of the armamentarium of the orthopedic surgeon in the treatment of biomechanical disorders of the knee and the hip. Osteotomy of the hip for osteoarthritis is less frequently performed than osteotomy of the knee. Abnormal distribution of load may be alleviated by osteotomy. Femoral head coverage may be improved with osteotomy of the pelvis, orientation of the femoral head may be improved with osteotomy of the proximal femur, and realignment of the load on the medial and lateral condyles of the tibia may be improved with osteotomy of the femur and/or the tibia. The most common procedure is high tibial osteotomy, sometimes referred to as **Coventry osteotomy,** which corrects varus malalignment of the knee by removal of a wedge of bone from the lateral side of the tibia. Other osteotomies are performed for residual deformity from healed fractures. These are tailored to the particular problem presented by the patient. Either intraarticular (ie, condylar osteotomy of the medial compartment [Figure 6–6]) or extraarticular osteotomies can be done to correct deformity.

A. High Tibial Osteotomy

Alleviation of abnormal stress through high tibial osteotomy prevents osteoarthrosis or, alternatively, reduces pain

caused by unicompartmental gonarthrosis. The procedure is indicated in relatively young (<55 years) patients who have unicompartmental degeneration with relative sparing of the patellofemoral joint. The knee should have a good ROM, preferably with no flexion contracture. The knee must be stable, with no demonstrated medial or lateral subluxation. The ideal patients are younger than 55 years, not obese, and wish to continue an active lifestyle, including activities such as skiing or tennis. Evaluation of the uninvolved compartment (either medial or lateral) may be accomplished by arthroscopy or with an MRI bone scan. The normal anatomic axis of 5–7 degrees (angle between the shaft of the femur and the shaft of the tibia) on the standing AP film must usually be overcorrected to 10 degrees. High tibial osteotomy is usually indicated for patients with medial gonarthrosis, although it can be performed in patients with a mild valgus malalignment (genu valgum) of less than 12 degrees. If malalignment is larger than this, it can be treated with a distal femoral supracondylar osteotomy. A high tibial osteotomy that results in a joint line that is not parallel to the ground indicates that the osteotomy should be performed through the distal femur. Lateral gonarthrosis from genu valgum is a relatively frequent result of lateral tibial plateau fractures, although rheumatoid osteoarthritis, rickets, and renal osteodystrophy may also produce this disorder.

A closing wedge proximal tibial osteotomy to treat varus malalignment is performed through a lateral hockey-stick incision or a straight lateral incision. Exposure of the lateral, anterior, and posterior aspects of the tibia is made, and a closing wedge osteotomy is performed. The proximal portion of this osteotomy is made parallel to the joint surface under image intensifier control (Figure 6–7). With the help of guide pins, the appropriate distal cut is made, as determined from preoperative standing radiographs, to provide the necessary correction, which in the average case is approximately 1 mm per degree of correction as measured on the lateral cortex. This technique should only be used to double-check previous calculations, however. Resection of the fibular head or the proximal tibiofibular joint allows correction of the valgus angle. Fixation can reliably be obtained with staples, and other commercial fixation devices are available. Care must be taken to avoid damage to the peroneal nerve. Medial opening wedge osteotomy is performed through a medial incision, using a plate to hold the correction. The opening wedge defect is bone grafted. Other problems that may be encountered include fracture of the proximal fragment or avascular necrosis of this fragment, which may occur if care is not exercised in performing the procedure. Preoperative planning and intraoperative navigation can aid in achieving appropriate alignment.

The results of high tibial osteotomy are not as predictable as unicompartmental knee replacement or total knee replacement. Although pain is relieved in a high percentage of patients, this relief deteriorates over time. Clinical reports indicate that approximately 65–85% of patients have

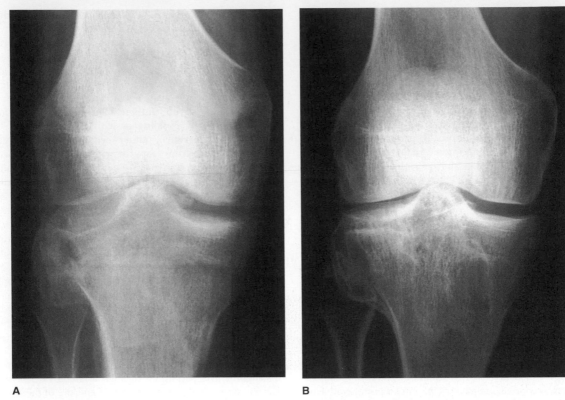

▲ Figure 6–6. An intraarticular osteotomy can be of benefit in tibial plateau fractures. **A:** Preoperative radiograph of an intracondylar fracture of the tibial plateau. **B:** Postoperative view after osteotomy of the lateral tibial condyle.

a good result after 5 years. Results of series vary because of the differences in patient population, surgical technique, and preexisting pathologic factors. The procedure should be considered in a patient who wants to maintain a more active lifestyle and would be willing to accept the possibility of some pain or loss of pain relief over time.

B. Osteotomy of the Hip

Certain unusual conditions of the hip can be treated with osteotomy to prevent or retard coxarthrosis. These include osteochondritis dissecans and other traumatic conditions that produce localized damage to the surface of the hip. Various biomechanical theories are proposed regarding the benefit of osteotomy of the pelvis and hip in decreasing the load on the hip. Although the theoretical arguments may be correct, in practical terms, the two reasons for performing this procedure are (1) a normal viable cartilage surface is moved to the weight-bearing area where previously there was degenerated, thinned articular cartilage; and (2) the biomechanical loads on the joints that cause pain are reduced. These can be reduced either through alteration of moment arms for muscles or, alternatively, by releasing or weakening

the muscles. Significantly lengthening or shortening a muscle reduces the force it can apply across a joint. In hip disorders, disease on one side of the hip joint cannot be addressed by an operation on the other side. For example, although it is tempting to use femoral osteotomy to treat acetabular dysplasia, only temporary relief may be obtained.

1. Treatment for acetabular dysplasia—Acetabular dysplasia as occurs in developmental dysplasia of the hip may be defined by the center edge angle. The normal center edge angle is 25–45 degrees; an angle of less than 20 degrees is definitely considered dysplastic (Figure 6–8). The anterior center edge angle can also demonstrate an acetabulum that is too open anteriorly; an angle of 17–20 degrees is considered the lower limit on the false profile view. There is also an increased acetabular index.

In individuals with a mature skeleton, limited pelvic osteotomies such as the Salter innominate or shelf procedure are not appropriate. These measurements are probably best considered in a three-dimensional view with CT.

To improve coverage and hip biomechanics significantly, an acetabular-reorienting procedure that also permits medialization is ideal. The Wagner spherical osteotomy

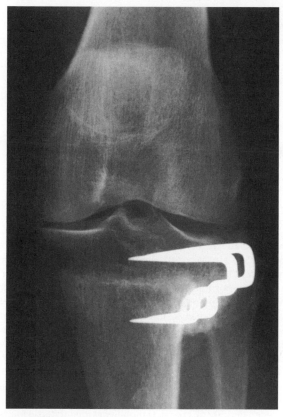

▲ **Figure 6–7.** High tibial osteotomy, showing staples holding the osteotomy in place.

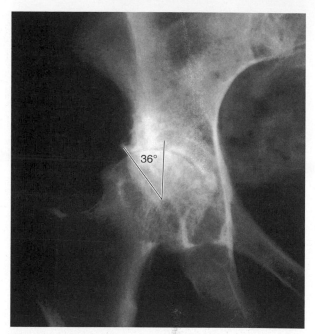

▲ **Figure 6–8.** Anteroposterior pelvis film demonstrating the center edge angle.

permits complete redirection of the acetabulum but does not permit medialization and is technically demanding. A triple osteotomy is useful in positioning the acetabulum but causes severe pelvic instability. The periacetabular osteotomy described by Ganz permits acetabular redirection and medialization but preserves the posterior column, minimizing instability.

2. Treatment of femoral disorders—Osteotomy of the femur can safely and reliably be performed in the intertrochanteric region, with the expectation of union. Osteotomy of the femoral neck is likely to compromise the blood supply to the femoral head as the deep branch of the medial femoral circumflex courses along the posterior aspect of the greater trochanter.

Intertrochanteric osteotomies of the femur of various types are described. The goal of osteotomy is removal of degenerated articular cartilage from the weight-bearing dome and replacement of it with more viable cartilage. This procedure may involve any of the three degrees of freedom: varus and valgus angle, internal and external rotation, and flexion and extension. It is necessary when planning these

procedures to be sure the osteotomy will provide an adequate ROM for the patient. These osteotomies have usefulness in very specific cases for osteoarthrosis, but their usefulness for osteonecrosis is extremely limited in the United States.

Feeley BT, Gallo RA, Sherman S, et al: Management of osteoarthritis of the knee in the active patient. *J Am Acad Orthop Surg* 2010;18:406. [PMID: 20595133]

Heijens E, Kornherr P, Meister C: The role of navigation in high tibial osteotomy: a study of 50 patients. *Orthopedics* 2009;32(Suppl 10):40. [PMID: 19835307]

Marker DR, Seyler TM, Ulrich SD, et al: Do modern techniques improve core decompression outcomes for hip osteonecrosis? *Clin Orthop Relat Res* 2008;466:1093. [PMID: 18392909]

Mont MA, Zywiel MG, Marker DR, et al: The natural history of untreated asymptomatic osteonecrosis of the femoral head: a systematic literature review. *J Bone Joint Surg Am* 2010;92:2165. [PMID: 20844158]

Santore RF, Turgeon TR, Phillips WF 3rd, et al: Pelvic and femoral osteotomy in the treatment of hip disease in the young adult. *Instr Course Lect* 2006;55:131. [PMID: 16958446]

Sherman C, Cabanela ME: Closing wedge osteotomy of the tibia and the femur in the treatment of gonarthrosis. *Int Orthop* 2010;34:173. [PMID: 19830426]

Sierra RJ, Trousdale RT, Ganz R, et al: Hip disease in the young active patient: evaluation and nonarthroplasty options. *J Am Acad Orthop Surg* 2008;16:689. [PMID: 19056918]

Van den Bekerom MP, Patt TW, Kleinhout MY, et al: Early complications after high tibial osteotomy: a comparison of two techniques. *J Knee Surg* 2008;21:68. [PMID: 18300676]

JOINT SALVAGE PROCEDURES

1. Arthrodesis

Arthrodesis is the creation of a bony union across a joint. The creation of a fibrous union across a joint with no motion is ankylosis. With bony union across a joint, motion of one bone on another is eliminated, relieving pain caused by arthritis. Although ankylosis may prevent observable motion, micromotion may be associated with significant pain. Ankylosis or arthrodesis may occur spontaneously, as in infection or ankylosing spondylitis, or may be surgically produced. The functional results of spontaneous arthrodesis are not ideal because the patient typically holds the joint in the position that causes minimum pain, which frequently is an inappropriate position for function. Although surgical arthrodesis can be created in almost any joint, including the spine, the most common joints fused are the ankle, knee, shoulder, and hip. The technique used in any of the joints follows the same general pattern. The articular surfaces are denuded of remaining articular cartilage and then placed together in the optimal position of function after shaping to achieve maximum contact between the two opposing surfaces. Bone grafting is frequently used, and some form of fixation, either internal (plates, rods, or screws) or external (external fixators or a cast), is used to immobilize the arthrodesis site in the optimal position (Table 6–5). After adequate healing, the rehabilitation process is begun. Multiple techniques of arthrodesis have been described for each joint.

▶ Ankle Arthrodesis

The orthopedic community generally considers arthrodesis of the tibiotalar joint to be a good operation for treatment of tibiotalar arthrosis. A well-done ankle arthrodesis results in freedom from pain and nearly normal walking ability. Perhaps the main reason that the ankle arthrodesis is regarded so highly, however, is that other options, such as total ankle replacement, are less viable.

The indications for ankle arthrodesis are as follows:

1. Degenerative arthrosis
2. Rheumatoid arthritis
3. Posttraumatic arthritis
4. Avascular necrosis of the talus
5. Neurologic disease resulting in an unstable ankle
6. Neuropathic ankle joint

The relative contraindications include degenerative joint disease in the subtalar and midtarsal joints.

The ankle arthrodesis can be performed through an anterior, lateral, or medial approach, and even posterior approaches are described. Arthroscopic techniques are now employed. The most common techniques are probably external fixation or internal screw fixation to achieve compression. Preparation of the ankle for arthrodesis is performed as mentioned earlier. Positioning of the ankle is important, with the talus in a neutral position or at an angle of 5 degrees of dorsiflexion. The midtarsal joints have a greater ROM in plantar flexion than in dorsiflexion, resulting in a more flexible foot. The talus is also displaced slightly posteriorly to make it easier for the patient to roll the foot over at the completion of the stance phase. A varus position is to be avoided because this restricts mobility at the midtarsal joints.

Nielsen KK, Linde F, Jensen NC: The outcome of arthroscopic and open surgery ankle arthrodesis: a comparative retrospective study on 107 patients. *Foot Ankle Surg* 2008;14:153. [PMID: 19083634]

Table 6–5. Optimal position of joints after arthrodesis.

Joint	Angle	Length	Other Consideration
Ankle	0° dorsiflexion 0–5° valgus of hindfoot 5–10° external rotation	Slight shortening	Talus displaced posteriorly
Knee	15° flexion 5–8° flexion	Slight shortening	—
Shoulder	20–30° flexion 20–40° abduction (lateral border of scapula) 25–40° internal rotation	—	Patient's hand should be able to touch the head and face
Hip	25° flexion 0–5° abduction (measured between the shaft and a line through the ischia) 0–5° external rotation	Slight shortening	Do *not* destroy abductor mechanism

Knee Arthrodesis

Knee arthrodesis is seldom done for primary problems and generally done as the last resort for other problems. Indications for the procedure include infection, such as tuberculosis, neuropathic joint secondary to syphilis or diabetes, and loss of quadriceps function. The latter is a relative indication for arthrodesis because joint mobility can be maintained without quadriceps function, and joint stability can be obtained through the use of orthosis, which locks the joint in the fully extended position but can be unlocked for sitting. Although knee arthrodesis is usually successful and provides pain-free weight bearing, it is associated with other problems, especially in tall people. Sitting in airplanes, movie theaters, and even automobiles may be difficult. The most common indication for knee arthrodesis at the present time is failed total knee arthroplasty, usually because of infection. In a patient who wishes to maintain an active lifestyle, such as hunting on rough ground or performing manual labor, a knee arthrodesis is a viable alternative. The relative contraindications include bilateral disease or a problem such as an above-knee amputation of the other leg. In such a case, it would be extremely difficult for a person to arise from a chair with an arthrodesis on the contralateral side.

The technique of arthrodesis varies with the problem being treated. After infection, particularly when it is associated with total knee replacement, bone loss is often moderate to severe. Severe cases of bone loss may require distraction osteogenesis to achieve enough bone to prevent disabling shortening. This technique can also be used to get fusion of the femur to the tibia. Cancellous bone from the distal femur and proximal tibia may be nearly nonexistent, and external fixation may be necessary to obtain adequate immobilization for arthrodesis. For less severe cases, intramedullary rod fixation may be indicated, particularly if the infection is under control. Similarly, use of double plates at 90 degrees is a viable method of immobilization. Frequently, iliac crest bone grafting is necessary to stimulate healing. Although bone loss often makes it necessary to shorten the extremity, some shortening (2–3 cm) is desirable to prevent a circumduction gait after fusion. The knee should be positioned at 10–15 degrees of flexion and at the normal valgus alignment of 5–8 degrees, if possible.

Parvizi J, Adeli B, Zmistowski B, et al: Periprosthetic joint infection: treatment options. *Orthopedics* 2010;33:659. [PMID: 20839679]

Spina M, Gualdrini G, Fosco M, et al: Knee arthrodesis with the Ilizarov external fixator as a treatment for septic failure of knee arthroplasty. *J Orthop Traumatol* 2010;11:81. [PMID: 20425133]

Elbow Arthrodesis

Elbow arthrodesis is an uncommon procedure. Loss of elbow motion may be particularly disabling. Thus, the indications for arthrodesis are few, and few are performed because fusion causes severe functional limitations. To perform activities of daily living, a flexion arc of 100 degrees from 30 degrees of extension to 130 degrees of flexion is required. A range of 100 degrees for pronation and supination is also required. Painful arthrosis in a patient who is willing to accept the tradeoff between stability and loss of motion is the indication for arthrodesis. Salvage of infectious processes, such as tuberculosis or fungus or bacterial infections after joint replacement, are also indications for arthrodesis.

Several techniques are described, but the relative rarity of the operation prevents recommendation of one particular method. One report recommends screw fixation. Resection of the radial head may be necessary to allow for pronation and supination. The position of fusion is 90 degrees.

Gallo RA, Payatakes A, Sotereanos DG: Surgical options for the arthritic elbow. *J Hand Surg Am* 2008;33:746. [PMID: 18590859]

Irvine GB, Gregg PJ: A method of elbow arthrodesis: brief report. *J Bone Joint Surg Br* 1989;71:145. [PMID: 2914994]

Morrey BF, Askew LJ, Chao EY: A biomechanical study of normal elbow motion. *J Bone Joint Surg Am* 1981;62:872. [PMID: 7240327]

Shoulder Arthrodesis

Paralysis of the deltoid muscle and sepsis after an arthroplasty are possible indications for shoulder arthrodesis. Rarely, arthrodesis may be used to stabilize the shoulder after failed reconstruction procedures. Obtaining fusion may be a relatively difficult process because of the very long lever arm on the shoulder joint. This is accentuated by the position of fusion, which optimally places the arm in abduction, forward flexion, and internal rotation. In the correct position of fusion, the hand can reach the mouth. Before the advent of comprehensive internal fixation devices, intraarticular and extraarticular arthrodeses were performed to provide a reasonable probability of obtaining fusion.

Rigid internal fixation with a plate and screws can be done without postoperative external immobilization. The patient is placed in the lateral decubitus position. The incision is made over the spine of the scapula, over the acromion, and down the lateral aspect of the humerus. The surface of the glenohumeral joint and the undersurface of the acromion are cleaned of residual cartilage and cortical bone to provide as much contact as possible with the arm in the appropriate position (see Table 6–5). A broad bone plate or pelvic reconstruction plate is then used to fix the humerus to the scapula. The bone plate is fixed to the spine of the scapula and the shaft of the humerus and bent into the appropriate position. Additional fixation may be obtained by placing another plate posteriorly. Bone grafting may be necessary for defects. Rigid fixation must be obtained. After surgery, a soft dressing is used until pain is controlled. A shoulder spica cast is preferred for immobilization by some surgeons. Exercises are begun to gently obtain scapular motion if no cast is used.

A modification of this technique that uses an external fixator to neutralize forces on interfragmentary screws has good results. Functional results are varied and depend on the position of fusion. Overhead work or work with the arm abducted is not possible. Excessive internal and external rotation must be avoided.

Johnson CA, Healy WL, Brooker AF Jr, et al: External fixation shoulder arthrodesis. *Clin Orthop Relat Res* 1986;211:219. [PMID: 3769260]

Safran O, Iannotti JP: Arthrodesis of the shoulder. *J Am Acad Orthop Surg* 2006;14:145. [PMID: 16520365]

Scalise JJ, Iannotti JP: Glenohumeral arthrodesis after failed prosthetic shoulder arthroplasty. Surgical technique. *J Bone Joint Surg Am* 2009;91:30. [PMID: 19255198]

▶ Hip Arthrodesis

Arthrodesis of the hip, as of other joints, produces a relatively pain-free stable joint that allows the patient to perform heavy labor. The disadvantage of hip arthrodesis in a young person who performs heavy labor is that over a period of time, degenerative disk disease of the lumbar spine and degenerative arthrosis of the ipsilateral knee frequently occur, even with optimal position of the arthrodesis. In fact, an indication for converting a hip fusion to a total hip arthroplasty is incapacitating back or knee pain.

The most obvious indication for arthrodesis of the hip is tuberculosis. Chronic osteomyelitis is a relative indication. Contraindications to arthrodesis include limited motion of the ipsilateral knee or degenerative arthrosis of the ipsilateral knee, as well as significant degenerative lumbar spine disease and arthrosis of the contralateral hip. Perhaps the biggest problem in performing a hip arthrodesis in a patient with adequate indications is obtaining agreement from the patient. Because joint replacement offers mobility, early rehabilitation, and a less extensive operation, patients are reluctant to consider the potential problems of hip arthrodesis. This is particularly true when total hip arthroplasty is performed in professional athletes, permitting some of them to continue in sports. Because of these factors, hip arthrodesis is now a relatively uncommon operation.

Multiple techniques are described for performing hip arthrodesis. Truly rigid fixation is difficult to achieve, and cast immobilization after surgery is usually needed. During the fusion procedure, care should be taken to preserve the abductors, so future reconstructive procedures may be performed if desired. The crucial aspect of the operation is fusing the hip in the appropriate position. The optimal position is slight flexion (25 degrees) from the normal position of the pelvis and spine, slight external rotation (5 degrees), and neutral abduction and adduction. Previously, the hip was placed in abduction, producing a very abnormal gait with additional stress on the lumbar spine. A position of neutral to slight abduction minimizes this problem because the body's center of gravity when the patient is in a one-legged stance is moved closer to the foot. Too much flexion makes both walking and lying in bed difficult, and too little flexion makes sitting difficult. Too much external rotation forces the knee joint to move in a plane oblique from that defined by the collateral and cruciate ligaments.

Beaule PE, Matta JM, Mast JW: Hip arthrodesis: current indications and techniques. *J Am Acad Orthop Surg* 2002;10:249. [PMID: 15089074]

Stover MD, Beaulé PE, Matta JM, et al: Hip arthrodesis: a procedure for the new millennium? *Clin Orthop Relat Res* 2004;418:126. [PMID: 15043103]

2. Resection Arthroplasty

Resection arthroplasty, or excisional arthroplasty, is a procedure that is applied primarily to the hip, the elbow, and, more recently, the knee. Resection arthroplasty, or a modification called **fascial arthroplasty,** was a procedure used in the elbow for many years. Resection arthroplasty of the hip is also called **Girdlestone pseudoarthrosis** and dates back to 1923. Resection arthroplasty of the knee is a relatively new procedure that is used when infection compromises total knee replacement. Similarly, Girdlestone pseudoarthrosis is performed with increasing frequency as an intervening, sometimes permanent treatment for infection following total hip arthroplasty.

▶ Resection Hip Arthroplasty

Resection arthroplasty of the hip produces a relatively pain-free joint with reasonably good motion. It is indicated as a primary procedure when ankylosis causes the hip to be placed in an unsuitable position; such patients would otherwise be at high risk for dislocation or infection with a total hip arthroplasty. Spinal cord injury, head injury, and, perhaps, severe Parkinson disease would be diagnoses that might warrant primary resection arthroplasty. Disadvantages of the procedure result from lack of mechanical continuity between the femur and the pelvis; this causes an abnormal gait and the need for support with a cane or other device, and shortening occurs with each step. Patients who previously had infection following total hip replacement usually have the most stable hip joints because dense scar tissue has formed. The procedure can be very helpful in reambulating wheelchair-bound patients in whom peroneal care is very difficult.

For infection compromising total hip replacement, resection arthroplasty is accomplished by removing all of the cement, the prosthesis, any necrotic bone, and the soft tissue.

In primary resection arthroplasty, the procedure is more of a reconstructive procedure in which the femoral head and neck are removed flush with the intertrochanteric line and the capsule is reconstructed to help provide some stability of the hip. Traction with a pin in the tibia is frequently used for variable periods to maintain leg length.

▶ Resection Knee Arthroplasty

Resection arthroplasty of the knee has a much less satisfactory functional result. After removal of an infected knee prosthesis, there is usually significant bone loss and the knee is quite unstable. Bracing improves the condition only modestly, and the patient still requires crutches or a walker to ambulate.

▶ Resection Elbow Arthroplasty

Resection arthroplasty or fascial arthroplasty of the elbow is one means of managing ankylosis after trauma or infection. Resection arthroplasty may be performed for failure of total elbow arthroplasty resulting from sepsis. Resection arthroplasty in the patient with rheumatoid osteoarthritis should be discouraged because one of the problems associated with the procedure is instability. The rheumatoid patient frequently depends on the upper extremity to ambulate with walking aids. Interpositional arthroplasty, using fascia or split-thickness skin grafts, was thought to reduce resorption of bone, but the additional benefit of the interpositional tissue is doubtful. Although resection arthroplasty frequently relieves pain, instability is a major problem and bracing is required in most cases. With the availability of elbow arthroplasty, this procedure is rarely performed.

Cheung EV, Adams R, Morrey BF: Primary osteoarthritis of the elbow: current treatment options. *J Am Acad Orthop Surg* 2008;16:77. [PMID: 18252838]

Manjon-Cabeza Subirat JM, Moreno Palacios JA, Mozo Muriel AP, et al: Functional outcomes after resection of the hip arthroplasty (Girdlestone technique). *Rev Esp Geriatr Gerontol* 2008;43:13. [PMID: 18684383]

JOINT REPLACEMENT PROCEDURES

1. Hemiarthroplasty

Hemiarthroplasty is the replacement of only one side of a diarthrodial joint. The procedure is indicated for displaced fractures of the femoral neck or four-part fractures of the humeral head, but there are other indications in adult reconstructive surgery. In both the shoulder and the hip, osteonecrosis may result in collapse of the humeral or femoral articulating surface, with sparing of the glenoid or acetabulum. In the hip, nonunion of the femoral neck after open reduction and internal fixation may also be an indication for endoprosthetic replacement. In either joint, pathologic fracture or tumor may be an indication. Contraindications

include active infection, rheumatoid arthritis, and possibly the patient's age. Endoprosthetic replacement in a young individual is certain to result, with time, in destruction of the articular surface that contacts the prosthesis. This may, however, take many years, and the patient may have a serviceable joint in the intervening period.

The choice of prosthesis depends on factors such as life expectancy, cost, and physiologic demand. For the shoulder, a cemented prosthesis should probably be modular to permit conversion to total shoulder replacement at a later date without removal of the stem, should that become necessary. Similar concerns for the hip apply. The femoral head can be replaced with a unipolar or bipolar prosthesis. The bipolar prosthesis allows motion to occur between the acetabulum and the prosthesis, as well as between the prosthesis and the articulating surface of the metal femoral head. This articulation is metal or ceramic on plastic and certain to produce debris from wear that may be detrimental to the durability of the hip prosthesis. Selection of a monopolar prosthesis, however, must not compromise conversion of the hemiarthroplasty to a total hip arthroplasty, should this become necessary. Hemiarthroplasty of the hip has been shown to be preferable to a total hip replacement in cases of displaced, intracapsular femoral neck fracture. The operative technique is quite similar to that of total joint replacement for each joint. The main difference in the hip is that the capsule is usually repaired after hemiarthroplasty. A posterolateral approach is most commonly used in the hip, although an anterolateral approach may be preferred in a patient with associated mental problems that may limit postoperative cooperation. If the posterolateral approach is used in such patients, a knee immobilizer may be necessary to prevent hip flexion that might lead to dislocation.

2. Total Joint Arthroplasty

Joint replacement surgery became a viable treatment for arthritic afflictions of joints when the low-friction hip arthroplasty was developed by Sir John Charnley in the 1960s. This procedure consisted of the articulation of a metal femoral head on an ultrahigh-molecular-weight polyethylene (UHMWPE) acetabular component, with both components fixed in place with acrylic cement (polymethylmethacrylate [PMMA]). The long-term results are quite satisfactory, and the concept is now applied to other joints with variable success. Knee replacement, shoulder replacement, and elbow replacement now have satisfactory results and are routine when the indications for surgery are appropriate. Other arthroplasties, such as the ankle, wrist, and first metatarsophalangeal joint, are less successful. In fairness, the application of technology to these joints is not at the level applied to other joints. Success of all arthroplasties depends on the skill of the surgeon, the surgeon's understanding of the basic biomechanics underlying the joint function, the design of the prosthesis, and the technical equipment used to insert the prosthesis.

The design of the prosthesis is an evolutionary process that depends on laboratory and clinical experience. Hip replacement surgery, performed often, is highly successful. Less frequently performed arthroplasties, such as elbow replacement, are associated with less clinical and laboratory experience.

▶ Total Hip Arthroplasty

The original Charnley total hip arthroplasty was a stainless steel femoral prosthesis with a small collar, a rectangular cross section, and a 22-mm femoral head. The acetabular component was a UHMWPE cup. Both components were cemented into place with acrylic bone cement. Since then, an entire industry has evolved to produce new designs for hip components, including different head sizes (22, 25, 25.4, 28, 32, 35, and 36 mm); different femoral component lengths (ranging from 110 to 160 mm for standard prostheses); different cross sections (square, round, oval, I-beam); a porous coating for bone ingrowth attachment; and metal backing for the acetabulum (cemented or porous coated). The two generic designs that evolved from experience with bone attachment technique are the porous ingrowth and cement fixation prostheses.

A variant of total hip replacement, hip surface replacement, was popularized in the 1980s, but there were problems with design, which resulted in a high failure rate and caused it to be withdrawn from the market. Those designs used a spherical metal shell cemented on the femoral side with a polyethylene (UHMWPE) shell cemented on the acetabular side. The impetus for surface replacement is preservation of bone stock and lower dislocation rate, which has encouraged their use in younger patients. With the advent of metal on metal bearings, surface replacement has again become an alternative to total hip replacement. The current designs use a cemented, spherical shell with a small stem on the femoral side and an ingrowth metal shell on the acetabular side. Early results have been promising, but one design has been pulled from the market due to wear problems.

A. Indications

The indications for hip arthroplasty are incapacitating arthritis of the hip combined with appropriate physical and radiographic findings. The historical data that justify consideration of hip replacement surgery include pain requiring medication stronger than aspirin, inability to walk more than a few blocks without stopping, pain following activity, pain that wakes the patient at night, difficulty with shoes and socks or foot care such as cutting nails, and difficulty in climbing stairs. It is good practice to use a clinical rating score to evaluate these historical data (Table 6–6).

Physical examination typically demonstrates a limited ROM, pain at extremes of motion, a positive Trendelenburg test, a limp, and groin or anterior thigh pain with active straight leg raising.

Radiographs demonstrate loss of joint space and other findings consistent with the cause of the disorder.

Noteworthy features requiring special considerations for surgery are dysplasia of the acetabulum, protrusio acetabuli, and proximal femoral deformity or the presence of metal implants from previous operations.

After consideration of the lifestyle requirements of the patient, the surgeon may suggest this procedure as a means of alleviating pain, which is the main indication for hip replacement surgery. Other reconstructive procedures should be considered, including arthrodesis, osteotomy, and hemiarthroplasty. When selecting a procedure, one should consider the patient's goals in terms of work and leisure activity. A young person who performs heavy labor and has unilateral traumatic arthritis may be best served by arthrodesis, unless a change to a more sedentary occupation is anticipated. A 50-year-old bank executive who does not ski, play tennis, or ride horses but does swim and bicycle will probably have the best results with hip arthroplasty.

A choice must be made between cemented and uncemented arthroplasty, with the uncemented acetabular component nearly universally indicated. Its advantages include a consistently pain-free result, long-lasting fixation, and modularity to permit latitude in selecting head size and acetabular polyethylene component offset designs. Its disadvantages include the need for metal backing of the polyethylene liner, which may increase wear, and the possibility of dissociation of the plastic component from the metal. A cemented acetabular component manufactured from UHMWPE is usually reserved for an individual with a life expectancy of 10 years or less. The indications for an uncemented femoral component vary with the surgeon but usually depend on the age of the patient and the quality of bone, with younger patients or patients with type A or B bone most likely to benefit from the porous-coated prosthesis. The surface replacement is an alternative to total hip replacement with a cemented femoral component and ingrowth acetabular component. Past problems with surface replacement and the reports of serum metal ion increases suggest caution in recommending this device.

B. Surgical Technique

Certain aspects of hip replacement surgery apply to all arthroplasty techniques, including cement technique and bone surface preparation.

1. Posterolateral approach—The most common approach for total hip arthroplasty is the posterolateral approach. After administration of anesthesia and placement of a thromboembolic stocking and intermittent compression stocking on the unaffected limb, the patient is rolled into the lateral decubitus position, with the affected side superior. Draping should leave the entire leg free and extending above the iliac crest. Kidney rests are used to support the pelvis at the pubis and the sacrum, and bony prominences should be protected. The incision is outlined on the skin before the skin is completely covered with an adhesive drape. By flexing the hip to 45 degrees, the incision can be made in line with

Table 6–6. Harris hip evaluation (modified).

I. Pain (44 possible)
  A. None or ignores it...
  B. Slight, occasional, no compromise in activities..44
  C. Mild pain, no effect on average activities, rarely moderate pain; with unusual activity may take aspirin.........40
  D. Moderate pain, tolerable, but makes concessions to pain; some limitation of ordinary activity or work;
     may require occasional pain medicine stronger than aspirin..30
  E. Marked pain, serious limitation of activities..20
  F. Totally disabled, crippled, pain in bed, bedridden...10
                                                                                                                             0
II. Function (47 possible)
  A. Gait (33 possible)
    1. Limp
       a. None..11
       b. Slight..8
       c. Moderate...5
       d. Severe...0
    2. Support
       a. None..11
       b. Cane for long walks...7
       c. Cane most of the time..5
       d. One crutch...3
       e. Two canes..2
       f. Two crutches..0
       g. Not able to walk (specify reason)..0
    3. Distance walked
       a. Unlimited...11
       b. Six blocks...8
       c. Two or three blocks..5
       d. Indoors only...2
       e. Bed and chair...0
  B. Activities (14 possible)
    1. Stairs
       a. Normally without using a railing...4
       b. Normally using a railing..2
       c. In any manner..1
       d. Unable to do stairs...0
    2. Shoes and socks
       a. With ease...4
       b. With difficulty..2
       c. Unable...0
    3. Sitting
       a. Comfortably in ordinary chair 1 hour...5
       b. On a high chair for one-half hour..3
       c. Unable to sit comfortably in any chair...0
    4. Enter public transportation...1
  C. Range of Motion   R   L
     Flexion
     Flexion contracture   ____   ____
     Abduction   ____   ____
     Adduction   ____   ____
     External rotation   ____   ____
     Internal rotation   ____   ____
  D. Location of pain
     Groin
     Thigh   ____   ____
     Buttock   ____   ____

the femur from approximately 10 cm proximal to the tip of the trochanter to 10 cm distal to the tip of the trochanter.

Alternatively, with the hip in the extended position, the incision is made from 10 cm distal to the tip of the trochanter extending proximally along the line of the trochanter and then curving posteriorly at approximately a 45-degree angle for another 10 cm. The incision is deepened to show the fascia lata and the gluteus maximus. An incision is made in the fascia lata directly lateral and extended proximally into the gluteus maximus, which is split in line with its fibers. A Charnley retractor is placed, and fat overlying the external rotators is removed. After putting the femur into internal rotation, the external rotators (piriformis, gemelli, obturator internus, and quadratus femoris) are tagged with sutures for reattachment and removed from their attachments at the trochanter. The gluteus minimus is separated from the capsule and preserved and protected, and a capsulectomy is performed. Alternatively, portions of the posterior capsule can be reflected for later reattachment. If the patient is not paralyzed with nondepolarizing muscle relaxant agents, excision of the capsule with electrocautery signals whether the sciatic nerve is particularly closely applied to the posterior of the acetabulum. The sciatic nerve must be identified and protected throughout the procedure if there is electrical transmission. Internal rotation of the flexed hip dislocates the hip, and the femoral head is delivered into the operative field. Using an appropriate template, the femoral head is resected with an oscillating saw. The femur is then externally rotated, and Taylor retractors are placed anteriorly and posteriorly to permit visualization of the acetabulum. The acetabulum is medialized, if appropriate, when medial osteophytes are present. Anterior osteophytes, if present, are removed under direct visualization. Reaming of the acetabulum is performed until a good bed of bleeding subchondral bone is obtained; progressive reamers are usually used. At this point, techniques diverge based on whether a cemented or an uncemented cup is used.

If a cemented cup is used, multiple holes with a diameter of $1/4$–$3/8$ in are drilled in the acetabulum to provide firm cement interdigitation. One of the commercially available techniques that prevents bottoming out of the acetabular cup should be used, so the medial cement mantle will be adequate. The position of the cup is determined with trials, using the native acetabulum for guidance and radiograph if there is any concern about positioning. The cup is cemented into place after the acetabular bone is prepared with pulsatile lavage, epinephrine-soaked sponges, and pressurization of the cement.

If an uncemented cup is used, reaming progresses to a diameter 1–2 mm smaller than the actual size of the cup to be implanted. The cup is impacted into place, ensuring appropriate positioning. Fixation is achieved with screws or pegs, as specified by the manufacturer. A trial plastic component is inserted, and attention is returned to the femur.

The hip is internally rotated, flexed to approximately 80 degrees, and adducted, so the cut femoral neck is presented to the surgeon. Homan retractors may be used to help elevate the amputated femoral neck into the wound. A box chisel is then used to remove the femoral neck laterally. The canal is broached with a curet to provide an indication of the direction of the intramedullary canal. The femoral canal is then broached with increasing sizes of broaches, until all weak cancellous bone is removed. The prosthesis size is determined, and a cement restrictor is placed 2 cm distal to the final position of the stem tip. The canal is prepared for cementing with pulsatile lavage, medullary canal brushing, and sponges soaked with hydrogen peroxide or epinephrine. The cement is prepared and centrifuged or vacuum mixed and inserted into the femoral canal with a cement gun. The cement is pressurized, and the prosthesis is inserted into appropriate anteversion (approximately 10 degrees) and held in position until the cement cures. When the appropriate broach, as indicated by preoperative templating, is reached, a trial femoral prosthesis is inserted, the neck length is checked, and the prosthesis is reduced into position. ROM is tested at 90 degrees of flexion and should be stable to 40–45 degrees of internal rotation. External rotation to 40 degrees in the fully extended position must be obtained without impingement on the femoral neck posteriorly. Proper myofascial tension is assessed by telescoping the hip at 45 degrees (approximately 3 or 4 mm). Proper leg length is usually achieved when the rectus femoris tightness (flexion of the knee with the hip extended) is similar to prior to surgery. A further check on leg lengths can be made by comparing the center of the femoral head preoperatively with the proximal tip of the trochanter to trochanter-prosthesis center distance with the prosthesis in place. Measuring devices are designed to measure leg lengths, but up to 1 cm of discrepancy can still occur. An extended lip on the UHMWPE component may provide additional stability but may form a fulcrum on which the head may be levered out. The prosthesis trial is removed, and the permanent polyethylene component is put into place in the acetabular metallic shell. The femoral canal is then prepared for cementing.

After the cement hardens, a trial femoral head is used to put the hip through a second ROM. The optimal neck length is selected, and the appropriate prosthetic component is impacted into place. When combining modular components held together with a Morse-type taper, the manufacturers' components should not be mixed. The bore in the femoral head is placed on the trunnion and twisted and impacted into place with several sharp blows. The acetabulum is cleaned of debris, the femoral head is reduced, and the wound is closed. The external rotators are reattached with sutures placed through bone while the hip is in external rotation and abduction. The fascia is closed with interrupted sutures.

The design and insertion technique of the uncemented femoral components are somewhat variable and therefore are not described here, but a typical anatomic design uncemented hip is shown in Figure 6–9. This type of stem is inserted after reaming and broaching to size.

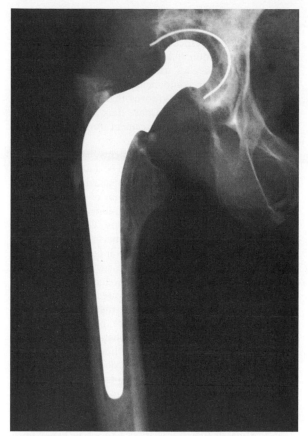

▲ **Figure 6–9.** Radiograph of a standard design cemented arthroplasty with Co/Cr-polyethylene bearing surface.

Abbreviated mini incisions for the posterolateral approach to the hip are described. These generally use a small portion of the routine incision but are carefully placed to optimize visualization of the hip. One such technique places the incision posterior to the trochanter, about 8–10 cm in total length, with 4–5 cm proximal to the tip and 4–5 cm distal to the tip of the trochanter. This technique is becoming more prevalent among surgeons.

2. Lateral approach—The lateral approach to the hip is performed with a trochanteric osteotomy after the fascia of the tensor fascia lata and gluteus maximus are entered. The patient may be in the supine position with a bump under the hip or in the lateral position. Prior to osteotomy, the trochanter is mobilized, and the trochanteric osteotomy is performed with an osteotome or a Gigli saw. The gluteus minimus is peeled off the capsule as the trochanter is mobilized proximally. After capsulectomy, the femoral head is dislocated anteriorly. The procedure is essentially identical from this point on until the trochanter is reattached. Various

modifications of trochanteric osteotomy techniques are described. The abductor mechanism is extremely important in preserving the stability of the hip as well as the gait. Thus, extreme care must be taken to reattach the trochanter when the procedure is completed, so reliable union is achieved. Even in the best of hands, approximately one in 20 trochanters fails to unite, although the number of people who have disability or pain from a fibrous union is much lower. If wires are used to reattach the trochanter, they should be biocompatible with the prosthetic component, and a minimum of three should be used to achieve adequate fixation.

Trochanteric osteotomy is seldom used except for anatomic variations such as previous fracture that make other approaches difficult.

3. Anterolateral approach (Watson-Jones approach)—The interval between the gluteus medius muscle and the tensor fascia lata is used proximally to gain access to the femoral neck and hip joint. The patient is in the supine position, with a bump under the buttock. The skin incision follows the shaft of the femur distally and curves slightly anteriorly proximally. The fascia is incised in line with the skin incision and proximally splits the interval between the tensor fascia lata and the gluteus medius. The tensor fascia lata is then retracted anteriorly, and the gluteus medius is retracted superiorly and laterally. Because the fibers of the gluteus medius and minimus tend to run anteriorly, particularly in the osteoarthritic hip with destruction and shortening, these fibers must be released to provide access to the hip joint. The hip is externally rotated. The anterior capsule is incised, and the hip joint can then be dislocated. Osteotomy of the femoral neck proceeds at the appropriate level. Capsulotomy is performed, retractors are placed to provide acetabular exposure, and hip replacement is performed. The femur during this procedure is externally rotated. Care must be taken in exposing the acetabulum to prevent damage to the femoral nerve and femoral muscles.

4. Other approaches and techniques—Many variations of standard approaches are used for hip replacement including minimally invasive anterior, posterior, and anterolateral, with proponents espousing the benefits of each technique. The anterior, between the tensor fascia lata and sartorius muscles, and anterolateral approaches seem to offer the advantages of lower dislocation rate and ease of obtaining correct leg length. However, lateral femoral cutaneous nerve palsies are a problem. The posterior approaches may have a higher dislocation rate. Satisfactory results can be obtained with any approach in the hands of an experienced surgeon. Data have shown that proper prosthetic placement, especially the acetabular component, is critical to long-term survival of the implant. This is particularly true for ceramic-on-ceramic and metal-on-metal bearing surfaces. To achieve optimal placement of components, computer-aided surgical navigation has become available and is being used on a trial basis by many surgeons. These techniques can significantly lengthen surgical times, require additional or extended incisions, and increase costs as a balance to the gains in accuracy.

C. Implants

The two basic types of total hip replacement are cemented and uncemented. The bearing surfaces for both are the same, either cobalt chromium alloy, ceramic (alumina or zirconia), or an oxidized zirconium surface (which is chemically a ceramic zirconia surface), articulating with a UHMWPE bearing surface. The femoral stem replacement may be cobalt chromium or titanium alloy, either of which is also used for the metal backing of the acetabulum. Titanium is poorly suited to cemented applications in hip arthroplasty because it is less stiff than cobalt-chrome (and stainless steel), and therefore transmits greater stresses to the cement column.

The femoral component should be designed to provide intrinsic torsional stability without having sharp edges that would create stress concentration sites in the bone cement. A matte surface should be created to allow some mechanical interlocking with the cement, although currently this is controversial, and some surgeons recommend a polished surface. Adequate offset is necessary to restore the mechanical advantage of the abductors.

The choice of material for the femoral head is a trade-off between cost and theoretical advantages. The harder, wettable surface of ceramic heads theoretically results in less production of debris from wear and longer service of the hip replacement without loosening, but the cost is two to three times that of an equivalent-sized cobalt chromium (Co/Cr) head. The ceramic head also has a small chance of fracture, which can have significant ramifications for the patient, requiring another surgical procedure to correct the problem. Thus, in most individuals undergoing total hip arthroplasty, a Co/Cr head is probably optimal. In younger patients, the increased cost of a ceramic head may be warranted. At a higher cost than the Co/Cr, but lower than the ceramic femoral head, is the oxidized zirconium head which will not fracture, but may offer the advantages of lower wear. Femoral heads are available now in 22-, 26-, 28-, 32-, and 36-mm sizes. One clinical investigation of total hip replacements showed that 26- and 28-mm heads are associated with the least amount of linear and volumetric wear. A head of 22 mm may be necessary for patients with smaller acetabular sockets to provide adequate thickness of the polyethylene bearing surface. A minimum of 6 mm, preferably 8 mm or more, is suggested to lower the contact stress on the polyethylene and thereby reduce wear.

New bearing surfaces for the articulation of the hip joint are becoming popular. The possibilities include ceramic on ceramic (COC), Co/Cr on Co/Cr (metal on metal [MOM]), and ceramic or Co/Cr on radiation cross-linked polyethylene. The COC and MOM couples have been shown to be very sensitive to surgical placement of the acetabular component. More verticality of the cup can lead to higher wear, and squeaking of the bearing surface has been seen in a significant percentage of cases, a higher rate in COC than MOM. The impetus for this change is the possibility of lower wear debris. These articulation couples require long-term follow-up to determine if they will live up to their promise.

No evidence justifies use of a metal backing on the cemented acetabular component. Other design considerations to avoid are deep grooves that might evolve into cracks in the PMMA. The surface must be rough enough to allow the cup to bond to the cement through mechanical interlock.

Uncemented acetabular components have a spherical outer surface with at least one hole to permit the surgeon to determine if the prosthesis is fully impacted into place. The shell should have a minimum of 3 mm of metal to reduce the risk of fatigue failure. Cobalt chromium alloy or titanium alloy appears to be equally efficacious. The inner surface should lock the polyethylene in some fashion to reliably limit rotation and dissociation. The inner surface should be the mate of the polyethylene outer surface to reduce the chance of cold flow of the plastic as well as wear from relative motion. Recommended materials are listed in Table 6–7.

Design considerations for the uncemented femoral component are unclear at present. Use of porous coating, hydroxyapatite, or tricalcium phosphate coating is driven by manufacturing concerns and prosthesis strength requirements rather than an understanding of the biologic principles of hip replacement. Three design factors are important: (1) If a prosthesis is excessively stiff in relation to the bone to which it is attached, proximal osteopenia may result from "stress shielding" or "stress bypassing" of the bone; (2) approximately anatomic shape is appropriate to maximize the bone–prosthesis contact and reduce contact stress; and (3) stiffer prostheses seem to be associated with more pain in the thigh. Therefore, strategies to reduce stiffness seem appropriate. These factors are addressed by using titanium alloy as opposed to cobalt chromium alloy, but other factors may surface to affect this choice. Creating slots or grooves to reduce the torsional and bending stiffness also seems to be effective in reducing stiffness and resulting thigh pain.

D. Complications

Any major surgery is associated with a certain incidence of complications, which is certainly true for total hip arthroplasty. The surgeon must recognize these complications in a timely manner and treat them appropriately. The most common complications include deep venous thrombosis (DVT), fracture or perforation of the femoral shaft, infection, instability (dislocation), heterotopic bone formation, and nerve palsies.

1. Deep venous thrombosis—Although some morbidity results from DVT, the real risk is pulmonary embolism, which is occasionally fatal. The incidence of DVT is high, but the incidence of fatal pulmonary emboli fortunately is low, in the range of 0.3%. The high incidence of DVT during hip replacement surgery is related to femoral vein damage from

Table 6–7. Preferred materials for total hip replacement.

Component	Material	Alternative Material
Uncemented femoral component	Titanium alloy	Cobalt chromium alloy
Cemented femoral component	Cobalt chromium alloy (forged)	Cast cobalt chromium alloy, titanium alloy
Femoral head	Cobalt chromium alloy	Zirconia, alumina, oxidized zirconium alloy
Cemented acetabulum bearing surface	UHMWPE component (no metal backing)	Metal shell with UHMWPE liner (revision)
Uncemented acetabulum bearing surface	UHMWPE with metal ingrowth outer shell	Ceramic or metal bearing surface with ingrowth outer shell
Acetabulum ingrowth	Titanium alloy, cobalt chromium	—
surface for acetabular shell	Cobalt chromium alloy	

UHMWPE, ultrahigh-molecular-weight polyethylen.

manipulation or retraction, intraoperative or postoperative venous stasis caused by immobility and limb swelling, and a hypercoagulable state directly resulting from the surgical trauma to the patient. Certain factors are recognized as predisposing the patient to higher risk for DVT, including a prior history of pulmonary embolus, estrogen treatment, preexisting cancer, older (>60 years) age of the patient, and length of the operative procedure, one factor that is under the surgeon's control.

Pharmacologic and mechanical measures are used to reduce the risk of DVT. The American College of Chest Physicians recommends at least 10 days of pharmacologic prophylaxis with low-molecular-weight heparin, fondaparinux, or warfarin. Recently, the U.S. Food and Drug Administration (FDA) approved rivaroxaban, an oral thrombin inhibitor, for DVT prophylaxis, which may become a standard for DVT prophylaxis. The National Institutes of Health Consensus Conference concluded that mechanical measures such as intermittent pneumatic compression (IPC) provide adequate prophylaxis for patients who are mobilized quickly, whereas anticoagulation therapy is recommended for those expected to undergo prolonged bed rest. Recent studies suggest that adequate mechanical measures may be used for postoperative prophylaxis, which is accomplished with a portable IPC device. Because DVT can lead to a catastrophic outcome, preventive measures are indicated starting in the presurgical area. The patient should wear an antiembolic stocking on the unaffected extremity, and both extremities can be treated with intermittent pneumatic compression during the operative procedure. Following surgery, a low-molecular-weight heparin (enoxaparin or dalteparin) is the treatment of choice. Patients who develop pulmonary embolus should receive routine treatment with heparin followed by warfarin.

2. Nerve palsies—Three degrees of nerve injury are recognized. In order of increasing severity, these are neurapraxia,

in which conduction is disrupted; axonotmesis, in which the neuron is affected but not the myelin sheath; and neurotmesis, in which the nerve is completely disrupted, as in laceration. In total hip arthroplasty, the most common injuries are neurapraxia and axonotmesis. Neurotmesis is unlikely to occur, except when severe scar tissue predisposes the nerve to laceration. Early nerve recovery (days to weeks) indicates neurapraxia; while longer recovery (months) indicates axonotmesis.

Nerve palsies after total hip arthroplasty are relatively infrequent, but the incidence increases as the complexity of the surgical procedure increases. The sciatic nerve is most commonly involved, with the peroneal division of the sciatic nerve at the greatest risk (80% of cases). The femoral nerve is involved less frequently. An early study indicated an overall prevalence of 1.7%, with total hip arthroplasty for congenital hip dysplasia having a rate of 5.2% and for osteoarthrosis 1%, but a subsequent review suggested that the overall rate of palsy was reduced to approximately 1%. Revision surgery was associated with a rate of 3.2%. The type of injury most likely to produce nerve palsy is stretching or compression, although other mechanisms, such as ischemia, intraneural hemorrhage, dislocation of the femoral component, and cement extrusion, are also suggested as causes.

Nerve injury may be prevented by identifying high-risk cases, protecting the sciatic nerve from compression, and evaluating the sciatic nerve for possible stretching before the wound is closed. Stretching the sciatic nerve by as little as 2 cm increases the risk of palsy significantly. Palpation of the sciatic nerve for tautness with the hip and knee extended and with the hip flexed and knee extended (straight leg raising test) indicates whether there is danger of stretching the sciatic nerve. Shortening the femoral neck is one means of addressing this problem. If any doubt exists about whether stretching occurred, the patient should be placed in the hospital bed following operation with the hip extended and the knee flexed to relieve tension of the nerve, until the patient is awake and function of the nerve can be monitored.

Management of nerve palsy is generally conservative, with observation when the nerve is known to be in continuity and not stretched. Electromyograms and nerve conduction studies may be helpful but may not show changes until 3 weeks after injury. Recovery of some motor function in the hospital heralds a good prognosis, and if complete return is to occur, it does so by 21 months, according to one study.

3. Vascular complications—Significant vascular complications are reported to occur in approximately 0.25% of total hip replacements. These may be caused by placement of retractors and acetabular screws (the safest screw location is in the anterior and superior quadrant of the acetabulum) and by damage to atherosclerotic vessels. Early recognition is important in these injuries.

4. Fracture or perforation—The typical fracture associated with total hip arthroplasty involves the femoral shaft, but other fractures do occur. Fatigue fractures of structures such as the pubic ramus may occur following increased activity after hip replacement relieves pain. The intraoperative problem of fracture or perforation of the femur is relatively uncommon in primary arthroplasty. Perforation may occur in disorders such as sickle cell anemia and osteopetrosis or following previous internal fixation. These conditions may have resulted in sclerotic bone, which may direct the broach astray. Perforations are relatively easily managed by extending the prosthesis past the area of perforation. This distance is generally considered to be two femoral diameters for a perforation with a cemented arthroplasty, but longer distances may be necessary with uncemented arthroplasties, depending on the size of the perforation. An alternative is to use a structural allograft held in place with cerclage wires. In either case, cancellous bone grafting is prudent to facilitate healing.

After total hip arthroplasty, the stress state of the bone is definitely changed, and there is a stress concentration area at the tip of the prosthesis. Fractures in the periprosthetic area are relatively common. These fractures are classified as type A, involving the greater or lesser trochanter; type B1, B2, B3, around or just below the stem, with the stem well fixed (B1), stem loose (B2), or poor bone stock in the proximal femur (B3); or type C, well below the stem. Type A fractures are treated nonoperatively unless the cause is osteolysis, which may predispose the femur to more serious injury. Type B and C fractures are generally treated surgically. Revision is usually the treatment of choice if the prosthesis demonstrates loosening on plain radiographs. Bone grafting is generally necessary with bone deficiencies, and bicortical onlay grafting techniques may be necessary with poor bone stock. Open reduction and internal fixation may be indicated if the prosthesis is tight (types B1 and C), but generous bone grafting and careful observation are necessary to ensure healing. Fracture fixation devices applied in the vicinity of the femoral component may be tenuous, and these devices

must not compromise the integrity of the cement mantle or prosthesis.

5. Dislocation following total hip arthroplasty—The incidence of dislocation following total hip arthroplasty varies somewhat from series to series, but ranges from 1% to 8% and averages 2–2.5%. Several factors are associated with higher rates of dislocation, including female sex of the patient and nonunion of the trochanteric osteotomy, revision surgery, and use of the posterior approach. Dislocation after revision surgery in one series was 10% after the first revision and 26.7% after two or more revisions. An ununited trochanter after revision was associated with a 25% rate of dislocation.

Factors important in preventing dislocation are proper placement of components, adjustment of myofascial tension, component design, and patient compliance. Variables found to have no statistically significant effect on the dislocation rate include the ROM of the hip and the femoral head size. However, a 32-mm head has a theoretic advantage over a 28-mm head because a neck of the same diameter would impinge earlier with a 28-mm head and when dislocation is a concern, larger heads are generally recommended, especially in revision situations. At the time of surgery, the myofascial tension is tested by traction on the femur. Displacement of 1 cm or more suggests an increased probability of dislocation after surgery.

The risk of dislocation after total hip arthroplasty diminishes as time passes without dislocation. A first dislocation often occurs within 6 weeks following surgery and is frequently a result of patient noncompliance with postsurgical guidelines. For a first dislocation, closed reduction is used, and careful assessment of the cause of dislocation should be made. If component position appears to be adequate, bracing for 3 months is recommended, along with careful explanation of hip dislocation precautions to the patient. Alternatively, removal of the acetabular component with replacement by a bipolar into the reamed acetabulum may be the best salvage procedure. Recurrent dislocation should be examined carefully for cause, with radiographs taken to evaluate the abduction and anteversion of the cup as well as the anteversion of the femoral head (Figure 6–10). Examination under fluoroscopy may reveal impingements, and push-and-pull films may reveal inadequate myofascial tension.

After careful evaluation of the cause(s) of dislocation, surgical correction may be undertaken. Possible solutions include reorienting the offset lip of the acetabulum, changing the anteversion or abduction of the acetabulum, changing the anteversion of the femoral component, or advancing the trochanter to tighten the muscle envelope. Failure of these methods may require the use of a constrained acetabulum to prevent dislocation. This treatment should be considered a last resort because the reduced ROM resulting from the design of these cups can predispose the patient to dislocation as a result of levering out of the cup from neck impingement. Long-term bracing is a possible solution for approximately 5%, but trochanteric osteotomy is now seldom used in primary hip replacement. The percentage of patients who develop symptoms from this complication is smaller. Usually, migration of less than 1 cm is not associated with functional symptoms or pain.

The rate of nonunion after revision surgery is much higher, as much as 40%, particularly if there has been nonunion following the primary procedure. Diminished function, as evidenced by weakness in abduction and a limp that cannot be compensated for with a cane, is an indication for an attempt at reattachment of the trochanter. The surfaces should be freshened and rigidly fixed together; bone grafting may be necessary. Subperiosteal release of the iliac wing muscles may be necessary to allow the trochanter to be reattached to the femur.

Pain after trochanteric nonunion may be the result of a painful pseudoarthrosis or, alternatively, of fixation wires that may form a painful bursa.

8. Heterotopic ossification—The incidence of significant heterotopic ossification after total hip arthroplasty is 5% or 10%, although it is present to a lesser degree in perhaps 80% of patients. Definite risk factors include previous heterotopic ossification, ankylosing spondylitis, diffuse idiopathic skeletal hyperostosis or spinal ostosis (Forestier disease), unlimited hip motion preoperatively, head injury, and male sex of the patient. Other possible risk factors include trochanteric osteotomy, interoperative fracture, bone grafting, or localized muscle damage or hematoma.

Heterotopic bone is classified by either the Brooker or the Mayo classification (Table 6–8). Patients identified as being at risk for heterotopic ossification should undergo prophylactic treatment, careful surgical treatment, wound drainage, and irrigation of the wound prior to closing. In patients at risk, low-dose radiation, 6–8 cGy within a 1 day before surgery or the first 3 days after surgery, prevents grade 3 or 4 heterotopic ossification. Indomethacin given postoperatively for 7–21 days is effective, although it may

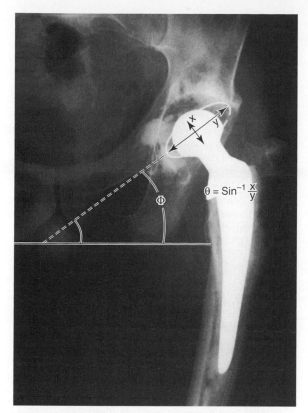

▲ **Figure 6–10.** Approximate determination of the abduction-adduction angle and angle of anteversion of the cup. Exact measurement requires careful control of the direction of the x-ray beam.

$$\theta = \operatorname{Sin}^{-1} \frac{x}{y}$$

recurrent dislocation in a patient with limited goals for activity. Recurrent dislocation causes significant anxiety, which encourages patients to seek surgical correction. The recurrence rate in such patients is as high as 20% after surgical correction.

6. Leg-length discrepancy—During hip replacement surgery, an attempt is made to maintain or correct the preoperative length of the affected leg, so it is equal to the unaffected leg. This goal, however, is sometimes incompatible with (and therefore subservient to) myofascial tension in the ligamentously lax individual. Excessive lengthening is a potential cause of damage to nerve or vascular structures. Computer-assisted navigation or intraoperative radiography offers the best opportunity to achieve equal leg lengths, although other intraoperative measurement systems can be used. None are fail-safe. Hence, most surgeons advise their patients that the leg may be longer or shorter than normal after operation.

7. Trochanteric nonunion—The rate of trochanteric nonunion after a primary total hip arthroplasty was

Table 6–8. Heterotopic bone classification systems.

St age	Mayo Classification	Brooker Classification
I	≤5 mm	Islands of bone
II	<50% bridging laterally	Bone spurs ≥1 cm gap
III	>50% bridging laterally	Bone spurs <1 cm
IV	Apparent ankylosis	Apparent ankylosis

Reprinted, with permission, from Brooker AF, Bowerman JW, Robinson RA, et al: Ectopic ossification following total hip replacement. *J Bone Joint Surg Am* 1973;55:1629; and Morrey BF, Adams RA, Cabanela ME: Comparison of heterotopic bone after anterolateral, transtrochanteric, and posterior approaches for total hip arthroplasty. *Clin Orthop Relat Res* 1984;188:160.

be poorly tolerated by some patients. Early studies indicate that the bone inhibition is a COX-1 function, suggesting that COX-2 inhibitors may not prevent heterotopic bone. Diphosphonates are not effective in prevention of heterotopic ossification and should not be used. Indomethacin may not be optimal for prophylaxis in uncemented total hip arthroplasty because ingrowth may be retarded. Irradiation may cause problems if ingrowth components are not appropriately shielded.

Brooker grade 1 or 2 heterotopic ossification does not influence the outcome of total hip arthroplasty, whereas restricted ROM and pain may occur in patients with more severe grade 3 or 4 heterotopic ossification. If heterotopic ossification causes symptoms (pain, decreased ROM), surgical excision may be considered after the ossification is fully mature. Irradiation and NSAIDs are recommended postoperatively to prevent recurrence. Patients with ankylosing spondylitis have an increased chance of heterotopic ossification with arthroplasty, and in one series, the incidence of heterotopic ossification following total knee arthroplasty in patients with ankylosing spondylitis was 20%.

9. Infection—Prevention of infection after total hip arthroplasty is important because of the grave consequences. In the first few weeks after surgery, irrigation and debridement with retention of the prosthesis is possible. Afterward, the only way to treat an infected total hip arthroplasty is to remove the components and control the infection with antibiotics. Reinsertion of the components is then required 1.5–6 months later.

An innovation in the treatment of infected total hips and knees is the prosthetic antibiotic-loaded acrylic cement (PROSTALAC) technique. The prostheses are removed, sterilized, and reinserted as press-fit components with a layer of antibiotic-impregnated bone cement covering all surfaces except the bearing surface. This procedure is performed at the initial meticulous debridement to provide a spacer for subsequent, definitive joint replacement.

Prevention is much more desirable than subsequent treatment of infection. Total joint arthroplasty implants are such large foreign bodies that all reasonable prophylactic measures should be employed. Laminar flow and ultraviolet lights are used in operating rooms to reduce the number of viable particles per volume of air in the room. Because bacteria are shed from people, keeping the number of people in an operating room to a minimum and reducing the exposed skin area may be beneficial. Antimicrobial therapy may be the single most important prophylaxis against infection. Good surgical technique and minimal operating times also contribute to lowering of infection rates. Infections occurring 6 weeks to 3 months after surgery probably originate from intraoperative contamination. Careful surveillance in this period for signs of infection, including pain, elevated white blood cell count, fever, and wound drainage, allows for early identification of deep wound infection, and early debridement is then indicated to eradicate the infection.

Similarly, large hematomas should be debrided because they may cause chronic drainage and constitute a culture media for infectious agents. One report indicates that prophylactic antibiotics given in the period before and immediately after significant dental procedures may be beneficial in preventing hematogenous infection of total joints. Probably any broad-spectrum antibiotic would provide adequate prophylaxis; the dental profession has specific recommendations. There is a growing body of information that indicates that patients who are obese undergoing total hip arthroplasty are at increased risk of infection and other complications in the perioperative period. Obesity is defined as a BMI (mass in kilograms divided by the height in meters squared) over 30 kg/m^2, whereas overweight is 25–30 kg/m^2. Diabetes, which is frequently present in obese patients, is also a risk factor for infection.

Barrack RL, Harris WH: The value of aspiration of the hip joint before revision total hip arthroplasty. *J Bone Joint Surg Am* 1993;75:66. [PMID: 8419393]

Beaule PE, Mussett SA, Medley JB: Metal-on-metal bearings in total hip arthroplasty. *Instr Course Lect* 2010;59:17. [PMID: 20415363]

Browne JA, Bechtold CD, Berry DJ, et al: Failed metal-on-metal hip arthroplasties: a spectrum of clinical presentations and operative findings. *Clin Orthop Relat Res* 2010;468:2313. [PMID: 20559767]

Callaghan JJ, Albright JC, Goetz DD, et al: Charnley total hip arthroplasty with cement: minimum twenty-five year follow-up. *J Bone Joint Surg Am* 2000;82:487. [PMID: 10761939]

Colwell CW, Froimson MI, Mont MA, et al: Thrombosis prevention after total hip arthroplasty: a prospective, randomized trial comparing a mobile compression device with low-molecular-weight heparin. *J Bone Joint Surg Am* 2010;92:527. [PMID: 20194309]

Daniel J, Ziaee H, Kamali A, et al: Ten-year results of a double-heat-treated metal-on-metal hip resurfacing. *J Bone Joint Surg Br* 2010;92:20. [PMID: 20044674]

DeHart MM, Riley LH: Nerve injuries in total hip arthroplasty. *J Am Acad Orthop Surg* 1999;7:101. [PMID: 10217818]

Dorr LD, Faugere MC, Mackel AM, et al: Structural and cellular assessment of bone quality of proximal femur. *Bone* 1993;14:231. [PMID: 8363862]

Dowsey MM, Choong PF: Early outcomes and complications following joint arthroplasty in obese patients: a review of the published reports. *ANZ J Surg* 2008;78:439. [PMID: 18522562]

Farrell CM, Springer BD, Haidukewych GJ, et al: Moro nerve palsy following primary total hip arthroplasty. *J Bone Joint Surg Am* 2005;87:2619. [PMID: 16322610]

Fransen M, Neal B, Cameron ID, et al: Determinants of heterotopic ossification after total hip replacement surgery. *Hip Int* 2009;19:41. [PMID:19455501]

Geerts WH, Bergqvist D, Pineo GF, et al: Prevention of venous thromboembolism: ACCP evidence-based clinical practice guidelines (8th edition). *Chest* 2008;133:381s. [PMID: 18574271]

Harris WH: Traumatic arthritis of the hip after dislocation and acetabular fractures: treatment by mold arthroplasty. *J Bone Joint Surg Am* 1969;51:737. [PMID: 5783851]

Hummel MT, Malkani AL, Yakkanti MR, et al: Decreased dislocation after revision total hip arthroplasty using larger femoral head size and posterior capsular repair. *J Arthroplasty* 2009;24(6 Suppl):73. [PMID: 19577890]

Jarrett CA, Ranawat AS, Bruzzone M, et al: The squeaking hip: a phenomenon of ceramic-on-ceramic total hip arthroplasty. *J Bone Joint Surg Am* 2009;91:1344. [PMID: 19487511]

Kelly SJ, Robbins CE, Bierbaum BE, et al: Use of a hydroxyapatite-coated stem in patients with Dorr Type C femoral bone. *Clin Orthop Relat Res* 2007;465:112. [PMID: 17704696]

Langton DJ, Jameson SS, Joyce TJ, et al: Early failure of metal-on-metal bearings in hip resurfacing and large-diameter total hip replacement: a consequence of excess wear. *J Bone Joint Surg Br* 2010;92:38. [PMID: 20044676]

Lester DK, Helm M: Mini-incision posterior approach for hip arthroplasty. *Orthop Traumatol* 2001;4:245. [No PMID]

Lewinnek GE, Lewis JL, Tarr R, et al: Dislocations after total hip replacement arthroplasties. *J Bone Joint Surg Am* 1970;60:217. [PMID: 641088]

Moskal JT Capps SG: Improving the accuracy of acetabular component orientation: avoiding malposition. *J Am Acad Orthop Surg* 2010;18:286. [PMID: 20435879]

Parvizi J, Pulido L, Slenker N, et al: Vascular injuries after total joint arthroplasty. *J Arthroplasty* 2008;23:1115. [PMID: 18676115]

Platzer P, Schuster R, Aldrian S, et al: Management and outcome of periprosthetic fractures after total knee arthroplasty. *J Trauma* 2010;68:1464. [PMID: 20539190]

Platzer P, Schuster R, Luxl M, et al: Management and outcome of interprosthetic femoral fractures. *Injury* 2011;42:1219. [PMID: 21176899]

Schmalzried TP, Noordin S, Amstutz HC: Update on nerve palsy associated with total hip replacement. *Clin Orthop Relat Res* 1997;344:188. [PMID: 9372771]

Smith DE, McGraw RW, Taylor DC, et al: Arterial complications and total knee arthroplasty. *J Am Acad Orthop Surg* 2001;9:253. [PMID: 11476535]

Van den Bekerom MP, Hilverdink EF, Sierevelt IN, et al: A comparison of hemiarthroplasty with total hip replacement for displaced intracapsular fracture of the femoral neck: a randomized controlled multicentre trial in patients aged 70 years and over. *J Bone Joint Surg Br* 2010;92:1422. [PMID: 20884982]

Waldman BJ, Mont MA, Hungerford DS: Total knee arthroplasty infections associated with dental procedures. *Clin Orthop Relat Res* 1997;343:164. [PMID: 9345222]

Walter WL, Yeung E, Esposito C: A review of squeaking hips. *J Am Acad Orthop Surg* 2010;18:319. [PMID: 20511437]

Wixson RL: Computer-assisted total hip navigation. *Instr Course Lect* 2008;57:707. [PMID: 18399618]

▶ Revision Total Hip Arthroplasty

The clinical success of revision total hip arthroplasty procedures historically was greatly inferior to the results of primary hip arthroplasty procedures. Loosening rates from 13% to 44% of cemented femoral revision procedures were reported at follow-up times of less than 5 years.

Improved techniques of cementing femoral stems led to improved results with cemented femoral revision. Pressurization of cement delivered, in a doughy stage, with a cement gun; pulsatile lavage; and an intramedullary plug permitted reproducible creation of adequate cement mantles. Only 14% of revised cemented femoral components were loose radiographically in one series after an average of 6 years. Other series indicate a revision rate of approximately 10% at 10 years, which is much improved from earlier series but inferior to those obtained with primary cemented stems.

Cementless reconstructions of failed femoral components were developed in response to the early high rates of failure with cemented revision procedures. However, early cementless revision series were generally unsuccessful, with failure rates of 4–10% at follow-ups of less than 4 years. The use of proximally porous coated stems with inadequate stabilization, in the setting of deficient femoral bone stock, led to unreliable bone ingrowth fixation. Encouraging reports were obtained with modular proximally coated stems, such as the S-ROM (Johnson and Johnson, Raynham, MA) prosthesis, and extensively porous coated stems, such as the AML and Solution (Depuy, Warsaw, IN). Re-revision rates from 1.5% to 6% were achieved with use of these types of cementless femoral components at follow-ups from 5 to 8.4 years.

In the situation where inadequate femoral bone stock exists, the use of allograft bone is advocated. For extended loss of proximal femoral bone stock, cementing a smooth tapered femoral stem in a bed of impacted particulate allogeneic bone produces promising short-term clinical results. When deficiency of proximal bone stock is severe, use of structural femoral allografts may be required, and short-term reports suggest good clinical results.

Similar to early experience with cemented revisions of the femoral component, acetabular revision with cement was generally unsuccessful. Because of the difficulty of interdigitating cement into a sclerotic and often deficient acetabular bone stock, failure rates of loosening were reported from 53–93% at follow-ups from only 2–4.5 years.

The introduction of cementless porous-coated acetabular implants for revision of failed cemented cups greatly facilitated early clinical results. Large hemispherical cementless acetabular implants can accommodate most bone defects encountered after removal of failed cemented cups. Where an adequate press-fit cannot be obtained, adjuvant fixation of the implant with screws or spikes can provide adequate stability to permit bone ingrowth fixation. Re-revision rates are reported from 0% to 1.6% with follow-up of 2–4 years.

Where inadequate bone stock of the acetabulum precludes reconstructions with conventional hemispherical implants, structural allografts fixed to the pelvis with screws can provide acceptable middle-term results. Other alternatives include the use of eccentric-shaped cementless implants and cemented reconstructions with particulate allografting and antiprotrusio cages.

Fink B, Grossmann A, Schubring S, et al: A modified transfemoral approach using modular cementless revision stems. *Clin Orthop Relat Res* 2007;462:105. [PMID: 17496558]

Haddad FS, Rayan F: The role of impaction grafting: the when and how. *Orthopedics* 2009;32:9. [PMID: 19751009]

Hooper GJ, Rothwell AG, Stringer M, et al: Revision following cemented and uncemented primary total hip replacement: a seven-year analysis from the New Zealand Joint Registry. *J Bone Joint Surg Br* 2009;91:451. [PMID: 19336803]

Issack PS, Nousiainen M, Beksac B, et al: Acetabular component revision in total hip arthroplasty. Part I: cementless shells. *Am J Orthop* 2009;38:509. [PMID 20011740]

▶ Total Knee Arthroplasty

A. Indications

As with other joints, the primary indication for total knee arthroplasty is pain. Absolute contraindications to total knee arthroplasty include active sepsis, absence of an extensor mechanism, and a neuropathic joint. Relative contraindications include a patient's young (<40 years) age, heavy demand for activity, or a patient being unreliable.

When both hips and knees are involved with painful arthritis, the joint causing the most discomfort should be replaced first. If hips and knees are equally painful, hip arthroplasty should precede knee arthroplasty. Rehabilitation following total hip arthroplasty is easier and less affected by a painful knee than vice versa. Additionally, motion of the hip joint greatly facilitates surgery for the knee.

B. Implants

Early designs of total knee arthroplasty were developed in Europe and may be categorized as constrained or resurfacing. Constrained devices consisted of fixed hinges, and resurfacing devices relied on ligaments for stability. Constrained devices predictably loosened, although they were used primarily in severe bone or ligamentous deficiency states. Early resurfacing implants were flat, roller pin–shaped implants or unicondylar devices that replaced only the medial or lateral compartment. Early knee replacements did not resurface the patellofemoral joints.

Contemporary total knee replacements represent a convergence of two major designs developed in the United States during the early 1970s: the total condylar and the duopatellar prostheses. The total condylar prosthesis had a femoral component made of Co/Cr and an all-polyethylene tibial component with a central peg. Excision of the posterior cruciate ligament was required because the entire surface of the tibial plateau was resurfaced. The patellar component was a dome-shaped polyethylene implant. All components were fixed with acrylic cement.

The duocondylar knee replacement was the forerunner of the duopatellar prosthesis and did not resurface the patellofemoral joint. Extension of the anterior flange of the Co/Cr femoral component provided an articulation surface for an all-polyethylene dome-shaped patellar component. The tibial component was originally designed with separate medial and lateral runners, allowing preservation of the central insertion of the posterior cruciate ligament. Later, the two components were joined together, but a cutout was made posteriorly to permit retention of the posterior cruciate ligament.

Retention of the posterior cruciate ligament permitted increased flexion over that with the total condylar design because the normal femoral rollback during knee flexion was retained. Shifting of the center of rotation posteriorly during knee flexion greatly improves the lever arm of the quadriceps mechanism. The ability to climb stairs was superior when the cruciate ligament was retained. Central to the design of a cruciate ligament–retaining prosthesis is avoidance of excessive constraint by the tibial surface to permit rollback.

To overcome limitations in flexion and stair-climbing function, the total condylar prosthesis was modified with a cam mechanism (posterior-stabilized condylar prosthesis). The central cam design permits substitution of the function of the posterior cruciate ligament, providing a mechanical recreation of femoral rollback.

The differences in ROM and stair-climbing function achieved with cruciate-retaining and posterior-stabilized knee replacements are now considered negligible. Arguments in favor of the posterior-stabilized implant include technical ease in reconstructing severely deformed knees and less shear force at the articular bearing because sliding is reduced. The arguments in favor of cruciate-retaining designs are reduction of bone–cement interface forces because of less constraint, improved stability in flexion, less removal of bone from the intercondylar region, and absence of patellofemoral impingement syndrome (formed by scar tissue in the intercondylar recess of the posterior stabilized femoral component).

Problems with high-contact, stress-inducing fatigue wear of the polyethylene surfaces stimulated a new design concept in knee replacement. This design uses a polyethylene component that can move in relation to the tibial base plate. Thus, the surface of polyethylene in contact with the femoral component can be made to be more conforming because it can change positions during flexion and extension of the knee. Two types have evolved: the rotating platform, which only allows rotation of the polyethylene around an axis approximating the axis of the tibia, and variations on the "meniscal bearing" knee. In this design, the individual medial and lateral poly components can rotate (tibial axis) and translate (AP direction), or the entire poly plateau can rotate and translate in the AP direction. The latter concept seems to better address the biomechanical aspects of the knee, but results are early or limited on all designs.

C. Surgical Technique

Total knee replacement surgery is greatly facilitated by use of a thigh tourniquet. Following exsanguination of the lower limb with an elastic wrap, the tourniquet is inflated to an adequate pressure, usually ~300 mm Hg. An anterior midline skin incision is made, followed most commonly by a deep medial parapatellar approach. The lateral flap containing the patella is everted to allow exposure of the tibiofemoral joint. Remnants of menisci and anterior cruciate ligament are excised, with careful release of contracted soft-tissue structures as needed.

Instrumentation systems guide the surgeon to create bone cuts with a saw that match the prosthetic fixation surface and reproduce anatomic alignment of the knee joint. Typically, in the coronal plane, the tibial plateau is cut horizontally to be at a right angle with the shaft of the tibia. The distal femur is usually cut at 5–7 degrees of valgus from the shaft of the femur. Such bone cuts provide a neutral mechanical alignment in the coronal plane so a line can be drawn from the center of the femoral head, through the middle of the knee joint, and through the center of the ankle joint. In the sagittal plane, the femoral cut is at right angles to the femoral shaft, but the tibial cut is made with 3–5 degrees of posterior slope. Slight external rotation of the femoral component allows symmetric tension of collateral ligaments during knee flexion and facilitates tracking of the patellar component.

Retention or sacrifice of the posterior cruciate ligament depends on the design of the implant used. When the cruciate ligament is sacrificed, usually bone from the intercondylar notch is removed to accommodate a box that houses the cam mechanism. Other alternative designs can prevent posterior translation of the tibia on the femur. When the patellar surface is replaced, a saw is used to create a flat surface with symmetric bone thickness. Inadequate resection predisposes to subluxation because excessive extensor mechanism length is used, and the lateral ligamentous structures are relatively tightened. Many patellar components are 10 mm thick; thus, adequate resection must be almost 10 mm, within the limits of the anatomy of the patella. At least 10 mm and preferably 15 mm of patella (AP thickness) should remain. Patellar tracking is assessed by using trial components and ranging the knee from full extension to full flexion. In knees with valgus deformity, it is common to have lateral subluxation of the patella. In such cases, a careful lateral retinacular release that preserves the superior lateral geniculate vessels is performed. Positioning femoral and tibial components in slight external rotation and positioning the patellar implant slightly medially on the patellar bone surface also improves tracking.

After appropriate trials are used to confirm accurate sizes of the components as well as ligamentous stability, cementing is performed. Careful cleansing of the bone surfaces with pulsatile lavage facilitates interdigitation of doughy-stage methylmethacrylate cement. The prosthetic components must be seated in the correct orientation, and excess acrylic cement must be removed. Before closure of the knee, it is prudent to lavage fragments of bone and cement and release the tourniquet to obtain hemostasis. At surgery, little bleeding is seen in the flexed knee. Thus, many surgeons close the wound and maintain the knee in flexion for periods up to 24 hours to decrease blood loss.

D. Clinical Results

Long-term results of contemporary cemented total knee arthroplasty designs are excellent. Survivorship of the total condylar prosthesis is calculated to be 90–95% at 15 years. Excellent functional results of posterior stabilized total knee replacements are also reported, with a 12-year survival rate of 94% for functional prostheses. Similarly, excellent function and only a 1% rate of loosening of the tibial or femoral component were reported with a cruciate ligament–retaining knee replacement when followed up at 10–14 years. Cementless designs have not consistently achieved the results of the cemented arthroplasties. Primary patella resurfacing is generally preferred as the best treatment path, although many surgeons prefer to leave the native patella unresurfaced.

E. Complications

Complications are infrequent with total knee arthroplasty but include many of the same problems encountered with total hip arthroplasty. Additional problems arise from wound healing, fracture, extensor mechanism problems, and stiffness of the knee.

1. Deep vein thrombosis—DVT is common following knee arthroplasty, occurring in more than 50% of patients in one study. Further, 10–15% of patients develop DVT in the contralateral leg after unilateral knee arthroplasty. The use of the tourniquet during surgery does not have a clear detrimental effect on thrombus formation. The incidence of pulmonary embolism is lower than that reported in hip arthroplasty. This may be caused by the greater propensity to form calf thrombi after total knee arthroplasty; these thrombi may be less likely to cause emboli than thigh thrombi. Antithrombotic prophylactic measures include use of pulsatile compression stockings and administration of warfarin or low-molecular-weight heparin.

2. Wound problems—Wound problems can arise from incision-related issues and from patient-related risk factors. The skin incision should optimally be midline and longitudinal, and the skin should have minimal undermining. Preexisting skin incisions should be used when possible. Because wound healing is crucial to the success of the procedure, preoperative plastic surgery consultation may be beneficial if multiple scars, burns, or previous irradiation to the skin are present. Patient-related risk factors include chronic corticosteroid use, obesity, malnutrition, tobacco use, diabetes, and hypovolemia.

Treatment of wound problems depends on the type of problem. Drainage of serous fluid that does not clear in 5–7 days is an indication for open debridement. Hematoma formation (without drainage) is treated nonoperatively unless there are signs of impending skin necrosis or compromise of ROM. Small areas of superficial necrosis at the wound edge are treated with routine local wound care. Full-thickness soft-tissue necrosis places the joint space at high risk of infection and must be treated aggressively. Debridement with flap closure is frequently required. The medial gastrocnemius flap is useful because the tissue necrosis is frequently medial.

Prevention of wound problems through careful planning, gentle handling of soft tissues, and patient education to minimize risk factors is preferable to subsequent treatment of the problems.

3. Nerve palsy—Nerve palsies are a rare complication of total knee arthroplasty. The peroneal nerve is believed to be at increased risk for injury from surgery performed on valgus knees with flexion contractures or other significant deformity, ischemia from stretching small vessels in the surrounding soft tissue, and compression resulting from a tight dressing or splint. The risk is reported to be approximately 0.6%.

4. Femoral fracture—Notching of the anterior femoral cortex may predispose to distal femoral fracture. A technical error, notching can be prevented by careful femoral sizing before use of the anterior distal femur cutting block and by avoidance of posterior displacement or extension of the cutting block. Use of an intramedullary stem extension is advised if notching occurs. Fracture of the medial or lateral condyle may occur, particularly in patients with poor bone stock, such as those with rheumatoid osteoarthritis or osteoporosis or in patients with cruciate-sacrificing femoral components. Large intercondylar boxes in these prostheses can cause weakening of the distal femur. Similarly, tibial plateau fractures can occur because of osteopenia or even through stress concentration sites caused by pins used to fix tibial cutting blocks. These are treated by internal fixation, if needed, in combination with extended intramedullary stems to bypass the fracture site.

5. Patellar and other extensor mechanism complications—Many patellar and extensor mechanism problems can be prevented by careful surgical technique because many of these arise from technical problems during surgery, such as quadriceps (or patellar) tendon rupture or avulsion, patellofemoral instability, and patella fracture. Vigilance during exposure of a stiff knee to avoid excessive tension on the extensor mechanism is important. Useful techniques to avoid avulsion include a V turndown quadricepsplasty, quadriceps "snip," tibial tubercle osteotomy, and placement of a Steinmann pin in the tubercle to prevent excessive traction on the patellar tendon. Treatment of the disruption is similar to the treatment in a normal knee. The patellar tendon is attached to bone, and the repair is protected with a wire around the patella and through the tibial tubercle, holding the patella at the correct length from the tibial tubercle.

This repair complicates the postoperative ROM regimen, at least to some extent. The incidence ranges from 0.2% to 2.5%. Patellar complications include maltracking, loosening of the patellar component, fractures, and impingement. The patellofemoral forces are among the highest anywhere in the body, and avoidance of intraoperative technical errors may minimize patellar complications. Patellar tracking should be assessed intraoperatively during flexion and extension of the prosthetic knee. Lateral patellar subluxation or dislocation may be caused by internal rotation of the femoral or tibial component, as well as a tight lateral patellar retinaculum. Careful release of the lateral patellar retinaculum may correct maltracking. Subluxation can predispose to patellar component loosening, as can abnormal stress caused by uneven patellar bone resection. Excessive bone resection and avascularity, caused by damage to the superior lateral geniculate artery during lateral release, can predispose to fractures. When using a posterior stabilized prosthesis, maintaining the inferior pole of the patella within 10–30 mm of the joint line may prevent impingement syndrome, which is characterized by pain or clicking when peripatellar synovial scar tissue impinges against the intercondylar box of the femoral component during flexion and extension.

In some studies, patellar complications are the cause for as many as half of the knee revisions performed. For this reason, some surgeons do not resurface the patella when the appearance is relatively normal. Because most patellofemoral replacement problems are attributed to technical errors, inferior prosthetic design, and excessive loads, replacement will probably become more prevalent as these problems are resolved.

6. Knee stiffness—Knee stiffness is a common problem in the early postoperative period. Methods to reduce stiffness include physical therapy (active or active-assisted ROM) and continuous passive motion (CPM). The CPM machine moves the knee through a preset passive ROM. This modality is generally accepted and even liked by patients but does not affect the final ROM or reduce hospital stay. An acceptable ROM is 90–95 degrees of flexion with less than 10 degrees of flexion contracture, but the activities of daily living, such as getting out of a chair or climbing stairs, should be painless. Postoperative stiffness should generally subside by 6–8 weeks after surgery, and improvement in ROM should occur for 1 year with most gain in the first 3 months. The preoperative ROM is an important indicator of the ROM to be expected postoperatively.

Prevention of significant flexion contracture at the time of surgery and in the early postoperative period is important because improvement with manipulation is unrewarding. Manipulation with or without steroid injection can be beneficial in the first 3 months. Arthroscopic debridement may be necessary after intraarticular fibrosis occurs. Decreases in ROM after initial gains should alert the surgeon to possible infection, reflex sympathetic dystrophy, or mechanical problems, such as loose components or interposed soft tissue.

Baker PN, Khaw FM, Kirk LM, et al: A randomized, controlled trial of cemented versus cementless press-fit condylar total knee replacement: 15-year survival analysis. *J Bone Joint Surg Br* 2007;89:1608. [PMID: 18057361]

Colwell CW, Chen PC, D'Lima D: Extensor malalignment arising from femoral component malrotation in knee arthroplasty: effect of rotating bearing. *Clin Biomech* 2011;26:52. [PMID: 20869142]

Dennis DA, Berry DJ, Engh G, et al: Revision total knee arthroplasty. *J Am Acad Orthop Surg* 2008;16:442. [PMID: 18664633]

Gandhi R, Tsvetkov D, Davey JR, et al: Survival and clinical function of cemented and uncemented prostheses in total knee replacement: a meta-analysis. *J Bone Joint Surg Br* 2009;91:889. [PMID: 19567852]

Hahn SB, Lee WS, Han DY: A modified Thompson quadricepsplasty for stiff knee. *J Bone Joint Surg Br* 2000;82:992. [PMID: 11041587]

Helmy N, Anglin C, Greidanus NV, et al: To resurface or not to resurface the patella in total knee arthroplasty. *Clin Orthop Relat Res* 2008;466:2775. [PMID: 18726657]

Meneghini RM, Hanssen AD: Cementless fixation in total knee arthroplasty: past, present, and future. *J Knee Surg* 2008;21:307. [PMID: 18979934]

Patel J, Ries MD, Bosic KJ: Extensor mechanism complications after total knee arthroplasty. *Instr Course Lect* 2008;57:283. [PMID: 18399592]

Swan JD, Stoney JD, Lim K, et al: The need for patella resurfacing in total knee arthroplasty: a literature review. *ANZ J Surg* 2010;80:223. [PMID: 20575947]

► Total Shoulder Arthroplasty

A. Indications

The primary indication for shoulder arthroplasty is persistent pain resulting from the loss of articular cartilage and incongruent joint surfaces (ie, arthritis) that has failed nonsurgical management. The most common etiologies are osteoarthritis, rheumatoid osteoarthritis, posttraumatic arthritis, cuff arthropathy, and dislocation arthropathy. Both total shoulder arthroplasty and hemiarthroplasty diminish pain. Hemiarthroplasty can be done with either a traditional stemmed humeral prosthesis or a humeral resurfacing prosthesis with similar outcomes. The humeral resurfacing prosthesis preserves bone stock, but a traditional stemmed humeral prosthesis is still best when there is humeral head bone loss that prevents the resurfacing prosthesis from being well secured. Another reason that a hemiarthroplasty is done rather than a total shoulder arthroplasty is when there is significant erosion of the glenoid beyond the base of the coracoid. This can occur in osteoarthritis but is more commonly seen in rheumatoid osteoarthritis.

Decision making in shoulder arthroplasty depends on many factors, including the integrity of the rotator cuff, capsulolabrum, and articular surfaces. Traditional total shoulder arthroplasty is not indicated in those with arthritis and who also have a torn rotator cuff that cannot be repaired at surgery. Most commonly, this is encountered in a patient who has tolerated a rotator cuff tear for many years and developed arthritis as a result. This occurs as the humerus comes to be positioned superior on the glenoid and the normal compression of the humeral head into the concavity of the glenoid, termed concavity compression, is lost. In this situation, a glenoid prosthesis would be subject to eccentric loading and a "rocking-horse effect," which is thought to be the reason for its unacceptably high rates of loosening. Shoulder instability is not usually corrected by traditional total shoulder arthroplasty alone. In other words, performing a total shoulder arthroplasty in a shoulder that dislocates will often result in dislocation of the shoulder arthroplasty. This is because the total shoulder arthroplasty can correct damage to the articular surfaces but does not correct damage to the capsulolabrum.

The combination of a severe rotator cuff tear, joint osteoarthritis, and superior position of the humeral head on the glenoid is called cuff arthropathy and is usually associated with poor shoulder function. Surprisingly, there are some individuals with cuff arthropathy who have full ROM and little weakness. In these patients, a shoulder hemiarthroplasty is effective in diminishing pain. But when the shoulder function is poor such that the individual is unable to lift the arm against gravity, sometimes called "pseudoparalysis," a reverse shoulder prosthesis may be best. With this design, the socket is placed on the humerus and the ball is placed on the glenoid. This prosthesis not only diminishes pain but also is a substitute for the torn rotator cuff, and function is improved postoperatively.

Contraindications to shoulder arthroplasty include infection, neuropathic arthropathy, and the absence of a functional deltoid.

B. Surgical Technique

A deltopectoral surgical approach is performed, with careful retraction of the conjoined tendon medially to avoid injury to the musculocutaneous nerve. Current techniques require incision of the subscapularis, and this can be done in three different manners: incision of its tendon 1 cm lateral to the insertion, detaching the tendon off the lesser tuberosity, or detaching the tendon with osteotomy of the lesser tuberosity. Osteotomy may provide opportunity for the best repair at the end of the procedure. Because there is often loss of external rotation motion in patients with shoulder arthroplasty, the subscapularis can be lengthened by attaching the tendon more medially on the lesser tuberosity or even at the edge of the humeral osteotomy. Likewise, a coronal Z-plasty of the tendon can be done to increase external rotation afterward. Many surgeons choose to incise the biceps tendon at the supraglenoid tubercle (ie, biceps tenotomy) to improve exposure. It can be tenodesed at the end if the surgeon chooses. The axillary nerve is palpated along the inferior border of the subscapularis to avoid injury. The anterior capsule is incised along with the subscapularis tendon, and some surgeons choose to resect it to improve ROM in external rotation, and then the humeral head is dislocated anteriorly with extension and external rotation of the arm and is delivered out of the wound. The humeral head is resected at the head–neck junction, while the remainder of the rotator cuff insertions remain intact. Preparation of the humeral intramedullary canal is followed by insertion of a trial stemmed humeral component in about 30 degrees of retroversion. The appropriate thickness of the humeral head is determined, and head components are trialed. Attention then moves to the glenoid. The humeral stem may be left in place to tamponade bleeding and to diminish the chances of the humerus being damaged during glenoid preparation. The humerus is displaced posteriorly using a humeral head retractor, such as a Fukuda retractor, for exposure of the glenoid. Motorized reamers or a burr are used to remove a small amount of bone so that bleeding cortical bone remains for support of the glenoid component. With osteoarthritis, there is often posterior glenoid wear necessitating removal of more anterior than posterior bone to restore normal glenoid version and provide an optimal surface for implanting the glenoid component. Using large, bulk bone grafts or cement in this situation to fill an uncontained posterior glenoid defect is not recommended. Depending on the prosthesis to be used, holes are then drilled or a keel is burred for implantation of a cemented, all-polyethene glenoid component. Keeping the glenoid bone as dry as possible during cementing is a challenge. The humeral component can be implanted with or without cement, and the subscapularis tendon is repaired. A biceps tenodesis may be done at this time as well.

C. Implants

Basically, there are four types of shoulder arthroplasty: humeral resurfacing prostheses with either a very small stem or no stem at all, stemmed hemiarthroplasty, total shoulder arthroplasty, and reverse total shoulder arthroplasty.

Hemiarthroplasty can be done with a humeral resurfacing prosthesis that has survivorship similar to stemmed hemiarthroplasty. Humeral resurfacing prostheses necessitate sufficient humeral head bone stock for reaming and implantation. When there is severe humeral head deformity from large osteochondral lesions or sequelae of severe humeral head fractures, for example, resection of the humeral head and implantation with a stemmed hemiarthroplasty are best. Also, in the hands of most surgeons, the humeral resurfacing prostheses do not allow adequate exposure for a glenoid component to be implanted, and a stemmed humeral component may be best.

Current total shoulder arthroplasties have nonconstrained surfaces and stemmed humeral components. These prosthetic designs incorporate modular components and sufficient sizes to accommodate differences in anatomy found in the general population. Humeral stem surfaces are available with either cemented or cementless designs. The glenoid components are all-polyethene and are pegged or keeled for cemented implantation. Metal-backed glenoid

prostheses have failed at high rates. In reverse total shoulder arthroplasty, the socket is placed on the humerus, the ball is placed on the glenoid, and the surfaces are more constrained than in traditional total shoulder arthroplasty. The glenoid components have cementless designs and the humeral stem comes in both cemented and uncemented designs.

D. Clinical Results

Outcomes in pain relief after shoulder arthroplasty are similar to those after hip and knee arthroplasty. Total shoulder arthroplasty alleviates about 90% of pain. There is not as much pain relief with hemiarthroplasty; pain is diminished by about two thirds. Although easier for the surgeon to perform, surprisingly, revision is more common after hemiarthroplasty done for glenohumeral osteoarthritis than total shoulder arthroplasty. Primarily for this reason, hemiarthroplasty may not be as cost-effective as total shoulder arthroplasty. Outcomes after shoulder arthroplasty are similar for those with osteoarthritis and rheumatoid arthritis.

Results after shoulder arthroplasty are not as good in younger patients as the elderly. There are many possible reasons for this, but most likely, higher activity demands and posttraumatic etiologies in younger patients result in less satisfactory results.

Improvements in function after shoulder arthroplasty are not as good as relief of pain. The best predictors of ROM and strength after shoulder arthroplasty are the ROM and strength present before surgery. Mild to moderate gains can be expected, but the patient with poor ROM and strength is likely to have persistent deficits postoperatively. Better improvements in ROM and strength can be expected in the patient with cuff arthropathy and pseudoparalysis who undergoes reverse total shoulder arthroplasty. Then restoration of about two thirds of normal ROM and strength in elevation is common.

Complications after shoulder arthroplasty are equal or less than after hip or knee arthroplasty. Today, the most common "complication" of shoulder arthroplasty is a rotator cuff tear. This occurs because rotator cuff tears are common in patients in this age group; having had a shoulder arthroplasty does not diminish the chances of a rotator cuff tear occurring. Another complication is aseptic loosening and occurs more commonly at the glenoid than the humeral prosthesis. Radiolucent lines occur around the all-polyethene glenoid component and depend on the type of prosthesis. It is more common in keeled than pegged designs. Radiolucent lines at the glenoid component are much more common than the rate of revision. Less common complications include fracture, nerve injury, instability, venous thrombosis, deep vein thrombosis, pulmonary emboli, and infection. Infection may be less than that after hip and knee arthroplasty (<0.5%) and may be due to the excellent blood supply and musculature surrounding the joint. Complications are greater in reverse total shoulder arthroplasty compared to traditional shoulder arthroplasty and are as high as 25% for primary procedures and 40% for revision procedures.

Contraindications to total shoulder arthroplasty include active shoulder infection, poor bone stock that precludes fixation of the prosthesis, the absence of a deltoid function, and neuropathic arthropathy as occurs, for example, with a cervical syrinx.

Edwards TB, Labriola JE, Stanley RJ, O'Connor DP, Elkousy HA, Gartsman GM: Radiographic comparison of pegged and keeled glenoid components using modern cementing techniques: a prospective randomized study. *J Shoulder Elbow Surg* 2010;19:251. [PMID: 20185072]

Farmer KW, Hammond JW, Queale WS, Keyurapan E, McFarland EG: Shoulder arthroplasty versus hip and knee arthroplasties: a comparison of outcomes. *Clin Orthop Relat Res* 2007;455:183. [PMID: 16980898]

Fox TJ, Cil A, Sperling JW, et al: Survival of the glenoid component in shoulder arthroplasty. *J Shoulder Elbow Surg* 2009;18:859. [PMID: 19297199]

Guery J, Favard L, Sirveaux F, Oudet D, Mole D, Walch G: Reverse total shoulder arthroplasty. Survivorship analysis of eighty replacements followed for five to ten years. *J Bone Joint Surg Am* 2006;88:1742. [PMID: 16882896]

Levy O, Copeland SA: Cementless surface replacement arthroplasty (CSRA) for osteoarthritis of the shoulder. *J Shoulder Elbow Surg* 2004;13:266. [PMID: 15111895]

Mather RC 3rd, Watters TS, Orlando LA, Bolognesi MP, Moorman CT 3rd: Cost effectiveness analysis of hemiarthroplasty and total shoulder arthroplasty. *J Shoulder Elbow Surg* 2010;19:325. [PMID: 20303459]

Mulieri P, Dunning P, Klein S, Pupello D, Frankle M: Reverse shoulder arthroplasty for the treatment of irreparable rotator cuff tear without glenohumeral arthritis. *J Bone Joint Surg Am* 2010;92:2544. [PMID: 21048173]

Saltzman MD, Mercer DM, Warme WJ, Bertelsen AL, Matsen FA 3rd: Comparison of patients undergoing primary shoulder arthroplasty before and after the age of fifty. *J Bone Joint Surg Am* 2010;92:42. [PMID: 20048094]

Scalise JJ, Ciccone J, Iannotti JP: Clinical, radiographic, and ultrasonographic comparison of subscapularis tenotomy and lesser tuberosity osteotomy for total shoulder arthroplasty. *J Bone Joint Surg Am* 2010;92:1627. [PMID: 20595569]

▶ Total Elbow Arthroplasty

A. Indications

Like other arthroplasties, the main indication for total elbow arthroplasty is persistent pain resulting from the loss of articular cartilage and incongruent joint surfaces (ie, arthritis) that has failed nonsurgical management. Etiologies include rheumatoid arthritis, osteoarthritis, and posttraumatic arthritis. However, total elbow arthroplasty is also done for distal humeral nonunions and severe comminuted distal humeral fractures, especially in the elderly. For young active patients, especially those with limited elbow motion, debridement using either an arthroscopic or open technique

or interpositional arthroplasty may be best. However, it should be remembered that these are salvage procedures because they neither eliminate pain nor restore full function and are not indicated in those with preoperative instability. These procedures are for patients who are not ready to accept the limitations of a total elbow arthroplasty. Results after total elbow arthroplasty are best in elderly patients and those with rheumatoid arthritis, in part because these individuals are happy to once again use their elbows for activities of daily living.

B. Surgical Technique

Attention to the soft tissue, including the triceps insertion, collateral ligaments, and the ulnar nerve, is essential during total elbow arthroplasty. The direct posterior approach can be used when a semiconstrained prosthesis is used but requires dissection of the posterior skin from the underlying tissue and detachment of the triceps tendon. Careful soft-tissue handling and repair of the triceps tendon afterward are essential to avoid skin necrosis and weakness of the triceps muscle. The Bryan posteromedial approach is also used for implantation of semiconstrained devices. The surgical plane is between the medial triceps and forearm flexors proximally and between the flexor carpi ulnaris and flexor carpi radialis distally. This allows direct visualization of the ulnar nerve and facilitates transposition of the nerve. Great care should be taken when elevating the triceps from its insertion on the olecranon so that it remains in continuity with the forearm fascia. With this approach, total elbow arthroplasty can be done without detachment of the triceps. Release of the collateral ligaments is required. Because integrity of the collateral ligaments is vital when a nonconstrained device is used, the Kocher posterolateral approach may be best because it allows preservation of the ulnar collateral ligament. This ligament provides the major restraint against valgus forces in the flexed elbow. The surgical plane is between the anconeus and extensor carpi ulnaris muscles distally and proximally between the triceps and brachioradialis muscles.

C. Implants

Today's total elbow arthroplasty designs have less constraint, permitting more normal elbow kinematics than in the past. Both unconstrained and semiconstrained prostheses diminish pain, and complications are similar. The two currently available types of total elbow arthroplasty include semiconstrained and resurfacing nonconstrained prostheses. Semiconstrained prostheses have stems on both the humerus and the ulna and a linked hinge that provides stability. Excision of the radial head is usual during implantation. They are not a simple hinge and, instead, have been called a "sloppy hinge" by some, hence their name semiconstrained. This lessened constraint has resulted in much better survivorship; highly constrained total elbow arthroplasty prostheses failed due to loosening. Dislocation is not a concern with semiconstrained prostheses. Semiconstrained prostheses are best when there is instability or loss of bone stock. In theory, nonconstrained implants load the prosthesis less and yield less aseptic loosening. Because stability is not conferred from the prosthesis, they should not be used in cases of ligamentous instability or loss of bone stock.

Radial head prostheses have long been available for severe fractures of the radial head. They may also be an aid in providing stability in the elbow with a comminuted radial head fracture. Short-term results are excellent and remain good over 10 years, although arthritis of the capitellum, radiolucencies along the stem, and other problems occur; long-term follow-up is needed. Hemiarthroplasty is now available for severe fractures of the distal humerus. Early outcomes are encouraging.

D. Clinical Results

Total elbow arthroplasty has survivorship that may be as high as 85% at 10 years, but patient selection, compliance, and age are critical factors to success. In patients who have had a total elbow arthroplasty for posttraumatic arthritis, failure is much more common. Failure is also more common in younger patients, under 65 years of age. Outcome is similar in elderly patients who have had total elbow arthroplasty for treatment of osteoarthritis and rheumatoid osteoarthritis. Total elbow arthroplasty reliably improves functional ROM and strength in most patients. Even in those with ankylosis after posttraumatic arthritis, improvements of about 80 degrees of ROM occur in the flexion and extension arc.

Complications are more common than with other total joint arthroplasties, and the short-term complication rate (within the first year) may be as high as 10%. Complications include aseptic loosening, joint instability, fracture, ulnar neuropathy, wound complications, venous thrombosis, pulmonary emboli, and infection. Ulnar neuropathies do not usually require an additional procedure, paresthesias are usually transient, and motor weakness is rare. Many patients with rheumatoid osteoarthritis have ulnar neuropathy before surgery, and the total elbow arthroplasty may not have contributed significantly to postoperative symptoms. Aseptic loosening, metallosis, severe polyethylene bushing wear in semiconstrained devices, instability in nonconstrained devices, and infection are reasons for revision. For aseptic loosening, revision with a longer stemmed prosthesis usually suffices. Impaction bone grafting into the endosteal canal of the distal humerus or proximal ulna is also an option. Polyethylene bushing wear is diagnosed from diminished space between the humeral and ulnar components on radiographs.

Contraindications to total elbow arthroplasty include active shoulder infection, poor bone stock that precludes fixation of the prosthesis, neuropathic arthropathy as occurs for example with a cervical syrinx, and the absence of biceps and triceps function.

Ali A, Shahane S, Stanley D: Total elbow arthroplasty for distal humeral fractures: indications, surgical approach, technical tips, and outcome. *J Shoulder Elbow Surg* 2010;19(2 Suppl):53. [PMID: 20188269]

Celli A, Morrey BF: Total elbow arthroplasty in patients forty years of age or less. *J Bone Joint Surg Am* 2009;91:1414. [PMID: 19487519]

Cook C, Hawkins R, Aldridge JM 3rd, Tolan S, Krupp R, Bolognesi M: Comparison of perioperative complications in patients with and without rheumatoid arthritis who receive total elbow replacement. *J Shoulder Elbow Surg* 2009;18:21. [PMID: 19095171]

Kokkalis ZT, Schmidt CC, Sotereanos DG: Elbow arthritis: current concepts. *J Hand Surg Am* 2009;34:761. [PMID: 19345885]

Krenek L, Farng E, Zingmond D, Soohoo NF: Complication and revision rates following total elbow arthroplasty. *J Hand Surg Am* 2011;36:68. [PMID: 21193128]

Larson AN, Morrey BF: Interposition arthroplasty with an Achilles tendon allograft as a salvage procedure for the elbow. *J Bone Joint Surg Am* 2008;90:2714. [PMID: 19047718]

Shore BJ, Mozzon JB, MacDermid JC, Faber KJ, King GJ: Chronic posttraumatic elbow disorders treated with metallic radial head arthroplasty. *J Bone Joint Surg Am* 2008;90:271. [PMID: 18245585]

Skyttä ET, Eskelinen A, Paavolainen P, Ikävalko M, Remes V: Total elbow arthroplasty in rheumatoid arthritis: a population-based study from the Finnish Arthroplasty Register. *Acta Orthop* 2009;80:472. [PMID: 19562563]

Throckmorton T, Zarkadas P, Sanchez-Sotelo J, Morrey B: Failure patterns after linked semiconstrained total elbow arthroplasty for posttraumatic arthritis. *J Bone Joint Surg Am* 2010;92:1432. [PMID: 20516319]

Wada T, Isogai S, Ishii S, et al: Debridement arthroplasty for primary osteoarthritis of the elbow. *J Bone Joint Surg Am* 2005;87-A:95. [PMID: 15743851]

▶ Total Ankle Arthroplasty

The total ankle arthroplasty was under development for many years as a result of the success with total joint replacement of the knee and the hip. Initial designs met with modest short-term success and caused almost an abandonment of the procedure because of the comparison to ankle arthrodesis. The longevity of total ankle joint replacements has been somewhat erratic for a variety of reasons. The articular surface that must be replaced is unlike any other joint, and thus experience cannot be carried directly from the knee or the hip to the ankle. Joint loads and requirements are less well characterized, and surgical technique is less well developed and, therefore, less reliable. For these reasons, total ankle replacement had been a developmental procedure indicated for patients with low activity demand and the need for ankle motion. In 2006, the FDA approved two new and improved designs that have renewed interest in this procedure.

Total ankle replacement is desirable because of the drawbacks of ankle arthrodesis, which include a significant pseudoarthrosis rate of 10–20%, despite extended cast immobilization to achieve arthrodesis. Furthermore, arthrodesis results in osteopenia and diminished motion in the subtalar and midtarsal joints. The additional stress on these joints from the ankle arthrodesis predisposes them to degenerative changes over the long term, as is seen frequently above and below the arthrodesis in other joints such as the cervical spine, the lumbar spine, and the hip.

Chou LB, Coughlin MT, Hansen S Jr, et al: Osteoarthritis of the ankle: the role of arthroplasty. *J Am Acad Orthop Surg* 2008;16:249. [PMID: 18460685]

Guyer AJ, Richardson G: Current concepts review: total ankle arthroplasty. *Foot Ankle Int* 2008;29:256. [PMID: 18315988]

Raikin SM, Kane J, Ciminiello ME: Risk factors for incision–healing complications following total ankle arthroplasty. *J Bone Joint Surg Am* 2010;92:2150. [PMID: 20842156]

▶ Evaluation of Painful Total Joint Arthroplasty

A certain degree of adaptation and accommodation is possible in the normal joint, allowing it to last for a lifetime in most persons. After replacement of a diseased joint by a metal-and-plastic artificial joint, no remodeling or accommodation is possible. Loosening of the interface between bone and prosthesis is possible and, indeed, may be inevitable. In addition, during and subsequent to the implantation process, bacteria may find their way into a prosthetic joint, causing pain or loosening. Implantation of a new joint markedly alters the stress state in the bone, particularly with uncemented prostheses, and a certain amount of pain may result. The presence of the new joint is likely to alleviate pain markedly, and the patient's activity level may increase, resulting in bone remodeling around the prosthesis or at a remote site or even fatigue fractures. All of these problems may result in a painful arthroplasty. Evaluation is complicated by the presence of the artificial joint, which introduces several new variables when compared with a normal arthritic joint. The same process of evaluation is used as with an arthritic joint; a history is obtained, physical examination is performed, and laboratory data are obtained.

A. History

Referred pain from other sources must be ruled out, particularly with the shoulder and the hip, where referred pain from the lumbar and cervical spine may confuse the picture. A history of pain radiating into the shoulder with motion of the neck, for example, may be helpful in this process. Pain related to activity of the affected joint, as compared with pain all the time, is an important fact, with constant pain or night pain suggesting chronic infection. Pain in the hip or knee that occurs with the first few steps but then improves somewhat with further ambulation is likely to be caused by loosening of the prosthesis. This pain probably arises from a fibrous membrane between the prosthesis and bone, which, with weight bearing, compresses and provides better contact, thereby lessening the pain. A history of swelling, redness, fevers, or chills must be obtained, which is suggestive of an infectious etiology for the painful joint. Also suggestive of infection is excessive drainage or delayed wound healing or skin necrosis in the postoperative period of the initial implantation.

B. Physical Examination

The same tests are performed as for an arthritic joint to evaluate the location, magnitude, and severity of pain.

C. Workup

1. Laboratory findings—Laboratory data may be helpful. The ESR (>35–40 mm/h) or C-reactive protein (CRP) (>0.7) points toward an infected arthroplasty; with the knee, a lower ESR does not rule out infected arthroplasty. A complete blood count is also sometimes helpful in demonstrating an elevated white blood cell count.

These data are less helpful in the early postoperative period. The CRP will be elevated after surgery and should trend to normal by 6 weeks after surgery. The ESR rises after surgery, peaks at about 2 weeks after surgery, and returns to normal by 6 months after surgery. The skin temperature is elevated due to inflammation after surgery and averages 4.5°C higher than the normal knee at 2 weeks and slowly decreases to within 1°C at 6 months after surgery.

2. Arthrographic evaluation—Arthrographic evaluation may be helpful by showing dye penetration into the cement–bone interface, prosthesis–bone interface, or prosthesis–cement interface. The most important aspect of arthrographic evaluation is the fluid obtained for culture and for cell count and differential. A high percentage of polymorphonuclear leukocytes (>90%) is highly suggestive of infection, despite a low cell count or negative culture. Arthrographic evaluation is mainly indicated when infection is suspected because there is a risk of contaminating the joint as well as the possibility of obtaining false-positive and false-negative cultures. Another important aspect of arthrographic evaluation is the pain response to injection of lidocaine into the joint. Alleviation of essentially all pain when weight bearing is attempted after injection localizes the problem to the affected joint.

3. Indium-labeled white blood cell scan—Bone scans have little value immediately after surgery. Significant bone remodeling is present, which continues for several months. Bone scans may not be helpful until 6 months to 1 year after surgery. At that point, increased uptake indicates bone remodeling and loosening or infection of the prosthesis.

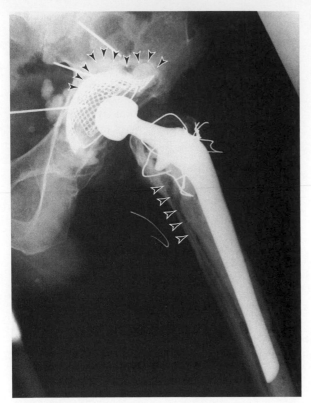

▲ **Figure 6–11.** Radiograph of radiolucent lines around an acetabular component.

The indium-labeled white blood cell scan can be useful immediately after surgery or in the face possible acute infection.

This nuclear medicine study uses the patient's polymorphonuclear leukocytes, which are labeled with radioactive indium and injected back into the patient. It may be quite beneficial in localizing acute infectious processes but is frequently not helpful in the evaluation of chronic infection.

4. Plain radiographs—Radiographic examination is the single most useful test in the evaluation of nonseptic loosening. Important signs are radiolucent lines adjacent to the prosthesis or cement, particularly if they are 2 mm or greater or are becoming enlarged on serial radiographs (Figure 6–11). Fracture of the cement and change in position of the component are indications of loosening.

Honsawek S, Deepaisarnsakul B, Tanavalee A, et al: Relationship of serum IL-6, C-reactive protein, ESR and knee skin temperature after total knee arthroplasty: a prospective study. *Int Orthop* 2011;35:31. [PMID: 21203883]

Lee SC, Jung KA, Yoon JY, et al: Analysis of synovial fluid in culture-negative samples of suspicious periprosthetic infections. *Orthopedics* 2010;33:725. [PMID: 20954662]

▶ Treatment of Infected Total Joint Arthroplasty

Definitive evidence of a septic total joint arthroplasty forecasts a poor prognosis for the patient. The infectious process is either acute or chronic, and the infection is either gram negative or gram positive. Either the components are tightly fixed to bone or one or more of the components is loose. In acute infection with tightly fixed components, most surgeons debride the joint without removing the components and treat the infection locally and with systemic antibiotic therapy. A chronically infected or loose prosthesis is usually treated with removal of the prosthesis, local wound care, and systemic antimicrobial therapy. Therapy for an acutely infected, firmly fixed prosthesis varies according to surgeon preference.

There is general concurrence that thorough debridement of the joint, synovectomy, removal of necrotic material, and copious irrigation are necessary at the time of debridement. Because of the potential presence of glycocalyx, surfaces of the prosthesis available for inspection are scrubbed with Dakin solution, which dissolves the glycocalyx. Removable components are removed, and the undersurfaces are cleaned with Dakin solution. New polyethylene components are inserted if available; if this is not possible, the old polyethylene prosthesis is scrubbed with Dakin solution and reinserted. To prevent superinfection, the wound must be tightly closed. To help eradicate the existing infection, however, irrigation and drainage must be continued. One suitable method is that described by Jergesen and Jawetz, in which small volumes of antibiotic solution are instilled into the joint twice a day, and the joint is sealed off for 3 hours, followed by 9 hours of suction (Figure 6–12). This protocol begins 24 hours after surgery, during which time suction drainage is maintained. The instillation-suction system is maintained for 10 days. At the end of the course of

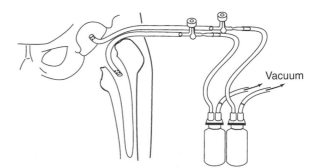

▲ **Figure 6–12.** Schematic diagram of the Jergesen system of instillation of antibiotics. The antibiotics can be varied depending on the susceptibility of the infecting bacteria (fungus). The amount instilled is approximately 5 mL per tube plus the dead space from the valve to the joint.

irrigation and instillation, a culture is aspirated from the joint after one antibiotic instillation. This system can also be used for osteomyelitis and routine joint infections. Antibiotics are continued for an appropriate period of time (usually 6 weeks) after the tubes are withdrawn.

In cases of loose prostheses, little alternative is available except to remove the prosthesis. A similar system of instillation and suction is then used, using the same protocol. If reimplantation is likely after infected total knee prosthesis, an antibiotic cement block is used to separate the bone ends and maintain a potential joint space. An alternative to the cement block is the PROSTALAC system as described earlier. This technique has the benefit of maintaining hip or knee joint muscle length and elasticity. In patients in whom reimplantation is planned, the ESR is followed monthly until it is normal without antibiotic therapy. In patients with rheumatoid osteoarthritis or other disorders in which the rate may be elevated, 6 months is an appropriate time to wait for possible recrudescence of the infection. At this point, either an aspiration arthrogram or a Craig needle biopsy is used to obtain specimens for culture. If these are negative, reimplantation surgery is planned.

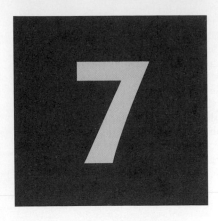

7

Orthopedic Infections: Basic Principles of Pathogenesis, Diagnosis, and Treatment

Richard L. McGough, III, MD

Dann Laudermilch, MD

Kurt R. Weiss, MD

ESSENTIALS OF DIAGNOSIS

Orthopedic infections are common entities. Orthopedic infections can arise de novo, even in healthy hosts. Orthopedic infections are unfortunately a common surgical complication as well. Like all surgical complications, the only way to avoid encountering infection is to either ignore the problem or not to perform surgery in the first place. Otherwise, infections can and will occur. Infections, especially iatrogenic and nosocomial infections, are receiving increasing attention and visibility in the lay press. There is no shortage of popular media describing individual or institutional infectious complications and a rapidly evolving movement by the Centers for Medicare and Medicaid Services (CMS) to not reimburse institutions for the treatment of nosocomial infection. For this reason, infection prevention, recognition, and prompt attention are of paramount importance.

The most essential element of diagnosis is an appropriate index of suspicion. Orthopedic infections are frequently subtle, and without a high level of suspicion, treatment will be delayed. Diagnosis is especially difficult for postoperative wounds for a variety of reasons. The first and most important reason for this difficulty is denial: the quality of our work becomes questioned, and the path of least resistance is to deny that a problem exists. This is especially dangerous in the postoperative situation and in compromised hosts. Prompt treatment may salvage the index procedure, and patients with decreased physiologic reserve may possess the reserve to overcome a developing infection but not an established one. A second difficulty with postoperative wounds is the overlapping qualities of subcutaneous hematomas, delayed wound healing, and frank infection. Many postoperative wounds can be slow to heal without being infected. Likewise, different individuals will demonstrate differing levels of swelling, erythema, and tissue warmth in an uncomplicated postoperative course based simply on body habitus, coagulation status, or skin complexion. Our mandate to "do no harm" becomes most difficult in the complex patient who

is most threatened, as unnecessary returns to the operating room for unsubstantiated infectious concerns may subject the patient to further risk. Accurate diagnosis remains difficult, as most signs of infection are subjective.

In the first century AD, Celsus described the quartet of calor (warmth), dolor (pain), rubor (redness), and tumor (swelling) as the essential quartet of infection. Two millennia later, these clinical clues are still the "vital signs" of infection. Beyond this, infection should be suspected in patients who are "going the wrong direction" after treatment. More intensive investigations, as detailed later by general category, are warranted in these individuals.

Any discussion of orthopedic infections varies tremendously based on etiology, because, for example, pediatric osteomyelitis is a very different entity than periprosthetic knee infections. Detailed discussions of specific infections are given in topical areas within this book. For the purposes of this chapter, different types of orthopedic infections will be discussed in general categories.

GENERAL CONSIDERATIONS

As alluded to earlier, orthopedic infections can be broadly divided into two categories. The first is spontaneous infection, where no orthopedic surgical intervention has occurred, and some combination of factors contributes to the infection. This encompasses pediatric and adult osteomyelitis, as well as spontaneous soft-tissue infections. The second broad category is that of postoperative or posttraumatic infections. These occur when the soft-tissue envelope has been breached either deliberately (postoperative infections) or traumatically. In modern trauma care, infection can often be attributed to both, as after surgical stabilization of open fractures.

▶ Pediatric Osteomyelitis

Spontaneous osteomyelitis is a common entity in children. It may occur at any time from birth to adulthood, but generally possesses a decreasing incidence into adolescence, after which it is possible but becomes much rarer (see Clinical Corollary #1). The pathogenesis of pediatric osteomyelitis is thought to be due to the watershed nature of the metaphyseal vascularity, with a low-flow, centripetal system of vascularity. This allows normally encountered blood pathogens a microenvironment in which they may multiply isolated from most circulating lymphocytes, thereby evading initial immune surveillance. The most common pathogen is *Staphylococcus aureus,* followed by group A *Streptococcus* and *Haemophilus influenzae.* Patients suffering from sickle cell anemia have an unusual propensity for *Salmonella* infections.

Upon multiplication, bacteria produce matrix metalloproteinases, which degrade the surrounding cancellous bone and allow abscess formation. The abscess further disrupts an already poor blood supply and shields bacteria from the immune response. This devascularization causes osteonecrosis and formation of a *sequestrum,* which is a radiographic hallmark of osteomyelitis. This sequestrum is seen as an area of hyperdense, necrotic bone surrounded by lysis on plain radiographs. The rate of progression depends on how robustly the host can respond to the infection. If the host is able to mount a response and surround the sequestrum, it will be encapsulated by a rim of living, immunocompetent bone called an *involucrum.* If, on the other hand, the infection spreads with enough vigor that the host bone cannot contain it, bacteria will continue to multiply. The abscess will enlarge and eventually destroy the surrounding cortex. This will cause a purulent response that will produce a very aggressive radiographic appearance, mimicking Ewing sarcoma (see Clinical Corollary #1). The purulent material will raise the surrounding periosteum, create a *Codman triangle,* and produce a permeative appearance in the subjacent cortex, and may even form a soft-tissue mass.

Clinically, children with acute osteomyelitis typically appear ill. Many, if not most, will have a febrile response greater than 38.5°C. Nearly all will complain of localized pain and swelling and, in lower extremity cases, will present with an inability or unwillingness to ambulate. If the area of infection occurs beneath the adjacent joint capsule, an acute septic joint may occur with substantial pain, resistance to motion, and effusion. Radiographs may demonstrate the features described earlier and, in the case of joint sepsis, will have evidence of effusion. Laboratory analysis generally demonstrates leukocytosis with a left shift to greater than 70% neutrophils. Erythrocyte sedimentation rates (ESRs) will be elevated, as will C-reactive protein (CRP) levels. Laboratory results are especially important in the differential diagnosis of pediatric osteomyelitis because radiographs can easily be confused with pediatric sarcomas, especially Ewing sarcoma.

A. Clinical Corollary #1

Patient 1 is a healthy 15-year-old male student athlete who noted the onset of pain, swelling, and cramping in his left thigh 1 month before presentation. He denied any trauma. These symptoms gradually worsened to the point of his being unable to attend school. He also developed fevers, chills, night sweats, and malaise. Radiographs and a magnetic resonance imaging (MRI) scan were obtained by a community physician, and he was subsequently referred to a tertiary medical center.

X-rays were essentially normal (Figures 7–1 to 7–5), but MRI scan revealed extensive bone marrow infiltration and a large soft-tissue mass involving nearly the entire circumference of the femur (Figures 7–6 to 7–10). The differential diagnosis at this point included bone neoplasm versus infection. The patient was sent for a computed tomography (CT) scan–guided biopsy. The CT scan suggested intramedullary abscess formation and showed air within the soft tissues (Figure 7–11). Laboratory evaluation showed a white blood cell count of 14.0×10^3 cells/mL with 79.4% neutrophils. ESR and CRP were 114 mm/h and 22.31 mg/dL, respectively, consistent with infection. Biopsy revealed acute inflammatory cells and bacteria, further substantiating the diagnosis.

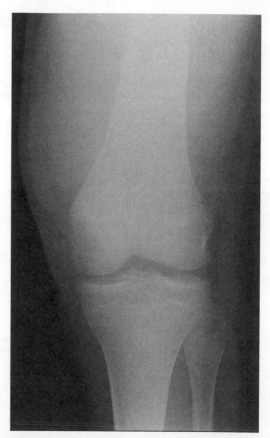

▲ **Figure 7–1.** Anteroposterior knee for Patient 1. Beside the suggestion of a soft-tissue mass, there are no obvious destructive changes to the bone.

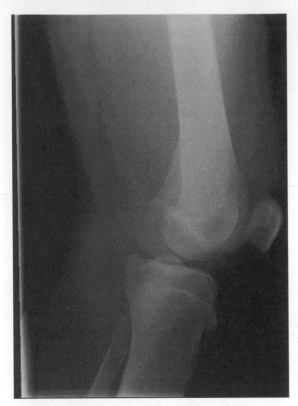

▲ **Figure 7–2.** Lateral knee for Patient 1.

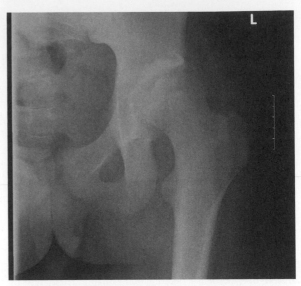

▲ **Figure 7–4.** Anteroposterior hip for Patient 1.

The patient was taken to the operating room where a lateral approach to the femur was made. Copious amounts of purulent material were encountered, and the soft tissues were extensively irrigated and debrided. A 4-cm × 2-cm ovoid hole was made in the lateral cortex of the femur, and flexible reamers were passed into the proximal and distal femur. Antibiotic beads containing 1 g of tobramycin and 3 g of vancomycin per 40 g of polymethylmethacrylate (PMMA) were placed in

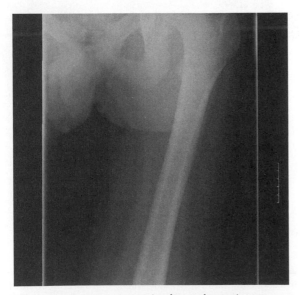

▲ **Figure 7–3.** Anteroposterior femur for Patient 1.

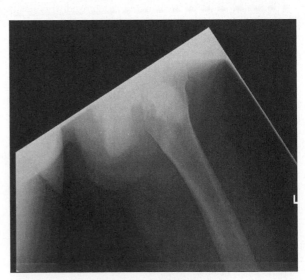

▲ **Figure 7–5.** Lateral femur for Patient 1.

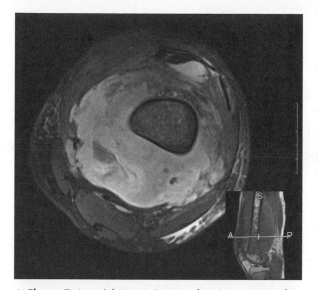

▲ **Figure 7–6.** Axial T2 MRI image of Patient 1. Note the extensive marrow involvement and nearly circumferential involvement of the femur.

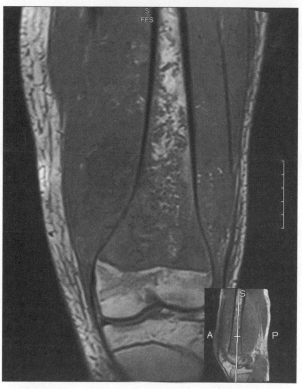

▲ **Figure 7–8.** Coronal T1 MRI image of Patient 1.

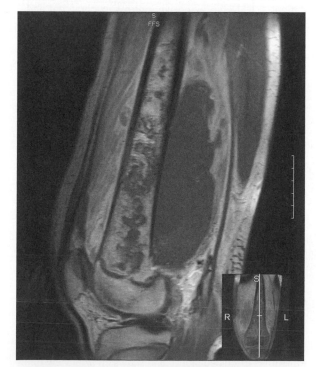

▲ **Figure 7–7.** Sagittal T1 MRI image of Patient 1.

the intramedullary canal (Figures 7–12 to 7–15). Operative cultures from the purulent material, soft tissue, and bone reamings were all positive for methicillin-sensitive *S. aureus*, and the patient was placed on intravenous therapy with continuous-infusion oxacillin for 6 weeks under the supervision of a musculoskeletal infectious disease consultant.

Subsequent to the completion of systemic antibiotic therapy, he was taken back to the operating room for removal of the antibiotic beads, irrigation, and repeat intraoperative cultures of the bone and soft tissues. These cultures were all negative. At the most recent follow-up, his knee motion was normal. The laboratory parameters had normalized with an ESR of 3 mm/h and a CRP of less than 0.1 mg/dL.

▶ Adult Osteomyelitis

Adult osteomyelitis is fortunately rare. As the growing child reaches skeletal maturity, the metaphyseal bone vascularity changes, and the pediatric venous sinusoids are eliminated. This produces improved blood flow, decreasing the prevalence of spontaneous osteomyelitis. Most cases of adult osteomyelitis are therefore a result of skin penetration, either deliberate or accidental. A few cases merit special mention.

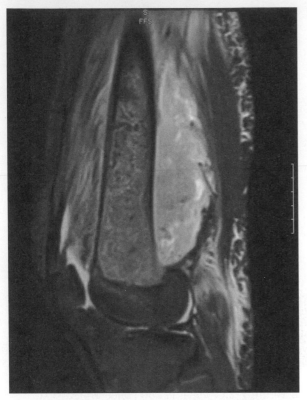

▲ **Figure 7–9.** Sagittal T2 MRI image of Patient 1. Note the extensive marrow involvement and nearly circumferential involvement of the femur.

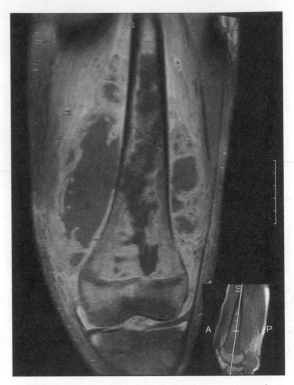

▲ **Figure 7–10.** Coronal fat-saturated MRI image of Patient 1. Note the extensive marrow involvement and nearly circumferential involvement of the femur.

Aside from accidental or surgical trauma, most cases of adult osteomyelitis occur in individuals who are unable to maintain a normal soft-tissue envelope over subjacent bone. This occurs with disturbing frequency in paraplegics and diabetics, as the normal protective sensation over bony prominences (sacrum, femora, ischial tuberosities, calcanei, and metatarsals) is disrupted. This leads to pressure sores, which, if untreated, will progress to the bone. Once the bone is exposed to air, its vascularity is compromised and osteomyelitis occurs. This form of osteomyelitis is much more chronic than that seen in children, and the symptomatology is quite different. Because many of these individuals are insensate, pain is not a prominent finding. Also, the acute purulent response found in the pediatric case is rarely present, instead manifesting as open, draining sinuses. Infectious indices (ESR/CRP) may demonstrate increased values, but a leukocytosis with left shift is generally absent. Individuals with this condition may persist for years or even decades with osteomyelitis, having no symptoms until developing squamous cell carcinoma (Marjolin ulcer) within the sinus tract.

The situation is quite different in patients who are immunocompromised. Patients who are suffering from human

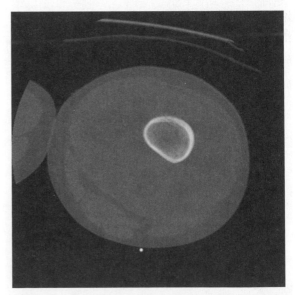

▲ **Figure 7–11.** This image was obtained at the time of Patient 1's CT-guided biopsy and shows an axial view of his thigh. There is a suggestion of air in the soft tissues, which supports the diagnosis of infection rather than tumor.

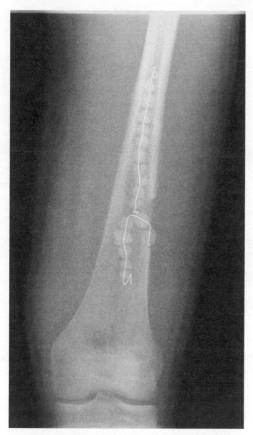

▲ **Figure 7–12.** Orthogonal view 1 of Patient 1's femur after debridement, irrigation, intramedullary reaming, and the placement of antibiotic beads. The beads were subsequently removed after 6 weeks of intravenous antibiotic therapy, and Patient 1's clinical examination improved tremendously. He has returned to limited participation in sports.

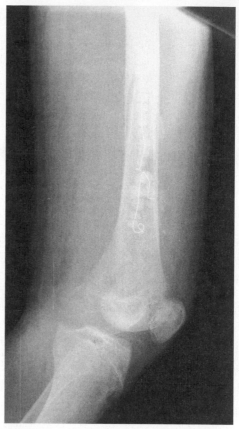

▲ **Figure 7–13.** Orthogonal view 2 of Patient 1's femur after debridement, irrigation, intramedullary reaming, and the placement of antibiotic beads. The beads were subsequently removed after 6 weeks of intravenous antibiotic therapy, and Patient 1's clinical examination improved tremendously. He has returned to limited participation in sports.

immunodeficiency virus (HIV) or acquired immunodeficiency syndrome (AIDS), who have undergone solid organ or bone marrow transplantation, or who are undergoing cytotoxic chemotherapy may develop acute osteomyelitis. The hallmark of this disease is pain without an obvious source, and this symptom may occur anywhere in the involved bone. This condition may also produce spontaneous joint sepsis, most commonly in the sternoclavicular and sacroiliac joints. Immunocompromised individuals with osteomyelitis will present with pain and fever but will lack leukocytosis, as the dysfunctional immunity producing the osteomyelitis precludes an adequate immune response. Infectious indices are rarely useful, as many of these individuals have other causes of inflammation that will confound these nonspecific test parameters. A very high index of suspicion is required to make this diagnosis, as plain radiographs will likely only demonstrate osteopenia and MRI scanning shows only bony edema on T2-weighted sequences. Generally no abscess forms within the bone. In this instance, prompt diagnosis can be critical because patients do not possess the immunologic reserve to fight a fulminant infection.

Collinet-Adler S, Castro CA, Ledonio CG, Bechtold JE, Tsukayama DT: *Acinetobacter baumannii* is not associated with osteomyelitis in a rat model: a pilot study. *Clin Orthop Relat Res* 2011;469:274. [PMID: 3008889]

A. Clinical Corollary #2

Patient 2 is a 33-year-old man with a chief complaint of steadily increasing left thigh pain for 1 month. He denied any trauma or constitutional symptoms. He had a negative

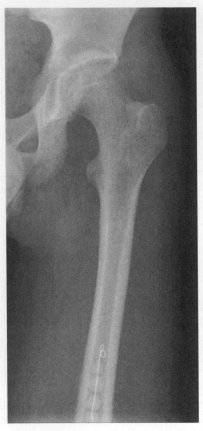

▲ **Figure 7–14.** Orthogonal view of Patient 1's femur after debridement, irrigation, intramedullary reaming, and the placement of antibiotic beads. The beads were subsequently removed after 6 weeks of intravenous antibiotic therapy, and Patient 1's clinical examination improved tremendously. He has returned to limited participation in sports.

medical and surgical history but had a social history of heavy drug abuse. He was initially seen at a community hospital where radiographs suggested a permeative lesion in the lateral cortex of the left femur (Figure 7–16). He was subsequently transferred to a tertiary medical center for further management.

At the tertiary medical center, he was found to be afebrile with stable vital signs. Laboratory evaluation disclosed a white blood cell count of 12.4×10^9 cells/L with 70.5% neutrophils and a platelet count of 524×10^3 cells/mL. His ESR and CRP were both elevated at 66 mm/h and 1.96 mg/dL, respectively.

CT scan and MRI scan were obtained. CT scan showed changes in the femur consistent with sequestrum formation, and MRI scan revealed intense soft-tissue edema around the lesion. A presumptive diagnosis of tumor versus infection was made (Figures 7–17 to 7–20).

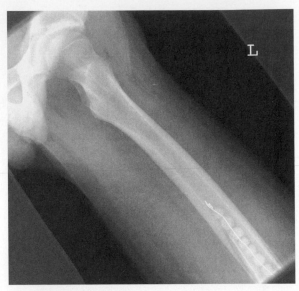

▲ **Figure 7–15.** Orthogonal view of Patient 1's femur after debridement, irrigation, intramedullary reaming, and the placement of antibiotic beads. The beads were subsequently removed after 6 weeks of intravenous antibiotic therapy, and Patient 1's clinical examination improved tremendously. He has returned to limited participation in sports.

The patient was subsequently taken to the operating room where an open biopsy of the left femur and the surrounding tissues was performed. Pathology on frozen section was consistent with acute infection and the diagnosis of osteomyelitis with soft-tissue involvement was made. The muscle around the femur was thoroughly debrided, and the femur itself was likewise debrided with rongeurs, curettes, and a high-speed burr (Figure 7–21). Cultures from the musculature, periosteum, bone, and intermedullary canal were all obtained. After copious irrigation, a strand of antibiotic beads containing 1 g of tobramycin and 3 g of vancomycin per 40 g of PMMA was made and placed next to the femur (Figure 7–22). The wound was closed in layers. Postoperative radiographs showed obliteration of the abnormal bone (Figure 7–23).

All operative cultures were positive for methicillin-resistant *S. aureus* (MRSA). The patient was placed on oral antibiotic therapy with linezolid for 6 weeks with plans to remove his antibiotic beads and perform a repeat irrigation and debridement after the completion of antibiotic therapy.

Hamzaoui A, Salem R, Koubaa M, et al: *Escherichia coli* osteomyelitis of the ischium in an adult. *Orthop Traumatol Surg Res* 2009;95:636. [PMID: 19944663]

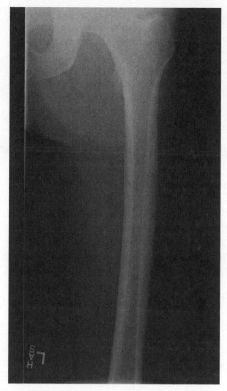

▲ **Figure 7–16.** Anteroposterior projection of Patient 2's femur. Note the poorly defined, permeative lesion in the lateral diaphyseal cortex. This was concerning for infection or a bone neoplasm.

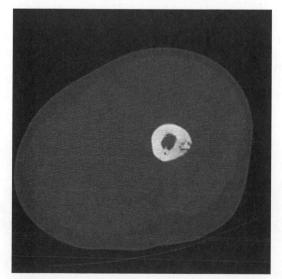

▲ **Figure 7–17.** Axial CT image suggests the presence of a sequestrum within the lateral cortex of the femur.

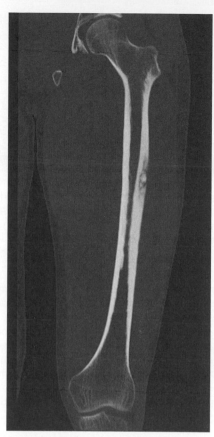

▲ **Figure 7–18.** Coronal CT image suggests the presence of a sequestrum within the lateral cortex of the femur.

▶ Adult Spontaneous Soft-Tissue Infections

Soft-tissue infections are common. Admissions to medical services for cellulitis, a common skin infection, are frequent in most hospitals. These conditions may occur in the setting of medical comorbidities, such as venous stasis, diabetes, obesity, or immunocompromise. They are generally treated with antibiotics alone, and rarely is surgical intervention necessary.

Deep, abscess-producing skin infections in adults are usually the result of skin penetration. This occurs either due to trauma, iatrogenic skin penetration, or intravenous drug use. These causes are sometimes obvious, as in the case of intravenous drug use, but may be difficult to ascertain, as in septic olecranon bursitis. Bursitis is often presumed to be due to trauma, as the extensor surface of the elbow is frequently traumatized. Surgical treatment of simple abscesses with irrigation and drainage as well as wound packing or vacuum-assisted closure generally yields satisfactory results.

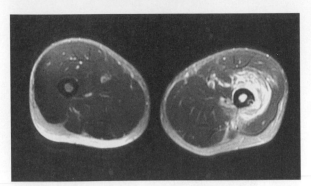

▲ **Figure 7–19.** Axial MRI image illustrating the dramatic difference between the affected and nonaffected limbs. The image also shows a substantial soft-tissue component to the process.

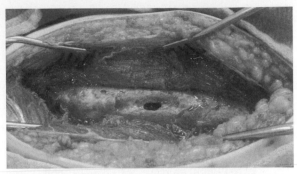

▲ **Figure 7–21.** Intraoperative view of Patient 2's femur after biopsy, culture, thorough curettage, and burring of the abnormal bone in the lateral cortex. Bone and soft tissue were sent for pathologic and microbiologic testing. All samples were positive for methicillin-resistant *Staphylococcus aureus* infection and negative for neoplasm.

Occasionally, intravenous drug abusers can present with a mixed picture of both bone and soft-tissue infection (see Clinical Corollary #2).

Severe, spontaneous, deep soft-tissue infections, those occurring below the fascia, are decidedly rarer, and tend to occur in individuals with some form of immunocompromise. While the often publicized "flesh-eating bacteria" seen in necrotizing fasciitis may infect immunocompetent hosts, those with an immune-compromised comorbidity are at much greater risk. These individuals are generally as follows: patients who are neutropenic secondary to cytotoxic chemotherapy, those suffering from HIV/AIDS, or those with other, frequently autoimmune, diseases that render the normal tissues susceptible to bacteria in the environment. In immunocompromised individuals, the typical signs of infection may be absent, and the patient may simply manifest a high fever (>38.5°C), tenderness, and erythema. Advanced imaging with MRI may demonstrate only edema within the affected area because the patient often does not have adequate immunity to form an abscess. These patients are at great risk, and surgical debridement coupled with broad-spectrum antibiotics may be lifesaving.

Because of the vascular nature of muscle, pyomyositis in immunocompetent individuals is rare. Etiologically, pyomyositis is different than simple abscess formation; in pyomyositis, the bacteria occlude the small vascular inflow into the muscle, producing necrosis. This avascular bed is an

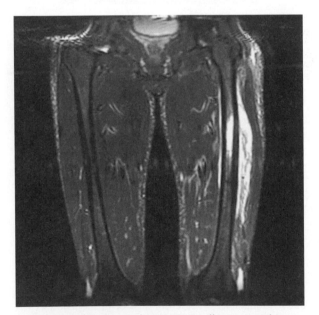

▲ **Figure 7–20.** Coronal MRI image illustrating the dramatic difference between the affected and nonaffected limbs. The image also shows a substantial soft-tissue component to the process.

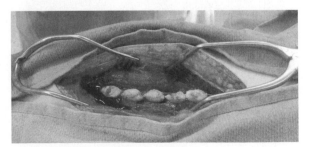

▲ **Figure 7–22.** A strand of antibiotic-impregnated beads were placed after copious irrigation with antibiotic-containing pulse lavage fluid.

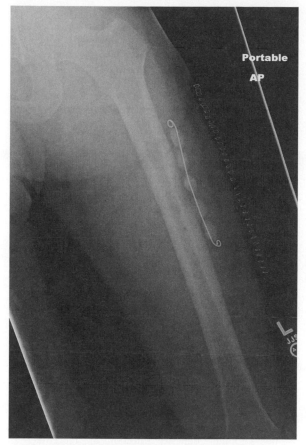

▲ Figure 7–23. Postoperative anteroposterior (AP) radiograph of Patient 2's femur. Note the removal of the permeative lateral bone (see Figure 7–16 for comparison).

ideal culture medium for bacteria, and liquefactive necrosis occurs. Treatment of pyomyositis is more extensive than many soft-tissue infections because all necrotic material must be thoroughly removed before the infection can be controlled. Serial debridement and adjunctive intravenous antibiotics are the mainstays of treatment, as initial debridement often fails to remove all necrotic material.

Necrotizing fasciitis is the most dreaded deep soft-tissue infection. Classically caused by *Clostridium perfringens*, it can become a rapidly progressive, life-threatening event. Necrotizing fasciitis caused by other organisms may not present with as fulminant a course and may more closely mimic cellulitis or other soft-tissue infections. Necrotizing fasciitis is a clinical diagnosis: although MRI may demonstrate T2 enhancement of the fascia, this finding is extremely nonspecific, and the clinician acting on the clinical findings will yield a much more timely diagnosis. Clinically, the patients are quite ill, with fever, malaise, and localized pain. Signs of systemic sepsis may be present, with mental status

changes, tachycardia, or even hypotension. Palpation of the affected area demonstrates a swollen, boggy texture to the skin and soft tissues. The skin may also be hypermobile, similar to after a fasciocutaneous injury. Bullous changes may also occur.

Treatment of necrotizing fasciitis is time dependent. Time should not be wasted obtaining confirmatory diagnostic tests, as these are rarely specific enough to change the clinical diagnosis, and substantial delays may be limb or life threatening. Surgical treatment is extensive and requires debridement of *all* affected skin and fascia. In fulminant cases, soft-tissue reconstruction is generally required. Debridement to healthy, vascularized skin is mandatory, and debridement of the subjacent muscle may be required. The presence of myonecrosis may make amputation necessary, and the performance of a high amputation such as a hip disarticulation or forequarter amputation may be necessary as a lifesaving measure.

JOINT INFECTIONS

▶ Prosthetic Joint Infections

Prosthetic infection after arthroplasty is a dreaded complication of this procedure, which is performed with increasing frequency in our aging population. With the number of arthroplasties projected to increase dramatically, treating prosthetic infections may become a full-time profession for some orthopedic surgeons. The costs of this treatment are extensive and, when multiplied by our aging population, may become astronomical.

Prosthetic infections are divided into three categories. The first is an acute infection following surgery. In this case, the patient will demonstrate fever, increasing pain, erythema, and poor wound healing. Distinguishing a typical postoperative knee wound from an acutely infected postoperative knee wound is an art, and the gravity of ignoring the infection must be balanced with the morbidity of a return to the operating theater. Fortunately, acute sepsis following arthroplasty is rare (<1%), and most of these situations may be salvaged by aggressive and timely debridement and polyethylene exchange, followed by intravenous antibiotics.

A more difficult problem to distinguish is the subacute prosthetic infection. In this case, a well-functioning, painless arthroplasty becomes acutely painful, warm, and effusive. At times, a suggestive history such as recent dental infection, skin trauma to the ipsilateral limb, or an unrelated invasive procedure may be elicited. If the aforementioned constellation of symptoms has been occurring for only a short period of time (generally <2 or 3 weeks), the joint may be salvaged with aggressive surgical debridement, intravenous antibiotics, and polyethylene exchange. Removal of the bacterial exudate (glycocalyx or biofilm) with Dakin's solution from the prosthetic surfaces may be helpful.

The most common variety of prosthetic infection is a chronic infection. This occurs when a well-functioning joint of intermediate to long duration (>3 months, but perhaps years after the index procedure) becomes painful, warm, and effusive. Sinus tracts may form in the adjacent skin, leading to chronic drainage. In this situation, the infection has generally been present for weeks to years, and bacterial colonization and biofilm formation have organized on the joint surface. Many surgeons attempt a debridement and polyethylene component exchange if the components are tightly fixed. When the components are loose, or if permanent suppression is planned, the affected joint should generally be removed and replaced with antibiotic-containing bone cement. The patient is then treated with systemic antibiotics for several (usually 6) weeks. If sterilization occurs, as determined by normal CRP and ESR laboratory values and a normal aspirate culture, replantation may then be contemplated.

Traumatic Infections

Traumatic infections are unfortunately common, and their incidence corresponds directly to the energy imparted by the injury. The maxim that "an open fracture is a soft-tissue injury that happens to have a broken bone in it" is true, as devitalized, devascularized tissue becomes rapidly colonized upon exposure to air, soil, or other materials. To minimize the risk of traumatic infection, all open fractures should be treated urgently with thorough debridement and skeletal stabilization. This allows devitalized tissues to declare themselves so that subsequent surgeries facilitate complete removal of all abnormal tissue. Despite the most meticulous care, open fractures may still become infected, and this problem is much more prevalent in certain anatomic locations. Clearly the tibia, a subcutaneous bone throughout much of its circumference, is the most at risk, and modern trauma care often combines soft-tissue reconstruction with bony stabilization to minimize the risk of osteomyelitis.

Septic Arthritis

Nonprosthetic septic arthritis is unusual in adults. Most commonly, a history of penetrating injury will be elicited. Septic arthritis can also be seen in immunocompromised individuals without trauma. Septic arthritis with a past history lacking trauma or immunocompromise is decidedly rare, and a more common crystalline arthropathy, such as gout, is more often the culprit.

Pathologically, a native joint is relatively resistant to infection. While cartilage itself is avascular, the synovium and joint capsule are richly vascularized and provide ample protection from infection. Children can develop septic arthritis from penetration of bacteria from a nearby osteomyelitis due to the configuration of the joint capsule, allowing bacteria to enter the joint space. In adults, osteomyelitis in proximity rarely occurs. This is fortunate, as the sequelae of septic arthritis can be devastating and can lead to rapid joint destruction. Bacterial matrix metalloproteases can rapidly degrade the articular cartilage, leading to severe cartilage damage and end-stage arthrosis.

Clinically, patients present with severe pain, effusion, and resistance to joint motion. Warmth and redness of the surrounding skin may also be present. Unless an osteomyelitis in proximity is also present, both plain radiographs and MRI scanning will reveal only a joint effusion. Arthrocentesis demonstrates an exudative effusion, with a leukocyte count greater than 50×10^9 cells/L. Bacterial cultures are frequently positive, with *Staphylococcus* species the most frequent causative organisms.

Treatment of septic arthritis is time dependent and demands a high index of suspicion. Awaiting final culture results in a patient with a purulent effusion may cause irreversible joint damage. Debate exists regarding the means of surgical treatment, with open synovectomy being the traditional procedure. Arthroscopic irrigation and debridement may allow more thorough visualization and lavage of all joint surfaces but is more technically demanding. All patients with septic arthritis are treated with antibiotics following surgery, frequently a short intravenous course. Results of this depend on both the cause of the infection and the amount of joint destruction that has occurred.

PATHOGENESIS

General

All clinical infections must be considered as a conflict between the attacking microbes' ability to cause disease and the host's immune defenses. Infections are more likely to occur if the organisms are more virulent and if the inoculum is larger. Conversely, an infection is less likely if the host has a greater ability to eradicate the pathogens or if the host has fewer deficits that encourage infection. Additionally, the pathogenesis of infection involving foreign materials and osteomyelitis are discussed.

Organisms

Although the musculoskeletal system may be infected by any infectious agent, the vast majority of infections are bacterial (Table 7–1). *S. aureus, Streptococcus,* and *H. influenzae* are the most common causes of acute hematogenous osteomyelitis in children. The most common causes of septic arthritis are *Neisseria gonorrhoeae, S. aureus,* and group A *Streptococcus.* Septic arthritis is less often caused by gram-negative organisms, including *Escherichia coli, Pseudomonas aeruginosa, Klebsiella, Enterobacter, Serratia, Proteus,* and *Salmonella.* Uncommon bacterial organisms include *Borrelia burgdorferi* (Lyme disease), *Mycobacterium tuberculosis, Brucella,* and the anaerobes *Clostridium* and *Bacteroides.* Unusual organisms that may preferentially infect immunocompromised patients include fungi (*Blastomyces, Cryptococcus, Histoplasma, Sporotrichum,* and

Table 7–1. Common offending organisms in orthopedic conditions.

Disease	Offending Organism
Acute hematogenous osteomyelitis in children	*Staphylococcus aureus, Streptococcus,* and *Haemophilus influenzae*
Septic arthritis	Most common: *Neisseria gonorrhoeae, S. aureus,* and group A *Streptococcus* Less common: *Escherichia coli, Pseudomonas aeruginosa, Klebsiella, Kingella, Enterobacter, Serratia, Proteus,* and *Salmonella* Uncommon bacterial organisms: *Borrelia burgdorferi* (Lyme disease), *Mycobacterium tuberculosis, Brucella,* and the anaerobes *Clostridium* and *Bacteroides*
Patients with immunocompromise	Fungi: *Blastomyces, Cryptococcus, Histoplasma, Sporotrichum,* and *Coccidioides* Atypical *Mycobacterium* species: *kansasii, avium-intracellulare, fortuitum, triviale,* and *scrofulaceum* *Campylobacter, Peptostreptococcus,* and *Propionibacterium*

Coccidioides) and atypical mycobacteria (*Mycobacterium kansasii, M. avium-intracellulare, M. fortuitum, M. triviale,* and *M. scrofulaceum*).

Brook I: Microbiology and management of joint and bone infections due to anaerobic bacteria. *J Orthop Sci* 2008;13:160. [PMID 18392922]

Peterson MC: Rheumatic manifestations of *Campylobacter jejuni* and *C. fetus* infections in adults. *Scand J Rheumatol* 1994;23:167. [PMID: 8091140]

The increase in the immunocompromised population due to the success of solid organ transplants and advancements in the treatment of HIV/AIDS and autoimmune disorders has increased the spectrum of bacteria that can cause musculoskeletal infection. Likewise, an increase in the number of antibiotic-resistant organisms presents a difficult, constantly evolving challenge in the eradication of infection. MRSA can infect bones, joints, soft tissues, and surgical implants. Other common bacterial species have become more resistant to a variety of drugs, delaying the proper treatment of infection and decreasing the number of antibiotics that can be used effectively. For instance, *Acinetobacter baumannii* is a pan-resistant bacterial strain that can cause severe lung and soft-tissue infections. Its role

in clinically significant osteomyelitis is unknown, although some evidence suggests that it may be of limited importance.

▶ Host Factors

A given host may have several factors that promote or defend against infection. Comorbid medical conditions and compromised immunity play a role in the establishment of infectious disease. The presence (or lack) of implanted devices affects infection risk and treatment strategies. Nutritional status and acute nutritional requirements also play a role.

A. Comorbid Diseases and Host Immunity

Comorbid diseases that are known to contribute to infection risk include diseases such as diabetes mellitus, obesity, peripheral vascular disease, chronic renal and liver disease, cancer, autoimmune diseases, and AIDS. Iatrogenic causes, often as a treatment for other diseases, include the use of cytotoxic chemotherapy, corticosteroids, and inhibitors of inflammatory molecules (such as inhibitors of tumor necrosis factor-alpha). Diabetes mellitus has been shown to increase the risk of infection following surgeries, including total joint surgery, spinal surgeries, and foot and ankle surgery. The role that diabetes plays in infectious disease pathogenesis is related to vascular disease, as well as the effects of high glucose, which can cause granulocyte dysfunction. Obesity, often associated with diabetes, has also been shown in some studies to be an independent risk factor for infection.

B. Nutrition and Infection

Nutritional status must be thought of in terms of host requirements. In an adult with static requirements, poor nutrition may develop due to a variety of medical issues, including advanced age, alcoholism, renal disease, chronic diseases, cancer, malabsorption, and other infirmities. It is also necessary to consider the nutritional requirements of patients who have increased nutritional physiologic demand. These patients at baseline may have been well nourished. However, a significant event (such as trauma) may increase their nutritional requirements and cause a relative nutritional deficiency. Laboratory testing for nutritional deficiency includes levels of transferrin (normal, 70–850 mg/dL), serum albumin (normal, 3.4–5.0 g/dL), total lymphocyte count (normal, $0.8–3.65 × 10^3$ cells/µL), and prealbumin (normal, 18–38 mg/dL). Values below those shown may indicate malnutrition and consequent immunocompromise.

C. Foreign Material

All biomaterials commonly used for total joint arthroplasty increase the incidence of *S. aureus* infections. In contrast, biomaterials appear to have no effect on *E. coli* and *Staphylococcus epidermidis* infections except when polymethylmethacrylate is used, in which case the incidence rises markedly.

D. Biofilms

Adherence of bacteria to the surface of implants is promoted by a polysaccharide biofilm called glycocalyx that acts as a barrier against host defense mechanisms and antibiotics. In addition, this film makes culture of organisms difficult, even with the use of special techniques. Hence, other approaches must be taken for culture and treatment. Mixing antibiotics such as vancomycin and gentamicin into PMMA cement can theoretically lower the risk of infection from cemented metal joint replacements, presumably by killing surface bacteria before they produce glycocalyx. Before a glycocalyx is produced, the bacteria undergo a process referred to as quorum sensing. Quorum sensing dispersion is a technique under development that might allow clinicians to disrupt a biofilm, therefore making it susceptible to treatment. As stated, the formation of biofilm makes cultures unreliable. Other means, such as the polymerase chain reaction, have been employed to diagnose infection.

Collinet-Adler S, Castro CA, Ledonio CG, Bechtold JE, Tsukayama DT: *Acinetobacter baumannii* is not associated with osteomyelitis in a rat model: a pilot study. *Clin Orthop Relat Res* 2011;469:274. [PMID: 3008889]

Lauderdale KJ, Malone CL, Boles BR, Morcuende J, Horswill AR: Biofilm dispersal of community-associated methicillin-resistant *Staphylococcus aureus* on orthopedic implant material. *J Orthop Res* 2010;28:55. [PMID: 19610092]

PREVENTION

▶ Overview

Prevention of infection starts long before the operative date, continues both during and after surgery, and is influenced by multiple factors and personnel. As discussed previously, medical comorbidities influence the pathogenesis of infection. It follows that the management and prevention of such comorbidities will contribute to infection prevention. Multiple physician and patient factors contribute to medical optimization of comorbidities before surgery. Preoperatively, factors such as nutrition, MRSA colonization, preoperative hygiene, and bathing can contribute to infection risk. Perioperative and intraoperative factors such as proper prepping, operative room sterility, appropriate use of antibiotics, closure material choice, and minimization of intraoperative time can help prevent infection. Finally, optimizing postoperative factors including postoperative antibiotics, management of blood glucose levels, and choices regarding blood transfusions can also positively affect infection rates.

▶ Preoperative Optimization

A. Medical Comorbidities

Some medical comorbidities (and their necessary treatment) represent nonmodifiable risk factors for infection, whereas other present an opportunity for preoperative optimization. Rheumatoid arthritis (RA) provides an excellent example. Individuals with RA have an increased risk of infection, both from the disease and its treatment. Surgeons working in concert with the patient's rheumatologist can optimize the treatment of RA while decreasing the risk of poor operative outcomes, including infection. This approach to medical comorbidity management can be applied to other diseases as well.

Obesity, for instance, represents a modifiable risk factor that is becoming a more frequently encountered condition in developed countries, especially in the United States. In the total joint literature, obesity has been shown to be associated with an increased risk of infection. An increase of 5 points in body mass index (BMI) has been shown to be associated with a 50% increase in the odds ratio for acquiring a prosthetic joint infection. In the spine literature, obese patients have an odds ratio of 2.2 relative to nonobese patients. The surgeon must be aware of the association between obesity and infection and work with patients to decrease their risk of infection. Unfortunately, weight loss can be extremely difficult, especially in patients with orthopedic conditions. Gastric bypass therapy may be necessary before orthopedic intervention, especially in patients with a BMI greater than 45. This, unfortunately, produces relative malnutrition.

Bosco JA 3rd, Slover JD, Haas JP: Perioperative strategies for decreasing infection: a comprehensive evidence-based approach. *J Bone Joint Surg Am* 2010;92:232. [PMID: 20048118]

Chen S, Anderson MV, Cheng WK, Wongworawat MD: Diabetes associated with increased surgical site infections in spinal arthrodesis. *Clin Orthop Relat Res* 2009;467:1670. [PMID: 2690748]

Dowsey MM, Choong PF: Obesity is a major risk factor for prosthetic infection after primary hip arthroplasty. *Clin Orthop Relat Res* 2008;466:153. [PMID: 2505299]

Dowsey MM, Choong PF: Obese diabetic patients are at substantial risk for deep infection after primary TKA. *Clin Orthop Relat Res* 2009;467:1577. [PMID: 2674158]

Howe CR, Gardner GC, Kadel NJ: Perioperative medication management for the patient with rheumatoid arthritis. *J Am Acad Orthop Surg* 2006;14:544. [PMID: 16959892]

Jämsen E, Varonen M, Huhtala H, et al: Incidence of prosthetic joint infections after primary knee arthroplasty. *J Arthroplasty* 2010;25:87. [PMID: 19056210]

Moucha CS, Clyburn T, Evans RP, Prokuski L: Modifiable risk factors for surgical site infection. *J Bone Joint Surg Am* 2011;93:398. [PMID: 21325594]

Olsen MA, Nepple JJ, Riew KD, et al: Risk factors for surgical site infection following orthopaedic spinal operations. *J Bone Joint Surg Am* 2008;90:62. [PMID: 18171958]

B. Nutrition

The overall health of a given host's immune system influences susceptibility to infection. Indeed, malnutrition can lead directly to immune dysfunction. A recent review highlights the importance of recognizing and correcting patient nutrition. Testing for nutritional status should include albumin (normal, 3.4–5.0 g/dL), total lymphocyte count (normal, $0.8–3.65 \times 10^3$ cells/μL), and transferrin (normal, 70–850 mg/dL) levels. Supplementation to correct deficiency of both macro- and micronutrients should be accomplished preoperatively.

Katona P, Katona-Apte J: The interaction between nutrition and infection. *Clin Infect Dis* 2008;46:1582. [PMID: 18419494]

C. *Staphylococcus aureus* Decolonization/ Preoperative Bathing

It has been clear for some time that certain organisms possess an increased potential to cause severe infections. *S. aureus* is one such bacterium. Attempts to thwart infection with *S. aureus* have led to the development of preoperative decolonization protocols designed to eradicate *S. aureus* from the skin flora before the patient undergoes surgery. At certain institutions, adult reconstruction surgeons have begun to screen the nares of patients preoperatively. One protocol uses nasal cultures 2–4 weeks before surgery. If positive for *S. aureus*, patients apply nasal mupirocin twice daily and take chlorhexidine baths for the 5 days immediately prior to surgery. This has been shown to decrease the rate of *S. aureus* infections, as well as the overall rate of surgical site infections. Similar protocols have been used to prevent infections in other surgical disciplines, prompting the Cochrane group to conclude that nasal mupirocin is effective in preventing infections. Conversely, a separate Cochrane review demonstrated that chlorhexidine baths alone did not change the incidence of infection as compared to washing preoperatively with regular soap and water.

Hacek DM, Robb WJ, Paule SM, Kudrna JC, Stamos VP, Peterson LR: *Staphylococcus aureus* nasal decolonization in joint replacement surgery reduces infection. *Clin Orthop Relat Res* 2008;466:1349. [PMID: 2384050]

Rao N, Cannella B, Crossett LS, Yates AJ Jr, McGough R 3rd: A preoperative decolonization protocol for staphylococcus aureus prevents orthopaedic infections. *Clin Orthop Relat Res* 2008;466:1343. [PMID: 2384036]

Rao N, Cannella BA, Crossett LS, Yates AJ Jr, McGough RL 3rd, Hamilton CW: Preoperative screening/decolonization for *Staphylococcus aureus* to prevent orthopedic surgical site infection prospective cohort study with 2-year follow-up. *J Arthroplasty* 2011;26:1501. [PMID: 21507604]

van Rijen M, Bonten M, Wenzel R, Kluytmans J: Mupirocin ointment for preventing *Staphylococcus aureus* infections in nasal carriers. *Cochrane Database Syst Rev* 2008;4:CD006216. [PMID: 18843708]

Webster J, Osborne S: Preoperative bathing or showering with skin antiseptics to prevent surgical site infection. *Cochrane Database Syst Rev* 2007;2:CD004985. [PMID: 16625619]

▶ Perioperative and Intraoperative Factors
A. Prepping

Preparing the patient for surgery requires many steps once the patient has arrived in the operating theatre. The first decision in regard to infection control is whether or not to remove hair. The three options for hair removal are shaving, clipping, and depilatory creams. Alternatively, the hair can be left intact. Traditionally, it has been taught that shaving is inferior, a finding that is supported by a recent Cochrane review. However, no difference was found between removing the hair using the other two approaches and leaving the hair intact. The next step that influences infection control involves the selection of prepping solution. Options include iodophor or chlorhexidine gluconate–based solutions. Furthermore, these can be aqueous or alcohol based. Alcohol-based chlorhexidine gluconate solutions are superior to other preparation solutions when the outcome measure is simply positive cultures from the operative field. However, the extent to which these cultures correlate with an eventual surgical site infection is not clear. Interestingly, in urologic surgery, other preparation solutions have been shown to be superior. This is ostensibly the result either of a statistical phenomenon or a different bacterial milieu in this patient population that responds differently to a given preparation solution. A Cochrane review from 2004 failed to show any significant difference between different preparation solutions.

Edwards PS, Lipp A, Holmes A: Preoperative skin antiseptics for preventing surgical wound infections after clean surgery. *Cochrane Database Syst Rev* 2004;3:CD003949. [PMID: 15266508]

Ostrander RV, Botte MJ, Brage ME: Efficacy of surgical preparation solutions in foot and ankle surgery. *J Bone Joint Surg Am* 2005;87:980. [PMID: 15866959]

Saltzman MD, Nuber GW, Gryzlo SM, Marecek GS, Koh JL: Efficacy of surgical preparation solutions in shoulder surgery. *J Bone Joint Surg Am* 2009;91:1949. [PMID: 19651954]

B. Antibiotics

The use of preoperative antibiotics within 1 hour of surgery is standard, routine, and required for adherence to national Surgical Care Improvement Project (SCIP) protocols. Recommendations for antibiotic timing, duration, selection, and redosing include the following: administration of a first-generation cephalosporin within 1 hour of surgical initiation, use of clindamycin or vancomycin if patient is allergic to cephalosporin, and maintenance of antibiotics for no more than 24 hours total unless infection is suspected or confirmed. A proposed adjunct to systemic antibiotics involves the use of local antibiotics, namely gentamicin. Two separate studies used a rat injury model to show improved bactericidal activity in vivo. Results are yet to be demonstrated in a human, randomized controlled trial.

Cavanaugh DL, Berry J, Yarboro SR, Dahners LE: Better prophylaxis against surgical site infection with local as well as systemic antibiotics. An in vivo study. *J Bone Joint Surg Am* 2009;91:1907. [PMID: 2714810]

Prokuski L: Prophylactic antibiotics in orthopaedic surgery. *J Am Acad Orthop Surg* 2008;16:283. [PMID: 21553797]

Yarboro SR, Baum EJ, Dahners LE: Locally administered antibiotics for prophylaxis against surgical wound infection. An in vivo study. *J Bone Joint Surg Am* 2007;89:929. [PMID: 17473127]

C. Operating Room Sterility

Sterility in the operating theater is the responsibility of anyone who enters the room. This includes the surgical team, the anesthesiology team, the nursing team, the scrub technician team, and the medical equipment team. Lapses in sterile technique can undoubtedly increase bacterial exposure to the patient. However, other factors also contribute, namely the sterility of the air in which the surgery is performed. Ultraviolet (UV) lighting has long been tried as an attempt to reduce the bacterial content of the air. A recent study demonstrated a decreased incidence of surgical site infections with use of UV light in the operating theater. In addition, the sterility of the air and the direction of the air flow are also controllable factors in the operating room. For many years, both vertical and horizontal airflow systems, combined with a variety of filters, have been employed to theoretically lower the risk of surgical site infections. Despite these efforts over many years, there is still no clear consensus on whether such systems decrease, make no difference, or actually increase the risk of airborne contamination.

Brandt C, Hott U, Sohr D, Daschner F, Gastmeier P, Ruden H: Operating room ventilation with laminar airflow shows no protective effect on the surgical site infection rate in orthopedic and abdominal surgery. *Ann Surg* 2008;248:695. [PMID: 18948793]

Owers KL, James E, Bannister GC: Source of bacterial shedding in laminar flow theatres. *J Hosp Infect* 2004;58:230. [PMID: 15501339]

Ritter MA, Olberding EM, Malinzak RA: Ultraviolet lighting during orthopaedic surgery and the rate of infection. *J Bone Joint Surg Am* 2007;89:1935. [PMID: 17768189]

Stocks GW, O'Connor DP, Self SD, Marcek GA, Thompson BL: Directed air flow to reduce airborne particulate and bacterial contamination in the surgical field during total hip arthroplasty. *J Arthroplasty* 2011;26:771. [PMID: 20851565]

Stocks GW, Self SD, Thompson B, Adame XA, O'Connor DP: Predicting bacterial populations based on airborne particulates: a study performed in nonlaminar flow operating rooms during joint arthroplasty surgery. *Am J Infect Control* 2010;38:199. [PMID: 19913327]

D. Closure

The two main options for closure of a surgical wound are sutures and staples. A recent meta-analysis combined the outcomes of six different studies. Despite the methodologic limitations inherent in this meta-analysis, it suggests that closure with staples increases the risk of infection. When closing deep layers with suture, the nature of the filament can be considered. Traditional teaching is that monofilament closure decreases the risk of infection because theoretically, braided sutures provide a greater surface area for microbial contamination than monofilament sutures. This is likely merely anecdotal, however, as no studies have demonstrated superiority of one closure material over another regarding infection. Adherence to good surgical tissue handling techniques including atraumatic closure technique, maintenance of full-thickness fasciocutaneous flaps, and avoidance of excessive tissue undermining or devascularization are likely substantially more important than the choice of closure material.

Smith TO, Sexton D, Mann C, Donell S: Sutures versus staples for skin closure in orthopaedic surgery: meta-analysis. *BMJ* 2010;340:c1199. [PMID: 20234041]

E. Postoperative Blood Glucose Control

It is well known that diabetes is a risk factor for surgical site infections. However, the consequence of poor perioperative glucose control in terms of surgical site infection is less clear. Recent literature suggests that poor control of postoperative hyperglycemia substantially increases the risk of surgical site infection.

Ata A, Lee J, Bestle SL, Desemone J, Stain SC: Postoperative hyperglycemia and surgical site infection in general surgery patients. *Arch Surg* 2010;145:858. [PMID: 20855756]

CLINICAL FINDINGS

Despite 2500 years of medical progress, the aforementioned cardinal signs of inflammation described by originally recorded by the Roman encyclopedist Celsus in the first century AD are still our primary means of diagnosing infection. In immunocompetent hosts, many, if not all, of the signs will be present in acute infection. In the postsurgical setting, wound drainage, whether purulent, bloody, or clear, may also indicate that an infectious process is occurring. The postsurgical setting is the most difficult, however, because the signs mentioned earlier are significant for inflammation in general and are not specific for infection. Distinguishing between a routine postoperative wound, a poorly healing postoperative wound, a hematoma, or an infection can be extremely difficult.

In the postoperative situation, infection may be diagnosed by a clinical scenario that does not improve with time. After surgery, pain, swelling, and erythema usually decrease over a period of days to weeks. If, instead of improving, the symptoms of inflammation increase, infection may be present.

Laboratory studies may help to distinguish infection from other diagnoses. The presence of a high white blood cell count, especially if the percentage of neutrophils is greater than 70% of the total, suggests infection. Leukocytosis is not sensitive for localized infection, however, and has greater sensitivity with systemic disease than with a localized problem. An increased ESR is another sensitive, but nonspecific marker. The ESR will increase any time inflammation is present, dramatically reducing its utility in the postoperative situation or in any scenario wherein multiple inflammatory etiologies may be present. An increase in the serum CRP is somewhat more specific for infection, but not specific enough to act on in the absence of other signs or symptoms. The CRP generally increases very rapidly in the presence of infection and then begins to decrease after 48–72 hours. The ESR takes much longer to normalize, often peaking over a period of several days and decreasing much more slowly. Abnormalities in these lab values are corroborative of, but not diagnostic of, a musculoskeletal infection.

DIFFERENTIAL DIAGNOSIS

Infection, the great masquerader, generally is part of an extensive differential diagnosis. In fact, the diagnosis of infection is frequently confounded by many other medical conditions, most of them quite common.

Infection is frequently confused with trauma. In the early stages of a healing contusion, the soft-tissue hematoma mimics an abscess. Adding the complication that hematomas may subsequently become infected only serves to further confuse the clinical scenario. The increasing prevalence of anticoagulation for a number of cardiac or other medical comorbidities renders even the most trivial trauma capable of producing substantial bleeding. Furthermore, metabolizing blood products may yield a febrile response, placing the clinician in a position of possibly operating on a hematoma in an anticoagulated patient or ignoring a large soft-tissue infection in an individual who is substantially medically compromised.

Many musculoskeletal neoplasms may be confused with infections. Most soft-tissue sarcomas produce swelling and may produce pain to palpation. Their heterogeneous imaging characteristics on MRI scan have led numerous surgeons into a "simple irrigation and debridement" that unfortunately enters a sarcoma, thus producing substantial bleeding and possible oncologic compromise. Radiographically, osteosarcoma may look nearly exactly like osteomyelitis. Both produce permeative bony changes with substantial new bone formation. Both are painful and produce swelling. Both occur in the metaphyses of children. Similarly, Ewing sarcoma produces permeative bony changes mimicking those produced by purulence. Because Ewing sarcoma, lymphoma, and osteomyelitis are composed of small blue cells without matrix, all may resemble frank purulence at the time of debridement. The orthopedic oncologist's admonition to "send every infection to pathology and culture every tumor" was born of this confusion.

Fortunately, needle biopsy may assist in narrowing this differential diagnosis without the potential for causing harm. Unless the patient is septic and in extremis, most suspected infections can be simply aspirated, either with or without radiographic imaging guidance. This approach has multiple advantages:

1. Infections composed of purulent material can be aspirated, and appropriate cultures can be obtained quickly, easily, and before the administration of antibiotics.

2. Needle aspiration is unlikely to cause bleeding complications, even in anticoagulated patients. Hemostasis is almost always achievable using direct pressure, and the patient's coagulopathy may be corrected before any necessary surgical interventions.

3. In cases where sarcoma enters the differential diagnosis, needle biopsy may not only obtain purulent samples (if infection is present), but will also allow pathologic diagnosis. Although there is current debate regarding whether needle tracks should be excised at the time of sarcoma surgery, excising a needle track is always easier than a surgical incision and does not have the potential complication of an improperly placed incision.

Other inflammatory conditions also mimic infection. Because the physical signs of infection are the signs of inflammation, the two can present nearly identically. Aseptic myonecrosis, as seen in statin-induced myonecrosis, is remarkably similar to infection, with pain, inflammation, and swelling. Diabetic myonecrosis may behave like infection as well. Tumoral calcinosis, as seen in patients with renal insufficiency, produces soft-tissue masses with pain and skin changes, also mimicking abscesses.

COMPLICATIONS

The complications of infection may be truly grave. In situations of systemic sepsis, failure to adequately treat both the local and systemic manifestations of infection may lead to the patient's demise. Similarly, clostridial fasciitis may become rapidly progressive, causing massive tissue loss, loss of limb, or even death. If the patient's system fails to clear or suppress either prosthetic infection or osteomyelitis, amputation may be required to control local disease. Even with successful treatment, infection may lead to substantial loss of tissue, function, social status, and income for the affected patient.

One specific complication of chronic infection is the development of squamous cell carcinoma (a "Marjolin ulcer"). This occurs when any chronically (generally of >20 years' duration) draining infection causes enough irritation to the surrounding skin to cause the development of an invasive carcinoma. Because this becomes a potentially life-threatening situation in the face of limb salvage that has failed to control the baseline infection, amputation is often the treatment of choice.

Bauer T, David T, Rimareix F, Lortat-Jacob A: Marjolin's ulcer in chronic osteomyelitis: seven cases and a review of the literature [French]. *Rev Chir Orthop Reparatrice Appar Mot* 2007;93:63. [PMID: 17389826]

TREATMENT

Treatment of orthopedic infections generally involves a multimodality and often multidisciplinary approach. Although simple skin infections such as cellulitis or folliculitis may respond completely with medical treatments alone, deep orthopedic infections generally require both surgical and medical intervention. The presence of nonimmunocompetent materials, such as dead bone or metal prostheses, frequently mandates a more aggressive approach as the blood flow required for successful antibiotic treatment is obviously not present.

▶ Pediatric Osteomyelitis

Pediatric osteomyelitis is primarily a surgical disease. The slow, sinusoidal blood flow within the metaphyses allows bacteria to multiply in the region (see General Considerations). Once a sequestrum has formed, this necrotic substrate provides a perfect medium for bacterial growth. Infection will progress until an involucrum forms or the bone is entirely destroyed.

Surgery consists of draining the infected bone and removing any sequestrum, if present. If no sequestrum is present, the bone may be opened with a high-speed burr, gouges, drill, or osteotome, and the purulent material drained. If the adjacent joint is also involved, it may be opened, drained, and irrigated. A deep drain is usually placed within the bone and/or joint and left until drainage ceases. Intravenous antibiotics are then instituted and tailored to the culture results, if positive. Four to six weeks of treatment are generally sufficient to produce a cure.

▶ Adult Osteomyelitis

Treatment of adult osteomyelitis is often much more difficult than the pediatric variety. Often the comorbidities surrounding the orthopedic condition are chronic and may only be optimized rather than eliminated. Adult osteomyelitis also requires much more aggressive surgical and medical treatment than the pediatric condition.

Like pediatric osteomyelitis, treating adult osteomyelitis absolutely requires the removal of all necrotic bone. This is frequently much more difficult, as areas of necrosis may be extensive and removal of all dead bone may produce large,

segmental bony defects. Similarly, extensive areas of poorly vascularized, fibrotic, or necrotic soft tissue may be present, requiring thorough debridement.

Careful preoperative planning is required. The extent of bony involvement can be estimated preoperatively using CT scanning, as necrotic bone is frequently sclerotic and hyperdense with this modality. If a segmental defect is anticipated or if circumferential debridement would yield a bone at substantial risk for pathologic fracture, stabilization will be necessary. For small defects or situations where a limited number of debridements is anticipated, stabilization using intramedullary nail or plate fixation may be ideal. For larger defects or situations where multiple debridements are necessary, external fixation either using standard or thin wire (Ilizarov) techniques may be ideal. This allows skeletal stabilization with access to the soft tissues. External fixation may ultimately be revised to internal fixation once the infection is eradicated or used as definitive fixation after grafting or bone transport.

Planning for soft-tissue reconstruction is also necessary. Draining sinuses, necrotic tissue, and poorly vascularized areas should be thoroughly and radically debrided. This generally yields soft-tissue defects that require plastic surgical reconstruction, either with rotational or free tissue transfers.

Adult osteomyelitis secondary to pressure phenomena provides a special case (see General Considerations). In this situation, patients are either mentally or physically inhibited from perceiving or responding to pressure. If the pressure sore extends to the bone, osteomyelitis occurs by definition. Bone biopsy is not necessary for diagnosis in this case but may be useful to tailor antibiotic treatment. Surgical treatment, if necessary based on patient wishes, life expectancy, and comorbidities, is often radical with removal of large portions of the sacrum, pelvis, or proximal femur. Plastic reconstruction is generally necessary.

Antibiotic treatment for adult osteomyelitis is often multimodal. Using two or even three agents in combination can facilitate penetration into involved tissues and can help to limit side effects and toxicities. Obtaining a culture from a deep source is very important for speciation, and patients with chronic draining sinuses are often given an antibiotic holiday for several days to weeks to allow deep cultures to grow. Deep tissue cultures are both more sensitive and specific than culture swabs. Culturing sinus tracts or purulent drainage is of no benefit and may cause harm and confusion.

▶ Adult Soft-Tissue Infections

Soft-tissue infections that result from intravenous or subcutaneous drug abuse may be treated by incision and drainage, possibly with open packing and systemic antibiotics. More severe infections, especially in immunocompromised individuals, require much more aggressive treatment. All abscess cavities must be thoroughly opened, and all necrotic tissue removed. Broad-spectrum antibiotics are generally used, and multiple agents may be used in combination, depending on the clinical scenario. Successful treatment demands an immunocompetent host, so any immunomodulating agents should be discontinued. Leukocyte proliferation growth factors may be contemplated in neutropenic hosts.

Treatment of neutropenic myonecrosis is especially difficult. In this scenario, a neutropenic host presents with fever, severe pain, and cellulitis. MRI generally fails to reveal any abscess or other surgical condition, as the host does not possess enough immune function even to create an abscess. Broad-spectrum antibiotics are instituted, as in any neutropenic fever protocol, but will fail to reduce fevers or eliminate erythema. If the patient's condition continues to deteriorate without another source, the area of erythema should be opened, and the subjacent muscle examined surgically. Frequently, the muscle will be completely necrotic, but *without* the liquefactive necrosis encountered in the pyomyositis of immunocompetent individuals. Debridement must continue until adequate bleeding and viable muscle are appreciated. The entire necrotic portion of the compartment must be removed. In severe cases, the entire compartment will be necrotic, and all vessels leading into the muscle will have clotted due to bacterial thrombi. This appearance is not dissimilar to that found in advanced compartment syndrome, with patent major vessels and compromised muscular branches. Unlike in compartment syndrome, the entire compartment must be removed as a lifesaving measure.

Prosthetic Infections

As previously mentioned, the treatment of prosthetic joint infection depends on the acuity of the infection from the time of surgery or the inciting event. Early (within 4–6 weeks of surgery or within a few days of an invasive procedure) infections can be treated with surgical irrigation and exchange of the bearing surfaces. After this course of treatment, the surgeon must maintain a high level of vigilance, because this limited approach may not be successful. In chronic infections (months to years after implantation with no inciting event), the surgeon must assume that biofilm has contaminated the metal prosthesis and cannot be salvaged. If the patient is able to tolerate a staged revision and systemic antibiotics, this is the treatment with the greatest chance of success. If the patient cannot tolerate a staged revision due to comorbidities, the options include chronic antibiotic suppression and amputation. As the population ages, joint arthroplasties increase in frequency, and bacterial resistance continues to evolve, prosthetic infections will continue to challenge orthopedic surgeons.

Traumatic Infections

Traumatic infections are an especially difficult problem because they combine the infection risks inherent in any orthopedic surgery as well as the contamination of the traumatic event. The mainstays of modern treatment are prompt, thorough debridement of devitalized tissue and rigid fixation. Not surprisingly, the risk of infection is directly proportional to the degree of soft-tissue damage imparted by the injury. The host's functional capacity, regenerative capacity, nutrition, and overall health also affect the risk of infection. Although the surgeon has no control over the magnitude of the trauma or the health of the host, the surgeon has complete control over the quality of the debridement and fixation, and therefore must maximize these. The optimal treatment of traumatic infections often involves a multidisciplinary team including orthopedic surgeons, plastic surgeons, and infectious disease specialists. Indeed, the literature suggests that patients treated with a multidisciplinary approach have better outcomes than those who are not.

Cierny G 3rd, DiPasquale D: Treatment of chronic infection. *J Am Acad Orthop Surg* 2006;14:S105. [PMID: 17003180]

Copley LA: Pediatric musculoskeletal infection: trends and antibiotic recommendations. *J Am Acad Orthop Surg* 2009;17:618. [PMID: 19794219]

Duzgun AP, Satir HZ, Ozozan O, Saylam B, Kulah B, Coskun F: Effect of hyperbaric oxygen therapy on healing of diabetic foot ulcers. *J Foot Ankle Surg* 2008;47:515. [PMID: 19239860]

Forsberg JA, Potter BK, Cierny G 3rd, Webb L: Diagnosis and management of chronic infection. *J Am Acad Orthop Surg* 2011;19(Suppl 1):S8. [PMID: 21304049]

Noel SP, Courtney HS, Bumgardner JD, Haggard WO: Chitosan sponges to locally deliver amikacin and vancomycin: a pilot in vitro evaluation. *Clin Orthop Relat Res* 2010;468:2074. [PMID: 2895824]

Prokuski L: Treatment of acute infection. *J Am Acad Orthop Surg* 2006;14(10 Spec No.):S101. [PMID: 17003179]

Stinner DJ, Noel SP, Haggard WO, Watson JT, Wenke JC: Local antibiotic delivery using tailorable chitosan sponges: the future of infection control? *J Orthop Trauma* 2010;24:592. [PMID: 20736801]

Ziran BH, Rao N, Hall RA: A dedicated team approach enhances outcomes of osteomyelitis treatment. *Clin Orthop Relat Res* 2003;414:31. [PMID: 12966273]

PROGNOSIS

It is virtually impossible to predict the prognosis of musculoskeletal infections as a whole because the ultimate success of treatment depends on enumerable variables, as we have indicated many times within this chapter. Host factors (age, nutrition, comorbidities, anatomic location), pathogen factors (organism type and virulence), and physician factors (index of suspicion, quality of technique, available resources) all impact tremendously on the patient's outcome. However, the principles of musculoskeletal infection treatment are the same in every instance. A high index of suspicion, correct interpretation of laboratory and clinical data, thorough surgery when indicated, optimization of host factors, and pathogen-specific antibiotic therapy are the pillars of treatment for musculoskeletal infections. In all instances, adherence to these principles will maximize the patient's prognosis.

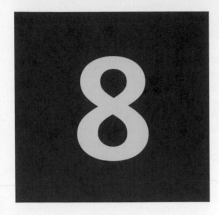

Foot and Ankle Surgery

Jeffrey A. Mann, MD
Loretta B. Chou, MD
Steven D. K. Ross, MD

BIOMECHANIC PRINCIPLES OF THE FOOT AND ANKLE

The primary role of the foot and ankle is locomotion. Therefore, it is critical for the clinician treating disorders of the foot and ankle to have the knowledge and understanding of the anatomy and biomechanic principles of the foot and ankle. The following is a limited discussion of the biomechanic principles governing the foot and ankle during the gait cycle. Once these principles are familiar and understood, it will enable the clinician to make diagnoses of problems that affect the anatomy and function of the foot and ankle.

▶ Gait

Gait is the orderly progression of the body through space while expending as little energy as possible. As the body moves through a gait cycle, muscle forces are generated actively to counteract the passive effects of gravity on the body. To accommodate these forces, the foot is flexible at the time of heel strike to allow for absorption of impact of the body against the ground. However, at the end of stance phase, the foot becomes rigid at toe-off, when it must assist in moving the body forward. The magnitude of the forces on the foot increases significantly as the speed of gait increases. For example, when an individual is walking, the initial force with which the foot meets the ground is approximately 80% of body weight. With jogging, the force increases to approximately 160%. Also, the peak force against the foot during walking is 110% of body weight, and for jogging 240%. This marked increase contributes to some of the injuries seen in runners.

▶ The Walking Cycle

Gait analysis has been described in Chapter 1, but further detail of the role of the foot and ankle are described here (Figures 8–1 and 8–2). An important component of the physical examination is observation of the patient during the walking cycle. This will help the physician with the cause of a gait anomaly. For example, an equinus deformity from spasticity or contracture will cause the toe to make initial contact with the ground rather than the heel. Furthermore, at 7% of the gait cycle, the foot is usually flat on the ground, but spasticity or contracture of the Achilles tendon causes this to be delayed. At 12% of the cycle, the opposite foot toes off and the swing phase begins. Heel rise of the standing foot begins at 34% of the cycle as the swinging leg passes the standing limb. With spasticity, heel rise may occur earlier, and in contrast, with gastrocsoleus weakness, heel rise will be later. Heel strike of the opposite foot occurs at 50% of the cycle, ending the period of single-limb support; and may occur sooner if there is weakness of the contralateral gastrocsoleus muscle. Toe-off of the opposite foot occurs at 62% of the cycle, at the beginning of the swing phase. These markers of the gait cycle should be kept in mind when observing gait, so pathologic conditions may be identified.

▶ Motions of the Foot and Ankle

The majority of dorsiflexion and plantar flexion occurs through the ankle joint. The subtalar joint allows for inversion (varus) and eversion (valgus). Next, adduction, which is movement toward the midline, and abduction, which is movement away from the midline, occurs through the transverse tarsal joint (talonavicular and calcaneocuboid joints). Supination and pronation are used in describing combinations of movements, but unfortunately, these terms are sometimes used in the literature interchangeably. Supination is a combination of plantar flexion of the ankle joint, inversion of the subtalar joint, and adduction of the transverse tarsal joint. Pronation is the exact opposite movement: dorsiflexion of the ankle joint, eversion of the subtalar joint, and abduction of the transverse tarsal joint. The nomenclature may also be confusing when such terms as forefoot varus and forefoot valgus are used (Figure 8–3). Forefoot varus or valgus is an anatomic deformity that is observed when the hindfoot is placed in neutral position. Neutral position is achieved when the calcaneus is aligned with the long axis of

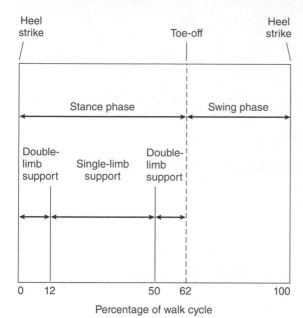

▲ Figure 8–1. Phases of the walking cycle. Stance phase constitutes approximately 62% and swing phase 38% of the cycle. (Reproduced with permission, from Mann RA, Coughlin MJ: *The Video Textbook of Foot and Ankle Surgery.* Medical Video Productions, 1991.)

the tibia and the head of the talus is covered with the navicular bone. Forefoot varus deformity is present when the lateral aspect of the forefoot is in greater plantar flexion than the medial aspect. With a flexible deformity, the foot lies flat on the floor during stance, but with a fixed deformity, excessive weight is borne on the lateral side of the foot. As a result, as the weight passes onto the forefoot, the calcaneus goes into valgus position, and this may result in lateral impingement

of the calcaneus against the fibula if severe. In forefoot valgus deformity, the medial side of the foot has greater plantar flexion than the lateral side and results in excessive weight bearing by the first metatarsal head. To accommodate for this deformity, the calcaneus assumes a varus position, which may result in a feeling of instability at the ankle joint.

Mechanisms of the Foot During Weight Bearing

During gait, the foot is flexible at heel strike to absorb the impact of striking the ground. As a result, the subtalar joint literally collapses into a position of valgus, causing internal rotation of the tibia and resulting distally in unlocking of the transverse tarsal (talonavicular and calcaneocuboid) joint. This allows the foot to be flexible. During this part of the gait cycle of heel strike, the anterior compartment muscle group is the only muscles that are active. The anterior compartment muscles control the initial rapid plantar flexion following heel strike by an eccentric or lengthening contraction. The flexibility of the foot is greatest at approximately 7% of the cycle. As the body passes over the foot in foot flat, the heel up begins to rise and then forces the metatarsophalangeal joints into extension. As this occurs, the foot is converted into a rigid lever that supports the body at the time of toe-off. The mechanisms that bring about conversion of the foot from a flexible to a rigid structure are (1) the tightening of the plantar aponeurosis, the windlass mechanism; (2) the progressive external rotation of the lower extremity, which begins at the pelvis and is passed distally across the ankle joint into the subtalar joint; and (3) the stabilization of the transverse tarsal joint, which results from the progressive inversion of the subtalar joint.

Joints of the Foot and Ankle

A. Ankle Joint

The ankle joint is the articulation of the talus with the tibia and fibula and has a range of motion (ROM) of 15 degrees of dorsiflexion to 55 degrees of plantar flexion. There is also a small amount of motion in the transverse plane, approximately 15 degrees. The anterior compartment muscles of the leg, the tibialis anterior and the toe extensors, control the amount of plantar flexion of the ankle joint at the time of heel ground contact to 10% stance. These muscles are responsible for dorsiflexion of the foot and ankle during swing phase. Any weakness or pathology affecting the anterior compartment may result in a footslap at heel strike and a dropfoot during swing phase. The greatest force across the ankle joint during walking is calculated to be approximately 4.5 times body weight, which occurs at 40% of the walking cycle.

B. Subtalar Joint

The subtalar joint is the articulation between the talus and the calcaneus. There are three components of this joint, the

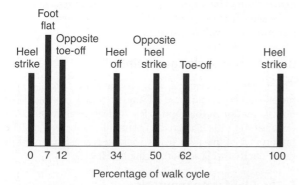

▲ Figure 8–2. Events of the walking cycle. (Reproduced, with permission, from Mann RA, Coughlin MJ: *The Video Textbook of Foot and Ankle Surgery.* Medical Video Productions, 1991.)

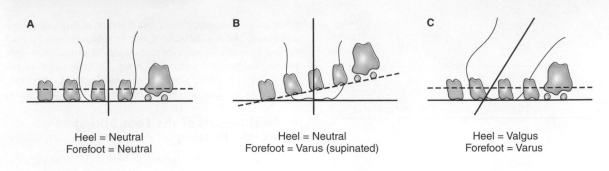

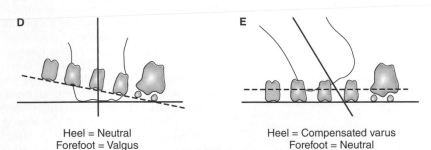

▲ **Figure 8–3.** Biomechanics of foot pressure. **A:** Normal alignment: forefoot perpendicular to heel. **B:** Forefoot varus (uncompensated): lateral aspect of forefoot plantar flexed in relation to medial aspect. **C:** Forefoot varus (compensated): with the forefoot flat on the floor, the heel assumes a valgus position. **D:** Forefoot valgus (uncompensated): medial aspect of forefoot plantar flexed in relation to lateral aspect. **E:** Forefoot valgus (compensated): with the forefoot flat on the floor, the heel assumes a varus position. (Reproduced, with permission, from Mann RA, Coughlin MJ: *The Video Textbook of Foot and Ankle Surgery.* Medical Video Productions, 1991.)

posterior, middle, and anterior facets. The most important and largest of these facets is the posterior facet. Through the subtalar joint, inversion of approximately 20 degrees and eversion of approximately 5–10 degrees occurs. These motions are brought about by the tibialis posterior muscle (inversion) and the peroneus brevis (eversion). During the walking cycle at initial ground contact, eversion is a passive mechanism and occurs because of the shape of the articulations and their ligamentous support. Inversion occurs both actively and passively at the time of toe-off. Active control is achieved by the gastrocsoleus and posterior tibial muscles, and passive inversion occurs by the action of the plantar aponeurosis, the external rotation of the lower extremity, and the oblique metatarsal break.

C. Talonavicular Joint and Calcaneocuboid Joint

The talonavicular and calcaneocuboid joints functionally act as a single joint, also called the transverse tarsal joint. The transverse tarsal joint is responsible for adduction and abduction, 15 degrees and 10 degrees, respectively. The head of the talus is firmly seated into the navicular at the time of toe-off, adding stability to the foot. Also, the stability of the transverse tarsal joint is controlled by the position of the subtalar joint. When the subtalar joint is in an inverted position, the axes of these two joints are nonparallel, giving rise

to increased stability of the hindfoot. When the calcaneus is in an everted position at the time of heel strike, these joints are parallel to one another, thereby giving rise to increased flexibility of these joints (Figure 8–4). An important aspect of this position is that when the position of a subtalar arthrodesis is determined, careful alignment into 5–7 degrees of the subtalar joint will maintain the foot's flexibility and ability to walk. However, if the subtalar joint is placed in a malposition of hindfoot varus, the transverse tarsal joint will be locked. The resulting foot will be stiff, and the patient will have difficulty with walking.

D. Metatarsophalangeal Joints

The metatarsophalangeal joint is the articulation of the metatarsal head and base of the proximal phalanx. The normal motion at this joint is 50–70 degrees of dorsiflexion (extension) to 15–25 degrees of plantar flexion (flexion). The importance of this joint in the walking cycle is discussed in detail the following section on the first toe.

E. The Plantar Aponeurosis

Although the plantar aponeurosis is not an articulation per se, it probably plays the predominant role in the overall stability of the foot. The plantar aponeurosis originates from the

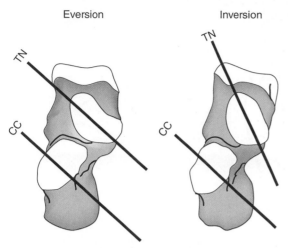

Eversion   Inversion

▲ **Figure 8–4.** The function of the transverse tarsal joint as described by Elftman demonstrates that when the calcaneus is in eversion, the resultant axes of the talonavicular (TN) and calcaneocuboid (CC) joints are parallel or congruent. When the subtalar joint is in an inverted position, the axes are incongruent, giving increased stability to the midfoot. (Reproduced, with permission, from Mann RA, Coughlin MJ: *The Video Textbook of Foot and Ankle Surgery*. Medical Video Productions, 1991.)

tubercle of the calcaneus and inserts on the base of the proximal phalanges (Figure 8–5). During gait, the metatarsophalangeal joints extend at the last half of the stance phase. The plantar aponeurosis forces the metatarsal heads into a plantarward direction, which raises the longitudinal arch, and this is known as a windlass mechanism. Additionally, the plantar aponeurosis increases the effect that a tensile force in the Achilles tendon has on the tensile force in the plantar fascia. The result is a rigid foot that allows for the body to push-off during gait. Also, this mechanism helps to invert the subtalar joint, thereby increasing the rigidity of the foot for push-off.

F. Gait Abnormalities

Common disorders of gait are described.

1. Pes planus deformity—Pes planus is a decreased longitudinal arch. This may occur when the patient has hypermobility of the joints and the foot is too flexible. As a result, the gait pattern is abnormal; there is excessive valgus of the hindfoot and, in severe cases, breaking down of the longitudinal arch. The forefoot becomes abducted at the beginning of the gait cycle, and there is increased weight-bearing surface on the plantar aspect of the foot. This may cause easy fatigability because of the lack of adequate support of the longitudinal arch.

2. Cavus deformity—A cavus deformity is an excessive elevation of the longitudinal arch. Frequently, there is an associated decrease in the motion the foot, and the hindfoot is in varus while the forefoot is in valgus. Also, the toes may assume a claw deformity. Clinical examples of this deformity are Charcot-Marie-Tooth disease, poliomyelitis, and sometimes chronic stage compartment syndrome of the leg. The overall effect is decreased surface area for weight bearing. Furthermore, claw toe deformities may reduce contact with the ground more. As a result, the gait pattern is abnormal, and increased pressure on the heel at heel strike is seen. With the progression of gait, there is increased pressure of the lateral plantar aspect of the foot and the first metatarsal head.

3. Dropfoot gait—Weakness of the anterior tibialis muscle or a common peroneal nerve palsy may result in a dropfoot gait. These patients lack ankle dorsiflexion, and so the ankle plantar flexes at the ankle joint. When walking, these patients adopt a steppage-type gait. This gait pattern is manifested by increased flexion of the hip and knee to enable the swinging leg to clear the ground. If this compensatory mechanism does not occur, the patient may catch the toes on the ground and fall.

4. Equinus gait—An equinus contracture can occur if there is anterior compartment weakness, which results in uncompensated pull of the gastrocsoleus complex. Also, equinus contracture may be caused by a stroke or head injury, trauma to the lower extremity, or a congenital deformity, and it often is associated with tightness of the posterior capsule. The ankle is fixed in plantar flexion throughout the entire gait cycle. This gait pattern is characterized by forefoot floor contact only. The heel does not touch the ground. The anterior loading of the foot results in a back knee thrust, which may, over a long period of time, result in a hyperextension deformity of the knee. A weak quadriceps muscle may accentuate this problem.

Baker R, McGinley JL, Schwartz MH, et al: The gait profile score and movement analysis profile. *Gait Posture* 2009;30:265. [PMID: 19632117]

Biga N: Clinical examination of the foot and the ankle. Data collection and interpretation of the pathogenic causal sequence of disorders. *Orthop Traumatol Surg Res* 2009;95:41. [PMID: 19427281]

Jenkyn TR, Anas K, Nichol A: Foot segment kinematics during normal walking using a multisegment model of the foot and ankle complex. *J Biomech Eng* 2009;131:034504. [PMID: 19154075]

Lee JH, Sung IY, Yoo JY: Clinical or radiologic measurements and 3-D gait analysis in children with pes planus. *Pediatr Int* 2009;51:201. [PMID: 19405916]

Mann RA: Biomechanics of the foot and ankle. In: Mann RA, Coughlin MJ, eds: *Surgery of the Foot and Ankle*, New York: Mosby-Year Book; 1993.

Orendurff MS, Schoen JA, Bernatz GC, Segal AD, Klute GK: How humans walk: bout duration, steps per bout, and rest duration. *J Rehabil Res Dev* 2008;45:1077. [PMID: 19165696]

Yamaguchi S, Sasho T, Kato H, Kuroyanagi Y, Banks SA: Ankle and subtalar kinematics during dorsiflexion-plantarflexion activities. *Foot Ankle Int* 2009;30:361. [PMID: 19356362]

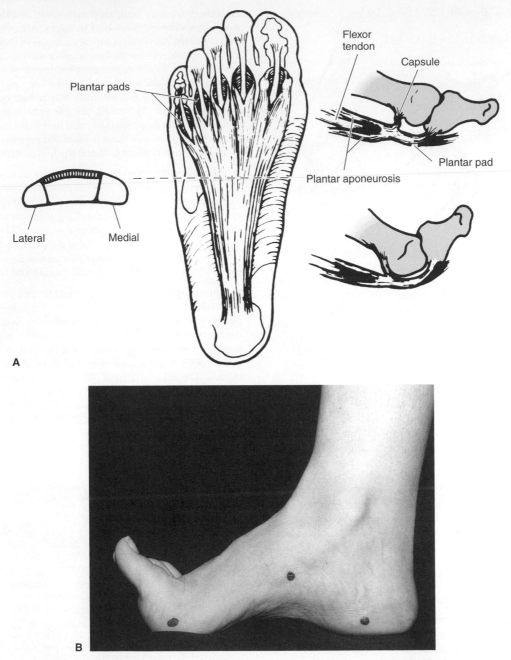

▲ **Figure 8–5.** Windlass mechanism. **A:** The plantar aponeurosis, which arises from the tubercle of the calcaneus, divides and inserts into the base of each of the proximal phalanges. **B:** Dorsiflexion of the metatarsophalangeal joints wraps the plantar aponeurosis around the metatarsal head, depressing the metatarsal heads and elevating the longitudinal arch. (Reproduced with permission, from Mann RA, Coughlin MJ: *The Video Textbook of Foot and Ankle Surgery.* Medical Video Productions, 1991.)

DEFORMITIES OF THE FIRST TOE

▶ Biomechanic Principles

The first metatarsophalangeal joint functions mainly as a weight-bearing structure and stabilizer of the medial aspect of the longitudinal arch. The static stability of the first metatarsophalangeal joint is provided by the collateral ligaments and the strong plantar plate, which consists of the plantar aponeurosis and the joint capsule. Added dynamic stability is provided by the abductor hallucis and adductor hallucis muscles, which insert along the medial and lateral sides of the metatarsal head, respectively. No muscle inserts into the metatarsal head per se, and therefore, it is suspended in a sling of muscles and tendons. This allows the metatarsal head to be pushed in a medial or lateral direction, depending on the deviation of the proximal phalanx.

The plantar aponeurosis forces the metatarsal heads into plantar flexion during the last third of the stance phase of the walking cycle. The hallux experiences greater pressure as it is transferred from the metatarsal heads to the toes (see Figure 8–5). If this windlass mechanism for the hallux is lost as occurs in a bunion deformity, pressure is no longer transferred to the toes but remains beneath the metatarsal heads. Metatarsalgia results from this transfer of load, especially beneath the lesser metatarsal heads. The second metatarsal frequently bears the load because the weight-bearing ability of the first metatarsal is disrupted.

Changes to the normal biomechanics of this joint may result in a transfer lesion, which is a hyperkeratotic lesion under the lesser metatarsal heads. The most common cause is a surgical procedure that disrupts this mechanism, such as a Keller arthroplasty. In this procedure, the base of the proximal phalanx is removed, thereby disrupting the insertion of the plantar aponeurosis into the hallux. Also, prosthetic replacement of the first metatarsal joint will result in loss of this mechanism. Metatarsal osteotomy with excessive shortening (>5–7 mm) or dorsiflexion of the first metatarsal may also cause this problem.

▶ Normal Anatomy

The first metatarsophalangeal joint is complex. It is made up of the articular surface of the metatarsal head and the base of the proximal phalanx, along with the two sesamoid bones plantarly. The sesamoids are connected by an intersesamoidal ligament, separated by a bony crista, and lie within the dual tendons of the flexor hallucis brevis. Medially and laterally, the collateral ligaments stabilize the metatarsophalangeal joint, and toward the plantar surface, they blend with the adductor and abductor hallucis tendons along the lateral and medial sides of the joint. Further toward the plantar surface, the sesamoids are stabilized by the firm attachment of the encapsulating plantar aponeurosis, which inserts into the base of the proximal phalanx. Plantar to the sesamoids passes the flexor hallucis longus tendon. Dorsally,

the extensor hallucis longus tendon is stabilized by a medial and lateral hood mechanism similar to that present in the hand, and the extensor digitorum brevis muscle inserts into the proximal phalanx along the lateral aspect of the joint. Normal motion of the metatarsophalangeal joint consists of dorsiflexion and plantar flexion.

1. Hallux Valgus

Hallux valgus is also known as a bunion deformity (ICD-9 735.0). It is a complex deformity that includes lateral deviation of the proximal phalanx and the resultant medially directed pressure exerted against the metatarsal head. The medial eminence becomes prominent as the proximal phalanx drifts into a valgus position. With chronic deformity, the medial joint capsule becomes attenuated, and the lateral joint capsule becomes contracted. As the metatarsal head is pushed medially, the sesamoids, which are firmly anchored by the adductor hallucis tendon and transverse metatarsal ligament, slowly erode the crista. This allows for lateral subluxation of the sesamoids from directly plantar to the first metatarsal. With the lateral deviation of the hallux, the extensor hallucis longus and flexor hallucis longus assume a lateral position and contribute to the lateral forces on the hallux. With a severe deformity, both the extrinsic and intrinsic muscles lie lateral to the longitudinal axis of the first metatarsophalangeal joint, thereby further enhancing the deformity. As the deformity progresses, pronation of the hallux occurs because attenuation of the weakest portion of the capsule (the dorsomedial aspect) allows the abductor hallucis tendon to slide beneath the metatarsal head and rotate the proximal phalanx into a position of pronation. More rapid progression of the deformity may occur in a small percentage of patients whose first metatarsocuneiform joint demonstrates a significant degree of instability.

▶ General Considerations

The incidence of hallux valgus deformity is 10 times greater in women than in men. The incidence is also significantly higher in shod populations than unshod ones. The conclusion can therefore be made that a major contributing cause of hallux valgus deformity is wearing constricting shoes. Other factors that may contribute to hallux valgus are familial history of bunions, bilateral involvement, female gender, a long first ray, an oval or curved metatarsophalangeal joint articular surface, spasticity, and systemic disease such as rheumatoid arthritis. Furthermore, hallux valgus deformity is not associated with chronic tightness of the Achilles tendon or gastrocnemius, increased first ray mobility, bilaterality, or pes planus.

▶ Clinical Findings

A. Symptoms and Signs

The most common symptom is pain over the medial eminence. Patients also complain of pain in the joint and pain under the second metatarsal head (transfer lesion or meta-tarsalgia). The deformity may prevent shoewear, and the activity limitation may be part of the constellation of symptoms. The patient's occupation, sports activities, and typical shoewear should be noted.

A complete evaluation is performed on both lower extremities with the patient undressed from the knees to the toes. The patient is instructed to stand and walk. The posture of the foot is noted as well as the position of the hallux and lesser toes. The skin is evaluated for erythema, swelling, ulceration, or callosities. The ROM is checked for the ankle, subtalar, transverse tarsal, and metatarsophalangeal joints. The neurovascular status of the foot is carefully assessed, noting absent pulses and venous stasis changes. If there is compromise of the vascularity, then vascular studies may be obtained. Doppler studies are obtained if there is any question regarding the circulatory status of the foot. It is important to note the ROM of the first metatarsophalangeal joint in the deformed and corrected position. The amount of motion limitation will give the surgeon insight into the degree of surgical correction that can be obtained at the joint without impairing motion of the joint. The first metatarso-cuneiform joint is examined for hypermobility by stabilizing the medial cuneiform and ranging the first metatarsal dorso-medially and plantolaterally.

B. Imaging Studies

Weight-bearing radiographs of the foot are important to evaluate the type and severity of the hallux valgus deformity. Radiographic evaluation of the first metatarsophalangeal joint includes:

1. The hallux valgus angle: The angle created by the inter-section of the lines that longitudinally bisect the proximal phalanx and first metatarsal. A normal angle is less than 15 degrees (Figure 8–6).

2. The 1,2 intermetatarsal angle: The angle created by the intersection of the lines bisecting the first and second metatarsal shafts. A normal angle is less than 9 degrees (Figure 8–6).

3. The distal metatarsal articular angle: The angle of the distal articular surface of the first metatarsal to the long axis of the metatarsal. Normal is less than 10 degrees of lateral deviation.

4. Congruency of the first metatarsophalangeal joint: A congruent joint has no lateral subluxation of the proximal phalanx in relation to the first metatarsal head, and an incongruent joint has lateral subluxation of the proximal phalanx on the metatarsal head (Figure 8–7).

5. The first metatarsocuneiform joint: The angle is based on the distal articular surface of the medial cuneiform and the longitudinal axis of the first metatarsal. Excessive medial deviation may indicate that hypermobility may be present.

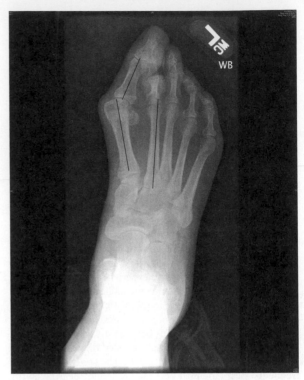

▲ **Figure 8–6.** Anteroposterior weight-bearing radiograph of a patient with a symptomatic hallux valgus deformity. Lines drawn show hallux valgus angle and 1,2 intermetatarsal angle.

6. Arthrosis of the metatarsophalangeal joint has joint space narrowing, subchondral sclerosis, and osteophyte formation.

7. The medial eminence: The characteristics are evaluated, especially size, as measured from the sagittal groove on the medial aspect of the first metatarsal shaft.

8. The hallux valgus interphalangeus is present when there is lateral deviation of the proximal or distal phalanx, or both, in relation to a line drawn across the base of the proximal phalanx. Normal is less than 10 degrees of lateral deviation.

▶ Treatment

A. Nonoperative Treatment

As with all forefoot disorders, proper shoewear is important for successful conservative management. The patient should be encouraged to wear shoes of adequate size and shape. This simple form of management may relieve most symptoms. Padding is helpful to alleviate symptoms associated with the bunion deformity. Pads may be placed in the first web space or over the median eminence to help take

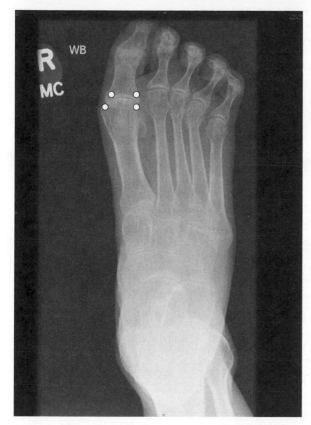

▲ **Figure 8–7.** Example of an incongruent first metatarsophalangeal joint, with mild lateral subluxation.

pressure off a painful median eminence. Pads are also available that can be placed underneath the metatarsal heads to take pressure off painful calluses or sesamoids. In some patients, custom orthotic devices are helpful. These, too, will decrease pressure in symptomatic areas. Patients who fail these treatment options may consider surgical treatment to correct the deformity. An operation is not performed for cosmetic reasons or to allow patients to wear fashionable shoes, but rather to correct a symptomatic structural deformity.

Juvenile hallux valgus deformity is considered a different entity than adult hallux valgus. These patients may be challenging to treat, but as a general rule, nonoperative management should be continued until growth is completed, after which surgery may be considered. Extra care must be taken into consideration in the juvenile population where cosmetic appearance may play a greater role in the patient's or parents' desire for surgery. Hallux valgus surgery is generally contraindicated in high-performance athletes or dancers until they are no longer able to perform at the level necessary to continue in their vocation or avocation. Premature surgery in these individuals may diminish their special abilities.

B. Surgical Treatment

1. Algorithm for surgical treatment—The patient's symptoms, the physical signs, and the radiographic findings must be taken into account in determining the best operation for that patient. It must be emphasized that there is not a single procedure appropriate for all hallux valgus deformities. Preoperative planning with all these considerations is important.

The following factors need to be considered in the decision-making process:

1. Patient's chief complaint

2. Physical findings

3. Degree of hallux valgus and intermetatarsal angle

4. Distal metatarsal articular angle

5. Congruency or incongruency of the metatarsophalangeal joint

6. Presence of arthrosis of the joint

7. Degree of pronation of the hallux

8. Age of the patient

9. Circulatory status

10. Patient expectations for outcome of operation

The algorithm in Figure 8–8 divides hallux valgus deformities into three main groups: those with a congruent joint, those with an incongruent joint, and those associated with degenerative joint disease. The algorithm lists the operative procedure that may best correct the deformity within each classification. Although no one scheme is all inclusive, this algorithm is helpful in organizing the treatment plan.

The first step is to evaluate the first metatarsophalangeal joint for congruency. A congruent metatarsophalangeal joint generally requires excision of the large and symptomatic medial eminence, and the joint does not require realignment. For a mild to moderate deformity, a chevron osteotomy with or without an Akin procedure yields good to excellent results.

With an incongruent joint, the proximal phalanx is subluxed laterally on the metatarsal head. The operative procedure necessitates that the proximal phalanx be reduced onto the metatarsal head. The procedure of choice depends on the severity of the deformity (see Figure 8–8).

If the first metatarsocuneiform joint is hypermobile, a distal soft-tissue procedure with a metatarsocuneiform arthrodesis (Lapidus procedure) may be indicated. With a severe hallux valgus deformity, a greater than 45- to 50-degree hallux valgus angle, and degenerative joint disease, arthrodesis of the joint is indicated. If routine hallux valgus repair is attempted in the patient with advanced arthrosis, stiffness of the metatarsophalangeal joint frequently results. Use of a prosthetic replacement, as a general rule, does not produce a satisfactory long-term result, particularly in active individuals.

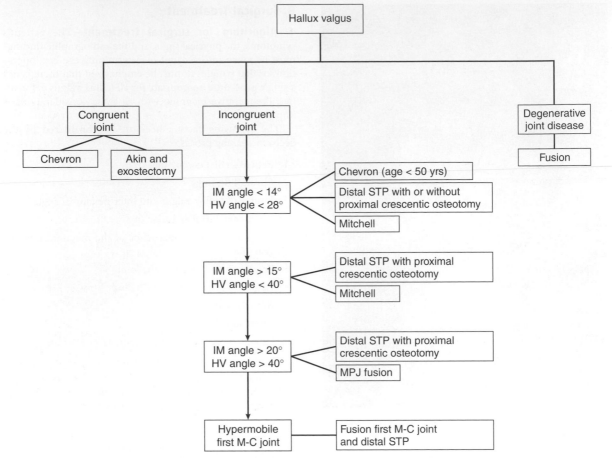

▲ **Figure 8–8.** Algorithm for hallux valgus deformities. M-C, metatarsocuneiform; MPJ, metatarsal phalangeal joint; STP, soft-tissue procedure. (Redrawn, with permission, from Mann RA, Coughlin MJ: *The Video Textbook of Foot and Ankle Surgery*. Medical Video Productions, 1991.)

2. Surgical procedures

A. DISTAL SOFT-TISSUE PROCEDURE—The McBride procedure was a commonly performed operation (CPT 28292). It was modified by DuVries, followed by additional modifications, and is now called the distal soft-tissue procedure. The procedure used by itself is appropriate in mild hallux valgus deformities, where the intermetatarsal angle is less than 12–13 degrees and the hallux valgus angle is less than 30 degrees. Within this range of deformity, a satisfactory outcome can usually be anticipated from this procedure.

The distal soft-tissue procedure involves a medial incision to expose the metatarsophalangeal joint. The joint is inspected, and the medial eminence is removed 1–2 mm just medial to the sagittal sulcus and in line with the medial aspect of the metatarsal shaft. A second incision in the first interspace allows for releasing the soft-tissue contracture on the lateral side of the metatarsophalangeal joint. These structures include the lateral joint capsule, the adductor hallucis

tendon, and the transverse metatarsal ligament (Figure 8–9). Once released, the medial side of the joint is plicated to hold the toe in correct alignment. Postoperatively, the patient is maintained in a firm compression dressing in the correct alignment, and the dressing is changed on a weekly basis for 8 weeks. During this period, the patient is permitted to ambulate in a postoperative shoe.

The most common complication consists of recurrence of the deformity, usually because the deformity was too severe to be corrected by the procedure. In these cases, a metatarsal osteotomy added to the distal soft-tissue procedure completes the correction.

Hallux varus deformity is a medial deviation of the proximal phalanx on the metatarsal head, a complication that may occur in approximately 5–7% of cases. This deformity is usually a result of excessive excision of the medial eminence or fibular sesamoidectomy, which causes joint instability. Occasionally, the medial joint capsule is overplicated or the

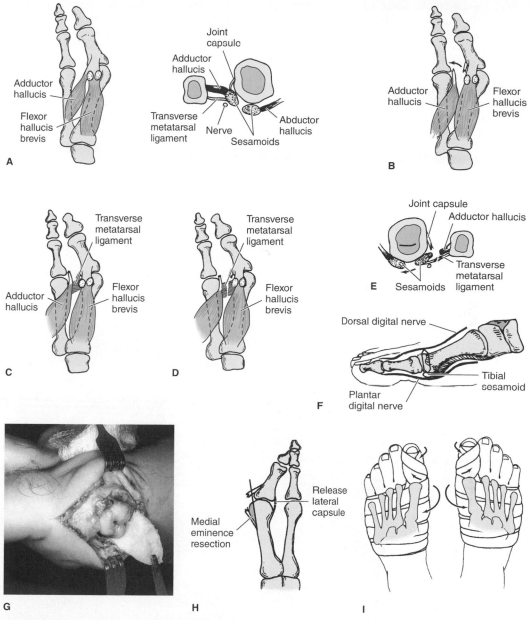

▲ **Figure 8–9.** Total soft-tissue procedure. **A:** The adductor tendon inserts into the lateral aspect of the fibular sesamoid and into the base of the proximal phalanx. **B:** The adductor tendon was removed from its insertion into the lateral side of the fibular sesamoid and base of the proximal phalanx. **C:** The transverse metatarsal ligament is passed from the second metatarsal into the fibular sesamoid. **D:** The transverse metatarsal ligament was transected. **E:** The three contracted structures on the lateral side of the metatarsophalangeal joint were released. **F:** The medical capsular incision begins 2–3 mm proximal to the base of the proximal phalanx, and a flap of tissue measuring 3–8 mm is removed. **G:** The medial eminence is exposed by creating a flap of capsule that is based proximally and plantarward. **H:** The medial eminence is removed in line with the medial aspect of the first metatarsal. **I:** The postoperative dressings are critical. Note that the metatarsal heads are firmly bound with the gauze, and the great toe is rotated so as to keep the sesamoids realigned beneath the metatarsal head. This necessitates dressing the right great toe in a counterclockwise direction and the left great toe in a clockwise direction when one is standing at the foot of the bed. (Reproduced, with permission, from Mann RA, Coughlin MJ: *The Video Textbook of Foot and Ankle Surgery.* Medical Video Productions, 1991.)

lateral joint capsule fails to attain adequate strength. Mild hallux varus deformity, up to 7–10 degrees, usually is of no clinical significance unless the joint is also hyperextended.

B. DISTAL SOFT-TISSUE PROCEDURE WITH PROXIMAL METATARSAL OSTEOTOMY

A proximal metatarsal osteotomy (CPT 28296) will increase the correction of the distal soft-tissue procedure. A proximal metatarsal osteotomy will correct an increased 1,2 intermetatarsal angle, such as a deformity greater than 12–13 degrees, whereas the distal soft-tissue procedure alone cannot. Realignment of the fixed bony deformity present between the first and second metatarsals permits the combined procedure to be used for deformities with up to 50 degrees of hallux valgus and a 25-degree intermetatarsal angle.

The distal soft-tissue procedure is performed, as previously described. Another incision, based over the base of the first metatarsal, is made. A crescentic-shaped saw blade is used to create a crescentic osteotomy, in which the concavity is directed proximally (Figure 8–10). This enables the surgeon to rotate the metatarsal head laterally as the metatarsocuneiform joint is pushed in a medialward direction. This usually results in approximately 2–3 mm of lateral displacement of the osteotomy site. A single cancellous screw placed from the distal fragment into the proximal aspect allows for stable fixation. A popular osteotomy is a chevron cut, or various oblique cuts, opening or closing wedge osteotomies.

Postoperatively, the treatment is the same as for the distal soft-tissue procedure, with 8 weeks of dressing changes and immobilization in a postoperative shoe. As a general rule, cast immobilization is not necessary.

The long-term postoperative results following the distal soft-tissue procedure with proximal osteotomy result in greater than 90% patient satisfaction. The addition of the osteotomy does create an increased risk of complications, but this risk is reported to be uniformly low. Dorsiflexion of the osteotomy site may occur but is usually not of clinical significance. Nonunion of the osteotomy is rare (<1% of cases). Excessive lateral displacement of the metatarsal head can result in hallux varus deformity, which is more resistant to treatment than when osteotomy is not included.

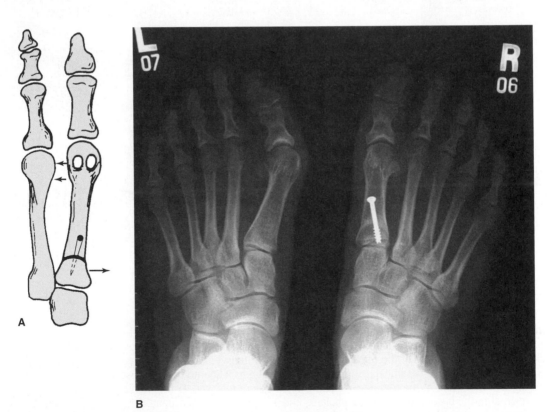

▲ **Figure 8–10. A:** The osteotomy site is reduced by pushing the proximal fragment medially with a small freer while pushing the metatarsal head laterally. This locks the lateral side of the osteotomy site so the internal fixation can be inserted. (Reproduced, with permission, from Mann RA, Coughlin MJ: *The Video Textbook of Foot and Ankle Surgery.* Medical Video Productions, 1991.) **B:** Anteroposterior postoperative radiographs of a case of proximal crescentic osteotomy. The patient underwent the same procedure to the contralateral foot.

C. CHEVRON OSTEOTOMY—The chevron osteotomy is the most common bunion procedure in the United States (CPT 28296). It is indicated for mild to moderate hallux valgus deformities. The procedure is used in deformities when the hallux valgus angle is less than 30 degrees and the 1,2 intermetatarsal angle is less than 12 degrees. The distal metatarsal articular angle should be less than 12 degrees, or complete correction will not be obtained. The operative procedure is based on lateral translation of the metatarsal head, along with plication of the medial joint capsule. The osteotomy is performed through a medial incision to allow removal of the medial eminence. Then, a chevron-shaped cut with the apex based distally is made with a small sagittal saw. The metatarsal head fragment is translated laterally approximately one third of the width of the metatarsal head, or 3–4 mm. The medial bony prominence created by the shift of the metatarsal head is excised and the medial joint capsule plicated. The osteotomy site is fixed with a pin or a screw (Figure 8–11).

Postoperatively, the foot is firmly bandaged for 6–8 weeks in corrected alignment, and the patient is permitted to ambulate in a postoperative shoe. If a pin was used for fixation, it is removed after 4–6 weeks.

Radiographic improvement is seen with high patient satisfaction. In addition, a greater than 10-year follow-up showed consistent improvement with time. There was no difference between patients younger and older than 50 years; patients had equally positive outcomes. However, if the indications are stretched to include more severe deformities, then results may not be satisfactory, with a recurrence or incomplete correction. The most serious complication, occurring in 0–20% of cases, is avascular necrosis of the metatarsal head, which is probably the result of extensive stripping of the soft tissue surrounding the head, especially laterally. The major blood supply to the metatarsal head is from the plantar lateral corner of the metatarsal neck. Therefore, care must be used when performing the saw cut, and the saw should be removed once the osteotomy is completed so as to not injure the vessels on the lateral aspect of the metatarsal head. As with any type of osteotomy, the distal fragment is capable of migrating either too far laterally or medially, giving rise either to hallux varus deformity or recurrent hallux valgus deformity. Occasionally, arthrofibrosis of the joint is noted, resulting in significant joint stiffness.

D. AKIN PROCEDURE—The Akin procedure is useful as an adjunct to a bunion procedure of the first metatarsal (CPT 28298). It involves a medial closing-wedge osteotomy at the base of the proximal phalanx to correct the hallux interphalangeal component of the deformity. It is commonly used with simple excision of the median eminence or with a chevron osteotomy to correct a mild to moderate hallux valgus deformity with a congruent joint. The Akin procedure is indicated for a hallux valgus deformity of less than 25 degrees, with an intermetatarsal angle of 12 degrees or less.

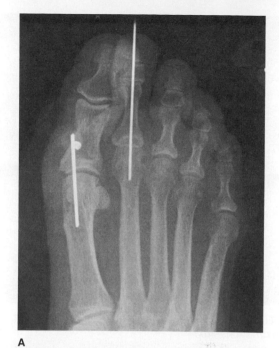

A

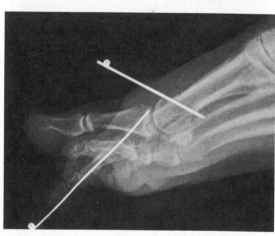

B

▲ **Figure 8–11. (A)** Anteroposterior and **(B)** lateral radiographs of a chevron osteotomy.

Through a medial incision, the base of the proximal phalanx and the median eminence are exposed. After removing the median eminence in line with the metatarsal, a small sagittal saw is used to remove a wedge of bone from the medial aspect of the proximal phalanx. The osteotomy is closed down and stabilized internally with sutures or wires or externally with a Kirschner wire (K-wire) (Figure 8–12). Dressings are applied for 6–8 weeks postoperatively. Patients may ambulate in a postoperative shoe until the osteotomy has healed.

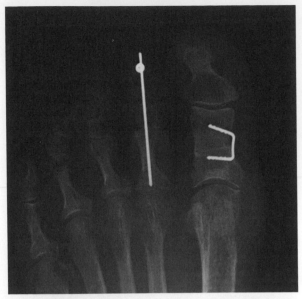

▲ **Figure 8–12.** Radiograph of an Akin osteotomy of the proximal phalanx.

E. KELLER PROCEDURE—The Keller procedure is seldom indicated as a hallux valgus procedure (CPT 28292). It is reserved for the older, less active patient; in a patient prone to skin problems; or in the case of an arthritic joint.

This procedure is contraindicated in an active person because of its known complications.

The procedure involves excision of the base of the proximal phalanx to decompress the metatarsophalangeal joint. Along with the procedure, the medial eminence is removed, and then the intrinsic muscle attachments are repaired to the remaining stump of bone (Figure 8–13). A Kirschner wire is drilled through the toe as a stabilizer until the toe heals and scar tissue forms, approximately 4–6 weeks. Postoperatively, the patient is permitted to ambulate in a postoperative shoe, and dressings are changed for 6 weeks.

Results in the older (>65 years) patient with low functional demand are satisfactory. If the procedure is used in a younger patient, there is instability and loss of weight bearing by the first metatarsophalangeal joint because the base of the proximal phalanx was removed. There is significant loss of foot function, and a transfer lesion may develop beneath the second metatarsal head because the great toe no longer carries adequate weight. The metatarsophalangeal joint develops into a cocked-up deformity with some varus malalignment.

F. ARTHRODESIS OF THE FIRST METATARSOPHALANGEAL JOINT—Arthrodesis of the first metatarsophalangeal joint is used in treatment of severe hallux valgus deformities (CPT 28750) with concomitant advanced degenerative arthrosis of the joint or as a salvage procedure following a previously failed surgical attempt to realign the metatarsophalangeal joint. Also, patients with deformities in which the proximal phalanx is subluxed more than 50% of the

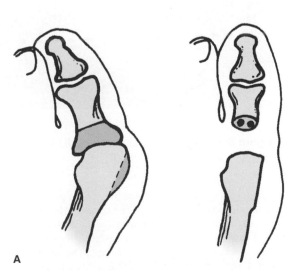

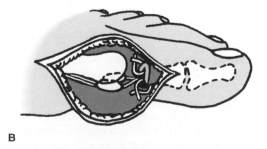

A **B**

▲ **Figure 8–13.** Keller procedure. **A:** The medial eminence is removed in line with the medial aspect of the metatarsal shaft. The proximal third of the proximal phalanx is removed. **B:** An attempt is made to reapproximate the plantar and medial capsular structures to the remaining base of the proximal phalanx. (Reproduced, with permission, from Mann RA, Coughlin MJ: *The Video Textbook of Foot and Ankle Surgery* Medical Video Productions, 1991.)

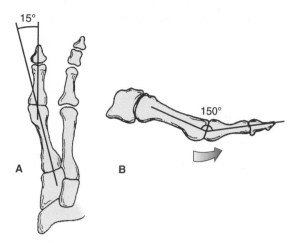

▲ **Figure 8–14.** Arthrodesis of the first metatarsophalangeal joint. **A:** The joint is placed into approximately 10–15 degrees of dorsiflexion in relation to the floor, which is approximately 25–30 degrees of dorsiflexion in relation to the first metatarsal shaft. (Reproduced, with permission, from Mann RA, Coughlin MJ: *The Video Textbook of Foot and Ankle Surgery.* Medical Video Productions, 1991.)

metatarsal head or who have significant stiffness of the metatarsophalangeal joint should be considered for fusion.

The procedure is performed through a dorsal longitudinal incision, and the joint surface is removed with a sagittal saw to yield two flat surfaces. Alternatively, a dome-shaped reamer may be used to create a ball-and-socket type of configuration. The arthrodesis site is stabilized with an interfragmentary screw and a dorsal plate or Steinmann pins if the bone quality is poor and inadequate screw fixation results. As with any fusion, the position of the arthrodesis is critical; the joint should be placed in 15 degrees of valgus and 10–15 degrees of dorsiflexion in relation to the ground or the plantar aspect of the foot. In relation to the first metatarsal shaft, which is inclined plantarward approximately 15 degrees, it should be in approximately 30 degrees of dorsiflexion (Figures 8–14 and 8–15). Any pronation that is present must also be corrected at the same time.

The patient may ambulate on the heel while wearing a postoperative shoe and progress to full weight bearing in the postoperative shoe until radiographic union is seen, generally in 12 weeks. The unreliable patient may be treated in a short leg walking cast.

The most common complication of arthrodesis of the first metatarsophalangeal joint is malposition. If the toe is not placed into adequate dorsiflexion or valgus, excessive stress occurs against the interphalangeal joint, which may result in a painful arthritic condition of the joint. The fusion rate is 90–95%. In cases of severe hallux valgus deformities, the arthrodesis will correct the hallux valgus angle as well as the increased 1,2 intermetatarsal angle; thus, the need for a

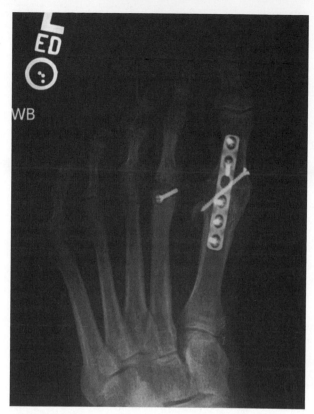

▲ **Figure 8–15.** Radiograph of a patient with a first metatarsophalangeal arthrodesis for degenerative arthritis and severe hallux valgus deformity.

proximal osteotomy is unnecessary. Occasionally, the degree of valgus and dorsiflexion is correct but the toe is left in a pronated position, which results in pressure along the medial side of the interphalangeal joint and possible discomfort.

The patient's gait following arthrodesis of the first metatarsophalangeal joint in proper alignment is improved in propulsive power, weight-bearing function of the foot, and stability during gait. These patients are able to roll over the fusion site in an ordinary store-bought shoe, and they may expect to return to normal activities. Squatting is the only activity that is difficult because the toe must be in full dorsiflexion when this activity is carried out. Patients are able to return to most types of athletic activities, although at a somewhat slower pace.

2. Hallux Rigidus

▶ General Considerations

Hallux rigidus is the name for arthrosis of the first metatarsophalangeal joint (ICD-9 715.17). It is a common entity and frequently affects patients at a much younger age than arthritis of other joints. Hallux rigidus is seen in patients from their thirties onward. The reason why arthritis of this joint is seen in younger patients is unclear but may be associated with an unrecognized chondral injury to the metatarsal head. It is also associated with hallux valgus interphalangeus, bilateral involvement in those with a family history, and female gender. Hallux rigidus is not associated with elevatus, first ray hypermobility, a long first metatarsal, Achilles tightness, abnormal foot posture, symptomatic hallux valgus, adolescent onset, shoe wear, or occupation.

► Clinical Findings

A. Symptoms and Signs

Patients complain primarily of pain of the first metatarsophalangeal joint, especially with extension. Also, the dorsal eminence may prevent shoewear and have associated swelling and redness. Weight bearing and sports activities exacerbate the pain.

B. Imaging Studies

Weight-bearing radiographs of the foot demonstrate arthritic changes, including loss of joint space, subchondral sclerosis, and the presence of osteophytes, especially on the dorsal aspect of the metatarsal neck.

C. Conservative Management

Conservative treatment consists of nonsteroidal anti-inflammatory drugs (NSAIDs) and wearing a stiff-soled shoe with a deep toe box. An orthotic device with a Morton's extension or a carbon fiber plate would be beneficial. Both of the devices prevent extension in late stance phase. A rocker-bottom shoe would also be helpful. In older (>60 years), sedentary patients, these measures are usually adequate. In more active individuals, however, surgical treatment is usually indicated.

D. Surgical Treatment

There are multiple described surgical treatment options for hallux rigidus. Of these, the simplest is a cheilectomy (CPT 28289) and is indicated in patients with mild to moderate arthrosis but who have a large dorsal osteophyte. Approximately one fourth to one third of the dorsal metatarsal head is excised with an osteotome (Figure 8–16). The medial and lateral osteophytes are also debrided, and a thorough synovectomy of the joint is performed. Postoperatively, patients regain up to 50% of their dorsiflexion and have improvement of their total motion. More than 90% of patients have improvement of pain, ability to wear shoes, and increased physical abilities. This procedure is less likely to have a favorable outcome on joints with advanced arthritis.

A Keller procedure is a resection arthroplasty and may be useful in older, less active patients, but it has a high rate of complications, as previously discussed. Prosthetic replacement of the arthritic first metatarsophalangeal joint can be used in older, lower demand patients but has high rates of failure in younger, more active individuals.

First metatarsophalangeal joint arthrodesis is a predictable and durable procedure. The drawback is lost motion at the joint. However, patients can remain quite active with a first metatarsophalangeal joint fusion as described previously.

3. Sesamoid Disorders

► General Considerations

The sesamoid bones are plantar to the first metatarsal head and are part of the first metatarsophalangeal joint complex. Sesamoid disorders can be painful as they are in the weight-bearing part of the foot. Fractures, osteonecrosis, arthritis, and subluxation can affect the sesamoids. A puzzling entity is called sesamoiditis (ICD-9 733.99), which means inflammation of the sesamoids, but it encompasses painful sesamoids without an etiology.

► Clinical Findings

A. Symptoms and Signs

The patient complains of pain directly under the first metatarsophalangeal joint that is worse with weight-bearing activities. The history may be significant for a trauma to the toe causing a fracture, but most commonly, the pain has an insidious onset.

Manual palpation of the area will reveal which sesamoid is affected, medial or lateral. Also, during the physical examination, postural abnormalities of the foot that may be contributing to the condition are evaluated. For example, hallux valgus deformity may cause a subluxation of the sesamoid from its normal articulation with the plantar aspect of the metatarsal head, causing pain, whereas pes cavus may result in greater pressure under the sesamoids, leading to symptoms.

B. Imaging Studies

Radiographs of the weight-bearing foot are taken and include a skyline or sesamoid view, which is a tangential view of the sesamoid metatarsal head articulation. On the anteroposterior view, subluxation of the sesamoids lateral to the first metatarsal head can be present with hallux valgus deformities. On the skyline view, fragmentation can be seen in cases with osteonecrosis, and joint space narrowing and osteophyte formation are seen with osteoarthritis. Displaced fractures are easy to determine, but nondisplaced fractures may be difficult to distinguish from a bipartite sesamoid that is a normal finding. A magnetic resonance imaging (MRI) or bone scan may be helpful in the case of normal radiographs to diagnose osteonecrosis or sesamoiditis.

C. Treatment

Acute injuries involving the sesamoid can be treated with a course of cast immobilization, sometimes non–weight bearing. A toe plate on the cast will provide greater immobilization and support. For chronic problems, a stiff-soled postoperative-type shoe may be used, and a soft felt pad can

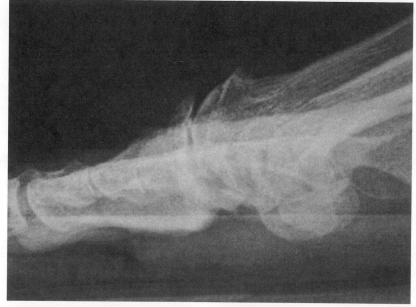

A

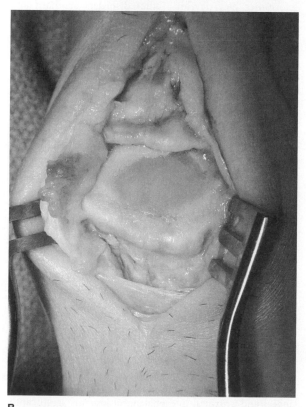

B

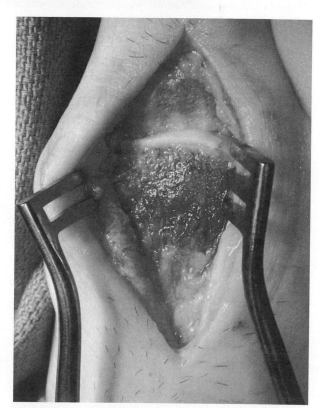

C

▲ **Figure 8–16. A:** Preoperative lateral radiograph of a patient with hallux rigidus. **B:** Intraoperative photograph of the dorsal osteophyte. **C:** Following removal of the osteophyte. **D:** Extension of the first metatarsophalangeal joint is 70 degrees, and confirms adequate resection of the first metatarsal head.

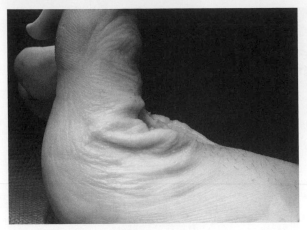

D

▲ **Figure 8–16.** (Continued)

be placed just proximal to the sesamoids to take the pressure off the involved area. If needed, an orthotic device with a metatarsal pad or bar will relieve sesamoid pressure. Usually the majority of symptoms resolve in a matter of weeks, although some degree of discomfort may persist for several months. If 6–12 months of conservative treatment does not relieve the symptoms, the affected sesamoid can be removed via sesamoidectomy, which relieves the pain. There is the possibility of transferring pain to the remaining sesamoid.

Brodsky JW, Baum BS, Pollo FE, Mehta H: Prospective gait analysis in patients with first metatarsophalangeal joint arthrodesis for hallux rigidus. *Foot Ankle Int* 2007;28:162. [PMID: 17296132]

Coughlin MJ, Jones CP: Hallux valgus: demographics, etiology, and radiographic assessment. *Foot Ankle Int* 2007;28:759. [PMID: 17666168]

Coughlin MJ, Jones CP: Hallux valgus and first ray mobility. A prospective study. *J Bone Joint Surg Am* 2007;89:1887. [PMID: 17768183]

Goucher NR, Coughlin MJ: Hallux metatarsophalangeal joint arthrodesis using dome-shaped reamers and dorsal plate fixation: a prospective study. *Foot Ankle Int* 2006;27:869. [PMID: 17144945]

Lee KM, Ahn S, Chung CY, Sung KH, Park MS: Reliability and relationship of radiographic measurements in hallux valgus. *Clin Orthop Relat Res* 2012;470:2613. [PMID: 22544667]

Lin J, Murphy GA: Treatment of hallux rigidus with cheilectomy using a dorsolateral approach. *Foot Ankle Int* 2009;30:115. [PMID: 19254504]

Malal JJ, Shaw-Dunn J, Kumar CS: Blood supply to the first metatarsal head and vessels at risk with a chevron osteotomy. *J Bone Joint Surg Am* 2007;89:2018. [PMID: 17768200]

Okuda R, Kinoshita M, Yasuda T, Jotoku T, Shima H: Proximal metatarsal osteotomy for hallux valgus: comparison of outcome for moderate and severe deformities. *Foot Ankle Int* 2008;29:664. [PMID: 18785415]

Potenza V, Caterini R, Farsetti P, et al: Chevron osteotomy with lateral release and adductor tenotomy for hallux valgus. *Foot Ankle Int* 2009;30:512. [PMID: 19486628]

Pydah SK, Toh EM, Sirikonda SP, Walker CR: Intermetatarsal angular change following fusion of the first metatarsophalangeal joint. *Foot Ankle Int* 2009;30:415. [PMID: 19439141]

Usuelli F, Palmucci M, Montrasio UA, Malerba F: Radiographic considerations of hallux valgus versus hallux rigidus. *Foot Ankle Int* 2011;32:782. [PMID: 22049864]

DEFORMITIES OF THE LESSER TOES

The most common disorders of the lesser toes are mallet toe, hammer toe, and claw toe deformities. Understanding the etiology is important in effective treatment of the deformity. Some of the causes include inflammatory arthritis, trauma, congenital abnormalities, or neuromuscular disorders. There may be anatomic factors, such as a wide foot, a long second ray, or postural abnormalities of the foot. However, the most common etiology is long-standing, ill-fitting shoewear. A narrow toe box with a high heel places abnormal forces on the lesser toes. With chronic wear, deformities may develop. Other disorders are hard and soft corns and metatarsophalangeal joint subluxation or dislocation. Patients may complain of pain and difficulty with shoewear. Importantly, patients with neuropathy may develop ulcerations over the bony prominences of these deformities, such as the proximal interphalangeal joint in a hammer toe or claw toe deformity.

▶ **General Considerations**

The anatomic structures that stabilize the metatarsophalangeal joint on the plantar aspect are the plantar capsule, plantar aponeurosis (plantar plate), and medial and lateral collateral ligaments. While on the dorsal aspect of the metatarsophalangeal joint, the extensor digitorum longus and brevis tendons and the extensor hood or sling make up the extensor mechanism. The extensor mechanism allows for dorsiflexion of the metatarsophalangeal joint. In addition, this mechanism can extend the distal interphalangeal and proximal interphalangeal joints if the proximal phalanx is in a neutral or plantar-flexed position. On the plantar aspect, the interossei and lumbricals lines of action pass plantarward to the axis of the metatarsophalangeal joint, and thus flex the metatarsophalangeal joint. Also, the flexor digitorum brevis flexes the distal interphalangeal joint, and the flexor digitorum longus muscle flexes the proximal interphalangeal joint. When the metatarsophalangeal joint is hyperextended, the ability of the extensor hood to extend the distal interphalangeal and proximal interphalangeal joints is significantly diminished. Chronic hyperextension of the metatarsophalangeal joint eventually leads to fixed flexion deformities at the interphalangeal joints. A fixed deformity is significantly more symptomatic than a flexible deformity.

1. Mallet Toe Deformity

A mallet toe is a flexion deformity of the distal interphalangeal joint, and it may be fixed or flexible. In most cases, the second toe is involved, because it is the longest toe.

▶ Clinical Findings

A. Symptoms and Signs

The patient complains of pain either on the dorsum of the distal interphalangeal joint or on the tip of the toe from striking the ground. The affected area may have a callus. Patients with peripheral neuropathy may present with an ulcer. The nail may develop a deformity with chronic trauma from pressure from the shoe or ground.

Physical examination includes a complete evaluation of both feet, including the neurovascular status. To diagnose a flexible mallet toe, the ankle is brought into plantar flexion. If the deformity corrects and then recurs when the ankle is placed into dorsiflexion, the mallet toe is flexible. However, with a fixed deformity, ankle motion does not affect the deformity.

B. Imaging Studies

Weight-bearing radiographs of the foot are obtained to show the deformity of the distal interphalangeal joint.

▶ Treatment

A. Conservative Management

The patient should be educated to wear a shoe with a wide toe box to accommodate the deformed toe. An extra-depth shoe may be needed to decrease pressure on the deformity. A small felt pad may be placed on the shoe liner, just proximal to the deformity, to prevent the tip of the toe from striking the ground.

B. Surgical Treatment

A flexible mallet toe can be treated by releasing the flexor digitorum longus tendon. This can be accomplished under a

digital block, and a small incision on the plantar aspect of the toe at the level of the middle phalanx allows for releasing the flexor tendon. This treatment is usually effective.

With a fixed mallet toe deformity, the toe must be treated with a condylectomy. Under digital or ankle block anesthesia, a dorsal elliptical incision over the distal interphalangeal joint exposes the distal aspect of the middle phalanx. The head and neck of the middle phalanx are removed with a small bone cutter. A 0.045-inch K-wire is used to hold the reduction for 4 weeks (Figure 8–17).

Generally, good resolution of symptoms and deformity results. Persistent deformity or recurrence may occur if contracture of the flexor digitorum longus tendon was not appreciated prior to surgery or insufficient bone was removed from the middle phalanx to decompress the deformity adequately.

2. Hammer Toe Deformity

A hammer toe is flexion contracture of the proximal interphalangeal joint (ICD-9 735.4), and it may be fixed or flexible. It is frequently associated with varying degrees of hyperextension of the metatarsophalangeal joint, and there may be an associated flexion deformity of the distal interphalangeal joint. Occasionally, the distal interphalangeal joint has an extension deformity.

▶ Clinical Findings

A. Symptoms and Signs

Like the mallet toe, patients complain of pain and difficulty with shoewear. The pain is localized to the dorsal aspect of the proximal interphalangeal joint or on the plantar aspect of the affected metatarsal head. Physical examination evaluates both lower extremities, noting if the deformity is fixed or flexible. Also, the metatarsophalangeal joints are inspected for joint abnormalities, most commonly hyperextension deformities. Callus formation or even an ulcer may be present over the extensor surface of the proximal interphalangeal

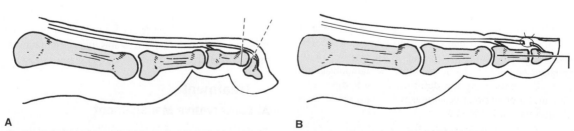

A   **B**

▲ **Figure 8–17.** Mallet toe repair. **A:** Resection of condyles of the middle phalanx. **B:** Intramedullary K-wire fixation. (Reproduced, with permission, from Mann RA, Coughlin MJ: *The Video Textbook of Foot and Ankle Surgery.* Medical Video Productions, 1991.)

joint, where the deformity rubs against the shoe. If the metatarsophalangeal joint is involved, then correction may be needed to fully correct the hammer toe. It is important to evaluate any deformity involving the hallux; a hallux valgus deformity may be part of the cause of a hammer toe deformity. If this is the case, then the hallux valgus deformity requires correction to provide space for the second toe to be reduced into corrected alignment.

B. Imaging Studies

Weight-bearing radiographs of the foot will reveal arthrosis of the joint. The radiographs will confirm the clinical findings of the proximal interphalangeal flexion deformity, hyperextension deformity at the metatarsophalangeal joint, and hallux valgus deformity. It is important to fully evaluate the entire forefoot and all its joints when planning a procedure.

▶ Treatment

A. Conservative Management

As with mallet toes, patients may benefit from shoe wear that accommodates the deformity. The shoe should have a wide toe box and may be of extra depth. Over-the-counter toe sleeves and pads can alleviate pain in the affected areas, especially around callosities. With more severe deformities, shoewear becomes more difficult. Hence, nonoperative management becomes more difficult. This is especially true with a severe hallux valgus deformity or claw toe deformity.

B. Surgical Treatment

The operative procedure to correct the hammer toe deformity depends on whether it is a fixed or flexible deformity. Additionally, deformity of the metatarsophalangeal joint needs to be corrected concomitantly, and finally, the hallux deformity, if present, must be addressed. This will provide a space for the second toe to be placed in correct alignment.

1. Flexible hammer toe deformity—A flexible hammer toe deformity can be treated with a Girdlestone flexor tendon transfer. A small plantar incision is made to harvest the flexor digitorum longus. The tendon is split in half, and each portion is brought up subcutaneously on each side of the proximal phalanx through a dorsal longitudinal incision. The tendon segments are sutured into the extensor hood mechanism with the toe held in approximately 5 degrees of plantar flexion and the ankle in plantar flexion (Figure 8–18). This causes the long flexor tendon to act as an extensor of the interphalangeal joints and a flexor of the metatarsophalangeal joint, thereby correcting the deformity. A soft dressing is applied, and a postoperative shoe is worn for 4 weeks, after which ambulation is allowed.

2. Fixed hammer toe deformity—A fixed hammer toe deformity requires a bony procedure to correct the flexion contracture. This is accomplished with the DuVries proximal phalangeal condylectomy (CPT 28285). This procedure is identical to that described for treatment of the mallet toe deformity, but occurs at the proximal interphalangeal joint instead of the distal interphalangeal joint (Figure 8–19). Clinical results show a majority of patients were satisfied and a low risk of recurrence of deformity.

3. Complications—The main complication observed with either procedure is inadequate correction of the deformity, usually because of failure to appreciate a contracture of the flexor digitorum longus tendon at the time of surgery. In the DuVries condylectomy, inadequate bone may have been resected.

3. Claw Toe Deformity

A claw toe deformity involves hyperextension of the metatarsophalangeal joint and flexion of the interphalangeal joint. The deformity may be flexible or fixed. Patients complain of pain and difficulty with shoewear. Patients with a neuromuscular disorder frequently will have severe fixed deformities. The pain experienced by patients is over the dorsal aspect of the interphalangeal joints from pressure against the shoe. Also, they have pain on the plantar aspect of the metatarsal heads because the metatarsal heads are forced into plantar flexion from the extended toe. In contrast to hammer toe or mallet toe deformities, which usually involve a single toe, claw toe deformity usually involves all of the lesser toes. An associated deformity of the great toe may occur as well.

▶ Clinical Findings

A. Symptoms and Signs

Physical examination is performed in a similar manner to mallet and hammer toe deformities. With claw toe deformities, the metatarsal heads are palpated because the fat pad may be displaced distally and the skin beneath the metatarsal heads may be atrophic. Callosities may be present on the extensor surface of the proximal interphalangeal joints and on the plantar aspect of the metatarsophalangeal joints.

B. Imaging Studies

As previously described, radiographs of the foot confirm the severity of the deformity, which is present at the metatarsophalangeal and interphalangeal joints. The posture of the entire foot needs to be evaluated, looking for the presence of a cavus-type foot deformity, characterized by increased dorsiflexion pitch of the calcaneus and increased plantar flexion of the first metatarsal.

▶ Treatment

A. Conservative Management

The goal of nonoperative treatment is to decrease the pressure on the claw toe deformities. This is best accomplished with an extra-depth shoe. A custom orthotic device of soft material will help pad the painful metatarsal heads. Flexible mild deformities

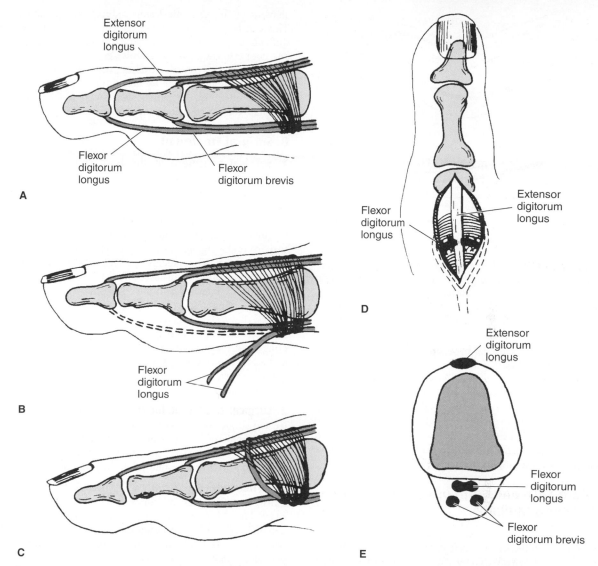

▲ **Figure 8–18.** Flexor tendon transfer for flexible hammer toe deformity. **A:** Lateral view of lesser toe. **B:** The long flexor is detached from its insertion and delivered through the proximal plantar wound. It is split longitudinally along the median raphe. **C:** Each limb is transferred dorsally on either side of the proximal phalanx and secured on the dorsal aspect. **D:** Dorsal view after tendon transfer. **E:** Cross section showing flexor digitorum longus tendon in sheath. (Reproduced, with permission, from Mann RA, Coughlin MJ: *The Video Textbook of Foot and Ankle Surgery*. Medical Video Productions, 1991.)

can be treated with shoe inserts placed immediately proximal to the metatarsophalangeal joints. These can have the effect of balancing the extensors and flexors of the toes.

B. Surgical Treatment

The operative procedure is determined by the flexibility of the deformity. A flexible claw toe can be treated with the Girdlestone flexor tendon transfer. The extensor tendons must be lengthened to correct the hyperextension of the metatarsophalangeal joints to realign to neutral plantar flexion. Also, a capsulotomy and release of the medial and lateral collateral ligaments may be necessary.

A concomitant fixed hammer toe deformity requires a DuVries proximal phalangeal condylectomy in addition to the Girdlestone tendon transfer procedure. Postoperative management for the patient with claw toe deformity is the same as discussed earlier for hammer toe deformity.

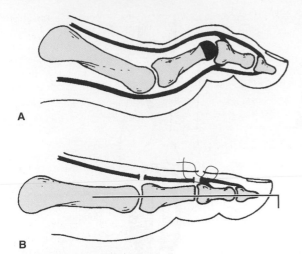

A

B

▲ **Figure 8–19.** Fixed hammer toe repair. **A:** Resection of the head of the proximal phalanx. **B:** Intramedullary K-wire fixation. (Reproduced, with permission, from Mann RA, Coughlin MJ: *The Video Textbook of Food and Ankle Surgery.* Medical Video Productions, 1991.)

Following this surgical procedure, no active motion of the toes occurs. The toes are usually well aligned in a plantigrade position. The marked deformity of the proximal interphalangeal joints is relieved so they no longer strike the top of the shoe. The main problems that can occur after surgery are (1) failure to correct a fixed hammer toe deformity adequately by use of the tendon transfer and (2) failure to release the fixed deformity adequately at the metatarsophalangeal joint, resulting in recurrence of the deformity.

4. Hard Corn and Soft Corn (Clavus Durum and Clavus Mollum)

A corn is a keratotic lesion that can develop over a bony prominence on the lesser toes from excessive pressure on the skin such as shoewear (ICD-9 700). A hard corn frequently involves the dorsal and lateral aspect of the fifth toe, over the bony prominence of the lateral condyle of the proximal phalanx, whereas a soft corn presents in the web space, and it is so named because maceration results from moisture between the toes. The soft corn may occur anywhere along the toe where a bony prominence is present, but it is seen mostly in the fourth web space between the base of the proximal phalanx of the fourth toe and the medial condyle of the head of the proximal phalanx of the fifth toe. In a severe case, an ulceration or local infection may occur because of the extent of the maceration.

▶ **Treatment**

A. Conservative Management

Decreasing the pressure on the affected toes will help improve symptoms. This can be accomplished with shoewear with a large toe box to relieve this pressure. Local debridement or shaving of the keratotic lesion reduces pain temporarily. This can be performed by the patient; however, it may be difficult in older patients because of decreasing flexibility and poor eyesight. Skin compromise, especially in the diabetic patient, must be avoided. At times, soft pads or lamb's wool can be placed around the toe to minimize pressure on the involved area, but the patient must wear a shoe with an adequate toe box to accommodate such modalities.

B. Surgical Treatment

1. Surgical treatment of the hard corn—A hard corn on the fifth toe can be simply treated surgically by excising the distal aspect of the proximal phalanx. Sometimes, the dorsolateral part of the proximal portion of the middle phalanx also needs to be removed. The operation is performed through a longitudinal incision dorsally to avoid a painful scar from chafing against the shoe. The extensor tendon is split, the collateral ligaments cut, and the condyle exposed. With a bone cutter, the distal portion of the proximal phalanx is generously removed and the edges smoothed with a rongeur. Following closure, a compression dressing is applied for several days. The toe is taped to the adjacent fourth toe for 8 weeks, and the patient may ambulate in a postoperative shoe. Long-term results show a high level of patient satisfaction and a low recurrence rate. Removal of excessive bone is the major complication, which causes the small toe to become too floppy, creating a nuisance for the patient.

2. Surgical treatment for the soft corn—Soft corns are treated surgically by making an incision over the lesion and using a small rongeur to remove the underlying bony excrescence. This is a simple procedure and almost invariably results in satisfactory resolution of the problem.

3. Syndactyly—Syndactyly is a procedure in which the fourth and fifth toes are connected by removing the web space skin and suturing the two toes together. This will eliminate the problem of a soft corn in the web space. Also, a soft corn can be treated with a condylectomy of the prominent part of the phalanx. This procedure can only be performed if there is no sign of significant maceration, ulceration, or infection. If there is compromise of the skin, then a syndactyly is indicated.

5. Subluxation and Dislocation of the Metatarsophalangeal Joint

In more severe deformities of the lesser toes, dorsal subluxation or dislocation of the metatarsophalangeal joint may occur. The plantar structures of the plantar plate, collateral ligaments, and plantar capsule become incompetent, and the toe assumes a dorsal position. A hammer toe or mallet toe may be associated with the subluxation or dislocation. Patients complain of pain over the dorsal interphalangeal joint from pressure from shoewear or on the plantar aspect of the metatarsal head. Keratosis can form under the plantar metatarsal head from increased weight-bearing pressure.

General Considerations

The most commonly affected toe is the second, and it is usually associated with a hallux valgus deformity. The pressure of the deformed hallux causes the second toe to sublux or dislocate. Less commonly, a nonspecific synovitis, isolated to the metatarsophalangeal joint and usually involving the second metatarsophalangeal joint, can result in a dislocation. The patient notes some discomfort and swelling around the metatarsophalangeal joint that eventually resolves, usually in 3–6 months. Then an ensuing deformity is noted, with subluxation and possibly dislocation of the joint. Other causes of subluxation and dislocation are direct trauma, rheumatoid or psoriatic arthritis, and neuromuscular disorder.

A somewhat more difficult deformity is a medially or laterally deviated toe. The most common toe is the second because of its prevalence with hallux valgus deformities. With the bunion pressing on the second toe, it can sublux or dislocate and then deviate medially. This deformity may be the result of a steroid injection into the joint. With such a deformity, shoewear is problematic. Patients must wear sandals or an extra-depth shoe to accommodate the deformity.

Clinical Findings

A. Symptoms and Signs

Patients present with complaints of pain, deformity, and difficulty with shoewear. Swelling may be present. The pain is directly at the joint, on the plantar aspect of the metatarsal head, or over the dorsal aspect of the interphalangeal joint. On examination, the patient is evaluated with the patient in a standing and sitting position. The affected metatarsophalangeal joint is palpated for active synovitis, flexibility of the joint, and degree of subluxation. An anterior drawer test is performed on the affected joint to determine its stability. This is performed by holding the proximal phalanx between the examiner's fingers and moving it dorsally and plantarward, similar to a Lachman test of the knee. Also, the hallux is noted for any deformity, namely a hallux valgus deformity, as this is frequently associated with crossover of the second toe on the first toe.

B. Imaging Studies

Weight-bearing foot radiographs allow for evaluation of the severity of the subluxation or frank dislocation. Also, the hallux valgus deformity is evaluated, and changes about the articular surface of the joint are observed. Patients with rheumatoid arthritis usually have multiple joint abnormalities.

Treatment

A. Conservative Management

Patient education is an important first step to conservative management. A wide toe box shoe to accommodate the patient's deformity is often helpful. If needed, a total contact soft orthotic device will relieve pressure on the metatarsal head. The shoewear may need to be adjusted to accommodate an insert. For nonspecific synovitis, a cortisone injection may be beneficial; however, only three injections are given, and at least 1 month is allowed between injections. If the patient cannot be accommodated adequately with these modalities, surgical intervention may be indicated. A significant hallux valgus deformity indicates the need for correction to make a space for second toe correction. Failure to treat both problems results in recurrence.

B. Surgical Treatment

The subluxed metatarsophalangeal joint with a flexible hammer toe is treated by releasing the dorsal contracture of the extensor tendons, joint capsule, and collateral ligaments. A Girdlestone flexor tendon transfer, as previously described, will maintain the correction. Also, tenodesis of the plantar plate may be a treatment option. If a fixed hammer toe is present, a proximal phalanx condylectomy is added to the procedure. A dislocation of the metatarsophalangeal joint is a more severe deformity and requires some bony element. The soft tissues, including the extensor tendons, joint capsule, and collateral ligaments, are incised. In addition, a synovectomy of the metatarsophalangeal joint is performed, and finally, the distal third of the metatarsal head is excised to allow reduction of the joint. Accompanying hammer toe procedures are performed to correct the invariably present fixed hammer toe.

A 0.062-inch K-wire is used to stabilize the correction for 4–6 weeks. After pin removal, the toe is taped for several weeks. This procedure results in significant joint stiffness and possible resubluxation of the joint.

For severe deformities such as dislocation of the metatarsophalangeal joint, a bony procedure is added. This is achieved with an osteotomy at the level of the metatarsal neck (CPT 28308). The osteotomy is performed through a hockey stick incision over the dorsal joint, and the saw blade is placed at the dorsal aspect of the metatarsal head and aimed proximally. The saw blade is kept parallel to the plantar aspect of the foot to result in a long oblique osteotomy. A 1-mm saw blade is used for most osteotomies. A thicker saw blade, 2 mm, is used when more than 5 mm of shortening is required or with a plantar inclination of less than 19 degrees. Once the osteotomy is complete, the metatarsal head is allowed to slide proximally to the appropriate level that will allow the joint to reduce. The amount of shortening is usually between 4.0 and 6.0 mm. The osteotomy is fixed with a single 2.5-mm or smaller diameter cortical screw.

If necessary, a hammer toe procedure may be added to fully correct the deformity. Good to excellent results have been reported, but there is limited follow-up and number of cases. There can be reduction in pain, improvement of function, and resolution of intractable plantar keratosis, without the complication of joint stiffness as occurs with the previously described procedures. Complications from this procedure are stiffness, redislocation, plantar penetrating hardware, and floating-toe deformity (extension contracture of the metatarsophalangeal joint causing the toe not to touch the ground).

A crossover toe is difficult to treat. Generally, the deformity is more severe, and radiographs show a dislocated second or third metatarsophalangeal joint with medial or lateral deviation. The operative treatment realigns the toe with soft-tissue release of the contracted tendons and ligaments medially or laterally, depending on the deformity. For more severe deformities, a bony procedure is added. This can be accomplished with a closing-wedge osteotomy at the base of the proximal phalanx or an oblique distal metatarsal osteotomy, previously described for treatment of dorsally subluxated metatarsophalangeal joints. The technique is identical, but some soft-tissue balancing may need to be added to the procedure to correct the medial/lateral deviation.

Garg R, Thordarson DB, Schrumpf M, Castaneda D: Sliding oblique versus segmental resection osteotomies for lesser metatarsophalangeal joint pathology. *Foot Ankle Int* 2008;29:1009. [PMID: 18851817]

Grimes J, Coughlin M: Geometric analysis of the Weil osteotomy. *Foot Ankle Int* 2006;27:985. [PMID: 17144965]

Hofstaetter SG, Hofstaetter JG, Petroutsas JA, Gruber F, Ritschl P, Trnka HJ: The Weil osteotomy: a seven-year follow-up. *J Bone Joint Surg Br* 2005;87:1507. [PMID: 16260668]

Kaz AJ, Coughlin MJ: Crossover second toe: demographics, etiology, and radiographic assessment. *Foot Ankle Int* 2007;28:1223. [PMID: 18173985]

Lui TH, Chan LK, Chan KB: Modified plantar plate tenodesis for correction of claw toe deformity. *Foot Ankle Int* 2010;31:584. [PMID: 20663424]

REGIONAL ANESTHESIA FOR FOOT AND ANKLE DISORDERS

Regional anesthesia is an important component of foot and ankle surgery because most procedures are performed in the outpatient setting. The nerve block can be administered by the surgeon. Many operations distal to the ankle can be performed without general anesthesia, which can eliminate the possible complications of central nervous system depression. In addition, the postoperative opioid requirements are significantly reduced.

▶ Digital Block

A. Indications

A digital block is ideal for operations involving the toes. These may include procedures for nail disorders, correction of hammer toe or mallet toe, tendon releases, and some metatarsophalangeal joint procedures.

B. Technique

Short- and longer-term anesthesia is provided by digital block using a 1:1 mixture of 1% lidocaine hydrochloride and 0.25% bupivacaine. A short 25-gauge needle is used to inject approximately 1.5 mL on either side of the toe within the subcutaneous layer between the skin and deeper fascia. The needle is then passed toward the plantar aspect of the toe to anesthetize the digital nerves. Both sides of the toe should be anesthetized. Anesthesia should be administered before the operative site is prepared to allow the approximately 15 minutes necessary for the block to take effect before starting a procedure.

▶ Ankle Block

A. Indications

Ankle block anesthesia is useful for forefoot and midfoot procedures. These can include bunionectomies, neuroma excision, metatarsal osteotomies, and tarsometatarsal arthrodeses. Also, ankle block anesthesia is preferred to multiple digital blocks for ipsilateral multiple toe procedures. Ankle block anesthesia is appropriate for more proximal procedures, such as hindfoot arthrodesis or ankle arthroscopy.

B. Technique

An ankle block anesthetizes the posterior tibial nerve, superficial branch of the deep peroneal nerve, sural nerve, saphenous nerve, and superficial peroneal nerve. The posterior tibial nerve requires a larger 3-cm, 22- or 25-gauge needle and approximately 7–10 mL of a 1:1 mixture of 1% lidocaine hydrochloride and 0.25% bupivacaine. The landmark for the posterior tibial nerve behind the malleolus is approximately two finger breadths proximal to the tip of the malleolus and along the medial border of the Achilles tendon (Figure 8–20). The needle is inserted perpendicular to the shaft of the tibia until the posterior cortex of the tibia is palpated with the tip of the needle. The needle is then withdrawn approximately 2 mm. Approximately 5 mL of anesthetic agent is injected into this area after aspiration is done to confirm that the needle is not in a vessel. The deep peroneal nerve is injected at the level of the navicular. The extensor hallucis and extensor digitorum longus tendons are palpated at this site, and the deep peroneal nerve is just lateral to the dorsalis pedis artery. The 25-gauge needle is inserted and advanced to bone and then withdrawn 1–2 mm, aspiration is attempted, and approximately 5 mL of anesthetic is injected. The saphenous nerve is identified one to two finger breadths proximal to the tip of the medial malleolus and just posterior to the saphenous vein. A 25-gauge needle is inserted and 5 mL of anesthetic injected. The sural nerve is blocked approximately 1–1.5 cm distal to the tip of the lateral malleolus and can often be palpated in the subcutaneous fat. A 25-gauge needle is inserted and approximately 5 mL of anesthetic injected. The superficial peroneal nerve branches are blocked starting two finger breadths proximal and anterior to the tip of the lateral malleolus, and the injection is carried out below the subcutaneous veins but above the long extensor tendons in

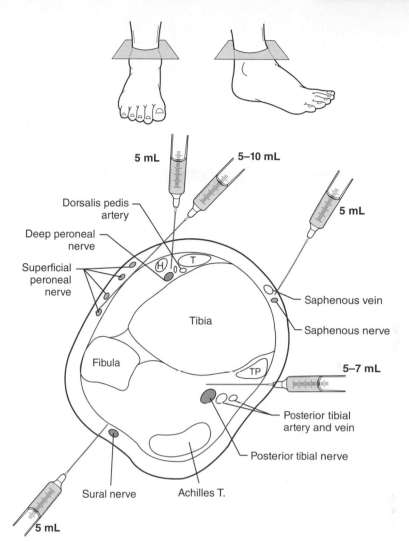

▲ Figure 8–20. Anesthetic technique for ankle block. H, extensor hallucis longus tendon; T, tibialis anterior tendon; TP, tibialis posterior tendon. (Reproduced, with permission, from Delgado-Martinez AD, Marchal-Escalona JM: Supramalleolar ankle block anesthesia and ankle tourniquet for foot surgery. *Foot Ankle Int* 2001;22:836.)

a ring-type block. Approximately 5 mL of anesthetic agent is used. The anesthesia for ankle block takes effect within 15–20 minutes.

▶ Popliteal Block

A. Indications

The popliteal block can be used for most major foot or ankle procedures. These include ankle arthrodesis, hindfoot arthrodesis, calcaneal osteotomy, tarsometatarsal arthrodesis, posterior tibial tendon reconstruction, and surgical treatment of calcaneal or ankle fractures. The nerve block can be used with general anesthesia, sedation, or as the sole anesthetic technique. If a thigh tourniquet is required, then a general anesthetic may be added. The popliteal nerve block has low morbidity, high success rate, long analgesia, and can be administered by the orthopedic surgeon.

B. Technique

The patient is placed in the lateral decubitus position with a pillow between the knees. The landmarks to block the tibial nerve in the popliteal fossa are the lateral and medial

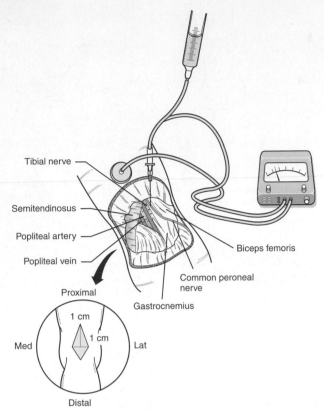

▲ **Figure 8–21.** Anesthetic technique. The popliteal block is performed with the needle tip inserted 7–8 cm above the popliteal crease and 1 cm lateral to the midline. (Reproduced, with permission, from Rongstad KM, Mann RA, Prieskorn D, et al: Popliteal sciatic nerve block for postoperative analgesia. *Foot Ankle Int* 1996;17:378).

epicondyles of the femur and the medial and lateral belly of the gastrocnemius. The puncture site is at the idle of the line connecting the epicondyles (Figure 8–21) where the nerve stimulator set at 1.2 mA is inserted vertically to locate the tibial nerve. At a penetration depth of 2–3 cm, a contraction is found, and the needle is advanced until plantar flexion and inversion occurs. The output of the stimulator is decreased gradually to 0.5 mA. Following aspiration, a test dose of 1 cc is placed of 0.5% bupivacaine. The test dose should cause a pause of muscle contraction, and the remaining 29 cc of 0.5% bupivacaine is injected with intermittent aspiration. The peroneal nerve is located at the head of the fibula and the neurostimulator with an output of 1.2 mA, causing dorsiflexion and eversion of the foot. The output is reduced to 0.5 mA to confirm the proximity of the nerve, and 3–5 cc of bupivacaine is injected. Finally, the saphenous nerve is located at the level of the tibial tubercle. The area infiltrated is between the tibial tubercle and the proximal

gastrocnemius muscle. Approximately 3–5 mL of 0.5% bupivacaine is used.

Alternatively, a perineural catheter can give up to 72 hours of postoperative pain relief compared to 13–16 hours with a single-shot popliteal block. The block can be performed with the patient supine. The stimulating needle is placed anterior to the biceps femoris tendon at the superior pole of the patella level, angling 45 degrees (Figure 8–22). The nerve stimulator is used to confirm placement, and a test dose of 1 cc of anesthetic is placed. Then a standard block of 20 cc of 0.5% bupivacaine is placed. The catheter is connected to a pain pump to infuse the local anesthetic dose depending on the patient's weight. The pain pump begins infusion at 6 hours postoperatively and then is removed by a visiting nurse at 72 hours. Another method for the sciatic popliteal block is with localization with ultrasound guidance, with the needle insertion at the separation of the tibial nerve and common peroneal nerve.

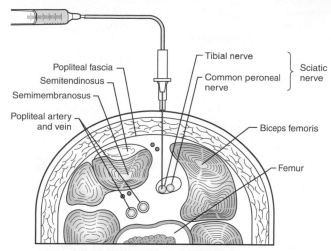

▲ **Figure 8–22.** Anesthetic technique for the popliteal block. The needle top is positioned to localize the sciatic nerve, and aspiration ensures no vascular penetration. (Reproduced, with permission, from Rongstad KM, Mann RA, Prieskorn D, et al: Popliteal sciatic nerve block for postoperative analgesia. *Foot Ankle Int* 1996;17:378.)

Calder JD, Elliot R, Seifert C: Technical tip: lateral popliteal sciatic nerve block with continuous infusion for foot and ankle surgery. *Foot Ankle Int* 2007;28:1106. [PMID: 17923066]

Grosser DM, Herr MJ, Claridge RJ, Barker LG: Preoperative lateral popliteal nerve block for intraoperative and postoperative pain control in elective foot and ankle surgery: a prospective analysis. *Foot Ankle Int* 2007;28:1271. [PMID: 18173991]

Herr MJ, Keyarash AB, Muir JJ, Kile TA, Claridge RJ: Lateral trans-biceps popliteal block for elective foot and ankle surgery performed after induction of general anesthesia. *Foot Ankle Int* 2006;27:667. [PMID: 17038275]

Sala-Blanch X, de Riva N, Carrera A, López AM, Prats A, Hadzic A: Ultrasound-guided popliteal sciatic block with a single injection at the sciatic division results in faster block onset than the classical nerve stimulator technique. *Anesth Analg* 2012;114:1121. [PMID: 22366843]

Samuel R, Sloan A, Patel K, Aglan M, Zubairy A: The efficacy of combined popliteal and ankle blocks in forefoot surgery. *J Bone Joint Surg Am* 2008;90:1443. [PMID: 18594091]

Varitimidis SE, Venouziou AI, Dailiana ZH, Christou D, Dimitroulias A, Malizos KN: Triple nerve block at the knee for foot and ankle surgery performed by the surgeon: difficulties and efficiency. *Foot Ankle Int* 2009;30:854. [PMID: 19755069]

METATARSALGIA

Metatarsalgia is a general term for pain arising from the metatarsal head region. The center of pressure during normal gait is initially applied to the heel and progresses along the plantar aspect of the foot. For more than 50% of the stance time, the pressure is concentrated beneath the metatarsal head area. This extended period of pressure can cause bothersome pain. A precise diagnosis is necessary in metatarsalgia to direct treatment toward the specific cause.

► Etiologic Findings

Metatarsalgia encompasses a broad spectrum of conditions with various causes arising out of the anatomic structures in the area. It may be associated with abnormalities of the metatarsal head subluxation or dislocation of the metatarsophalangeal joints, systemic diseases, dermatologic lesions, soft-tissue disorders, or iatrogenic causes. Table 8–1 lists the various causes of metatarsalgia and the differential diagnoses that should be considered in evaluating these patients.

► Clinical Findings

A. Symptoms and Signs

The clinical evaluation begins with a careful history directed toward delineating the precise location of the pain. The physical examination of the foot and lower extremity begins with the patient standing. Any deformities of the toes are noted, such as clawing of the toes, a long second ray, or swelling around any of the joints. The patient should be evaluated for a postural problem of the foot, such as a flat foot or cavus foot. The plantar aspect of the foot is carefully evaluated for evidence of callus formation. The metatarsal heads are palpated individually to assess for generalized plantar fat pad atrophy, a prominent fibular condyle, synovitis, or possibly a transfer lesion beneath a metatarsal head resulting from previous forefoot surgery.

B. Imaging Studies

The radiographic evaluation includes weight-bearing anteroposterior, lateral, and oblique views of the foot. Occasionally, the so-called skyline view of the metatarsal heads (obtained with the metatarsophalangeal joints in dorsiflexion) is

Table 8–1. Causes of metatarsalgia.

Bone causes
    Prominent fibular condyle of the metatarsal head
    Long metatarsal
    Morton foot
    Hypermobile first ray
    Posttraumatic malalignment of metatarsals
    Abnormal foot posture such as forefoot varus or valgus, cavus foot,
        or equinus deformity
    Systemic disease, rheumatoid arthritis, psoriatic arthritis

Dermatologic lesions
    Wart, seed corn, hyperkeratosis of the skin

Soft-tissue disorders
    Atrophy of the plantar fat pad
    Sequelae of a crush injury
    Plantar scars secondary to trauma or surgery

Metatarsophalangeal joint disorders
    Subluxed or dislocated joint
    Freiberg infraction
    Nonspecific synovitis

Iatrogenic causes
    Residuals of metatarsal surgery
    Transfer lesion due to previous surgery
    Hallux valgus surgery (eg, shortening or dorsiflexion of the metatarsal)

helpful to evaluate their overall alignment, particularly in cases resulting from previous surgery, by demonstrating the height of the metatarsal heads. MRI can be useful in the diagnosis of metatarsalgia, such as distinguishing among a neuroma, cyst, bursa, or synovitis.

▶ Treatment

A. Conservative Management

Conservative management is directed at relieving the pressure beneath the area of maximum pain. Initially, the patient must obtain a shoe of appropriate style and adequate size to allow an orthotic device to be inserted. A lace-type shoe with a soft sole material and an adequate toe box is appropriate. High-heeled shoes, loafers, or tight shoes are inappropriate because they have decreased volume for the foot and may cause increased pressure against the involved area. As a general rule, the softer the orthotic device, the more comfortable is the patient. A hard acrylic orthotic device is not particularly comfortable for the patient and should usually be avoided.

B. Surgical Treatment

The surgical management of metatarsalgia depends on the cause and is discussed in different sections of this chapter. In general, pain from a bony prominence can be relieved by a partial ostectomy or osteotomy, dermatologic lesions such as warts can often be burned off with liquid nitrogen or excised, or pain caused by a subluxated metatarsophalangeal joint can be corrected with tendon transfer. The outcome

depends on the severity of the problem and the type of surgical intervention required for correction.

KERATOTIC DISORDERS OF THE PLANTAR SKIN

Keratotic disorders of the foot usually manifest in plantar callosities and are also called intractable plantar keratosis (ICD-9 700). These occur as a result of friction and increased pressure over bony prominences. Some plantar callosity is normal, but if it becomes excessive, it can be painful and disabling.

▶ General Considerations

Many of the intractable plantar keratoses arise from the bony abnormalities of the forefoot. These abnormalities are listed in Table 8–1.

▶ Clinical Findings

A. Symptoms and Signs

The patient's history will reveal the affected area on the foot and the severity of pain. In addition, the past medical history is important, as past operations and medical disorders may be part of the etiology. The patient's work, type of activities, shoewear, how often the callus needs to be trimmed, and the type of orthotic devices used are all important in a complete history. The physical examination, however, is the most important single factor in the diagnosis of intractable plantar keratoses. First, the overall posture of the foot needs to be evaluated to determine whether the condition is the result of a postural abnormality. This is accomplished with the patient undressed from both knees down and standing. Findings can involve a rigid plantar-flexed first metatarsal that could cause a diffuse callus beneath the first metatarsal head, or a hypermobile first ray that fails to support the medial forefoot may result in generalized callus formation beneath the second and third metatarsal heads. Another type of deformity is a varus posture of the forefoot (the lateral aspect of the foot in greater plantar flexion than the medial aspect), which may result in callus formation beneath the fifth metatarsal head. Also, note the type of callus. A diffuse callus is usually associated with a long metatarsal. The callus may have arisen after trauma or surgery in which an adjacent metatarsal was dorsiflexed, thereby increasing the weight-bearing load of the metatarsal. In contrast, a distinct well-localized lesion beneath the metatarsal head is often caused by a prominent fibular condyle of the metatarsal head of the second or third metatarsal. A callus on the bottom of the foot must be differentiated from a plantar wart, which can occasionally mimic a plantar callosity. Shaving the lesion reveals bleeding from end arteries in a plantar wart, whereas a keratotic lesion consists only of hyperkeratotic tissue.

▶ B. Imaging Studies

Weight-bearing anteroposterior, oblique, and lateral radiographs of the foot will generally reveal abnormalities seen clinically. These include hallux valgus, hammer toe, claw toe, and varus deformity.

Treatment

A. Conservative Management

Debridement or trimming of the intractable plantar keratosis can provide some relief, albeit temporary. Directing the treatment to the underlying deformity will bring long-term benefit. This can be achieved by decreasing the direct pressure or friction from the callosities. A shoe that is made of soft material and accommodates the size and shape of the foot will provide some relief of pain and disability. This usually involves a lace-up type shoe with adequate padding. Inexpensive padding and soft inserts can be found over the counter and will benefit many patients. With some patients and deformities, however, a total contact orthotic device can be effective (Figure 8–23). It is usually made of soft material and redistributes the weight bearing from bony prominences that cause the callosities.

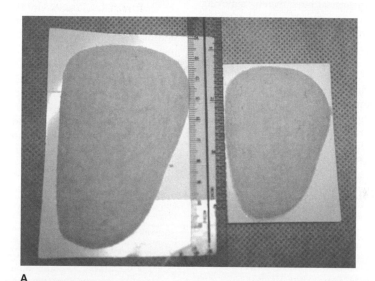

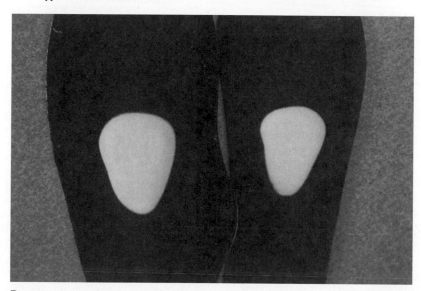

▲ **Figure 8–23. A:** A metatarsal pad may help redistribute weight bearing and relieve symptoms. **B:** Soft, over-the-counter, felt metatarsal pads are effective in decreasing pressure under the metatarsal heads. These can be adhered to a shoe insert to allow for use in multiple shoes. (Reproduced, with permission, from Mann RA, Coughlin MJ: *The Video Textbook of Foot and Ankle Surgery.* Medical Video Productions, 1991.)

B. Surgical Treatment

Operative procedures for intractable plantar keratoses are determined by the underlying deformity. One of the most common problems is a prominent fibular condyle of the metatarsal head. It occurs most frequently underneath the second metatarsal but may also be found underneath the third and fourth metatarsals. The prominence is approached through a dorsal hockey stick incision over the metatarsophalangeal joint, and the toe is plantar flexed to expose the plantar aspect of the metatarsal head (CPT 28288). An osteotome is used to excise 30% of the plantar condyle of the metatarsal head, thereby removing the sharp bony prominence (Figure 8–24). This procedure results in predictable pain relief of the affected toe, although 5–10% of patients develop a transfer lesion beneath the adjacent metatarsal head.

A diffuse callus beneath the second metatarsal that is the result of a dorsiflexed or hypermobile first metatarsal can be treated with dorsiflexion osteotomy done at the base of the second metatarsal. If the lesion is the result of an excessively long metatarsal, it may be shortened to the level of a line drawn between the adjacent metatarsal heads, thereby reestablishing a smooth metatarsal pattern. If the callus is a result of a dislocated metatarsophalangeal joint, such as in a claw toe deformity, the joint must be reduced, using one of the techniques previously described. Correction of the joint alignment will decrease the plantar against the metatarsal head. All of these surgical procedures to eliminate a callus are fairly successful, although the possibility of a transfer lesion developing is approximately 5–10%.

The tibial sesamoid can be prominent and an underlying callosity can form. This is treated through a medial approach, and the plantar third of the sesamoid is shaved down. This alleviates the callus in almost all cases, with the only significant complication being caused by inadvertent disruption of the plantar medial cutaneous nerve during the surgical approach to the sesamoid.

Keratoses can occur about the fifth metatarsal head. If it occurs on the lateral aspect of the forefoot, the deformity may be a bunionette, also called tailor's bunion. A diffuse callus beneath the fifth metatarsal head can be treated with a midshaft metatarsal osteotomy to bring it out of its plantar-flexed position, which usually alleviates the condition. It is unusual for a transfer lesion to occur beneath the fourth metatarsal head. If the bony prominence is on the lateral aspect of the foot rather than the plantar aspect, then an osteotomy of the fifth metatarsal head will correct the deformity. A chevron type osteotomy can be made and the head is translated medially (Figure 8–25).

Finally, a subhallux sesamoid can cause a small callus on the plantar aspect of the interphalangeal joint of the great toe. Treatment is simply surgical excision of the sesamoid, and good results can be expected with little or no disability.

Davys HJ, Turner DE, Helliwell PS, Conaghan PG, Emery P, Woodburn J: Debridement of plantar callosities in rheumatoid arthritis: a randomized controlled trial. *Rheumatology (Oxford)* 2005;44:207. [PMID: 15479752]

Menz HB, Zammit GV, Munteanu SE: Plantar pressures are higher under callused regions of the foot in older people. *Clin Exp Dermatol* 2007;32:375. [PMID: 17425648]

DIABETIC FOOT

Approximately 22 million people in the United States are diabetic, and foot problems are the most common cause for hospitalization, accounting for 20% or more of all inpatient days in this population. More than half of all nontraumatic amputations are performed on diabetics. One report showed a 68% incidence of foot disorders in a large diabetic clinic, and the cost of care of these problems approaches $100 million per year. Treatment of the diabetic who presents with foot problems can be complex and require a team approach, involving the primary care physician, vascular surgeon, orthopedic surgeon, infectious disease specialist, orthotist, diabetic nurse specialist, and, whenever possible, the patient's family members.

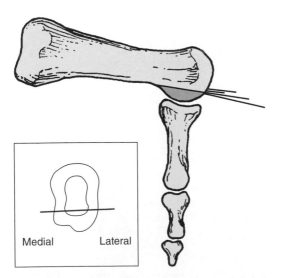

▲ **Figure 8–24.** A plantar condylectomy is performed with resection of one fourth to one third of the plantar surface of the metatarsal head. (Reproduced, with permission, from Mann RA, Coughlin MJ: *The Video Textbook of Foot and Ankle Surgery.* Medical Video Productions, 1991.)

► Pathophysiologic Findings

Diabetes is a metabolic disorder that involves all the organ systems. Those of primary interest to the orthopedist are integumentary with the risk of ulceration, neurologic

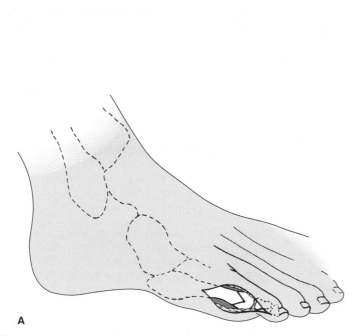

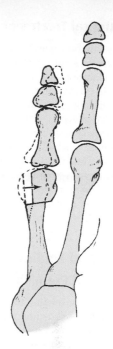

A

B

▲ **Figure 8–25. A:** Lateral view of chevron fifth metatarsal osteotomy. **B:** Diagram following completion of this procedure. (Reproduced, with permission, from Mann RA, Coughlin MJ: *The Video Textbook of Foot and Ankle Surgery.* Medical Video Productions, 1991.)

with the loss of protective sensation, vascular with diminished perfusion, and immunologic with limited ability to fight infection. The most frequent problem faced by the diabetic is breakdown of the skin of the foot (Figure 8–26). The cause of foot ulcers is multifactorial but stems

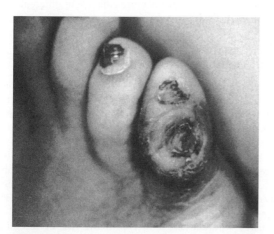

▲ **Figure 8–26.** Ulceration over the dorsolateral aspect of the fifth toe as the result of pressure from a shoe. (Reproduced, with permission, from Mann RA, Coughlin MJ: *The Video Textbook of Foot and Ankle Surgery.* Medical Video Productions, 1991.)

from diminished sensation resulting from neuropathic disease. Unappreciated local stresses are placed on the skin externally by poorly fitting shoes and internally by skeletal deformity. Autonomic neuropathy causes dry skin and cracks in the dermis, which may become portals of entry for infection. Reactive hyperemia, which normally helps to clear infections, is blunted by autonomic neuropathy. Motor neuropathy affects the intrinsic muscles of the foot and may lead to claw toe deformities with metatarsal heads and proximal interphalangeal joints becoming prominent and predisposed to ulcerations. Hyperglycemia can impair wound healing strength as well as damage vascular endothelium, which is a precursor to atherosclerosis and leads to diminished extremity blood flow and limited healing potential. Elevated blood glucose levels over a long period also lead to glycation of the body's proteins and is commonly measured by hemoglobin A1c. Glucose covalently binds to lysine in proteins in a reversible process. It is felt that the addition of glucose molecules changes the flexibility of tissues, especially fibrous tissue, making tissues such as skin less able to handle sheer stresses. The neuropathy in diabetics is due to the loss of myelinated and unmyelinated nerve fibers. Other factors that affect healing in diabetics include nutritional deficiencies, diminished ability to protect oneself due to diabetic encephalopathy and diminished cognition, and lowered resistance to infection.

► History

When a diabetic patient presents to an orthopedist, there are four areas of impact: ulcers and their prevention, amputations, Charcot arthropathy, and toenail abnormalities. With an infected foot ulceration, it is essential to obtain a history that will help delineate why the ulcer occurred and how to optimize the patient's healing potential. A past history of foot surgery is sought, previous or current antibiotic usage is detailed, and any recent trauma to the foot is noted. A history is taken about the severity of the patient's diabetes, including how long ago the diabetes was diagnosed, whether the patient is taking insulin, their recent level of control, what other organ systems are involved, and the degree of neuropathy that is present in the patient's feet.

► Clinical Findings

A. General Examination

Examination of the diabetic patient should begin with inspection of the shoe for internal and external wear patterns. The leg and foot are inspected for overall appearance of the skin, hair growth, perfusion, pulses, and color.

B. Foot Examination

Any bony prominences are recognized as areas of potential skin breakdown. The most common prominences are located at the apex of deformities such as under the metatarsal heads, on the dorsum of the proximal interphalangeal joints, under the medial sesamoid, at the base of the fifth metatarsal, under the medial arch in the Charcot foot, and over the medial eminence of the hallux. Neurologic examination should test for the presence of protective sensation, as defined by the patient's ability to feel the 10-g Semmes-Weinstein monofilament as well as motor function. Ulcers should be carefully documented and evaluated for evidence of infection in the adjacent soft tissues. Wounds should be measured for length, width, and depth, in addition to documenting their location. Open wounds should be probed with a sterile Q-tip or other appropriate instrument to evaluate the extent of involvement of deeper structures, such as tendons, joints, and bone. A positive probe to bone test usually indicates the presence of osteomyelitis.

C. Vascular Findings

Vascular evaluation is essential to ensure that the patient has adequate perfusion to allow healing. Patients with palpable pedal pulses and normal capillary filling have adequate blood supply and usually do not require further vascular evaluation. For patients with less perfusion, one method of assessing the overall potential for healing of foot lesions in a diabetic is the ischemic index. This index is obtained by dividing the blood pressure measurement in the brachial artery by that in the dorsalis pedis and posterior tibial arteries, as measured by Doppler ultrasound with a calf cuff. If the index is 0.45 or greater, there is a 90% chance that a foot ulcer will heal. Lower indices are an indication for a vascular surgery consultation. It must be kept in mind, however, that falsely elevated values of blood pressure in the foot may result from calcification of major blood vessels. Thus, apparent vascular insufficiency in the light of an adequate ischemic index also warrants a vascular surgery consultation. A laser Doppler study can also be beneficial in assessing local skin perfusion. This information can be used to help predict the patient's response to surgical intervention.

D. Imaging Studies

Radiographic studies should include weight-bearing radiographs of both feet and ankles as indicated. Plain radiographs can help identify bony prominences that predispose the patient to ulcer formation, and osteomyelitis or changes consistent with a neuropathic foot may be identified. Early Charcot (neuropathic) joint changes may be difficult to differentiate from osteomyelitis. The four D's of neuropathic joints are helpful in delineating more advanced cases: debris, destruction, dislocation, and densification.

The presence of bony infection may be delineated on serial radiographs as progressive osteolysis, realizing that changes on plain films are late findings and suggesting that the infection has been present for weeks. A technetium bone scan is sensitive in detecting early osteomyelitis but is quite nonspecific. MRI can demonstrate bone and soft-tissue changes, such as edema or the extent of an abscess cavity, and can be helpful distinguishing Charcot changes from osteomyelitis. The recent addition of ring positron emission tomography (PET) scans is more effective in differentiating osteomyelitis from Charcot changes.

► Classification and Treatment of Diabetic Foot Ulcers

The Rancho Los Amigos Hospital classification of diabetic foot ulcers is based on the depth of tissue affected and extent of the foot involved. Treatment choice depends on the grade of ulcer (Figure 8–27). Table 8–2 shows treatment based on classification of foot ulcers.

As a general rule in treating infections of the foot, a balance must be struck between salvage of tissue and foot function. A healed amputation at a more proximal level is more advantageous to the patient than leaving a marginally viable area of the foot that requires constant wound care.

Large wounds heal slowly with the risk of secondary infection and, if possible, should not be left to heal by secondary intention. Split-thickness skin grafts, especially on the sole of the foot or over an amputation site, are prone to breakdown.

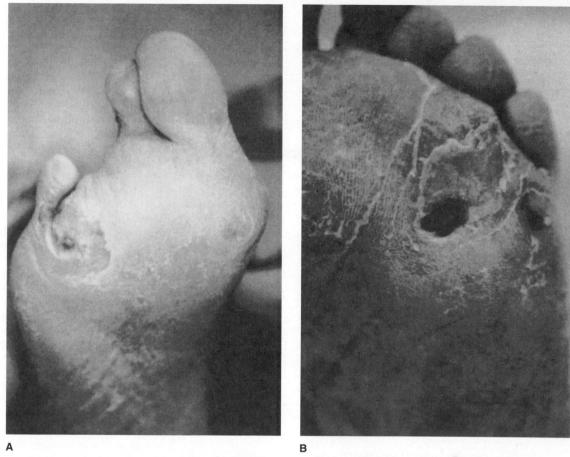

A   B

▲ **Figure 8–27.** Comparison of **(A)** grade 1 and **(B)** grade 2 ulcers (new depth and ischemia classification). Note the exposed deep tissues of the grade 2 ulcer. (Reproduced, with permission, from Brodsky JW: The diabetic foot. In Mann RA, Coughlin MJ, eds: *Surgery of the Foot and Ankle,* 6th ed. St. Louis: Mosby-Year Book; 1993.)

A. Surgical Treatment for Relieving Bony Prominences

As previously stated, a major goal of treatment in the ulcerated or "at risk" foot is to relieve bony prominences that cause pressure on the skin. Treatment consists of measures to relieve the pressure. There are many appropriate measures to relieve pressure on the skin from the outside. Examples include extra-depth shoes for claw toes and accommodative foot orthoses with metatarsal pads to relieve pressure under a prominent metatarsal head. If these measures fail or are inappropriate, the pressure should be relieved from the inside by correcting the bony deformity. These prominences are located at several common sites.

The hallux may have a prominence beneath the metatarsal head, on the plantar-medial aspect of the interphalangeal joint, or over the median eminence secondary to a bunion deformity. A prominence caused by the medial sesamoid can be relieved by complete or partial removal of the sesamoid. If this does not adequately relieve the prominence, a dorsiflexion osteotomy or resection of the metatarsal head can be performed. Ulcers found over the plantar-medial aspect of the interphalangeal joint can often be relieved by simple excision of the prominent medial condyles or by resection of the entire joint. If this ulcer is associated with limited metatarsophalangeal extension, then a cheilectomy or metatarsophalangeal arthroplasty may be appropriate to allow the toe to extend further during the toe-off phase of gait and thus decrease the pressure on the skin under the interphalangeal joint. A prominence over the median eminence can be addressed with a routine bunion procedure.

The diabetic patient is subject to claw toe deformities resulting from motor neuropathy, causing prominences under the metatarsal heads and over the dorsum of the

Table 8–2. Classification and treatment of diabetic foot ulcers.

Grade	Classification	Treatment
0	Foot is "at risk" for developing ulcer. Skin remains intact, but underlying bone deformity places foot at risk for skin breakdown.	Proper footwear plus other preventive measures such as patient education and surgical correction as described in text.
1	Lesion affects skin only.	Outpatient dressing changes or total contact cast. Antibiotics usually not necessary.
2	Deep lesions that involve underlying tendons, bones, or ligaments (Figure 8–28).	Surgical debridement and hospitalization for aggressive wound care and intravenous antibiotics. Goal is conversion to grade 1 ulcer.
3	Abscess or osteomyelitis present as complication of ulcer.	Emergency surgery for drainage of acute infection. Wound often left open, with dressing changes performed until definitive closure or amputation is done at a later date.
4	Gangrene is present in the toes or forefoot.	Appropriate amputation.
5	Entire foot is gangrenous.	Appropriate amputation.

proximal interphalangeal joints. Depending on the severity, treatment varies from reduction of the metatarsophalangeal joints and proximal interphalangeal arthroplasties to resection of the metatarsal heads and interphalangeal fusions.

A collapsed longitudinal arch from Charcot changes causes the classic rocker-bottom foot with prominences along the plantar and medial aspects of the midfoot. This can be addressed with a simple exostectomy for a mild deformity that is stable, or an appropriate osteotomy and arthrodesis for a more complex deformity or when there is progressive instability.

B. Treatment of Osteomyelitis

Osteomyelitis is a common complication present in a grade 3 diabetic foot ulcer. The infection is seldom eradicated without surgical debridement of the bone. Frequently, more radical treatment than simple exostectomy is required. For example, infection of a proximal phalanx is usually treated by resection of the phalanx. Osteomyelitis of the metatarsal

may require ray amputation if more than just the head is involved. If multiple metatarsals are infected, a transmetatarsal amputation is often the best treatment with the reminder to always consider lengthening the tendoachilles to decrease load on the residual forefoot.

Osteomyelitis of the midfoot is often a complication of a collapsed Charcot foot. The treatment options for such an infection include wide local debridement with exostectomy or a more proximal amputation. Similarly, osteomyelitis of the calcaneus can be treated with a partial calcanectomy or a more proximal amputation.

Treatment of ulcers should make sense. A patient with a superficial wound with good blood supply, minimal infection, and protective sensation would be treated with topical wound care, a shoe to accommodate the dressing, and limited activity to control swelling. A patient with an infected deep wound with osteomyelitis and nonreconstructable dysvascularity would probably be best served with early amputation. Of course, each patient is unique and deserves an evaluation of all organ systems to develop an appropriate treatment plan.

Wound dressings should try to mimic skin. They should try to provide a healing environment that is bacteria free, warm, moist, strain free, nontoxic, and well oxygenated. There is nothing that will provide all of these. Dressings should be chosen based on the needs of the wound, possibly needing infection control and debridement in the initial phases but later only requiring protection and absorption of wound drainage. The gold standard for treating plantar ulcers is a total contact or healing cast. This protective cast provides wound protection, edema control, and a moist environment, and has been shown to decrease plantar loading to the ulcer. When the wound is draining, they do require frequent changing or the odor can be intolerable.

Biologic wound healing products that provide wound healing factors can be helpful in the patient with marginal healing potential. Larger wounds, especially those with considerable drainage, can benefit from vacuum-assisted closure where a constant negative suction pressure is applied to a sealed wound, thereby decreasing its size and pulling away wound drainage.

There are a small number of patients who are marginal wound healers who will benefit from hyperbaric oxygen treatment. When placed at two atmospheres of pure oxygen, the serum becomes supersaturated and has been shown to benefit some patients who receive serial treatments.

C. Charcot Foot

A Charcot joint is also referred to as a neuropathic, neurotrophic, or neuroarthropathic joint. Diabetes is by far the leading cause of Charcot joints. A Charcot foot is characterized by destruction of joint surfaces, fractures often accompanied by dislocations of one or more joints in a patient with inappropriate pain response. The requirements are an active patient who has neuropathy and adequate blood supply. The pathophysiology is not fully understood, but there are two theories. The neurotraumatic theory says that cumulative mechanical strains in a patient with inadequate sensory protection leads to stress fractures that are progressive because the patient does not have adequate sensory feedback to limit their activity. The neurovascular theory suggests that there is a neurally initiated vascular reflex that leads to juxtaarticular osteopenia weakening the bone in this area while glycation of the joint capsule causes stiffness. These factors, when combined with mechanical stress, can lead to the fracture dislocations that are commonly seen. There are probably elements of both of these theories that are contributing to Charcot arthropathy.

There are three stages in Charcot arthropathy as defined by Eichenholtz. Stage 1 is the acute inflammatory phase where there is swelling, redness, and increased warmth. Radiographs would likely show fractures and dislocations, and the involved area would be unstable. The concern in this stage would be to rule out infection. If the patient is neuropathic with good blood supply and has an acute, red, hot, swollen foot without an ulcer or a history of an ulcer in that area, it is probably Charcot arthropathy and not infection. Hematogenous osteomyelitis is very rare, and infections in the foot are usually introduced locally through the skin. Stage 2 is the subacute phase where there are signs of healing, less swelling and warmth, and radiographic signs of new bone formation. Stage 3 is the chronic phase with consolidation and resolution of inflammation. Typical locations include the midfoot, with the creation of the rocker-bottom foot deformity as the arch collapses, and the hindfoot and the ankle, with the risk of collapse into varus or valgus that can lead to pressure ulcerization.

1. Principles of treatment—There are several important principles to follow in the treatment of Charcot joints. The primary goal is to limit joint destruction and preserve a stable plantigrade foot that will protect the soft tissues and prevent ulceration.

2. Treatment of acute phase—For a patient who presents in the acute phase of Charcot joint, the initial treatment should be immobilization and elevation of the foot. This can best be achieved with a non–weight-bearing total contact cast for patients who can be placed in a plantigrade position. The skin must be checked at weekly intervals initially to look for breakdown. Surgery is rarely attempted on the acute Charcot foot, unless necessitated by the inability to obtain a stable plantigrade position. Even in patients who will require acute stabilization to obtain a plantigrade foot, it is best to allow the swelling and inflammation to diminish by offloading and immobilization prior to surgical intervention. Once the acute phase subsides and the fractures heal, immobilization can be accomplished by means of an ankle-foot orthosis or other appropriate removable support. Custom-made shoes can then be fitted to accommodate for the bony prominences.

3. Treatment of subacute phase—In this phase, the foot has stabilized, and there is no ongoing bony destruction. Operations address the bony prominences that have been created by Charcot destruction and collapse. Often, simple removal of a prominence is all that is required, and sometimes, fusion of one or several joints is necessary. One of the most common foot deformities is a collapsed arch and rocker-bottom deformity from subluxation of multiple joints in the midfoot. Usually, an exostectomy of the prominent bones on the plantar aspect of the midfoot is sufficient. Alternatively, an osteotomy and arthrodesis of the midfoot can be performed to realign the foot and reconstitute the arch in cases where a simple exostectomy is inadequate (Figure 8–28). There is usually a contracture of the ankle plantar flexors, and this deforming force may need to be released as part of this procedure. This procedure has a high complication rate and an extended time to achieve union. In the case of Charcot involvement of the ankle joint, the goal is a stable and plantigrade foot, which often requires arthrodesis. Retrograde intramedullary nailing has been shown to be successful in achieving union but also has significant complication rates.

Andros G: Diagnostic and therapeutic arterial interventions in the ulcerated diabetic foot. *Diabetes Metab Res Rev* 2004;20(Suppl 1): S29. [PMID: 15150810]

Gil H, Morrison WB: MR imaging of diabetic foot infection. *Semin Musculoskel Radiol* 2004;8:189. [PMID: 15478022]

Hopfner S, Krolak C, Kessler S, et al: Preoperative imaging of Charcot neuroarthropathy in diabetic patients: comparison of ring PET, hybrid PET, and magnetic resonance imaging. *Foot Ankle Int* 2004;25:890. [PMID: 15680102]

Lowery NJ, Woods JB, Armstrong DG, et al: Surgical management of Charcot neuroarthropathy of the foot and ankle: a systematic review. *Foot Ankle Int* 2012;33:113. [PMID: 22381342]

Pinzur M: Surgical versus accommodative treatment for Charcot arthropathy of the midfoot. *Foot Ankle Int* 2004;25:545. [PMID: 15363375]

Strauss M: The orthopaedic surgeon's role in the treatment and prevention of diabetic foot wounds. *Foot Ankle Int* 2005;26:5. [PMID: 15680112]

Wagner FW Jr: A classification and treatment program for diabetic, neuropathic, and dysvascular foot problems. *Instr Course Lect* 1979;28:143. [No PMID]

DISORDERS OF THE TOENAILS

Toenail problems, in younger diabetics, usually involve trauma, such as stubbing the toe or, more frequently, improper nail care, which can contribute to ingrown toenails. This is usually the result of tearing off a toenail, which leaves the nail too short and predisposes it to become ingrown.

Toenail problems in the older age group are more varied, including an incurvating nail, a thickened hypertrophied

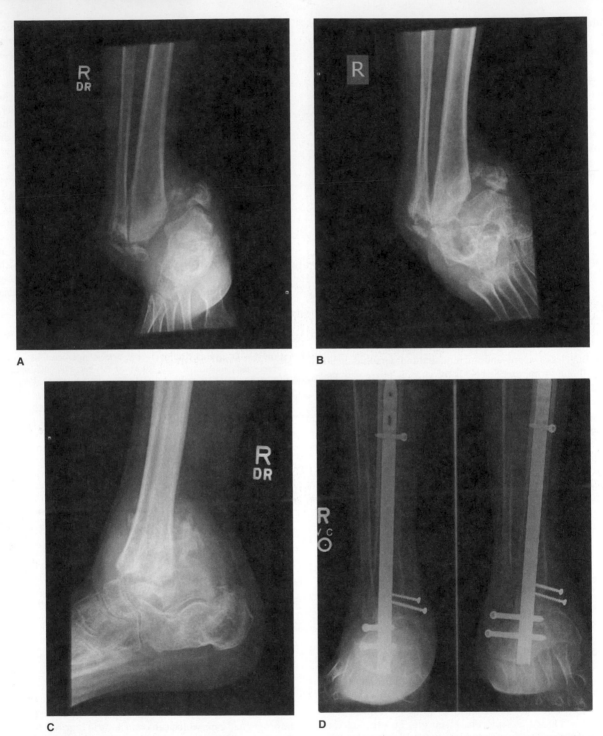

▲ **Figure 8–28. A–C:** This is a 35-year-old neuropathic insulin-dependent type I diabetic who complains of pain and instability of his ankle when walking. There is marked destruction of the ankle with severe instability and deformity that is not treatable with bracing. **D, E:** The ankle is stabilized with an arthrodesis using intramedullary fixation and returns the patient to an ambulatory status requiring a rocker-bottom shoe and an accommodative insert.

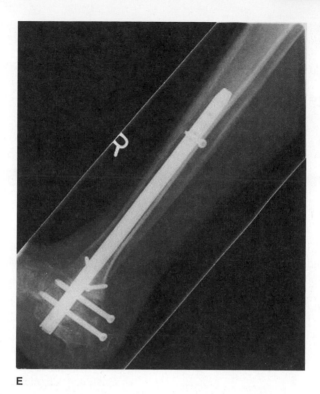

E

▲ **Figure 8–28.** (Continued)

nail associated with a chronic fungal infection, an ingrown nail resulting from improper nail cutting, and on rare occasions, a subungual exostosis.

▶ Etiologic Findings

The anatomy of the toenail is demonstrated in Figure 8–29. The nail unit consists of four components: the proximal nail fold, the nail matrix, the nail bed, and the hyponychium. The area in which most of the problems occur is the lateral or medial nail groove, where an ingrown nail occurs at the level of the nail bed or hyponychium.

▶ Clinical Findings

A. Symptoms and Signs

The history of most nail problems is not complex and usually quickly defines the nature of the problem.

1. Infection of the toenails—Infection of the toenails usually begins slowly, with erythema and swelling along the margin of the nail, followed by increasing pain and drainage, and finally the development of granulation tissue, usually in response to the foreign body reaction to the nail itself.

2. Mycotic nail—In the case of the mycotic (fungal) nail, there is usually a long, slow history of development of deformation of the nail, often with medial or lateral deviation of the nail, marked hypertrophy, and increased pain when wearing shoes. At times, an incurvated nail condition develops in which one or both edges of the nail slowly curve inward, resulting in pinching of the nail plate. This may cause a localized infection, or it may be that just the sheer pressure of the nail against the skin is the cause of the pain.

3. Subungual exostosis—The patient who develops subungual exostosis usually notes pain evolving beneath the toenail over a long period. Erosion of the nail from below occurs because of the pressure of the exostosis against the nail itself. Often, the patient does not seek help until there is actual breakdown of the tissue, giving rise to a rather ugly appearing lesion that seems much more ominous than the condition itself.

B. Imaging Studies

Radiographs are necessary when evaluating a toenail problem for subungual exostosis, which is clearly seen with a lateral view. In patients with long-standing infected ingrown

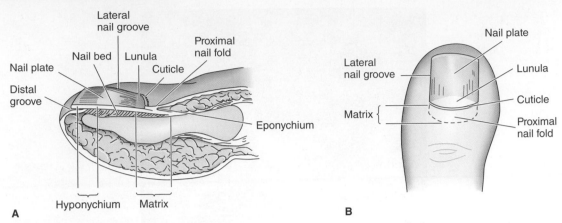

▲ **Figure 8–29. A:** Cross section of the toe demonstrates the components of the toenail and supporting structures. **B:** The proximal nail is covered by the proximal nail fold and cuticle. The lunula is the main germinal area. (Reproduced, with permission, from Mann RA, Coughlin MJ: *The Video Textbook of Foot and Ankle Surgery.* Medical Video Productions, 1991.)

toenails, a radiograph can be important to rule out underlying osteomyelitis.

▶ Treatment

A. Conservative Management

1. Chronic ingrown toenail—For the chronic ingrown toenail, the margin of the nail is removed to relieve the pressure of the nail against the skin. This procedure, along with local care and occasionally systemic antibiotics, usually permits the condition to resolve. It is important, however, to explain to the patient the necessity of permitting the nail to grow out over the ungual labia to depress it and prevent the ingrown nail from recurring.

2. Chronic onychophosis of the nail—Chronic onychophosis of the nail must be kept debrided. If an ingrown nail occurs, the margins must be trimmed to relieve the pressure against the skin.

3. Subungual exostosis—Subungual exostosis that is symptomatic is treated by excision.

B. Surgical Treatment

1. Ingrown toenail—The surgical management of the recurrent ingrown toenail consists of the Winograd procedure. In this procedure, the medial or lateral margin of the offending nail plate is removed along with the underlying nail matrix. The nail matrix is removed as thoroughly as possible to prevent the possible growth of a nail horn, which occurs in about 5% of cases. The nail matrix can be removed by sharp dissection or ablated with a laser or treated with phenol to kill the nail matrix.

2. Chronic infection—If there is severe distortion of the nail caused by chronic infection, the nail and the nail bed can be removed in their entirety. This usually results in a horny base where the nail existed, and this is often a satisfactory outcome. The terminal Syme amputation can be carried out to eliminate the nail and matrix completely (Figure 8–30). Although results are usually satisfactory, some patients do not like the appearance of the toe or absence of the toenail because of its somewhat bulbous appearance. The terminal Syme procedure can be carried out under digital block in most patients. An elliptical incision is made over the distal end of the toe, removing the nail and its matrix in their entirety. The distal portion of the distal phalanx is removed and the edges smoothed, thus shortening the toe. The tip of the toe is defatted and loosely sutured. In this manner, the nail is completely removed, and soft tissue covers the area of the former nail bed. The only significant complication associated with this procedure is the regrowth of some nail matrix beneath the healed flap, which will result in an inclusion cyst that must be drained and the residual nail matrix excised.

3. Subungual exostosis—Surgical management of subungual exostosis requires lifting the nail, identification of the exostosis, and complete removal of the exostosis and its stalk. The dissection must be carefully carried out and the entire exostosis removed to prevent recurrence. The nail bed is repaired to cover the defect.

Baran R, Dawber RPR: *Diseases of the Nails and Their Management.* Oxford, United Kingdom: Blackwell Scientific Publications, Osney Mead; 1984.

Kayalar M, Bal E, Toros T, Ozaksar K, Gürbüz Y, Ademoğlu Y: Results of partial matrixectomy for chronic ingrown toenail. *Foot Ankle Int* 2011;32:888. [PMID: 22097165].

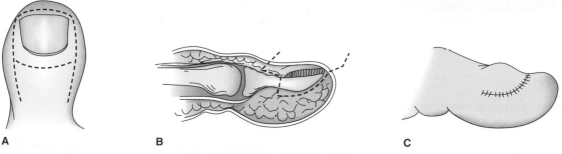

▲ **Figure 8–30.** Syme amputation of toenail. **A:** Elliptical or rectangular incision is centered over the nail bed and matrix. **B:** The distal half of the distal phalanx is resected. **C:** Excess skin is resected, and skin edges are approximated. (Reproduced, with permission, from Mann RA, Coughlin MJ: *The Video Textbook of Foot and Ankle Surgery.* Medical Video Productions, 1991.)

NEUROLOGIC DISORDERS OF THE FOOT

1. Interdigital Neuroma (Morton Neuroma)

An interdigital neuroma is a painful affliction involving the plantar aspect of the forefoot. It usually involves the third interspace and is characterized by a well-localized area of pain on the plantar aspect of the foot that radiates into the web space. The symptoms are usually aggravated by ambulation and relieved by rest. As a rule, wearing a tight-fitting shoe aggravates the pain, and walking barefoot often relieves it.

▶ Etiologic Findings

The precise cause of interdigital neuroma has not been determined. It occurs in women about 10 times more frequently than men, and, as a result, high-fashion shoewear has been implicated. Several studies demonstrate that the changes in the nerve appear to occur just distal to the transverse metatarsal ligament. This finding has given rise to the hypothesis that the neuroma results from the constant traction of the nerve against the ligament as the toes are brought into a dorsiflexed position, a theory that would explain the higher incidence in women wearing high-heeled shoes. Although this condition is called interdigital neuroma, it is not a true neuroma. The pathologic changes involve actual degeneration of the nerve fibers associated with deposition of amorphous eosinophilic material that is felt to be consistent with an entrapment neuropathy (Figure 8–31).

▶ Clinical Findings

A. Symptoms and Signs

Patients with an interspace neuroma usually present with a complaint of localized pain in the metatarsal head region that is increased by walking and relieved by rest and removing the shoe. Palpation of the involved interspace produces sharp pain that often radiates into the toes. There can be a palpable mass, and squeezing the forefoot, thereby narrowing the intermetatarsal space while compressing the mass, often reproduces the patient's symptoms. If this maneuver produces a snapping sensation, it is referred to as a Mulder click. The third interspace is more frequently involved than the second, and it is extremely rare to have involvement of the first or fourth web space. Pain over the metatarsophalangeal joint itself is caused by disease involving the metatarsophalangeal joint, and it is important to distinguish pain in the interspace from pain associated with pathology in the metatarsophalangeal joint. The differential diagnosis of metatarsalgia includes avascular necrosis (Freiberg), synovitis due to mechanical instability, synovial cysts, or even referred pain from tarsal tunnel compression or lumbar disk disease.

B. Imaging Studies

Radiographs are not helpful in the diagnosis of an interdigital neuroma but may reveal pathology at the metatarsophalangeal

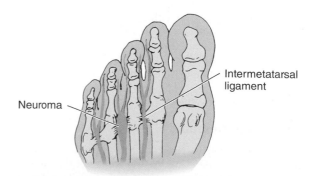

Neuroma

Intermetatarsal ligament

▲ **Figure 8–31.** An interdigital neuroma impingement occurs beneath the intermetatarsal ligament. (Reproduced, with permission, from Mann RA, Coughlin MJ: *The Video Textbook of Foot and Ankle Surgery.* Medical Video Productions, 1991.)

joint as the cause of the patient's symptoms. There are several reports regarding the use of ultrasound to evaluate the presence of nerve enlargement, but this is very user dependant. MRI can be used effectively but is rarely necessary.

▶ Treatment

A. Conservative Management

Conservative management begins with wearing a wider, soft-soled shoe to accommodate the foot without mediolateral compression and lowering the heel. A soft metatarsal support is placed in the shoe proximal to the area of the neuroma, thereby spreading the metatarsal heads and lifting them. Approximately one third of patients will respond to this treatment. Steroid injection into the web space can be helpful in resolving the symptoms but is not without the hazard of local fat atrophy, which can lead to diminished padding under the metatarsal heads or local skin thinning and discoloration.

B. Surgical Treatment

Surgical excision of the nerve is indicated if conservative treatment fails. A dorsal incision is made in the midline of the involved web space and carried down to the transverse metatarsal ligament, which is cut. The nerve is noted to lie just beneath the transverse metatarsal ligament. A nerve that is quite thickened is reassuring evidence that the correct diagnosis has been made; however, a nerve of normal thickness should still be removed if the clinical diagnosis of neuroma has been made from other evidence. The nerve is delivered into the interspace by plantar pressure and is freed up distally and proximally, transected proximal to the metatarsal head, and then dissected out distally, where it is cut just past its bifurcation. Care is taken not to disrupt the surrounding fatty tissue or intrinsic muscles. A compression dressing is used for 3 weeks after routine wound closure, and ambulation is permitted in a postoperative shoe. Decreased sensation in the toes on either side of the web space is expected postoperatively. Approximately 80% of patients are totally satisfied with the results of the procedure, whereas 20% obtain little or no relief. The precise cause of this failure rate is a bit of an enigma. Obviously in some patients, the diagnosis was incorrectly made and the metatarsophalangeal joint was actually involved.

C. Recurrent Neuroma

A recurrent neuroma is indeed a true surgical bulb neuroma that has resulted following the transection of the common digital nerve on the plantar aspect of the foot. True neuritic symptoms occur in some cases in which transection was not proximal enough or the nerve became adherent and trapped beneath the metatarsal head. Careful percussion of the plantar aspect to elicit the Tinel sign can frequently localize the

cut end of the nerve (bulb neuroma). If the severed nerve can be clinically well localized, reexploration for the neuroma is carried out either through a dorsal or plantar approach. The neuroma is identified and transected to a more proximal level or implanted into muscle, and symptoms are relieved in 60–70% of patients.

2. Tarsal Tunnel Syndrome

Tarsal tunnel syndrome is a compressive or traction neuropathy of the posterior tibial nerve as it passes behind the medial malleolus. The tarsal tunnel is formed by the fibro-osseous tunnel resulting from the flexor retinaculum as it wraps around the posterior aspect of the medial malleolus (Figure 8–32). Tarsal tunnel syndrome causes poorly localized dysesthesias on the plantar aspect of the foot. The symptom complex is often aggravated by activity and relieved by rest. Some patients complain mainly of nocturnal dysesthesias.

▶ Etiologic Findings

Tarsal tunnel syndrome may arise from a space-occupying lesion within the tarsal tunnel (eg, a ganglion, synovial cyst, or lipoma) or distally against one of the two terminal branches: the medial or lateral plantar nerve. It occasionally follows severe trauma to the lower extremity probably because of edema or scarring. Other causes are severe venous varicosities, tenosynovitis, or a tumor within the nerve. Traction neuropathy can occur in patients who have an excessively valgus hindfoot position, especially those that are unstable. As the patient walks, the posterior tibial nerve is subjected to stretching as it courses around the

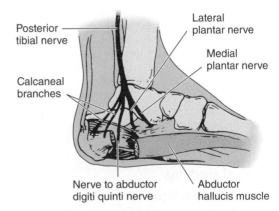

▲ **Figure 8–32.** Posterior tibial nerve and major branches. (Reproduced, with permission, from Mann RA, Coughlin MJ: *The Video Textbook of Foot and Ankle Surgery.* Medical Video Productions, 1991.)

convex side of the deformity. In more than half of the cases, however, the precise cause cannot be determined.

▶ Clinical Findings

A. Symptoms and Signs

The diagnosis is entertained after obtaining a history of paresthesias or burning in the posterior tibial nerve distribution. Careful evaluation of the patient in the standing and sitting positions is necessary to check posture and increased fullness, thickening, or swelling in the involved tarsal tunnel area. Careful percussion may elicit a Tinel sign over the posterior tibial nerve in the tarsal tunnel or distally along the divisions of the posterior tibial nerve (the medial calcaneal nerve and medial and lateral plantar nerves).

Muscle weakness is usually not observed, but loss of sensation and two-point discrimination may be occasionally detected.

Electrodiagnostic studies should be carried out to help confirm the diagnosis of tarsal tunnel syndrome. Nerve conduction velocities along the medial plantar nerve to the abductor hallucis muscle (latency <6.2 ms) and of the lateral plantar nerve to the abductor digiti quinti (latency usually <7 ms) should be within 1 ms of each other, otherwise indicating nerve compression in the tarsal tunnel. Motor-evoked potentials that demonstrate a decreased amplitude and increased duration are also felt to be indicative of tarsal tunnel syndrome. The most accurate study for tarsal tunnel syndrome appears to be sensory nerve conduction velocity, although this is also the least reproducible study.

The definitive diagnosis of tarsal tunnel syndrome should be based on (1) the clinical history of ill-defined burning, tingling pain in the plantar aspect of the foot; (2) positive physical findings of Tinel sign along the course of the nerve; and (3) electrodiagnostic studies. If all three factors are not positive, the diagnosis of tarsal tunnel syndrome should be suspect. MRI may be quite useful in demonstrating the presence of a space-occupying lesion.

▶ Treatment

A. Conservative Management

Tarsal tunnel syndrome should be managed with anti-inflammatory medications and an occasional steroid injection into the tarsal tunnel area. Aspiration and injection of a cyst or ganglion may be attempted but are rarely successful. Immobilization in a polypropylene ankle-foot orthosis may also be useful especially in the patient with unstable valgus who is suffering from a traction injury to the nerve.

B. Surgical Treatment

Surgical intervention can be considered if conservative management fails. Approximately 75% of patients operated on for tarsal tunnel syndrome are satisfied with the result. The other 25% may continue to have varying degrees of discomfort. The surgical release uses an incision behind the medial malleolus that is carried distally to about the level of the talonavicular joint. The investing retinaculum is exposed and released. The posterior tibial nerve is identified proximal to the tarsal tunnel area and carefully traced distally behind the medial malleolus. The division into its three terminal branches is identified. Because the medial calcaneal branch passes from the posterior aspect of the lateral plantar nerve, the dissection should be carried out along its dorsal aspect. There may be one or more medial calcaneal branches. The medial plantar nerve should be traced distally until it passes through the fibro-osseous tunnel in the abductor hallucis muscle. The lateral plantar nerve should be traced behind the abductor hallucis muscle until it passes toward the lateral aspect of the foot. A preoperative Tinel sign distal to the tarsal tunnel area requires that the area be carefully explored to determine whether there is a ganglion or cyst within the tendon sheath as a cause of the tarsal tunnel syndrome.

Postoperatively, a compression dressing is applied and weight bearing is prohibited for 3 weeks, before progressive ambulation is permitted.

The results following tarsal tunnel release depend on the pathology that is found at the time of surgery. Removal of a space-occupying lesion usually relieves all of the symptoms. Involvement of a single nerve branch, such as the medial or lateral plantar nerve, also portends good results after surgery. If more diffuse pain is felt throughout the foot before surgery and no definite constriction on the nerve is found at exploration, only one half to two thirds of patients can be expected to experience pain relief. Patients with traction neuropathy due to the unstable valgus foot are treated by correction of the instability, usually with arthrodesis, and not with soft-tissue tarsal tunnel release.

3. Traumatic Neuromas about the Foot

A traumatic neuroma about the foot presents a difficult problem in management because footwear can cause constant irritation of the neuroma. The most frequent cause of traumatic neuroma in the foot is previous surgery. Despite caution in making incisions about the foot, many lesser and occasionally major nerve trunks can be injured. The dorsal aspect of the foot is most frequently involved (Figure 8–33).

▶ Clinical Findings

The clinical evaluation begins with a careful history of the problem and an evaluation of the area involved to determine the precise location of the neuroma, which is essential for proper treatment. Rarely is any type of electrodiagnostic study indicated, and radiographs are not usually necessary.

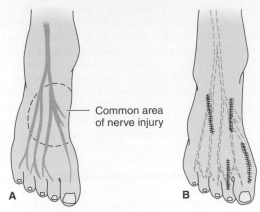

▲ **Figure 8–33. A:** Common area of traumatic nerve entrapment. **B:** Frequent incisions that may lead to entrapment of dorsal sensory nerves. (Reproduced, with permission, from Mann RA, Coughlin MJ: *The Video Textbook of Foot and Ankle Surgery.* Medical Video Productions, 1991.)

▶ Treatment

A. Conservative Management

Attempts to relieve pressure on the neuroma with a large shoe or a carefully designed pad may be of benefit. Occasionally a cortisone injection into the area may help, particularly when a small nerve is involved. Surgical intervention is indicated if conservative measures fail.

B. Surgical Treatment

Careful planning must be undertaken prior to the excision of a traumatic neuroma. The exact location of the neuroma and the area of sensitivity proximal to it must be determined. The incision must be made as precisely as possible to identify the neuroma and trace the nerve proximally into an area that would not be affected by pressure from shoes and boots. The neuroma is excised, leaving enough nerve to bring the cut end into an area of minimal pressure. The cut end is buried into an excavation in bone, if possible, or beneath a muscle such as the extensor digitorum brevis muscle. When carrying out a resection of the sural nerve, it is important, particularly in an individual who wears heavy work boots, that the end of the nerve is brought proximally enough so that the top of the boot will not press upon the nerve, resulting in continued symptoms.

The results following resection of a traumatic neuroma are quite variable. Initial relief from removing the traumatic neuroma is routine, but unless the nerve is buried where it will not be exposed to pressure, the symptoms may recur in time. It is therefore preferable to bury the end of the nerve into bone, if possible. Resection of most neuromas will accentuate a sensory deficit, but this is usually not a significant clinical problem.

4. Entrapment of the Sensory Branch of the Deep Peroneal Nerve

Osteophyte formation at the talonavicular or metatarsocuneiform joint may entrap the sensory branch of the deep peroneal nerve as it passes beneath the extensor retinaculum. Patient complaints are of dysesthesias on the foot or difficulty in wearing shoes, depending on the location of the entrapment.

The sensory branch of the deep peroneal nerve passes onto the dorsum of the foot between the extensor hallucis longus and extensor digitorum longus tendons. It continues beneath the extensor retinaculum, coursing along the dorsal surface of the talus and navicular, and more distally across the metatarsocuneiform joints. Osteophyte formation at any point along the course of the nerve may cause sufficient pressure against the nerve to cause an entrapment problem.

▶ Clinical Findings

A. Symptoms and Signs

The clinical evaluation begins with a careful history regarding the patient's complaint of dysesthesias over the dorsum of the foot. The physical examination demonstrates tingling along the course of the sensory branch of the deep peroneal nerve, which radiates into the first web space. Often the precise location of the nerve entrapment can be identified by careful palpation and by rolling the nerve across the involved bony prominence.

B. Imaging Studies

Radiographs usually reveal the offending osteophytes, often along the area of the talonavicular or metatarsocuneiform joints. Placing a radiographic marker at the area of maximum tenderness can help to identify the offending bony prominence.

▶ Treatment

A. Conservative Management

Conservative management consists of attempting to keep the pressure off the involved area, either by padding the tongue of the shoe or by trying to create a pad that will not put pressure directly on the nerve. If these measures fail, decompression of the nerve will usually bring about satisfactory resolution of the condition.

B. Surgical Treatment

Depending on the area of entrapment (talonavicular or metatarsocuneiform), a slightly curved incision is made and carried down through the retinaculum to expose the nerve. Great caution must be taken during the approach so that the nerve is not inadvertently damaged. The nerve is carefully lifted off of its bed, exposing the osteophytes, which are removed with a rongeur. The bone surfaces are coated with bone wax prior to laying the nerve back on its bed. After wound closure in layers, the foot is immobilized for approximately 3 weeks in a postoperative shoe.

The results following release of the sensory portion of the deep peroneal nerve are usually satisfactory. Because the nerve itself usually is not damaged by the entrapment, a favorable outcome is expected.

Gould JS: Tarsal tunnel syndrome. *Foot Ankle Clin* 2011;16:275. [PMID: 21600447]

Hassouna H, Singh D: Morton's metatarsalgia: pathogenesis, aetiology and current management. *Acta Orthop Belg* 2005;71:646. [PMID: 16459852]

RHEUMATOID FOOT

The foot is involved in 90% of patients with long-standing rheumatoid arthritis, and the involvement is almost always bilateral. The forefoot is most commonly involved and often contains the first joints to be affected, but deterioration of the subtalar joint has been noted in about 35% of patients and of the ankle joint in about 30%.

▶ Etiologic Findings

The changes in the forefoot are caused by chronic synovitis, which destroys the supporting structures about the metatarsophalangeal joints. The joint capsules are distended and the ligaments destroyed. When these structures no longer function to provide stability for the joint, progressive dorsal subluxation and eventual dislocation of the metatarsophalangeal joints occur. As the metatarsophalangeal joints progress from subluxation to dislocation, the plantar fat pad is drawn distally, and the base of the proximal phalanx eventually comes to rest on the metatarsal head. Thus, the metatarsals are forced into a position of plantar flexion, which results in significant callus formation beneath the metatarsal heads. The changes at the metatarsophalangeal joints result in imbalance of the intrinsic muscles, and severe hammer toe and claw toe deformities usually result.

Significant midfoot and hindfoot pathology is also found in patients with rheumatoid arthritis. A severely flattened longitudinal arch can result from long-standing subtalar joint involvement with subluxation. Pain with less severe deformity is present in isolated talonavicular involvement of the midfoot.

▶ Clinical Findings

A. Symptoms and Signs

The clinical evaluation of the rheumatoid patient begins with a careful history of the disease and the medications the patient is taking and an attempt to ascertain whether the disease process is currently in an active or a quiescent stage. It is important to obtain some indication of the patient's wound-healing capacity in the foot or elsewhere in the body.

The vascular status of the foot and quality of the skin are noted. The feet are assessed with the patient standing, which will often demonstrate marked deformities of multiple joints or localized involvement of only one or two joints. The patient is then seated, and a careful evaluation of all the joints about the foot and ankle is carried out to determine precisely the degree to which they are affected. Careful palpation of the metatarsophalangeal joints will often demonstrate the degree of the synovial activity as well as the degree of stability of the joints. The plantar aspect of the foot is inspected for the callus formation and past or present ulcerations. Flattening of the longitudinal arch and any hindfoot valgus are evaluated with a careful assessment of joint stability to determine the risk of deformity progression.

B. Imaging Studies

Radiographs help to assess the number of joints involved and the degree of involvement. Bilateral involvement is frequently asymmetric. Standing radiographs are beneficial in assessing the effect of joint stability on the severity of deformity.

▶ Treatment

A. Conservative Management

Conservative management includes medical management, carried out by the patient's rheumatologist. The patient with sufficient deformity should wear an extra-depth shoe with a soft accommodative liner to reduce pressure on the metatarsal heads and the toes, which may be severely contracted dorsally. Frequently, the patient is quite comfortable in this shoe and does not require further treatment. With significant hindfoot involvement, an ankle-foot orthosis may be required to help relieve pain by providing adequate stabilization.

B. Surgical Treatment

The main goal of surgical management of the forefoot is to create a stable foot that will alleviate the pain beneath the metatarsal head region (Figure 8–34). Arthrodesis of the first metatarsophalangeal joint is the procedure most commonly used, with the joint placed in approximately 15 degrees of dorsiflexion in relation to the floor and approximately 15 degrees of valgus position. The lesser metatarsophalangeal joints are corrected by release of the soft-tissue contracture and resection arthroplasty. The metatarsal heads are excised to decompress the metatarsophalangeal joints, and the fat pad is brought back down onto the plantar aspect of the foot by realigning and securing the plantar plates of the joints under the residual metatarsals. The hammer toes can be corrected by closed osteoclasis, which often results in satisfactory realignment. Open hammer toe procedures are

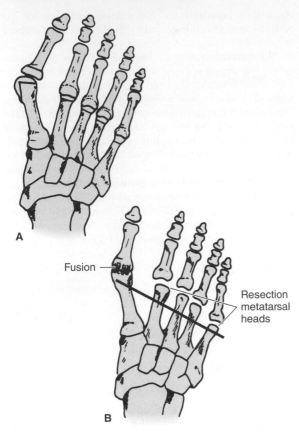

▲ Figure 8–34. A: Resection of metatarsal heads.
B: Symmetric resection of metatarsal heads minimizes recurrence of intractable plantar keratoses. (Reproduced, with permission, from Mann RA, Coughlin MJ: *The Video Textbook of Foot and Ankle Surgery.* Medical Video Productions, 1991.)

also very effective in correcting residual deformities. The toes and metatarsophalangeal joint area are stabilized with longitudinal Kirschner wires postoperatively for approximately 4 weeks.

The results of this rheumatoid forefoot repair are most gratifying in that about 90% of patients will be satisfied with the results. There are few complications, although the blood supply to the toes is always of concern because the procedure is extensive. Occasionally, wound healing is delayed, particularly if the patient is taking high dosages of corticosteroids or antimetabolite drugs.

Hindfoot and ankle disease is usually managed medically unless there is instability and progressive deformity. Orthotic support or bracing can be beneficial, but if the deformity is increasing and the patient's thin skin cannot tolerate further pressure, then surgical stabilization with

arthrodesis is necessary. If only a single joint is involved with the rheumatoid process, a less extensive procedure is carried out. For isolated talonavicular rheumatoid arthritis with no significant deformity of the arch, an isolated talonavicular fusion is adequate. If significant deformity is present because of subtalar joint subluxation, a triple arthrodesis is required. Ankle joint involvement is treated with ankle joint fusion or total ankle arthroplasty. The details of the surgical procedures are described elsewhere in this chapter.

Cracchiolo A III: Surgery for rheumatoid disease. Part I. Foot abnormalities in rheumatoid arthritis. *Instr Course Lect* 1984; 33:386. [No PMID]

Jaakkola J, Mann R: A review of rheumatoid arthritis affecting the foot and ankle. *Foot Ankle Int* 2004;25:866. [PMID: 15680099]

Loveday DT, Jackson GE, Geary NP: The rheumatoid foot and ankle: current evidence. *Foot Ankle Surg* 2012;18:94. [PMID: 22443994]

Wechalekar MD, Lester S, Proudman SM, et al: Active foot synovitis in patients with rheumatoid arthritis: applying clinical criteria for disease activity and remission may result in underestimation of foot joint involvement. *Arthritis Rheum* 2012;64:1316. [PMID: 22135142]

HEEL PAIN

Heel pain can be caused by several distinct entities. When evaluating the patient for heel pain, the clinician must attempt to define as precisely as possible the location and, hence, the cause of the pain.

The causes of heel pain are presented in Table 8–3. The causes are quite variable and need to be carefully defined, so that the proper treatment can be chosen.

Table 8–3. Causes of heel pain.

Causes of plantar heel pain
Plantar fasciitis
Atrophy of heel pad
Posttraumatic (eg, calcaneal fracture)
Enlarged calcaneal spur
Neurologic conditions such as tarsal tunnel syndrome or entrapment of nerve to abductor digiti quinti
Degenerative disk disease with radiation toward heel
Systemic disease (eg, Reiter syndrome, psoriatic arthritis)
Acute tear of plantar fascia
Calcaneal apophysitis
Causes of posterior heel pain
Retrocalcaneal bursitis
Achilles tendinitis
Haglund deformity
Degeneration of Achilles tendon insertion

Clinical Findings

A. Symptoms and Signs

The clinical evaluation begins with a careful history of the onset and location of the pain. The patient's activities and types of footwear that aggravate and relieve the pain are discussed. Specific inquiry regarding radiation of pain proximally in the lower extremity may suggest lumbar disk disease as the cause. Patients active in sports should be questioned regarding significant changes in their level of activity because heel pain often is the result of increased stress on the foot.

The cause of the patient's heel pain can usually be determined by palpating the area of maximum tenderness.

Plantar fasciitis, the most common cause of plantar heel pain, usually has an area of maximum tenderness along the plantar medial aspect of the heel, which corresponds to the origin of the plantar fascia at the medial calcaneal tuberosity. In most cases, the pain is most severe with the first steps upon arising. The pain is usually aggravated by dorsiflexion of the toes, the so-called windlass stretch, because this applies more tension on the damaged plantar fascia.

Achilles tendonitis/tendinosis typically occurs at one of two discreet sites: at the calcaneal insertion or centered 3.0–4.0 cm proximal to the insertion. Insertional Achilles tendonitis/tendinosis is characterized by pain and swelling that is increased by activity. There is usually tenderness in the posterior midline with local increased warmth. Noninsertional Achilles tendonitis/tendinosis is usually associated with a thickened tendon and often quite severe tenderness to palpation of the thickened area in the midportion of the tendon. Both of these are more degenerative than true inflammatory processes and more properly referred to as tendinosis.

Heel pain can also be caused by inflammation of the retrocalcaneal bursa, which sits between the tendoachilles and the posterior calcaneus and is often associated with the Haglund heel deformity.

Tarsal tunnel syndrome with involvement of the medial calcaneal branches should be investigated by careful percussion of the posterior tibial nerve. Evidence of degenerative disk disease requires careful testing of motor function and sensation more proximally in the calf.

B. Imaging Studies

Radiographs may demonstrate calcaneal spur formation or calcification at either the insertion of the Achilles tendon or the origin of the plantar fascia. Alternatively, the posterosuperior aspect of the calcaneus may be too prominent and protrude into the Achilles tendon, a condition known as Haglund disease or Haglund deformity, with the symptoms coming from the inflamed retrocalcaneal bursa. A bone scan will sometimes reveal increased activity diffusely about the calcaneus, as may be seen in systemic diseases such as Reiter syndrome, or a discreet area of uptake, as in a stress fracture. MRI scan may help to delineate the degree of the Achilles tendon degeneration present in cases of Achilles tendinosis and can help to identify rupture of the tendon if this is in question.

Treatment

A. Conservative Management

The conservative management of heel pain depends on the specific cause. Because many causes are related to abnormal stress on the foot, the basic principles involve reducing the stress on the involved area. Activity modification, footwear with a softer, more resilient heel, and use of a soft orthotic device under the longitudinal arch to relieve some of the pressure on the region of pain can be helpful. NSAIDs are often useful, as is physical therapy to teach stretching exercises of the Achilles tendon and plantar fascia. Plantar fasciitis is treated initially with stretching exercises, soft cushioned heel shoes, NSAIDS if they are tolerated, and avoidance of strong toe-off activities such as running and jumping. The use of a night splint to help keep the Achilles tendon and plantar fascia stretched often relieves the acute pain patients experience when they first get up in the morning. Patients who are refractory to treatment may benefit from a steroid injection into the plantar fascia origin, although there is a risk of plantar fascia rupture. Cast immobilization has also been shown to benefit these refractory patients. Recently there is some evidence that injection of platelet-rich plasma may be of benefit to these refractory patients.

In general, the treatment of heel pain is often prolonged, requiring a great deal of patience on the part of the physician and patient. It is important to explain to the patient the nature of the problem and the fact that it is often a chronic condition that requires many months to resolve.

Achilles tendinosis is treated with stretching exercises, activity modification, NSAIDs, and a heel lift. If these modalities are inadequate, then bracing or casting will provide more strain relief to the damaged tissue.

B. Surgical Treatment

Patients with plantar fasciitis, in whom symptoms cannot be controlled after 9–12 months of conservative management, may become candidates for surgery. The options include orthotripsy or surgical release of the medial half of the plantar fascial origin. With surgical release, the success rate is approximately 75%. Caution must be exercised with the approach to the medial side of the heel to avoid damage to the medial calcaneal branch of the posterior tibial nerve. Disruption of this nerve will cause an area of heel numbness and possibly a troublesome neuroma along the medial side of the heel. An endoscopic approach for plantar fascia release has been described in patients who do not have a plantar heel spur that requires removal. Orthotripsy, while less invasive, still has conflicting literature as to its effectiveness.

Surgical treatment of Achilles tendinosis is offered if 6–9 months of conservative measures do not help to eliminate symptoms. Insertional Achilles tendinosis is treated with debridement of degenerative tendon and excision of bone spurs with repair of the Achilles insertion. If a Haglund deformity is present, it is also resected. Noninsertional Achilles tendinosis is treated with debridement of degenerative tendon. In either case, if the majority of the tendon is nonviable, it must be repaired, often requiring a graft such as the flexor hallucis longus tendon transfer.

Bader L, Park K, Gu Y, O'Malley MJ: Functional outcome of endoscopic plantar fasciotomy. *Foot Ankle Int* 2012;33:37. [PMID: 22381234]

Baxter DE, Pfeffer GB: Treatment of chronic heel pain by surgical release of the first branch of the lateral plantar nerve. *Clin Orthop Relat Res* 1992;279:229. [PMID: 1600660]

Goff JD, Crawford R: Diagnosis and treatment of plantar fasciitis. *Am Fam Physician* 2011;84:676. [PMID: 21916393]

Murphy GA, Pneumaticos SG, Kamaric E, et al: Biomechanical consequences of sequential plantar fascia release. *Foot Ankle Int* 1998;19:149. [PMID: 9542985]

Ragab EM, Othman AM: Platelets rich plasma for treatment of chronic plantar fasciitis. *Arch Orthop Trauma Surg* 2012; 132:1065. [PMID: 22555761]

ARTHRODESIS ABOUT THE FOOT AND ANKLE

▶ General Considerations

A. Goals of Arthrodesis

Arthrodesis is surgical fixation of a joint to obtain fusion of the joint surfaces. Arthrodesis about the foot and ankle can be effective in achieving the following goals:

1. Elimination of joint pain

2. Correction of deformity

3. Stabilization of the foot or ankle when adequate muscle function or ligamentous support is lacking, as in residual poliomyelitis or the acquired flat foot due to peritalar instability

4. Restoration of function by salvaging a situation in which no reasonable reconstructive procedure is available, as in fusion of the first metatarsophalangeal joint after failed hallux valgus repair

B. Principles of Arthrodesis

An arthrodesis about the foot and ankle requires adherence to these general principles:

1. To be effective, the arthrodesis must produce a plantigrade foot.

2. Broad, cancellous bony surfaces must be placed into apposition.

3. The arthrodesis site should be stabilized with rigid internal fixation, preferably with interfragmentary compression.

4. When correcting malalignment of the foot, it is imperative that the hindfoot be placed into 5–7 degrees of valgus and the forefoot in neutral position with regard to abduction, adduction, pronation, and supination.

5. The surgical approaches should be carried out in such a way as to minimize the risk of damage to the nerves.

C. Effects of Arthrodesis on Joint Motion

Following ankle arthrodesis, residual dorsiflexion and plantar flexion movement occurs within the subtalar and transverse tarsal joints, and additional, compensatory motion may develop over time. Arthritic changes in these joints may become symptomatic following ankle arthrodesis, and in time, extension of the fusion may be required.

The subtalar joint and transverse tarsal joints must be viewed as a joint complex similar to the universal joint of a car. Movement in these joints is interrelated. After subtalar arthrodesis, inversion and eversion are lost, but transverse tarsal joint motion in dorsiflexion and plantar flexion remains. Arthrodesis of the talonavicular joint, however, will eliminate most of the subtalar joint motion because rotation must occur around the head of the talus for subtalar motion to occur.

A triple arthrodesis eliminates the subtalar and transverse tarsal joint motion, causing increased stress on the ankle joint and the midtarsal joints distal to the fusion site. A small percentage of patients will develop degenerative changes in the ankle joint following triple arthrodesis. It is imperative, therefore, to carefully evaluate the ankle joint prior to carrying out a triple arthrodesis.

Arthrodesis of the tarsometatarsal joints will not significantly affect motion of the foot and ankle, but a certain degree of stiffness is noted through the midtarsal area following this fusion. Fusion of the first metatarsophalangeal joint places added stress on the interphalangeal joint of the great toe, particularly with poor alignment. Although up to 40% of patients may develop degenerative changes in this joint, they are rarely of clinical significance.

D. Disadvantages of Arthrodesis

Although arthrodesis is an effective reconstructive tool, the resulting loss of motion places increased stress on the surrounding joints, making them more prone to developing arthritis or worsening preexisting degenerative changes. Thus, correction of a problem without arthrodesis is preferable whenever possible, such as with an osteotomy, tendon transfer, or both.

▶ Ankle Fusion

A. Indications

The main indications for ankle arthrodesis are the following:

1. Arthrosis of the ankle joint usually secondary to a previous ankle fracture, although primary arthrosis does occur

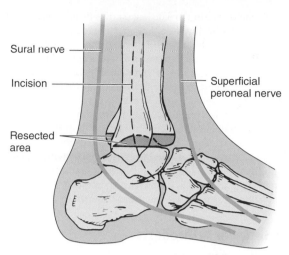

▲ **Figure 8–35.** Technique for ankle arthrodesis. Skin incision is laced between superficial peroneal nerve and sural nerve. (Reproduced, with permission, from Mann RA, Coughlin MJ: *The Video Textbook of Foot and Ankle Surgery.* Medical Video Productions, 1991.)

2. Arthritis secondary to rheumatoid disease

3. Instability with malalignment of the ankle joint as the result of an epiphyseal injury or previous fracture

B. Technique

The surgical approach preferred by the authors is a transfibular approach (Figure 8–35). The incision begins along the fibula, approximately 10 cm proximal to the tip of the fibula, and is carried distally along the shaft of the fibula and then curves toward the base of the fourth metatarsal. In this way, the incision avoids the sural nerve posteriorly and the superficial peroneal nerve dorsally. The flaps that are created are full thickness, to lessen the possibility of wound healing problems. The dissection is carried across the anterior aspect of the ankle joint, to the medial malleolus and along the lateral aspect of the neck of the talus. Posteriorly, the fibula and the posterior aspect of the ankle joint are exposed, while distally, the subtalar joint and sinus tarsi area are exposed. The fibula is removed approximately 2 cm proximal to the joint, after which the residual cartilage and subchondral bone are removed from the distal tibia (Figure 8–36). This cut should be made as perpendicular as possible to the long axis of the tibia and should extend to the medial malleolus but not through it. The foot is placed into a plantigrade position and a cut made in the dome of the talus parallel to the cut in the tibia, thereby creating two flat surfaces and correcting any malalignment. At this point, the ankle should be aligned in neutral position, insofar as dorsiflexion and plantar flexion are concerned, and at about 5 degrees of valgus. The degree of rotation should be equal to that of the opposite extremity,

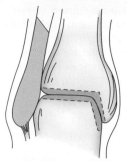

▲ **Figure 8–36.** The fibula is excised approximately 2–2.5 cm proximal to the ankle joint, and the distal portion of the tibia is cut, producing a flat cut perpendicular to the long axis of the tibia. (Reproduced, with permission, from Mann RA, Coughlin MJ: *The Video Textbook of Foot and Ankle Surgery.* Medical Video Productions, 1991.)

which is usually 5–10 degrees of external rotation. If the two joint surfaces do not easily oppose each other, it is because the medial malleolus is too long, and the malleolus should be exposed through a dorsomedial incision and the distal centimeter removed.

The two flat surfaces should now be in total apposition, with little or no pressure being exerted. Temporary fixation is obtained by inserting two 0.062-inch K-wires. Interfragmentary compression is gained with at least two 6.5-mm cancellous screws. These screws should be placed to gain adequate interfragmentary compression (Figure 8–37). Following insertion of the screws, there should be rigid fixation of the arthrodesis site. Because the joint surfaces are fully opposed, there is no room for bone grafting. In the immediate postoperative period, a firm compression dressing

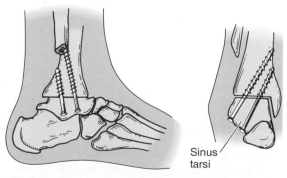

▲ **Figure 8–37.** Diagram demonstrating placement of the 6.5-mm screws across the arthrodesis site. (Reproduced, with permission, from Mann RA, Coughlin MJ: *The Video Textbook of Foot and Ankle Surgery.* Medical Video Productions, 1991.)

incorporating plaster splints is applied. After swelling is decreased, a short leg cast is applied and weight bearing is not allowed for 6 weeks. Weight bearing is then allowed with the short leg cast in place for another 6 weeks. Arthrodesis generally occurs following 12 weeks of immobilization.

C. Complications

Nonunion of the ankle joint, although uncommon, does occur. Using the surgical technique described earlier, a fusion rate of 90% can be anticipated. If nonunion occurs, bone grafting and further internal fixation may be required.

Malalignment of the ankle joint with the foot in too much internal rotation is poorly tolerated and often requires revision surgery. Excessive plantar flexion causes a back knee thrust and eventually some knee discomfort; excessive dorsiflexion causes increased stress on the heel (that can usually be treated with adequate padding); varus deformity may cause subtalar joint instability; excessive valgus causes stress on the medial aspect of the knee joint.

It is extremely important not to place any pin or screw across the subtalar joint for fear of damaging the posterior facet, which may lead to arthrosis.

D. Special Considerations

Avascular necrosis of the talus requires excision and tibiocalcaneal fusion or a fusion that bypasses the necrotic bone. Bone grafting may also be necessary when attempting to carry out a fusion after a severely comminuted pilon fracture because there are often defects that affect stability due to the previous crushing of cancellous bone.

▶ Total Ankle Arthroplasty

Total ankle arthroplasty is an alternative to ankle arthrodesis for painful arthrosis of the ankle joint. Advantages include maintenance of some ankle joint motion with a more normal gait and thus less stress on adjacent joints. Unfortunately the disadvantages of the procedure are that it is technically difficult with a steep learning curve, there is a higher complication rate than with arthrodesis, and the long-term survival rate is unknown. The intermediate-term survival rate of the Agility total ankle reported by Saltzman suggests that the outcome is durable in selected patients. The procedure is performed through an anterior incision in all of the implants that are currently available in the United States (ie, the Agility, the Salto-Talaris, and the INBONE), all of which are two-part implants (Figure 8–38). There are several other prostheses, including the STAR, the Mobility, and the Hintegra, used primarily in Europe that have reported promising early results; these are three-part implants with a polyethylene mobile bearing. There is the expectation that these newer designs will eventually be approved by the U.S. Food and Drug Administration (FDA) and become available in the United States. Studies to date have shown no advantage to the mobile bearing implants, although there is the possibility of less polyethylene wear; the disadvantage is the potential for instability of the mobile bearing. There is general consensus that the ideal patient is older, thin, and less active, but there are no clinical data that specifically support this. Proponents of arthroplasty have suggested that their patients may be able to have a more active lifestyle than those with arthrodesis, but there are no studies that actually look at this question. There are studies that show that patients after arthroplasty have a greater ability to perform light recreational activities such as swimming, biking, and hiking than they did before surgery. Survey data suggest that physicians recommend that arthrodesis patients participate in low-impact sports.

▶ Subtalar Arthrodesis

A. Indications

The main indications for subtalar arthrodesis are the following:

1. Arthrosis of the subtalar joint, usually following a calcaneal fracture, but occasionally for primary arthrosis of the joint

2. Varus or valgus deformity secondary to rheumatoid arthritis

3. Varus deformity secondary to residual clubfoot or possibly following compartment syndrome

4. Unstable subtalar joint secondary to poliomyelitis, a neuromuscular disorder, or tendon dysfunction such as posterior tibial tendon dysfunction

5. Symptomatic talocalcaneal coalition without secondary changes in the talonavicular or calcaneocuboid joints

B. Technique

The incision for subtalar arthrodesis begins at the tip of the fibula and is carried distally toward the base of the fourth metatarsal. As the incision is deepened, the sural nerve or one of its branches should be carefully noted and retracted. Small "twigs" of nerve may be present that unfortunately may be cut and give rise to a painful neuroma. The sinus tarsi area is exposed by reflecting the extensor digitorum brevis muscle distally. The use of a lamina spreader in the subtalar joint will enhance the exposure.

The articular cartilage is removed from the joint surfaces, which include the middle and posterior facets. The bony joint surfaces are then deeply feathered or scaled using a small osteotome. These cuts through the subchondral bone will greatly enhance the possibility of fusion. The area around the floor of the sinus tarsi and anterior process region can be carefully shaved to obtain local bone graft for the fusion.

The alignment of the subtalar joint is critical. It must be aligned into approximately 5–7 degrees of valgus position,

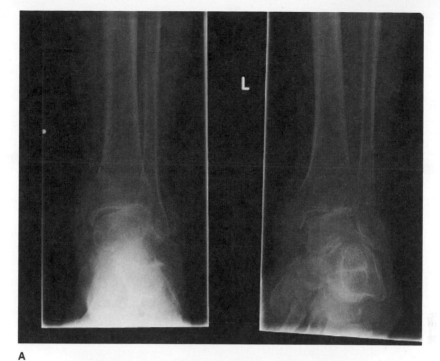

A

B

▲ **Figure 8–38. A, B:** This is a 60-year-old man with progressive ankle arthritis associated with instability. **C, D:** The same patient after ankle arthroplasty and ligament reconstruction.

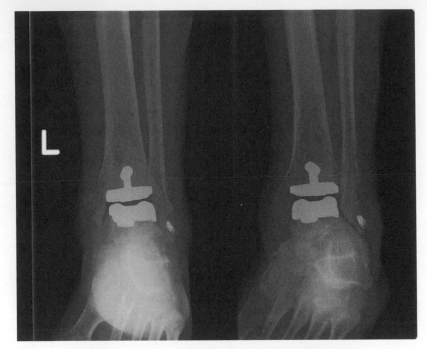

C

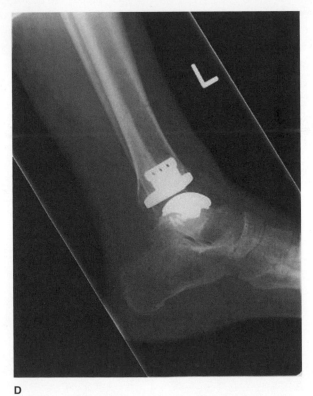

D

▲ **Figure 8–38.** (Continued)

producing a supple transverse tarsal joint. If it is placed in varus position, the foot is stiff and the patient will walk on the side of the foot.

Rigid fixation of the subtalar joint is achieved by using a 7-mm cannulated interfragmentary screw starting at the posterior tip of the calcaneus and passing into the body or neck of the talus. The guide pin is first placed up into the posterior facet, the subtalar joint is then manipulated into proper alignment, and the guide pin is passed into the talus. The alignment of the screw is verified on radiograph, and the screw inserted.

Following adequate internal fixation, the local bone graft is packed into the sinus tarsi area. Additional bone may be obtained from the area of the medial malleolus, the proximal tibia, or occasionally the iliac crest, although the latter site significantly adds to the morbidity of the procedure.

Postoperatively, a firm compression dressing incorporating plaster splints is applied. A short leg cast is applied, and weight bearing is not allowed for 6 weeks. The cast is changed, and weight bearing is not allowed for another 6 weeks. Twelve weeks of immobilization generally achieves an arthrodesis.

C. Complications

Nonunion of the subtalar joint is uncommon, although it can occur. Careful surgical technique and heavy scaling of the joint surfaces can help to prevent this complication. If nonunion occurs, bone grafting and added fixation are required to attempt to achieve a solid union.

Misalignment of the subtalar joint may also be a complication. An excessive valgus deformity following subtalar fusion may result in impingement laterally against the fibula or peroneal tendons. It will also cause excessive stress along the medial aspect of the midfoot and occasionally the knee joint. A varus deformity of the subtalar joint imparts rigidity to the transverse tarsal joint, resulting in stiffness of the forefoot. This also increases pressure along the lateral aspect of the foot, particularly in the area of the base of the fifth metatarsal.

D. Special Considerations

The patient with rheumatoid arthritis or posttraumatic complications may have lateral subluxation of the calcaneus in relation to the talus, which usually requires computed tomography (CT) scanning for identification. The calcaneus must be displaced medially at operation to align it with the lateral aspect of the talus and place it under the tibia in a proper weight-bearing position. If the calcaneus is fused with significant lateral deviation, the abnormal alignment places added stress on the ankle and midfoot region.

Special attention to the peroneal tendons is necessary when a subtalar arthrodesis is done to correct an old calcaneal fracture. Protrusion of the lateral wall of the body of the calcaneus

from the healed fracture results in impingement on the peroneal tendons beneath the fibula. This protrusion must be carefully excised when the subtalar fusion is carried out, so that the lateral aspect of the talus and calcaneus are in line. Further, the peroneal tendon sheath should be dissected subperiosteally off the calcaneus to provide tendon sheath to protect the peroneal tendons from the raw, bony surface of the calcaneus.

Occasionally a bone block distraction arthrodesis of the subtalar joint is performed in cases of severe deformity after a calcaneus fracture. If the talus has assumed a horizontal position because of flattening of Böhler's angle, this can cause limited ankle joint dorsiflexion. Placing a tricortical block of iliac crest into the posterior facet of the subtalar joint will help to improve the overall alignment of the hind foot and regain ankle joint dorsiflexion.

► Talonavicular Arthrodesis

A. Indications

Talonavicular arthrodesis is indicated in the following conditions:

1. Posttraumatic injury, rheumatoid arthritis, or primary arthrosis

2. Unstable talonavicular joint secondary to rupture of the posterior tibial tendon and the peritalar ligaments, and rheumatoid arthritis

3. In conjunction with double or triple arthrodesis of the hindfoot

B. Technique

The talonavicular joint is approached through a medial or dorsomedial incision that starts in the region of the naviculocuneiform joint and extends to the neck of the talus. The soft tissues are stripped from around the joint and the articular cartilage removed with a curet or curved osteotome. Distraction of the joint by placing a towel clip into the navicular often facilitates exposure and debridement of the joint. Correct alignment of the talonavicular joint is extremely critical because this fusion essentially eliminates motion in the subtalar joint. The fusion position of the subtalar joint is 3–5 degrees of valgus with the forefoot in a plantigrade position (Figure 8–39). After the foot has been properly aligned to correspond to the opposite foot, fixation of the joint is carried out. Proper alignment of this joint is particularly critical when treating the laterally subluxed talonavicular joint in the patient with a ruptured posterior tibial tendon. The internal fixation is carried out by using interfragmentary compression with a single large screw (6.5 mm) or two smaller screws (4.0 mm) or by using multiple staples.

Postoperatively, the patient is immobilized in a non-weight-bearing cast for 6 weeks followed by a weight-bearing cast for an additional 6 weeks.

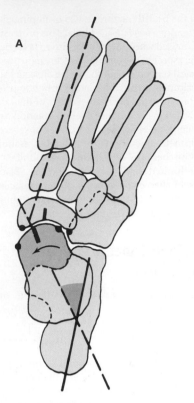

A

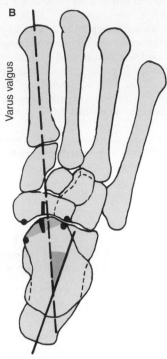

B

Varus valgus

Flatfoot deformity

Long axis of talus
through first metatarsal

▲ **Figure 8–39.** Talonavicular fusion. **A:** Changes that occur in the talonavicular joint with a flatfoot deformity. Note that the head of the talus deviates medially as the forefoot deviates laterally into abductions. **B:** The forefoot was brought into adduction so the navicular is once again centered over the head of the talus. (Reproduced, with permission, from Mann RA, Coughlin MJ: *The Video Textbook of Foot and Ankle Surgery.* Medical Video Productions, 1991.)

The talonavicular joint has a relatively high incidence of nonunion, which is probably the result of the difficulty in exposing the joint. If the joint is also approached medially to gain additional exposure, the surfaces can be well scaled, and the fusion rate should approach 90%.

C. Complications

Complications of nonunion and misalignment are similar to those discussed for subtalar joint fusion.

D. Special Considerations

An isolated talonavicular joint fusion will usually produce a satisfactory result, particularly in relatively sedentary patients older than 50 years. In younger, more active individuals with no other affliction (eg, rheumatoid arthritis), consideration should be given to including the calcaneocuboid joint at the same time to obtain a more stable transverse tarsal joint and enhance the fusion of the talonavicular joint through added stability.

▶ Double Arthrodesis (Calcaneocuboid and Talonavicular Joints)

A. Indications

In recent years, double arthrodesis has evolved as a procedure that provides the same degree of stability to the foot as a triple arthrodesis (Figure 8–40). By locking the transverse

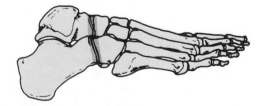

▲ **Figure 8–40.** Double arthrodesis consisting of a talonavicular and calcaneocuboid fusion. (Reproduced, with permission, from Mann RA, Coughlin MJ: *The Video Textbook of Foot and Ankle Surgery.* Medical Video Productions, 1991.)

tarsal joint (calcaneocuboid and talonavicular), further subtalar motion is prevented because these three joints function together. This procedure is also indicated in the younger, active patient in whom an isolated talonavicular fusion is contemplated because it gives added stability to the foot.

Indications for double arthrodesis are as follows:

1. Arthrosis of the talonavicular and calcaneocuboid joints (eg, following trauma)

2. Unstable talonavicular and calcaneocuboid joint following rupture of the posterior tibial tendon or neuromuscular disease when a flexible subtalar joint is present

3. Arthrosis of the talonavicular joint or calcaneocuboid joint in an active individual, usually younger than 50 years of age, to give the midfoot a greater degree of stability

B. Technique

The talonavicular joint is approached through a medial or dorsomedial incision, as previously described, and the calcaneocuboid joint is approached through the same incision along the lateral side of the foot as was described for subtalar fusion. Once these joints are exposed, the joint surfaces are denuded of articular cartilage and the subchondral bone is heavily feathered.

The alignment when carrying out a double arthrodesis is extremely critical because once this fusion has been achieved, the subtalar joint or the transverse tarsal joints no longer move. Therefore, the foot must be placed into a plantigrade position prior to the fixation of the arthrodesis site. The desired position is 5 degrees of valgus of the calcaneus, neutral abduction and adduction of the transverse tarsal joint, and correction of any forefoot varus that is present. This alignment creates a plantigrade foot. The fixation of the talonavicular joint is done first with the insertion of a screw (6.5 mm) or screws (4 mm) or possibly the use of multiple staples. The calcaneocuboid joint is then fixed the same way. Postoperative care is the same as for other foot fusions.

C. Complications

Complications of nonunion and malalignment are similar to those discussed for subtalar joint fusion.

▶ Triple Arthrodesis

The triple arthrodesis is a fusion of the talonavicular, calcaneocuboid, and subtalar joints (Figure 8–41). In the past, it was the procedure of choice for all hindfoot problems, before isolated fusions became more accepted. Now, this procedure is still commonly used when limited fusions are inadequate.

A. Indications

Indications for triple arthrodesis are as follows:

1. Arthrosis secondary to trauma involving the subtalar, talonavicular, or calcaneocuboid joints

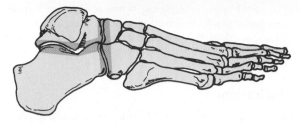

▲ **Figure 8–41.** Diagram of a triple arthrodesis. (Reproduced, with permission, from Mann RA, Coughlin MJ: *The Video Textbook of Foot and Ankle Surgery.* Medical Video Productions, 1991.)

2. Arthrosis or instability of the talonavicular or calcaneocuboid joints in association with a fixed deformity of the subtalar joint

3. Instability of the foot secondary to posterior tibial tendon dysfunction with a fixed subtalar joint that cannot be realigned by a double arthrodesis

4. Unstable hindfoot secondary to poliomyelitis, nerve injury, or rheumatoid arthritis

5. Symptomatic, unresectable calcaneonavicular bar

6. Malalignment of the hindfoot secondary to trauma such as a crush injury or compartment syndrome

B. Technique

The triple arthrodesis is carried out as previously described for subtalar fusion and talonavicular fusion. The foot is fixed after manipulation back into a plantigrade position (3–5 degrees of valgus of the subtalar joint), neutral position as far as abduction and adduction of the transverse tarsal joint, and correction of forefoot varus. Postoperative care is the same as for subtalar fusion.

C. Complications

The main complication is failure of fusion of one of the joints, but this is uncommon, as the successful fusion rate exceeds 90%. The talonavicular joint is most likely to have nonunion. Malalignment of the foot or forefoot may require revision and technically is a difficult procedure. The sural nerve may become entrapped or disrupted through the lateral approach.

▶ Tarsometatarsal Arthrodesis

Arthrodesis in the tarsometatarsal area may involve a single tarsometatarsal joint, usually the first joint, or multiple joints. The fusion mass not infrequently will extend proximally to include the intertarsal bones and sometimes even the naviculocuneiform joints. A careful determination of the involved joints is important when considering a tarso-metatarsal fusion for a patient with posttraumatic disorders. At times, in addition to the plain radiograph, a CT scan and bone scan may be necessary to help in precisely defining the involved area.

A. Indications

The indications for a tarsometatarsal fusion are as follows:

1. Hypermobility of the first metatarsocuneiform joint associated with a hallux valgus deformity in a small percentage of patients with a bunion deformity

2. Arthrosis involving one or more of the tarsometatarsal joints either resulting from trauma or as a primary disease process

3. Arthrosis associated with a deformity resulting from an old Lisfranc fracture-dislocation

B. Technique

The surgical approach to the first metatarsocuneiform joint is through a dorsomedial longitudinal incision to expose the joint. If multiple joints are involved, the second incision is centered over the second metatarsal, through which the lateral side of the first and all of the second and third metatarsocuneiform joints can be adequately viewed (Figure 8–42). The incision must be sufficiently long to permit adequate exposure of the joints and must be extended proximally if the navicu-locuneiform joints are going to be fused as well. Cautious dissection is necessary, as there are numerous superficial nerves as well as the neurovascular bundle (dorsalis pedis and superficial branch of the deep peroneal nerve) passing over the area of the second metatarsocuneiform joint in this approach. If the fourth and fifth metatarsocuboid joints are to be fused, then a third longitudinal incision is made over this area to enable adequate exposure. The articular cartilage is carefully removed from the tarsometatarsal and intertarsal joints, depending on the extent of the fusion mass. The bones are heavily feathered to create a good environment for healing. If a deformity is present (usually an abduction deformity of the foot or possibly dorsiflexion), it should be corrected. The first metatarsocuneiform joint is aligned and fixed using 4-mm cancellous screws or a dorsomedial plate. Interfragmentary longitudinal compression of the other joints is obtained to prevent possible nonunion. The screw pattern found to be most useful for the first metatarsocuneiform joint is one brought from the dorsal aspect of the cuneiform directed distally, and a second screw from the dorsal aspect of the metatarsal base directed proximally, crossing the metatarsocuneiform joint. Care must be taken to also correct any dorsiflexion or abduction deformity that is present.

Postoperatively, the joint is placed in a short leg, non–weight-bearing cast for 6 weeks and then in a weight-bearing cast for another 6 weeks.

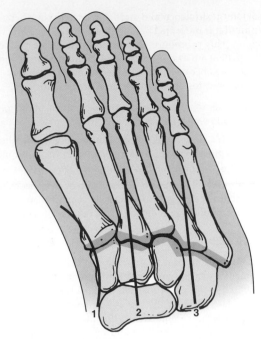

▲ **Figure 8–42.** Longitudinal incisions used for a tarsometatarsal arthrodesis. (Reproduced, with permission, from Mann RA, Coughlin MJ: *The Video Textbook of Foot and Ankle Surgery.* Medical Video Productions, 1991.)

C. Complications

The possibility of nonunion exists, but with interfragmentary compression, this risk is minimized. If nonunion occurs, bone grafting may be required as well as improved internal fixation. When multiple tarsometatarsal joints are fused, there is a moderate amount of swelling and tension placed against the incisions. It is critical postoperatively to use a compression dressing to minimize the risk of swelling and prevent possible wound sloughing. If sloughing occurs, it must be treated appropriately, and occasionally, skin grafting is required.

A tarsometatarsal fusion involving multiple joints may cause a plantar callus because one of the metatarsals has been placed in a position of too much plantar flexion. Osteotomy at the base of the metatarsal may be necessary to realign the metatarsal.

Staples should be avoided as a means of internal fixation of the tarsometatarsal joints because they have a tendency to cause dorsiflexion of the metatarsals, which could result in transfer pressure problems under the uninvolved metatarsal heads.

▶ First Metatarsophalangeal Joint Arthrodesis

See the discussion of hallux valgus at the beginning of the chapter.

Interphalangeal Joint Arthrodesis (Hallux Arthrodesis)

A. Indications

Interphalangeal joint arthrodesis is usually indicated for the following problems:

1. Arthrosis, usually secondary to trauma or occasionally following a first metatarsophalangeal joint arthrodesis

2. Stabilization of the interphalangeal joint when carrying out a transfer of the extensor hallucis longus into the neck of the first metatarsal (first toe Jones procedure)

B. Technique

The interphalangeal joint is approached through a dorsal transverse incision centered over the joint. Usually, an ellipse of skin is removed, exposing the ends of the involved joints. Using a small power saw, the end of the distal portion of the proximal phalanx and the proximal portion of the distal phalanx are removed, placing the distal phalanx into approximately 5–7 degrees of plantar flexion and 3–4 degrees of valgus position. Internal fixation is achieved by using a longitudinal screw (4 mm) or crossed K-wires, or both.

A postoperative shoe is used, with weight bearing allowed but avoiding the toe-off phase of gait until fusion occurs, usually in 8 weeks.

C. Complications

Nonunion of interphalangeal joint fusion is uncommon. If it does occur, it often is asymptomatic and does not require treatment. If it is symptomatic, usually the fusion will need to be revised because the area is too small for adequate bone grafting.

Barg A, Tochigi Y, Amendola A, Phisitkul P, Hintermann B, Saltzman CL: Subtalar instability: diagnosis and treatment. *Foot Ankle Int* 2012;33:151. [PMID: 22381348]

Buck P, Morrey BF, Chao EY: The optimum position of arthrodesis of the ankle. *J Bone Joint Surg Am* 1987;69:1052. [PMID: 3656947]

Carr JB, Hansen ST, Benirschke SK: Subtalar distraction bone block fusion for late complications of os calcis fractures. *Foot Ankle Int* 1988;9:81. [PMID: 3066724]

Klein SE, Putnam RM, McCormick JJ, Johnson JE: The slot graft technique for foot and ankle arthrodesis in a high-risk patient group. *Foot Ankle Int* 2011;32:686. [PMID: 21972763]

Reinhardt KR, Oh LS, Schottel P, Roberts MM, Levine D: Treatment of Lisfranc fracture-dislocations with primary partial arthrodesis. *Foot Ankle Int* 2012;33:50. [PMID: 22381236]

Saltzman CL, Mann RA, Ahrens JE, et al: Prospective controlled trial of STAR total ankle replacement versus ankle fusion: initial results. *Foot Ankle Int* 2009;30:579. [PMID: 19589303]

Segal AD, Shofer J, Hahn ME, Orendurff MS, Ledoux WR, Sangeorzan BJ: Functional limitations associated with end-stage ankle arthritis. *J Bone Joint Surg Am* 2012;94:777. [PMID: 22552666]

Valderrabano V, Pagenstert G, Horisberger M, et al: Sports and recreation activity of ankle arthritis patients before and after total ankle replacement. *Am J Sports Med* 2006;34:993. [PMID: 16452268]

CONGENITAL FLATFOOT

Congenital flatfoot is the term used to describe a flatfoot present since birth. The condition may not be apparent during the early years of life but is usually identified toward the end of the first or during the second decade. The typical asymptomatic flexible flatfoot is probably a normal variant of the longitudinal arch. This deformity must be differentiated from the symptomatic flexible or more rigid flatfoot, which usually will become symptomatic in the early teen years and is often caused by a tarsal coalition. A tarsal coalition is the union of two or more tarsal bones, usually occurring between the calcaneus and the navicular or between the talus and the calcaneus. This process is a congenital failure of segmentation between the bones of the hindfoot. Coalitions are usually not symptomatic until adolescence, with symptoms brought on by increasing stiffness of the hindfoot as the cartilaginous coalition begins to ossify. These individuals have a fairly flexible foot until adolescence, when the foot often becomes somewhat more rigid and symptomatic.

The patient with a tarsal coalition will frequently present with a peroneal spastic flatfoot, usually around the age of 10–12 years. The theory is that the foot is locked in a valgus position by the peroneal muscle spasm that is trying to immobilize the painful peritalar joints. The navicular bone usually forms from three ossification centers inside the original cartilage, and occasionally, the medial center fails to coalesce with the main body, leaving a synchondrosis that is called an accessory navicular. Flatfoot associated with an accessory navicular bone usually becomes symptomatic in the early to mid teenage years and may be unilateral or bilateral.

Residual congenital deformity from conditions such as clubfoot or congenital vertical talus is present from birth and is discussed in Chapter 10, "Pediatric Orthopedic Surgery."

The patient with generalized dysplasia such as Marfan syndrome or Ehlers-Danlos syndrome may present with flatfoot. A generalized ligamentous laxity will be present from the time of birth, and the diagnosis is usually already known.

Clinical Findings

A. Symptoms and Signs

The clinical evaluation begins with the patient in a standing position. In all cases of congenital flatfoot, the longitudinal arch flattens when the patient is standing. In the case of tarsal coalition with peroneal spastic flatfoot, the calcaneus is in a severe fixed valgus position. A tarsal coalition or an accessory navicular may be unilateral, as well as the residuals of a congenital deformity such as clubfoot or congenital vertical talus. The symptomatic and asymptomatic flexible flatfoot and the generalized dysplasias are present bilaterally.

The physical examination of these patients is extremely important. The asymptomatic flexible flatfoot will usually demonstrate a satisfactory range of motion and no contracture of the Achilles tendon. The symptomatic flexible flatfoot, however, will almost invariably demonstrate an equinus contracture. To adequately test for tightness of the Achilles tendon, the head of the talus is covered with the navicular, after which the foot is brought up into dorsiflexion with the knee extended. If the foot is brought into dorsiflexion, permitting lateral subluxation of the talonavicular joint, the examiner often is fooled into thinking that dorsiflexion is adequate when indeed it is not.

The patient with tarsal coalition usually demonstrates restricted hindfoot motion secondary to peroneal spasm and to the cartilaginous or bony bar. The peroneal tendons can actually be felt to be bow-strung behind the fibula, not permitting any passive or active inversion of the subtalar joint to occur. On occasion, clonus can be elicited. As a rule, stressing of these joints causes the patient increased discomfort. In flatfoot associated with an accessory navicular, pain is present over the prominence. Frequently, stressing of the posterior tibial tendon aggravates the condition. The patient with residual congenital deformity often demonstrates a certain degree of stiffness of the foot and, not infrequently, varying degrees of deformity of the remainder of the foot. The patient with generalized dysplasia demonstrates marked hypermobility of all the joints, with no contractures whatsoever.

B. Imaging Studies

The radiographic evaluation is useful in differentiating the various types of flatfoot. In almost all cases, the lateral view shows a lack of normal dorsiflexion pitch of the calcaneus, which is approximately 20 degrees or more. In symptomatic flexible flatfoot, the calcaneus may even be in a mild degree of equinus position. On the lateral radiograph, a line drawn through the long axis of the talus and first metatarsal will demonstrate an angle of more than 30 degrees in severe flatfoot, 15–30 degrees in moderate flatfoot, and 0–15 degrees in mild flatfoot (Figure 8–43).

The calcaneonavicular coalition is best observed on an oblique radiograph and is identified as a bridge from the anterior process of the calcaneus to the inferior lateral aspect of the navicular. The subtalar or talocalcaneal bar is best demonstrated on a CT scan taken in the coronal plane. Flatfoot associated with an accessory navicular demonstrates the accessory bone along the medial side of the navicular, but occasionally a medial oblique view is necessary to outline the size of the fragment. In a patient with a residual congenital deformity, such as a clubfoot or congenital vertical talus, the changes about the foot will often be sufficient to make the diagnosis fairly obvious. The patient with generalized

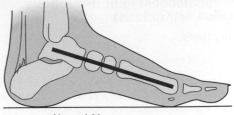

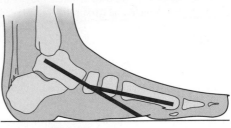

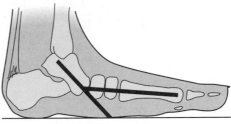

▲ **Figure 8–43.** Measurement of flatfoot deformity by using the lateral talometatarsal angle: 0 degrees, normal; 1–15 degrees, mild; 16–30 degrees, moderate; and >30 degrees, severe. (Reproduced, with permission, from Bordelon RL: Correction of hypermobile flatfoot children by molded insert. *Foot Ankle* 1980;1:143.)

dysplasia often demonstrates complete collapse of the longitudinal arch.

▶ Treatment

A. Conservative Management

Conservative management is undertaken for congenital flatfoot deformities. A longitudinal arch support may benefit the patient but is usually not necessary for the asymptomatic flexible flatfoot. For symptomatic flexible flatfoot, a semirigid longitudinal arch support and Achilles stretching exercises may be of some benefit.

The tarsal coalition can be treated conservatively with a short leg walking cast, followed by a polypropylene ankle-foot orthosis or a University of California Biomechanics Laboratory (UCBL) insert. If adequate pain relief is achieved, further treatment is not necessary. Flatfoot with an accessory navicular may respond to modification of the shoe to relieve some of the pressure from the involved area. Occasionally, the use of a longitudinal arch support will relieve the pressure.

Residual flatfoot resulting from congenital problems can be treated with an ankle-foot orthosis or UCBL insert if symptomatic. The patient with generalized dysplasia usually does not require any treatment at all.

B. Surgical Management

Surgical procedures are never appropriate for asymptomatic flatfoot. Symptomatic flexible or semiflexible flatfoot occasionally is treated surgically, particularly if equinus contracture is observed after age 5 or 6 years. A significant equinus contracture may benefit from lengthening of the Achilles tendon. A lateral column lengthening procedure, such as an Evans calcaneal osteotomy, is indicated in cases of symptomatic flexible flatfoot that have failed conservative management. This procedure helps to correct heel valgus and forefoot abduction and should be done as late into growth as possible to avoid disturbing open growth centers. Rarely should a triple arthrodesis be carried out because this leaves a young patient with a very stiff foot.

A tarsal coalition that does not respond to conservative management may require resection. The surgical approach to the calcaneonavicular bar is identical to that of the subtalar joint. The bar is carefully outlined and then resected in its entirety. Talocalcaneal coalitions are resectable throughout the adolescent years, if less than 20% of the posterior facet of the subtalar joint is involved or if the coalition is confined only to the middle facet. More extensive involvement of the subtalar joint in an adolescent or any bar in an adult patient is an indication for subtalar arthrodesis. The approach is through a medial incision centered over the middle facet, and caution is taken to carefully reflect the tendons and posterior tibial nerve. The extent of the coalition is identified, and it is resected to expose the area of normal-appearing articular cartilage. Bone wax is applied to the edges or a free fat graft is inserted to prevent re-formation of the bar. Flatfoot associated with an accessory navicular may require excision of the accessory navicular and plication of the posterior tibial tendon (Kidner procedure). This fairly successful operation is usually carried out during the late adolescent years.

Residual congenital deformity or generalized dysplasias usually will not require surgical management. In severe cases, a triple arthrodesis is indicated after the foot has matured.

Coleman S: *Complex Foot Deformities in Children.* Philadelphia, PA: Lea and Febiger; 1983.

Evans D: Calcaneo-valgus deformity. *J Bone Joint Surg* 1979;57:270. [PMID: 1171869]

Zaw H, Calder JD: Tarsal coalitions. *Foot Ankle Clin* 2010;15:349. [PMID: 20534361]

ACQUIRED FLATFOOT DEFORMITY

Acquired flatfoot deformity is a condition affecting a foot that at one time had a normal functioning longitudinal arch. Over time, the arch progressively flattens, often causing the foot to become symptomatic. This deformity is different from congenital flatfoot deformity, present since birth. Acquired flatfoot deformity in the adult may be caused by the following conditions:

1. Posterior tibial tendon dysfunction
2. Arthrosis of the tarsometatarsal joints, which may be primary or secondary to a previous Lisfranc fracture or dislocation
3. Charcot changes in the midfoot resulting from a peripheral neuropathy
4. Talonavicular collapse resulting from trauma or rheumatoid arthritis

Acquired flatfoot deformities are complex deformities that affect different areas of the midfoot and hindfoot. The deformities may include dorsal subluxation of the talonavicular joint and tarsometatarsal joints, abduction of the forefoot, valgus deformity of the hindfoot, or all three. The extent of the deformity varies widely and is usually progressive. Depending on the etiology, acquired flatfoot deformity may affect a patient bilaterally.

Clinical Findings

A. Symptoms and Signs

A careful history is important to help distinguish among differing causes of acquired flatfoot deformity. Usually, no specific traumatic event is recalled by the patient who presents with dysfunction of the posterior tibial tendon. In approximately half of patients with tarsometatarsal joint arthrosis, a Lisfranc fracture-dislocation has occurred, whereas the other half has primary arthrosis. The patient with Charcot foot usually gives a relevant history of the cause of the peripheral neuropathy, such as diabetes. The patient with collapse of the talonavicular joint gives a history of prior trauma to the talus or navicular or has rheumatoid arthritis, which causes disruption of the spring ligament complex.

The physical examination begins by observing the foot with the patient standing, observing for unilateral or bilateral flattening of the longitudinal arch. Varying degrees of abduction of the forefoot and hindfoot valgus should also be evaluated.

The patient with posterior tibial tendon dysfunction demonstrates little or no active inversion strength. Usually, the posterior tibial tendon is thick and swollen, and there is increased warmth and pain to palpation over the tendon sheath. When the patient is asked to stand on tiptoe, the involved calcaneus remains in valgus position rather than inverting, as normally occurs. When the patient is viewed from the posterior aspect, more toes are visible laterally on the involved foot than the uninvolved foot, commonly known as the "too many toes sign."

Arthrosis of the tarsometatarsal joints creates a deformity of abduction of the forefoot with varying degrees of dorsi-flexion, giving rise to a rather prominent medial cuneiform. Not infrequently, palpable osteophytes are present on the dorsal and plantar aspect of the tarsometatarsal joints.

A Charcot foot presents with varying degrees of swelling and deformity. In the early stages, the foot demonstrates generalized swelling and increased warmth, with loss of sensation in a stocking-glove distribution. Deformity may vary from a mild flat foot to a severe rocker-bottom deformity. It is important to palpate for bony prominences on the medial and plantar aspects of the foot that make it at risk for ulcerations.

In the patient with rheumatoid arthritis, most of the changes occur within the talonavicular joint. In this case, the head of the talus is often palpable on the plantar medial aspect of the foot. When the subtalar joint is more involved, a fixed hindfoot valgus deformity is usually present as well.

The posttraumatic deformity may vary, depending on precisely which joints are involved. If trauma led to a collapse of the navicular, the longitudinal arch is flattened with little forefoot abduction, and the head of the talus is often palpable on the plantar medial aspect of the foot. There is usually little or no motion in the hindfoot and midfoot joints.

B. Imaging Studies

Radiographs usually differentiate the cause of the problem. In the patient with posterior tibial tendon dysfunction, there is sagging of the talonavicular joint and abduction of the navicular on the head of the talus. The patient with tarso-metatarsal joint arthrosis demonstrates typical degenerative changes at the affected joints, along with varying degrees of lateral and dorsal subluxation of the joints. Patients with Charcot foot demonstrate characteristic changes seen in a neuropathic joint, including dramatic bone destruction and joint dislocations (Figure 8–44). The patient with rheumatoid

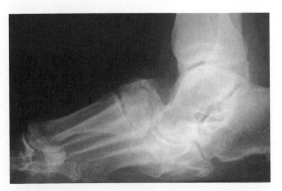

▲ **Figure 8–44.** Charcot midfoot changes resulting in joint dislocations and a rocker-bottom deformity of the foot.

arthritis demonstrates the typical destructive changes observed with this disease process, with joint space narrowing but little osteophyte formation.

▶ Treatment

A. Conservative Management

Conservative management is aimed at providing support to the longitudinal arch and ankle with a polypropylene ankle-foot orthosis (AFO). The orthosis must be shaped to accommodate any prominences that might be present. Unfortunately, these prominences present the potential for skin breakdown, particularly in the neuropathic foot. A rocker-bottom-type shoe with an adequate toe box is sometimes indicated to give the patient a smoother gait pattern.

B. Surgical Treatment

The surgical management of these various conditions is specific for each problem. Posterior tibial tendon dysfunction with a satisfactory ROM of the joints of the hindfoot and midfoot can be treated with reconstruction of the posterior tibial tendon, using a flexor digitorum longus tendon transfer. A calcaneal osteotomy is performed as well, if a significant valgus deformity of the heel is present. Alternatively, a lateral column lengthening, consisting of a calcaneal-cuboid distraction arthrodesis, can be used to correct a flexible flatfoot with significant abduction of the forefoot. When a fixed deformity is present in the hindfoot or forefoot, a triple arthrodesis is indicated.

The patient with Charcot foot is treated in a short leg cast until the acute process subsides, after which a polypropylene AFO is used. Occasionally, a bony prominence that continues to cause skin breakdown may be excised to permit the patient to use an AFO. In extreme rocker-bottom deformities, midfoot correction with an osteotomy may be required. The rheumatoid patient usually requires stabilization of the involved area with an isolated talonavicular fusion if little deformity is present, or a triple arthrodesis if there is a hindfoot or midfoot deformity.

The posttraumatic foot with involvement of the talonavicular joint requires a triple arthrodesis. The fusion may need to be extended distally to include the naviculocuneiform joints if arthrosis is present at these joints.

The patient with arthrosis of the tarsometatarsal joints responds well to surgical management by realigning the foot and carrying out arthrodesis of the involved joints.

Bolt PM, Coy S, Toolan BC: A comparison of lateral column lengthening and medial translational osteotomy of the calcaneus for the reconstruction of adult acquired flatfoot. *Foot Ankle Int* 2007;28:1115. [PMID: 18021579]

Brodsky JW, Charlick DA, Coleman SC, Pollo FE, Royer CT: Hindfoot motion following reconstruction for posterior tibial tendon dysfunction. *Foot Ankle Int* 2009;30:613. [PMID: 19589306]

Deland JT: Adult-acquired flatfoot deformity. *J Am Acad Orthop Surg* 2008;16:399. [PMID: 18611997]

Ellis SJ, Williams BR, Wagshul AD, Pavlov H, Deland JT: Deltoid ligament reconstruction with peroneus longus autograft in flatfoot. *Foot Ankle Int* 2010;31:781. [PMID: 20880481]

Grier KM, Walling AK: The use of tricortical autograft versus allograft in lateral column lengthening for adult acquired flatfoot deformity: an analysis of union rates and complications. *Foot Ankle Int* 2010;31:760. [PMID: 20880478]

Lin JL, Balbas J, Richardson G: Results of non-surgical treatment of stage II posterior tibial tendon dysfunction: a 7- to 10-year follow up. *Foot Ankle Int* 2008;29:781. [PMID: 18752775]

O'Connor K, Baumhauer J, Houck JR: Patient factors in the selection of operative versus nonoperative treatment for posterior tibial dysfunction. *Foot Ankle Int* 2010;31:197. [PMID: 20230697]

CAVUS FOOT

Cavus foot deformity is characterized by an abnormal elevation of the longitudinal arch, with resulting decrease in the plantar weight-bearing area and stress concentrated on the metatarsal heads. The condition may be aggravated by clawing of the toes, further reducing the forefoot weight-bearing area. Generalized stiffness of the joints is common, causing the patient to avoid prolonged use of the foot.

► Etiologic Findings

The various causes of cavus foot deformity include the following:

1. Anterior horn cell disease, such as poliomyelitis, diastematomyelia, and spinal cord tumor

2. Nerve disorders, such as Charcot-Marie-Tooth disease and spinal dysraphism

3. Muscular diseases, such as muscular dystrophy

4. Long tract and central diseases, such as Friedreich ataxia and cerebral palsy

5. Idiopathic conditions, such as residual clubfoot, arthrogryposis, and cavus foot of undetermined cause

6. Posttraumatic disorders following injuries, such as compartment syndrome or crush injury

► Anatomy

Cavus foot deformity is extremely variable in its presentation, from a mild to extremely severe degree of cavus. The types of deformities can be classified based on localizing of the area of deformity.

A. Posterior Cavus Deformity

This deformity mainly involves the calcaneus, which has a dorsiflexion pitch angle of greater than 40 degrees measured on a weight-bearing lateral radiograph. Normally, the dorsiflexion pitch to the calcaneus is approximately 20 degrees. Some degree of varus deformity of the heel is usually present as well.

B. Anterior Cavus Deformity

In anterior cavus deformity, there is a forefoot equinus deformity with the hindfoot in a neutral position. The anterior cavus may be localized, mainly involving the first and second metatarsal, or it may be more global, with the entire forefoot in a position of plantar flexion. Some degree of adduction of the forefoot is usually present.

C. Combined Cavus Deformity

In a combined cavus deformity, which is the most severe, there are both anterior and posterior components.

► Clinical Findings

A. Symptoms and Signs

A careful history regarding the onset of the condition and progression is important. A detailed family history should also be obtained because idiopathic cavus deformity does tend to run in families. Progression of deformity should be ascertained, particularly in the adolescent, because it may indicate a spinal cord abnormality or neoplasm. Activity level and ambulation should also be carefully evaluated as markers of progression of neural or muscular disease.

The degree of deformity of the foot must be examined with the patient in a standing position. This also reveals any evidence of atrophy of the calf muscles, as seen in Charcot-Marie-Tooth disease, clubfoot, or arthrogryposis. The active and passive ROM of the joints of the foot and ankle should be carefully measured. The muscle strength of each muscle must be carefully evaluated, especially if considering a tendon transfer. The degree of deformity and flexibility of the rearfoot, forefoot, metatarsophalangeal joints, and lesser toes must be ascertained. The presence of a tight plantar fascia should also be noted. The lateral ankle ligaments must be evaluated for integrity because they often become stretched out with long-standing varus heel deformity.

B. Imaging Studies

Weight-bearing radiographs of the foot and ankle are obtained to help classify the type of cavus deformity and formulate a treatment plan. Any degree of arthrosis or varus tilting of the talus in the ankle mortise is also evaluated.

► Treatment

A. Conservative Management

Conservative care is tailored to the severity of the cavus deformity. Mild deformities may only require a softer-soled shoe. Significant clawing of the lesser toes may require an extra-depth shoe. A custom-made Plastazote liner with a built-in arch support helps decrease the stress on the metatarsal heads. A significant motor deficit may require an AFO to stabilize the ankle. Most cases of cavus foot can be managed with conservative modalities.

B. Surgical Treatment

Surgical treatment for the cavus foot is aimed at correcting the site of the deformity. The most frequent pattern consists of plantar flexion of the first metatarsal, contracture of the plantar fascia, and varus deformity of the calcaneus. These problems respond to release of the plantar fascia, dorsiflexion osteotomy of the first and perhaps second metatarsal, and lateral closing-wedge osteotomy (Dwyer procedure) of the calcaneus to correct the varus deformity. Fusion of the joints is avoided to maintain as much flexibility of the foot as possible (Figure 8–45).

A more severe deformity involving dorsiflexion of the calcaneus can be treated with sliding osteotomy of the calcaneus (Samilson procedure), correcting any varus deformity with a lateral closing-wedge osteotomy and releasing the plantar fascia (Figure 8–46). Forefoot deformity is treated with osteotomy of the first and sometimes second

metatarsal. In some patients, transfer of the peroneus longus tendon into the brevis and lengthening of the posterior tibial tendon provides dynamic muscle balance for the foot.

Severe deformities not amenable to procedures that retain joint motion require triple arthrodesis. A Siffert beak-type triple arthrodesis corrects the deformity because the navicular is mortised under the head of the talus to help reduce the elevation of the longitudinal arch (Figure 8–47). A first metatarsal osteotomy may need to be added to the procedure as well.

The lesser toes may have either fixed or flexible claw toe deformities. Flexible deformity often responds to release of the extensor tendons and a Girdlestone flexor tendon transfer. If a fixed deformity is present, a DuVries phalangeal condylectomy corrects the hammer toe, followed by extensor tendon release and the Girdlestone procedure.

Hyperextension of the first metatarsophalangeal joint is corrected by interphalangeal arthrodesis of the hallux and transfer of the extensor hallucis longus tendon into the neck of the first metatarsal (Jones procedure).

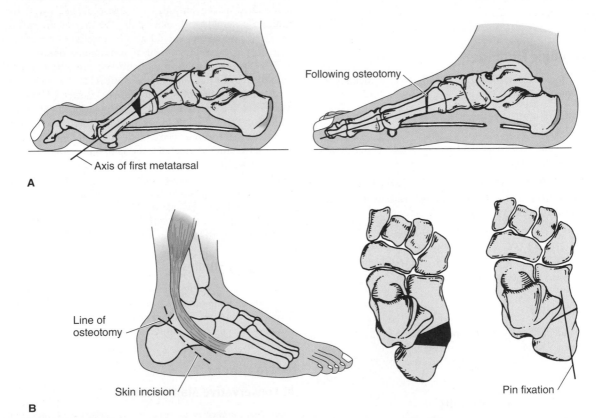

A

B

▲ **Figure 8–45.** Technique for correction of cavus foot. **A:** For first metatarsal osteotomy, a dorsally based wedge of bone was removed approximately 1 cm distal to the metatarsocuneiform joint. The plantar fascia was released. Dorsiflexion of the osteotomy site helps correct the cavus deformity by flattening the arch. **B:** Heel varus is corrected by a closing-wedge calcaneus osteotomy. (Reproduced, with permission, from Mann RA, Coughlin MJ: *The Video Textbook of Foot and Ankle Surgery.* Medical Video Productions, 1991.)

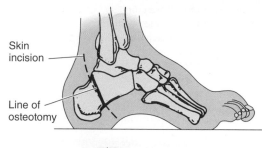

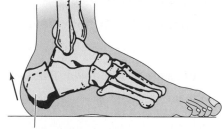

Skin incision

Line of osteotomy

Dorsal displacement of posterior calcaneus

▲ **Figure 8–46.** Techniques of calcaneal osteotomy. In the treatment of pes cavus, the osteotomy permits the calcaneus to be moved into a more dorsal position and, if necessary, to be closed laterally to correct heel varus. (Reproduced, with permission, from Mann RA, Coughlin MJ: *The Video Textbook of Foot and Ankle Surgery*. Medical Video Productions, 1991.)

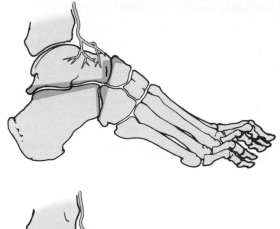

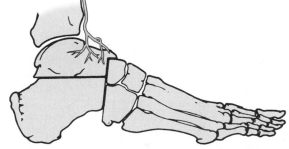

▲ **Figure 8–47.** A diagram of a beak-type triple arthrodesis. This mortises the navicular underneath a portion of the head of the talus to allow rotation of the distal portion of the foot, permitting flattening of the longitudinal arch and correction of the cavus deformity. (Reproduced, with permission, from Mann RA, Coughlin MJ: *The Video Textbook of Foot and Ankle Surgery*. Medical Video Productions, 1991.)

Breusch SJ, Wenz W, Döderlein L: Function after correction of a clawed great toe by a modified Robert Jones transfer. *J Bone Joint Surg Br* 2000;82B:250. [PMID: 10755436]

Giannini S, Ceccarelli F, Benedetti MG, et al: Surgical treatment of adult idiopathic cavus foot with plantar fasciotomy, naviculocuneiform arthrodesis, and cuboid osteotomy. A review of thirty-nine cases. *J Bone Joint Surg Am* 2002;84-A(Suppl 2):62. [PMID: 12479341]

Siffert RS, del Torto U: "Beak" triple arthrodesis for severe cavus deformity. *Clin Orthop Relat Res* 1983;181:64. [PMID: 6641068]

Sammarco GJ, Taylor R: Cavovarus foot treated with combined calcaneus and metatarsal osteotomies. *Foot Ankle Int* 2001;22:19. [PMID: 11206819]

Vienne P, Schoniger R, Helmy N, Espinosa N: Hindfoot instability in cavovarus deformity: static and dynamic balancing. *Foot Ankle Int* 2007;28:96. [PMID: 17257547]

Ward CM, Dolan LA, Bennett L, Morcuende JA, Cooper RR: Long-term results of reconstruction for treatment of a flexible cavovarus foot in Charcot-Marie-Tooth disease. *J Bone Joint Surg Am* 2008;90:2631. [PMID: 19047708]

ORTHOTIC DEVICES FOR THE FOOT AND ANKLE

Orthotic devices are used to redistribute stresses on the foot as it makes contact with the ground and to accommodate for abnormal function of defective muscles or ligaments.

This is achieved by controlling the posture of the foot and padding certain areas to relieve pressure and provide increased comfort for the foot. Orthoses are also used to limit motion in arthritic joints, making them less painful. The orthotic device may be attached to the sole of the shoe, may be inserted inside the shoe as an insole, may cup the foot (UCBL insert), or may extend across the ankle to hold the entire foot and ankle in place (AFO).

▶ Orthotic Shoe Sole Devices

A variety of heel and sole corrections are available to accommodate foot postural abnormalities. A medial or lateral heel or sole wedge (or a combination of both) can help control excessive pronation or supination from weak tendons, ligamentous instability, or fixed deformities. A wide heel is used to increase the stability of the subtalar joint. A rocker sole helps stabilize the forefoot in the case of a fracture or arthritis and also aids a patient with an ankle fusion to allow a more normal gait pattern.

Orthotic Insole Devices

Insole orthotic devices can be used for flexible deformities to alter the posture of the foot and for fixed deformities to redistribute stress. The simplest device is a soft liner for a shoe or boot made out of a high-density foam material. Other simple orthoses include a soft felt pad to relieve pressure on the metatarsal heads or a combination of materials to produce a more rigid support to help control a forefoot deformity such as forefoot varus or valgus deformity. Orthotic devices take up space in the shoe, and the patient may need a larger or deeper shoe.

University of California Biomechanics Laboratory Insert

The principle of the UCBL insert is to correct a foot deformity such as flatfoot by stabilizing the calcaneus in neutral position and molding the orthosis to block abduction of the forefoot. Posting along the medial aspect may compensate for forefoot varus. In theory, this orthotic device is excellent for controlling the rearfoot and forefoot, but two caveats apply to the use of this device. The first is that the foot must be flexible because correction of a rigid deformity is impossible. The second is that a bony prominence can chafe against the polypropylene material, resulting in pain or skin breakdown over the prominence.

Ankle-Foot Orthosis

An AFO is a molded polypropylene device that passes along the posterior aspect of the calf and then onto the plantar aspect of the foot to the metatarsal heads. Alterations are made in a variety of ways to accommodate the patient's problem. Ankle problems such as arthrosis or dorsiflexion weakness require adequate rigidity to eliminate ankle joint motion. An orthosis for a subtalar joint problem should have enough flexibility to provide ankle joint motion but must be rigid enough to immobilize the subtalar joint. When the problem involves the transverse tarsal joint, the AFO can be fabricated to permit some ankle joint motion but maintain immobilization of the transverse tarsal joint area, usually by blocking abduction of the forefoot. When managing tarsometatarsal arthritis, the footpiece is carried to the tips of the toes. Again, a significant fixed bony deformity results in pressure points, making fitting of the device difficult. If the patient has loss of sensation, careful construction and padding are essential to minimize the risk of ulcers forming over a bony prominence. In cases of marked instability or discomfort, an anterior shell can be added to the AFO, and the brace is extended proximally to create a patellar tendon bearing surface.

Double Upright Orthosis

The double upright orthosis with a hinged ankle may be used when individuals require stability but are engaged in physically demanding activities. The double upright orthosis is somewhat more cumbersome than the AFO but provides rigid immobilization. The hinge mechanism of the ankle joint may be changed, depending on the nature of the patient's problem. The ankle joint can be free, which allows dorsiflexion and plantar flexion to occur, or it can be fixed to prevent plantar flexion past 90 degrees. This brace can be modified with a spring load to provide dorsiflexion for the patient with dropfoot resulting from paralysis but should not be used for the patient with spasticity because it may accentuate the spasticity.

Prescriptions for Orthotic Devices

The following are typical prescriptions for orthotic devices.

A. Metatarsalgia or Atrophy of Plantar Fat Pad

1. Treatment—A full-length well-molded orthosis for metatarsal arch support is used to relieve pressure under the metatarsal heads. Soft insole material should be used.

2. Explanation—In the treatment of metatarsalgia or atrophy of the plantar fat pad, a full-length orthosis is needed that is molded to the plantar aspect of the foot and built up just proximal to the metatarsal heads to relieve pressure on them. The material should be soft to provide extra cushioning for the foot.

B. Ruptured Posterior Tibial Tendon With Moderately Severe Flexible Flatfoot Deformity

1. Treatment—AFO with trim-line cut to permit 30% ankle joint motion is molded to reestablish the longitudinal arch and built up on the lateral aspect of the footpiece to block abduction of the forefoot.

2. Explanation—With a moderately advanced flexible flatfoot deformity, an in-shoe orthotic device alone does not provide sufficient support; the AFO is needed to provide adequate stability. Some ankle joint motion is included, which makes ambulation more comfortable for the patient. The longitudinal arch is molded to support the foot in a plantigrade position, and the lateral aspect of the AFO is built up to prevent the forefoot from moving into an abducted position. By blocking abduction, the amount of pressure needed beneath the longitudinal arch to prevent it from collapsing is decreased.

C. Posterior Tibial Tendon Insufficiency With Mild Flatfoot Deformity and 5 Degrees of Forefoot Varus Deformity

1. Treatment—Use a well-molded longitudinal arch support, with a 5-degree varus post and a 3-degree medial heel lift.

2. Explanation—Insufficiency of the posterior tibial tendon that has not produced a significant foot deformity can be treated with a well-molded longitudinal arch support. The 5-degree varus forefoot post compensates for the fixed forefoot varus, and the 3-degree heel lift likewise helps tilt the hindfoot from valgus deformity closer to neutral position.

D. Dropfoot Secondary to Peroneal Nerve Injury

1. Treatment—An AFO with a full footpiece is molded to the longitudinal arch.

2. Explanation—A dropfoot secondary to a peroneal nerve injury responds well to an AFO with a full footpiece. The footpiece supports the toes so they do not drop and makes it easier for the patient to put on shoes.

E. Diabetic Neuropathy With Clawfoot Deformity

1. Treatment—An extra-depth shoe with a molded Plastazote liner is backed with a Pelite material.

2. Explanation—The patient with clawfoot deformity requires a shoe that has extra height in the toe box. The extra-depth shoe provides enough room for the toes, so they do not chafe against the top of the shoe. The molded Plastazote liner is an excellent means of providing full contact to the plantar aspect of the foot. Plastazote has a tendency to bottom out, as it were, and by backing the material with a Pelite liner or some comparable material, the life expectancy of the Plastazote is extended significantly.

Brodsky JW, Pollo FE, Cheleuitte D, Baum BS: Physical properties, durability and energy-dissipation function of dual-density orthotic materials used in insoles for diabetic patients. *Foot Ankle Int* 2007;28:880. [PMID: 17697652]

Collins N, Bisset L, McPoil T, Vicenzino B: Foot orthoses in lower limb overuse conditions: a systematic review and meta-analysis. *Foot Ankle Int* 2007;28:396. [PMID: 17371668]

DiLiberto FE, Baumhauer JF, Wilding GE, Nawoczenski DA: Alterations in plantar pressure with different walking boot designs. *Foot Ankle Int* 2007;28:55. [PMID: 17257539]

Guillebastre B, Calmels P, Rougier P: Effects of rigid and dynamic ankle-foot orthoses on normal gait. *Foot Ankle Int* 2009;30:51. [PMID: 19176186]

Janisse DJ, Janisse E: Shoe modification and use of orthoses in treatment of foot and ankle pathology. *J Am Acad Orthop Surg* 2008;16:152. [PMID: 18316713]

Neville C, Lemley FR: Effect of ankle-foot orthotic devices on foot kinematics in stage II posterior tibial tendon dysfunction. *Foot Ankle Int* 2012;33:406. [PMID: 22735283]

LIGAMENTOUS INJURIES ABOUT THE ANKLE JOINT

Ankle ligament injuries represent the most common musculoskeletal injury; therefore, accurate assessment and treatment of these injuries are important. The lateral collateral ligament complex is most commonly injured, but damage to other important structures around the ankle joint should not be overlooked, as discussed in this section.

▶ Functional Anatomy

The lateral collateral ligament structure of the ankle consists of three distinct ligamentous bands: the anterior and posterior talofibular ligaments (ATFL and PTFL) and the calcaneal fibular ligament (CFL).

When the ankle joint is in plantar flexion, the ATFL is positioned in line with the fibula and therefore placed under stress with an inversion injury and will be damaged. Conversely, when the ankle joint is in dorsiflexion, the CFL is positioned in line with the long axis of the fibula and is therefore subject to injury. If the applied stress is severe, both the ATFL and the CFL may be torn, no matter the position of the ankle joint. The syndesmosis ligament complex tethers the tibia and fibula together and is injured by an external rotational force to the foot. The deltoid ligament is the sole medial stabilizer of the ankle joint. An isolated deltoid ligament injury can occur with an eversion or external rotation force on the foot. The deltoid ligament can also sustain injury in conjunction with a syndesmosis ligament injury, with lateral ankle sprains, or with a concomitant fibula fracture (known as a Maisonneuve fracture).

▶ Clinical Findings

A. Classification

Lateral collateral ankle ligament injuries are divided into three degrees of severity. A grade I sprain is confined to the ATFL and demonstrates no instability. A grade II sprain involves injury to both the ATFL and CFL, with mild laxity of one or both ligaments. A grade III sprain involves injury and significant laxity of both the ATFL and CFL.

B. Symptoms and Signs

A past history of injuries of the ankle and problems with chronic ankle ligament instability should be ascertained. A careful physical examination is important to evaluate the degree of involvement of each ligament and to rule out injury to any adjacent bony or soft-tissue structures. The ATFL, PTFL, CFL, and syndesmosis ligaments are palpated for tenderness. To rule out fractures, pain should be elicited in the area of the distal fibula, the anterior process of the calcaneus, the lateral process of the talus, and at the base of the fifth metatarsal. Other areas where an injury must be ruled out include the subtalar joint and the peroneal tendon sheath.

A patient with significant medial joint pain with or without lateral ligament pain should be evaluated for an injury to the deltoid ligament complex, the posterior tibial tendon, and the medial talar dome. Assessment of ankle ligament stability requires clinical and radiographic stress examinations. To perform an anterior drawer maneuver, which tests stability of the ATFL, the ankle is placed in 30 degrees of equinus, and the ankle is pulled in an anterior and slightly internally rotated direction (Figure 8–48). A feeling of subluxation is present if a significant ligament injury has occurred. A talar tilt maneuver

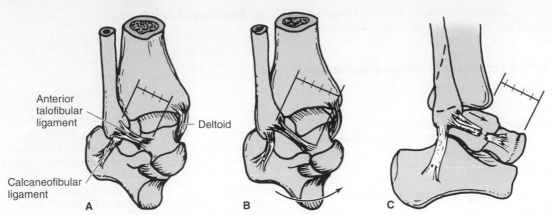

▲ **Figure 8–48.** Mechanics of carrying out a stress test of the lateral ankle ligaments. **A:** Normal anatomic alignment, which demonstrates the checkrein effect of the anterior talofibular ligament on the talus. **B:** The stress test for the calcaneofibular ligament is carried out by firmly inverting the calcaneus. **C:** The anterior talofibular ligament is tested by placing the ankle joint in neutral position and applying an anterior pull with slight medial rotation. (Reproduced, with permission, from Mann RA, Coughlin MJ, eds: *Surgery of the Foot and Ankle*, 6th ed. St. Louis: Mosby-Year Book; 1993.)

is performed by placing an inversion stress on the heel. With the foot in plantar flexion, this tests the stability of the ATFL. With the foot in neutral or dorsiflexion, a talar tilt maneuver tests the stability of the CFL. If clinical instability is suggested by either maneuver, radiographic confirmation can be performed, with comparison to the unaffected ankle.

Deltoid ligament insufficiency may cause a feeling of instability and giving way, affecting the medial aspect of the ankle joint. Stress examination is performed by pulling the foot laterally and into valgus while stabilizing the distal tibia.

Injury to the syndesmosis ligament complex is suspected if the region between the distal anterior tibia and fibula is tender to palpation. If extensive swelling is present more than 2 cm proximal to the ankle joint, syndesmosis rupture is a strong possibility. Pain elicited by squeezing the tibia and fibula together in the midcalf is diagnostic of a syndesmosis ligament tear. A syndesmosis ligament injury is also suspected if external rotation of the foot is painful or if lateral translation of the talus in the ankle mortise occurs with direct lateral force on the foot.

C. Imaging Studies

Standard anteroposterior, lateral, and oblique radiographs of the ankle should be obtained to rule out a fracture of the fibula, talus, or calcaneus. If ligament laxity is suggested on clinical examination, stress radiographs should be obtained. An anteroposterior view is taken while a talar tilt maneuver is performed, and a lateral view is taken while an anterior drawer maneuver is performed. More than 10 degrees of tilt and more than 5–7 mm of anterior drawer are considered abnormal.

If a syndesmosis ligament injury is suspected, careful attention must be paid to the joint spaces to rule out widening of the ankle mortise. If instability is suspected, a stress radiograph is performed by externally rotating the foot with the tibia held still.

MRI or CT scan may be helpful in some instances if there is a high index of suspicion for an accompanying injury. Osteochondral injuries to the talus should be ruled out with an MRI scan. If a talus or calcaneus fracture is suspected, either MRI or CT scan may be of benefit.

▶ Treatment

A. Conservative Management

Acute grade I ligament tears are treated with a lateral stabilizing ankle brace, ice, and avoidance of painful activities. Immediate full weight bearing is allowed, as are non–weight-bearing physical activities, such as bicycling and swimming. The brace can be discontinued in 1 month.

Grade II ligament tears are treated with protected weight bearing and a lateral stabilizing ankle brace. The patient can begin non–weight-bearing exercise (stationary bicycle) after 7 days, along with peroneal strengthening exercises. Weight-bearing exercise (jogging) may resume after 2–4 weeks.

In a grade III ligament tear, the ankle is immobilized with a removable walking cast for 3–4 weeks. This is followed by a period of physical therapy consisting of ROM exercises, peroneal strengthening, and proprioception training using a biomechanical ankle platform system (BAPS) board.

Treatment of isolated deltoid ligament sprains depends on the severity of the injury and is similar to lateral ligament injuries. Mild injuries can be treated with immediate mobilization and rapid return to activity, whereas more severe injuries should be casted for 3–4 weeks.

Syndesmosis ligament tears, if mild, can be treated with weight bearing in a cast or brace and close follow-up to assess for widening of the ankle joint mortise. If the interosseous membrane is damaged, as evidenced by massive swelling of the leg proximal to the ankle joint, treatment depends on the radiographic appearance of the ankle. If the mortise has not widened, the patient is kept on a non–weight-bearing regimen in a cast for 6 weeks, with close radiographic follow-up. If initial or follow-up radiographs show a widened mortise, the patient requires surgical repair of the syndesmosis ligaments with temporary screw placement until the ligaments heal.

B. Surgical Treatment

The surgical treatment of an acute ligamentous injury is indicated only for the occasional elite athlete. Most ligamentous injuries, even grade III sprains, heal sufficiently with no significant disability if properly treated, as just described. However, even less severe ankle sprains may cause chronic pain or functional instability if left untreated.

The indication for a lateral ligament reconstruction is functional ligament instability. A patient with ligament instability complains of recurrent sprains that occur with sports activities or even with activities of daily living, despite 4–6 months of physical therapy and use of a lateral stabilizing brace. A patient with functional ligament instability also complains of difficulty walking on uneven ground. This history must be found in conjunction with physical examination findings of ligament instability.

Although many lateral ankle reconstruction procedures are described for chronic lateral ankle ligament instability, a Broström repair is generally the procedure of choice. The Broström procedure is a soft-tissue ligamentous repair in which the ATFL and CFL are plicated and reattached to their anatomic positions (Figure 8–49). The repair is reinforced by bringing up a portion of the inferior extensor retinaculum. The Broström procedure is highly effective and has lower morbidity than other procedures that harvest the peroneus brevis tendon. In patients who have severe and long-standing laxity or have failed a Broström repair, revision surgery with an allograft or autograft tendon is indicated.

Chronic lateral ankle pain following an ankle sprain may be caused by a previously undiagnosed condition rather

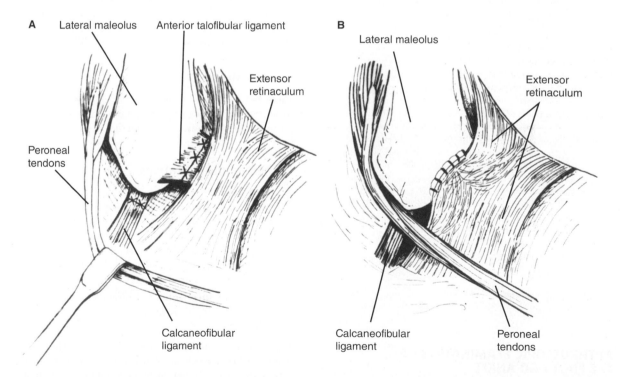

▲ **Figure 8–49.** Modified Broström anatomic reconstruction. **A:** Imbrication of anterior talofibular and calcaneofibular ligaments. **B:** Imbrication of inferior extensor retinaculum to reinforce the repair. (Reproduced, with permission, from Coughlin MJ, Mann RA, eds: *Surgery of the Foot and Ankle*, 7th ed. St. Louis: Mosby; 1999. Modified from Renstrom PA, Trevino S, eds: *Operative Techniques in Sports Medicine*, Vol. 2. New York: W.B. Saunders; 1994.)

than chronic ankle instability. The differential diagnosis for chronic ankle pain is similar to that following an acute injury and also includes subtalar joint instability, subtalar joint chondral damage or synovitis, and dislocating or torn peroneal tendons. Impingement of scar tissue in the lateral gutter between the talus and fibula may also cause chronic lateral ankle pain. In addition to a careful physical examination, an MRI or CT scan may be helpful for distinguishing among these possible causes of pain.

Surgical treatment may help relieve symptoms of chronic lateral ankle pain, once an accurate diagnosis is made. Chondral or osteochondral fractures involving the ankle or subtalar joints can be treated with arthroscopic or open debridement or pinning. Subtalar joint instability is addressed with a Broström procedure. A fracture of the anterior or lateral process of the talus is either removed if it is small or fixed if it is a large fragment. Tears or dislocations of the peroneal tendons are repaired or stabilized. Scar tissue in the lateral gutter can be treated with arthroscopic debridement.

Chronic instability of the deltoid ligament or syndesmosis ligament is uncommon but can occur after an untreated injury. Diagnosis of either condition is made with stress radiographs. Treatment usually requires a free tendon graft to reconstruct the damaged ligament, with the addition of internal fixation for chronic syndesmosis tears.

Ferkel RD, Chams RN: Chronic lateral instability: arthroscopic findings and long-term results. *Foot Ankle Int* 2007;28:24. [PMID: 17257534]

Hubbard TJ, Kramer LC, Denegar CR, Hertel J: Contributing factors to chronic ankle instability. *Foot Ankle Int* 2007;343-354. [PMID: 17371658]

Klitzman R, Zhao H, Zhang LQ, Strohmeyer G, Vora A: Suture-button versus screw fixation of the syndesmosis: a biomechanical analysis. *Foot Ankle Int* 2010;31:69. [PMID: 20067726]

Maffulli N, Ferran NA: Management of acute and chronic ankle instability. *J Am Acad Orthop Surg* 2008;16:608. [PMID: 18832604]

Panchbhavi VK, Vallurupalli S, Yang J, Andersen CR: Screw fixation compared with suture-button fixation of isolated Lisfranc ligament injuries. *J Bone Joint Surg Am* 2009;91:1143. [PMID: 19411463]

Pihlajamaki H, Hietaniemi K, Paavola M, Visuri T, Mattila VM: Surgical versus functional treatment for acute ruptures of the lateral ligament complex of the ankle in young men: a randomized controlled trial. *J Bone Joint Surg Am* 2010;92:2367-2374. [PMID: 20833874]

Zalavras C, Thordarson D: Ankle syndesmotic injury. *J Am Acad Orthop Surg* 2007;15:330. [PMID: 17548882]

ARTHROSCOPIC EXAMINATION OF THE FOOT AND ANKLE

Arthroscopy is an important tool for use in diagnosis and treatment of foot and ankle disorders. With developments in instrumentation, more ankle joint conditions can be treated arthroscopically. Arthroscopy of the subtalar joint is also

Table 8–4. Proven indications for ankle arthroscopy.

Loose body removal
Irrigation and debridement for infection
Shaving of small osteophytes
Debridement of localized general synovitis
Debridement of osteochondral fractures
Debridement of osteochondritis dissecans lesions
Debridement of soft-tissue impingement

now an accepted method for diagnosing and treating some subtalar joint abnormalities.

▶ Advantages of Ankle Arthroscopy Over Ankle Arthrotomy

Arthroscopy of the ankle joint offers distinct advantages over open exploration of the ankle. The entire joint can be visualized using the arthroscope, including the lateral and medial gutters and the posterior aspect of the joint. Dynamic studies can be performed to stress ligaments or identify areas of soft-tissue or bony impingement. Furthermore, the low morbidity of arthroscopy allows rapid rehabilitation.

▶ Indications

Table 8–4 lists the indications for ankle joint arthroscopy. In addition, arthroscopic examination can be used as a diagnostic tool in some instances when the precise cause of ankle pain remains in question.

A. Therapeutic Indications

1. Loose bodies—Intraarticular loose bodies are generally easy to identify and remove arthroscopically. These bony or cartilaginous fragments may occur as a result of a single incident or repetitive trauma, or they may represent a fragment of an osteochondritis dissecans lesion. They cause pain or locking symptoms of the ankle and are diagnosed on plain radiographs, CT, or MRI scan.

2. Ankle joint infection—Arthroscopic irrigation, drainage, and synovectomy is an excellent method of treating ankle joint infections.

3. Synovitis—Synovitis may be present as a result of inflammatory arthritis (rheumatoid arthritis) or neoplastic diseases (pigmented villonodular synovitis), following trauma, or for unknown reasons (idiopathic). Whether the synovitis is localized or diffuse, arthroscopic debridement of inflamed synovium often relieves symptoms. Synovectomy is more easily and thoroughly performed arthroscopically.

4. Osteophyte formation—Repetitive trauma or early osteoarthritis can lead to osteophyte formation on the anterior lip of the tibia and the neck of the talus. These lesions can cause pain and limited ankle joint dorsiflexion and can be removed arthroscopically with a high-speed burr.

5. Other lesions within the joint—Chondral or osteochondral lesions, whether caused by trauma or osteochondritis dissecans, can be treated arthroscopically. This may involve debridement of loose cartilage flaps, drilling of subchondral bone, or pinning of large osteochondral fragments.

Patients who present with ankle pain over the anterolateral joint line and a history of a severe ankle sprain or recurrent sprains may have impingement of scar tissue in the lateral gutter between the talus and fibula. This entity responds well to arthroscopic debridement of scar tissue from the lateral gutter.

6. Ankle arthrodesis—Techniques for arthroscopically assisted ankle arthrodesis are well detailed, and several published studies discuss this method. The technique causes less morbidity and allows a shorter time to fusion than open methods of ankle fusion. But this is a technically demanding procedure and cannot be used to correct any joint deformity.

7. Ankle arthritis—Arthroscopic debridement of the arthritic ankle joint is not beneficial for generalized arthritis but may help for localized degenerative changes accompanied by early osteophyte formation.

8. Ankle fractures—Arthroscopically assisted fixation of ankle fractures is described and potentially allows for more accurate realignment of the joint surfaces and identification of chondral lesions that might otherwise be missed. However, the use of arthroscopy in the treatment of most routine ankle fractures is probably not indicated.

B. Diagnostic Indications

Ankle arthroscopy can be a valuable diagnostic tool when the cause of symptoms remains unclear (Table 8–5). Chronic ankle pain or swelling that remains refractory to conservative measures and was not diagnosed by conventional imaging studies may warrant arthroscopic exploration to help make a diagnosis. Chondral damage and inflamed synovium are examples of symptomatic lesions that may not be demonstrated on imaging studies, including MRI. Patients with episodes of locking, stiffness, or instability for which a cause cannot be found may be aided by diagnostic ankle arthroscopy. Loose bodies, cartilage flaps, or arthrofibrosis may be contributing to such symptoms, all of which can be treated arthroscopically (see Table 8–5).

▶ Technique of Ankle Arthroscopy

The patient is placed supine on the operating table with the foot positioned to allow access from all directions. This can be achieved with the foot placed off the edge of the bed or with the thigh held flexed in a well-padded thigh holder (Figure 8–50). General or spinal anesthesia is necessary for full relaxation of the extremity.

The use of distraction greatly enhances arthroscopic procedures, providing better views of the structures of the joint and allowing tools to be introduced into the joint. Noninvasive distractors with padded straps over the foot and heel are most commonly used (see Figure 8–50). Invasive distractors require placement of pins or screws through the tibia proximally and the calcaneus or talus distally. Stronger distraction forces can be obtained in this manner, but the morbidity is higher when using an invasive distractor.

Most ankle arthroscopies are performed using two anterior portals: anterolateral and anteromedial. A posterolateral portal may be helpful for use as outflow or to access the posterior aspect of the joint. Thorough knowledge of the anatomy of the tendons, nerves, and vessels is essential to prevent damage to any of these structures with

Table 8–5. Refractory conditions diagnosed by arthroscopy.

Chondromalacia
Synovitis
Locking of the joint
Chronic stiffness
Instability
Loose bodies
Cartilage flaps
Arthrofibrosis

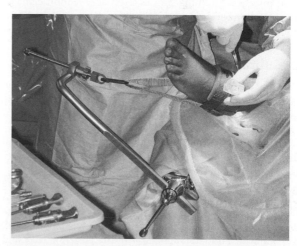

▲ **Figure 8–50.** Soft strap type of distractor used during ankle arthroscopy.

portal placement. The anterolateral portal is placed just lateral to the tendon of the peroneus tertius muscle, taking care to avoid branches of the superficial peroneal nerve. The anteromedial portal is placed just medial to the anterior tibial tendon, taking care to avoid the saphenous nerve and vein. The posterolateral portal is placed just lateral to the Achilles tendon, to avoid damage to the sural nerve.

Initially, the entire joint is explored systematically, to ensure that abnormalities are not overlooked. The cartilaginous surfaces of the talus and tibia are thoroughly examined for osteochondral defects, unstable cartilage flaps, and areas of softening. The medial and lateral gutters are explored, paying special attention to tibiotalar and talofibular articulations. The synovium is inspected for inflammation. Ligamentous structures are identified, specifically the deltoid and talofibular ligaments, which are observed closely for signs of laxity while varus and valgus forces are applied. Loose bodies are carefully searched for, especially in the anterior and posterior recesses of the joint. The presence of osteophytes on the distal tibia and talar neck is also evaluated.

After a thorough diagnostic examination, surgical procedures are performed. These include synovial biopsy or synovial resection, removal of loose bodies, debridement of abnormal cartilaginous surfaces with subchondral drilling, and removal of bone spurs.

Postoperatively, a compression dressing is applied with a posterior splint for 5–7 days to allow the portals to heal. Weight bearing is then progressed as tolerated, and activities are advanced to normal.

▶ Complications

Although several complications are reported, the most common is nerve damage in the form of hypesthesias or neuroma formation associated with portal placement. Postoperative joint infection, draining sinuses, arterial or tendon damage, and infections at the sites of distraction pins are all described but are very uncommon complications of ankle arthroscopy.

▶ Subtalar Joint Arthroscopy

The subtalar joint is technically challenging for arthroscopy, given its complex shape and the difficulty distracting the joint. Subtalar joint arthroscopy is indicated for several conditions involving the subtalar joint. Talocalcaneal interosseous ligament tears, chondral lesions, synovitis, and focal degenerative changes may respond to arthroscopic debridement of the subtalar joint.

For subtalar joint arthroscopy, the patient can either be placed supine with a bump under the ipsilateral hip or in the lateral decubitus position. Two portals are used over the anterolateral subtalar joint, approximately 1.5 cm apart. The anterior and lateral portions of the posterior facet and the interosseous ligament can be visualized from these

portals. A third portal is placed posterolaterally, for outflow and for visualization of the posterior aspect of the joint. The references here provide additional details about the technique of subtalar joint arthroscopy.

Bonasia DE, Rossi R, Saltzman CL, Amendola A: The role of arthroscopy in the management of fractures about the ankle. *J Am Acad Orthop Surg* 2011;19:236. [PMID: 21464216]

Gougoulias NE, Agathangelidis FG, Parsons SW: Arthroscopic ankle arthrodesis. *Foot Ankle Int* 2007;28:695. [PMID: 17592700]

Gras F, Marintschev I, Muller M, et al: Arthroscopic-controlled navigation for retrograde drilling of osteochondral lesions of the talus. *Foot Ankle Int* 2010;31:897. [PMID: 20964969]

Mologne TS, Ferkel RD: Arthroscopic treatment of osteochondral lesions of the distal tibia. *Foot Ankle Int* 2007;28:865. [PMID: 17697650]

Van Dijk CN, van Bergen CJ: Advancements in ankle arthroscopy. *J Am Acad Orthop Surg* 2008;16:635. [PMID: 18978286]

Scholten PE, Sierevelt IN, Van Dijk CN: Hindfoot endoscopy for posterior ankle impingement. *J Bone Joint Surg Am* 2008;90:2665. [PMID: 19047712]

▼ TENDON INJURIES

Tendon injuries about the foot and ankle are common causes of disability because large forces are acting on these tendons in a repetitive fashion during walking, running, and athletic activities. The tendons cross the ankle joint at an acute angle, which further predisposes them to injury. Injury to tendons may be caused by acute trauma, such as in Achilles tendon ruptures, or by chronic strain, such as in posterior tibial tendon dysfunction.

ACHILLES TENDON INJURIES

Achilles tendon abnormalities are extremely common, especially among active men and women between 30 and 50 years of age. The primary disorders are Achilles tendinitis, either insertional or noninsertional, and Achilles tendon ruptures. Achilles tendinitis was previously discussed in the section on heel pain.

1. Achilles Tendon Rupture

▶ Pathogenesis

The mechanism of injury is usually mechanical overload from an eccentric contraction of the gastrocsoleus muscle complex. This occurs as a sudden, forceful dorsiflexion of the foot as the gastrocsoleus is contracted. The tear usually occurs 3–6 cm proximal to the insertion of the Achilles tendon, at the site of its poorest blood supply. At times, a history of intermittent pain in the tendon is elicited, suggestive of a prior tendinitis. The typical patient is between

30 and 50 years of age and a recreational athlete. These factors suggest that insufficient conditioning of the musculotendon unit plays a role in many injuries. The most common sports activities leading to Achilles tendon ruptures are basketball, racket sports, soccer, and softball.

► Clinical Findings

A. Symptoms and Signs

The patient describes sudden pain in the calf after attempting a pushing-off movement, often accompanied by an audible pop. Immediate weakness is noted in the affected leg. On physical examination, a palpable defect is often present in the tendon. Ankle plantar flexion is markedly weak compared with the unaffected side. A positive Thompson test, diagnostic of complete Achilles tendon rupture, is performed with the patient prone and the affected knee bent 90 degrees. Squeezing the calf causes plantar flexion of the foot if the Achilles tendon is intact or partially torn but not if there is complete rupture of the tendon.

B. Imaging Studies

Plain radiographs are not helpful in diagnosing Achilles tendon tear, unless there is an avulsion off the calcaneus with a fragment of bone, an uncommon condition. MRI is extremely sensitive in diagnosing this disorder and in determining if some tendon remains in continuity (Figure 8–51). However, MRI is rarely needed because physical exam is usually diagnostic of Achilles tendon rupture.

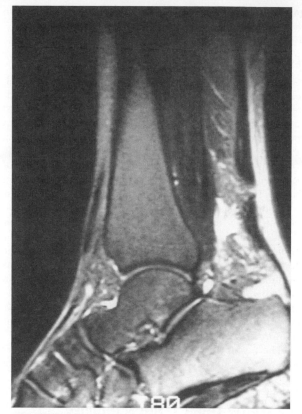

▲ **Figure 8–51.** MRI of Achilles tendon rupture.

► Treatment

Methods for treating Achilles tendon rupture include primary repair, using open or percutaneous techniques, or cast immobilization. Surgical repair is recommended for active individuals, in the case of a rerupture, or if the injury is older than 2 weeks.

Cast treatment for Achilles tendon ruptures is recommended for more sedentary individuals, patients who are at increased risk of developing wound problems, or high-risk surgical patients. The primary risk of cast immobilization is a higher chance of rerupture. For the vast majority of patients, either treatment method results in a good outcome.

A. Nonsurgical Treatment

Once an acute rupture is diagnosed, the patient should be placed in a gravity equinus cast. A below-knee cast is adequate in a reliable patient. If there is a question of whether the tendon edges are properly apposed in the cast, an MRI scan can be done, although this is not routine. After 4 weeks, the cast is changed, with correction of approximately half of the previous equinus. Over the next 4 weeks, the patient is brought down to neutral with serial casts. Once at neutral, the patient is given a removable walking cast for 4 weeks. Supervised strengthening activities then begin.

B. Surgical Treatment

The surgical approach is on the medial side of the Achilles tendon sheath. The frayed edges of the tendon are debrided. The foot is positioned in equinus position equal to the resting equinus of the opposite ankle. Two heavy nonabsorbable sutures are woven through 3–4 cm of each tendon edge using a Bunnell or Kessler stitch. The repair can be reinforced with lighter, absorbable sutures at the site of the tear. If the plantaris tendon is intact, it can be harvested and used to reinforce the repair.

Postoperatively, a hard cast is used for 3 weeks, followed by a removable cast with adjustable ankle motion. Over the next 2–3 weeks, the joint should be gradually brought out of equinus. Weight bearing is then allowed, and ROM exercises are begun. The cast is discontinued at 6–8 weeks, and supervised strengthening exercises are performed.

The primary risk of surgical repair is wound healing problems, which occur in approximately 5% of patients.

A percutaneous method of Achilles tendon repair is listed in the references.

C. Treatment of Chronic Ruptures or Reruptures

Chronic Achilles tendon ruptures, more than 6 weeks old, or reruptures of previously treated injuries can be challenging reconstruction problems because of retraction and degeneration of the tendon ends. A number of different procedures are described to address this problem, including a variety of synthetic and interpositional grafts.

Small defects can be bridged by turning down a strip of gastrocnemius fascia, which is sutured into the distal tendon stump. Larger defects can be treated by using a V-Y lengthening of the gastrocnemius aponeurosis. If the deficit is too large for V-Y lengthening, transfer of the flexor hallucis longus tendon can be performed. The tendon of the flexor hallucis longus is transected distally in the foot, and the distal segment is tenodesed to the flexor digitorum longus to maintain flexion of the great toe. The proximal tendon is secured to the calcaneus through a drill hole or by using an absorbable anchor or screw. A central slip of the Achilles tendon is advanced to bridge the gap, and then the repair is reinforced by securing it to the flexor hallucis.

The postoperative course for these procedures includes 6 weeks of non–weight bearing and a total of 3 months of protection in a cast.

POSTERIOR TIBIAL TENDON INJURIES

This topic is covered in the section on acquired flatfoot deformities.

PERONEAL TENDON INJURIES

Peroneal tendon injuries fall into the categories of peroneal tendonitis, peroneal tendon tears, and peroneal tendon subluxation or dislocation.

1. Peroneal Tendonitis

▶ Pathogenesis

Inflammation of the peroneal tendons may be caused by acute trauma, inflammatory arthropathy conditions, or repetitive motion. Traumatic events that may induce tendonitis include a direct blow to the posterolateral ankle, a fracture of the calcaneus or fibula, or a severe inversion sprain of the ankle. Most tendonitis is caused by repetitive motion injury from recurrent rubbing of the peroneal tendons on the distal end of the fibula. Often there is an abnormal bony contour of the distal fibula or the peroneal tubercle. Tendonitis of the peroneus longus may be associated with abnormality of the os peroneum, a small sesamoid bone located in the tendon where it curves around the lateral border of the cuboid.

▶ Clinical Findings

A. Symptoms and Signs

The patient complains of pain over the lateral aspect of the ankle, made worse with activity and improved with rest and NSAIDs. The onset may be insidious, or it may be associated with an acute injury. Physical examination usually demonstrates pain located along the course of the peroneal tendons. Pain and weakness are noted with resisted eversion of the foot.

B. Imaging Studies

An MRI scan may help distinguish between tendonitis and a tendon tear, although small tears may not be identified on an MRI.

▶ Treatment

A. Nonsurgical

If symptoms are mild, the recommended treatment includes NSAIDs, activity modification, and an ankle brace. Four to 6 weeks of cast immobilization are used for more advanced symptoms or for patients who do not respond to initial treatment. Occasionally, a diagnostic injection with bupivacaine is given into the tendon sheath.

B. Surgical

Operative intervention is recommended for patients who fail conservative treatment. The tendon sheath is explored, inflamed synovium is removed, and the tendons are carefully explored to look for tears or degenerative lesions. Postoperatively, early ROM is encouraged.

2. Peroneal Tendon Tears

▶ Pathogenesis

The majority of peroneal tendon tears are attritional in nature, caused by mechanical irritation within the fibular groove. The peroneus longus tendon, which lies posterior, places pressure on the brevis tendon. Also, a sharp lateral edge of the fibula may predispose to a longitudinal split of the tendons. Laxity of the tendon sheath and subluxation of the tendons out of the fibular groove may contribute to tears as well. Acute tears of the peroneal tendons may occur with a sudden, severe stress to the ankle, but usually there is some degree of preexisting degeneration within the tendon.

▶ Clinical Findings

Clinical presentation is similar to that of peroneal tendonitis, but with a more acute onset of pain and swelling along the tendon sheath.

Treatment

A. Nonsurgical

Initial treatment is similar to that of peroneal tendonitis, but it is less likely to result in resolution of symptoms if a tear is present.

B. Surgical

Surgical repair of a peroneal tendon tear is indicated when nonoperative treatment fails to relieve symptoms. At surgery, both tendons are carefully examined, the fibula is explored for sharp edges, and the tendon sheath is evaluated for laxity. Small areas of the tendon that demonstrate significant degeneration are removed. The remainder of the tendon is repaired with nylon or polypropylene suture. Postoperatively, the ankle is immobilized for 4 weeks; then weight bearing and gentle ROM are allowed.

3. Peroneal Tendon Subluxation and Dislocation

▶ Pathogenesis

Peroneal tendon dislocation is caused by a sudden forceful dorsiflexion motion of the ankle combined with a simultaneous strong contraction of the peroneal musculature. This mechanism injures the superior peroneal retinaculum, which holds the peroneal tendons in place along the posterior border of the distal fibula. The retinaculum is either stripped off the fibular periosteum or avulsed with a small piece of fibular cortex. This permits the creation of a false pouch and laxity of the retinaculum, allowing the peroneal tendons to dislocate anteriorly. If this condition goes unrecognized, either the tendons remain dislocated, or they relocate with the propensity for recurrent subluxation or dislocation.

▶ Clinical Findings

A. Symptoms and Signs

The patient usually recalls an acute episode of trauma and frequently the sensation of the tendon dislocating. Pain and swelling are localized to the peroneal tendon sheath around the tip of the fibula. With recurrent subluxation or dislocation, the tendons are felt to pop out of place. On examination, resisted eversion of the ankle elicits pain and may cause the tendons to subluxate. Unfortunately, many acute peroneal tendon dislocations go unrecognized as lateral ankle sprains.

B. Imaging Studies

Radiographs may show a small piece of bone lateral to the distal fibula, indicative of avulsion of the retinaculum. MRI scan usually details the injury well if careful attention is paid to this area.

Treatment

A. Nonsurgical

Treatment of acute peroneal tendon dislocations consists of casting in plantarflexion and inversion for 4 weeks, followed by a walking cast for an additional 2 weeks. Cast treatment has at least a 50% failure rate. Once a tendon is chronically dislocated or recurrently subluxates, only surgical treatment will keep it in position.

B. Surgical

Surgical repair is recommended for an athletic individual following an acute dislocation of the peroneal tendons. It is also recommended for patients with recurrent dislocation if their physical activities are significantly restricted. The procedure consists of repairing the superior peroneal retinaculum to the fibula, either through drill holes or with suture anchors. In the case of attenuated retinaculum caused by chronic dislocations, the repair can be reinforced with a strip of Achilles or by rerouting the calcaneofibular ligament over the tendons. At the time of surgical repair, the tendons are inspected for tears and the contour of the posterior fibular groove is evaluated. If a shallow groove is noted, a bony procedure to deepen the groove is necessary to prevent recurrent dislocations. Postoperatively, the patient is immobilized in a cast for 6 weeks.

ANTERIOR TIBIAL TENDON RUPTURE

▶ Pathogenesis

Rupture of the anterior tibial tendon occurs infrequently, and most often in patients older than 60. The mechanism is either chronic rubbing against the inferior edge of the extensor retinaculum or rubbing against an exostosis at the first metatarsocuneiform joint. The rupture usually occurs at the distal 2–3 cm of tendon. Nondegenerative traumatic ruptures of the anterior tibial tendon are rare.

▶ Clinical Findings

A. Symptoms and Signs

Patients with a degenerative rupture present with complaints of pain and swelling over the anterior ankle. They sense the foot slapping down, or they may be catching their toes on the ground when they walk. Patients frequently present after the symptoms have been bothersome for several months. Physical exam is notable for weakness of ankle dorsiflexion, often with a palpable mass over the anterior ankle joint.

B. Imaging Studies

If the diagnosis is in doubt, MRI scan can accurately determine if the tendon is ruptured.

Treatment

A. Nonsurgical

In the case of a less active patient, nonsurgical treatment appears to give equal functional results to surgical repair. Cast immobilization is followed by long-term use of an AFO.

B. Surgical

Acute tendon rupture in an active individual should be surgically repaired. Chronic ruptures that are symptomatic usually require reconstruction using an extensor tendon graft or tendon transfer because the distal stump is usually too degenerated to perform a primary repair.

Chiodo CP, Glazebrook M, Bluman EM, et al: American Academy of Orthopedic Surgeons clinical practice guideline on treatment of Achilles tendon rupture. *J Bone Joint Surg Am* 2010;92:2466. [PMID: 20962199]

Chiodo CP, Glazebrook M, Bluman EM, et al: Diagnosis and treatment of Achilles tendon rupture. *J Am Acad Orthop Surg* 2010;18:503. [PMID: 20675643]

Courville XF, Coe MP, Hecht PJ: Current concepts review: non-insertional Achilles tendinopathy. *Foot Ankle Int* 2009;30:1132. [PMID: 19912730]

Irwin TA: Current concepts review: insertional Achilles tendinopathy. *Foot Ankle Int* 2010;31:933. [PMID: 20964977]

Ogawa BK, Thordarson DB: Current concepts review: peroneal tendon subluxation and dislocation. *Foot Ankle Int* 2007;28:1034. [PMID: 17880883]

Philbin TM, Landis GS, Smith B: Peroneal tendon injuries. *J Am Acad Orthop Surg* 2009;17:306. [PMID: 19411642]

Reddy SS, Pedowitz DI, Parekh SG, Omar IM, Wapner KL: Surgical treatment for chronic disease and disorders of the Achilles tendon. *J Am Acad Orthop Surg* 2009;17:3. [PMID: 19136422]

Sammarco VJ, Sammarco GJ, Henning C, Chaim S: Surgical repair of acute and chronic tibialis anterior ruptures. *J Bone Joint Surg Am* 2009;91:325. [PMID: 19181976]

OSTEOCHONDRAL LESIONS OF THE TALUS

Osteochondral lesions of the talus (OLTs) are defects of cartilage and subchondral bone in the talar dome. More sophisticated imaging techniques allow for precise diagnosis of OLTs, and advanced arthroscopic and open methods are available to treat this difficult problem.

Pathogenesis

OLTs, also known as osteochondritis dissecans lesions, are generally located in one of two areas on the talar dome: either posteromedial or anterolateral. The more common posteromedial lesions are usually deeper lesions involving subchondral bone. Their origin is thought to involve ischemia, often with an episode of trauma exacerbating the underlying condition. Anterolateral lesions are a result of a single traumatic episode or repetitive trauma from lateral ankle sprains. These lesions tend to be purely cartilaginous.

Clinical Findings

A. Symptoms and Signs

Patients usually present with several months of ankle pain following a routine ankle sprain. Sometimes they recount a history of recurrent sprains to the ankle. The pain is usually located over the anterior aspect of the ankle on the side of the lesion, but it may be diffuse. Occasionally, there is a sensation of locking in the ankle when a loose flap of cartilage is present. A high index of suspicion is necessary because OLTs can be misdiagnosed as a chronic ankle sprain, as discussed in the section on ligamentous injuries about the ankle joint.

B. Imaging Studies

Radiographs are often normal in OLTs. MRI scan is the imaging procedure of choice for determining the size, location, and extent of bony or cartilaginous involvement (Figure 8–52).

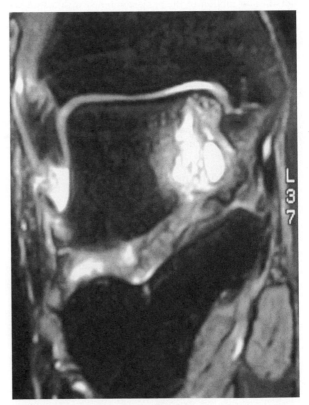

▲ **Figure 8–52.** MRI scan of extensive osteochondral lesion of the talus.

▶ Treatment

A. Nonsurgical

A 6-week trial of cast immobilization is warranted if the MRI scan shows no evidence of a displaced bone or cartilage fragment.

B. Surgical

The surgical treatment method depends on the type of lesion. Acutely displaced lesions can be reduced and pinned with an absorbable pin by either open or arthroscopic methods. Purely cartilaginous lesions are curetted to a stable rim and drilled to stimulate vascular ingrowth and fibrocartilage formation. OLTs with significant bony involvement require bone grafting in addition to drilling and curettage. A medial malleolar osteotomy is required to access a posteromedial lesion. If a bony lesion has intact overlying cartilage, drilling and bone grafting can be performed under radiographic guidance through the talus, thereby sparing the overlying cartilage. Postoperatively, patients are kept non–weight bearing for 4 weeks, but early ROM is encouraged.

New techniques were developed for larger lesions or ones that fail curettage and drilling. Osteochondral autograft or allograft plugs can be used to replace bone and cartilage defects. Autograft plugs are generally harvested from the ipsilateral knee. Intermediate-term follow-up data show good results in most patients following this technique. Autologous chondrocyte implantation is also used to a limited extent for OLTs.

Easley ME, Latt D, Santangelo JR, Merian-Genast M, Nunley JA: Osteochondral lesions of the talus. *J Am Acad Orthop Surg* 2010;18:616. [PMID: 20889951]

Elias I, Raikin SM, Schweitzer ME, Besser MP, Morrison WB, Zoga AC: Osteochondral lesions of the distal tibial plafond: localization and morphologic characteristics with an anatomical grid. *Foot Ankle Int* 2009;30:524. [PMID: 19486630]

Gortz S, De Young AJ, Bugbee WD: Fresh osteochondral allografting for osteochondral lesions of the talus. *Foot Ankle Int* 2010;31:283. [PMID: 20371013]

Haene R, Qamirani E, Story RA, Pinsker E, Daniels TR: Intermediate outcomes of fresh talar osteochondral allografts for treatment of large osteochondral lesions of the talus. *J Bone Joint Surg Am* 2012;94:1105. [PMID: 22717829]

Hahn DB, Aanstoos ME, Wilkins RM: Osteochondral lesions of the talus treated with fresh talar allografts. *Foot Ankle Int* 2010;31:277. [PMID: 20371012]

Mitchell ME, Giza E, Sullivan MR: Cartilage transplantation techniques for talar cartilage lesions. *J Am Acad Orthop Surg* 2009;17:407. [PMID: 19571296]

Raikin SM: Fresh osteochondral allografts for large-volume cystic osteochondral defects of the talus. *J Bone Joint Surg Am* 2009;91:2818. [PMID: 19952243]

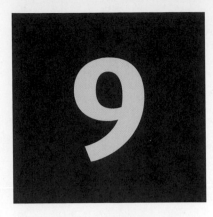

Hand Surgery

Michael S. Bednar, MD

Terry R. Light, MD

Randy Bindra, MD, FRCS

Function of the Hand

The hand is a vital part of the human body, allowing humans to directly interact with their environment. The functional capabilities of the hand are many because the hand is ultimately an end organ of the human mind. The hand's enormous capacity for adaptability allowed primitive humans to make stone tools and modern humans to pilot complex aircraft.

The human hand is capable of prehension, which involves approaching an object, grasping it, modulating and maintaining grasp, and ultimately releasing the object. When a power grasp is used, the object is pushed by the flexed fingers against the palm while the thumb metacarpal and proximal phalanx stabilize the object. When an object is held with a precision pinch pattern, the object is secured between the pulps of the thumb and index fingers or index and middle fingers.

The hand can touch objects or other human beings while sensing temperature, vibration, and texture. This quality of tactile gnosis is sophisticated enough to allow blind individuals to read the pattern of small elevations that distinguish one Braille letter from another. The hand is also an instrument of communication, whether by making a gesture, playing a musical instrument, drawing, writing, or typing.

General Considerations in Treatment of Hand Disorders

Treatment of hand disorders requires an understanding of normal anatomy and its common variations. Treatment usually attempts to restore the normal anatomy, but when that is not possible, the goal should be restoration of maximal function. The aesthetic appearance of the hand is vital because the hand is usually uncovered and exposed to the scrutiny of others and to the owner. Imperfections are often a source of embarrassment. Effective treatment requires a mature balancing of the need for optimal function and normal appearance of the hand. Complex reconstruction that restores prehension but results in a hideous appearance of the hand is ineffective if the patient is so reluctant to

expose the hand that he or she avoids using it. Conversely, a functionless stiff finger leading to awkward motion of an otherwise supple hand may cause the patient more embarrassment than amputation.

DIAGNOSIS OF DISORDERS OF THE HAND

History

When a patient seeks evaluation of a hand disorder, the physician should ask many general questions as well as questions specific to hand function and injury. The chief complaint as perceived by the patient should be summarized in one or two sentences. The patient's hand dominance, age, gender, and occupation should be noted, as well as any hobbies that require hand dexterity or strength. The approximate date of onset of symptoms should be recorded. If injury is the cause of discomfort, the exact date and mechanism of injury should be noted and whether the injury occurred at the workplace. The patient should be questioned about prior treatment and his or her perception of its effectiveness.

Complaints should then be further detailed, such as the nature of pain (sharp, aching, dull, or burning), whether night symptoms are present, aggravating and relieving factors, and whether the pain is worse upon awakening in the morning or after a full day of work. The patient should be asked whether symptoms include numbness or tingling, which would indicate a neurologic problem rather than a mechanical one. Specific motor difficulties, such as difficulty in writing or unscrewing jar tops, should be noted. If the patient complains principally of unilateral symptoms, the examiner should ask whether similar symptoms are occurring on the opposite side. Finally, because the hand is an exposed area of the body, the impact of altered appearance should be discussed.

The medical history should include any prior hand injuries and any systemic diseases such as rheumatoid arthritis (RA) or other inflammatory arthropathies, diabetes, other endocrine disorders, renal disease, or vascular disease. Women of childbearing age should be questioned about recent pregnancies. A careful history suggests the correct diagnosis in approximately 90% of patients with hand problems.

▶ Examination of the Hand

A. General Examination

Examination of the hand should begin with observation. Vascular condition can be assessed by noting the color of the fingers. Some hint of nerve function can be obtained by observing sudomotor function as revealed by sweatiness of the finger pulps. The extent and timing of injury are suggested by the degree of swelling and ecchymosis. The posture of the digits and the wrist may signal tendon or bone disruption. Normally, a cascade of increased digital flexion is noted when ulnar digits are observed next to radial digits (Figure 9–1).

A diagram of the hand is often helpful in documenting the abnormality. Lumps, laceration sites, previous scars, amputated fingers, and areas of decreased sensation can be noted on the diagram.

Next, the hand, wrist, and forearm are gently palpated. The temperature and moisture of the fingers should be noted. Circulation is assessed by capillary refill; when the skin is blanched in the paronychial region, circulation should return within 3 seconds. Areas of tenderness on palpation are carefully noted.

B. Range of Motion

The passive and active range of motion (ROM) of the shoulder, elbow, forearm, wrist, and hand are evaluated. The normal ROM of the wrist and fingers is indicated in Table 9–1. In documenting ROM, active extension should be to the left and active flexion to the right. When the range of passive extension and flexion is different from that of active motion, the passive ROM values are noted in parentheses next to the corresponding active ROM values. The ROM of a stiff proximal interphalangeal joint could thus be recorded as 20/70 (15/80), indicating an arc of active motion from 20 to 70 degrees and a passive arc of motion from 15 to 80 degrees.

C. Muscle Function

The integrity of individual muscles should be documented. The flexor digitorum profundus to each finger is tested by stabilizing the middle phalanx and asking the patient to flex the distal interphalangeal joint (Figure 9–2). The flexor digitorum superficialis of each finger is tested by keeping all fingers except the one to be tested in full extension. The patient is then asked to flex the finger being evaluated at the proximal interphalangeal joint (Figure 9–3). The function of the flexor pollicis longus is tested by asking the patient to flex the interphalangeal joint of the thumb.

The function of the extrinsic extensors is tested by asking the patient to extend the metacarpophalangeal joints of the

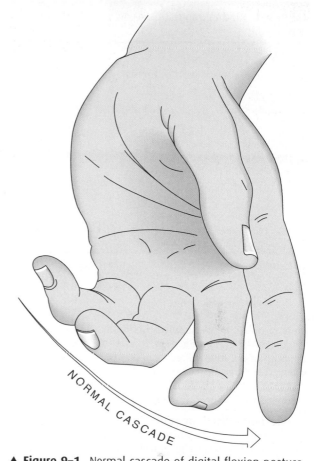

▲ **Figure 9–1.** Normal cascade of digital flexion posture. When the wrist is in slight extension and the fingers are at rest, there is progressively less flexion from the little finger to the index finger. (Reproduced, with permission, from Carter PR: *Common Hand Injuries and Infections.* New York: WB Saunders; 1983.)

fingers. If the examiner simply asks the patient to open the hand, the proximal and distal interphalangeal joints may be extended by contraction of the intrinsic muscles, which may mislead the examiner to conclude that digital extension is normal. Interosseous muscle function is screened by asking the patient to abduct the fingers. The examiner assesses the strength of muscle force while palpating the contraction of the hypothenar and the first dorsal interosseous muscles.

D. Sensory Function

Examination of sensory function requires evaluation of the integrity of the median, ulnar, and radial nerves as well as the component proper digital nerves to each side of each finger. Each of the major nerves has an autogenous sensory zone:

Table 9–1. Normal range of motion in joints of arm and hand.

Elbow: Extension and flexion 0°/135°
Forearm: Supination and pronation 90°/90°
Wrist: Flexion and extension 80°/70°   Radial deviation and ulnar deviation 20°/30°

Finger
  MP: Extension and flexion 0°/90°
  PIP: Extension and flexion 0°/110°
  DIP: Extension and flexion 0°/65°

Thumb
  CMC: Extension and flexion 50°/50°
     Abduction and adduction 70°/0°
  MP: Extension and flexion—variable, up to 0°/90°
  IP: Extension and flexion—variable, up to 0°/90°

CMC, carpometacarpal; DIP, distal interphalangeal; IP, interphalangeal; MP, metacarpal phalangeal; PIP, proximal interphalangeal.

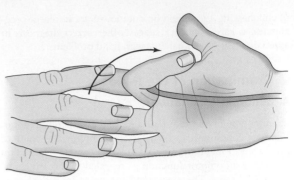

▲ **Figure 9–3.** Testing of flexor digitorum superficialis integrity. If the proximal interphalangeal joint can be actively flexed while the adjacent fingers are held completely extended, the sublimis tendon is not severed. (Reproduced, with permission, from American Society for Surgery of the Hand: *The Hand: Examination and Diagnosis,* 2nd ed. Philadelphia: Churchill Livingstone; 1983.)

an area of the hand supplied predominantly by that nerve (Figure 9–4). The autogenous zone of the median nerve is the pulp of the index finger, whereas the ulnar nerve exclusively carries sensory fibers from the pulp of the little finger. The skin on the dorsum of the first web space is innervated by the superficial branch of the radial nerve.

1. Two-point discrimination—The integrity of each digital nerve may be evaluated using either a blunt-tipped caliper or an unfolded paper clip to test two-point discrimination.

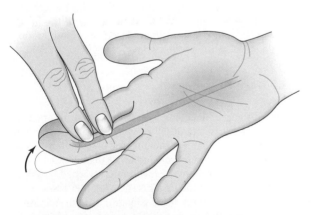

▲ **Figure 9–2.** Testing of flexor digitorum profundus integrity. If the distal interphalangeal joint can be actively flexed while the proximal interphalangeal joint is stabilized, the profundus tendon is not severed. (Reproduced, with permission, from American Society for Surgery of the Hand: *The Hand: Examination and Diagnosis,* 2nd ed. Philadelphia: Churchill Livingstone; 1983.)

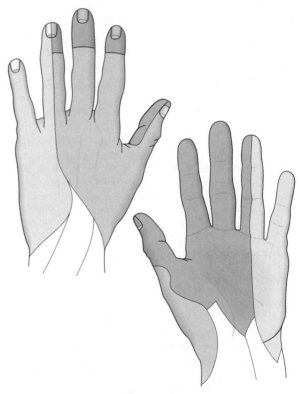

▲ **Figure 9–4.** Sensory distribution in the hand. Light shading, ulnar nerve; medium shading, radial nerve; darkest shading, median nerve. (Reproduced, with permission, from Way LW, ed: *Current Surgical Diagnosis and Treatment,* 10th ed. Stamford, CT: Appleton & Lange; 1994.)

The two points of the testing instrument are held apart at a measured distance. The examiner alternates between touching the skin with one or two points. The points may be either touched (static two-point discrimination) or longitudinally moved (moving two-point discrimination) against the skin on either the radial or ulnar side of the finger. The points should be pressed against the finger until the skin just begins to blanch. The two-point discrimination value is the smallest distance between the two points that the patient can correctly detect in two out of three trials. Because of the increased sensory cues provided by movement, moving two-point discrimination has a value less than or equal to static two-point discrimination. Static two-point discrimination is normal if the distance is less than 7 mm, impaired if 7–14 mm, and absent if 15 mm or greater.

E. Motor Function

Examination of motor function may be organized by considering groups of muscles within specific nerve domains (Table 9–2). Proximally, the median nerve innervates the pronator teres, flexor carpi radialis, palmaris longus, and flexor digitorum superficialis muscles. The anterior interosseous nerve branch of the median nerve innervates the flexor digitorum profundus of the index and middle fingers, flexor pollicis longus, and pronator quadratus muscles. The motor branch of the median nerve to the thenar musculature innervates the opponens pollicis, abductor pollicis brevis, and superficial portion of the flexor pollicis brevis. The index- and long-finger lumbricals are innervated by median motor fibers running with the sensory nerve branches of the median nerve to the index and middle fingers.

Table 9–2. Innervation of the hand and forearm.

Median nerve
  Proximal median nerve: pronator teres, flexor carpi radialis, flexor digitorum superficialis
  Anterior interosseous nerve: flexor pollicis longus, index and middle flexor digitorum profundus, pronator quadratus
  Distal median nerve: index and middle lumbrical, opponens pollicis, abductor pollicis brevis, flexor pollicis brevis

Ulnar nerve
  Proximal ulnar nerve: flexor carpi ulnaris, ring and small flexor digitorum profundus
  Distal ulnar nerve: flexor digiti minimi, abductor digiti minimi, opponens digiti minimi, volar and dorsal interossei, flexor pollicis brevis, adductor pollicis, ring and small lumbricals

Radial nerve: brachioradialis, extensor carpi radialis longus, supinator, anconeus

Posterior interosseous nerve: extensor carpi radialis brevis, extensor digitorum communis, extensor indicis proprius, extensor digiti minimi, extensor carpi ulnaris, abductor pollicis longus, extensor pollicis longus, extensor pollicis brevis

The ulnar nerve innervates the flexor carpi ulnaris and flexor digitorum profundus of the ring and little fingers proximally. Within the hand, the ulnar nerve innervates the hypothenar musculature, flexor digiti quinti, and abductor digiti quinti. The deep motor branch of the ulnar nerve innervates the dorsal and palmar interosseous muscles, lumbricals to the ring and little fingers, deep portion of the flexor pollicis brevis, and adductor pollicis muscles.

The radial nerve innervates the triceps, brachioradialis, extensor carpi radialis longus and brevis, supinator, and anconeus muscles. The posterior interosseous division of the radial nerve then distally innervates the extensor digitorum communis, extensor indicis proprius, extensor digiti minimi, extensor carpi ulnaris, abductor pollicis longus, and extensor pollicis longus and brevis.

Muscle strength should be graded according to the Medical Research Council of Great Britain grading system based on a scale of 0 to 5, with 5/5 being normal strength, 4/5 less than normal strength but with ability to resist a fair amount of resistance, 3/5 resistance against gravity, 2/5 resistance with gravity eliminated, and 1/5 only a trace or flicker of contraction without significant motion.

▶ Diagnostic Studies

A number of studies may be helpful in establishing the proper diagnosis in a patient with hand or wrist pain or disorders. The choice of technique should be based on a careful history and physical examination.

A. Imaging Studies

In most instances, radiographic evaluation includes posteroanterior (PA) and lateral films. The importance of obtaining a true lateral radiograph of the finger and wrist cannot be overemphasized because many disorders, particularly interphalangeal joint subluxation and carpal instability, are not evident on oblique views. Oblique views may be useful in defining phalangeal fracture patterns. Tangential views are useful in assessing a carpometacarpal boss. The carpal tunnel view may allow visualization of a fracture of the hook of the hamate.

Stress views allow assessment of ligamentous stability. This is particularly useful in the evaluation of collateral ligament stability of the thumb metacarpophalangeal joint.

Ligamentous stability of the wrist may also be evaluated by radial and ulnar deviation views and by clenched-fist grip views. Grip views and ulnar deviation views may demonstrate a gap between the scaphoid and the lunate that is not apparent on simple PA and lateral studies.

B. Electrodiagnostic Studies

Electrodiagnostic studies include both nerve conduction studies and electromyography. Nerve conduction studies measure both motor (proximal to distal) and sensory (distal to proximal) conduction. Electromyography allows evaluation of muscle function.

C. Computed Tomography Scan

A computed tomography (CT) scan allows excellent three-dimensional views of the joints of the hand and wrist and is critical to evaluation of joints such as the distal radioulnar joint. The relationship of the distal ulna to the sigmoid notch should be viewed in pronation, neutral, and supination. CT scanning may be helpful in evaluating displacement as well as healing of scaphoid fractures and in surgical planning of distal radius fractures.

D. Magnetic Resonance Imaging

Magnetic resonance imaging (MRI) provides visualization of soft-tissue structures such as ligaments and tendons. The integrity of the transverse carpal ligament may be evaluated, which is particularly helpful in patients with persistent symptoms following carpal tunnel release. Evaluation of tumors and avascular necrosis is also facilitated by MRI. MRI scans also allow visualization of many triangular fibrocartilage complex and intercarpal ligament tears.

E. Bone Scan

The technetium-99 methylene diphosphonate (MDP) bone scan is a useful physiologic test in the evaluation of unexplained hand or wrist pain. This test can rule out bone involvement and can be used to localize inflammatory processes for further study with CT or MRI scans (Figure 9–5).

F. Wrist Arthroscopy

Arthroscopic examination of the wrist allows for direct visualization of articular surfaces, wrist ligaments, and the triangular fibrocartilage complex. The effect of stress maneuvers on intercarpal kinematics may be directly observed. Wrist arthroscopy is particularly helpful in the debridement or repair of the triangular fibrocartilage complex tears. Partial tears of either the scapholunate or lunotriquetral ligaments may be debrided. Intraarticular fracture of the distal radius may be anatomically aligned and pinned under direct observation.

Bernstein MA, Nagle DJ, Martinez A, et al: A comparison of combined arthroscopic triangular fibrocartilage complex debridement and arthroscopic wafer distal ulna resection versus arthroscopic triangular fibrocartilage complex debridement and ulnar shortening osteotomy for ulnocarpal abutment syndrome. *Arthroscopy* 2004;20:392. [PMID: 15067279]

Cerezal L, del Pinal F, Abascal F, et al: Imaging findings in ulnar-sided wrist impaction syndromes. *Radiographics* 2002;22:105. [PMID: 11796902]

Kocharian A, Adkins MC, Amrami KK, et al: Wrist: improved MR imaging with optimized transmit-receive coil design. *Radiology* 2002;223:870. [PMID: 12034961]

Morley J, Bidwell J, Bransby-Zachary M: A comparison of the findings of wrist arthroscopy and magnetic resonance imaging in the investigation of wrist pain. *J Hand Surg* 2001;26B:544. [PMID: 11884109]

Potter HG, Weiland AJ: Magnetic resonance imaging of triangular fibrocartilage complex lesions. *J Hand Surg Am* 2002;27:363. [PMID: 11901408]

Slutsky DJ: Wrist arthroscopy through a volar radial portal. *Arthroscopy* 2002;18:624. [PMID: 12098124]

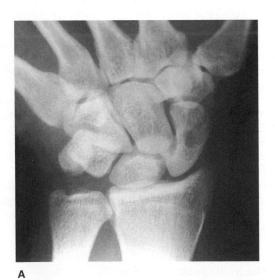

A

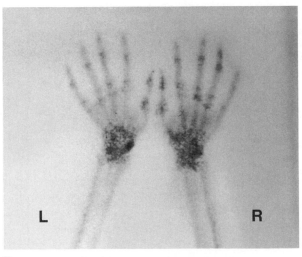

B

▲ **Figure 9–5.** Radiograph **(A)** and bone scan **(B)** demonstrating increased activity in the region of the scaphoid in a woman with a symptomatic cyst.

SPECIAL TREATMENT PROCEDURES FOR HAND DISORDERS

1. Replantation

Replantation is the reattachment of a body part that was totally severed from the body, without any residual soft-tissue continuity. Revascularization is the reconstruction of damaged blood vessels to prevent an attached but ischemic body part from becoming necrotic.

► Initial Care of Patient

Effective treatment of the patient and the ischemic or detached body part requires appropriate initial care and prompt referral to a surgeon at a center capable of mobilizing resources for early surgical care. The initial treating physician should place the amputated part in a sponge soaked with either normal saline or Ringer's lactate solution. The wrapped part should then be placed into a plastic bag, which is sealed and immersed in an ice-water solution. Under no circumstances should the amputated part be placed directly into ice water or exposed to dry ice.

A tourniquet is usually not required to control bleeding. A compressive dressing should be applied to the amputation stump. No attempt should be made to ligate bleeding vessels because it might compromise subsequent neurovascular repair. If the amputated part is not cooled, ischemia is poorly tolerated and successful revascularization is unlikely after 6 hours. Cooled parts may be replanted up to 12 hours after injury.

► Indications and Contraindications

Replantation is indicated for severed thumbs or multiple digits, transmetacarpal hand amputations, wrist- or distal forearm-level amputations, and amputations of almost any body part in a child. In more proximal levels of amputation, only sharp or moderately avulsed parts can be considered for replantation. The more proximal the amputation, the greater the amount of ischemic muscle mass and the more urgent the need for revascularization.

Contraindications to replantation include severely crushed or mangled parts; multilevel amputation; amputations in patients with arteriosclerotic vessels; amputations in patients with other serious injuries or diseases; and amputations with prolonged warm ischemic times, particularly at proximal levels.

In adults, replantation of a single finger proximal to the insertion of the flexor digitorum superficialis is usually contraindicated because of the poor functional outcome due to stiffness. Limited motion in these replanted fingers is caused by simultaneous zone 2 flexor digitorum superficialis and profundus tendon disruption, phalangeal fracture, and extensor tendon disruption. Replantation at this level may be considered in children or for aesthetic reasons.

► Surgical Procedure

The preferred method of anesthesia is axillary or supraclavicular block because this technique provides a sympathetic block resulting in vasodilation. The surgical sequence of replantation begins with a wide surgical exposure that allows identification and isolation of arteries, veins, and nerves. The soft tissue is then meticulously debrided. The bone is shortened and securely internally fixed with sufficient stability to allow institution of early postoperative motion.

The extensor tendons are repaired first and then the flexor tendons. Anastomosis of one or preferably two arteries is then performed, followed by repair of the nerves and anastomosis of the veins. Two veins should be repaired for each artery repaired. Skin should be closed loosely, with care taken to approximate soft tissue over repaired vessels and nerves.

In replantations proximal to the distal forearm, fasciotomies of all muscle compartments should be performed at the time of replantation. The patient undergoing proximal replantation should be returned to the operating room in 48–72 hours, so the wound may be reevaluated and any additional necrotic tissue debrided.

► Postoperative Care

Postoperatively, the hand is protected in a loose, bulky dressing. Anticoagulation should be given in the perioperative period to diminish the likelihood of anastomosis thrombosis. Low-molecular-weight dextran for 5–7 days and aspirin are among the recommended regimens. Some patients, particularly children, may require sedation to decrease early postoperative arterial spasm. Vasospastic agents such as nicotine, caffeine, theophylline, and theobromine should be restricted for the first few weeks after replantation or revascularization. The patient should be placed on a broad-spectrum antibiotic for 5–7 days. Clinical monitoring of the replanted or revascularized part may be supplemented with a pulse oximeter, laser Doppler, or temperature probe.

In those replanted or revascularized parts that show impending failure by change in color, capillary refill, or tissue turgor, the dressing should be loosened. Hand position should be changed to relieve pressure on the part. Patients may be given a heparin bolus of 3000–5000 U. The patient must be kept well hydrated and the room warm. If no improvement is seen after 4–6 hours, the patient may be returned to the operating room for exploration of the anastomoses. Vascular revision is most successful when carried out within 48 hours of injury.

Technical problems involving vascular anastomoses are most often caused by thrombosis, an ill-placed suture occluding the lumen, poor proximal flow secondary to spasm, or undetected intimal vessel damage. If vascular damage is found, a larger segment of the vessel should be resected and a vein graft interposed. If failure appears secondary to poor venous outflow, the intermittent application of leeches (*Hirudo* species) for 1–5 days may provide transient venous drainage while adequate venous drainage is reestablished.

▶ Prognosis

Approximately 85% of replanted parts remain viable. Sensory recovery with two-point discrimination of 10 mm or less occurs in approximately 50% of adults. Patients with viable replanted or revascularized parts often complain of cold intolerance during the first 2 or 3 years after replantation. ROM in replanted digits largely depends on the level of injury and averages approximately half of the normal side.

In most children, normal sensation is regained after digital replantation, and the epiphyseal plates remain open and achieve approximately 80% of normal longitudinal growth. Although the functional results are more promising in children, the viability rate is lower in children because of the greater technical demands of the small vessel anastomoses and the greater sympathetic tone.

Because nerves transected in the proximal arm must regenerate over the considerable length of the limb, only limited motor return is seen in the forearm and hand in proximal limb replantations in adults. One potential benefit of a proximal upper limb replantation may be converting a traumatic above-elbow amputation to an assistive limb with elbow control. Replantation may provide dramatic restoration of hand function when the level of initial amputation is either in the distal forearm or at the wrist level (Figure 9–6).

2. Amputation

The purpose of amputation is to preserve maximal function consistent with bone loss and to achieve an aesthetically acceptable appearance. Due to the common muscle belly of the flexor digitorum profundus muscles, one stiff finger can compromise flexion of other digits—the quadriga effect. Amputation of a stiff and insensate finger can improve function of the entire hand. Priority should be given to preserving functional length, minimizing scar and joint contractures, and preventing the development of symptomatic neuromas.

▶ Phalangeal Amputation

Digital amputation may be carried out through a phalanx or an interphalangeal joint. If the amputation is through the proximal or distal interphalangeal joint, the distal articular surface is reshaped to remove the palmar condylar prominences. If the normal insertion of a tendon was amputated, the tendon should be pulled distally, severed proximally, and allowed to retract. The flexor and extensor tendons should never be sewn over the amputation bone end to provide soft-tissue coverage. Nerves should be identified, gently drawn distally, and transected proximally to prevent the development of a neuroma adherent to the skin scar. If possible, the thick well-padded skin of the palmar surface of the finger should be used to cover the amputation stump. A nontender, shortened, well-padded digit is preferable to a poorly covered, slightly longer, tender digit.

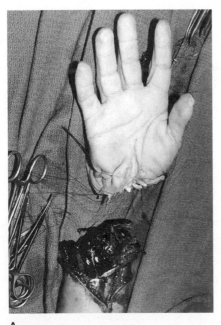
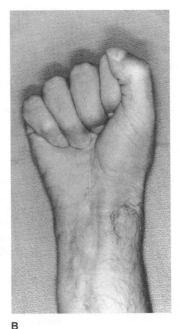
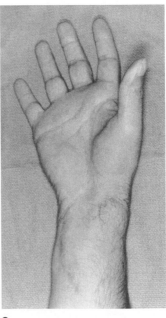

A　　　　　　　　　　　　**B**　　　　　　　　　　　　**C**

▲ **Figure 9–6.** Replantation of hand. Intraoperative view **(A)**. Following operation, flexion **(B)** and extension **(C)** are restored.

Ray Resection

Amputations through the proximal portion of the proximal phalanx or at the metacarpophalangeal joint of the index or little finger may leave an unsightly bony prominence on the border of the palm, and amputations at a similar level in the middle or ring finger may create an awkward interdigital gap that allows small objects to fall through the palm. Ray resection of a digit's phalanges and metacarpal may be employed to close traumatic wounds, remove dysfunctional or dysesthetic digits, or treat malignant tumors. The aesthetic and functional advantages of ray resection must be balanced against the loss of palm breadth and, hence, diminution of grip strength.

Index ray resection creates a normal-appearing web between the middle finger and the thumb. Similarly, resection of the little-finger metacarpal leaves a smooth ulnar contour. Little-finger ray resection is contraindicated in patients who prefer maximal grip strength over cosmesis. Resection of the middle- or ring-finger ray should be accompanied by either soft-tissue coaptation or metacarpal transposition. Resection of the middle ray through the proximal metacarpal metaphysis allows transposition of the corresponding distal portion of the index ray to the middle-ray position (Figure 9–7). Ring-finger ray resection may be closed by either osteotomizing the little-finger metacarpal and moving it to the ring-finger base or by pulling the little finger radialward across the hamate by tight repair of the deep transverse intermetacarpal ligament between the middle and little fingers.

Adani R, Marcoccio I, Castagnetti C, et al: Long-term results of replantation for complete ring avulsion amputations. *Ann Plast Surg* 2003;51:564. [PMID: 14646649]

Melikyan EY, Beg MS, Woodbridge S, et al: The functional results of ray amputation. *J Hand Surg* 2003;8:47. [PMID: 12923934]

Nuzumlali E, Orhun E, Ozturk K, et al: Results of ray resection and amputation for ring avulsion injuries at the proximal interphalangeal joint. *J Hand Surg* 2003B;28:578. [PMID: 14599832]

Wilhelmi BJ, Lee WP, Pagensteert GI, et al: Replantation in the mutilated hand. *Hand Clin* 2003;19:89. [PMID: 12683449]

Yu JC, Shieh SJ, Lee JW, et al: Secondary procedures following digital replantation and revascularisation. *J Plast Surg* 2003B; 56:125. [PMID: 12791355]

DISORDERS OF THE MUSCULATURE OF THE HAND

Anatomy

Control of digital posture requires a complex balance of extrinsic and intrinsic muscle forces. Extrinsic muscles have their origin outside of the hand and their insertion on the hand or carpus, whereas intrinsic muscles have both origin

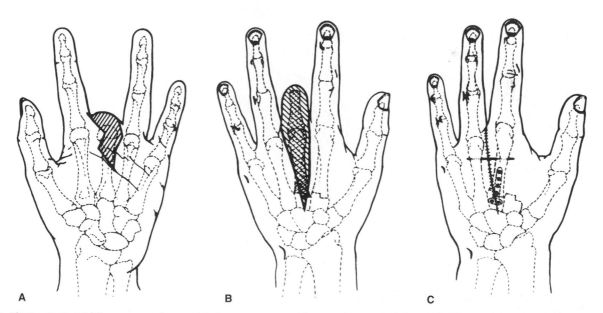

▲ **Figure 9–7.** Middle-ray resection and index-ray transposition. **A:** Converging chevron incisions reduce palmar skin and soft-tissue redundancy. **B:** Corresponding step-cut osteotomies are fashioned in both the index and middle metacarpal proximal metaphyses. **C:** The transposed index finger is fixed to the middle finger with a plate and further stabilized with K-wire into the ring-finger metacarpal. (Reproduced, with permission, from Chapman MW, ed: *Operative Orthopaedics*, Vol. 2, 3rd ed. Philadelphia: J.B. Lippincott; 2001.)

and insertion within the hand. Extrinsic muscles are either flexors or extensors, and intrinsic muscles contribute to both digital flexion and extension.

A. Extrinsic Extensor Muscles

The extrinsic extensors run through six different fibro-osseous retinacular compartments at the wrist level (Figure 9–8A). The first (most radial) compartment contains the abductor pollicis longus and the extensor pollicis brevis. The abductor pollicis longus has multiple slips that insert at the base of the thumb metacarpal and radially abducts the thumb, whereas the extensor pollicis brevis inserts on the dorsum of the proximal aspect of the proximal phalanx of the thumb and actively extends the metacarpophalangeal joint of the thumb.

The second extensor compartment contains the extensor carpi radialis longus and the extensor carpi radialis brevis.

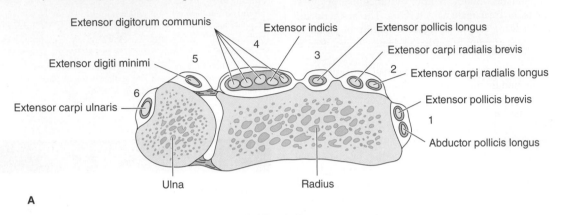

A

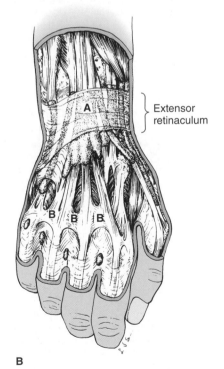

B

▲ **Figure 9–8.** The six dorsal compartments of the wrist. **A:** Cross-section of pronated right wrist viewed from distal to proximal. (Reproduced, with permission, from Reckling FW, et al: *Orthopaedic Anatomy and Surgical Approaches.* St. Louis: Mosby-Year Book; 1990.) **B:** Dorsal view. A, extensor retinaculum over the compartments; B, juncturae tendinum (conexus intertendineus). (Reproduced, with permission, from Way LW, ed: *Current Surgical Diagnosis & Treatment,* 10th ed. Stamford, CT: Appleton & Lange; 1994.)

The extensor carpi radialis longus, inserting on the index metacarpal, dorsiflexes and radially deviates the wrist, and the extensor carpi radialis brevis, inserting into the base of the middle metacarpal, provides balanced wrist dorsiflexion.

The third compartment contains the extensor pollicis longus, which runs longitudinally down the forearm through the third compartment and turns abruptly radialward about Lister tubercle, a dorsal prominence on the distal radius. Because its insertion is on the distal phalanx, the extensor pollicis longus provides forceful extension of the thumb interphalangeal joint. The oblique course of the extensor pollicis longus tendon provides a substantial adduction component to the pull of the extensor pollicis longus.

The fourth extensor compartment contains the extensor indicis proprius lying deep to the four tendons of the extensor digitorum communis, whereas the fifth compartment contains the extensor digiti quinti. These three muscles each have a role in digital extension at the metacarpophalangeal, proximal interphalangeal, and distal interphalangeal joints of the fingers. The principal bony insertion of the extrinsic digital extensors is on the dorsal proximal aspect of the middle phalanx. Metacarpophalangeal joint extension is provided by extrinsic extensor force transmitted through the sagittal bands. Distal interphalangeal joint extension is achieved through the conjoined lateral bands that are composed of tendinous slips from the extrinsic and intrinsic tendons.

The extensor indicis proprius inserts on the index finger ulnar to the extensor digitorum communis. The extensor digitorum communis inserts on the index, middle, ring, and, in some cases, little fingers. The extensor digiti quinti tendon inserts on the little finger ulnar to the extensor digitorum communis insertion.

The extensor carpi ulnaris tendon runs through the sixth compartment and inserts at the base of the little finger metacarpal. It provides wrist extension and ulnar deviation.

The extensor digitorum communis tendons of the middle, ring, and little fingers are tethered together by juncturae tendinum over the dorsum of the hand proximal to the metacarpophalangeal joint (Figure 9–8B). The extensor indicis proprius tendon may be recognized at the wrist level as possessing the most distal muscle belly of any of the digital extensor tendons.

The digital extensor tendons are stabilized over the midline of the metacarpophalangeal joint by their attachment to sagittal band fibers (Figure 9–9). The sagittal band fibers insert onto the volar proximal phalanx and onto the lateral borders of the volar plate. The sagittal band fibers form a sling that allows proximal extrinsic extensor tension to be transmitted to the proximal phalanx, permitting metacarpophalangeal joint extension without a tendinous insertion onto the proximal phalanx. By holding the extrinsic extensor tendon balanced over the prominence of the metacarpal head, the sagittal bands normally keep the extrinsic extensor as far as possible away from the center of rotation of the metacarpophalangeal joint, thereby giving it the greatest mechanical efficiency. With rupture or attenuation of the sagittal band fibers, the extrinsic extensor tendon can sublux to the ulnar side of the metacarpal head causing ulnar deviation of the finger.

B. Extrinsic Flexor Muscles

The extrinsic finger flexors are the flexor digitorum profundus and the flexor digitorum superficialis. The flexor digitorum profundus inserts on the proximal volar aspect of the distal phalanx, flexing the distal interphalangeal joint as well as the proximal interphalangeal and metacarpophalangeal joints. The flexor digitorum superficialis acts as a flexor of the proximal interphalangeal and metacarpophalangeal joints. It lies palmar to the flexor digitorum profundus tendon in the palm, splits at the level of the metacarpophalangeal joint, and passes dorsal to the flexor digitorum profundus tendon before inserting into the sides of the middle phalanx. Although the extrinsic flexors provide metacarpophalangeal joint flexion, this occurs only after most of their excursion is expended flexing the interphalangeal joints.

C. Intrinsic Muscles

The intrinsic muscles that control finger posture are the dorsal and palmar interossei, lumbricals, and hypothenar muscles. These muscles are responsible for primary flexion, abduction, and adduction of the metacarpophalangeal joints and primary extension of the proximal interphalangeal and distal interphalangeal joints.

The index finger is abducted by the first dorsal interosseous muscle and adducted by the first palmar interosseous muscle. The middle finger is radially abducted by the second dorsal interosseous muscle and ulnarly abducted by the third dorsal interosseous muscle. The ring finger is adducted by the second volar interosseous muscle and abducted by the fourth dorsal interosseous muscle. The little finger is adducted by the third volar interosseous muscle and abducted by the abductor digiti quinti muscle.

The first, second, and fourth dorsal interossei have both superficial and deep muscle bellies, with the superficial belly giving rise to a tendon of insertion on the proximal phalanx tubercle. The deep muscle belly inserts into the hood of the dorsal aponeurosis and thus contributes to metacarpophalangeal joint flexion and proximal and distal interphalangeal joint extension. The third dorsal interosseous usually has a single muscle belly, which inserts into the dorsal hood apparatus. The insertion of the volar interosseous muscles is also into the hood apparatus (see Figure 9–9).

All interosseous muscles course palmar to the axis of motion of the metacarpophalangeal joint and dorsal to the transverse intermetacarpal ligament. Their tendinous insertions are into the lateral band fibers, which pass dorsal to the axis of motion of the proximal and distal interphalangeal joints. When the metacarpophalangeal joint is flexed, the interossei are less effective in extending the interphalangeal

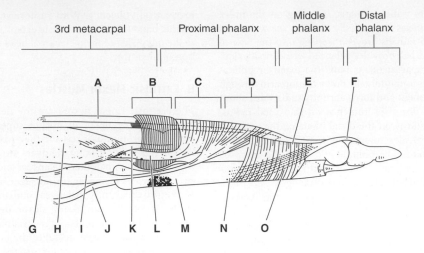

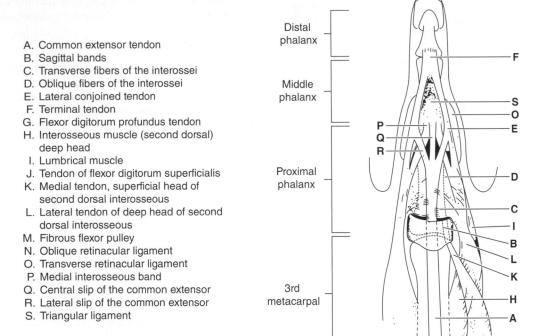

A. Common extensor tendon
B. Sagittal bands
C. Transverse fibers of the interossei
D. Oblique fibers of the interossei
E. Lateral conjoined tendon
F. Terminal tendon
G. Flexor digitorum profundus tendon
H. Interosseous muscle (second dorsal)
   deep head
I. Lumbrical muscle
J. Tendon of flexor digitorum superficialis
K. Medial tendon, superficial head of
   second dorsal interosseous
L. Lateral tendon of deep head of second
   dorsal interosseous
M. Fibrous flexor pulley
N. Oblique retinacular ligament
O. Transverse retinacular ligament
P. Medial interosseous band
Q. Central slip of the common extensor
R. Lateral slip of the common extensor
S. Triangular ligament

▲ **Figure 9–9.** Extensor hood mechanism. The dorsal hood apparatus provides points of insertion of both extrinsic extensors and intrinsic muscles of the hand. (Modified and reproduced, with permission, from Way LW, ed: *Current Surgical Diagnosis & Treatment,* 10th ed. Stamford, CT: Appleton & Lange; 1994.)

joints than when the metacarpophalangeal joint is in extension or slight flexion.

The four lumbrical muscles insert into the radial lateral band of the dorsal hood aponeurosis of each finger. The lumbricals originate from the flexor digitorum profundus

tendons of the corresponding finger. Their course is more volar than that of the dorsal or palmar interosseous muscles because they lie palmar to the transverse intermetacarpal ligament. The lumbrical muscles modulate flexor and extensor digital tone and may have a role in digital proprioception.

Contraction of the profundus muscle belly draws the profundus tendon proximally and shifts the lumbrical origin proximally, thereby increasing tension on the dorsal hood fibers that extend the proximal and distal interphalangeal joints. Contraction of the lumbrical muscle draws the proximal profundus distally and reduces tension on the flexor digitorum profundus at the distal interphalangeal joint, so that distal interphalangeal joint extension is facilitated.

The abductor digiti quinti, like the first, second, and fourth interossei, has two tendons of insertion. One of these tendons inserts directly onto the bone of the abductor tubercle along the ulnar aspect of the little finger proximal phalanx, and the other insertion is into the dorsal hood apparatus. The flexor digiti quinti inserts onto the ulnar tubercle at the base of the proximal phalanx but does not insert into the dorsal hood apparatus. The primary function of the flexor digiti quinti is flexion of the metacarpophalangeal joint.

D. Dorsal Hood Apparatus

The dorsal hood apparatus, frequently referred to as the extensor mechanism, is the confluence of intrinsic and extrinsic tendon insertions on the dorsal aspect of the finger (see Figure 9–9). Through dorsal hood attachments, the extrinsic extensor muscles extend the metacarpophalangeal joint, the intrinsic muscles flex the metacarpophalangeal joint, and both the intrinsic and extrinsic muscles extend the proximal and distal interphalangeal joints.

Extension of the metacarpophalangeal joint is achieved through the action of the extrinsic extensor tendons pulling through the sagittal band sling mechanism, which lifts up the proximal phalanx. Flexion of the metacarpophalangeal joint is achieved both by the tendinous insertion of the intrinsics on the proximal phalanx and by a similar sling effect created by oblique fibers of the intrinsic mechanism blending into the hood, which flexes the metacarpophalangeal joint. Additionally, the flexor digitorum profundus and superficialis secondarily flex the metacarpophalangeal joint.

Extension of the proximal interphalangeal joint is achieved through the action of the central slip, which is the bony insertion of the extrinsic digital extensors on the middle phalanx. In addition, the intrinsic muscles contribute to proximal interphalangeal joint extension through medial slips from the lateral band, which run centrally to insert on the proximal dorsal aspect of the middle phalanx as part of the central slip.

Distal interphalangeal joint extension is achieved through both intrinsic and extrinsic forces pulling through the radial and ulnar conjoined lateral bands, which merge to form the terminal tendon insertion. The intrinsic contribution to the conjoined lateral band is through its insertion into the lateral band. The extrinsic contribution to distal interphalangeal joint extension occurs through lateral slip fibers that diverge from the central slip over the dorsum of the proximal phalanx and join the lateral band to form the conjoined lateral band. The conjoined lateral bands from the radial and ulnar side converge distally as the terminal tendon inserting on the distal phalanx.

DISRUPTION OF EXTENSOR MUSCLE INSERTIONS

1. Sagittal Band Disruption

▶ Anatomy and Clinical Findings

The sagittal band fibers transmitting extrinsic extensor power may be disrupted by laceration or, more often, may become attenuated because of underlying synovitis of the metacarpophalangeal joint, as occurs in RA. When the sagittal band fibers along either the radial or ulnar aspect of the dorsal hood become attenuated, the extensor tendon may sublux into the valley between the adjacent metacarpal heads. Because the subluxed extrinsic extensors are mechanically less effective at extending the metacarpophalangeal joint, full active extension of this joint may be lost. This phenomenon occurs commonly in RA. It also may result from tearing of the sagittal band fibers with torquing activity such as occurs in the middle finger with pitching a baseball.

▶ Treatment

An acute tear of the radial sagittal band may be treated by splinting. If this is ineffective, surgical repair may be indicated. Chronic injuries are treated by releasing the ulnar sagittal band and recentralizing the extensor tendon by placing a strip of the tendon around the radial collateral ligament.

2. Boutonnière Deformity

▶ Anatomy and Clinical Findings

When the central slip is disrupted by laceration or closed rupture or elongated by synovitis of the proximal interphalangeal joint, the direct bony insertion of the extrinsic extensors on the middle phalanx is lost. When the insertion of the medial slips from the lateral band is also lost, active proximal interphalangeal joint extension is lacking. The finger is rapidly drawn into a position of proximal interphalangeal joint flexion as the unopposed motion of the flexor digitorum sublimis and profundus draws the finger into flexion (Figure 9–10). The lateral bands migrate apart as the finger is flexed and are drawn into a progressively more palmar position, eventually coming to lie palmar to the axis of flexion of the joint. In the subluxed position, the lateral bands become a deforming force contributing to the tendency of the finger to flex at the proximal interphalangeal joint.

With central slip disruption, the force normally transmitted through the central slip to the middle phalanx from both extrinsic extensor and intrinsic muscles bypasses the proximal interphalangeal joint and is refocused on the distal interphalangeal joint, amplifying the force of extension of

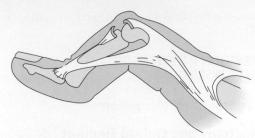

▲ **Figure 9–10.** Boutonnière deformity caused by loss of active proximal interphalangeal extension secondary to loss of the central slip insertion on the proximal dorsal middle phalanx. (Reproduced, with permission, from Way LW, ed: *Current Surgical Diagnosis & Treatment,* 10th ed. Stamford, CT: Appleton & Lange; 1994.)

this joint and hyperextending it. Because the distal interphalangeal joint is relatively resistant to active flexion, contraction of the flexor digitorum profundus muscle primarily flexes the proximal interphalangeal joint and is relatively ineffective in flexing the distal interphalangeal joint, unless the proximal interphalangeal joint is supported in maximal extension. The digit eventually assumes the boutonnière deformity posture of proximal interphalangeal joint flexion and distal interphalangeal joint hyperextension.

▶ **Treatment**

Because the proximal interphalangeal joint is at the center of the complex balance of the intrinsic and extrinsic forces, restoration of proper balance and tension on the central slip may be technically difficult. When the central slip is acutely lacerated, it should be directly repaired and the joint pinned in full extension for 3–6 weeks to protect the integrity of the repair. Closed ruptures of the central slip, if diagnosed acutely, should be treated with 6 weeks of splinting of the proximal interphalangeal joint in full extension. When diagnosis is delayed even a few weeks, a fixed flexion contracture of the proximal interphalangeal joint is usual.

Surgical treatment of closed rupture of the central slip in a finger that develops a fixed flexion contracture is frequently disappointing because the surgical procedure must both release the contracture on the palmar aspect of the joint and augment proximal interphalangeal joint extension on the dorsal aspect. A better strategy employs prolonged splinting to diminish the extent of the fixed proximal interphalangeal joint flexion contracture. Among the variety of splints available for this, the Capener splint and the Joint Jack splint are particularly useful. Serial casting of the finger with a circumferential digital cast that is changed every few days may also be helpful in bringing the proximal interphalangeal joint into extension. During the period of splinting, the patient should be instructed to carry out active flexion of the distal interphalangeal joint, with the middle phalanx supported in extension. Care should be taken to assure

that splints and casts allow distal interphalangeal joint flexion. Once full proximal interphalangeal joint extension is achieved, splinting should be continued full time for an additional 6–12 weeks. In many instances, this achieves sufficient tightening of the central slip to permit satisfactory active proximal interphalangeal joint extension.

If active extension cannot be restored with prolonged splinting, several operative interventions may be considered. The first, a Fowler type of tenotomy, obliquely divides the dorsal hood apparatus over the middle phalanx, proximal to the terminal tendon insertion. This diminishes distal interphalangeal joint hyperextension and may improve active proximal interphalangeal joint extension by refocusing intrinsic and extrinsic forces at the more proximal joint.

Alternatively, other surgical techniques attempt to more directly augment proximal interphalangeal joint extension, either by shortening the central slip or by mobilizing portions of one or both lateral bands. Although such techniques may increase active extension of the joint, they often do so at the loss of full proximal interphalangeal joint flexion.

3. Mallet Finger

▶ **Anatomy and Clinical Findings**

The mallet finger deformity is characterized by a loss of active distal interphalangeal joint extension with full passive ROM evident. The mallet finger reflects the loss of normal extensor force transmission via the terminal tendon insertion onto the distal phalanx. The unopposed flexor digitorum profundus pulls the distal joint into flexion (Figure 9–11). The usual mechanism of injury involves sudden passive flexion of the actively extended distal interphalangeal joint. Disruption of the terminal tendon may be entirely confined to the tendon or may involve an avulsed fracture fragment from the dorsal lip of the distal phalanx proximal articular surface.

Because the avulsed fragment includes the terminal tendon insertion, the clinical appearance of soft tissue and bony mallet fingers is similar. The distal joint rests in flexion, a posture that cannot be actively changed. Full passive extension of the distal interphalangeal joint is possible.

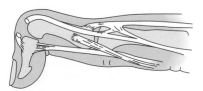

▲ **Figure 9–11.** Mallet finger deformity is secondary to loss of terminal tendon insertion on the distal phalanx. (Reproduced, with permission, from Way LW, ed: *Current Surgical Diagnosis & Treatment,* 10th ed. Stamford, CT: Appleton & Lange; 1994.)

Treatment

A radiograph should be obtained to determine whether a fracture is present and, if the dorsal fragment is large, whether the distal phalanx is subluxed palmarward. If the joint is congruent, splinting is recommended even if a small articular surface fracture site gap persists. The distal interphalangeal joint should be splinted in extension continuously for 8 weeks, and the finger may then be tested. If residual drooping of the distal joint is noted, an additional 2–4 weeks of splinting are required.

Kalainov DM, Hoepfner PE, Hartigan BJ, et al: Non-surgical treatment of closed mallet finger fractures. *J Hand Surg Am* 2005;30: 580. [PMID: 15925171]

INTRINSIC PLUS AND INTRINSIC MINUS POSITIONS

Together, the interossei and lumbricals flex the metacarpophalangeal joints and extend the proximal and distal interphalangeal joints. Hence, the posture of the hand in which the metacarpophalangeal joints are flexed and the proximal and distal interphalangeal joints are extended is known as the intrinsic plus position (Figure 9–12). This is an ideal position for splinting the hand because the collateral ligaments of the metacarpophalangeal and interphalangeal joint are taut, and because it is also ideal for immobilization of most hand injuries, it is termed the *position of safety* or *position of advantage*.

The normal excursion of the intrinsic muscles is sufficient to allow simultaneous passive positioning of the metacarpophalangeal joints in extension while the proximal and distal

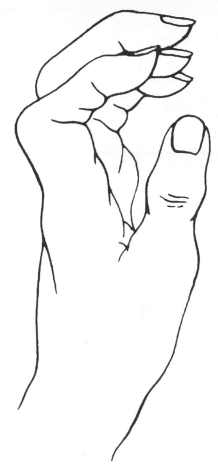

▲ **Figure 9–13.** Intrinsic minus position secondary to low median and ulnar nerve palsies.

interphalangeal joints are flexed. This posture, known as the intrinsic minus position, requires full excursion of the relaxed intrinsic muscles (see Figure 9–12; Figure 9–13). When the intrinsic muscles are paralyzed, the hand tends to assume the intrinsic minus posture, sometimes referred to as a clawhand. Although the extrinsic extensors have fibers that can provide proximal and distal interphalangeal joint extension in the hand with competent intrinsic muscles, in the intrinsic minus hand, their excursion is expended in unopposed metacarpophalangeal joint hyperextension. Thus, the hand devoid of intrinsic power is unable to achieve active extension of the proximal and distal interphalangeal joints, unless the metacarpophalangeal joint is flexed by other means.

Treatment

Surgical correction of the intrinsic minus hand must either prevent passive hyperextension of the metacarpophalangeal joint or restore active control of metacarpophalangeal

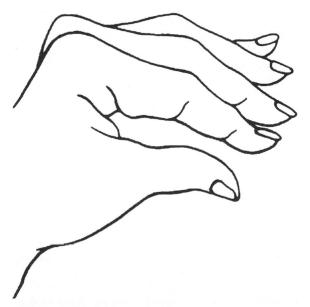

▲ **Figure 9–12.** Intrinsic plus position.

joint flexion. This may be achieved either by tenodesis or capsulodesis across the metacarpophalangeal joint or by an active tendon transfer. Once metacarpophalangeal joint hyperextension is prevented, the extrinsic extensors usually can effectively open the hand by extending the proximal and distal interphalangeal joints. If active proximal interphalangeal joint extension is not possible through the extrinsic extensors when the metacarpophalangeal joint is flexed, then tendon transfer for metacarpophalangeal joint flexion should be inserted into the digital lateral bands. This augments proximal interphalangeal joint extension and provides metacarpophalangeal joint flexion.

INTRINSIC MUSCLE TIGHTNESS

▶ Anatomy and Clinical Findings

When the lumbricals and interossei become contracted and overly tight, the limitation of their excursion does not permit full simultaneous metacarpophalangeal joint extension and interphalangeal joint flexion. The intrinsic tightness test was originally described by Finochietto and later by Bunnell (Figure 9–14). It is accomplished by first determining that the metacarpophalangeal and interphalangeal joints each have a full range of passive joint motion in a reduced position. The metacarpophalangeal joint is then passively held in an extended position while the examiner attempts to flex the proximal and distal interphalangeal joints passively. If full passive flexion of the proximal and distal interphalangeal joints is not possible in this position, the intrinsic muscles are deemed tight.

Causes of intrinsic muscle tightness include conditions as diverse as RA, neurologic dysfunction secondary to closed head injury, and crush injury of the hand.

▶ Treatment

Surgical treatment of intrinsic tightness may be carried out as an isolated procedure or in combination with metacarpophalangeal joint reconstruction. The intrinsic force is diminished either by intrinsic muscle tenotomy or by resection of a triangular segment of one or both lateral bands. The intrinsic tightness test may be used intraoperatively to judge the adequacy of intrinsic muscle release.

SWAN-NECK DEFORMITY

▶ Anatomy and Clinical Findings

Swan-neck deformity is characterized by hyperextension of the proximal interphalangeal joint and flexion of the distal interphalangeal joint (Figure 9–15). The pathophysiology of swan-neck deformity involves either primary or secondary stretching or disruption of the volar plate's restraint on proximal interphalangeal joint hyperextension. Synovitis of the proximal interphalangeal joint secondary in patients with RA may distend the joint and thus render the volar

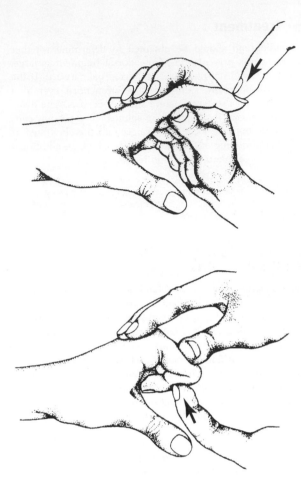

▲ **Figure 9–14.** Intrinsic tightness test is performed by flexing the proximal interphalangeal joint with the metaphalangeal joint extended and flexed. Tightness to proximal interphalangeal flexion occurs with the metaphalangeal joint extended. (Reproduced, with permission, from Green DP, ed: *Operative Hand Surgery*, 2nd ed. Philadelphia: Churchill Livingstone; 1988.)

plate ineffective in preventing proximal interphalangeal joint hyperextension. Overly forceful intrinsic muscle contraction (as occurs with an intrinsic plus deformity) transmits an abnormally high force through the central slip, hyperextending the proximal interphalangeal joint. When the proximal interphalangeal joint is hyperextended, the dorsal hood apparatus is relatively ineffective in extending the distal interphalangeal joint, allowing the distal interphalangeal joint to fall into flexion.

In some fingers, a fixed extension contracture or ankylosis of the proximal interphalangeal joint may occur as a consequence of swan-neck deformity. In other fingers, the proximal interphalangeal joint remains supple but the finger is locked in a hyperextended posture.

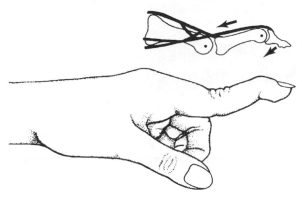

▲ **Figure 9–15.** Swan-neck deformity. (Reproduced, with permission, from American Society for Surgery of the Hand: *The Hand: Examination and Diagnosis,* 2nd ed. Philadelphia: Churchill Livingstone; 1983.)

▶ Treatment

Surgical treatment of swan-neck deformity secondary to intrinsic tightness requires diminishing intrinsic muscle force, usually through resection of a triangle of the proximal lateral band and dorsal hood. A new checkrein to proximal interphalangeal joint extension is created, either through tenodesis of one slip of the flexor digitorum superficialis or tenodesis in which one of the lateral bands is rerouted volar to the center of rotation of the proximal interphalangeal joint, recreating the sagittal oblique retinacular ligament.

Bruner S, Wittemann M, Jester A, et al: Dynamic splinting after extensor tendon repair in zones V to VII. *J Hand Surg* 2003B; 28:224. [PMID: 12809652]

▼ DISORDERS OF THE TENDONS OF THE HAND

FLEXOR TENDON INJURY

▶ Anatomy

The extrinsic flexors of the finger consist of the flexor digitorum profundus and the flexor digitorum superficialis. The flexor digitorum profundus originates from the proximal ulna and the interosseous membrane. In the forearm, it divides into two muscle groups: the most radial component supplying the index finger and the ulnar component supplying the middle, ring, and little fingers. The flexor digitorum profundus and flexor pollicis longus muscles form the deep compartment of the volar forearm. As the flexor digitorum profundus and flexor pollicis longus tendons travel through the carpal tunnel, they occupy the floor of the carpal tunnel.

The tenosynovial sheath of the flexor pollicis longus is continuous with the radial bursa; the tenosynovial sheath to the little finger is continuous with the ulnar digital bursa. In some patients, these two bursae communicate, allowing a so-called horseshoe abscess to spread between the thumb and little finger if infection occurs in the flexor tendon sheath of either one of these digits.

The lumbricals originate from the radial side of the index, middle, ring, and little fingers in the palm. The profundus tendon passes through the bifurcation of the flexor digitorum superficialis before inserting into the proximal palmar base of the distal phalanx. The innervation of the flexor digitorum profundus of the index and middle fingers is through the anterior interosseous branch of the median nerve, whereas the profundus of the ring and little fingers is innervated by the ulnar nerve. The flexor digitorum profundus provides digital flexion at both the proximal and distal interphalangeal joints.

The flexor digitorum superficialis has two heads: The radial head originates from the proximal shaft of the radius, and the humeral ulnar head originates from the medial humeral epicondyle and coronoid process of the ulna. Each digit has a corresponding independent superficialis muscle. As the superficialis tendons pass through the carpal tunnel, the tendons of the middle and ring fingers are more superficial and central than those of the index and little fingers. In the proximal aspect of the finger, the flexor digitorum superficialis tendon bifurcates around the flexor digitorum profundus at the beginning of the A2 pulley. The flexor digitorum superficialis tendon slips then reunite distally at the Camper chiasm, with approximately half of the fibers staying on the ipsilateral side and half crossing to the contralateral side of the finger. The tendon then inserts via radial and ulnar slips into the proximal metaphysis of the middle phalanx. The entire flexor digitorum superficialis muscle receives innervation from the median nerve. The primary function of the superficialis is digital flexion at the proximal interphalangeal joint.

The flexor pollicis longus originates from two heads: The radial head takes origin from the proximal radius and interosseous membrane, and an accessory head originates from the coronoid process of the ulna and from the medial epicondyle of the humerus. In the palm, the flexor pollicis longus tendon transverses between the abductor pollicis brevis and the flexor pollicis brevis. The flexor pollicis longus inserts into the proximal base of the thumb distal phalanx and is innervated by the anterior interosseous branch of the median nerve. The flexor pollicis longus flexes both the interphalangeal and metacarpophalangeal joints of the thumb.

As the flexor tendons pass distal to the metacarpal neck, they enter the fibroosseous tunnel, or digital flexor sheath. The fibroosseous tunnel extends distally to the proximal aspect of the distal phalanx. The tendinous sheath consists of annular pulleys, which provide mechanical stability, and cruciate pulleys, which provide flexibility (Figure 9–16). The

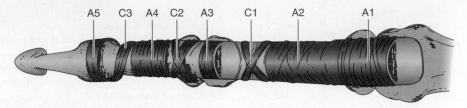

▲ **Figure 9–16.** Annular (A) and cruciate (C) pulley locations.

first, third, and fifth annular pulleys (A1, A3, and A5) are located over the metacarpophalangeal, proximal interphalangeal, and distal interphalangeal joints, respectively, and the second and fourth pulleys (A2 and A4) are situated over the middle portion of the proximal and middle phalanges. The A2 and A4 pulleys are the most essential in maintaining the mechanical advantage of the flexor tendons.

The tenosynovium that lines the fibroosseous tunnel supplies both nutrition and lubrication to the poorly vascularized flexor tendons. Proximal to the sheath, the tendons are well vascularized by the peritenon. Within the sheath, tendon vascularity is supplied via the vincula system: the vinculum longus and brevis.

Following injury, the flexor tendon heals through both extrinsic and intrinsic mechanisms. Extrinsic tendon healing occurs via cells brought to the site of repair by ingrowth of capillaries and fibroblasts; formation of adhesions follows at the repair site. Intrinsic healing occurs from tenocyte within the tendon. The goal of flexor tendon repair and postoperative care is to encourage both intrinsic and extrinsic healing without the formation of thick adhesions, which would limit tendon excursion and ultimately result in restricted motion of the finger.

▶ **Clinical Findings**

The time since injury as well as the mechanism of injury (sharp open injury versus closed avulsion injury) should be noted in the history.

A. Normal Cascade of Fingers

The resting posture of the fingers should be observed. Disruption of the normal cascade of increasing flexion in the relaxed fingers as one moves from the index finger to the little finger should arouse suspicion of tendon disruption (Figure 9–17).

B. Normal Tenodesis Phenomenon

Tendon integrity may also be evaluated by taking advantage of the normal tenodesis positioning of the digits, which occurs as the wrist is passively brought through a ROM. Normally, as the wrist is dorsiflexed, the digital extensors relax and the finger flexors become taut, passively flexing the fingers in the normal cascade pattern. When the muscles of the proximal forearm are squeezed, the fingers normally flex involuntarily.

C. Testing of Individual Tendons

Isolated testing of the superficialis and profundus tendons is employed to determine the integrity of each tendon (see Figures 9–2 and 9–3). Because the flexor digitorum superficialis of the little finger is not independent of the ring finger in many individuals, either because of cross connections between the two tendons or because of congenital absence of the tendon, it may be impossible from clinical examination to detect injury to the flexor digitorum superficialis tendon

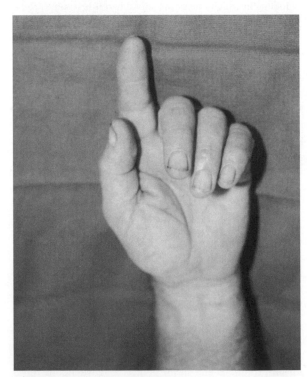

▲ **Figure 9–17.** If the index finger remains extended when the hand is at rest, its flexor tendons are severed.

of the little finger. The strength of flexion should be noted as each of the tendons is tested. If the patient is able to flex the finger but experiences pain with flexion and is unable to generate full power against resistance, a partial flexor tendon injury should be suspected.

▶ Treatment

Functional outcomes are equivalent if the repair is done the day of injury (primary repair) or within the first 7–10 days after the injury (delayed primary repair).

Because repair requires proper visualization of both ends of the tendon, the wound may need to be electively extended. The tendon ends must be gently retrieved because trauma to the flexor tendon sheath creates adverse scarring. Tendons should not be grasped along their tenosynovial surfaces. The A2 and A4 pulleys should be preserved. A maximum of 1 cm may be debrided from the tendon ends without compromising eventual digital extension. A core suture of either 3-0 or 4-0 braided synthetic material is secured to coapt tendon ends (Figure 9–18).

The flexor tendon repair is strengthened by employing four strands of suture across the repair site rather than two.

A running 6-0 nylon epitendinous suture completes the tendon repair. The role of flexor tendon sheath repair remains controversial.

Because the results and complications of flexor tendon repair vary by level of injury, five zones of injury are defined (Figure 9–19). Zone I extends from the insertion of the profundus on the distal phalanx to the insertion of the flexor digitorum superficialis on the middle phalanx. The tendon may be directly repaired if the distal stump is large enough, or it may be reinserted to bone. Care must be taken not to advance the tendon more than 1 cm.

Zone II, which extends from the proximal portion of the A1 pulley to the insertion of the superficialis tendon, is the most problematic region of injury because it contains both the profundus and superficialis tendons in a relatively avascular region. Care must be taken to preserve the vincular blood supply. When both the superficialis and profundus tendons are divided, it is preferable to repair both tendons because greater digital independence of motion may be achieved with a somewhat lower risk of tendon rupture during the rehabilitation period. Repair of the superficialis tendon as well as the profundus tendon also diminishes the likelihood of proximal interphalangeal joint hyperextension deformity.

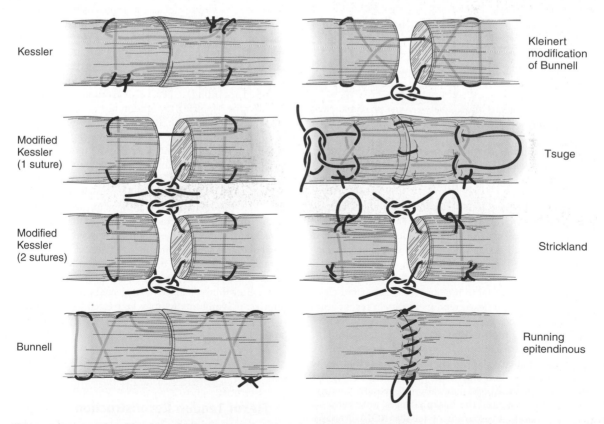

▲ **Figure 9–18.** Kessler sutures and other types of sutures for flexor tendon repair. (Reproduced, with permission, from Green DP, ed: *Operative Hand Surgery*, 2nd ed. Philadelphia: Churchill Livingstone; 1988.)

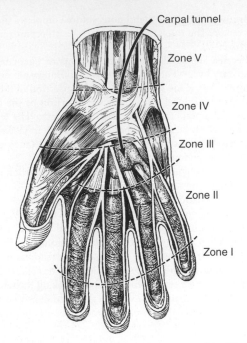

Carpal tunnel

Zone V

Zone IV

Zone III

Zone II

Zone I

▲ **Figure 9–19.** Flexor tendon injury zones. (Modified and reproduced, with permission, from Way LW, ed: *Current Surgical Diagnosis & Treatment,* 10th ed. Stamford: Appleton & Lange; 1994.)

Zone III injuries are located between the proximal edge of the A1 pulley and the distal edge of the transverse carpal ligament.

In zone IV injuries, the area beneath the transverse carpal ligament, a step-cut release and repair of the transverse carpal ligament should be performed to prevent flexor tendon bowstringing.

Zone I and II injuries of the thumb are handled similarly to those of analogous finger zones. In zone III of the thumb, it is difficult to access the flexor pollicis longus tendon as it passes through the thenar musculature. Options for treatment of injuries at this level include either primary tendon grafting or step-cut lengthening of the tendon in the forearm, so the repair is distal to the obscuring thenar muscles.

Improved results of flexor tendon surgery in recent years are substantially because of the evolution of postoperative therapy programs. Immobilization of the finger after tendon repair is appropriate only in very young or otherwise uncooperative patients. Following flexor tendon injury, the wrist should be immobilized at approximately 30 degrees of flexion, the metacarpophalangeal joints at approximately 45 degrees of flexion, and the interphalangeal joints at 0–15 degrees of flexion. A program of passive ROM exercises should be initiated that decreases the adhesions at the repair site and enhances intrinsic tendon repair. Passive motion

may be achieved either through rubber band splinting to flex the finger passively or by having the patient move the finger passively. At 4–6 weeks following repair, active flexion and extension exercises are allowed as splinting is discontinued. At 6–8 weeks, passive extension exercises and isolated blocking is encouraged. After 8 weeks, the patient may begin flexion against resistance.

When a four-strand repair is performed, active assisted motion is begun within the first 2 weeks. In this program, the wrist is extended and the fingers are passively flexed. The patient is then asked to flex the fingers actively to hold this position.

With four-strand techniques for flexor tendon repair, active motion can begin earlier than with a two-strand repair. In properly motivated and cooperative patients, an active hold program is begun during the first week. The therapist passively brings the hand into flexion and the patient is asked to maintain the position.

▶ Flexor Tendon Avulsion Injuries

The flexor tendon may be avulsed from its bony insertion, usually by forced extension of the finger while the finger is simultaneously actively flexed. An estimated 75% of flexor digitorum profundus avulsion injuries involve the ring finger. Such injuries commonly occur in football or rugby, when the athlete grabs an opponent's jersey and a finger is involuntarily extended as the opponent attempts to elude tackle.

Flexor digitorum profundus avulsion injuries may be classified according to the level of profundus tendon retraction. In type 1 injuries, the tendon retracts proximally from the sheath into the palm. Repair of these injuries should be performed within 10 days to avoid myostatic contracture, which will limit the ability to bring the tendon to its normal insertion without undue tension. In type 2 injuries, the tendon retracts to the level of the proximal interphalangeal joint. A small bony avulsion fragment may be seen on a lateral radiograph of the finger in these injuries. The tendon may be reinserted into the distal phalanx up to 6 weeks after injury. Type 3 injuries involve an osseous distal phalangeal avulsion fragment that is so large, it blocks retraction of the flexor digitorum profundus proximal to the A4 pulley. These injuries also may be repaired up to 6 weeks after injury. Missed or neglected profundus avulsion injuries, if symptomatic, may be treated by staged tendon reconstruction, distal interphalangeal joint arthrodesis, or tenodesis.

Moiemen NS, Elliot D: Primary flexor tendon repair in zone 1. *J Hand Surg Br* 2000;25:78. [PMID: 10763731]

▶ Flexor Tendon Reconstruction

Direct repair of a disrupted flexor tendon is not possible if there is loss of the tendon substance, long-standing myostatic contracture, or unresolved soft-tissue defects. If the flexor digitorum superficialis tendon is intact with a full active range of proximal interphalangeal joint motion, arthrodesis or tenodesis of the distal interphalangeal joint may be elected, creating a so-called superficialis finger. If the patient requires active motion at the distal interphalangeal joint, tendon grafting is necessary. Tendon grafting is usually indicated when neither flexor digitorum superficialis nor flexor digitorum profundus tendons can be repaired.

Primary tendon grafting may be performed when there is satisfactory skin coverage, full passive range of metacarpophalangeal and interphalangeal joint motion, an intact annular pulley system, minimal scarring in the sheath, adequate digital circulation, and at least one intact digital nerve. Possible donor tendon sources include the palmaris longus, plantaris, or toe extensor tendons. The palmaris longus and plantaris tendons are absent in a significant minority of individuals.

A. Surgical Procedure

The donor tendon graft is secured into the distal phalanx. The tendon graft is threaded beneath the flexor tendon sheath pulleys. The proximal attachment of the donor tendon to the profundus motor is performed either with a tendon weave or an end-to-end repair.

Establishing appropriate tension on the tendon graft is critical. If insufficient tension is placed on the tendon graft, a lumbrical plus deformity occurs. With this condition, as the patient pulls the proximal portion of the profundus tendon proximally, the lumbrical is placed under tension, and all of this tension is transmitted to the dorsal hood apparatus rather than to the flexor tendon graft. As a result, as the patient attempts to flex the finger, the finger paradoxically extends both the proximal and distal interphalangeal joints.

If the tendon graft tension is too tight, full extension is impossible. The results of primary tendon grafting are inferior to primary repair in similar circumstances.

Primary tendon repair is contraindicated if the fibroosseous sheath is extensively scarred or if critical pulleys are absent. Restoration of flexion in such situations requires a staged tendon reconstruction. In stage 1, the tendon remnants are excised from the sheath, and joint contractures are released. At a minimum, the A2 and A4 pulleys are reconstructed using a flexor tendon remnant, a tendon graft, or a strip of the wrist extensor retinaculum. A silicone rod similar in size to the anticipated tendon graft is secured to the distal phalanx and threaded through the sheath. Early passive ROM stimulates the development of a pseudosheath surrounding the silicone tendon rod.

The second stage of the procedure occurs at least 3 months after the initial procedure. Full digital passive ROM and soft-tissue equilibrium must be achieved before the second stage is undertaken. The silicone tendon rod is replaced with a tendon graft. The donor tendon is secured to the distal phalanx and to the donor motor in a manner similar to primary tendon grafting.

B. Complications

1. Adhesions—The most common complication following flexor tendon surgery is formation of adhesions between the repair site and the surrounding fibroosseous tunnel, which may occur despite an appropriate therapy program. Following flexor tendon repair or graft, tenolysis should be considered when active flexion is restricted, despite a normal passive ROM, in a wound that has reached soft-tissue equilibrium (usually at least 3 months since repair or reconstruction), in a motivated patient.

Ideally, tenolysis should be performed under local anesthesia with intravenous sedation. Elevation of skin flaps allows wide exposure of the sheath. Care is taken to preserve the annular pulleys while adhesions are released between the tendon and the sheath and between the tendon and the phalanges. Evaluation of the adequacy of lysis may be obtained by asking the patient under local anesthesia to flex the finger actively. If regional or general anesthesia is employed, the tendon must be identified at a more proximal level and traction applied to the tendon at this level to confirm the improvement in joint motion.

Active ROM exercise is begun within the first 24 hours after surgery. Electrical stimulation of the proximal muscle belly may facilitate early motion.

2. Tendon repair rupture—The second major postoperative complication of flexor tendon repair is rupture of the repair. When the rupture is promptly diagnosed, a second repair should be attempted because success rates approach those of uncomplicated primary repair. If rupture is not promptly diagnosed, the ruptured tendon ends must be resected, and either free tendon grafting or staged tendon reconstruction is necessary to restore active flexion.

3. Failure of staged reconstruction—If staged reconstruction fails, arthrodesis or amputation of the digit may be considered, particularly when accompanied by neurovascular compromise.

Beredjiklian PK: Biologic aspects of flexor tendon laceration and repair. *J Bone Joint Surg Am* 2003;85:539. [PMID: 12637445]

Beris AE, Darlis NA, Korompilias AV, et al: Two-stage flexor tendon reconstruction in zone II using a silicone rod and a pedicled intrasynovial graft. *J Hand Surg Am* 2003;28:652. [PMID: 12877856]

Slade JF, Bhargava M, Barrie KA, et al: Zone II tendon repairs augmented with autogenous dorsal tendon graft: A biomechanical analysis. *J Hand Surg Am* 2001;26:813. [PMID: 11561232]

TENOSYNOVITIS

Tenosynovitis may develop about any of the extrinsic flexor or extensor tendons, either throughout their course or, more commonly, at points of constraint by fibrous pulleys or retinacular sheaths.

1. de Quervain Tenosynovitis

▶ Clinical Findings

The abductor pollicis longus and extensor pollicis brevis tendons may become inflamed beneath the retinacular pulley at the radial styloid region. Symptoms are provoked by lifting activity in which the thumb is adducted and flexed while the hand is ulnarly deviated. Activities such as inflating a blood pressure cuff, picking up an infant out of a crib, or lifting a heavy frying pan off the stove may provoke pain along the radial aspect of the wrist.

Physical examination reveals tenderness directly over the first extensor compartment. A provocative maneuver, the Finkelstein test, is helpful in diagnosing this disorder (Figure 9–20).

▶ Treatment

Initial treatment includes either splinting or steroid injection. Immobilization limits extensor pollicis brevis tendon excursion using a forearm-based thumb spica splint, which prevents both wrist deviation and thumb carpometacarpal and metacarpophalangeal motion while allowing interphalangeal joint motion. Steroid injection into the first extensor compartment along the course of the extensor pollicis brevis may diminish swelling and pain.

If de Quervain tenosynovitis is unresponsive to conservative care, surgical release of the overlying retinaculum may be elected. Because most patients with symptomatic disease have more than one abductor pollicis longus slip, the extensor pollicis brevis tendon must be identified and decompressed. In some cases, the first extensor compartment is divided by a septum, creating two separate tendon sheaths. In such cases, the more dorsal component sheath must also be opened to allow unconstrained extensor pollicis brevis tendon gliding.

Extreme caution must be exercised in carrying out the skin incision and subcutaneous dissection in this region because injury to the sensory branch of the radial nerve as it runs over the first compartment is a troublesome complication that may overshadow any benefit from tendon decompression.

2. Flexor Tenosynovitis (Trigger Finger and Trigger Thumb)

▶ Clinical Findings

Flexor tenosynovitis or tenovaginitis is characterized by pain and tenderness in the palm at the proximal edge of the digital A1 pulley (Figure 9–21). Patients frequently note catching or triggering of the affected finger or thumb after forceful flexion. In more severe cases, the opposite hand must be used to force the finger or thumb passively into extension. In

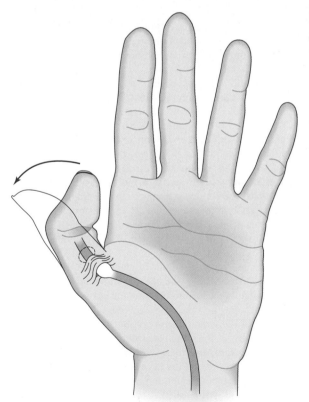

▲ **Figure 9–21.** Trigger thumb. (Reproduced, with permission, from American Society for Surgery of the Hand: *The Hand: Examination and Diagnosis,* 2nd ed. Philadelphia: Churchill Livingstone; 1983.)

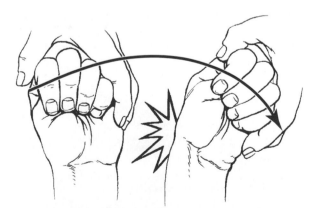

▲ **Figure 9–20.** Finkelstein maneuver. The patient's thumb is enclosed in the palm. The wrist is then abruptly deviated ulnarward by the examiner. In a positive test, pain is produced on the radial border of the wrist. (Reproduced, with permission, from Lister G: *The Hand: Diagnosis and Indications,* 3rd ed. Philadelphia: Churchill Livingstone; 1993.)

the most severe cases, the finger becomes locked in a flexed position. Triggering is often more pronounced in the morning than later in the day. Stenosing tenosynovitis is more common in diabetic patients than in nondiabetic patients. When multiple digits are involved, the possibility of diabetes should be considered.

Treatment

Most triggering digits may be successfully treated by long-acting steroid injection into the flexor sheath. To inject a trigger finger, the needle is inserted at the proximal palmar crease for the index finger and the distal palmar crease for the middle, ring, and small fingers. The needle enters the flexor tendon and pressure is applied to the plunger. The needle is slowly backed out until the needle is between the tendon and the tendon sheath, discerned by loss of plunger resistance. One milliliter of a combination of a short-acting anesthetic and steroid is given. The injection may be repeated if symptoms recur after an initially positive response to injection.

Surgical release of the A1 pulley is curative in digits refractory to steroid injection. Release is accomplished by directly exposing the pulley and incising its transversely oriented fibers longitudinally. The fibers of the A2 pulley must be spared to preserve effective digital flexion. Percutaneous release of the A1 pulley may be accomplished with a needle on the middle and ring fingers, especially if they actively lock. In patients with RA, the entire annular pulley system should be preserved to prevent further ulnar drift of the fingers. Triggering in these patients is treated by tenosynovectomy and excision of one slip of the flexor digitorum superficialis.

3. Flexor Carpi Radialis Tenosynovitis

Clinical Findings

Flexor carpi radialis tenosynovitis is characterized by pain with wrist motion, particularly active wrist flexion or passive wrist dorsiflexion. Marked tenderness is elicited on palpation of the skin overlying the tendon, particularly over the trapezium.

Treatment

Conservative care includes splinting the wrist in flexion and administration of oral anti-inflammatory medication. If these measures are ineffective, a long-acting steroid may be injected about the tendon at the trapezial level.

Surgical decompression of the flexor carpi radialis is considered if conservative measures are ineffective. Decompression unroofs the tendon sheath in the distal forearm and across the wrist. The fibroosseous sheath is further decompressed by resection of the palmar ulnar ridge of the trapezium overlying the tendon.

Finsen V, Hagen S: Surgery for trigger finger. *Hand Surg* 2003; 8:201. [PMID: 15002098]

Hwang M, Kang YK, Shin JY, et al: Referred pain pattern of the abductor pollicis longus muscle. *Am J Phys Med Rehabil* 2005;84:593. [PMID: 16034228]

Ragoowansi R, Acornley A, Khoo CT: Percutaneous trigger finger release: the "lift-cut" technique. *Br J Plast Surg* 2005;58:817. [PMID: 15936736]

Wilhelmi BJ, Snyder N 4th, Verbesey JE, et al: Trigger finger release with hand surface landmark ratios: an anatomic and clinical study. *Plast Reconstr Surg* 2001;108:908. [PMID: 11547146]

Zingas C, Failla JM, Van Holsbeeck M: Injection accuracy and clinical relief of de Quervain's tendinitis. *J Hand Surg Am* 1998; 22:89. [PMID: 9523961]

VASCULAR DISORDERS OF THE HAND

Anatomy

The blood supply to the hand is predominantly through the ulnar and radial arteries. The ulnar artery is larger than the radial artery and provides the primary arterial contribution to the hand. In most hands, the ulnar artery supplies the superficial palmar arch, which provides the principal blood supply to the common and proper digital arteries. The radial artery enters the hand by passing deep to the tendons of the first dorsal compartment across the anatomic snuffbox, dives palmarward between the bases of the first and second metacarpals, and forms the deep palmar arch. The median artery, a remnant of the embryologic vascular supply to the developing upper limb, contributes to the superficial palmar arch in 10% of patients.

The superficial palmar arch is located distal to the deep palmar arch. The arterial arch is complete, with total communication between the radial and ulnar arteries in 34% of hands and incomplete communication in 20%. The remaining hands have limited communication between the ulnar and radial arteries in varied configurations. The deep palmar arch runs alongside the motor branch of the ulnar nerve as it travels transversely just palmar to the proximal metacarpal shafts. The princeps pollicis artery is derived from the deep palmar arch in 98% of patients. The deep palmar arch also supplies the deep metacarpal arterial branches, which provide secondary blood flow to the digital arteries.

Clinical Findings

Patients with vascular insufficiency frequently complain of cold intolerance. When color changes occur, paleness or whiteness of the fingers is more suggestive of loss of inflow, whereas redness or bluish discoloration suggests inadequate venous return. Ulcerations of the tips of the fingers may denote ischemia.

The duration of vascular symptoms should be noted. If the abnormality is congenital in origin, changes in symptoms over time should be documented. The occupational history should record whether the patient uses vibrating tools or is subjected to repetitive blunt hand trauma during work. Occupations requiring outdoor work in all seasons (construction) or in a cold environment indoors (butchering) are noted. A history of trauma may suggest arterial or periarterial damage. Any sports activities that involve repeated trauma to the hand should be recorded; golfers, baseball catchers, and handball players are particularly at risk of closed vascular injury. Exposure to vasoconstrictive drugs such as beta-blockers and tobacco abuse should be noted. Other evidence of vascular disease should be sought, as well as diseases with vascular effects such as scleroderma or diabetes. Pulses are palpated, noting thrills or bruits.

A. Allen Test

The Allen test allows assessment of the extent of connection between the radial and ulnar arteries through the palmar arches. The examiner compresses both the radial and ulnar arteries at the wrist and then asks the patient to flex and extend the fingers repetitively. After the hand blanches, pressure is released from the radial artery while compression is maintained on the ulnar artery. The examiner observes how long it takes for each of the fingers to regain its pink color. The initial step is repeated with both vessels compressed, and the ulnar artery occlusion is then released while pressure is maintained on the radial artery. Again, examination of the reperfusion of the fingers reveals which digits are primarily supplied through the ulnar artery. In this fashion, the extent of interconnections between the radial and ulnar arteries may be assessed.

B. Diagnostic Studies

Noninvasive vascular diagnostic studies include Doppler scans, which detect the presence of flow; plethysmography, which determines the pulse volume difference between brachial and digital arteries; and cold stress testing, a technique that evaluates the effect of cold on arterial spasm. Invasive diagnostic procedures include arteriography, digital subtraction arteriography, and early-phase radionuclide scans.

ARTERIAL OCCLUSION

1. Arterial Trauma

▶ Clinical Findings

Partial or complete division of an artery may occur as the result of lacerations, acute injection trauma, or cannulation injuries. Hemorrhage from arterial disruption should initially be treated with direct pressure. Total arterial division must be repaired if distal vascularity is inadequate. Partial arterial injuries may bleed profusely because the lacerated vessel ends are tethered to one another and are unable to retract, constrict, and occlude further flow. Partial arterial injury may require resection with or without reconstruction to prevent the formation of aneurysms or arteriovenous fistulas. Injection injury may produce either spasm or occlusion.

▶ Treatment

The primary objective in treating arterial injuries is the restoration of adequate distal blood flow. Attempts may be made to remove distal clots with Fogarty catheters. If this is unsuccessful, clot-dissolving agents such as urokinase, local or systemic vasodilators, and stellate ganglion blocks may be employed to diminish vascular spasm. Care must be taken when using multiple agents to ensure they do not interfere with one another. For instance, use of urokinase after an axillary block may produce axillary artery hemorrhage, thereby compounding the problem.

2. Thrombosis

▶ Clinical Findings

The ulnar artery is the most common site of upper extremity arterial thrombosis. This entity, also known as ulnar hammer syndrome or hypothenar hammer syndrome, is most often the result of repetitive trauma to the hypothenar area of the hand. Patients may complain of a tender pulsatile mass on the ulnar side of the palm. In some instances, presenting symptoms reflect a low ulnar nerve palsy secondary to compression of the ulnar nerve by the aneurysm at the level of the Guyon canal. Distal vascular insufficiency may be evident in the ring and little fingers.

▶ Treatment

If evaluation demonstrates that all the fingers are well perfused by the radial artery alone, excision of the segment of the ulnar artery containing the aneurysm or thrombosed segment and ligation of the vessel ends is curative. Simple division of the vessel may confer a modest sympathectomy effect to the residual ulnar artery because sympathetic fibers surrounding the ulnar artery are disrupted at the time of vessel division. If, however, digital perfusion is inadequate after a vessel segment is resected and the tourniquet deflated, a segmental vein graft is required to reconstitute the ulnar artery.

3. Aneurysm

A distinction should be made between true and false aneurysms. In a true aneurysm, all layers of the arterial wall are involved. These aneurysms are usually caused by blunt trauma but may also be secondary to degeneration or infection. False aneurysms are characterized by partial wall involvement, with periarterial tissues forming a false wall lined by endothelium. False aneurysms are most common following penetrating trauma, such as stab wounds.

Both true and false aneurysms should be treated with resection. As discussed in the section about ulnar hammer syndrome, the necessity of vascular reconstruction is dictated by the adequacy of distal perfusion after tourniquet release.

VASOSPASTIC CONDITIONS

▶ Clinical Findings

Raynaud phenomenon, Raynaud disease, and Raynaud syndrome are often confused. Raynaud phenomenon is a condition in which pallor of the digits occurs with or without cyanosis on exposure to cold. Raynaud disease (primary Raynaud) is present when Raynaud phenomenon occurs without another associated or causative disease. Raynaud disease most commonly occurs in young (<40 years) women and is often bilateral, without demonstrable peripheral arterial occlusion. In severe cases, patients may develop gangrene or atrophic changes limited to the distal digital skin. Raynaud syndrome (secondary Raynaud) occurs when Raynaud phenomenon is associated with another disease, such as connective tissue disorders (systemic lupus erythematosus), neurologic disorders, arterial occlusive disorders, or blood dyscrasias.

▶ Treatment

All patients with Raynaud phenomenon experience cyclic episodes of digital pallor alternating with episodes of cyanosis and hyperemia. Treatment includes protection of the hands from cold by the use of gloves or mittens. Patients should be strongly encouraged to cease all cigarette or cigar smoking. Drug treatment attempts to diminish occlusive phenomena. Alpha-receptor blocking agents, nitroglycerin ointment, nifedipine, and other calcium channel blockers are effective in decreasing spasm. Botulinum toxin type A (Botox) injection around the neurovascular bundles in the palm can also help in patients who do not respond to medication. Digital artery sympathectomy, the surgical stripping of the periarterial tissue of the common digital artery over a short segment at the distal palmar level, may improve circulation to ischemic digits.

Balogh B, Mayer W, Vesely M, et al: Adventitial stripping of the radial and ulnar arteries in Raynaud's disease. *J Hand Surg Am* 2002;27:1073. [PMID: 12457360]

Neumeister MW, Chambers CB, Herron MS, et al: Botox therapy for ischemic digits. Plast Reconstr Surg 2009;124:191. [PMID: 19568080]

Ruch DS, Aldridge M, Holden M, et al: Arterial reconstruction for radial artery occlusion. *J Hand Surg Am* 2000;25:282. [PMID: 10722820]

Ruch DS, Holden M, Smith BP, et al: Periarterial sympathectomy in scleroderma patients: Intermediate-term follow-up. *J Hand Surg Am* 2002;27:258. [PMID: 11901385]

▼ DISORDERS OF THE NERVES OF THE HAND

PERIPHERAL NERVE INJURY

▶ Anatomy

Peripheral nerves consist of a mixture of myelinated and unmyelinated axons. Motor, sensory, and sympathetic fibers often travel together in a single nerve. Axons are grouped in bundles termed *fascicles,* which are surrounded by perineurium. The fine connective tissue between axons within a fascicle is called *endoneurium.* Fascicles are held together as a nerve by the epineurium. Nerves are considered monofascicular, oligofascicular, or polyfascicular, depending on the number of fascicles. The relationship between fascicles changes along the longitudinal course of the nerve. The degree of fascicular change decreases distally. The mesoneurium, which is the connective tissue surrounding the epineurium, facilitates longitudinal gliding of the nerve.

After a nerve is injured, a number of changes occur. The somatosensory cortex reorganizes so the area represented by the injured nerve diminishes. The cell body of the lacerated axon increases in size. The production of materials for repair of the cytoskeleton is increased, and the production of neurotransmitters decreases. At the proximal segment of the injured axon, further proximal degeneration occurs based on the severity of the injury. In the axon distal to the laceration, Schwann cells phagocytose the axon, allowing the surrounding myelin tube to collapse.

Within 24 hours of injury, axonal sprouting occurs from the proximal stump. Multiple axons in a fascicle form a regenerating unit. The number of axons in the unit decreases with time. Longitudinal growth of the regenerating nerve depends on the ability of the axons to adhere to trophic factors in the basal lamina of the Schwann cell. Changes also occur at the distal end of the nerve. At the motor endplate, the muscle fibers atrophy. The sensitivity and number of acetylcholine receptors increase as their location expands from pits to the entire length of the muscle fiber. If the muscle fiber is reinnervated, both old and new motor endplates become active. The recovery of strength is greatest after primary nerve repair, less vigorous after repair with nerve grafting, and weakest after direct implantation of the nerve end into muscle. Muscle reinnervation occurs only if the axon reaches the muscle within a year. In contrast, sensory receptors may be effectively reinnervated years after injury.

Nerve injures are classified into three types. (1) Neurapraxia is a conduction block that occurs without axonal disruption. Recovery is usually complete within days to a few months. (2) Axonotmesis describes an injury in which axonal disruption occurs, with the endoneurial tube remaining in continuity. The intact endoneurial tube provides the regenerating sprouting axons with a well-defined path to the end organs. Because axonal growth occurs at approximately 1 mm/day, recovery is good but slow. (3) Neurotmesis refers to transection of the nerve. Unless the nerve is repaired, the regenerating axons cannot find a suitable path and recovery does not occur. The frustrated sprouting axons form a neuroma at the distal end of the proximal segment of the lacerated nerve.

▶ Diagnostic Studies

Preoperative and postoperative assessment of motor and sensory function include quantitative measurement of pinch and grip strength, static and moving two-point discrimination, and vibration and pressure measurements. Two-point discrimination reflects innervation density, whereas vibration and pressure measurements gauge innervation threshold.

▶ Treatment

Nerve repair should be carried out with magnification and microsurgical technique. A tension-free repair provides the ideal environment for nerve regeneration. Tension at the repair site may be diminished by advancement of the nerve (ie, anterior transposition of the ulnar nerve for proximal forearm ulnar nerve laceration) or by limitation of joint motion. If a tension-free repair is impossible, nerve grafting is necessary to bridge the defect in the nerve. Frequently used donor nerves include the sural nerve, the anterior branch of the medial antebrachial cutaneous nerve, and the lateral antebrachial cutaneous nerve. Nerve defects of 2 cm

or less may be managed by placing and securing the severed ends of the nerve within a conduit or adjacent vein that permits the uninterrupted regeneration of axons from the proximal nerve end.

Primary repair is preferred to nerve grafting because the latter procedure requires two sites of nerve coaptation. Epineurial repair is usually performed under magnification, using 8-0 or 9-0 suture (Figure 9–22A). When a particular fascicular group (eg, motor branch of the median nerve) is recognized as mediating a specific function, it may be repaired separately (Figure 9–22B). Postoperative therapy may include motor and sensory reeducation to maximize the clinical result.

Primary nerve repair is indicated after a sharp nerve division occurs. After avulsion injuries, repair even by nerve grafting cannot be performed until the proximal and distal extent of injury is known. When closed nerve injury occurs, sensory and motor function is closely monitored. If no recovery is seen within 3 months, electrodiagnostic studies are carried out. If no electrical evidence of recovery is documented, the nerve is explored, and neurolysis, secondary nerve repair, or nerve grafting is accomplished.

COMPRESSIVE NEUROPATHIES

Compressive neuropathies are a group of nerve injuries that have common pathophysiology factors and occur at predictable sites of normal anatomic constraint. Nerve dysfunction

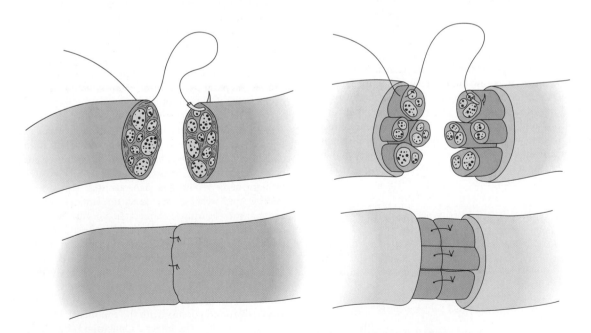

A. Epineurial repair   **B.** Group fascicular repair

▲ **Figure 9–22.** **A:** Schematic diagram of epineurial repair technique. **B:** Group fascicular repair technique.
(Reproduced, with permission, from Mackinnon SE, Dellon AL: *Surgery of the Peripheral Nerve.* New York: Thieme; 1988.)

is the result of neural ischemia in the compressed segment. Symptoms may resolve after release of the anatomic structures producing pressure on the nerve, particularly when compression is neither severe nor long standing.

1. Median Neuropathy

▶ Carpal Tunnel Syndrome

A. Anatomy

Compression of the median nerve within the carpal tunnel is the most common upper extremity compressive neuropathy. The carpal tunnel is that space along the palmar aspect of the wrist anatomically bounded by the scaphoid tubercle and the trapezium radially, the hook of the hamate and the pisiform ulnarly, the capitate dorsally, and the transverse carpal ligament palmarly (Figure 9–23).

B. Clinical Findings

Carpal tunnel syndrome is most often idiopathic. It is associated with pregnancy, amyloidosis, flexor tenosynovitis, acute or chronic inflammatory conditions, traumatic disorders of the wrist, endocrine disorders (diabetes mellitus and hypothyroidism), and tumors within the carpal tunnel.

Differential diagnosis includes compression of the median nerve or cervical roots in other anatomic locations. Diabetic neuropathy may produce symptoms similar to those of carpal tunnel syndrome, and patients with diabetic neuropathy may develop concomitant carpal tunnel syndrome.

1. Symptoms and signs—Most patients complain of numbness in the thumb and index and middle fingers, though many note that the entire hand feels numb. Pain rarely prevents the affected individual from falling asleep but characteristically awakens the patient from sleep after a number of hours. After a period of moving the fingers, most patients are able to return to sleep. Many patients complain of finger stiffness upon arising in the morning.

Discomfort or numbness, or both, may be incited by activities in which the wrist is held in a flexed position for a sustained period of time (eg, holding a steering wheel, telephone receiver, book, or newspaper). Discomfort and pain may radiate from the hand up the arm to the shoulder or neck. The patient may complain of clumsiness when trying to perform tasks such as unscrewing a jar top and may experience difficulty in holding on to a glass or cup securely.

Atrophy of muscles innervated by the median nerve is visible in severe long-standing cases but is uncommon in most cases of recent onset. Weakness of the abductor pollicis brevis muscle may be detected by careful manual muscle testing.

2. Provocative tests—Three provocative tests, the Phalen maneuver, the Tinel sign, and the wrist compression test,

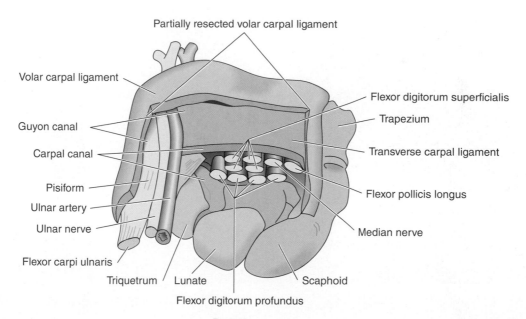

Partially resected volar carpal ligament

Volar carpal ligament

Guyon canal

Carpal canal

Pisiform

Ulnar artery

Ulnar nerve

Flexor carpi ulnaris

Triquetrum Lunate

Flexor digitorum profundus

Flexor digitorum superficialis

Trapezium

Transverse carpal ligament

Flexor pollicis longus

Median nerve

Scaphoid

Dorsal

▲ **Figure 9–23.** The Guyon canal and carpal tunnel and contents. (Cross section of supinated right wrist, viewed from proximal to distal.) Note the relationship between the transverse carpal ligament and the volar carpal ligament (partially resected). (Reproduced, with permission, from Reckling FW, Reckling JB, Mohn MP: *Orthopaedic Anatomy and Surgical Approaches.* St. Louis: Mosby-Year Book; 1990.)

are helpful in establishing the diagnosis of carpal tunnel syndrome.

A. TINEL SIGN—The Tinel sign is elicited by percussing the skin over the median nerve just proximal to the carpal tunnel; when it is positive, the patient complains of an electric or tingling sensation radiating into the thumb, index, middle, or ring fingers.

B. PHALEN MANEUVER—The Phalen wrist flexion sign, or Phalen maneuver, is usually positive in patients with carpal tunnel syndrome and is thought by many to be even more diagnostic than the Tinel sign. When this maneuver is performed, the elbow should be maintained in extension while the wrist is passively flexed (Figure 9–24). The time is then measured from initiation of wrist flexion to onset of symptoms; onset within 60 seconds is considered supportive of the diagnosis of carpal tunnel syndrome. Both the time to onset and the location of paresthesias should be recorded.

C. WRIST COMPRESSION TEST—Pressure over the median nerve proximal to the wrist provokes symptoms within 30 seconds. The test is confirmatory to other physical signs of median nerve compression.

3. Two-point discrimination test—Two-point discrimination is often diminished in the finger pulps of patients with carpal tunnel syndrome. Sensation in the radial aspect of the palm should be normal, however, because the palmar cutaneous branch of the median nerve does not pass through the carpal tunnel.

4. Imaging studies—Imaging studies are not routinely indicated for the management of carpal tunnel syndrome. MRI may be considered if a space-occupying lesion or tumor is suspected.

5. Electrodiagnostic studies—Nerve conduction velocities and electromyography help localize nerve compression to the wrist and evaluate residual neural and motor integrity. Nerve conduction velocity and electromyogram studies are indicated for patients who have failed conservative care and are considered candidates for surgery. A distal motor latency greater than 3.5–4.0 ms is the best indicator of carpal tunnel syndrome.

C. Treatment

1. Conservative measures—Because the pressure within the carpal tunnel increases if the wrist is held in sustained flexion (usual sleep posture) or sustained extension, the initial treatment of carpal tunnel syndrome should include a splint that maintains the wrist in a neutral position at night. Clinical improvement with this simple measure adds further support to the diagnosis of carpal tunnel syndrome. Activities that provoke symptoms may be modified with simple measures such as adjustment of keyboard height and rotation of repetitive job activities.

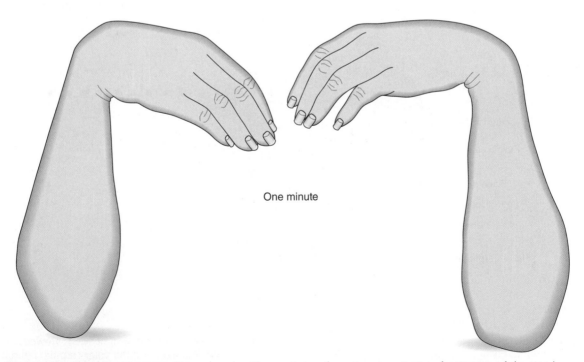

One minute

▲ **Figure 9–24.** Phalen maneuver. (Reproduced, with permission, from American Society for Surgery of the Hand: *The Hand: Examination and Diagnosis,* 2nd ed. Philadelphia: Churchill Livingstone; 1983.)

Injection of steroids into the carpal tunnel often decreases the inflammatory response around the flexor tendons and diminishes symptoms. To inject the carpal tunnel, a 25-gauge 1.5-inch needle is placed at the palmar wrist crease just ulnar to the palmaris longus tendon. If the palmaris longus is absent, a line along the radial border of the ring finger is drawn to the wrist crease. Before placing the needle, patients are told they may experience an electric shock sensation in the fingers. If this sensation occurs, the needle may be in the median nerve, and the injection should not be given. The needle is withdrawn and placed a few millimeters ulnar. When inserting the needle, first the skin is punctured, then a pop is felt as the needle passes through the transverse carpal ligament. A mixture of a short-acting anesthetic and steroid is injected. Transient relief of symptoms after injection suggests a greater likelihood of a favorable result after surgical decompression.

2. Surgical treatment—Patients unresponsive to conservative measures may benefit from surgical division of the transverse carpal ligament. This division may be accomplished through either direct open exposure or through an endoscopic approach. The open incision is made in the palm over the transverse carpal ligament, staying ulnar to the axis of the palmaris longus, along the longitudinal axis of the radial border of the ring finger. This incision avoids injury to the palmar cutaneous branch of the median nerve. After incising the palmar fascia longitudinally, the transverse carpal ligament is identified and sectioned longitudinally under direct observation. Endoscopic division of the transverse carpal ligament avoids a potentially tender palmar incision with either a single wrist portal proximal to the palm or with a combined proximal portal and short midpalmar portal along the axis of the open incision. Although some studies noted an earlier return to work activities after endoscopic release, the incidence of iatrogenic nerve and tendon injuries and late recurrence of symptoms from incomplete ligament division may be higher with endoscopic release than with open release. Both types of procedures are effective ways of treating carpal tunnel syndrome. The decision of which technique to use is based on the surgeon's experience. Endoscopic carpal tunnel release should not be used for treatment of recurrent carpal tunnel syndrome.

Patients are encouraged to actively move their fingers from the first postoperative day. Wrist motion is begun within the first week. Incisional tenderness often prevents patients from fully using their hands and returning to unrestricted work for the first 4–8 weeks. If patients have difficulty with hand function 3–4 weeks after surgery, a therapy program is prescribed consisting of desensitization, ROM, and strengthening.

▶ Pronator Syndrome
A. Anatomy

The median nerve may be compressed in the proximal forearm by one or more of the following structures: ligament of Struthers, lacertus fibrosus, pronator teres muscle, or proximal fibrous arch on the undersurface of the flexor digitorum superficialis muscle.

B. Clinical Findings

Patients with pronator syndrome complain of pain that is usually more severe in the volar forearm than in the wrist or hand. Pain usually increases with activity. Complaints of numbness in the thumb, index, middle, and ring fingers may initially suggest the possibility of carpal tunnel syndrome. Night symptoms, however, are unusual in cases of isolated pronator syndrome.

Examination may reveal sensory and motor deficits similar to those seen in carpal tunnel syndrome, but significant differences may be detected on careful evaluation. Dysesthesia may include the distribution of the palmar cutaneous nerve. The Tinel sign is positive at the forearm level rather than at the wrist. The Phalen maneuver does not provoke symptoms. Patients may experience pain with resistance to contraction of the pronator teres or flexor digitorum superficialis muscles tested by resistance to forearm pronation or to isolated flexion of the proximal interphalangeal joints of the long and ring fingers.

C. Treatment

Evaluation of symptomatic patients should include electrodiagnostic studies if a 6-week course of immobilization fails to effect improvement. Surgical treatment requires generous decompression of all potentially constricting sites.

▶ Anterior Interosseous Syndrome
A. Anatomy

The anterior interosseous nerve branch divides from the median nerve 4–6 cm below the elbow. This branch of the nerve innervates the flexor pollicis longus, flexor digitorum profundus of the index and middle fingers, and pronator quadratus muscles. The anterior interosseous nerve may be compressed by the deep head of the pronator teres, the origin of the flexor digitorum superficialis, a palmaris profundus, or the flexor carpi radialis. In addition, accessory muscles connecting the flexor digitorum superficialis to the flexor digitorum profundus proximally and Gantzer muscle (the accessory head of the flexor pollicis longus) may impinge on the anterior interosseous nerve.

B. Clinical Findings

Patients affected with anterior interosseous nerve syndrome complain of inability to flex either the thumb interphalangeal joint or the index-finger distal interphalangeal joint. In contrast to those with pronator syndrome, these patients do not complain of numbness or pain.

C. Treatment

Surgical decompression of the anterior interosseous nerve may be indicated when the syndrome does not spontaneously improve. All potentially compressing structures must be exposed and released.

2. Ulnar Neuropathy

▶ Cubital Tunnel Syndrome

A. Anatomy

The ulnar nerve is most commonly compressed at the cubital tunnel, along the medial side of the elbow. Compression may occur between the ulnar and humeral origins of the flexor carpi ulnaris or at the proximal border of the cubital tunnel because the nerve is tethered anteriorly with elbow flexion (Figure 9–25).

B. Clinical Findings

Patients affected with cubital tunnel syndrome most often complain of paresthesia and numbness involving the ring and little fingers. Because symptoms may be aggravated or provoked by sustained elbow flexion, patients may complain of increased symptoms while talking on the telephone. Many patients complain of being awakened at night by the symptoms, most often when sleeping with the elbows flexed. Patients whose exam demonstrates weakness of muscles innervated by the ulnar nerve may note clumsiness and lack of dexterity.

1. Provocative tests

A. **TINEL SIGN**—A positive Tinel sign is noted when percussion over the ulnar nerve at the elbow provokes paresthesias along the ulnar forearm and hand. The nerve may be noted to sublux over the medial epicondyle as the arm is brought into flexion.

B. **MOTOR STRENGTH**—Motor strength should be assessed both in intrinsic muscles innervated by the ulnar nerve (first dorsal interosseous muscle) and in extrinsic muscles innervated by the ulnar nerve (flexor digitorum profundus of the little finger).

C. **FROMENT SIGN**—With weakness of the ulnar nerve–innervated adductor pollicis muscle, a positive Froment sign may be observed. As the patient tries to hold a piece of paper placed between the thumb and the index finger, the thumb interphalangeal joint flexes in an attempt to substitute flexor pollicis longus activity for inadequate adductor pollicis strength.

D. **ELBOW FLEXION TEST**—The ulnar nerve may be rendered symptomatic by fully flexing the elbow with the wrist in the neutral position. The elbow flexion test, a provocative maneuver, is considered positive if paresthesia is elicited in the ring and little fingers within 60 seconds. The location of the paresthesia and the time between initiation of elbow flexion and the onset of symptoms should be recorded.

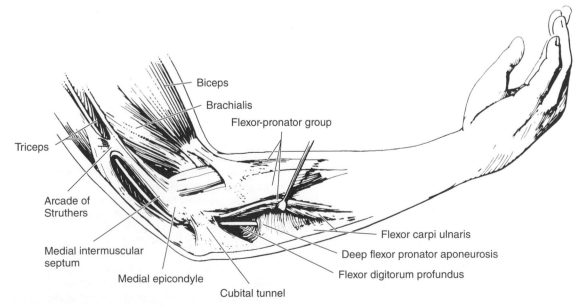

▲ **Figure 9–25.** Points of constriction of the ulnar nerve at the elbow. (From Amadio PC: Anatomic basis for a technique of ulnar nerve transposition. *Surg Radiol Anat* 1986;8:155; used, with permission, from Mayo Foundation.)

C. Treatment

1. Conservative treatment—Conservative treatment may include the use of an elbow pad to protect the nerve from trauma or a splint holding the elbow at approximately 45 degrees of flexion. The splint may be worn continuously or at night only, depending on the frequency and intensity of symptoms.

2. Surgical treatment—Electrodiagnostic studies should be obtained if conservative treatment does not alleviate the symptoms, particularly if motor weakness is evident. The reliability of nerve conduction studies at the elbow depends on the ability of the electromyographer to measure the length of the ulnar nerve accurately.

Numerous procedures are described to relieve ulnar nerve compression at the elbow. These include simple decompression of the ulnar nerve within the cubital tunnel or decompression with anterior transposition of the nerve subcutaneously, intramuscularly, or submuscularly into the flexor pronator mass. When the nerve is transposed, great care must be taken to excise the medial intermuscular septum proximally and to release the aponeurosis between the humeral and ulnar origins of the flexor carpi ulnaris distally, to avoid creating a new area of impingement.

An alternative surgical strategy involves decompression of the nerve and medial epicondylectomy. This technique removes the prominence against which the ulnar nerve is tethered with elbow flexion. After surgery, initial rehabilitation focuses on regaining elbow ROM. Strengthening begins at 4–6 weeks, and the patient is usually able to return to unrestricted work at 8–12 weeks.

▶ Ulnar Tunnel Syndrome

A. Anatomy

The ulnar nerve passes from the forearm into the hand through the Guyon canal (see Figure 9–23). The anatomic borders of the Guyon canal are the pisiform and pisohamate ligament ulnarly, the hook of the hamate and insertion of the transverse carpal ligament radially, and the volar carpal ligament forming the roof of the tunnel.

B. Clinical Findings

Examination should document ulnar nerve sensory and motor integrity. In contrast to the findings in cubital tunnel syndrome, the Tinel sign is positive at the wrist rather than at the elbow. Extrinsic motor function is normal. The region of compression should be delineated by electrodiagnostic studies. In some cases, MRI studies demonstrate a space-occupying lesion such as a ganglion compressing the nerve within the Guyon canal.

C. Treatment

When splinting is ineffective, surgical decompression should be considered. When symptoms exist in tandem with carpal tunnel syndrome, release of the transverse carpal ligament favorably alters the shape and size of the Guyon canal. Postoperative care is the same as following carpal tunnel release.

3. Radial Neuropathy

▶ Radial Tunnel Syndrome

A. Anatomy

The radial nerve may be rendered symptomatic if compressed in the region of the radial tunnel. Points of impingement along the radial tunnel, located at the level of the proximal radius, include fibers spanning the radiocapitellar joint, the radial recurrent vessels, the extensor carpi radialis brevis, the tendinous origin of the supinator (arcade of Frohse), and the point at which the nerve emerges from beneath the distal edge of the supinator.

B. Clinical Findings

Because radial tunnel syndrome often occurs in combination with lateral epicondylitis, the two diagnoses are frequently confused. Patients with radial tunnel syndrome experience pain over the midportion of the mobile wad (brachioradialis, extensor carpi radialis longus, and extensor carpi radialis brevis muscles), whereas the pain experienced by patients with lateral epicondylitis is located at or just distal to the lateral epicondyle. Patients with radial tunnel syndrome experience pain when simultaneously extending the wrist and fingers while the long finger is passively flexed by the examiner (positive long-finger extension test). Patients with radial tunnel syndrome often also experience pain with resisted forearm supination.

C. Treatment

Conservative treatment of radial tunnel syndrome includes measures to avoid forceful extension of the wrist and fingers. The wrist is splinted in dorsiflexion while the forearm is immobilized in supination. Persistent symptoms in spite of splinting may be treated by surgical decompression of the radial nerve. Concomitant lateral epicondylitis should be treated surgically at the same time that the radial nerve is decompressed.

▶ Posterior Interosseous Nerve Syndrome

A. Anatomy

The radial nerve splits into the posterior interosseous nerve and the superficial sensory branch of the radial nerve after passing anteriorly to the radiocapitellar joint. The posterior interosseous nerve then passes beneath the origin of the extensor carpi radialis brevis, radial recurrent artery, and arcade of Frohse. The posterior interosseous nerve is most commonly entrapped at the proximal edge of the supinator, although entrapment may also occur at either the middle or the distal edge of the supinator muscle.

B. Clinical Findings

In contrast to radial tunnel syndrome, patients with posterior interosseous nerve syndrome experience extrinsic extensor weakness. Pain may be less than that of patients with radial tunnel syndrome.

Paralysis may be either partial or complete. Because the brachioradialis, extensor carpi radialis longus, supinator, and often extensor carpi radialis brevis are innervated by the radial nerve proximal to the posterior interosseous nerve branch, these muscles are spared. Digital extension at the metacarpophalangeal joint is the principal deficit from loss of extensor digitorum communis, extensor indicis proprius, and extensor digit quinti function.

The differential diagnosis in a patient with spontaneous loss of digital extension should include the possibility of multiple tendon ruptures in addition to possible radial neuropathy, particularly in patients with RA. The tenodesis effect, in which the fingers extend as the wrist is passively flexed, is preserved in posterior interosseous nerve syndrome but absent if the extensor tendons are ruptured.

C. Treatment

Treatment of posterior interosseous nerve syndrome requires thorough decompression of the nerve. If motor recovery does not occur, tendon transfers restore digital extension.

4. Thoracic Outlet Syndrome

▶ Anatomy

The brachial plexus exits the base of the neck and upper thorax through the thoracic outlet. Anatomic boundaries of the outlet are the scalenus anterior muscle anteriorly, the scalenus medius muscle posteriorly, and the first rib inferiorly. Thoracic outlet syndrome, usually resulting from irritation of the C8- and T1-derived nerves, may be caused by a cervical rib, a fiber spanning from a rudimentary cervical rib, tendinous bands from the scalenus anterior to the medius muscles, or hypertrophic clavicle fracture callus. Poor posture with slumping shoulders and prolonged military brace position are both implicated as contributing factors.

▶ Clinical Findings

The symptoms of thoracic outlet syndrome are often vague. Symptoms may include pain in the C8-T1 dermatome, with a variable degree of intrinsic muscle weakness. Patients may experience vascular symptoms if the axillary artery is simultaneously being compressed in the thoracic outlet region.

A. Provocative Tests

1. Elevated stress test—Physical examination of the patient with suspected thoracic outlet syndrome should include an elevated stress test, in which the patient's shoulders are kept extended and the arm is externally rotated 90 degrees at the shoulder. The patient is then asked to open and close the hands with the arms elevated for 3 minutes. Reproduction of symptoms is suggestive of thoracic outlet syndrome.

2. Other tests—The Adson sign and the Wright test may be helpful in detecting vascular compression. In a positive Adson test, the radial pulse is obliterated when the patient holds a deep breath with the arm dependent and the head turned to the affected side. In the Wright test, the pulse is obliterated when the shoulder is abducted, externally rotated, and the head is turned away from the involved shoulder. In addition, this maneuver should reproduce the patient's symptoms. Physical examination should document C8 and T1 nerve root function: sensation along the inner border of the hand and forearm and hand intrinsic muscle strength.

B. Diagnostic Studies

Workup of the symptomatic patient should include radiographs of the cervical spine to rule out a cervical rib, electrodiagnostic studies to assess the function of the lower nerve roots, and Doppler studies of the arm in varied positions to assess compression of the axillary artery.

▶ Treatment

Initial treatment includes postural exercises. Patients who are unresponsive to conservative treatment or have demonstrable weakness may benefit from surgical resection of a cervical rib, resection of the first rib, or scalenotomy.

5. Cervical Root Compression

▶ Clinical Findings

Cervical spine root compression may result in complaints of hand pain or weakness. It is useful to inquire routinely about pain or limitation of motion of the cervical spine. If the patient was involved in an accident involving sudden neck flexion and extension, this should be noted. Cervical root compression may occur from a herniated cervical disk, cervical spondylosis, intervertebral foraminal osteophytes, or, rarely, a cervical cord tumor.

Patients with cervical root compression most often complain of pain in a radicular rather than a peripheral nerve distribution. Despite symptoms involving the hand, most patients, when carefully questioned, are able to distinguish pain that begins in the neck and radiates to the hand from pain that begins in the hand and radiates proximally to the neck. Pain may be exacerbated with neck motion (flexion and extension, lateral bending, or rotation), coughing, or sneezing.

A. Spurling Test

Physical examination of the patient with cervical radiculopathy frequently demonstrates either a decreased range of neck motion or pain with neck motion. Symptoms may be reproduced with axial compression on the patient's head (positive Spurling test). Detailed sensory and motor examination may reveal deficits in the domain of one or more roots.

B. Double-Crush Syndrome

The occasional simultaneous presentation of cervical radiculopathy with peripheral entrapment neuropathy is termed the *double-crush syndrome*. Whether compression at one level renders a nerve more vulnerable to compressive forces at a second level or whether such cases simply represent two common entities in the same extremity remains the subject of debate.

▶ Treatment

If a nerve is compressed at more than one location, the more symptomatic area is usually treated first. If both areas are equally symptomatic, the simpler of the two operations is chosen.

Lindley SG, Kleinert JM: Prevalence of anatomic variations encountered in elective carpal tunnel release. *J Hand Surg Am* 2003;28:849. [PMID: 14507518]

Morgenlander JC, Lynch JR, Sanders DB: Surgical treatment of carpal tunnel syndrome in patients with peripheral neuropathy. *Neurology* 1997;49:1159. [PMID: 9339710]

Naidu SH, Fisher J, Heistand M, et al: Median nerve function in patients undergoing carpal tunnel release: pre- and post-op nerve conductions. *Electromyogr Clin Neurophysiol* 2003;43:393. [PMID: 14626718]

Trumble TE, Diao E, Abrams RA, et al: Single-portal endoscopic carpal tunnel release compared with open release: a prospective, randomized trial. *J Bone Joint Surg Am* 2002;84:1107. [PMID: 12107308]

Upton AR, McComas AJ: The double crush in nerve entrapment syndromes. *Lancet* 1973;2:359. [PMID: 4124532]

▼ DISORDERS OF THE FASCIA OF THE HAND

DUPUYTREN DISEASE

Dupuytren disease is characterized by a nodular thickening on the palmar surface of the hand affecting the preexisting palmar fascia (Figure 9–26). It is a progressive condition, resulting from pathologic changes mediated by the myofibroblast. Dupuytren disease occurs most commonly in patients between 40 and 60 years of age. It is observed more often in men, in whom it appears earlier and is often more aggressive. Flexion contractures most frequently occur at the metacarpophalangeal joints but may also tether the proximal interphalangeal joint and, less commonly, the distal interphalangeal joint. The little and ring fingers and the thumb index web are the most commonly involved areas.

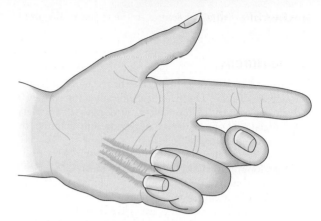

▲ **Figure 9–26.** Dupuytren contracture. (Reproduced, with permission, from American Society for Surgery of the Hand: *The Hand: Examination and Diagnosis,* 2nd ed. Philadelphia: Churchill Livingstone; 1983.)

Ectopic deposits may occur in the dorsum of the proximal interphalangeal joint (knuckle pads), the dorsum of the penis (Peyronie disease), and the plantar fascia of the foot (Ledderhose disease).

▶ Epidemiologic Factors

A number of predisposing factors are identified. The disease most commonly appears in patients of northern European ancestry and is occasionally encountered in Asians; it is rarer in other racial groups. Dupuytren disease is associated with epilepsy medications taken for seizure disorders and with alcoholism, smoking, and diabetes. The relationship of work and trauma to the development of the disease remains controversial. The most aggressive disease occurs in patients who have a family history of disease and in those who have onset of disease prior to 40 years of age. More severely involved patients may have extensive bilateral involvement and ectopic deposits on the dorsum of the hands and the feet. Although these patients often undergo surgery at an early age, both extension and recurrence of the disease are common.

▶ Anatomy

Dupuytren contracture distorts the anatomy of the palmar fascia. Flexion contractures of the metacarpophalangeal joint are caused by pathologic contracture of pretendinous bands at a superficial level. Contracture of the natatory ligaments produces web space contractures and scissoring of the fingers. The transverse fibers of the palmar aponeurosis remain uninvolved, except at the base of the thumb. In the fingers, the superficial volar fascia, lateral digital sheath, spiral band, and Grayson ligaments may contract alone or in combination to produce flexion contracture of the proximal interphalangeal joint. When a spiral band contracts, the digital nerve is often displaced palmarly to the band from proximal lateral to distal central in the region of the proximal phalanx.

Treatment

Nonsurgical treatment is ineffective in reversing or halting Dupuytren disease. The primary indication for surgery is a fixed contracture of more than 30 degrees at the metacarpophalangeal or any degree of flexion contracture at the proximal interphalangeal joint.

Surgical exposure may be achieved through either transverse or longitudinal skin incisions. A transverse incision across the distal palmar skin crease is useful when extensive palmar involvement is anticipated. Transverse incisions are usually sutured; if there is excessive tension, the wound may be left open to heal by secondary intention. When longitudinal exposure of the finger is needed, Brunner zigzag incisions are useful. An alternative is a longitudinal incision that is modified for closure by a series of Z-plasty flap transpositions.

The goal of surgical release is to achieve a regional fasciectomy or subtotal palmar fasciectomy that allows maximal untethered joint motion. A local fasciotomy may occasionally be elected in older, more debilitated patients with severe joint contractures.

Severe or recurrent proximal interphalangeal joint disease may occasionally be best treated with a salvage procedure, usually proximal interphalangeal joint arthrodesis. Amputation may be considered when profound stiffness or neurovascular compromise is present in patients with recurrent disease.

Enzymatic fasciotomy is an alternative to surgery for less severe forms of the disease. This is achieved by gently manipulating the finger into extension 24 hours after injection of a small amount of clostridial collagenase into the diseased cord.

Complications

The most common postoperative complication is hematoma, which may expand and compromise skin flaps and act as a nidus for infection. To diminish the possibility of postoperative hematoma, the tourniquet should be released and meticulous hemostasis obtained prior to wound closure. Tight skin closure should be avoided. If limited flap necrosis occurs, the affected regions should be treated by open dressing changes. If skin loss is extensive, skin graft application may be necessary to gain early wound closure.

Joint stiffness may occur, particularly after extensive surgical release of the long-standing fixed proximal interphalangeal joint. Extensive therapy is often necessary, consisting of both active and passive exercises and splinting.

Mild sympathetically mediated pain (reflex sympathetic dystrophy) is not uncommon. For patients who have a more severe form, hospitalization with elevation, sympathetic blocking agents, oral steroids, and intensive therapy may be necessary.

Prognosis

Contracture correction is usually maintained at the metacarpophalangeal joints. Recurrence is more common at the proximal interphalangeal joint, particularly when the extent of preoperative proximal interphalangeal joint contracture was more than 60 degrees. Long-term postoperative night splinting may diminish the extent of residual digital flexion contracture.

Forsman M, Kallioinen L, Kallioinen M, et al: Dupuytren's contracture; increased cellularity—proliferation, is there equality? *Scand J Surg* 2005;94:71. [PMID: 15865122]

Godtfredsen NS, Lucht H, Prescott E, et al: A prospective study linked both alcohol and tobacco to Dupuytren's disease. *J Clin Epidemiol* 2004;57:858. [PMID: 15485739]

Ketchum LD, Donahue TK: The injection of nodules of Dupuytren's disease with triamcinolone acetonide. *J Hand Surg Am* 2000;25:1157. [PMID: 11119679]

McFarlane RM: On the origin and spread of Dupuytren's disease. *J Hand Surg Am* 2002;27:385. [PMID: 12015711]

COMPARTMENT SYNDROMES

Compartment syndromes are a group of conditions that result from increased pressure within a limited anatomic space, acutely compromising the microcirculation and threatening the viability of the tissue within that space.

Recurrent or chronic compartment syndrome results from increased pressure within the compartment with a specific activity, most commonly in athletes during exercise. Symptoms of muscle weakness may be severe enough to stop the exercise activity despite the patient being asymptomatic between recurrences.

The Volkmann ischemic contracture is the result of an acute compartment syndrome in which fibrous tissue has replaced dead muscle. Because nerve injury is not always associated with this condition, sensation and intrinsic muscle function may be normal distal to the involved compartment. Because there is often no associated nerve injury, no sensory deficit or loss of motor function may be detected in the nerve domain distal to the involved compartment.

Etiologic Factors

The most common causes of compartment syndrome are fractures, soft-tissue crush injuries, arterial injuries either caused by localized hemorrhage or postischemic swelling, drug overdose with prolonged limb compression, and burn injuries. In most cases, fractures are closed or, if open, are grade 1 injuries, with only limited disruption of the compartmental soft-tissue envelopes.

The pathophysiology of compartment syndrome is a consequence of closure of small vessels. Increased compartment pressure increases the pressure on the walls of arterioles within the compartment. Increased local pressure also occludes small veins, resulting in venous hypertension within the compartment. The arteriovenous gradient in the region of the pressurized tissue becomes insufficient to allow tissue perfusion. Because the elevated pressure within the compartment is not high enough to occlude major arteries completely as they pass through the compartment, distal pulses usually remain strong despite increasing tissue ischemia in the affected soft-tissue compartment.

▶ Clinical Findings

The diagnosis of compartment syndrome is established predominantly on clinical findings. The clinician must have a high index of suspicion whenever a closed compartment has the potential for bleeding or swelling. Compartment syndromes are characterized by pain out of proportion to the initial injury. Pain is often persistent, progressive, and unrelieved by immobilization. Pain may be accentuated by passive stretching of the fingers. Diminished sensation may be noted in the distribution of the nerve whose compartment is being compressed. This phenomenon is believed to be secondary to nerve ischemia. A third sign is weakness and paralysis of muscles within the compartment. A fourth sign is tenseness of the compartment on palpation. Of the preceding signs and symptoms, pain with passive muscle stretching is the most sensitive in detecting compartment syndrome. Unless there is a vascular injury, distal pulses are preserved in compartment syndrome.

If the diagnosis of compartment syndrome is in question, the clinician is obligated to ascertain the pressure within the potential affected compartments. Various methods are available, including a portable hand-held pressure monitor or a simple modification of a mercury manometer connected to tubing and a three-way stopcock. Although the exact pressure threshold for requiring fasciotomy is controversial, fasciotomy should be strongly considered whenever the compartment pressure is more than 30 mm Hg in the forearm. Pressure measurements of the compartments of the hand are difficult to interpret. The decision to perform a fasciotomy of the hand or finger is based solely on clinical judgment.

▶ Treatment

Once the diagnosis of compartment syndrome is established, fasciotomy of the involved compartment should be performed as soon as possible because elevation of compartment pressure of more than 30 mm Hg for more than 8 hours is associated with irreversible tissue death. Prophylactic fasciotomy should also be considered in patients in whom ischemia is present for more than 4 hours. All patients undergoing forearm or arm replantation should have a fasciotomy performed at the time of the initial surgical procedure.

The volar compartment of the forearm is the upper extremity compartment most often requiring release (Figure 9–27A). The skin incision should extend from

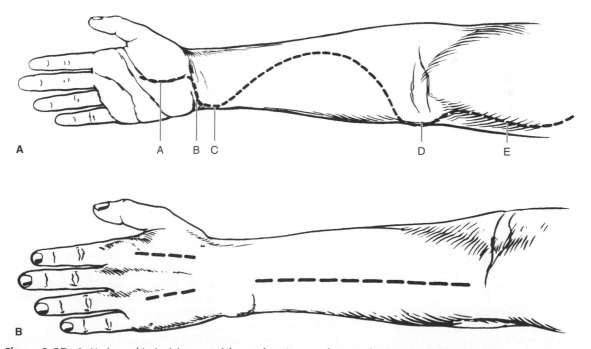

▲ **Figure 9–27. A:** Various skin incisions used for performing a volar arm fasciotomy. **B:** To decompress the dorsal and mobile wad compartments, straight incisions are preferred because fewer veins are damaged. (Reproduced, with permission, from Green DP, ed: *Operative Hand Surgery,* 2nd ed. Churchill Livingstone; 1988.)

the elbow to the carpal tunnel. The preferred skin incision extends from the medial side of the biceps and swings ulnarly toward the medial epicondyle. Care must be taken to incise the lacertus fibrosus at the elbow level. The incision may be extended in a radial direction to allow decompression of the mobile wad. In the distal half of the forearm, the incision runs along the ulnar border. The flap is designed to allow coverage of the median nerve in the distal forearm when the wounds are left open at the conclusion of the procedure. The incision is extended obliquely across the wrist to provide exposure of the carpal tunnel in the proximal palm.

An epimysiotomy of the individual superficial and deep compartment muscle bellies should be performed as needed. Care should be taken to ensure that the deep compartment musculature (the flexor pollicis longus and flexor digitorum profundus muscles) is completely decompressed. The skin incision should be partially closed over the median nerve in the hand and distal forearm. The proximal wound over muscle should be left open. The patient should be returned to the operating room within 48 hours for reevaluation. At the second surgery, dressings are changed, and secondary debridement is accomplished if nonviable muscle remains. In some instances, it is possible to close the wound secondarily; in most cases, split-thickness skin grafting of the residual skin defect is a safer alternative. Decompression of the dorsal forearm when necessary may be accomplished with a dorsal longitudinal incision (Figure 9–27B).

In the hand, the connections between compartments are limited; therefore, each compartment should be released individually. This may be accomplished by two longitudinal dorsal incisions over the index and ring metacarpals. Through these incisions, each of the interosseous compartments can be entered on both the radial and ulnar sides of each metacarpal. Separate volar incisions are needed when decompression of the thenar and hypothenar compartments is necessary on the palm of the hand.

In the finger, fasciotomy may be required for treatment of either severe trauma or snakebite injuries. Because compartment pressures in the finger are impossible to measure accurately, the indications for finger fasciotomy are based on the degree of swelling. Midaxial incisions along the ulnar side of the index, middle, and ring fingers and the radial side of the little finger and thumb allow satisfactory digital decompression. Care is taken to retract the neurovascular bundle palmarward, and the fascia between the neurovascular bundle and the flexor tendon sheath are then incised. Digital wounds are left open postoperatively, and wound closure is achieved either secondarily or with a split-thickness skin graft.

Botte MJ, Keenan MA, Gelberman RH: Volkmann's ischemic contracture of the upper extremity. *Hand Clin* 1998;14:483. [PMID: 9742427]

Dente CJ, Feliciano DV, Rozycki GS, et al: A review of upper extremity fasciotomies in a level I trauma center. *Am Surg* 2002;70:188. [PMID: 15663051]

Hovius SE, Ultee J: Volkmann's ischemic contracture. Prevention and treatment. *Hand Clin* 2000;16:647. [PMID: 11117054]

Ultee J, Hovius SE: Functional results after treatment of Volkmann's ischemic contracture: a long-term follow-up study. *Clin Orthop* 2005;431:42. [PMID: 15685054]

▼ FRACTURES AND DISLOCATIONS OF THE HAND

FRACTURES AND DISLOCATIONS OF THE METACARPALS AND PHALANGES

Fractures of the metacarpals and phalanges account for approximately 10% of all fractures. More than half of all hand fractures are work related. Fractures of the border digits, thumb, and little finger are most common. The most commonly fractured bone is the distal phalanx, accounting for 45–50% of all hand fractures.

▶ Clinical Findings

Description of a phalangeal or metacarpal fracture should include notation of the bone involved, the location within the bone (base, shaft, or neck) and whether the fracture is open or closed. Further determination should be made as to whether the fracture is displaced or nondisplaced, if it has an intraarticular component, and whether rotational or angular deformity is present.

Because rotational malalignment of a metacarpal or phalangeal fracture is difficult to evaluate from a radiograph, physical examination is essential. The patient is asked to flex actively the fingers individually and together. Nail rotation, finger orientation, and overlapping of the fingers are assessed. Associated vascular, nerve, and tendon injuries, as well as the adequacy of soft-tissue coverage, also should be evaluated.

▶ Treatment

Treatment of metacarpal and phalangeal fractures requires accurate diagnosis, reduction, and sufficient immobilization to maintain the fracture reduction, with early motion of the uninvolved fingers to prevent stiffness. Immobilization should usually place the hand in an intrinsic plus, or safe, position to avoid secondary joint contracture (see Figure 9–12). Immobilization should rarely exceed 3 weeks for phalangeal fractures or 4 weeks for metacarpal fractures. Because radiologic union usually lags behind clinical union in the hand, initiation of digital motion should not be delayed until radiologic union is visible. Prolonged immobilization increases the likelihood of residual stiffness.

The fixation required to maintain fracture reduction depends on the fracture characteristics. Stable fractures may be treated by either buddy taping the affected finger to an adjacent finger and allowing early motion or with a brief period of splint immobilization. Repeat radiographs at 7–10 days document maintenance of fracture reduction. Initially displaced unstable fractures that require closed reduction to achieve proper alignment require external immobilization with a cast or splint.

When external immobilization is impossible or unlikely to maintain fracture reduction, internal fixation is required. Internal fixation techniques useful in the management of hand fractures include Kirschner (K)-wire fixation, interosseous wiring, tension band wiring, interfragmentary screw fixation, or fixation with plates and screws. K-wire fixation is versatile but lacks the rigidity of other techniques. Additional stability may be achieved by combining K-wire fixation with tension band wires. Interfragmentary screws provide ideal fixation for long oblique fractures, in which the obliquity of the fracture is more than two times the diameter of the fractured bone. Plates and screws in the hand are particularly helpful in open metacarpal fractures with bone loss. When segmental bone loss occurs, initial treatment includes debridement of an associated open wound and maintenance of skeletal length with either internal or external fixation. After the soft-tissue coverage is established, bony graft reconstruction may be coupled with definitive internal fixation.

1. Physeal Fractures

Approximately a third of all fractures of the immature skeleton involve the epiphysis. Salter-Harris physeal fractures are divided into five types. Type 1 fractures, which shear through the growth plate without extension into the epiphysis or metaphysis, may be effectively treated with simple immobilization. Type 2 fractures, in which a metaphyseal fracture fragment is attached to the epiphysis, can usually be reduced in a closed fashion and immobilized with a splint. One of the more common type 2 fractures is the so-called extra octave fracture at the base of the proximal phalanx of the little finger, caused by forceful ulnar deviation of the finger. Reduction may be accomplished by metacarpophalangeal joint flexion and little-finger radial deviation. Type 3 and 4 fractures are intraarticular injuries. When displaced, these fractures require open reduction to achieve restoration of the articular surface and physis. Type 5 fractures are uncommon in the phalanges, occurring most often in the finger metacarpals as a result of axial compression. Type 5 crush injuries to the growth plate may provoke either partial or complete fusion of the physis and thereby result in late angular deformity or digital shortening.

2. Distal Phalanx Fractures

Distal phalangeal fractures occur most often in the middle finger and the thumb. These fractures usually result from a crushing injury, such as occurs with a misdirected hammer striking a thumb holding a nail or a protruding middle-finger distal phalanx caught in a closing door.

Precise reduction of distal phalangeal fracture fragments is not required in closed injuries, unless the articular surface is involved. Treatment consists of splinting the bone and distal interphalangeal joint for protection and pain relief. While the distal interphalangeal joint is splinted, motion should be encouraged at the metacarpophalangeal and proximal interphalangeal joints. Splint protection may be discontinued at 3 weeks.

Nail matrix injuries are often associated with open distal phalanx fractures. Proper treatment of these fractures requires removal of the nail, irrigation of the fracture and nail bed, and nail bed repair with fine absorbable sutures. Fracture reduction is usually accomplished by nail matrix repair and replacement of the nail. In rare cases, pin fixation of markedly displaced distal phalanx fractures may be required. After nail bed repair, either the original nail, a nail prosthesis, a piece of aluminum suture package, or a piece of gauze should be interposed between the nail roof and the nail bed to prevent synechia (adhesion) formation.

Displaced open distal phalangeal epiphyseal injuries are most often caused by flexion of the distal phalanx with the apex at the dorsal physis. The nail is often avulsed dorsal to the eponychia. Treatment requires nail removal, irrigation, reduction of the fracture, and nail bed repair. Failure to appreciate the open nature of a displaced type 1 fracture of the distal phalanx may result in osteomyelitis with growth arrest of the distal phalanx.

3. Proximal and Middle Phalanx Fractures

Angulation of fractures of the proximal and middle phalanges reflects the tendon forces inserting on the bone. The middle phalanx has an extensor force transmitted to it by the central slip attaching dorsally and proximally. The terminal extensor tendon inserts dorsally and distally into the terminal phalanx, providing a secondary dorsiflexion force. The flexor digitorum superficialis inserts volarly over the middle three fifths of the middle phalanx. Therefore, middle phalanx fractures that occur proximal to the flexor digitorum superficialis insertion angulate with the fracture apex dorsally; fractures that occur distal to the superficialis insertion angulate with the apex palmarly. Proximal phalangeal fractures tend to angulate with the apex palmarly because of the force of lateral bands that pass palmarward to the axis of the metacarpophalangeal joint and dorsalward to the axis of the proximal interphalangeal joint.

Adhesions involving the flexor or extensor tendons are a major complication of proximal and middle phalangeal fractures. Fracture displacement increases the likelihood of tendon adherence and limitation of joint motion. Malunion or malrotation of the fractures may require secondary correction.

Early appropriate treatment of these fractures attempts to prevent complications. In a stable nondisplaced or impacted fracture, only temporary splint protection is required, followed by dynamic splinting such as buddy taping to an adjacent finger. Radiographic follow-up is needed to document maintenance of the reduction. Patients who require closed reduction and immobilization should have the forearm, wrist, and injured digits as well as an adjacent digit immobilized in a plaster cast or gutter splint.

4. Metacarpal Fractures

▶ Metacarpal Head Fractures

Intraarticular fractures of the metacarpal head require open reduction and internal fixation if more than 20–30% of the joint surface is involved. Realigned articular fracture fragments may be held in place with either a K-wire or small screw. Fractures with marked comminution of the metacarpal head distal to the ligament origin may not be amenable to precise internal fixation and may be treated with early mobilization with distraction traction.

▶ Metacarpal Neck Fractures

Metacarpal neck fractures are most frequent in the little finger, although they may occur in any metacarpal. Metacarpal neck fractures result from a direct blow, either delivered to the hand or by the hand striking a solid object (animate or inanimate). Comminution of the volar cortex results in collapse deformity with apex dorsal angulation (Figure 9–28). Greater residual fracture angulation may be accepted in the ring and little fingers because the greater mobility in the ulnar carpometacarpal joints allows greater compensatory motion. The flexion and extension arc is 15 degrees in the ring-finger carpometacarpal joint and 30 degrees in the little finger.

Fracture site angulation of more than 10 degrees should not be accepted in the index and middle fingers. Fractures of the ring and little fingers with initial angulation of less than 15 degrees should be immobilized in a gutter splint for 10–14 days. When angulation is 15–40 degrees, reduction should be accomplished before an ulnar gutter splint immobilization is employed for 3 weeks. With angulation of more than 40 degrees, extensor lag may be noted at the proximal interphalangeal joint, and the patient may complain of a

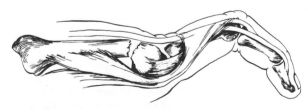

▲ **Figure 9–28.** Boxer's fracture. If the angulation in a metacarpal neck fracture is severe, clawing may result when the patient attempts to extend the finger. This is a good clinical test to supplement the evaluation of the severity of the angulation as seen radiographically. (Reproduced, with permission, from Rockwood CA Jr, et al, ed: *Fractures in Adults,* 3rd ed. Philadelphia: Lippincott; 1991.)

"marble" in the palm when making a fist. If closed reduction cannot be maintained, internal fixation may be employed.

▶ Metacarpal Shaft Fractures

Metacarpal shaft fractures result from a direct blow or crushing injury. Dorsal angulation of the fracture fragments is secondary to the interosseous muscle forces. The closer the fracture is to the carpometacarpal joints, the greater the lever arm and, hence, the less angulation can be tolerated. Less shortening occurs in isolated fractures of the middle and ring metacarpals than in the index or little fingers because the deep intermetacarpal ligaments of two adjacent rays tether the fractured metacarpal distally. Isolated metacarpal fractures may be treated with cast or splint immobilization for 4–6 weeks. Displaced metacarpal shaft fractures may be fixed percutaneously with a longitudinal pin or by percutaneously pinning the fractured metacarpal to an adjacent metacarpal. Skeletal fixation is essential if metacarpal rotational deformity cannot be corrected with closed means because modest metacarpal malrotation results in substantial digital overlap. Dorsal angulation of more than 10 degrees in index and middle metacarpals and more than 20 degrees in ring and little metacarpals, shortening of more than 3 mm, or multiple displaced metacarpal fractures should be treated with operative intervention. Long spiral fractures may be effectively fixed with multiple screws, and transverse fractures are usually most securely fixed with dorsally applied plates. When two or more metacarpals are simultaneously fractured, the splinting effect of the intact adjacent metacarpals is lost. Secure fixation with screws or plates should be employed in at least one of the multiple injured metacarpals.

5. Joint Injuries

▶ Distal Interphalangeal Joint

The most common intraarticular fracture of the distal interphalangeal joint is a bony mallet finger, in which a portion of the dorsal articular surface is avulsed by the extensor tendon. Most bony mallet injuries can be treated with splinting in extension for 6 weeks. Indications for fixation of these fractures are controversial. Internal fixation should be considered in fractures that include articular surface loss greater than 30% and subluxation of the joint.

Dislocation of the distal interphalangeal joint is uncommon without an associated fracture. Closed reduction with temporary splint protection allows early mobilization to begin within 7–10 days.

▶ Condylar Fractures

Condylar fractures may occur in either the proximal or middle phalanges. These fractures are most often athletic injuries. Anteroposterior, lateral, and oblique radiographs are necessary to identify the fracture fragments. If the injury is inadequately appreciated, angulation of the finger and joint incongruity may lead to stiffness, deformity. and early degenerative arthritis. Displaced fracture should be openly reduced and internally fixed if the condylar fracture is displaced by more than 2 mm. If both condyles are fractured, they must be precisely secured together and then secured to the phalangeal shaft. The collateral ligament insertion to the condyle must be preserved because it is the only blood supply to the fragment. Residual stiffness may be anticipated in complex condylar fractures.

▶ Proximal Interphalangeal Joint Dislocation and Fracture-Dislocation

Dorsal dislocations of the proximal interphalangeal joint are more common than palmar or lateral dislocations. Dorsal dislocations may be separated into three types (Figure 9–29). In type 1 dislocations, a hyperextension injury avulses the volar plate from the base of the middle phalanx, and the collateral ligaments partially split from the middle phalanx and the joint surface remains intact. Type 2 dislocations are dorsal dislocations similar to type 1 injuries, except that a larger portion of the collateral ligament is torn. In type 3 injuries, dorsal dislocation occurs with proximal retraction of the middle phalanx. A portion of the middle phalangeal palmar base may be sheared away. Stable fracture-dislocations are associated with fractures in which less than 40% of the middle phalanx base is fractured. Unstable fracture-dislocations have more than 40% bone fracture involvement and are associated with complete loss of collateral ligament stability.

Treatment of proximal interphalangeal joint dislocations depends on the dislocation type. Stable type 1 and 2 injuries should be treated by closed reduction and immobilization in a dorsal splint in 30 degrees of flexion for 1–2 weeks. After reduction and splinting, a radiograph should document the reduction. While in the splint, patients are encouraged to flex the proximal interphalangeal joint actively. After 2–3 weeks, the splint is removed. The finger may be buddy taped to an adjacent finger during sports for the next month.

Unstable fracture-dislocations should be treated with closed reduction. Considerable flexion (>75 degrees) may be necessary to achieve reduction. Again, radiographs must document congruent joint reduction. An extension block splint allows active proximal interphalangeal joint flexion while constraining extension. The splint is straightened by 10-degree increments each week until approximately 4 weeks after reduction, when splinting may be discontinued. If closed reduction cannot be achieved, open reduction is required. When a single large palmar articular fragment is present, internal fixation may be attempted. If the fragments are small and comminuted, the base of the middle phalanx can be reconstructed with similar-shaped osteochondral fragment harvested from the dorsal lip of the hamate bone to restore stability. Alternatively, the volar plate can be drawn into the joint with sutures to create an arthroplasty, or axial traction may be applied to allow early controlled passive joint motion.

Radial lateral proximal interphalangeal dislocation is six times more common than ulnar lateral interphalangeal dislocation. These dislocations are associated with avulsion of the volar plate, extensor mechanism, or a portion of the phalangeal base. After the joint is reduced, the residual joint stability should be assessed by observing the active ROM. Stable fracture-dislocations are immobilized at 5–10 degrees of flexion for 3 weeks, and then active ROM activities are allowed.

Palmar proximal interphalangeal dislocations are unusual. The condyle of the proximal phalanx may buttonhole between the central slip and the lateral bands. Closed reduction may be attempted by applying traction to the fingers after flexing both the metacarpophalangeal and proximal interphalangeal joints. If closed reduction

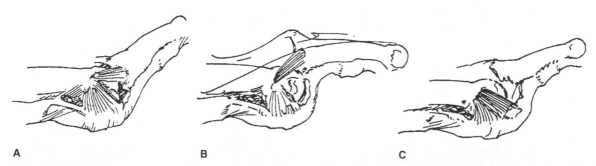

A   **B**   **C**

▲ **Figure 9–29.** Various dorsal dislocations of the proximal interphalangeal joint. **A:** Type 1 (hyperextension). The volar plate is avulsed, and an incomplete longitudinal split occurs in the collateral ligaments. The articular surfaces maintain congruous contact. **B:** Type 2 (dorsal dislocation). There is complete rupture of the volar plate and a complete split in the collateral ligaments, with the middle phalanx resting on the dorsum of the proximal phalanx. The proximal and middle phalanges lie in almost parallel alignment. **C:** Type 3 (fracture-dislocation). The insertion of the volar plate, including a portion of the volar base of the middle phalanx, is disrupted. The major portion of the collateral ligaments remains with the volar plate and flexor sheath. A major articular defect may be present.

is successful, the digit should be splinted in extension for 3–6 weeks to allow healing of the extensor mechanism. If closed reduction is unsuccessful, open reduction is necessary to free the condyle from the rent in the extensor mechanism.

Metacarpophalangeal Joint

Dorsal metacarpophalangeal dislocations most commonly involve either the index or little finger. The volar plate is ruptured proximally from the metacarpal by hyperextension injury. If the joint is subluxed and the volar plate has not yet become interposed in the joint, closed reduction may be achieved by flexion of the joint. Traction across the subluxated metacarpophalangeal joint can transform a reducible joint into an irreducible, dislocated joint. Once the joint dislocates, the volar plate becomes interposed between the dislocated articular surfaces. This injury, termed *complex* or *irreducible,* requires open reduction to extract the volar plate from between the articular surfaces (Figure 9–30). Open reduction may be accomplished through either a palmar or dorsal approach. If the palmar approach is used, care should be taken to avoid injury to the radial digital nerve of the index finger or the ulnar digital nerve of the small finger. The A1 pulley is incised to release the tension of the flexor tendons on the volar plate. If the dorsal approach is used, the volar plate is incised longitudinally to facilitate reduction.

Postoperatively, the metacarpophalangeal joint is immobilized in approximately 30 degrees of flexion for 3–5 days. Splinting that allows active motion is maintained for 3 weeks.

Although lateral dislocations of the metacarpophalangeal joint are rare, isolated radial collateral ligament ruptures may occur. These injuries should also be immobilized in

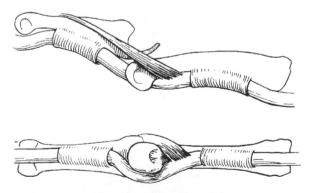

▲ **Figure 9–30.** Complex dislocation of the metacarpophalangeal joint. In the upper lateral diagram, the palmar plate is locked between the head of the metacarpal and the base of the proximal phalanx. In the lower diagram, an anterior view, the head of the metacarpal can be seen trapped between the flexor digitorum profundus on one aspect and the lumbrical on the other. (Reproduced, with permission, from Lister G: *The Hand: Diagnosis and Indications,* 3rd ed. Philadelphia: Churchill Livingstone; 1993.)

approximately 30 degrees of flexion for 3 weeks. The fingers should be protected from ulnar stress for an additional 3 weeks. Unstable index- and middle-finger radial collateral ligament tears may be surgically repaired.

Finger Carpometacarpal Joints

Sprains and fracture-dislocations may involve any of the carpometacarpal joints. Sprains of the index- and middle-finger carpometacarpal joints may occur with palmar flexion and torsion. If tenderness is localized to the carpometacarpal joint and careful radiographs fail to demonstrate fracture, a sprain may be diagnosed.

Treatment of acute sprain injuries consists of 3–6 weeks of immobilization. If localized pain persists, steroid injection may be considered. Chronic pain at the index middle trapezoid capitate joint may be treated with either carpal boss excision or arthrodesis of the carpometacarpal joint. Carpometacarpal fracture-dislocations of the ring and little fingers are usually secondary to direct or longitudinal blows. Dorsal dislocations are more common than volar dislocations. Oblique views with partial pronation and supination may be required to visualize the carpometacarpal joint clearly. Closed reduction may be achieved with longitudinal distraction. The reduction may be maintained by percutaneous K-wire fixation. When fracture-dislocation of the little-finger metacarpal articular surface shears off a fragment of the hamate, displacement of the metacarpal shaft is likely. Because of forces of the extensor carpi ulnaris and the hypothenar muscles, the metacarpal shaft tends to displace proximally and angulate palmarly. Longitudinal traction and percutaneous K-wire fixation of the ring- and little-finger metacarpals stabilize these fractures. Open reduction is necessary for an irreducible dislocation or for chronic fracture-dislocations. If the patient develops degenerative arthritis of the hamate metacarpal joint, arthrodesis of the ring- or small-finger carpometacarpal joint (or both) is well tolerated.

Thumb Metacarpophalangeal Joint

The most common injury to the metacarpophalangeal joint is sprain of the ulnar collateral ligament of the thumb (gamekeeper's thumb, skier's thumb). This injury occurs when the thumb is forced into radial deviation, stressing the ulnar collateral ligament. When the ulnar collateral ligament tears from its phalangeal insertion, the adductor aponeurosis may become interposed between the retracted ligament, preventing healing of the ligament to the proximal phalanx with closed treatment (Stener lesion). Evaluation of the integrity of the ligament may be made by radially stressing the flexed metacarpophalangeal joint under local anesthesia. Radial deviation that is more than 30 degrees from that of the opposite thumb is diagnostic of a totally disrupted, incompetent ligament.

Closed treatment of a partial ligament tear may be accomplished with a thumb spica splint for 3–4 weeks. Complete disruption of the ligament requires surgical exploration and reattachment to the bone. Avulsion of the ulnar collateral ligament may also occur with a bony fragment. If the fragment is greater than 15% of the articular surface or if the avulsed fragment is displaced more than 5 mm, open repair of the ligament is recommended.

Chronic symptomatic ulnar collateral ligament injuries may be repaired if the residual ligament is of sufficient quality. Supplementation of the repair with either tendon transfer or tendon grafting may be useful. In patients who develop traumatic arthritis or if ligament reconstruction is not deemed feasible, arthrodesis of the metacarpophalangeal joint is preferred.

▶ Thumb Carpometacarpal Joint

Four patterns of thumb metacarpal fracture are most commonly encountered.

A. Bennett Fracture

Bennett fracture is a fracture dislocation of the thumb basal joint in which the small volar ulnar fragment of the metacarpal articular surface remains attached to the anterior oblique ligament, and the remainder of the metacarpal articular surface and shaft is displaced proximally, radially, and into adduction in response to the force of the adductor pollicis and abductor pollicis longus muscles insertion on the metacarpal (Figure 9–31). Acute Bennett fractures may often be

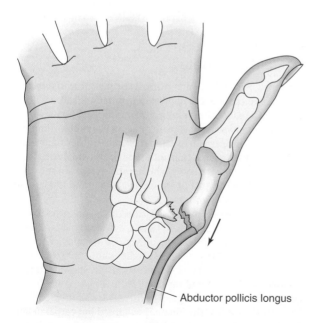

Abductor pollicis longus

▲ **Figure 9–31.** Bennett fracture. The first metacarpal shaft is displaced by the pull of the muscle. (Reproduced, with permission, from American Society for Surgery of the Hand: *The Hand: Examination and Diagnosis,* 2nd ed. Philadelphia: Churchill Livingstone; 1983.)

reduced by traction, abduction, and pressure on the proximal metacarpal, with slight pronation. The reduction may then be stabilized by percutaneous pin fixation through the metacarpal shaft into either the fragment or the trapezium. If satisfactory reduction cannot be achieved by closed means, open reduction and internal fixation is required.

B. Rolando Fracture

The Rolando fracture is a comminuted T or Y intraarticular fracture of the base of the thumb metacarpal. When large fragments are present, open reduction and internal fixation is possible. When the joint is highly comminuted, cast immobilization, traction, or limited open reduction and internal fixation with cast immobilization may be employed.

C. Extraarticular Fracture

Extraarticular fractures are less likely to develop traumatic arthritis than intraarticular fractures. Because of the mobility of the carpometacarpal joint of the thumb, up to 30 degrees of angulation can be accepted without functional loss.

D. Epiphyseal Fracture

Epiphyseal fractures of the thumb metacarpal are treated in a fashion similar to other Salter-Harris fractures.

Freeland AE, Lineaweaver WC, Lindley SG: Fracture fixation in the mutilated hand. *Hand Clin* 2003;19:51. [PMID: 12683446]

Kiefhaber TR, Stern PJ: Fractures dislocations of the proximal interphalangeal joint. *J Hand Surg Am* 1998;23:368. [PMID: 9620177]

Page SM, Stern PJ: Complications and range of motion following plate fixation of metacarpal and phalangeal fractures. *J Hand Surg Am* 1998;23:827. [PMID: 9763256]

WRIST INJURIES

▶ Scaphoid Injuries

The scaphoid is the most commonly fractured bone in the carpus. Anatomically, the scaphoid may be divided into proximal, middle, and distal thirds. The middle third is termed the *waist*. The scaphoid tubercle forms a distal volar prominence. Because the scaphoid articulates with four carpal bones and the radius, most of its surface is composed of articular cartilage, leaving little room for vascular perforation. Therefore, the vascular supply to the scaphoid comes through a narrow nonarticular region in the waist. Most of the blood supply to the scaphoid tuberosity enters distally. In approximately a third of fractures at the waist level, there is diminished flow to the proximal pole, which may result in ischemic necrosis of the proximal pole of the scaphoid. Almost 100% of proximal pole fractures develop ischemic or aseptic necrosis.

Middle third fractures account for approximately 70% of scaphoid fractures, proximal pole fractures for 20%, and distal pole fractures for the rest.

Cast immobilization is recommended in the treatment of all nondisplaced scaphoid fractures, defined as fractures with less than 2 mm of displacement and no fracture site angulation. On average, middle third fractures heal in 6–12 weeks, distal third fractures in 4–8 weeks, and proximal third fractures in 12–20 weeks. When initial radiographs demonstrate fracture displacement, open reduction and internal fixation is required to prevent malunion. Internal fixation is accomplished with either smooth K-wires or a buried headless compression screw. Because of the time to union in scaphoid fractures, some surgeons recommend primary fixation of these fractures even when nondisplaced. Newer studies demonstrate that percutaneous fixation of nondisplaced waist fractures decreases time to healing and shortens or eliminates the period of cast immobilization.

Delayed union may be treated with either prolonged casting or open reduction, curettage, and bone grafting. Nondisplaced ununited fractures may be treated by percutaneous screw fixation and injection of bone graft. If fracture site angulation or collapse is present, a cortical cancellous volar graft is employed to correct the deformity. The graft must be stabilized with either a buried compression screw or K-wires. If the proximal pole is avascular and no radiocarpal arthritis is present, revascularization of the scaphoid with a vascularized bone graft from the dorsal radius should be performed.

Once degenerative arthritis is evident at the radiocarpal joint, salvage procedures include proximal row carpectomy, scaphoid excision and midcarpal arthrodesis, and total wrist arthrodesis.

▶ Lunate and Perilunate Dislocations

Lunate and perilunate dislocations are the result of a powerful force causing disruption of the ligamentous support about the lunate. The mechanism of these injuries is usually dorsiflexion, ulnar deviation, and intercarpal supination. Mayfield defined four stages of disruption. Stage 1 injuries demonstrate disruptions of the scapholunate ligament. Stage 2 injuries also include tears of the ligaments dorsal to the lunate. In stage 3 injuries, the arc of disruption extends across the lunotriquetral ligament. Stage 4 injuries have total disruption of the entire lunate ligamentous support. The sequence of injuries is paralleled by a progression of clinical entities from scapholunate dissociation to perilunate dislocation to lunate dislocation.

When the entire carpus except the lunate dislocates and the lunate remains normally seated in the lunate fossa of the radius, the abnormality is termed *perilunate dislocation* (Figure 9–32). When the relationship between the carpus and the radius is maintained but the lunate is dislocated palmarward into the carpal tunnel, the condition is termed *lunate dislocation*. Both lunate and perilunate dislocations

imply disruption of ligamentous connections between the scaphoid and the lunate, between the capitate and the lunate, and between the lunate and the triquetrum. Although the lunate is bound to the scaphoid by the scapholunate ligament and to the triquetrum through the lunotriquetral ligament, the interval between the lunate and the capitate, known as the space of Poirier, lacks direct ligamentous connection.

A variant of perilunate dislocation is transscaphoid perilunate dislocation. With this injury, the arc of disruption passes through the scaphoid rather than the scapholunate ligament. The disruption then passes between the proximal scaphoid and the capitate, between the capitate and the lunate, and between the lunate and the triquetrum.

Intercarpal ligamentous disruptions heal if the normally connected bones are maintained in an anatomic relationship. Intercarpal dislocations should be reduced initially in a closed fashion. Reduction is usually achieved by longitudinal traction and direct pressure on the dislocated carpal bone or bones. Occasionally, anatomic alignment of the carpus can be achieved and maintained with closed reduction and cast application. In most instances, however, open reduction, pin fixation, and direct ligamentous repair are necessary to secure anatomic reduction. Surgical treatment of perilunate and lunate dislocations often requires both palmar and dorsal approaches. Through the dorsal approach, intercarpal alignment is visualized, adjusted, and stabilized. The palmar approach is employed to release the median nerve at the carpal tunnel and to repair the rent in the space of Poirier.

▶ Kienböck Disease

Kienböck disease results from ischemic necrosis of the lunate. The cause of the condition is the subject of extensive debate. The condition is more common in patients with a negative ulnar variance, in which the ulna is shorter than the radius. It is unclear whether the relatively shorter ulna alters and increases the force transmitted to the lunate through the lunate fossa of the radius or whether the altered stress causes the lunate to be shaped in a more triangular and less cuboid or trapezoidal configuration.

Kienböck disease may be classified based on the extent of collapse (Figure 9–33). Stage I disease demonstrates a linear compression fracture but an otherwise normal-appearing architecture and density. MRI studies show poor vascularity of the lunate in stage I (Figure 9–34). In stage II disease, the density is abnormal on plain films. By stage III, lunate collapse is present. Stage III disease is subdivided into stage IIIA, in which the lunate is collapsed but carpal height remains normal, and stage IIIB, in which the lunate is collapsed and carpal height is also abnormal. In stage IV wrists, extensive osteoarthritic changes are present.

The current recommendations for the treatment of Kienböck disease include radial shortening osteotomy for ulnar-negative or neutral variance when no carpal collapse

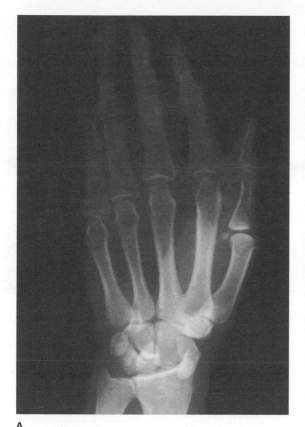

A

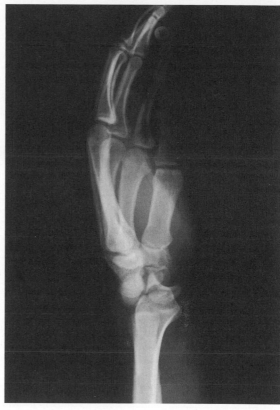

B

▲ **Figure 9–32.** Perilunate dislocation: Anteroposterior view **(A)**; lateral view **(B)**.

is present. If the patient initially demonstrates a positive ulnar variance, recommendations include either a capitate shortening osteotomy or an intercarpal arthrodesis of the scaphoid, trapezium, and trapezoid. A new technique restores the anatomic height of the lunate with a vascularized bone graft and additional cancellous bone. In stage IIIB and IV wrists, consideration is given to either proximal row carpectomy or wrist arthrodesis. Silicone replacement of the lunate is no longer advised for Kienböck disease.

▶ **Carpal Instability**

To evaluate the orientation of the carpus properly, true PA and lateral radiographs are required. The PA view should be obtained with the forearm positioned in neutral rotation to allow a precise standardized evaluation of the relationship between the distal radius and the distal ulna. When the ulna is shorter than the radius, the term *negative ulnar variance* is used, and when the ulna extends further distally than the radius, the term *positive ulnar variance* is used.

The PA radiograph should demonstrate the close relationship of the scaphoid and the lunate. Normally, the ossified portions of these two bones are separated by their abutting respective articular cartilage shells, creating a radiographic gap of 3 mm or less. In an adult a gap of more than 3 mm is considered abnormal and indicates separation of these two bones secondary to ligamentous disruption. When the scapholunate gap is abnormally wide on a standard radiograph, the abnormality is referred to as static scapholunate dissociation (Figure 9–35). When the standard PA radiograph is normal but an anteroposterior radiograph taken with the fingers squeezing tightly to form a fist reveals an abnormal gap, the condition is referred to as dynamic scapholunate dissociation.

The lateral radiograph should be obtained with the wrist in a neutral position, neither flexed nor extended. The lateral radiograph is often overlooked because of the projected superimposition of shadows. This normal overlapping allows measurement of a number of angles between bones. Normally, the middle metacarpal, capitate, lunate, and radius are collinear. The long axis of the radius is readily defined. Establishing the relationship of the scaphoid to the radius requires defining a line drawn along the most palmar portions of the distal and proximal poles of the scaphoid. The axes of the radius and the scaphoid intersect, forming the radioscaphoid angle (Figure 9–36). This angle is usually

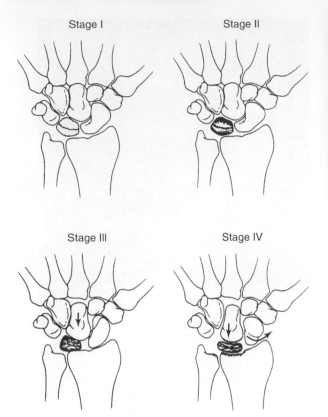

Stage I   Stage II

Stage III   Stage IV

▲ **Figure 9–33.** Staging of Kienböck disease (after Lichtman). Stage I: Routine radiographs (posteroanterior, lateral) are normal, but tomography may show a linear fracture, usually transverse through the body of the lunate. MRI confirms avascular changes. Stage II: Bone density increase (sclerosis) and a fracture line are usually evident on the posteroanterior radiograph. Posteroanterior and lateral tomograms demonstrate sclerosis, cystic changes, and often a clear fracture. There is no collapse deformity. Stage III: Advanced bone density changes are present, with fragmentation, cystic resorption, and collapse. The diagnosis is evident from posteroanterior radiograph. Tomograms (posteroanterior and lateral) show the degree of lunate infractionation and amount of fracture displacement. Proximal migration of the capitate is present, and there is mild to moderate rotary alignment of the scaphoid. Stage IV: Perilunate arthritic changes are present, with complete collapse and fragmentation of the lunate. Carpal instability is evident, with scaphoid malalignment and capitate displacement into the lunate space. (Reproduced, with permission, from Rockwood CA Jr, et al, eds: *Fractures in Adults,* 3rd ed. Philadelphia: Lippincott; 1991.)

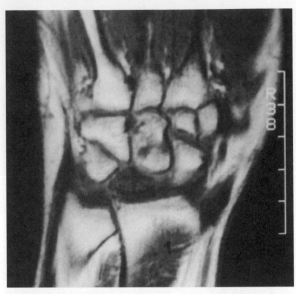

▲ **Figure 9–34.** MRI showing Kienböck disease.

between 40 and 60 degrees. When the angle is greater than 60 degrees, the scaphoid is abnormally flexed.

The orientation of the lunate viewed on the lateral radiograph is derived by first establishing a line between the most distal palmar and dorsal lips of the lunate. A second line is then drawn perpendicular to the first line, establishing the axis of the lunate. The angle between the radial and lunate axes (radiolunate angle) is normally less than 15 degrees.

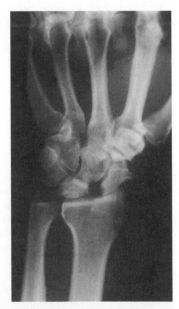

▲ **Figure 9–35.** Anteroposterior view of static scapholunate dissociation.

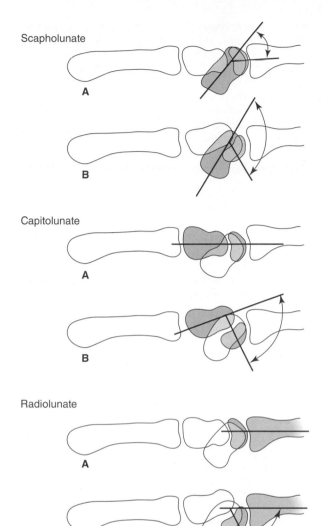

Scapholunate

A

B

Capitolunate

A

B

Radiolunate

A

B

▲ **Figure 9–36.** Carpal angle measurements are of considerable aid in identifying carpal instability patterns. A, normal angle; B, abnormal angle seen in dorsiflexion instability. The capitolunate angle should theoretically be 0 degrees with the wrist in neutral position, but the range of normal probably extends to as much as 15 degrees. The scapholunate angle may be the most helpful; an angle of greater than 80 degrees is definite evidence of dorsiflexion instability. The radiolunate angle is abnormal if it exceeds 15 degrees. (Reproduced, with permission, from Green DP, ed: *Operative Hand Surgery*, 2nd ed. Philadelphia: Churchill Livingstone; 1988.)

The orientation of the lunate seen on the lateral radiograph normally reflects a ligamentous balancing of the influences of the adjacent scaphoid and triquetrum. The scaphoid tends to tether the lunate into flexion through the scapholunate ligament, whereas the triquetrum tends to

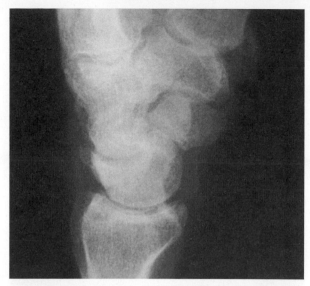

▲ **Figure 9–37.** Lateral radiograph of dorsal intercalated segment instability.

tether the lunate into extension (dorsiflexion) through the lunotriquetral ligament. When the scapholunate ligament is disrupted, the scaphoid tends to flex excessively, and the lunate, under the unopposed influence of the triquetrum, dorsiflexes (dorsal intercalated segment instability [DISI]) (Figure 9–37). When the lunotriquetral ligament is disrupted, the lunate, under the unopposed influence of the scaphoid, is flexed (volar intercalated segment instability [VISI]). The optimal treatment for DISI is currently an area of intense interest. Acute ligamentous disruption is usually treated with direct ligamentous reapproximation and repair. When ligamentous repair is not possible and articular surfaces are free of degenerative change, ligamentous reconstruction, dorsal capsular ligamentodesis, or intercarpal fusions may be considered.

Degenerative arthritis occurs in wrists subjected over time to loads applied to noncongruently articulating carpal bones. The scapholunate advanced collapse (SLAC) wrist pattern describes the evolution of degenerative arthritis resulting from disruption of the scapholunate ligament (Figure 9–38). The earliest evidence of degenerative change is seen at the radioscaphoid joint, and, with time, degenerative change progresses to include the capitate lunate articulation. When radioscaphoid change is present but the articular surface of the capitate retains its normal articular cartilage, proximal row carpectomy (removal of the scaphoid, lunate, and triquetrum) allows preservation of 50% of wrist motion as the capitate head shifts proximally to articulate within the lunate fossa of the distal radius. When degenerative change is present at the capitate-lunate portion of the midcarpal joints in addition to radioscaphoid change, the scaphoid may be excised and intercarpal fusion of the capitate, lunate, triquetrum, and hamate is accomplished. This selective osteotomy, performed in the diaphyseal ulna, and fixed with a plate and screws. After the wafer procedure, patients often complain of ulnar pain for a prolonged period (3–6 months). Approximately 50% of patients who have an ulnar shortening osteotomy require plate removal after osteotomy healing.

Another source of ulnar-sided wrist pain is a tear of the TFCC. Tears are divided into degenerative and traumatic types. Degenerative tears are usually related to ulnocarpal impaction. Traumatic tears usually occur after a twisting injury of the wrist. Central tears and tears near the attachment of the TFCC to the radius are usually treated with an arthroscopic debridement. Tears in the well-vascularized periphery of the TFCC are treated with either arthroscopic or open repair. After repair, patients are maintained in a long arm cast for 6 weeks to allow fibrocartilage healing.

Arthritis between the distal radius and ulna can be caused by traumatic, degenerative, or inflammatory disorders. Treatment consists of hemiresection or complete excision of the ulnar head (Darrach procedure). An alternative treatment, the Suave-Kapandji procedure, fuses the DRUJ and creates a pseudarthrosis of the distal ulna. This is particularly useful in the presence of ulnar translocation of the carpus.

Instability of the DRUJ is difficult to treat. Instability is usually the result of trauma, but it may occur after an excessive distal ulna resection. Treatment requires detection and correction of any degree of malunions in the radius or ulna. A number of soft-tissue operations are designed to stabilize the distal ulna, all with varying degrees of success.

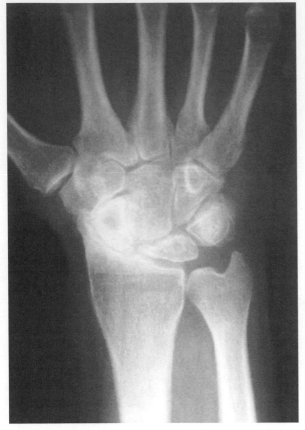

▲ **Figure 9–38.** Scapholunate advanced collapse pattern.

intercarpal fusion procedure provides motion through the residual radiolunate articulation. The ultimate salvage procedure, complete wrist fusion, provides reliable pain relief while permanently sacrificing wrist motion.

▷ Distal Radioulnar Joint

The distal radioulnar joint (DRUJ) is composed of two joints. The proximal and distal articulations of the ulna and radius allow forearm rotation. The ulna also articulates with the ulnar carpus through the triangular fibrocartilage complex (TFCC). Approximately 20% of the load from the hand to the forearm passes through the ulnocarpal joint. Problems at the DRUJ are related to one or both of these joints.

When the ulnar variance is positive, the patient may develop an ulnocarpal impaction syndrome. This often presents with pain on the ulnar side of the wrist, particularly with ulnar deviation. Radiographs may demonstrate degenerative changes of the distal ulna and cysts in the lunate. Treatment consists of shortening the ulna, accomplished by removing 2–3 mm of the ulnar head (wafer procedure) either by open method, by arthroscope, or by an ulnar-shortening

Adams BD, Berger RA: An anatomic reconstruction of the distal radioulnar ligaments for posttraumatic distal radioulnar joint instability. *J Hand Surg Am* 2002;27:243. [PMID: 11901383]

Aldridge JM III, Mallon WJ: Hook of the hamate fractures in competitive golfers: results of treatment by excision of the fractured hook of the hamate. *Orthopedics* 2003;26:717. [PMID: 12875568]

Berger RA: The anatomy of the ligaments of the wrist and distal radioulnar joints. *Clin Orthop* 2001;383:32. [PMID: 11210966]

Cohen MS, Kozin SH: Degenerative arthritis of the wrist: proximal row carpectomy versus scaphoid excision and four-corner arthrodesis. *J Hand Surg Am* 2001;26:94. [PMID: 11172374]

Gelberman RH, Salamon PB, Jurist JM, et al: Ulnar variance with Kienböck's disease. *J Bone Joint Surg Am* 1975;57:674. [PMID: 1150712]

Rettig ME, Kozin SH, Cooney WP: Open reduction and internal fixation of acute displaced scaphoid waist fractures. *J Hand Surg Am* 2001;26:271. [PMID: 11279573]

Shin AY, Bishop AT: Pedicled vascularized bone grafts for disorders of the carpus: scaphoid nonunion and Kienböck's disease. *J Am Acad Orthop Surg* 2002;10:210. [PMID: 12041942]

Shin AY, Weinstein LP, Berger RA, et al: Treatment of isolated injuries of the lunotriquetral ligament. A comparison of arthrodesis, ligament reconstruction and ligament repair. *J Bone Joint Surg Br* 2001;83:1023. [PMID: 11603516]

Slade JF III, Geissler WB, Gutow AP, et al: Percutaneous internal fixation of selected scaphoid nonunions with an arthroscopically assisted dorsal approach. *J Bone Joint Surg Am* 2003;85:20. [PMID: 14652390]

Steinmann SP, Bishop AT, Berger RA: Use of the 1,2 intercompartmental supraretinacular artery as a vascularized pedicle bone graft for difficult scaphoid nonunion. *J Hand Surg Am* 2002;27:391. [PMID: 12015712]

Szabo RM, Slater RR Jr, Palumbo CF, et al: Dorsal intercarpal ligament capsulodesis for chronic, static scapholunate dissociation: clinical results. *J Hand Surg Am* 2002;27A:978. [PMID: 12457347]

▼ FINGERTIP INJURIES

SOFT-TISSUE INJURIES

Because of the importance of the fingertip in providing a contact surface for sensate prehension, injuries to the fingertip may result in troublesome disability. The pulp of the fingertip is normally covered by tough, highly innervated skin, anchored to the phalanx by fibrous septa. The dorsum of the fingertip is composed of the nail and nail bed.

▶ Treatment

The goals in treatment of fingertip injuries are to provide adequate sensation, minimal tenderness, satisfactory appearance, and full joint motion. Preservation of length should be balanced with the other goals.

The choice of treatment depends on the size and location of the defect. The mechanism of injury (sharp, crushing, or avulsion), the presence of exposed bone, and the angle of soft-tissue loss are considered in planning treatment.

A. Open Wound Care

The simplest treatment is open wound care, which is indicated in most injuries in children and in defects of 1 cm² or less in adults. The wound is thoroughly cleansed. Bone is shortened so it is covered by soft tissue, and the length of the bone is the same as the length of the nail bed. Dressings are changed until the wound is healed. The disadvantages of the open method are the possibility of stump tenderness and prolonged healing time. Advantages include the ability to initiate movement immediately and to thus preserve full digital motion.

B. Composite Grafting

Replacement of the amputated part as a composite graft (skin and subcutaneous tissue) is indicated in children and selected adults with sharp distal amputations. When successful, this treatment gives the best appearance. The disadvantage, the unpredictable viability of the part, may result in recovery delayed by failure and secondary procedures.

C. Microvascular Replantation

Microvascular replantation is possible in selected sharp amputations distal to the distal interphalangeal joint.

Disadvantages include the expense of complex surgery and the time lost from work.

D. Primary Shortening and Closure

Primary bone shortening and closure are indicated when more than 50% of the distal phalanx is lost or the nail matrix is irreparably damaged. This one-stage procedure allows for immediate mobilization. In performing the procedure, the end of the distal phalanx bone should be trimmed to provide a tension-free soft-tissue closure. The nail bed should be trimmed as far proximal as the bone. If the nail bed is pulled over the end of the shortened bone, a hook-shaped nail results. Neurectomy of digital nerves under traction allows the nerve ends to retract into soft tissue proximal to the ultimate scar.

E. Skin Grafting

Skin grafting may also be employed to obtain closure if no bone is exposed. Split-thickness grafts may be placed on a less well-vascularized bed. Split-thickness grafts contract more than full-thickness grafts. As the graft shrinks, the area of sensory loss also shrinks. The appearance and durability of scar tissue may be less than ideal, however.

Full-thickness skin grafts provide more durable coverage and better appearance. Care should be taken to match the pigmentation of the skin at the donor and recipient sites. The ulnar border of the hand provides an ideal donor source. Full-thickness grafts require a better vascularized bed to assure survival.

F. Skin Flaps

Local advancement skin flaps are useful in the treatment of fingertip injuries.

1. V-Y advancement skin flaps—V-Y advancement skin flaps may advance palmar tissue or unite two lateral skin flaps. These skin flaps are helpful in the management of transverse or dorsal oblique amputations in which soft-tissue tip coverage is needed and further skeletal shortening deemed undesirable. Complete separation of the vertical septa between the skin and the bone is required to mobilize skin flaps for advancement. The septa between the flap and the proximal skin must then be divided. Traction on the flap helps differentiate the septa from vessels and nerves.

2. Moberg palmar advancement flap—Defects of up to 1.5 cm on the thumb may be covered by a palmar advancement flap, first described by Moberg. Bilateral midlateral incisions dorsal to the neurovascular bundles of the thumb allow mobilization of the flap from the flexor tendon sheath. The flap may be maximally advanced by flexion of the thumb interphalangeal joint. When additional coverage is required, the skin of the flap may be transversely divided at the metacarpophalangeal crease while the neurovascular bundles are preserved, the distal portion of the flap may be advanced further, and a skin graft may be placed between the distal flap and the proximal flap. Disadvantages of this flap include the possibility of interphalangeal joint flexion contracture and the potential for dorsal tip necrosis if dorsal vascular branches to the digit are injured.

3. Regional skin flaps—Regional skin flaps are considered when fingertip skin is lost but nail and bone are preserved.

A. Cross-finger flap—The cross-finger flap is the most commonly used distant flap. Skin is elevated from the dorsum of the adjacent finger, with care taken not to incise the extensor paratenon. The skin is then rotated palmarward and sewn to the palmar defect of the involved finger. The donor region on the donor finger is skin grafted. The transposed flap is divided from the donor finger after 2 weeks. Joint stiffness is a potential complication in both the donor and recipient digits. The creation of a defect on a normal digit is another disadvantage.

B. Thenar flap—The thenar flap may be used in children and young (<25 years) adults in whom the potential for joint stiffness is less. A flap of palmar skin is raised at the base of the thumb and applied to the injured tip of the flexed injured finger. More subcutaneous fat is transferred with a thenar flap than with a cross-finger flap. Thenar skin flaps usually result in good matching of color and texture with the pulp.

▼ NAIL BED INJURIES

▶ Clinical Findings

Nail bed injuries, often neglected, should be carefully attended to because the nail enhances sensibility, provides protection and fine manipulation of the finger, and gives the finger a normal appearance. The nail bed may be injured by subungual hematoma, nail matrix laceration, avulsion of the nail matrix from the nail fold, or complete loss of the nail matrix.

▶ Treatment

When a subungual hematoma involves more than 50% of the subungual area, the nail should be removed and the nail bed laceration repaired with fine absorbable suture or skin glue such as Dermabond. Either the nail is replaced or a dressing is placed under the nail fold to prevent synechia formation with resultant splitting of the nail. Nail bed defects are treated with split-thickness nail bed grafts taken from either an adjacent uninjured fingernail or a toenail.

When nail bed injuries occur with an open distal phalangeal fracture, pin fixation of the fracture may be considered because it stabilizes the nail bed repair.

Caution is required in the treatment of nail bed injuries in children, who often suffer injury from having a fingertip slammed in a door. The nail often lies dorsal to the nail fold, and a small subungual hematoma is noted. If a radiograph

is obtained, usually a physeal fracture of the distal phalanx is observed. Because the nail bed laceration communicates with the physeal fracture, this injury represents an open fracture and must be treated appropriately. The nail should be removed and the fracture site irrigated. An interposed portion of the nail bed often must be extracted from between the fragments of the physeal fracture. If the fracture is unstable, pin fixation facilitates nail bed repair. Failure to appreciate the open nature of this pediatric injury may result in osteomyelitis and physeal arrest of the distal phalanx.

Heistein JB, Cook PA: Factors affecting composite graft survival in digital tip amputations. *Ann Plast Surg* 2003;50:299. [PMID: 12800909]

Strauss EJ, Weil WM, Jordan C, Paksima N: A prospective, randomized, controlled trial of 2-octylcyanoacrylate versus suture repair for nail bed injuries. *J Hand Surg Am* 2008;33:250. [PMID: 18294549]

▼ THERMAL INJURY

ACUTE BURN INJURY

▶ Degree of Injury

A. First-Degree Burns

Burns are characterized by the depth of skin injury. First-degree burns involve only the epidermis. Patients usually present with swollen red areas, and care is symptomatic.

B. Second-Degree Burns

Second-degree burns involve both the epidermis and the superficial portion of the dermis. These burns may be identified by skin blistering and blanching of the skin when pressure is applied. Second-degree burns are subdivided into superficial and deep burns. Superficial second-degree burns are treated with topical antibiotics such as silver sulfadiazine. The extremity is elevated and the hand splinted in the intrinsic plus position. With the wrist in 30 degrees of extension, the metacarpophalangeal joint is flexed and the interphalangeal joints are extended. The thumb should be maintained in an abducted position to prevent contracture of the first web space. The patient should begin a vigorous therapy program emphasizing active ROM as soon as it is tolerated. Compression garments may reduce swelling and scar hypertrophy after reepithelialization.

In deep second-degree burns, excision of the remaining portion of the skin and application of a skin graft do not produce long-term results superior to those achieved with spontaneous healing. Therefore, the treatment of deep second-degree burns should be similar to that of superficial second-degree burns.

C. Third-Degree Burns

Third-degree burns involve the entire epidermis, dermis, and a portion of the subcutaneous region. These burns result in waxy dry regions often having a nontender central area, caused by burning of the neural tissue. Third-degree burns should be treated with excision within the first 3–7 days and a split-thickness skin graft applied to the involved areas.

D. Fourth-Degree Burns

In addition to involvement of the skin, fourth-degree burns involve deep tissues, including muscle, tendon, and bone. Often, the only effective treatment for these burns is amputation of the involved part, with appropriate soft-tissue coverage of the residual stump.

▶ Complications

A. Neurovascular Complications

The neurovascular status of the burned hand should be carefully monitored. Massive swelling necessitates release of compartments of the hand and forearm. Digital releases are best performed by longitudinal releases along the ulnar border of the index, middle, and ring fingers and along the radial border of the thumb and little finger. Longitudinal incisions on the dorsal hand allow decompression of interosseous muscle compartments. Incisions are made along the medial and lateral aspects of the arm and forearm.

B. Late Complications

1. Joint contractures—Joint contractures are the most common complications of upper extremity burns. At the elbow, these are most often flexion contractures. Treatment consists of soft-tissue release and either skin grafting of open regions or rotation of local skin flaps. Elbow motion may also be limited by the development of heterotopic ossifications. Excision of the ossification may be successful if delayed until the area of ossification has matured, often 1.5–2 years after the burn injury. Because the area of most intense heterotopic ossification is posteromedially, care must be taken to define and protect the ulnar nerve during elbow release surgery.

2. Wrist and hand contractures—Wrist contracture may tether the hand into either a flexed or extended position, depending on the region of the burn. In the fingers, burns usually involve the thin skin on the dorsum of the finger, often disrupting the central slip insertion onto the middle phalanx. The loss of active proximal interphalangeal joint extension combined with dorsal hand burns may result in development of a clawlike deformity, with flexion contractures of the proximal interphalangeal joints and hyperextension contracture at the metacarpophalangeal joint.

Treatment of metacarpophalangeal joint extension contracture usually requires release of the dorsal scar, addition

of a dorsal skin graft, and dorsal metatarsophalangeal joint capsular release. Proximal interphalangeal flexion contractures may also occur secondary to scarred volar skin. In such cases, soft-tissue release may be accomplished with either Z-plasty flap transposition or by palmar scar excision and full-thickness skin graft application. The most predictable treatment of severe proximal interphalangeal joint contracture in the burn patient is arthrodesis of the proximal interphalangeal joint.

Adduction contracture, the most common thumb deformity in the burned hand, may be difficult to resolve fully. The extent of release required depends on the degree of contracture. A modest adduction contracture may be effectively treated with Z-plasty of the thenar skin to regain adequate abduction in the first web space. With more severe contracture, release of the adductor pollicis from its origin or at its insertion and release of the first dorsal interosseous muscle origin from the thumb metacarpal may be required. If web space skin coverage is inadequate after muscle release, full-thickness skin grafting or local or distant skin flaps may be needed.

Ideally, first web space contracture should be avoided by carefully maintaining the first web space during the initial phases of burn treatment. When the extent of web space burn is severe and the normal first web cannot be maintained with dressings, an external fixator should be placed, spanning the thumb and index-finger metacarpals.

ELECTRICAL BURNS

The extent of injury in electrical burns is proportional to the amount of current that passes through the involved portion of the body. The Ohm law states that the amount of current is equal to the voltage divided by the resistance. Therefore, for a given voltage, those structures that have a lower resistance conduct a greater amount of current. The relative resistance of structures in the arm from least resistance to greatest resistance is as follows: nerve, vessel, muscle, skin, tendon, fat, and bone. Alternating current is more injurious than direct current. Because of its frequency, alternating current produces muscle tetany in the finger flexors, which may prevent the patient from releasing the grasped current source. The duration of contact plays a direct role in the severity of injury because a longer contact period results in more electrical energy passing through the body.

▶ Clinical Findings

The greatest current density occurs at the entrance and exit wounds, usually apparent as charred areas that are blackened and surrounded by a gray-white zone, an area of tissue necrosis in which the tissue is still intact but will die. These areas are surrounded by a red zone, in which there is a variable extent of vessel thrombosis, coagulation, and necrosis.

High-voltage, or arc, burns produce a greater thermal than electric injury. Arc burns may extend across flexor surfaces from the hand to the wrist or from the forearm to the arm. Arc burns are usually associated with a high temperature of 3000–5000°C.

It is difficult to assess precisely the extent of tissue necrosis in burn wounds at the time of initial presentation. All burn patients should be examined for fractures, particularly cervical spine fractures, because electrical burn patients were possibly thrown a distance by the current. The possibility of either compartment syndrome or concomitant peripheral nerve injury must also be considered. Patients should be admitted to an intensive care unit and monitored for cardiac arrhythmia, renal failure, sepsis, secondary hemorrhage, and neurologic complications to the brain, spinal cord, or peripheral nerves.

▶ Treatment

Treatment for upper extremity burns consists of initially debriding clearly nonviable tissue. The decision to carry out fasciotomy and nerve decompression should be guided by examination. A second debridement is performed 48–72 hours later, for tissue in the gray-white zones. Debridement should be continued every 48–72 hours until a stable wound is achieved. The extent of necrosis often appears to increase with each successive debridement. This phenomenon reflects both an underestimation of the extent of initial injury and progressive vascular thrombosis. After all necrotic tissue is debrided, reconstruction is accomplished with either local or distant skin flaps or amputation.

▶ Chemical Burns

The severity of chemical burns is directly proportional to the concentration and penetrability of the offending agent, the duration of skin exposure, and the mechanism of contact. Tissue destruction continues until either the chemical combines with tissue or the agent is neutralized by an applied secondary agent or washed from the skin surface. The mainstay of treatment of chemical burns of the skin is irrigation with water.

Two notable exceptions are burns resulting from hydrofluoric acid and from white phosphorous. Because hydrofluoric acid cannot be removed with water, calcium gluconate 10%, either applied to the skin as a gel or injected subcutaneously, is required to neutralize the acid. Patients with hydrofluoride burns experience severe pain seemingly out of proportion to the injury. White phosphorus burns, also refractory to water irrigation, are treated with 1% copper sulfate solution.

Iatrogenic chemical burns may occur with extravasation of chemotherapeutic agents administered intravenously. Chemotherapeutic agents are classified as vesicants, which include doxorubicin and vincristine and have a high probability of causing skin necrosis, and nonvesicants, which include cyclophosphamide. Management of both types of injury requires early surgical debridement of the region of extravasation. Secondary wound coverage may be obtained by either split-thickness skin grafting or skin flap coverage.

COLD INJURY (FROSTBITE)

▶ Clinical Findings

Frostbite occurs as the result of cellular injury when the cell membrane is punctured by ice crystals formed in the extracellular space. With the formation of ice crystals, osmotic gradients develop, leading to cell dehydration and electrolyte disturbances. Patients may develop severe vasoconstriction as a result of increased sympathetic tone. Vessel endothelial injury may cause thrombosis. With capillary endothelial damage, leakage occurs into the extracellular space, resulting in hemoconcentration and sludging within the capillary system.

Frostbite injuries may be classified as either superficial or deep. Superficial frostbite involves only the skin and usually heals spontaneously, whereas deep frostbite damages both the skin and subcutaneous structures (Figure 9–39). As with

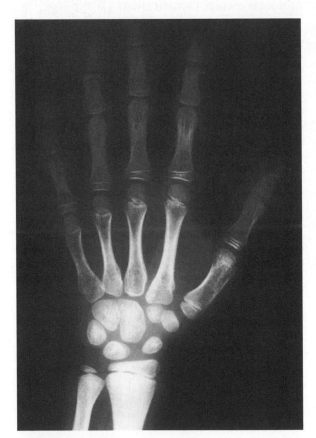

▲ **Figure 9–39.** Radiograph of deformities of the fingers of the left hand in a 12-year-old girl caused by frostbite incurred at 2 years of age. Note destruction of epiphyses of middle and distal phalanges of all fingers and deformity of epiphysis of proximal phalanx of little finger. Osseous changes in right hand were similar.

burn injuries, the depth of the area of necrosis is difficult to determine initially.

Treatment

The initial treatment of frostbite consists of rewarming the part and providing pain relief. The core body temperature should be restored and the frozen extremity rapidly rewarmed in a water bath at 38–42°C. Because rapid rewarming induces considerable pain, it should be delayed until adequate analgesia can be administered. After rewarming, treatment should include elevation of the hand, local wound care, and dressing changes. Frequent whirlpool debridement and active ROM exercises should be instituted. The role of anticoagulants and sympathectomy in increasing blood flow is controversial.

Long-Term Sequelae

Long-term sequelae depend on the extent of initial injury. Adult patients may develop osteoarthritis of the interphalangeal joints. Skeletally immature patients may develop epiphyseal destruction, with digital shortening, nail dysplasia, and joint destruction. Severe injuries may produce intrinsic muscle atrophy or vasospastic syndrome secondary to increased sympathetic tone. Vasospasm may lead to severe pain, coldness, or edema of the finger; trophic changes leading to decreased nail or hair growth; or Raynaud phenomenon. In severe injuries, mummification of nonviable portions of the fingers may become apparent. Amputation or surgical debridement of these mummified parts should usually be delayed 60–90 days, unless local infection develops. This delay allows maximal reepithelialization beneath the nonviable tissue.

Woo SH, Seul JH: Optimizing the correction of severe postburn hand deformities by using aggressive contracture releases and fasciocutaneous free-tissue transfers. *Plast Reconstr Surg* 2001;107:1. [PMID: 11176593]

HIGH-PRESSURE INJECTION INJURY

Injection machinery used in industry may create pressures of 3000–10,000 psi. The amount of pressure reflects both the design of the nozzle aperture and the distance between the nozzle and the finger. Virtually all patients who sustain injuries with pressures of over 7000 psi require amputation.

Clinical Findings

Injection injuries usually puncture the palmar digital pulp, track to the flexor tendon sheath, and fill the tendon sheath with the injected material. These injuries have a poor prognosis. Injections into the palm have a somewhat better prognosis because the site of the material is unconfined by fascial planes. Prognostic factors include the time interval from injury to treatment, as well as the amount and type of material injected. Whereas paint injection may cause more necrosis of the finger, grease injection more often leads to fibrosis of the finger. The amputation rate for paint injection injuries is approximately 60%; the rate for grease injection injuries is 20%.

The examiner must be wary of an innocuous-appearing entrance wound at the time of presentation. Initial pain may be modest but increases with time as more distal swelling and early necrosis occur.

Radiographic evaluation may be helpful if defining the extent of soft-tissue infiltration with identification of air within soft-tissue planes or if the material injected is radio-opaque such as lead-based paint.

Treatment

The effectiveness of corticosteroids administered every 6 hours remains controversial in the treatment of injection injuries. Patients should be operatively treated soon after the injury occurs. Thorough debridement of all injected material is easier when the injected material is pigmented. Nonpigmented materials such as kerosene or turpentine are considerably more difficult to remove thoroughly. The hand should be splinted in the safe position. Sympathetic blocks may be helpful in managing pain. Repeat debridement should be done if there is doubt about the adequacy of the initial procedure.

Although injection injuries may appear simple, these severe injuries compromise function and result in amputation. The seriousness of these injuries should be recognized at the time of presentation.

Christodoulou L, Melikyan EY, Woodbridge S, et al: Functional outcome of high-pressure injection injuries of the hand. *J Trauma* 2001;50:717. [PMID: 11303170]

Gutowski KA, Chu J, Choi M, et al: High-pressure hand injuries caused by dry cleaning solvents: case reports, review of the literature, and treatment guidelines. *Plast Reconstr Surg* 2003;111:174. [PMID: 12496578]

Luber KT, Rehm JP, Freeland AE: High-pressure injection injuries of the hand. *Orthopedics* 2005;28:129. [PMID: 15751366]

INFECTIONS OF THE HAND

Felon

A felon is an abscess of the pulp space of the distal phalanx. Vertical septa between the skin and the bone create small closed compartments within the pulp space. Infection

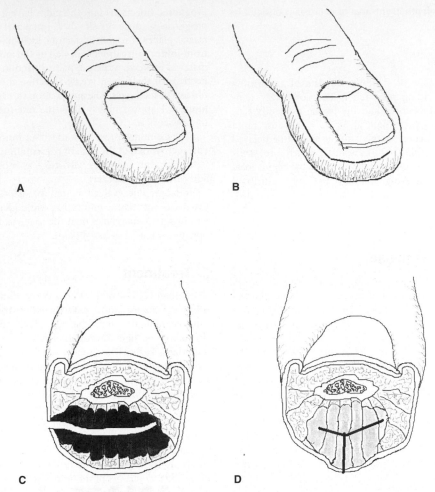

▲ **Figure 9–40.** Incisions for drainage of felons. **A:** Unilateral longitudinal approach that should be used for most felons. It is generally made on the ulnar side of the finger, unless it is the little finger, to preserve sensation. **B:** The hockey stick, or J, incision should be reserved for extensive or severe abscess or felon. **C:** The incision must decompress the longitudinal septa but should not go through and through. **D:** The felon that points volarly may be decompressed through a longitudinal midline incision, which is preferable because of less risk to sensory nerves. A transverse incision may also be made, but there is risk of damage to the digital nerves. (Courtesy of HB Skinner, © 2002.)

in this region produces localized erythema, swelling, and throbbing pain.

Treatment of these infections requires incision and drainage, with release of the vertical septa to decompress the pulp space completely (Figure 9–40). A drain is placed in the wound, the hand is elevated, and intravenous antibiotics are administered.

▶ Paronychia

Paronychia is the most common digital infection. The paronychia is the gutter along both the radial and ulnar borders of the fingernail. The eponychium is the roof of the nail over

the nail lunula. Paronychial infections may be classified as acute or chronic.

A. Acute Infection

Acute infections are most often caused by *Staphylococcus aureus*. These infections begin as a localized cellulitis, with erythema around the nail. Untreated, this cellulitis may progress to an abscess at the nail margin.

Treatment of early infection includes warm soaks and oral antibiotics. Once an abscess forms, incision and drainage are required. To debride the region adequately, either an incision is made in the abscess and the abscess is packed or a portion of the lateral nail is removed and the abscess is decompressed.

B. Chronic Infection

Chronic paronychial infections are most often caused by *Candida* species. These occur commonly in patients who work with their hands in water, such as bartenders or dishwashers. Patients may have repeated episodes of acute infection in addition to chronic infection.

Treatment of chronic infection may be accomplished by eponychial marsupialization, excision of a segment of the eponychia without incision of the nail roof. Simultaneous nail removal may increase the effectiveness of marsupialization.

▶ Web Space Abscess

Web space abscesses most often occur after palmar puncture wounds. The infection spreads from the palm along the path of least resistance to the dorsal web space. Treatment requires dorsal and palmar incision, drain placement, open wound care, and appropriate antibiotic coverage.

▶ Flexor Suppurative Tenosynovitis

Kanavel described four cardinal signs of acute suppurative tenosynovitis: (1) pain on passive digital extension; (2) flexed position of the digit; (3) symmetric swelling of the digit, which may include the palm; and (4) tenderness with palpation along the flexor tendon sheath. Acute suppurative tenosynovitis of the flexor pollicis longus sheath may extend into the thenar space. Likewise, infections in the flexor sheath of the little finger may extend into the ulnar bursa. In some patients, coalescence between the radial and ulnar bursas may allow infection to track in a horseshoe pattern, extending from the thumb to the little finger.

Treatment of acute suppurative tenosynovitis requires incision, irrigation, and drainage. Although an extensive midlateral incision may be used, limited incisions are preferred. Short incisions over the proximal (metacarpophalangeal joint region) and distal (distal interphalangeal region) margins of the flexor tendon sheath allow thorough sheath irrigation (Figure 9–41). The sheath is opened distally and a small tube (16-gauge catheter or number 8 pediatric feeding tube) is inserted. A drain is placed in the flexor sheath through the proximal wound. Irrigation of the finger is performed with 5 mL of saline injected every 2 hours. Intravenous antibiotics are administered, and the hand is elevated.

Two days after surgery, the dressing is changed. Swelling should be significantly decreased. The catheter is removed, and the patient is encouraged to begin active ROM exercises.

▶ Bite Injuries

Although bite wounds may initially appear harmless, a bite may inoculate deep tissues with virulent organisms.

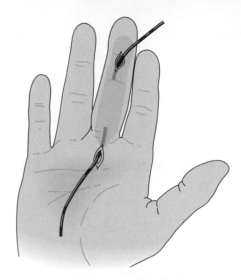

▲ **Figure 9–41.** Drainage and closed irrigation for flexor sheath infection. The antibiotic solution drips in through the distal catheter and drains out through the proximal one. (Reproduced, with permission, from Way LW, ed: *Current Surgical Diagnosis and Treatment,* 10th ed. Stamford, CT: Appleton & Lange; 1994.)

A. Cat and Dog Bites

Because the small puncture wounds of cat bites are more likely to be disregarded than the large tearing wounds of dog bites, late sequelae are more common after cat bites. Cat and dog bites frequently harbor *Pasteurella multocida,* an organism best treated with ampicillin, penicillin, or a first-generation cephalosporin. Acute animal bites may be treated with incision and drainage and an initial course of intravenous antibiotics in the emergency room followed by oral antibiotics.

B. Human Bites

Most human bite wounds result from a fist striking a tooth, which readily penetrates the skin, subcutaneous tissue, extensor tendon, and capsule of the metacarpophalangeal joint (Figure 9–42). Human bites often contain *Eikenella corrodens,* an organism best treated with penicillin or ampicillin. Human bite wounds should be excised and drained, and intravenous antibiotic therapy instituted. Arthrotomy of the metacarpophalangeal joint and irrigation are necessary if this injury is suspected.

C. Spider Bites

Although most spider bites are innocuous, the bite of a brown recluse spider requires early wide excision to control the locally injected toxin.

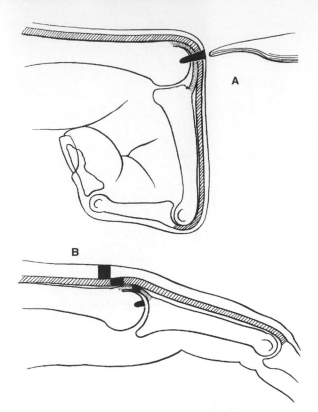

▲ Figure 9–42. Human bite wound of metacarpophalangeal joint. **A:** The tooth pierces the clenched fist of the attacker, penetrating skin, tendon, joint capsule, and metacarpal head. **B:** When the finger is extended by swelling and at surgery, the four puncture wounds do not correspond. (Reproduced, with permission, from Lister G: *The Hand: Diagnosis and Indications,* 3rd ed. Philadelphia: Churchill Livingstone; 1993.)

▶ Infection Caused by Unusual Organisms

A. Atypical Mycobacterial Infection

Mycobacterium marinum infection may present as a chronically inflamed finger that was punctured by the spine or a fin of a saltwater fish. Successful culture of the organism is difficult but is most likely at a temperature of 30–32°C. Antitubercular drug therapy is effective in treating and eradicating these infections.

B. Gram-Negative Infection

Because of the risk of a gram-negative infection following mutilating farm injuries or injuries with possible fecal contamination, these patients should be treated with broad-spectrum antibiotics.

C. Anaerobic Infection

When *Clostridium perfringens* infection occurs after hand injury, immediate wide fasciotomy and intravenous penicillin should be instituted. Hyperbaric oxygen therapy may be helpful. If infection cannot be adequately controlled, amputation may be necessary to avoid death.

The possibility of *Clostridium tetani* contamination must be remembered with any puncture wound. Initial evaluation of all patients with penetrating wounds must include questioning about tetanus inoculation. If inoculation is not up to date, antitoxin should be administered.

D. Gonorrhea

A patient who presents with an isolated septic joint or tenosynovitis without a history of puncture wound may have a hematogenous gonorrheal infection. Treatment consists of culturing the involved organism on the appropriate media and treatment with penicillin or tetracycline.

E. Necrotizing Fasciitis

The causative agent in necrotizing fasciitis is most commonly group A *Streptococcus* and can occur after a minor cut or abrasion. Patients with this infection are systemically very ill, and the infection spreads rapidly along fascial planes. Treatment consists of emergent wide surgical debridement to the fascia and appropriate antibiotics.

F. Herpetic Whitlow

Herpes simplex infections may involve the fingertips. They are most common in medical or dental personnel who care for the oral tracheal area and are also seen in small children. It may be difficult to distinguish herpetic lesions from acute bacterial infections of the fingers. Close examination reveals the presence of groups (crops) of vesicles, with surrounding erythema. Aspiration of a vesicle yields clear fluid. Serial viral titers confirm the diagnosis. Unlike bacterial infections, herpetic whitlow should not be incised but simply treated with splinting and elevation.

Connor RW, Kimbrough RC, Dabezies MJ: Hand Infections in patients with diabetes mellitus. *Orthopedics* 2001;24:1057. [PMID: 11727802]

Huish SB, de La Paz EM, Ellis PR 3rd, et al: Pyoderma gangrenosum of the hand: a case series and review of the literature. *J Hand Surg* 2001;26A:679. [PMID: 11466644.]

Karanas YL, Bogdan MA, Chang J: Community acquired methicillin-resistant *Staphylococcus aureus* hand infections: case reports and clinical implications. *J Hand Surg Am* 2000;25:760. [PMID: 1093220]

Perron AD, Miller MD, Brady WJ: Orthopedic pitfalls in the ED: fight bites. *Am J Emerg Med* 2002;20:114. [PMID: 11880877]

▼ ARTHRITIS OF THE HAND

OSTEOARTHRITIS

Osteoarthritis is a slowly progressive polyarticular disorder of unknown cause, predominantly affecting the hands and large weight-bearing joints. Clinically, osteoarthritis is characterized by pain, deformity, and limitation of motion. Focal erosions, articular cartilage space loss, subchondral sclerosis, cyst formation, and peripheral joint osteophytes are evident on radiographic examination.

▶ Epidemiologic Factors

The disease occurs commonly in older individuals, with approximately 80–90% of adults older than 75 years showing radiographic evidence of osteoarthritis. The strongest predictors of developing osteoarthritis of the hand are female gender, increasing age, and positive family history.

The most frequently involved joints in the hand are the distal interphalangeal joints, carpometacarpal joint of the thumb (Figure 9–43), and proximal interphalangeal joints.

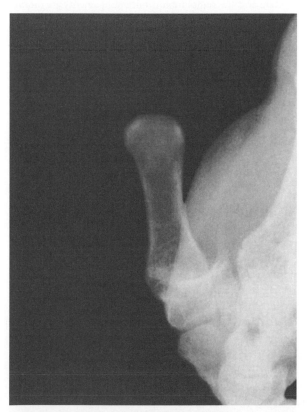

▲ **Figure 9–43.** Osteoarthritis of the carpometacarpal joint of the thumb.

The bony enlargements commonly seen in the osteoarthritic distal interphalangeal joint are referred to as Heberden nodes, whereas osteoarthritic enlargements at the proximal interphalangeal joint are known as Bouchard nodes.

Secondary osteoarthritis may develop in the hand as the result of trauma, avascular necrosis, prior inflammatory arthritis, or metabolic disorders.

▶ Clinical Findings

Patients with osteoarthritis of the hand often complain of activity-induced or work-related pain. Most patients experience periods of exacerbation and remission. Functional limitations result from pain, weakness, loss of motion, and deformity. Tenderness and enlargement of the distal and proximal interphalangeal joints are noted on examination. Axial compression of the thumb trapeziometacarpal with a circumduction motion (grind test) reproduces pain. As the disease progresses, radial subluxation of the thumb metacarpal on the trapezium may develop, leading to adduction deformity of the metacarpal.

▶ Treatment

Nonoperative treatment includes oral nonsteroidal anti-inflammatory drugs (NSAIDs), long-acting intraarticular steroid injection, and splint immobilization.

The primary indication for surgery is pain unresponsive to oral medication and splinting. Distal interphalangeal joint arthrodesis relieves pain, corrects deformity, and resolves joint instability. Because the severely arthritic distal interphalangeal joint is often stiff, the additional loss of motion occasioned by arthrodesis is usually tolerated well. The distal interphalangeal joint is fused in 10–15 degrees of flexion, a position in which the fingernail is parallel with the axis of the middle phalanx.

At the proximal interphalangeal joint, pain is the primary indication for surgery. Implant arthroplasty may be helpful in relieving pain and retaining motion in the ring and little fingers. The motion attained from implant arthroplasty is less in the proximal interphalangeal joints than in the metacarpophalangeal joints. Implant arthroplasty is usually avoided in the index- or middle-finger proximal interphalangeal joint because of residual instability to lateral or key pinch.

Arthrodesis effectively relieves pain at the proximal interphalangeal joint and provides pinch stability. The ideal position of arthrodesis varies from the radial to the ulnar digits. The index-finger proximal interphalangeal joint is usually fused at 40 degrees of flexion, the middle finger at 45 degrees, the ring finger at 50 degrees, and the little finger at 55 degrees.

At the trapeziometacarpal joint, conservative treatment includes a hand-based thumb spica splint with the interphalangeal joint left free, cortisone injections, and NSAIDs. Many patients with advanced degenerative changes on radiograph obtain good pain relief with conservative therapy.

The primary indication for surgery is persistent pain. Trapezium resection arthroplasty relieves pain at the trapeziometacarpal joint and allows retention of full metacarpal base motion. Either the distal half of the trapezium or the entire trapezium may be resected. A tendon interposition and sling are created using either the flexor carpi radialis or a slip of the abductor pollicis longus. The tendon may be threaded through a drill hole in the articular surface of the thumb metacarpal to suspend the thumb metacarpal. The remaining tendon is rolled into a so-called anchovy and placed in the space of the excised trapezium. This reconstruction prevents impingement of the metacarpal on the scaphoid. After surgery, the thumb is immobilized in a cast or splint for 6 weeks.

Arthrodesis of the thumb carpometacarpal joint is an alternative to trapeziectomy. With the joint fused, residual motion occurs at the scaphotrapezial joint, but notably patients are unable to lay their hand flat on a table. However, pain relief is excellent, and it may be the procedure of choice for a young laborer.

RHEUMATOID ARTHRITIS

RA is a chronic inflammatory disease of unknown cause. The combined effect of tenosynovitis and synovitis on joints and periarticular tissues results in progressive joint destruction and deformity. RA affects 0.3–1.5% of the population. Women are two to three times more commonly affected than men.

▶ Clinical Findings

Evaluation of the hand affected by RA requires care. The goal is to determine which of the patient's many problems—pain, weakness, or mechanical dysfunction—is most problematic. Evaluation detects tendon rupture, adherence, or triggering as well as nerve compression symptoms. The most common nerve compression syndromes involve compression of the median nerve at the wrist and compression of the radial nerve at the elbow. The appearance of rheumatoid nodules and ulnar drift deformity at the metacarpophalangeal joint may be disturbing aesthetically. Rheumatoid nodules, occurring in 20–25% of patients with RA, are not treated unless associated with erosion, pain, or infection.

▶ Treatment

The shoulder, elbow, forearm, wrist, and hand should be examined individually. The goal of surgical reconstruction is restoration of a functional upper extremity, not just a functional hand. Indications for surgical intervention include relieving pain, slowing the progression of disease, improving function, and improving appearance.

Surgical treatment may be classified as either preventive or corrective. Preventive options include tenosynovectomy and synovectomy. Corrective procedures include tendon transfers, nerve decompression, soft-tissue reconstruction, and arthrodesis.

Synovectomy is considered in patients who have pauciarticular persistent synovitis while under good medical control. Contraindications to synovectomy include rapidly progressive disease, multiple joint involvement, and underlying joint destruction.

A. Elbow Reconstruction

Synovitis of the elbow joint may cause pain, joint destruction, and radial nerve compression. Nodules or bursas are common over the olecranon. Surgical treatment of the rheumatoid elbow includes radial head excision and synovectomy. As the disease progresses, consideration may be given to total elbow arthroplasty.

B. Wrist Reconstruction

RA frequently involves the wrist and occurs in a predictable pattern. On the radial side of the wrist, the radioscaphocapitate and the radiolunototriquetral ligaments are attenuated, permitting rotatory displacement of the scaphoid. Scapholunate dissociation is followed by radiocarpal collapse.

On the ulnar side of the wrist, the ulnar carpal ligaments become attenuated, allowing the carpus to drift radially as the carpus translates ulnarward. Attenuation of the distal radioulnar joint allows the head of the ulna to displace dorsally, producing caput-ulnae syndrome. The extensor carpi ulnaris tendon displaces volarly. These changes lead to supination of the carpus on the radius, ulnar translocation of the carpus, and a concomitant radialward displacement of the metacarpals (Figure 9–44). The carpus may also dislocate volarly beneath the radius.

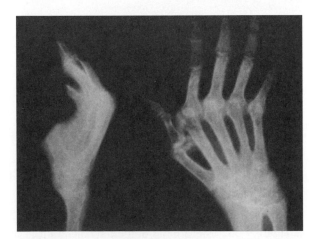

▲ **Figure 9–44.** Radialward displacement of the metacarpals in rheumatoid arthritis.

Surgical treatment consists of extensor tenosynovectomy, with transposition of the dorsal retinaculum over the wrist joint to reinforce the capsule, and wrist synovectomy. The extensor carpi ulnaris tendon can be relocated from a volar to a dorsal position.

If pain is present over the distal ulna or if rupture of the little or ring finger extensor tendon results from a sharp prominence of the distal ulna, then resection of the distal ulna is performed. Fusion of the rheumatoid wrist provides stability and may increase function. Either a total wrist arthrodesis or a radiolunate arthrodesis may be elected, depending on the extent of midcarpal joint involvement. With bilateral wrist involvement, replacement of one wrist and fusion of the other should be considered for functional preservation.

C. Hand Reconstruction

Triggering of the digits is a common problem caused by flexor tenosynovitis. The A1 pulley should not be incised in the treatment of rheumatoid trigger digits. Loss of the A1 pulley increases the tendency of the fingers to drift ulnarward. Instead, tenosynovectomy and excision of the ulnar slip of the sublimis tendon should be considered.

If flexor tendon rupture occurs, treatment may include tendon transfer, bridge grafting, or joint fusion. The flexor tendon that most commonly ruptures is the flexor pollicis longus because it rubs over an osteophyte on the volar aspect of the scaphotrapezial joint (Mannerfelt lesion). Extensor tendon ruptures are caused by attrition of the common extensor tendon of the ring and little fingers over the distal ulna (Vaughn-Johnson syndrome).

Treatment of the arthritic hand depends on the joints involved. The distal interphalangeal joint is usually best treated by arthrodesis. At the proximal interphalangeal joint, synovectomy may be performed if synovitis is isolated to the proximal interphalangeal joint without multiple joint involvement. Alternatives for the more involved joint are arthroplasty or arthrodesis.

At the metacarpophalangeal joint, inflammation of the synovium may cause the extensor mechanism to sublux ulnarly because of attenuation of the radial sagittal band. The mechanism may be relocated to improve function of the joint. For isolated joints without significant destruction, synovectomy may be performed. With more severe joint destruction, resection implant arthroplasty is required (Figure 9–45). Subluxation and ulnar drift alone are not absolute indications for arthroplasty if satisfactory function of the hand remains. Arthroplasty does not increase the ROM of the metaphalangeal joints, but it changes its arc. Because most patients have severe flexion and ulnar deviation of the joints, arthroplasty provides a more functional ROM, especially for grasping large objects. Because the implants fracture with extensive use, silicone arthroplasty is indicated only in the low-demand hand and is therefore better suited to rheumatoid than osteoarthritic patients.

1. Boutonnière deformity—In addition to arthritis, various finger deformities occur related to soft-tissue damage. At the proximal interphalangeal joints, the most common is boutonnière deformity. Because of proximal interphalangeal joint synovitis, the central slip is either elongated or ruptured, which allows the proximal interphalangeal joint to flex and the lateral bands to sublux volarly. As the lateral bands migrate below the proximal interphalangeal joint axis, they become active proximal interphalangeal flexors rather than extensors. In addition to increasing the proximal interphalangeal joint deformity, the relative shortening of the extensor mechanism leads to distal interphalangeal joint hyperextension. Treatment of mild boutonnière deformities, which are passively correctable, consists of synovectomy and splinting. Lateral band reconstruction may be considered to relocate the bands dorsal to the axis of rotation. Alternatively, tenotomy of the terminal slip may be done to allow relaxation of the extensor mechanism and prevent hyperextension of the distal interphalangeal joint. Once moderate deformity of the proximal interphalangeal joint occurs (30- to 40-degree flexion deformity, with a flexible joint and preservation of the joint space), consideration may be given to reconstruction of the central slip as well as lateral band reconstruction and terminal tendon tenotomy. In the final stage of boutonnière deformity, the joint deformity becomes fixed, and the best form of treatment is arthroplasty or fusion.

2. Swan-neck deformity—Swan-neck deformities consist of hyperextension at the proximal interphalangeal joint and flexion at the distal interphalangeal joint. The mechanism of swan-neck deformity is terminal tendon rupture or attenuation, with secondary hyperextension of the proximal interphalangeal joint resulting from overpulling of the central slip or proximal interphalangeal joint hyperextension caused by laxity of the volar plate, rupture of the flexor digitorum superficialis, or intrinsic tightness. The most common of these mechanisms is intrinsic tightness secondary to metacarpophalangeal joint synovitis.

Swan-neck deformities are divided into four stages. In stage 1, the joints are supple in all positions. Treatment consists of splinting, distal interphalangeal joint fusion, or soft-tissue reconstruction to limit proximal interphalangeal joint hyperextension. In stage 2, proximal interphalangeal flexion is limited because of intrinsic tightness. Intrinsic release with or without reconstruction of the metacarpophalangeal joint may be of benefit. In stage 3, proximal interphalangeal joint motion is limited in all positions, yet the joint is still preserved. Mobilization of the lateral bands may help relieve this deformity. Finally, in stage 4, the proximal interphalangeal joint is arthritic. Either proximal interphalangeal arthrodesis or arthroplasty should be considered for stage 4 joint destruction.

3. Synovitic metacarpophalangeal joint deformity—The metacarpophalangeal joints subluxes volarly and ulnarly

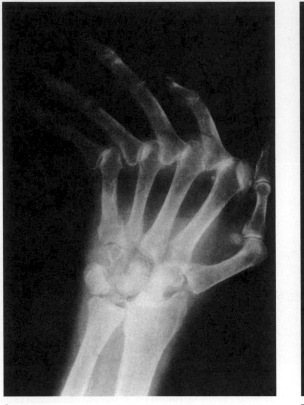

A

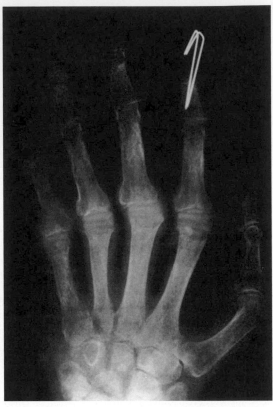

B

▲ **Figure 9–45. A:** Preoperative view of metacarpophalangeal joint in rheumatoid arthritis. **B:** Following resection arthroplasty.

in RA. This deformity results from synovial invasion of the collateral ligaments with secondary laxity, volar and ulnar forces that are normally present on the joint, augmentation of these forces by radial deviation of the wrist, attenuation of the radial sagittal band (allowing ulnar subluxation of the extensor tendon), and contracture of the intrinsic muscles. Treatment of the synovitic metacarpophalangeal joint consists of medical management and splinting. When the joint space is preserved, surgical synovectomy may provide symptomatic relief. Once moderate joint destruction or volar subluxation and ulnar deviation occurs, the decision about surgery is based on the function of the hand. When the patient is still able to use the hand for activities of daily living, splinting and other assistive aids are provided. Once loss of function is noted, metacarpophalangeal arthroplasty is considered. In performing metacarpophalangeal arthroplasty, the wrist deformity should first be corrected, and all soft-tissue releases required to relieve the subluxing forces should be performed. The radial collateral ligament of the index finger should be reconstructed, and the extensor tendon

should be relocated. Postoperatively, extensive splinting and therapy are required to hold the hand in proper position. Therapy utilizes an outrigger splint holding the wrist in dorsiflexion and the metaphalangeal joints in full extension and neutral radial-ulnar alignment. The splint is worn full time for 6 weeks and part time for 3 months. The patient wears a resting pan splint at night for 1 year.

D. Thumb Reconstruction

Three patterns of rheumatoid thumb deformities are defined. In type 1 deformity, the metacarpophalangeal joint is flexed while the interphalangeal joint is hyperextended and the thumb metacarpal is secondarily abducted. In type 2 and 3 deformities, carpometacarpal subluxation leads to metacarpal adduction. In type 2 deformities, interphalangeal joint hyperextension develops with metacarpophalangeal flexion, and in type 3 deformities, the metacarpophalangeal joint is hyperextended and the interphalangeal joint is flexed. Type 2 deformities are unusual. Type 1 deformities are usually initiated by synovitis of the metacarpophalangeal joint, leading to attenuation of the extensor pollicis brevis tendon, intrinsic muscle tightness, and ulnar and volar displacement of the extensor pollicis longus.

Treatment is based on the degree of progression. In type 1 deformities, if the metacarpophalangeal and interphalangeal joints are passively correctable, synovectomy and extensor reconstruction may be performed. If the metacarpophalangeal joint flexion deformity is fixed, arthrodesis or arthroplasty of the joint is considered. When fixed metacarpophalangeal flexion and interphalangeal extension deformities are present simultaneously, the interphalangeal joint is fused and the metacarpophalangeal joint is replaced with an arthroplasty or also undergoes arthrodesis.

Type 3 deformities are analogous to swan-neck deformities of the fingers. The carpometacarpal joint disease allows dorsal and radial subluxation of the joint, with secondary adduction contraction of the metacarpal and hyperextension of the metacarpophalangeal joint. Treatment with minimal metacarpophalangeal deformity (stage 1) or passively correctable metacarpophalangeal deformity (stage 2) consists of splinting and carpometacarpal arthroplasty or fusion. Once the metacarpophalangeal deformity becomes fixed (stage 3), first web release and carpometacarpal arthroplasty are required.

E. Surgical Priorities

When multilevel deformity is present, consideration should be given to combined procedures. If wrist and metacarpophalangeal deformities are both present, the wrist should be fused prior to or simultaneously with metacarpophalangeal joint reconstruction. When both metacarpophalangeal and proximal interphalangeal joint deformities are present, motion-preserving procedures such as arthroplasty should be carried out at the metacarpophalangeal joint. Treatment of concomitant proximal interphalangeal joint involvement depends on the stage of deformity. Mild to moderate proximal interphalangeal joint deformities can either be ignored or treated by closed manipulation and pin fixation. With severe deformity, arthrodesis of the proximal interphalangeal joint should be performed.

In all cases, attempts should be made to perform multiple procedures under a single anesthetic. These patients often require numerous operations for multiple joints of the upper and lower extremities, and surgical and rehabilitation time must be used judiciously.

▶ Other Inflammatory Arthritides

Other inflammatory conditions related to RA may affect the hand, producing joint destruction and deformity.

A. Juvenile Rheumatoid Arthritis

In juvenile rheumatoid arthritis (JRA), early epiphyseal closure occurs as a result of synovitis and increased periarticular blood flow. Narrowing of phalangeal and metacarpal medullary canals makes implant arthroplasty difficult. The metacarpophalangeal joints may deviate radially rather than ulnarly.

B. Arthritis Mutilans

In arthritis mutilans, axial shortening because of marked bone loss occurs while the soft-tissue envelope is preserved. Early joint fusion is required to avoid progressive bone loss.

C. Systemic Lupus Erythematosus

Systemic lupus erythematosus (SLE) affects periarticular soft tissue, resulting in joint laxity with secondary dysfunction. Synovitis is minimal in lupus, and therefore, the articular cartilage is preserved. Soft-tissue reconstruction is ineffective, and joint fusions are preferable to restore stability and function. The exception to this is the metacarpophalangeal joints, where implant arthroplasty may be appropriate, even though normal articular cartilage is sacrificed.

D. Psoriatic Arthritis

Psoriatic arthritis presents deformities similar to that of RA. The hand has a marked tendency to become stiff. In psoriatic arthritis, the metacarpophalangeal joints become stiff in extension, whereas in RA, these joints tend to become stiff in flexion.

Davis TR, Brady O, Dias JJ: Excision of the trapezium for osteoarthritis of the trapeziometacarpal joint: a study of the benefit of ligament reconstruction or tendon interposition. *J Hand Surg Am* 2004;29:1069. [PMID: 15576217]

Day CS, Gelberman R, Patel AA, et al: Basal joint osteoarthritis of the thumb: a prospective trial of steroid injection and splinting. *J Hand Surg Am* 2004;29:247. [PMID: 15043897]

Fulton DB, Stern PJ: Trapeziometacarpal arthrodesis in primary osteoarthritis: a minimum two-year follow-up study. *J Hand Surg Am* 2001;26:109. [PMID: 11172376]

Jain A, Witbreuk M, Ball C, et al: Influence of steroids and methotrexate on wound complications after elective rheumatoid hand and wrist surgery. *J Hand Surg Am* 2002;27:449. [PMID: 12015719]

▼ HAND TUMORS

Nearly all mass lesions in the hand or wrist are benign conditions. Foreign body granulomas, epidermoid inclusion cysts, and neuromas are usually related to prior trauma. Ganglions and fibroxanthomas arise adjacent to joints or tendon sheaths.

▶ Ganglion

Ganglions are the most common soft-tissue tumors of the hand and wrist. They are cystic structures filled with a

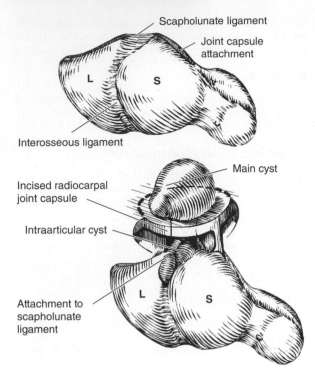

Scapholunate ligament

Joint capsule attachment

Interosseous ligament

Main cyst

Incised radiocarpal joint capsule

Intraarticular cyst

Attachment to scapholunate ligament

▲ **Figure 9–46.** The ganglion and scapholunate attachments are isolated from the remaining uninvolved joint capsule (not shown). (Reproduced, with permission, from Green DP, ed: *Operative Hand Surgery,* 2nd ed. Philadelphia: Churchill Livingstone; 1988.)

mucinous fluid but without a synovial or epithelial lining. In most cases, a stalk can be identified communicating between the cyst and an adjacent joint or tendon sheath. The most common locations for ganglions are the wrist, digital flexor sheath, and distal interphalangeal joint (Figure 9–46).

A. Dorsal Wrist Ganglion

Dorsal wrist ganglions arise from the dorsal capsule of the scapholunate joint. Small firm dorsal ganglions may be barely palpable but highly symptomatic, whereas large ganglions are often soft and only mildly symptomatic. Aspiration and steroid injection may provide transient symptomatic relief, but recurrence is frequent. Symptomatic lesions can be surgically excised, with expectation of cure if care is taken to excise the stalk of the lesion with a capsular base from the lesion's origin. Because these lesions arise from the dorsal portion of the scapholunate ligament, care must be taken to preserve the ligament's integrity to avoid an iatrogenic scapholunate dissociation. Alternatively, the ganglion can be excised using arthroscopic techniques especially to excise small ganglions that are located almost entirely within the wrist joint.

B. Palmar Wrist Ganglion

Palmar wrist ganglions present as swellings on the palmar radial aspect of the wrist, adjacent to the radial artery. These lesions arise from either the radioscaphoid or scaphotrapezial joint. Surgical resection of a symptomatic palmar radial ganglion requires mobilization and protection of the adjacent radial artery.

C. Flexor Sheath Ganglion

Flexor sheath ganglions present as firm pea-like lesions over the palmar aspect of the flexor sheath. The mass is usually between 3 and 8 mm in diameter and often so firm that it can be mistaken for a bone exostosis. Treatment of symptomatic lesions is accomplished with aspiration or excision.

D. Mucous Cyst

Mucous cysts are ganglions arising from the distal interphalangeal joint. The neck of the ganglion arises from either the radial or ulnar side of the terminal extensor tendon. Surgical excision must include debridement of the joint osteophyte. If the skin is thinned, a local rotation flap is required for soft-tissue coverage after excision.

E. Fibroxanthoma

Fibroxanthomas are also known as giant cell tumors of tendon sheath or tendon sheath xanthomas. These slowly enlarging, firm lesions are usually painless, often arising from an interphalangeal joint or the flexor tendon sheath. They are usually fixed to deep tissues, more often on the palmar aspect of the hand or finger. Surgical resection requires delineation of the entire mass and protection of digital nerves that may be displaced, compressed, or encircled by the tumor.

F. Epidermoid Inclusion Cyst

Epidermoid inclusion cysts are usually the result of previous trauma, such as a puncture wound, stab wound, or laceration. Epidermal cells become embedded in the subcutaneous tissue, gradually enlarging into a pearlike mass filled with toothpaste-like keratin. Eventually, the mass becomes noticeable, particularly when it is located over the palmar aspect of the pulp. Surgical treatment is excision of the mass without rupture.

G. Foreign Bodies

Foreign bodies may act as a nidus, inciting the development of a surrounding granuloma. This situation may be associated with a local inflammatory reaction or frank infection. Treatment consists of excision.

H. Neuromas

Neuromas, the bulbous enlargement of the distal end of a severed nerve, are a normal response to nerve transection.

Neuromas are inevitable in all amputations of the hand. If the neuroma enlargement of the distal end of the proximal segment of the transected nerve is in an area of palmar pulp contact, the lesion may be highly symptomatic. Treatment alternatives include neuroma revision or transposition of the neuroma to a location away from contact stress.

CONGENITAL DIFFERENCES

Congenital hand differences occur in approximately 1 in 1500 live births. The term *differences* is favored over the traditional terms *abnormality, anomaly,* or *malformation.* Many congenital hand differences are part of a well-delineated association or syndrome. The abnormality may suggest that other regions of the body or organ systems be evaluated. When an infant is seen with bilateral total absence of the radius and normal or very mildly hypoplastic thumbs, the possibility of thrombocytopenia with absent radius (TAR) syndrome should be considered and a platelet count obtained. Radial absence may also be associated with the VATER association, children with abnormalities that may include *v*ertebral, *a*nal, *t*racheal, *e*sophageal, and *r*enal defects.

A number of frequently encountered conditions such as cleft hand are inherited as autosomal-dominant traits. The expertise of an experienced geneticist is invaluable in providing counsel to families considering additional children and to patients wishing to know the likelihood that their offspring would be affected by the disorder.

The two most commonly encountered conditions are syndactyly and polydactyly. In white populations, syndactyly is more common, and in African American populations, polydactyly is the most commonly encountered congenital hand anomaly.

Syndactyly

Syndactyly, the webbing together of digits, is simple if soft tissue alone is involved and complex if bone or nails are joined (Figure 9–47). Surgical release of syndactyly requires the use of local flaps to create a floor for the interdigital web space and to partially surface the adjacent sides of the separated digits. Residual defects along the sides of the separated fingers are covered with full-thickness skin grafts. Surgery is indicated when the webbing occurs distal to the usual point of separation of the fingers and the webbing prohibits full use of the fingers. Surgery is usually performed at 6–12 months of age.

Polydactyly

Radial polydactyly is usually manifest as thumb duplication. When two thumbs are present in the same hand, they are rarely both normal in size, alignment, and mobility (Figure 9–48). The more ulnar thumb component is usually better developed than the more radial thumb component.

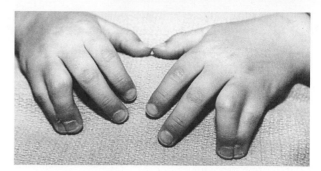

▲ **Figure 9–47.** Bilateral complex syndactyly of the ring and little fingers.

The level of bifurcation varies from a wide distal phalanx with two nails, to two digits each possessing a metacarpal and a proximal and distal phalanx. In the most common form of thumb duplication, a single broad metacarpal supports two proximal phalanges, each of which support a distal phalanx. Optimal reconstruction requires merging of elements of both component digits. Usually the ulnar thumb is maintained. If the duplication occurs at the metacarpophalangeal joint, the radial collateral ligament is preserved with the metacarpal and attached to the proximal phalanx of the ulnar thumb. Surgery is usually performed at 6–12 months

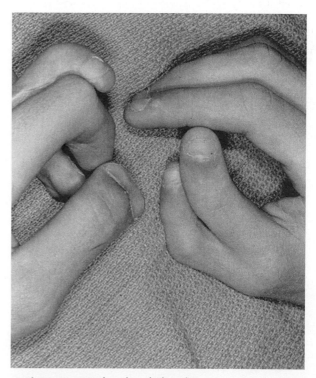

▲ **Figure 9–48.** Thumb polydactyly.

of age. Ulnar polydactyly, frequent in black children, may usually be treated by simple excision.

▶ Partial or Absent Structures

Absence or partial deficiency of the radius results in inadequate support of the hand and carpus. The unsupported hand angulates radially. Stretching of contracted radial soft-tissue structures is accomplished through repeat manipulation, casting, splinting, or distraction lengthening. The hand is then surgically reoriented onto the end of the ulna by a centralization procedure.

Mild hypoplasia of the thumb is treated by release of the first web space, metacarpophalangeal joint collateral reconstruction, and opponensplasty tendon transfer. More sever hypoplasia or absence of the thumb may be treated by pollicization of the index finger. This procedure shifts the index finger to the thumb position and repositions the index-finger extrinsic extensor tendons as well as the dorsal and palmar interosseous tendons to provide balanced control of the shifted digit.

Giele H, Giele C, Bower C, et al: The incidence and epidemiology of congenital upper limb anomalies: a total population study. *J Hand Surg Am* 2001;26:628. [PMID: 11466636]

McCarroll HR: Congenital anomalies: a 25-year overview. *J Hand Surg Am* 2000;25:1007. [PMID: 11119659]

Pediatric Orthopedic Surgery

10

George T. Rab, MD

The scope of pediatric orthopedics ranges from congenital anomalies to injuries in the adolescent. The pathophysiologic manifestations of many of these disorders differ from analogous adult problems because of the added dimension of growth. The physician's relationship with the pediatric patient generally occurs in the context of a protective family environment, in contrast to the more independent relationship the physician may form with an adult. The natural tendency for children to be active and the remarkable regenerative processes of the immature skeleton frequently make formal rehabilitation unnecessary following surgery or serious injury.

▶ Guidelines for Pediatric Orthopedics

The following rules may be helpful when applying general orthopedic principles to the child:

1. A growing bone normally tends to remodel itself toward the adult configuration. This process occurs faster in younger children and in deformities near the ends of bone. Remodeling is faster when deformity is in the plane of motion of the nearest joint.

2. Skeletal deformities worsen as abnormal growth continues (eg, following permanent damage to the growth plate), especially near rapidly growing areas such as the knee. This characteristic is exaggerated in younger children.

3. Children tolerate long-term immobilization better than adults and tend to recover soft-tissue mobility spontaneously following most injuries.

4. Fracture healing is usually more rapid and predictable in the actively growing skeleton than in the adult skeleton.

5. Joint surfaces in children are generally more tolerant of irregularity than those of the adult. Although degenerative arthritic changes may follow childhood injury,

there is often an asymptomatic interval of many decades before the process becomes clinically evident.

6. Many so-called deformities, such as metatarsus adductus, internal tibial torsion, genu valgum (knock-knee), and bowed legs, are actually physiologic variations that correct spontaneously with growth. For example, physiologic bowing is common and benign. It is typically symmetric, involves both the femur and tibia, and is most prominent in toddlers. It usually resolves by 2 years of age, but there is great variability. By age 36 months, almost all children will correct spontaneously. The clinician must distinguish between conditions that need no treatment and those requiring early intervention.

GROWTH DISORDERS

General skeletal growth is discussed in detail in Chapter 1.

1. Limb-Length Inequality

▶ Essentials of Diagnosis

- *Commonly asymptomatic difference in limb length must be detected to plan for appropriate treatment.*
- *Congenital anomalies may lead to significant inequality.*
- *Proper evaluation and planning allow optimal treatment during growth.*

▶ General Considerations

Limb-length inequality may reflect either a congenital deficiency or any of a wide variety of acquired conditions (Table 10–1). Posttraumatic physeal arrest occurs most commonly after injury in the distal medial tibia. Injuries of the distal femoral and distal ulnar physis have a high incidence of growth arrest as well. Upper extremities of unequal length are usually only of cosmetic interest and can easily

Table 10–1. Causes of limb-length inequality.

Infectious causes
Osteomyelitis
Septic arthritis
Neoplastic causes
Arteriovenous malformations
Hemangioma
Neuromuscular causes
Cerebral palsy
Isolated limb paralysis
Poliomyelitis
Traumatic causes
Malunion of long bones
Physeal injury
Other causes
Avascular necrosis of femoral head (and physis)
Congenital amputations
Legg-Calvé-Perthes disease

be compensated for by modifying clothing. In the lower extremities, however, length discrepancies may be severe enough—greater than 1 inch (2.5 cm)—to limit function and require treatment. Lesser discrepancies can be managed with a shoe lift.

▶ Clinical Findings

A. Symptoms and Signs

Most limb inequality in children is asymptomatic, even when severe. Marked deformity may cause a painless limp.

Clinical limb measurement is usually possible by checking for a level pelvis with the child standing on calibrated blocks under the short leg. Severe inequality may require alternate exam techniques.

B. Imaging Studies

All children should have an x-ray of the entire limb at initial visit to screen for anomalies and deformities. Scanograms (special leg-length films) are the standard for accurate measurement of inequality, but they can be inaccurate if the child moves. An option in older children is an anteroposterior (AP) pelvis with the child standing on clinically appropriate blocks under the short leg. Skeletal maturity is measured from wrist bone age films.

C. Calculation of Limb Length at Maturity

Clinical management of limb-length inequality in pediatric patients should include calculation of projected lengths at maturity. Several mathematical methods, based on skeletal age, gender, and normal growth rates, are available. The

following general rule can be used to estimate the extent of future growth: The average growth rates of the distal femur and proximal tibia are 10–12 mm/year and 5–6 mm/year, respectively, with growth continuing until bone age 14 in females and 16 in males.

▶ Treatment

A. Shoe Lift

A lift is rarely required in children, but adolescents may desire a lift. It generally may be ½ inch (1.27 cm) less than the measured difference in limb length.

B. Epiphysiodesis

The simplest surgical procedure to treat pediatric bone-length discrepancies is epiphysiodesis (surgical closure of the growth plate). In the longer limb, it involves curetting or drilling the physis or inserting small bone grafts across the medial and lateral edges of the plate. Epiphysiodesis is usually performed at the distal femoral physis, proximal tibial physis, or both, because they are rapidly growing and easily accessible surgically. The remaining open physes in the limb allow for continued growth but at a slower rate. The exact timing of epiphysiodesis is crucial to attaining equal limb lengths at skeletal maturity. Timing is calculated by the same method used to predict ultimate adult leg length. The effectiveness of epiphysiodesis requires that bone still be growing and that accurate data be collected on this growth for several years (ie, scanograms for leg-length measurement, skeletal age).

C. Femoral Shortening

If a child reaches the age when bone growth is insufficient to make epiphysiodesis practical, the long leg may be shortened at skeletal maturity by femoral shortening. This may be performed as an open procedure by removing a segment of femur and fixing the bone with a plate and screws. It may also be done as a closed procedure, using an intramedullary femoral rod introduced through a buttock incision for fixation. A cylindrical segment of femur is cut out of the bone using intramedullary saws, and the bone is pushed aside to allow the femur to shorten over the rod. The excised bone segment eventually resorbs.

D. Other Techniques

Leg-length inequalities projected to be 6 cm or more generally do not respond well to the previously described treatments, which in these cases may lead to unacceptably short stature or limb segments. Although some discrepancies are so severe that amputation of the foot and prosthetic fitting are required, techniques of bone lengthening are successful in treating these children (see Chapter 1).

Birch JG, Samchukov ML: Use of the Ilizarov method to correct lower limb deformities in children and adolescents. *J Am Acad Orthop Surg* 2004;12:144. [PMID: 15161167]

Inan M, Chan G, Littleton AG, Kubiak P, Bowen JR: Efficacy and safety of percutaneous epiphysiodesis. *J Pediatr Orthop* 2008;28:648. [PMID: 18724201]

Khakharia S, Bigman D, Fragomen AT, Pavlov H, Rozbruch SR: Comparison of PACS and hard-copy 51-inch radiographs for measuring leg length and deformity. *Clin Orthop Relat Res* 2011;469:244. [PMID: 20625949]

Paley D, Bhave A, Herzenberg JE, Bowen JR: Multiplier method for predicting limb-length discrepancy. *J Bone Joint Surg Am* 2000;82-A:1432. [PMID: 11057472]

Surdam JW, Morris CD, DeWeese JD, et al: Leg length inequality and epiphysiodesis: review of 96 cases. *J Pediatr Orthop* 2003; 23:381. [PMID: 12724605]

2. Dwarfism and Other Disorders of Growth

Orthopedic disorders (achondroplasia, multiple epiphyseal dysplasia) or other syndromes (Down syndrome, Marfan syndrome) often accompany dwarfism. The classification of skeletal syndromes and dysplasias is undergoing rapid change as knowledge is gained using molecular, biologic, and genetic techniques. In general, autosomal recessive genes code for enzymatic and biochemical defects and autosomal dominant gene defects cause structural deformities. An example of the latter is achondroplasia that results from mutation of fibroblast growth factor receptor 3 (FGFR3), a structural protein that results in the quantitative decrease in cartilage formation. The gene defects are inherited from one of the parents or are sporadic mutations. A detailed review of skeletal syndromes and dysplasias is outside the scope of this text; Table 10–2 lists some of these conditions and the major orthopedic problems associated with them.

INFECTIOUS PROCESSES

1. Hematogenous Osteomyelitis

▶ Essentials of Diagnosis

- *Limp, bone pain, fever, leukocytosis, and elevation of erythrocyte sedimentation rate (ESR) and C-reactive protein (CRP) characterize osteomyelitis.*
- *Methicillin-resistant* Staphylococcus aureus *(MRSA) osteomyelitis is increasingly common and may include serious life- and limb-threatening complications.*

▶ General Considerations

Osteomyelitis, an infection of bone tissue, usually occurs in the marrow cavity but sometimes affects the cortex as well. There is a predilection for metaphyseal involvement of long bones.

Table 10–2. Orthopedic involvement in selected syndromes and dwarfing conditions.

Achondroplasia
Short limbs; genu varum; exaggerated lumbar lordosis; spinal stenosis; ligamentous laxity
Apert syndrome
Foot deformities; hand and foot polydactyly
Arthrogryposis
Severe joint stiffness, contractures, and dislocations; resistant clubfoot
Cleidocranial dysplasia
Absent clavicles; coxa vara
Diastrophic dysplasia
Severe clubfoot; joint dislocations; joint stiffness; cervical kyphosis; scoliosis
Down syndrome
Cervical (C1–C2) instability; hip dislocation; ankle valgus; ligamentous laxity
Enchondromatosis
Asymmetric multiple enchondromas in long bones; limb-length inequality; angulation of long bones
Fibrous dysplasia
Multiple fibrous lesions in bone; limb bowing or shortening; occasional endocrine disorders
Larsen syndrome
Hip, knee, and radial head dislocations; severe cervical kyphosis and instability; scoliosis
Marfan syndrome
Scoliosis
Metaphyseal chondrodysplasia
Moderate dwarfing; genu varum; ligamentous laxity; cervical instability
Multiple epiphyseal dysplasia
Mild dwarfism; joint surface deformities with premature osteoarthritis; angular limb deformities
Multiple hereditary exostoses
Mild dwarfing; osteochondroma (external enlargements) at all long bone ends
Osteogenesis imperfecta
Bone fragility and multiple fractures; bowing of bones; scoliosis; mild to moderate dwarfing
Spondyloepiphyseal dysplasia
Severe dwarfing; coxa vara; genu valgum; scoliosis; odontoid hypoplasia, instability, and deformity

▶ Pathogenesis

In children, osteomyelitis is most commonly caused by hematogenous bacterial spread, frequently following an upper respiratory infection or partially treated distant infection. Direct inoculation of bacteria into an open fracture or

Table 10–3. Common pathogens in pediatric bone and joint infections.

Osteomyelitis
Group A *Streptococcus*
Salmonella (with sickle cell)
Staphylococcus aureus

Septic joint
Escherichia coli (neonatal)
Group A *Streptococcus*
Haemophilus influenzae (age 6–24 months) in non–HIB-immunized patients
Neisseria gonorrhoeae (adolescent)
Pneumococcus
Proteus (neonatal)
Staphylococcus aureus
Streptococcus faecalis (neonatal)

Soft-tissue infection
Escherichia coli (neonatal)
Group A *Streptococcus*
Proteus
Pseudomonas
Staphylococcus aureus
Streptococcus faecalis (neonatal)
Kingella kingae

penetrating wound can also lead to infection and may resemble other serious bacterial infections in children (Table 10–3).

Acute bacterial hematogenous osteomyelitis usually occurs in the metaphysis following sludging of bacteria-laden blood in the venous sinusoids. The majority of cases are caused by *Staphylococcus aureus*. As the infection progresses, edema fluid and infected purulent tissue invade the porous cortex and elevate the periosteum, which is highly resistant to infection because of its extreme vascularity. The pressure of the pus beneath the richly innervated periosteum causes localized pain. Eventually, if the infection is untreated, the periosteum itself ruptures, and infected tissue spills into the surrounding soft tissue or ruptures the skin (Figure 10–1).

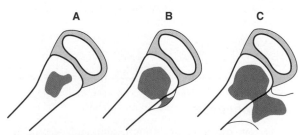

▲ **Figure 10–1.** Hematogenous osteomyelitis in children. Cellulitic phase **(A)** can exude through the cortex, raising periosteum **(B)**. Late rupture into soft tissues **(C)** is rare, unless infection is untreated.

The accumulated purulence in the marrow cavity and under the periosteum creates an efficient avascular culture medium in the cortex between them. This dead cortex is called a *sequestrum*, and, if it is large, surgical removal may be required to control the infection.

The elevated periosteum responds to infection by producing a shell of periosteal new bone called *involucrum*, which provides some stability to the infected bone and rarely becomes infected itself.

▶ Clinical Findings

Pain and tenderness at the infection site are universal signs, limping is common, and frequently the child is irritable. Fever and leukocytosis are common but not universal, and the ESR is almost always elevated, usually to 50 mm/hour or more. CRP is elevated. Children with MRSA infections may present with severe systemic illness and multisystem involvement. Although the diagnosis is usually clear, osteomyelitis should be suspected if a child has bone pain in the absence of other systemic signs but has recently received antibiotic treatment for other conditions.

▶ Imaging Studies

Clinical examination and routine x-rays are usually sufficient to make the diagnosis; occasionally, bone scans or magnetic resonance imaging (MRI) may be required to help localize lesions.

▶ Laboratory Findings

Elevation of ESR (>50 mm/hour) and CRP are typical of osteomyelitis.

▶ Treatment

A. Early Treatment

Treatment depends on the duration of symptoms, radiographic findings, and suspected or cultured organism. If the infection is detected early, no visible radiograph changes usually are apparent except for soft-tissue swelling. In that case, intravenous and, later, oral antibiotics may resolve the infection. Aspiration of the metaphysis should be done for culture before beginning antibiotic therapy. Up to 30–40% of cultures may be negative despite other clear evidence of bacterial infection; in that case, empirical treatment (usually with antistaphylococcal antibiotics) is appropriate.

B. Treatment for Advanced Infection or MRSA

In advanced cases, lytic defects or osteoporosis may be present, and periosteal reaction may be visible on radiograph; such cases require open drainage and debridement of the infected metaphysis. Antibiotic treatment must be continued until there is no evidence of residual infection because bacteria can survive in bone tissue that is not well perfused with antibiotic.

In such cases, a 3-month prolonged regimen of oral antibiotics minimizes the possibility of chronic osteomyelitis.

MRSA infections are more likely to require surgical drainage for mctaphyseal or subperiosteal abscesses, and multiple operative debridements may be necessary.

2. Septic Joint

Essentials of Diagnosis

- *Septic joints cause pain, limp, and refusal to move a joint.*
- *Aspiration of joint for culture, surgical drainage, and antibiotics are generally successful.*
- *Septic hip is a unique surgical emergency requiring urgent surgery.*

General Considerations

Septic arthritis in children, like osteomyelitis, usually is hematogenous in origin. The bacterial complications are similar to those seen in bone infections (see Table 10–3). Septic joints frequently follow upper respiratory infections; they may be delayed in onset by a week or more and may present in an attenuated form when a previous infection was partially treated.

Clinical Findings

The classic septic joint in a child presents a dramatic picture: The joint is splinted by muscle spasm, and motion of even a few degrees causes extreme pain. There may be effusion, but findings may be less striking if antibiotics were used in the recent past. During this acute inflammatory phase, children are more comfortable if the involved joint is immobilized.

Laboratory Findings

Although white blood cell counts and the ESR are usually elevated, the definitive diagnosis of septic joint requires aspiration and synovial fluid analysis. Sterile aspiration does not harm the joint and should be done immediately when the diagnosis is suspected. Aspiration of deep joints such as the hip may require radiographic control.

Synovial white blood cell counts range from 50,000/μL (in nonpyogenic infections such as *Neisseria gonorrhoeae*) to over 250,000/μL (*S. aureus*). This white cell response, with the concomitant high level of lysosomal enzyme release, is most destructive of articular cartilage in septic joints. Although synovial fluid cultures give definitive guidance for therapy, antibiotic treatment can initially be based on results of Gram staining. In addition, immunochemical tests may offer rapid identification of certain pathogens.

Imaging Studies

Most septic joints have normal radiographic findings or nonspecific signs of effusion or local tissue swelling. Late radiographic findings include subluxation, narrowing of joint space, and subchondral bone irregularity. MRI will demonstrate effusion or concurrent osteomyelitis or pyomyositis if present (see below).

Differential Diagnosis

Like osteomyelitis, septic joint may be mimicked by septic pyomyositis (almost always MRSA), with involvement of periarticular tissues with or without actual joint involvement.

Treatment

Treatment always includes drainage of the joint. In easily accessible joints, such as the finger or knee, certain low-grade infections may respond well to repeated aspirations. In most cases, however, surgical drainage by arthrotomy or arthroscopy is preferable.

Antibiotics easily cross the synovial membrane and are continued until the joint inflammation is resolved, usually for at least 3 weeks. Intravenous administration is used initially but may often be followed by oral medication once the temperature, ESR, and leukocyte count return to normal.

Hensinger RN: Impending danger: community-acquired methicillin-resistant *Staphylococcus aureus*. *J Pediatr Orthop* 2006;26:703. [PMID: 17065929]

Jagodzinski NA, Kanwar R, Graham K, Bache CE: Prospective evaluation of a shortened regimen of treatment for acute osteomyelitis and septic arthritis in children. *J Pediatr Orthop* 2009;29:518. [PMID: 19568027]

Kaplan SL: Acute hematogenous osteomyelitis in children: differences in clinical manifestations and management. *Pediatr Infect Dis J* 2010;29:1128. [PMID: 21099652]

3. Septic Hip

Septic hip is one of the true surgical emergencies in pediatric orthopedics. It must be differentiated from transient synovitis of the hip, which is a benign condition (see the section on transient synovitis of the hip).

Pathogenesis

Because of the unique structure and blood supply of proximal femur (Figure 10–2), purulence within the joint capsule can cause thrombosis of epiphyseal vessels and necrosis of the proximal femoral epiphysis. Neglected septic hips may subluxate or dislocate because of effusion and laxity caused by hyperemia. For these reasons, septic hip (or osteomyelitis of the proximal femur) always requires surgical drainage. Delay of even 4–6 hours may compromise the vascularity of the hip. An anterior approach is preferred to reduce the risk of vascular injury and subluxation.

Septic hip in a growing child is also a special orthopedic case because the femoral neck (which is intraarticular) is actually the anatomic metaphysis of the proximal femur. It is thus susceptible to hematogenous osteomyelitis, which may rupture into the hip joint and cause sepsis.

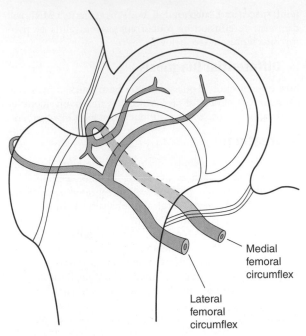

Medial
femoral
circumflex

Lateral
femoral
circumflex

▲ **Figure 10–2.** The blood supply of the proximal femur is unusual because the capsule interferes with the direct routing of blood vessels. The epiphyseal vessels emerge distal to the capsule and course up the surface of the femoral neck, rendering them susceptible to injury, thrombosis, or blockage by increased intraarticular pressure.

▶ **Differential Diagnosis**

A common clinical problem is the differentiation between septic hip and transient synovitis of the hip. Juvenile arthritis may occasionally be included in the differential. Table 10–4 highlights differences in the conditions.

Sultan J, Hughes PJ: Septic arthritis or transient synovitis of the hip in children: the value of clinical prediction algorithms. *J Bone Joint Surg Br* 2010;92:1289. [PMID: 20798450]

4. Puncture Wounds of the Foot

Sneakers and tennis shoes offer little protection from nail punctures of the plantar surface of the foot. The penetrating nail may carry *Pseudomonas* bacteria (which contaminate the soles of tennis shoes) into the plantar fascia, although one series found *S. aureus* or group A *Streptococcus* to be most common.

The symptoms of infection include redness, swelling, and pain that persist longer than 1 week. Surgical incision and drainage of the abscess and foreign body excision, when present (approximately one sixth of cases), are usually curative. Interestingly, prophylactic use of antibiotics does not seem to lessen the chance of developing late abscess. Late presentation is a marker for deep infection.

Eidelman M, Bialik V, Miller Y, Kassis I: Plantar puncture wounds in children: analysis of 80 hospitalized patients and late sequelae. *Isr Med Assoc J* 2003;5:268. [PMID: 14509132]

Schwab RA, Powers RD: Conservative therapy of plantar puncture wounds. *J Emerg Med* 1995;13:291. [PMID: 7673617]

5. Skeletal Tuberculosis

As in the adult, *Mycobacteria* organisms may invade the pediatric skeleton by hematogenous spread to bone or synovium while the initial pulmonary infection goes undetected. The most common sites of invasion are the hip and spine. Tuberculosis (TB) should be considered, and skin tests performed, in children suffering from chronic atypical musculoskeletal infections, particularly if the child is immunosuppressed.

Table 10–4. Clinical differential diagnosis of inflammatory hip conditions.

	Septic Hip	Transient Synovitis of Hip	Juvenile Arthritis of Hip
Pain	Severe	Moderate–severe	Moderate
Gait	Cannot walk	Limp or cannot walk	Limp
Fever	Common	No	No or low grade
Radiograph	Negative	Negative	Joint narrowing
WBC	Elevated	Normal	Normal–elevated
Aspirate	Turbid; 5000–250,000 WBC; bacteria present	Normal	25,000–50,000 WBC with monocytes
Treatment	Urgent surgical drainage; antibiotics	Symptomatic	Salicylates, rest, physical therapy

WBC, white blood cells.

Clinical Findings

Hip involvement with TB is characterized by a chronic limp associated with a flexion contracture. In addition, muscle atrophy of the thigh may be striking. Radiographic examination discloses osteoporosis, joint narrowing, and irregular erosions. Spine involvement typically has an indolent presentation. Unlike pyogenic infections of the spine, the disk space is usually preserved. Most commonly, the thoracic and lumbar spine are affected. It may include paraspinal abscess (best visualized by computed tomography [CT] scan or MRI), and if untreated, it can lead to vertebral destruction or kyphosis, which may be severe and lead to paralysis.

Laboratory Findings

Laboratory studies may be nonspecific.

Treatment

Treatment of skeletal TB consists of combination chemotherapy, with surgical debridement in resistant cases. Occasionally, surgical fusion of a joint may be required. Delayed presentation of spinal TB infection may result in neurologic compromise and a kyphotic deformity. Spinal surgery is occasionally indicated for deformity correction or failure of medical treatment.

Hosalkar HS, Agrawal N, Reddy S, et al: Skeletal tuberculosis in children in the Western world: 18 new cases with a review of the literature. *J Child Orthop* 2009;3:319. [PMID: 19543761]

6. Diskitis in Children

Diskitis is a low-grade inflammatory process involving the intervertebral disk, usually in the lumbar spine. It affects children at any age, although it is most frequent between 2 and 6 years of age. The disorder is caused by hematogenous bacterial seeding, with the most common cultures growing *S. aureus* from the disk aspirate. The classic presentation in a toddler is refusal to walk; pain is not a prominent symptom in this age group. Older children (up to early teen years) may have either back or abdominal pain.

Clinical Findings

Small children may have limitation of passive hyperextension of the spine (in the prone position) with no other findings. Older children have splinting of the paraspinous muscles and pain with percussion.

Laboratory Findings

The ESR may be normal or elevated; patients with an elevated ESR are more likely to have bacterial growth if cultures are done. Aspirate cultures may be negative in up to 40% of patients.

Imaging Studies

Radiographs at first are normal but eventually demonstrate disk space narrowing with sclerosis of adjoining endplates, best visualized on spot lateral views. Bone scan is positive in children with negative radiographs.

Treatment

Management depends on the severity of clinical findings because a large number of diskitis patients have self-limited disease and improve spontaneously. Children with sepsis or elevated ESR may benefit from disk aspiration and culture. Less ill children are usually treated with empirical antistaphylococcal oral antibiotics for 6 weeks. Pantaloon spica cast may occasionally be required for symptom relief. Long-term outcome is universally favorable, although occasional spontaneous fusion of the disk space occurs.

Early SD, Kay RM, Tolo VT: Childhood diskitis. *J Am Acad Orthop Surg* 2003;11:413. [PMID: 14686826]

Hamdy RC, Lawton L, Carey T, et al: Subacute hematogenous osteomyelitis: are biopsy and surgery always necessary? *J Pediatr Orthop* 1996;16:220. [PMID: 8742289]

Scott RJ, Christofersen MR, Robertson WW Jr, et al: Acute osteomyelitis in children: a review of 116 cases. *J Pediatr Orthop* 1990;5:649. [PMID: 2203820]

METABOLIC DISORDERS

Essentials of Diagnosis

- There is growth abnormality and weakening or bowing of long bones in children.
- There is widening, bowing, and cupping of the physes.
- Serum calcium, phosphorus, alkaline phosphate, blood urea nitrogen, and endocrine studies usually confirm the diagnosis.

1. Rickets and Rickets-Like Conditions

Nutritional rickets is a dietary deficiency of vitamin D that interferes with skeletal ossification. Although vitamin supplementation of food and milk has virtually eliminated the dietary form of rickets, there is still an increased frequency of nutritional rickets in the United States in children with dark skin pigmentation who are breast fed past 6 months of age without vitamin D supplementation. Nutritional rickets is rare in light-skinned children or those who are formula fed. Numerous rickets-like metabolic conditions persist with orthopedic consequences, however.

Renal Osteodystrophy

Renal osteodystrophy, a disorder of calcium, phosphorus, vitamin D, and parathyroid function in children with chronic renal disease, has potentially serious skeletal manifestations. In transplantation patients, the condition can be aggravated by chronic illness and antimetabolite or steroid usage.

Osteoporosis, leading to compression fractures of the spine, is a common complication. Delayed healing of fractures is also common. Inadequate metaphyseal ossification during skeletal growth results in wide, irregular cartilaginous growth plates, which tend to slip slowly, sometimes producing grotesque hip, knee, and ankle deformities. Such deformities are usually best treated only after transplantation or other improvement in renal status. Occasionally, severe functional disabilities may require osteotomy to correct deformity before renal transplantation. Healing may be delayed, however, and the condition may recur.

► Hypophosphatemic Rickets

Hypophosphatemic rickets (vitamin D–resistant rickets) is a dominant X-linked condition in which vitamin D production and metabolism are normal but renal tubular loss of phosphate interferes with skeletal ossification. The major manifestations are a mild-to-moderate decrease in stature and bowing of the lower extremities. The medical history usually discloses a parent or sibling with short stature and bowlegs.

A. Laboratory Findings

Serum phosphorus is reduced, and serum calcium is *normal*. This is because the disorder is caused by phosphorus excretion in the urine (detectible in 24-hour urine sample). Vitamin D levels are normal.

B. Imaging Studies

Characteristic widening of growth plates, funnel-like beaking of the metaphyses, and curvature of the femoral and tibial shafts, which are normally straight (Figure 10–3), are typical.

C. Treatment

Medical treatment with megadoses of vitamin D and phosphorus supplementation may not be curative. Functionally disabling deformities can be corrected by growth plate manipulation using hemiepiphyseodesis in younger children, or by multiple-level osteotomies, which usually require bilateral surgery. Because postosteotomy healing is delayed and recurrence of deformity is common during growth, such surgery should be postponed until adolescence, if possible.

Kocaoglu M, Bilen FE, Sen C, Eralp L, Balci HI: Combined technique for the correction of lower-limb deformities resulting from metabolic bone disease. *J Bone Joint Surg Br* 2011;93:52. [PMID: 21196543]

Novais E, Stevens PM: Hypophosphatemic rickets: the role of hemiepiphysiodesis. *J Pediatr Orthop* 2006;26:238. [PMID: 16557142]

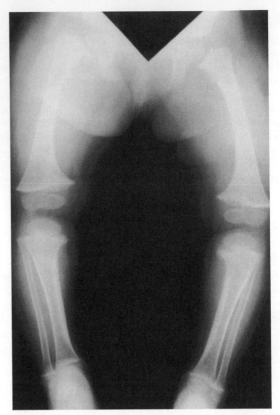

▲ **Figure 10–3.** Hypophosphatemic rickets. Radiographs demonstrate bowing of long bones and flared, irregular physes (see text).

Saland JM: Osseous complications of pediatric transplantation. *Pediatr Transplant* 2004;8:400. [PMID: 15265169]

Santos F, Carbajo-Pérez E, Rodríguez J, et al: Alterations of the growth plate in chronic renal failure. *Pediatr Nephrol* 2004; 20:330. [PMID: 15549411]

HIP DISORDERS

1. Transient Synovitis of the Hip

Transient synovitis of the hip is a benign, nontraumatic, self-limited disorder that mimics septic hip in clinical presentation. The physician confronting this condition must exclude septic hip, which is a surgical emergency.

Although the cause of transient synovitis is unclear, evidence suggests it is associated with immune responses to viral or bacterial antigens, mediated through the synovial membrane. Aseptic synovial fluid rapidly accumulates under pressure in the hip joint, and there may be severe pain from capsular distension. The fluid is resorbed within 3–7 days, with no long-term sequelae.

Clinical Findings

As with septic hip, upper respiratory tract infections often precede transient synovitis by a few days to 2 weeks. The hip contains excess synovial fluid and is held in flexion, abduction, and external rotation because this is the joint's position of maximum capacity. The joint may be sore and resistant to movement, but subluxation does not occur. Usually, the patient allows careful passive movement.

Laboratory Findings

Leukocytosis is absent, and ESR and CRP are not elevated. Synovial fluid does not show elevation of the white blood cell count, and bacterial cultures are negative.

Imaging Studies

Radiographs reveal only capsular swelling, and effusion may be detected on ultrasound. Although experienced physicians frequently suspect transient synovitis based only on clinical examination, aspiration of the hip following confirmation of needle position by radiograph or ultrasound is the safest approach.

Differential Diagnosis

The most important differential diagnosis is septic hip, which must be excluded. Also, early stages of Legg-Calvé-Perthes disease (see section on Legg-Calvé-Perthes disease) may include a synovitic stage that, until the development of characteristic radiograph findings, is indistinguishable from transient synovitis. No evidence indicates that transient synovitis leads to Legg-Calvé-Perthes disease itself. Typically, the pain is less severe than in transient synovitis, the children are a bit older (older than 4–5 years), and there is no history of recent illness.

Treatment

Treatment of transient synovitis includes simple analgesics and splintage, usually by bed rest, until symptoms resolve.

Sultan J, Hughes PJ: Septic arthritis or transient synovitis of the hip in children: the value of clinical prediction algorithms. *J Bone Joint Surg Br* 2010;92:1289. [PMID: 20798450]

2. Developmental Dysplasia of the Hip

Essentials of Diagnosis

- Certain infants (breech babies, babies with a family history, and females) are at higher risk for developmental dysplasia of the hip.
- Diagnosis is made *clinically* or by ultrasound.
- Early treatment gives the best results.

Developmental dysplasia of the hip is one of the most serious problems in pediatric orthopedics. The neonatal hip is a relatively unstable joint because the muscle is undeveloped, the soft cartilaginous surfaces are easily deformed, and the ligaments are lax. Exaggerated positioning in acute flexion and adduction in utero may occur, especially in breech presentation. This situation may cause excess stretching of the posterior hip capsule, which renders the joint unstable after delivery. Laxity may reflect family history or the presence of maternal relaxin hormone in the fetal circulatory system.

This relative instability may lead to asymptomatic subluxation (partial displacement) or dislocation (complete displacement) of the hip joint. Displacement of the femoral head in the infant is proximal (posterior and superior) because of the pull of the gluteal and hip flexor muscles. In the subluxated hip, asymmetric pressure causes progressive flattening of the posterior and superior acetabular rim and medial femoral head (*dysplasia* is the term to describe these structural deviations from normal).

In the completely dislocated hip, dysplasia also occurs because normal joint development requires concentric motion with normally mated joint surfaces. The shallow, deformed dysplastic joint surfaces predispose to further mechanical instability and the inexorable progression of the disorder.

Developmental dysplasia of the hip (DDH) occurs in approximately 1 in 1000 live births in whites, is less common in blacks, and may be more common in certain ethnic groups such as North American Indians. In all groups, this disorder is more likely if certain risk factors are present, such as positive family history, ligamentous laxity, breech presentation (and, by association, cesarean delivery), female gender, large fetal size, and first-born status. Dislocations may be bilateral but are more often unilateral and on the left side.

Clinical Findings

Reversal of dysplasia and subsequent normal hip development depend on early detection of DDH. Early detection is made more challenging by lack of a definitive test or finding on examination. Moreover, because this disorder is painless, there are no symptoms in the infant. Detection of bilateral dislocations may be particularly difficult.

Radiographs are usually not useful in newborn infants because the femoral head is composed of radiolucent cartilage. Ultrasound examination is helpful, but false-positive results are common before 8–10 weeks of age. The test is expensive, and interpretation requires comprehensive training. Thus, the best test for this disorder is careful physical examination at birth, repeated at each well-infant check until the child is walking normally. A high index of suspicion is mandatory, especially if risk factors are present.

A. Tests for Dysplasia

Several examination maneuvers require a quiet, relaxed infant and commonly produce false-negative findings.

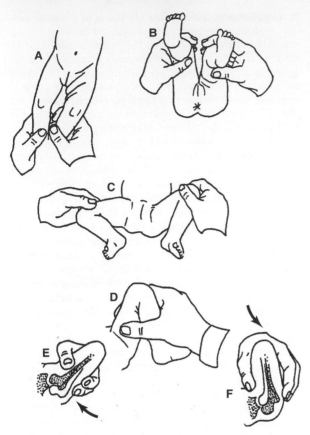

▲ Figure 10–4. Clinical examination of developmental dislocation of the hip. In all pictures, the child's left hip is the abnormal side. **A:** Asymmetric skin folds. **B:** Galeazzi test. **C:** Limitation of abduction. **D, E, F:** Ortolani and Barlow tests (see text).

Although it is imperative to detect subluxated or dislocated hips, it is also helpful to identify the very lax (unstable) but still located hip. This type of joint may either dislocate later or exhibit subtle dysplasia during growth that can cause premature osteoarthritis.

1. Asymmetric skin folds—A dislocated hip displaces proximally, causing the leg to be marginally shorter. This occasionally leads to the accordion phenomenon, with wrinkling of thigh skin folds. The most significant fold is between the genitals and gluteus maximus region. This test is not very reliable, frequently producing false-positive and false-negative results (Figure 10–4A).

2. Galeazzi test—With the child lying on a flat surface, flex the hips and knees so the heels rest flat on the table, just distal to the buttock (Figure 10–4B). A dislocated hip is signaled by relative shortening of the thigh compared with the normal leg, as shown by the difference in knee height level. This test

is almost always useless in children younger than 1 year and is negative if dislocation is bilateral.

3. Passive hip abduction—The flexed hips are gently abducted as far as possible (Figure 10–4C). If one or both hips are dislocated, the femoral head (the pivot point during abduction) is posterior, causing relative tightness of the adductor muscles. Asymmetric abduction or limited abduction (usually <70 degrees from the midline) is a positive finding. When the hip is lax (dislocatable but not dislocated), the abduction test is normal despite the presence of subluxation or dislocation.

4. Barlow test—A provocative test that picks up an unstable but located hip, the Barlow test is unsuitable for a dislocated hip. The flexed calf and knee are gently grasped in the hand, with the thumb at the lesser trochanter and fingers at the greater trochanter (knee flexion relaxes the hamstrings). The hip is adducted slightly and gently pushed posteriorly and laterally with the palm (Figure 10–4D, F). Detection of so-called pistoning, or the sensation of the femoral head subluxating over the posterior rim of the acetabulum, is a positive finding.

5. Ortolani test—This test detects hips that are already dislocated. The flexed limb is grasped as in the Barlow test. The hip is abducted while the femur is gently lifted with the fingers at the greater trochanter (Figure 10–4D, E). In a positive test, there is a sensation of the hip reducing back into the acetabulum. Reduction is felt but not heard: The old concept of a so-called hip click is incorrect. The Ortolani test may be negative at 2–3 months of age, even when the hip is dislocated, because of the development of soft-tissue contracture.

B. Imaging Studies

In the infant, diagnosis is made by physical examination alone, and radiographs are generally unnecessary. Dysplasia, instability, and dislocation may appear on ultrasound studies, which can allow visualization of hip contour and stability before ossification is present. Sonography is a dynamic examination that requires an experienced interpreter, and there can be false positives prior to 6–10 weeks of age. Radiographs may be used at any age, but the absence of ossified structures renders them inaccurate in the newborn. After 4–6 months, when the ossific nucleus appears in the femoral head, radiographs are more helpful. Because much of the skeleton is cartilaginous at this age, certain lines and angles may be drawn on radiographs to allow estimates of geometric parameters (Figure 10–5). These may suggest evidence of acetabular dysplasia (a more vertical slope of the acetabular roof, measured as the acetabular index), femoral dysplasia (small or absent ossification center in the femoral head), or lateral superior displacement of the femoral head.

Increased femoral anteversion (external rotation of the femoral head and neck) is often present in DDH but not

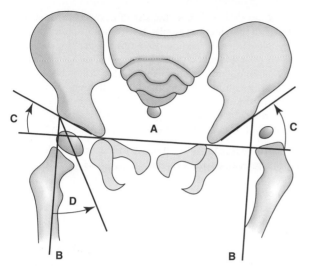

▲ **Figure 10–5.** Lines drawn for measurement in developmental dysplasia of the hip. In the figure, the patient's left hip (on the right of the figure) is the subluxated one. **A:** Hilgenreiner line is a horizontal line of the pelvis, drawn between the triradiate cartilages. The proximal femoral ossification center should be below this line. **B:** Perkins line is a vertical line (perpendicular to Hilgenreiner line) drawn down from the lateral edge of the acetabulum. The femoral head ossification center, as well as the medial beak of the proximal metaphysis, should fall medial to this line. **C:** The acetabular index is the angle between Hilgenreiner line and a line joining the acetabular center (triradiate) with the acetabular edge as it intersects Perkins line. It measures acetabular depth and should be below 30 degrees by 1 year of age and below 25 degrees by 2 years of age. **D:** The center-edge angle is the angle between Perkins line and a line joining the lateral edge of the acetabulum with the center of the femoral head. It is a measure of lateral subluxation that becomes smaller as the hip subluxates laterally. Normal is 20 degrees or greater.

visible. Increased anteversion may be seen as an increase in relative femoral neck valgus in the older child.

C. Detection of Dysplasia in the Older Child

As the infant grows older, many diagnostic maneuvers that are positive in a young infant become negative because soft-tissue changes accommodate the displaced structures. Thus, the Ortolani and Barlow signs can be negative, even in the face of grossly abnormal hip development, making detection particularly difficult (especially between 4 and 15 months of age). The first signs of developmental dysplasia may then not be recognized until the child begins to walk and demonstrates a waddling gait with excessive lumbar lordosis. Radiographs at this age are diagnostic.

▶ **Treatment**

Treatment of DDH should be initiated as soon as the diagnosis is suspected. Early treatment is generally successful, whereas a delay in treatment may result in permanent dysplastic changes. Exact treatment depends on patient age at presentation and degree of involvement. Regardless of age, treatment may fail, and the physician may need to institute a more complex treatment plan. The current recommendations described next.

A. Age 0–6 Months

A dislocated hip at this age may spontaneously reduce over 2–3 weeks if the hip is held in a position of flexion. This is best accomplished with the Pavlik harness (Figure 10–6), a canvas device that holds the hips flexed at 100 degrees and prevents adduction but does not limit further flexion. Movement in the harness is beneficial for the joint and helps achieve gradual spontaneous reduction and stabilization of the hip. Treatment with a Pavlik harness has a low risk of avascular necrosis (see section on avascular necrosis of the hip). This treatment should not be continued beyond

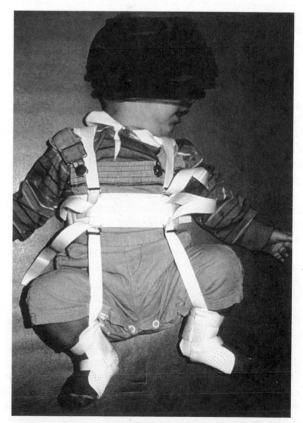

▲ **Figure 10–6.** The Pavlik harness, a device used for treatment of hip dislocation, subluxation, and dysplasia.

3–4 weeks if there is no improvement. The failure rate of the Pavlik harness is approximately 10%, necessitating more invasive treatment, such as closed or open reduction.

B. Age 6–12 Months (Before Walking)

Gentle manipulative reduction of the dislocation under a general anesthetic and maintenance of a located position for 2–3 months in a spica cast usually stabilizes the joint. Even after the hip is stable, any residual dysplasia must be treated by bracing or surgery. In the past, prereduction skin traction was thought to reduce the risk of avascular necrosis. It is now believed that adequate hip flexion and limited abduction in the spica cast are the most important safety factors, and most surgeons no longer use traction.

C. Age 12 Months to 2 Years

In toddlers or young children in whom closed reduction failed, open reduction of the hip is required. Severe flattening of the acetabulum with distortion of the normal spherical femoral head shape is found on opening the hip. The limbus (acetabular rim) may be flattened and inverted, and the ligamentum teres is always hypertrophic. Fibrofatty tissue occupying the center of the acetabulum must be removed. Femoral shortening osteotomy may be required at the time of open reduction to reduce soft-tissue tension and minimize the risk of avascular necrosis. After reduction, the position is maintained by capsular repair (capsulorrhaphy) and a cast, until stability is achieved. Prolonged bracing or surgery is often required to resolve the residual dysplasia that accompanies untreated dysplasia in this group of children.

D. Age Older Than 2 Years

Significant residual dysplasia is present in children with DDH who are untreated at this age. Dysplasia may also persist despite successful reduction performed by any method at an earlier age. The dysplasia may be accompanied by a limp, and radiographs show a high acetabular index (more vertical acetabular roof), increased valgus of the femoral neck, and subluxation of the femoral head.

Surgical correction of dysplasia creates a stable mechanical environment that permits remodeling to a more normal joint during growth. Treatment requires bony procedures, either on the acetabular or femoral sides of the joint, or on both sides. Acetabular procedures, such as the Salter or Pemberton osteotomies, improve the acetabular index and increase the mechanical stability of the joint.

Femoral osteotomy corrects the anteversion and femoral neck valgus that characterize femoral dysplasia. The exact selection of osteotomy site may be based on maximum radiographic dysplasia or on the individual surgeon's preference. All of the osteotomies require that the femoral head be spherical and the hip joint concentrically reduced before an attempt can be made to correct the dysplasia. In general, the

osteotomy should address the site of dysplasia, that is, acetabular dysplasia is not ideally treated with femoral osteotomy. Nevertheless, femoral osteotomy, if performed before 4 years of age, stimulates a dysplastic shallow acetabulum to remodel into a more normal shape. This occurs because the femoral osteotomy renders the hip joint more stable, thus allowing the normal mechanisms of growth to take over. Similarly, patients exhibit a progressive decrease in femoral dysplasia following successful acetabular osteotomy.

1. Salter osteotomy—Salter osteotomy is a surgical procedure to redirect the acetabulum in DDH (Figure 10–7). Animal models demonstrate that residual hip dysplasia is accompanied by acetabular malrotation and deficiency in the anterolateral acetabular rim. Salter osteotomy corrects this deficiency by rotating the acetabular region anteriorly and laterally.

The procedure is indicated in children 18 months to 10 years of age in whom concentric reduction of the hip was achieved. It is used to correct moderate acetabular dysplasia and can improve the acetabular index by 15 degrees. It may also be used to stabilize the hip at the time of open reduction. The pelvis above the hip joint is exposed subperiosteally. A transverse cut is made, using a wire saw, from the sciatic notch to the anteroinferior iliac spine, and the entire distal fragment (including the acetabulum) is spun on the pivot points of the notch and the pubic symphysis. This redirects the entire dysplastic acetabulum to a more horizontal stable position. A bone graft and pins hold the osteotomy open until it heals. A spica cast is used for 6 weeks to protect the graft during healing.

Salter osteotomy requires a second operation to remove the fixation pins. Because the geometric reorientation afforded is limited, there may be residual dysplasia. In addition, failure to achieve a concentric reduction before pelvic osteotomy usually renders the procedure ineffective.

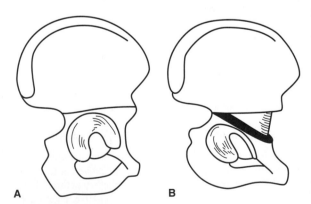

▲ **Figure 10–7.** Salter innominate osteotomy, used for managing acetabular dysplasia. After a transverse cut is made above the acetabulum **(A)**, the acetabular fragment is rotated forward and outward **(B)** to improve acetabular coverage.

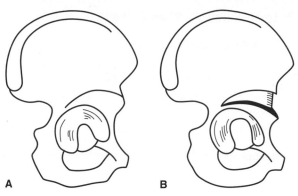

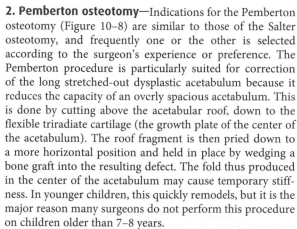

▲ **Figure 10–8.** Pemberton pericapsular iliac osteotomy. An osteotomy cut is made above the acetabulum down to the flexible triradiate cartilage **(A)**. The fragment is pried down to improve acetabular coverage and held with a bone graft **(B)**.

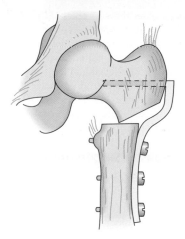

▲ **Figure 10–9.** Femoral osteotomy is performed at the intertrochanteric level and fixed with a plate and screws.

2. Pemberton osteotomy—Indications for the Pemberton osteotomy (Figure 10–8) are similar to those of the Salter osteotomy, and frequently one or the other is selected according to the surgeon's experience or preference. The Pemberton procedure is particularly suited for correction of the long stretched-out dysplastic acetabulum because it reduces the capacity of an overly spacious acetabulum. This is done by cutting above the acetabular roof, down to the flexible triradiate cartilage (the growth plate of the center of the acetabulum). The roof fragment is then pried down to a more horizontal position and held in place by wedging a bone graft into the resulting defect. The fold thus produced in the center of the acetabulum may cause temporary stiffness. In younger children, this quickly remodels, but it is the major reason many surgeons do not perform this procedure on children older than 7–8 years.

Like the Salter procedure, Pemberton osteotomy requires concentric reduction before it is performed. For the Pemberton osteotomy, the pelvis is exposed above the joint. Under radiographic guidance, a curved osteotome is used to cut the pelvic bone from the acetabular roof down to the triradiate cartilage (the central growth plate of the acetabulum). The flexible cartilage allows the fragment to be hinged down over the femoral head, producing a more horizontal acetabular roof. A bone graft from the upper ilium wedges into the osteotomy site to maintain correction, and a spica cast is used until healing, which takes approximately 6 weeks.

Rarely, early extrusion or graft collapse occurs, and transient stiffness may be seen in older children. Because there is no internal fixation, a second procedure is unnecessary.

3. Femoral osteotomy—Femoral osteotomy (Figure 10–9) may be used to correct severe increased femoral anteversion or coxa valga (a high neck-shaft angle), conditions that are sometimes seen in residual DDH.

The procedure is particularly indicated when radiographs taken with the hip in abduction and internal rotation show improvement in the overall congruency of the hip. Redirection of an anteverted, valgus hip stimulates spontaneous improvement in dysplastic acetabula in children younger than 4 years.

Femoral osteotomy is performed using a lateral approach, with the cut made across the intertrochanteric region of the femur. This site is chosen both because it is distal to the blood supply of the femoral head and because the cancellous bone heals easily. A metal blade-plate is placed in the proximal (femoral neck) fragment, usually after positioning with a provisional guidewire. The femoral neck fragment is rotated into a more horizontal position (varus) and is then internally rotated to correct excessive anteversion. The exact degree of correction is determined by preoperative radiograph positioning to achieve maximum congruence and correction of radiographic dysplasia. The plate portion is then clamped to the shaft of the bone and fixed with screws. A spica cast is usually used to supplement fixation.

After healing (6 weeks), the patient may resume walking. A Trendelenburg limp is common for 1–2 years after femoral osteotomy because of the geometric distortion of the relationship between the joint and insertion of the abductor muscles. This resolves as the femur remodels with growth and does not present a long-term problem.

4. Late salvage operations—After age 6–10 years, reduction and reconstruction of severely dysplastic or dislocated hips may be impossible. If acetabular coverage is poor but the joint is concentric, major reorientation of the acetabulum may be indicated. Salter osteotomy (see above) may be inadequate for this degree of reorientation, necessitating the addition of osteotomy cuts in the pubis and ischium to allow more aggressive repositioning of the joint surface (triple innominate osteotomy).

For children older than 10 years with hip pain and non-reconstructable joints, Chiari osteotomy reliably improves pain. After a slightly upwardly angled cut is made through the ilium just at the proximal edge of the hip capsule, the hip joint is medially displaced half the width of the iliac cut. After healing, the lateral protruding shelf of the ilium blends with the hip capsule to create a functional equivalent of an augmented hip socket, lined with the smooth capsule, which serves as part of the joint surface.

E. Complications of Surgery for DDH

1. Avascular necrosis of the hip—If a reduction maneuver for DDH was forceful or if there is tension in the soft tissues around the hip, the resulting compression of the joint may cause transient blockage of the blood supply to the femoral head. The subsequent death of the ossific nucleus and proximal growth plate of the femur (avascular necrosis) is a complication of treatment rather than of the disorder itself. A well-recognized cause of avascular necrosis is exaggerated forced abduction in the spica cast used after closed or open reduction. Avascular necrosis may be mild (involving a small fraction of the ossific nucleus), in which case it may go undetected and be of little significance. At the other extreme, avascular necrosis may lead to complete femoral head death and loss of future growth at the proximal physis. As it revascularizes, a dead femoral head may deform significantly, subluxate further, and require abduction bracing or osteotomy. Thus, it can cause leg-length inequality or early osteoarthritis of the hip. The best treatment for avascular necrosis is prevention.

2. Residual dysplasia and degenerative arthritis—No form of treatment uniformly resolves hip dysplasia, and residual dysplasia is common. It may lead to resubluxation or cause failure of remodeling. Older children are more prone to residual problems and may require repeat surgery to help resolve them. Dysplasia is a major cause of premature osteoarthritis of the hip.

Lehmann HP, Hinton R, Morello P, et al: Developmental dysplasia of the hip practice guideline: technical report. Committee on Quality Improvement, and Subcommittee on Developmental Dysplasia of the Hip. *Pediatrics* 2000;105:E57. [PMID: 10742378]

Rejholec M: Combined pelvic osteotomy for the bipartite acetabulum in late developmental dysplasia of the hip: a ten-year prospective study. *J Bone Joint Surg Br* 2011;93:257. [PMID: 21282768]

Walton MJ, Isaacson Z, McMillan D, Hawkes R, Atherton WG: The success of management with the Pavlik harness for developmental dysplasia of the hip using a United Kingdom screening programme and ultrasound-guided supervision. *J Bone Joint Surg Br* 2010;92:1013. [PMID: 20595124]

Weinstein SL, Mubarak SJ, Wenger DR: Developmental hip dysplasia and dislocation: part II. *Instr Course Lect* 2004;53:531. [PMID: 15116642]

3. Legg-Calvé-Perthes Disease

▶ Essentials of Diagnosis

- Legg-Calvé-Perthes disease is most common in children age 4–8 years and is largely self-healing.
- Flexion contracture and loss of abduction are uniform and characteristic.
- There may be a small subgroup of patients with Legg-Calvé-Perthes disease who benefit from surgical treatment.

Legg-Calvé-Perthes disease (LCP, Perthes disease) is a serious but mostly self-limited pediatric hip disorder. Although its cause is unknown, the disease is thought to be related to avascular necrosis of the hip. It affects children between 4 and 10 years of age and is somewhat more common in boys. Children with the disease are often small for their age and have retarded bone age. The disease is generally unilateral. Although bilateral LCP of the hips occurs in about 10% of cases, in patients with symmetric changes/stages, other conditions such as Gaucher disease or multiple epiphyseal dysplasia must be considered. Multiple epiphyseal dysplasia is most readily diagnosed by evaluation of other radiographs, in particular of the knee and, if confirmatory, of the spine to assess for spondyloepiphyseal dysplasia. Patients with multiple epiphyseal dysplasia generally have heights in the fifth percentile or below. Newer investigations suggesting that some cases of LCP might be related to a variety of transient or permanent hypercoagulation states are intriguing but not confirmed in multiple centers. Surprisingly, trauma is not considered a causative factor in LCP.

Although early radiographs may be negative, they eventually show fragmentation, irregularity, and collapse of part or the entire femoral head ossification center (Figure 10–10). The few pathologic specimens that were examined suggest that multiple rather than single episodes of avascular necrosis occur over a period of months. Early bone scans may show a filling defect corresponding to areas of necrosis, and MRI is typical of avascular necrosis. The disease has a characteristic course (see Figure 10–10). Initially, the avascular episodes are silent and the child is asymptomatic. As the disease progresses, the necrotic femoral epiphysis is revascularized. Osteoclasts remove dead bone while osteoblasts simultaneously lay down new bone on the dead trabeculae (a process known as creeping substitution). During this phase, the femoral head is mechanically weak. Fragmentation and collapse of the bony structure may then occur, causing geometric flattening and deformity of the ossific nucleus and femoral head. The newly replaced bone takes the shape of the collapsed head. At this point, continued growth may allow gradual remodeling and improvement of the femoral head shape until maturity. The symptomatic collapse phase rarely exceeds 1–1.5 years, but full revascularization and remodeling may continue silently for several years thereafter. Although cartilage is not specifically injured by the avascular events, hyperemia can

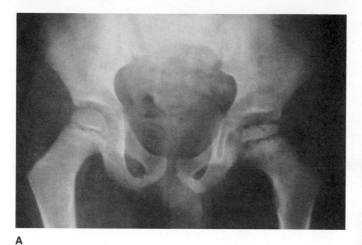

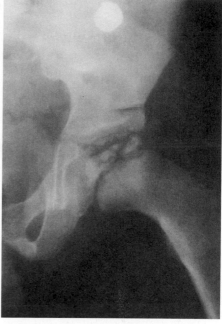

▲ **Figure 10–10.** Legg-Calvé-Perthes disease. **A:** Central necrotic fragment with collapse. **B:** Same patient after healing and partial remodeling.

cause articular cartilage thickening, ectopic ossification, and physeal damage that affects femoral neck growth.

▶ Clinical Findings and Classification

A. Symptoms and Signs

The initial presentation of LCP is usually a painless limp, with aching pain in older children. If pain is present, it may be mild and referred to the thigh or knee. Physical examination discloses atrophy of the thigh on the affected side and, usually, limited hip motion. The typical patient has a flexion contracture of 0–30 degrees, loss of abduction compared with the opposite side (in severe cases, no abduction beyond 0 degrees), and loss of internal rotation of the hip.

B. Imaging Studies

Radiographs may be negative at first, probably because the initial softening of the femoral head is sufficient to cause symptoms but insufficient to change the radiographic appearance of the femoral head. The eventual characteristic collapse of portions of the femoral head is diagnostic of the disease, however.

The exact extent of necrosis, which is estimated in fourths of the head using the Catterall classification (Figure 10–11), is helpful in determining whom to treat. This may require additional radiographs.

An alternative radiograph classification uses the lateral third of the femoral epiphysis (the so-called lateral pillar). Collapse of this structure suggests a poor prognosis for late deformity (class C), whereas maintenance of pillar height correlates with good long-term results (class A). Partial collapse suggests an intermediate prognosis (class B). The difficulty with all classification systems is their reproducibility and the need to delay until the collapse phase before the exact extent of involvement is clear.

There is little value in bone scans or MRI in the clinical management of LCP.

▶ Treatment Options

A. No Treatment

Age at presentation and range of motion (ROM) of the hip are the two most significant predictors of long-term outcome. Children with bone age less than 5 years and children who exhibit relatively minor involvement (less than half of the femoral head) rarely need treatment. In these children, so much of the femoral head is cartilage, and therefore unaffected by necrosis, that mechanical collapse does not markedly decrease sphericity. Also, younger children have tremendous remodeling potential, and minor collapse can be outgrown before maturity. Limited hip ROM may be due to muscle spasm early on, or synovitis; but in late disease, it may reflect incongruity of the joint. Older children who

AP   Frog-leg lateral

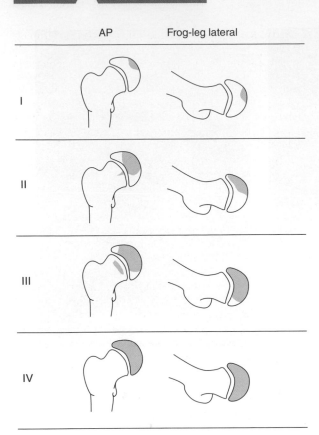

▲ **Figure 10–11.** The Catterall classification is used to determine probable course and prognosis of Legg-Calvé-Perthes disease. It is based on progressive involvement of approximate fourths of the femoral head. AP, anteroposterior.

exhibit some radiographic changes but have excellent ROM may require only observation and serial reexamination.

B. Nonoperative and Operative Treatment

The issues surrounding selection of patients with LCP who need treatment are as highly controversial as the treatment itself. Most experts agree that children who maintain excellent motion (particularly abduction greater than 30 degrees in the absence of flexion contracture) may not require intervention. In children older than 4–5 years with significant collapse or progressive loss of abduction, treatment is frequently recommended.

No evidence indicates that use of crutches or relief of weight bearing has any effect on femoral head collapse in this disease. For those children requiring it, however, treatment should minimize the effects of collapse and subluxation that often occur when the femoral head deforms. This is best achieved by abduction of the hip until subluxation resolves. The molding action of the acetabular shape is thought to

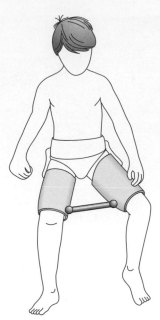

▲ **Figure 10–12.** Abduction bracing is one method used for ambulatory treatment of Legg-Calvé-Perthes disease.

help improve the contour of the collapsing femoral head. Abduction can be accomplished nonoperatively by holding the legs in abduction (Petrie) casts or using an ambulatory brace (Figure 10–12).

Operative procedures are advocated by some and include varus femoral osteotomy and Salter osteotomy, which were adapted from hip dysplasia treatment to control the subluxation seen in some cases of LCP. Healing usually occurs within 18 months. The best current investigations suggest that children over 8 years who have partial head collapse (lateral pillar B-C or Catterall III) may ultimately have better radiographic outcome if treated by surgery.

Despite many studies, there is still no consensus for the best method of treatment; some patients do well without treatment, whereas others have a poor result after aggressive treatment. Prognosis can often be predicted from the knowledge of certain factors (Table 10–5), with age being the most important.

Herring JA, Kim HT, Browne R: Legg-Calvé-Perthes disease. Part II: prospective multicenter study of the effect of treatment on outcome. *J Bone Joint Surg Am* 2004;86-A:2121. [PMID: 15466720]

Karol LA: Legg-Calvé-Perthes disease 100 years on: what have we learned? *J Am Acad Orthop Surg* 2010;18:643. [PMID: 21041798]

Kim HK: Legg-Calvé-Perthes disease. *J Am Acad Orthop Surg* 2010; 18:676. [PMID: 21041802]

Terjesen T, Wiig O, Svenningsen S: The natural history of Perthes' disease. *Acta Orthop* 2010;81:708. [PMID: 21067434]

Table 10–5. Factors in long-term prognosis for patients with Legg-Calvé-Perthes disease.

Relative Prognosis	Good	Poor
Age at diagnosis	<5 years	>8-9 years
Hip motion[a]	Maintained (abduction >30 degrees)	Stiff (abduction <15 degrees)
Extent of involvement	<50% of femoral head	>50% or total femoral head
Radiograph features	Little or no subluxation	Subluxation, lateral calcification

[a]During first year of treatment.

4. Slipped Capital Femoral Epiphysis

▶ **Essentials of Diagnosis**

- Slipped capital femoral epiphysis is most common in overweight children entering puberty.
- Early diagnosis and surgical management give the best results.

Slipped capital femoral epiphysis is an adolescent hip disorder characterized by displacement of the femoral head on the femoral neck through failure of the proximal femoral physis (growth plate). Displacement changes the geometry of the upper end of the femur and hinders hip function (Figure 10–13). This disorder is one of the main causes of premature osteoarthritis in young adults.

Slipped capital femoral epiphysis affects both male and female adolescents 11–13 years of age. In 30–40% of patients, the condition is bilateral, although both legs are not always affected simultaneously. The typical patient is overweight—often markedly so—and is in either late prepuberty or early

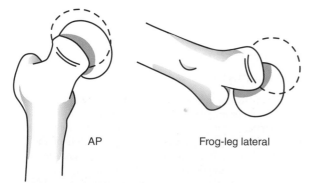

▲ **Figure 10–13.** Anteroposterior (AP) and frog-leg views of a slipped epiphysis. The dotted lines show the normal position of the femoral head.

puberty. Rarely, the patient is tall, asthenic, and rapidly growing.

This disorder occurs at a time when the cartilage physis of the proximal femur is thickening rapidly under the influence of growth hormone. The vigorous secretion of sex hormone has not yet begun, however, so the biological effect of sex hormones on closure and stabilization of the growth plate is absent. This combination of thick growth plate cartilage (weaker than bone and subject to shear), lack of sexual maturity (which would stabilize the physis), mechanical stress (caused by obesity), and the peculiar anatomic mechanics of the hip joint renders the growth plate susceptible to slippage.

The direction of the slip is always posterior and often medial, and the mechanical bases of chronic and acute disorders are the same. In chronic slipped capital femoral epiphysis, the most common form (90% of patients), the femoral head slips insidiously at the growth plate over the course of several months. In the acute form, the femoral head is suddenly displaced, a condition that can be superimposed on chronic changes. Displacement may occur during normal activity or following minor trauma.

Because slipped capital femoral epiphysis is a progressive disorder and the prognosis depends on the severity of the slippage, early detection and prompt treatment are imperative.

▶ **Clinical Findings**

A. Symptoms and Signs

There are two forms of the disorder: chronic and acute. The onset of chronic slipped capital femoral epiphysis is usually insidious, with a history of a painful limp for 1 to several months prior. The pain is characteristically aching and located in the thigh or knee rather than the hip. This referred pain to the knee is responsible for many misdiagnoses. Patients may be seen for knee pain and dismissed as normal after a negative knee examination and radiographs. A high index of suspicion is required to detect slipped capital femoral epiphysis in the obese limping adolescent complaining of knee pain. The change in hip ROM is usually diagnostic: loss of abduction and internal rotation of the hip are evident, although these may be difficult to identify in the grossly overweight child. There is almost always a characteristic obligatory external rotation of the hip when it is flexed because of the distorted hip anatomy caused by the disorder. The femoral head is posterior to its normal position, so the flexed hip must externally rotate to keep the head within the acetabulum.

Acute slipped capital femoral epiphysis is accompanied by severe pain and limping, which may render the patient immobile. The onset is sudden, following little or no trauma, and examination discloses a painful, guarded, restricted range of hip motion. An acute slip is analogous to an epiphyseal fracture. In its unstable form, the patient is unable to bear weight, and there is a high rate of avascular necrosis. In its stable form, the sudden increase in displacement is painful, but limited weight bearing is possible and the risk of avascular necrosis appears to be lower.

B. Imaging Studies

Slipped capital femoral epiphysis can be difficult to detect on standard AP radiographs (Figure 10–14). A frog-leg lateral view is the best for detecting mild forms because slippage is always posterior. A radiograph also shows changes suggesting acute or chronic forms, information that may be critical to management of the disorder.

Establishing the severity of slippage is important in determining treatment and prognosis. Severity is estimated by the percentage of femoral neck left exposed. Slippage of less than 25% of neck width is mild; 25–50% is moderate; and more than 50% is severe.

▶ Treatment

Slipped capital femoral epiphysis is usually a progressive disease that requires prompt surgical treatment. Because the changes in the chronic form occur so slowly, it is impossible to manipulate the femoral head into a better position. Treatment consists of fixing the slip in its current position and preventing progression. This is done by inserting one or more screws or pins across the growth plate, regardless of the severity of the slip (pinning in situ).

Following surgery, aching rapidly resolves, and during the remaining 2–3 years of skeletal growth, the extent of remodeling of the distorted proximal femur may be considerable, leading to an improved ROM.

Because of bilateral involvement, some surgeons recommend prophylactic screw fixation of the normal side at the time of initial treatment. This is particularly indicated in children ages 10 years and under.

Acute slips, if unstable, may be gently reduced before fixation, but the risk of further damage to the tenuous blood supply of the proximal femur and subsequent avascular necrosis is always significant. For this reason, many surgeons accept the position of an acute slip and pin it in situ.

In some cases, high-grade slipped capital femoral epiphysis does not remodel sufficiently with growth, despite treatment. In these cases, a residual, chronically painful limp is present, requiring correction by proximal femoral osteotomy. The osteotomy site may be at the level of the slip, which is mechanically effective but relatively risky for the blood supply. Alternatively, osteotomy can be performed at the trochanteric level; this is a safer procedure for correction of the functional deformity but does not resolve the exact anatomic deformity.

▶ Complications

A. Chondrolysis

In addition to the problems of impingement of the anterior metaphyseal prominence, which can impede motion, patients with slipped capital femoral epiphysis may rarely develop chondrolysis, a poorly understood degeneration of the hip articular cartilage. It may be painful and may progress to severe joint narrowing and degenerative changes within 6 months.

During chondrolysis, cartilage is replaced by fibrous tissue, the joint capsule thickens and contracts, and joint motion is lost. Typically, the joint stiffens in flexion, abduction, and external rotation. Radiographs reveal joint narrowing,

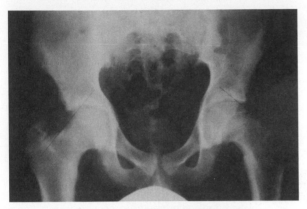

A

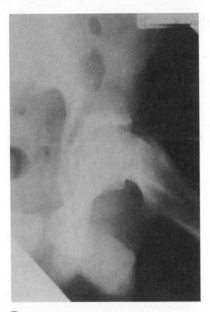

B

▲ **Figure 10–14.** Radiograph diagnosis of left slipped capital femoral epiphysis. **A:** Anteroposterior film shows subtle medial displacement of left epiphysis, best appreciated by drawing a line (Klein line) along the lateral side of the normal and abnormal femoral neck. The slipped epiphysis does not protrude lateral to this line. **B:** Frog-leg lateral radiograph clearly demonstrates posterior displacement.

irregularity, and subchondral sclerosis, as well as regional osteoporosis from disuse.

Chondrolysis can result from iatrogenic malposition (permanent penetration) of pins or screws used for fixation of slipped capital femoral epiphysis. Although brief penetrations during surgery are probably common and cause no complications, unrecognized permanent pin penetration is disastrous. Chondrolysis also appears without obvious penetration and occasionally is detected in patients before treatment begins.

Chondrolysis is treated by nonsteroidal anti-inflammatory drugs (NSAIDs), aggressive physical therapy and ROM exercises, and observation. Capsular release is sometimes useful in resistant cases. Approximately half of patients eventually recover satisfactory painless motion. The other half may require hip fusion for symptomatic relief.

B. Avascular Necrosis

Patients with an acutely slipped capital femoral epiphysis can develop avascular necrosis of the femoral head (see section on developmental dysplasia of the hip). These patients are usually teenagers so their hips lack potential for remodeling, and the prognosis is therefore poor. Yet, some patients with partial head involvement regain a painless hip after 1–2 years of symptoms. Some patients with painless but abnormal ROM may be treatable by intertrochanteric osteotomy to reorient the arc of motion. Long-term pain following avascular necrosis is treated by hip fusion.

▶ Prognosis

Slipped epiphysis is a major cause of early osteoarthritis. In general, the higher the degree of slip, the earlier the degenerative changes begin. In fact, a statistical increase in degenerative arthritis is evident even in the radiographically normal hip of patients with a contralateral slipped epiphysis. This suggests that subclinical bilateral involvement is more common than recognized.

Loder RT, Greenfield ML: Clinical characteristics of children with atypical and idiopathic slipped capital femoral epiphysis: description of the age-weight test and implications for further diagnostic investigation. *J Pediatr Orthop* 2001;21:481. [PMID: 11433161]

Peck D: Slipped capital femoral epiphysis: diagnosis and management. *Am Fam Physician* 2010;82:258. [PMID: 20672790]

Sankar WN, McPartland TG, Millis MB, Kim YJ: The unstable slipped capital femoral epiphysis: risk factors for osteonecrosis. *J Pediatr Orthop* 2010;30:544. [PMID: 20733417]

FOOT DISORDERS

1. Metatarsus Adductus

Metatarsus adductus (metatarsus varus) is the most common foot deformity in the newborn infant, occurring in 5 in 1000 live births, frequently bilaterally. Although it is usually isolated, several apparently unrelated deformities (such as DDH) are statistically more likely to occur in the presence of this disorder. The cause is unknown but might be related to so-called uterine packing.

▶ Clinical Findings

The hallmark of metatarsus adductus is medial deviation of the forefoot, with the apex of the deformity at the midtarsal region. The hindfoot is normal. A deep skin crease frequently is evident at the medial border of the foot, suggesting the deformity has been present for some time. The adducted forefoot usually can be passively corrected to a neutral position but occasionally is fairly rigid. Ankle motion is normal, without contracture of the gastrocnemius-soleus muscles.

▶ Treatment

Metatarsus adductus tends to be self-correcting. Even severe cases generally resolve by 12–18 months of age without treatment. Nevertheless, many orthopedists use passive stretching to reassure parents the child is being treated. There is no scientific evidence that passive correction and serial plaster casting will speed resolution of the disorder.

2. Congenital Clubfoot

▶ Essentials of Diagnosis

- Clubfoot is characterized by equinus, smaller foot size, smaller calf muscles, and stiffness of tarsal joints.
- Treatment with casting and minor surgical tenotomy is usually successful but technique dependent.
- Bracing for 1–4 years after cast correction improves the ultimate outcome.

Congenital clubfoot (equinovarus foot; talipes equinovarus) is a severe fixed deformity of the foot (Figure 10–15). It is characterized by fixed ankle plantar flexion (equinus), inversion and axial internal rotation of the subtalar (talocalcaneal) joint (varus), and medial subluxation of the talonavicular and calcaneocuboid joints (adductus). Severe cavus may be present, with a medial and plantar midfoot crease. Calf atrophy, while variable, is always present. Whether unilateral or bilateral, the deformity is more common in males, although when it occurs in females, it tends to be more severe.

The incidence in the newborn population is 1 in 1000, with increased risk for families in which even distant members have the deformity. There is considerable evidence that clubfoot is an inherited trait, but the disorder appears to reflect polygenetic expression, and exact inheritance patterns are unclear. Although most are isolated deformities and considered idiopathic, clubfoot may be present in association with a wide variety of syndromes that affect the musculoskeletal system.

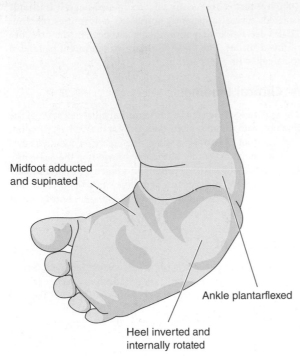

Midfoot adducted
and supinated

Ankle plantarflexed

Heel inverted and
internally rotated

▲ **Figure 10–15.** Clinical appearance of congenital right clubfoot.

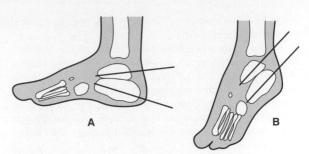

A   B

▲ **Figure 10–16.** Diagrammatic appearance of radiograph in clubfoot. **A:** Normal foot. **B:** Clubfoot.

▶ Clinical Findings

A. Symptoms and Signs

Clinical diagnosis of clubfoot is uncomplicated. Because it is a rigid deformity, clubfoot cannot be passively corrected the way metatarsus adductus can. Frequently, the foot is so severely internally rotated and inverted that the sole faces superiorly. Occasionally, the plantar flexion of the ankle is not obvious because the posterior tip of the calcaneus is small, high, and difficult to palpate. Clubfoot is always associated with a permanent decrease in calf circumference related to fibrosis of the calf musculature. This may not be obvious at birth but becomes more apparent after the child begins to walk.

Special attention should be paid to the presence of spine deformity, caudal dimpling, or midline spinal hairy patches, all of which may imply a neurogenic component. Thus, the examining physician should carefully search for features of other deformities or syndromes.

B. Imaging Studies

Increasingly, clubfoot is suspected from prenatal ultrasound examination. Radiographs are rarely of value in the initial clubfoot evaluation because the bones of the foot are minimally ossified at birth. Radiographs become more important if the physician is considering surgical intervention or if the child has reached walking age, and radiographs can quantify the completeness of correction achieved by casting or surgery.

The typical radiographic findings of incompletely treated clubfoot include the following features:

1. Presence of hindfoot plantar flexion

2. Lack of the normal angular relationship between the talus and calcaneus (so-called parallelism of talus and calcaneus)

3. Residual medial subluxation or displacement of the navicular on the talus and the cuboid on the calcaneus (Figure 10–16)

▶ Treatment

A. Manipulative Treatment

Clubfoot always requires treatment, which should begin at birth. The initial approach is passive manipulation and positioning to the corrected position. In the United States, the majority of orthopedists use serial manipulation and casting, usually at 1-week intervals in the first month of life, and at 1- to 2-week intervals thereafter if required. In other parts of the world, strapping (with adhesive tape) and splinting with a variety of braces are popular methods (in addition to serial casting) for maintaining the manipulated correction. When casting is performed, there is agreement that specific techniques are more likely to be successful. Even when the deformity responds to casting, there is usually sufficient Achilles tightness that a heel cord lengthening needs to be done at 4 weeks or later to facilitate cast correction.

The Ponseti method of casting has been widely adopted in many parts of the world as an effective cast protocol. In this method, a specific sequence of casts is applied weekly for 3–4 weeks, followed by early percutaneous Achilles tenotomy. After a brief additional period of casting, the foot position is maintained by use of a brace for up to 3 years, worn at nights and during naps.

B. Surgical Treatment

Most clubfeet are successfully treated with casting and limited release, but severe clubfeet (often associated with syndromes) may require more extensive surgery. Surgical correction of all clubfoot deformities is generally performed in one stage. At times, the casting corrects most of the midfoot deformity, and simple posterior release (ankle capsulotomy and Achilles tendon lengthening) are all that is required. Frequently, the surgeon must consider correction of the entire group of deformities through a comprehensive, extensive surgical approach.

One common approach uses the so-called Cincinnati incision, which extends from the navicular bone medially, around the superior portion of the heel, to the cuboid bone laterally (Figure 10–17). During surgery, the medial posterior tibial neurovascular bundle must be identified and protected. The tendons of the posterior tibialis, flexor digitorum longus, flexor hallucis longus, and Achilles tendon are Z-lengthened. The capsules of the talonavicular joint, subtalar (talocalcaneal) joint, and posterior ankle joint are released to allow repositioning of the bones of the hindfoot and midfoot.

The navicular is usually subluxated medially on the head of the talus and must be repositioned onto its normal location. The calcaneus is both inverted and internally rotated on the talus. This is corrected by manually derotating the subtalar joint and tilting the calcaneus back into a neutral position. These corrections are usually held in place after reduction by inserting small K-wires, which are removed after 4–6 weeks.

The ankle is repositioned by dorsiflexion to neutral prior to repair of the lengthened Achilles tendon. Postoperative casting allows the gaping capsule to reform with the bones of the clubfoot in their appropriate, corrected position.

C. Complications

Early complications of clubfoot surgery are rare, but the rate of recurrence within 3 years is 5–10%. Mild recurrence of deformity is fairly common, and even when deformity is permanently corrected, the foot always remains smaller and stiffer than normal and calf circumference is reduced. Families must be informed of this possibility early in treatment so they have realistic expectations about the outcome.

If surgical release is too aggressive, overcorrection with late heel valgus and an overlengthened heel cord can occur. There is broad agreement that a slightly underreleased clubfoot is much more functional than an overreleased one, and the trend to less surgery and more conservative treatment is currently strong.

Dobbs MB, Morcuende JA, Gurnett CA, et al: Treatment of idiopathic clubfoot: an historical review. *Iowa Orthop J* 2000;20:59. [PMID: 10934626]

Herzenberg JE, Radler C, Bor N: Ponseti versus traditional methods of casting for idiopathic clubfoot. *J Pediatr Orthop* 2002; 22:517. [PMID: 12131451]

Matos MA, de Oliveira LA: Comparison between Ponseti's and Kite's clubfoot treatment methods: a meta-analysis. *J Foot Ankle Surg* 2010;49:395. [PMID: 20610205]

Richards BS, Faulks S, Rathjen KE, Karol LA, Johnston CE, Jones SA: A comparison of two nonoperative methods of idiopathic clubfoot correction: the Ponseti method and the French functional (physiotherapy) method. *J Bone Joint Surg Am* 2008; 90:2313. [PMID: 18978399]

Zionts LE, Dietz FR: Bracing following correction of idiopathic clubfoot using the Ponseti method. *J Am Acad Orthop Surg* 2010;18:486. [PMID: 20675641]

Zionts LE, Zhao G, Hitchcock K, Maewal J, Ebramzadeh E: Has the rate of extensive surgery to treat idiopathic clubfoot declined in the United States? *J Bone Joint Surg Am* 2010;92:882. [PMID: 20360511]

3. Calcaneovalgus Foot

Calcaneovalgus foot is generally considered a uterine-packing problem in which the foot is markedly dorsiflexed at birth so the dorsum of the foot sits against the anterior surface of the tibia (Figure 10–18). The hindfoot is usually in moderate eversion (valgus) as well. Although some flexibility is present with the deformity, there is resistance to full motion, and most cases do not allow ankle plantar flexion beyond a right angle.

Despite its dramatic appearance, calcaneovalgus foot corrects spontaneously within 2–3 months. Although some orthopedists brace or apply serial casts and many recommend

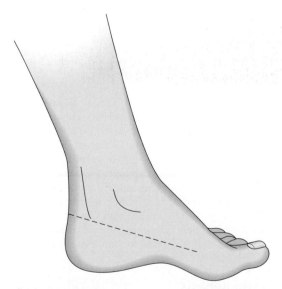

▲ **Figure 10–17.** Cincinnati incision used for surgical correction of clubfoot.

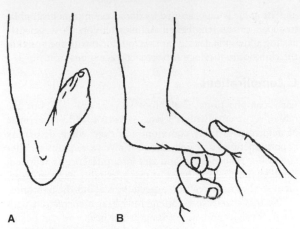

▲ **Figure 10–18.** Calcaneovalgus foot as it appears in relaxed position **(A)** and maximally plantar flexed **(B)**.

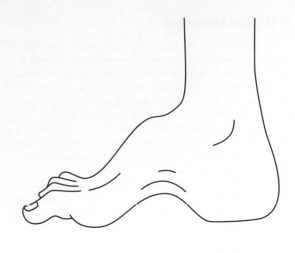

stretching exercises, all true calcaneovalgus feet resolve without treatment.

▶ Congenital Vertical Talus

Calcaneovalgus foot must be differentiated from a much rarer condition known as congenital vertical talus (congenital rocker-bottom foot, congenital complex pes valgus). In this deformity, although the foot appears to lie against the anterior tibia, the hindfoot is actually plantar flexed (positioned in equinus) because of contracture of the posterior calf muscles. To accommodate plantarflexion of the hindfoot and dorsiflexion of the forefoot, the midfoot joints (talonavicular and calcaneocuboid joints) must subluxate or dislocate dorsally.

Congenital vertical talus often accompanies genetic disorders, syndromes such as arthrogryposis, or neuromuscular disorders such as spina bifida. It is occasionally found in otherwise normal infants, however. Treatment is usually surgical, and casting frequently does not resolve the disorder.

4. Cavus Foot

Cavus foot is a foot with an abnormally high arch. Although it is difficult to ascribe a particular threshold of arching beyond which treatment is necessary, most deformities are dramatic enough to make diagnosis straightforward (Figure 10–19).

Cavus foot frequently accompanies hindfoot varus deformity (cavovarus foot), and there may be clawing of the toes and demonstrable weakness of ankle or foot muscles. In addition, calluses beneath the metatarsal heads and heel skin are common. Hindfoot varus in individuals with a cavovarus deformity is nonstructural if it can be corrected with the "block test," and surgical procedures directed at correcting the hindfoot deformity are not necessary. If the patient is symptomatic, the treatment of choice is plantar release with first metatarsal osteotomy and possible tendon transfers.

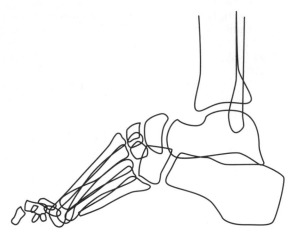

▲ **Figure 10–19.** Cavus foot: clinical appearance and radiographic appearance.

▶ Clinical Findings

One of the most common symptoms of cavus foot is anterior ankle pain, sometimes associated with toe walking. This paradoxical situation occurs because of the pathologic anatomy of the cavus foot. The forefoot is severely plantar flexed on the hindfoot, requiring marked ankle dorsiflexion to compensate. When the cavus becomes too severe, ankle dorsiflexion is blocked, leading to anterior ankle impingement and pain. The inability to dorsiflex further compromises forefoot clearance, and eventually, only the metatarsals can contact the floor. This can be misinterpreted as ankle plantarflexion contracture, leading to unnecessary (and possibly harmful) heel cord release.

▶ Pathogenesis

The cause of cavus foot is usually muscle imbalance in a growing foot. Thus, cavus is rarely found in early childhood

Table 10–6. Common neuromuscular causes of cavus foot.

Cerebral palsy
Charcot-Marie-Tooth disease
Compartment syndrome
Diastematomyelia
Friedrich ataxia
Muscular dystrophy
Spinal cord tumor
Spinal dysraphism (spina bifida)

but is fairly frequent after 8–10 years of age. Although intrinsic muscle weakness is a major cause of cavus foot, weakness of the peroneal or anterior tibialis muscles is also implicated. Cavus foot is rarely found in the absence of an underlying neuromuscular condition.

Cavus foot is a marker for neuromuscular disease. Diagnosis requires a thorough search for the underlying cause and may require neurologic consultation, spinal MRI, and electromyographic (EMG) studies. Table 10–6 lists common neuromuscular causes of cavus foot.

▶ Treatment

Conservative treatment of cavus foot includes accommodation by shoe modifications or inserts. These modalities do not actually correct the condition; severe deformity requires surgical correction by tendon transfers to restore muscle balance, by midfoot wedge osteotomy to correct bony deformity, or by triple arthrodesis (hindfoot fusion in a corrected position).

Schwend RM, Drennan JC: Cavus foot deformity in children. *J Am Acad Orthop Surg* 2003;11:201. [PMID: 12828450]

5. Pes Planus (Flatfoot)

Flatfoot refers to loss of the normal longitudinal arch of the medial foot. Many cases of flatfoot are inherited, and a careful family history may uncover other persons with the condition. The foot is usually flexible, so the arch appears when the foot is not bearing weight. Hindfoot valgus (heel eversion) is often present. In severe cases, flatfoot may be painful, but this aspect of the deformity is often overemphasized.

▶ Clinical Findings

Physical determination of the flexibility of the flatfoot requires careful examination. Subtalar motion is usually normal. In feet that exhibit a flat arch and valgus heel while standing, examination from the posterior aspect frequently discloses a normal arch and varus heel by muscle action when the patient stands on tiptoe. If these signs of a flexible flatfoot are not present, alternative diagnoses such as tarsal coalition (see section on tarsal coalition) should be considered. The physician should also look for painful plantar calluses.

▶ Imaging Studies

Standing radiographs disclose loss of the normal medial longitudinal arch and may show mild lateral subluxation of the talonavicular joint as well. In severe chronic cases, degenerative talonavicular spurring may be present.

▶ Treatment

Symptomatic treatment (shoe modifications, arch supports, and plantar inserts) is appropriate because no long-term treatment can alter the anatomic features of the disorder. Posterior tibial advancement, subtalar joint elevation or fusion, and elongation osteotomy of the lateral calcaneal neck are surgical options, but they may not provide reproducible, predictable resolution of the problem.

6. Tarsal Coalition

Tarsal coalition is a congenital connection between two or more tarsal bones. Coalitions may be fibrous, cartilaginous, or bony. Coalitions usually occur between two bones and are cartilaginous in early life but eventually ossify (or nearly ossify) as the foot matures. Frequently bilateral, coalitions often follow an autosomal dominant inheritance pattern.

The most common sites for tarsal coalition are between the calcaneus and the navicular laterally (Figure 10–20) and between the talus and the calcaneus medially.

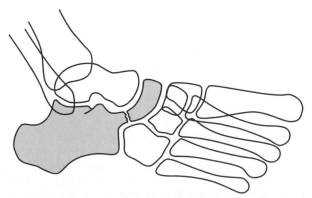

▲ **Figure 10–20.** Calcaneonavicular tarsal coalition is best seen on oblique radiograph projection.

▶ Clinical Findings

Symptoms of tarsal coalition may include foot pain and stiffness as the lesion begins to ossify during early adolescence. The resulting stiffness and abnormal intertarsal movement patterns in the hindfoot lead to progressive loss of subtalar motion and fixed valgus (eversion) of the heel. Tarsal coalition is often called peroneal spastic flatfoot because the peroneals appear to be protectively overactive. As the lesion matures, pain may diminish but stiffness increases, and the abnormal valgus posture persists.

This diagnosis should be suspected in adolescents with foot pain, valgus heel, and decreased subtalar motion.

▶ Imaging Studies

Lateral, anteroposterior, and oblique radiographs of the foot confirm the diagnosis of calcaneonavicular coalition, but special subtalar radiographs (Harris views), CT scan, or MRI may be necessary to delineate medial talocalcaneal lesions.

▶ Treatment

Not all coalitions require treatment. The decision to initiate treatment depends on the severity of pain, stiffness, and fixed valgus deformity. Conservative treatment consists of casting to reduce pain and peroneal spasm. If this fails, the coalition can be surgically resected and the resultant space filled with autologous fat or muscle to prevent recurrence. In late or neglected cases with pain or deformity, hindfoot fusion by triple arthrodesis is effective treatment for both symptoms.

Sankar WN, Weiss J, Skaggs DL: Orthopaedic conditions in the newborn. *J Am Acad Orthop Surg* 2009;17:112. [PMID: 19202124]

Yeagerman SE, Cross MB, Positano R, Doyle SM: Evaluation and treatment of symptomatic pes planus. *Curr Opin Pediatr* 2011;23:60. [PMID: 21169838]

7. Toe Deformities

Toe deformities occur as isolated conditions, in association with similar hand deformities, and as part of other syndromes. The more commonly found deformities are presented here, with mention of associated hand problems.

▶ Simple Syndactyly

Simple syndactyly, a connection of two or more toes, is the most common toe deformity. It is most common between the second and third toes. The webbing is usually complete. This disorder demonstrates a strongly familial inheritance pattern and causes no symptoms. It is rarely treated in the foot. In the hand, however, surgical separation is required to restore normal finger function.

▶ Polydactyly

Polydactyly is the presence of more than five digits on either the hands or the feet. It is frequently hereditary and often bilateral. Duplication of the thumbs may mirror duplication of the great toes, and both generally require surgical treatment. Both preaxial (duplication of medial toes and radial digits) and postaxial polydactyly (duplication of the lateral toes or ulnar digits) often accompany genetic syndromes and should prompt the physician to look for other symptoms. Treatment is by surgical excision at about 1 year of age; the actual surgery, particularly for medial duplications, may be complex.

8. Constriction Bands (Amniotic Bands) and Acrosyndactyly

During gestation, protein-laden amniotic material can condense around limb segments. These amniotic bands may indent delicate embryonic tissues, causing constriction rings or even necrosis and resorption of the distal segment (congenital amputation). Constriction bands may be isolated or associated with Streeter dysplasia. The syndactyly of Streeter dysplasia differs from simple syndactyly in that the distal, rather than proximal, web is obliterated (acrosyndactyly). It is thought to be an acquired, rather than hereditary, condition, caused by shearing of the delicate tips of the embryonic digits, followed by conjoined healing of distal digits. Although acrosyndactyly of the fingers must be released to allow independent function, acrosyndactyly of the toes is rarely symptomatic, and does not need treatment.

Constriction bands may be very deep and circumferential and occasionally must be released surgically by Z-plasty immediately after birth to avoid postnatal necrosis. Usually, only half of the circumference of a band is released at one time, to protect any remaining blood supply in the other half. Reports of successful one-stage resection and Z-plasty of constriction bands suggest that the remaining blood supply is probably subfascial and interosseous.

9. Adolescent Bunions (Hallux Valgus)

Although bunion (prominence of the medial metatarsophalangeal joint of the great toe) is rare in children, this troublesome deformity often requires treatment. It is frequently hereditary, usually seen in early adolescence, and almost always found in conjunction with a wide forefoot caused by varus (medial deviation) of the first metatarsal shaft (metatarsus primus varus). The wide forefoot allows severe lateral deviation of the great toe (hallux valgus), causing the prominent base of the great toe to rub against the inside of the shoe and create a painful bunion (Figure 10–21).

Although conservative measures may relieve discomfort, many adolescent bunions are progressive and require surgical management. Surgery must address each aspect of the deformity. The surgeon must trim the bunion, correct the varus

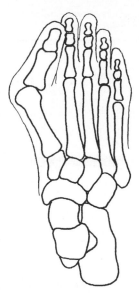

▲ **Figure 10–21.** Adolescent bunion (hallux valgus) is generally accompanied by a wide forefoot with splaying of the first metatarsal (metatarsus primus varus).

angulation of the first metatarsal by osteotomy, and centralize and balance the hallux valgus by lengthening the adductor hallucis muscle. There is a fairly high incidence of recurrence of the deformity following surgery.

Johnson AE, Georgopoulos G, Erickson MA, et al: Treatment of adolescent hallux valgus with the first metatarsal double osteotomy: the Denver experience. *J Pediatr Orthop* 2004;24:358. [PMID: 15205615]

TORSIONAL AND ANGULAR DEFORMITIES OF THE KNEE AND LEG

▶ Essentials of Diagnosis

- Most torsional deformities are benign and self-correcting with growth.
- Angular deformities at the knee, particularly genu varum, must be distinguished from more common physiologic variants, since they often need early treatment.

Torsional (rotational) and angular deformities are a major source of referrals to pediatric orthopedic surgeons (Figure 10–22). Most of these patients are young (<5 years) and have internal rotational deformities resulting in a so-called pigeon-toed gait.

The internal rotation, which can occur at the level of the thigh, leg (shin), or foot, is a cosmetic problem. Little evidence indicates that any of the so-called torsional deformities are harmful to the child or cause significant disability in the adult. Angular deformities (usually varus or valgus at

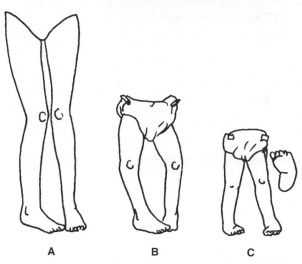

▲ **Figure 10–22.** The major causes of clinical in-toeing include increased femoral anteversion **(A)**, internal tibial torsion **(B)**, and metatarsus adductus **(C)**.

the knee) are also usually benign, although careful evaluation and workup, including radiographic or other imaging modalities, occasionally disclose conditions requiring treatment. Nevertheless, most torsional and angular deformities are physiologic variations of normal anatomy, and they correct spontaneously over time.

▶ Increased Femoral Anteversion

The normal femoral neck does not lie exactly in the frontal (coronal) plane but rather projects anteriorly from the plane at an angle called the angle of anteversion (Figure 10–23).

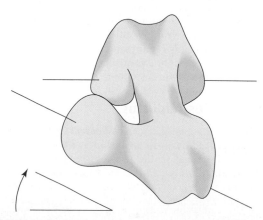

▲ **Figure 10–23.** The angle of anteversion describes the inclination of the femoral neck forward of (anterior to) the frontal plane.

Infants have anteversion of as much as 40 degrees, but this angle gradually reduces with growth, so normal adult femurs exhibit anteversion of 15 degrees. In some children, this gradual regression is slow or incomplete, causing the child to have excessive anteversion compared with an average child of the same age. This excessive anteversion produces a relative increase in internal femoral rotation, since the hip joint seeks to center itself regardless of the rotational profile of the femur. The clinical manifestation of this increased internal rotation and decreased external rotation of the hip is in-toeing during walking.

Observation of the walking child discloses internal rotation of the entire femur by the medial position of the patella. Although parents may consider this pigeon-toed gait unsightly, increased femoral anteversion is a normal variant that has no effect on function.

Increased femoral anteversion gradually decreases, with improvement in in-toeing, until 9–11 years of age. Subsequently, persistent in-toeing in the adult becomes more likely. Increased femoral anteversion requires no treatment.

▶ Internal Tibial Torsion

Some infants are born with a relatively dramatic internal twisting (torsion) of the tibia that makes the foot and ankle appear markedly rotated inward, relative to the axis of the knee. This internal tibial torsion is usually bilateral, frequently familial, and inevitably a normal variant in the wide torsional range seen in infants.

Internal tibial torsion can be clinically measured by comparing the bimalleolar axis (imaginary line connecting the medial and lateral malleoli of the ankle) with the frontal plane of the knee as determined by the position of the patella.

Torsion of 30–40 degrees is not uncommon in the newborn. When the child starts to walk, torsion can cause significant in-toeing, which, in turn, causes excessive tripping.

With growth, internal tibial torsion spontaneously resolves, and normal foot position and walking eventually occur. Some children improve by 24 months of age but may require up to 4 years for full resolution of the torsion. Internal tibial torsion requires no treatment. There is no scientific evidence that braces or shoe modifications alter the natural correction of the deformity.

▶ Metatarsus Adductus

Metatarsus adductus may cause apparent in-toeing in the young child, leading to its inclusion as a torsional deformity. It is described in the previous section on the foot (Table 10–7).

Staheli LT, Corbett M, Wyss C, King H: Lower-extremity rotational problems in children. Normal values to guide management. *J Bone Joint Surg Am* 1985;67:39. [PMID: 3968103]

Table 10–7. In-toeing summary.

	Metatarsus Adductus	Internal Tibial Torsion	Internal Femoral Torsion (Increased Femoral Anteversion)
Age at resolution	12 months	3–4 years	9–10 years
Leg position	Femur and tibia normal	Patella forward; foot/ankle internally rotated	Patella internally rotated
Hip examination	Normal	Normal	Internal rotation exceeds external rotation

▶ Bowlegs, Knock-Knee, and Genu Varum

Many infants have bilateral symmetric bowing of the legs, which may persist in the first 1–2 years of walking before developing into an exaggerated knock-kneed condition. The knock-knee is most dramatic at 3–6 years of age when it is known as physiologic genu valgum. At this time, the anatomic angle may be as high as 15–20 degrees of valgus. The genu valgum then gradually remodels spontaneously to the adult average value of 5–7 degrees of valgus.

Bowing of the legs in infants and excessive valgus of the knees in children 6 years of age are normal phenomena that require no treatment, although parents may have to be reassured that the condition is benign. The rare case of bowing that persists beyond 3 years of age may require further evaluation or treatment. Following are disorders that cause bowing.

A. Internal Tibial Torsion

Internal tibial torsion may masquerade as bowing when the child walks with the feet forward and the knees rotated externally rather than internally. As the laterally facing knees flex, they give the appearance of bowlegs. Careful physical examination discloses internal tibial torsion, which spontaneously resolves by 4 years of age. As the torsion corrects, the apparent bowlegs disappear.

B. Blount Disease

Also known as tibia vara, Blount disease is a poorly understood loss of medial tibial physeal growth that causes progressive bowing of the leg (Figure 10–24). It may occur as early as 3 years of age and can be bilateral or unilateral. If unilateral, the condition may be suspected earlier because it is obvious by comparison with the other leg. Excessive loading of the knee by early walking in heavy children with physiologic bowing of the legs may contribute to the development

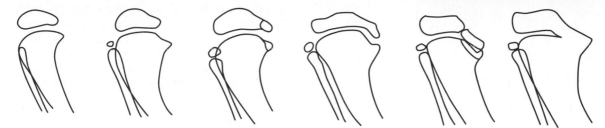

▲ **Figure 10–24.** The Langenskiöld diagrammatic classification of radiographic changes in Blount disease (infantile tibia vara). The higher grades are associated with permanent closure of the medial tibial physis, which leads to progressive varus and internal rotation deformity with growth.

of Blount disease, but this is not proven. It occurs in all racial groups but is particularly common in blacks and Hispanic children.

Diagnosis of Blount disease is based on radiographic evidence of decreased medial tibial physeal growth. Later, the medial articular surface is distorted and the medial physis fuses. This causes progressive angular deformity to develop as the lateral growth plate continues elongating while the medial side is tethered.

Spontaneous resolution of adolescent tibia vara is uncommon but can occur in mild cases. Although some orthopedists recommend bracing to assist the process, there is no consensus that this is necessary or effective.

Severe or progressive cases of Blount disease require surgical correction by tibial osteotomy to regain the normal physiologic valgus angle of the knee. Surgery reduces the physiologic load on the medial tibial plateau and may allow normal growth. Slight overcorrection of the bowing often ensures load reduction, and the resulting valgus slowly resolves as the child grows.

Surgical treatment early in life is now popular, and many orthopedists recommend osteotomy after 3–4 years of age if radiographic changes are present. In early cases, surgical correction may cause reversal before there is permanent growth arrest that would require physeal bridge resection and/or repeated osteotomies. Once physeal bridging occurs, however, there is no alternative to repeated surgical correction of angular deformity and leg-length inequality until growth ceases at maturity. Surgical elevation of the medial tibial plateau is a procedure that is occasionally necessary in individuals with early-onset Blount disease but is not indicated for individuals with late-onset Blount disease. Distal femoral varus deformity is commonly present and must be addressed as well. Controlled studies of the issues involved in treatment of Blount disease by bracing and surgery are not available.

C. Rickets

Metabolic disorders of calcium intake (nutritional rickets) can decrease the rate of calcification and ossification of physeal cartilage, causing the development of softer bones that are prone to bowing. Vitamin and calcium dietary supplements have virtually eliminated nutritional rickets in the United States. Hypophosphatemic rickets was discussed earlier in the section on metabolic bone disease.

Jones JK, Gill L, John M, Goddard M, Hambleton IR: Outcome analysis of surgery for Blount disease. *J Pediatr Orthop* 2009; 29:730. [PMID: 20104154]

Rab GT: Oblique tibial osteotomy revisited. *J Child Orthop* 2010; 4:169. [PMID: 20234769]

▶ Tibial Bowing and Pseudarthrosis

The tibia has a propensity to exhibit congenital angular deformities (bowing of the tibial shaft), which, although rare, are significant. The direction of the bowing is important in both diagnosis and prognosis and usually detectable at birth. Bowing direction is described by the apex of the bow, not the direction of displacement of the distal part (Figure 10–25).

A. Congenital Posteromedial Bowing of Tibia

Congenital posteromedial bowing of the tibia is a unilateral birth deformity of the distal fourth of the tibia. The apex of the bow is posteromedial, and often a skin dimple is present over the area. Because of the angle of bowing (often approximately 50 degrees) and the proximity to the ankle joint, the clinical appearance often mimics calcaneovalgus foot. The spatial position of the ankle joint, however, not the foot itself, is responsible for the deformity. Radiographs of posteromedial bowing disclose the curvature of the distal tibia, often with sclerosis in the underlying section of bone.

Despite its dramatic appearance, posteromedial tibial bowing corrects spontaneously in all cases. Some recommend casting to bring the dorsiflexed foot down to plantigrade position, but because the actual deformity is not related to the foot, this advice is not logical: Patients who are never casted resolve as quickly as those who are.

The tibial curvature remodels enough by 3 years of age that the limb appears cosmetically straight, although some

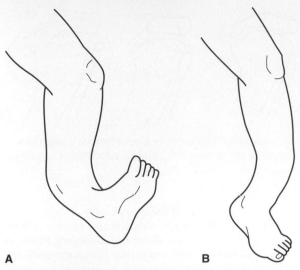

▲ **Figure 10–25.** The major types of tibial bowing.
A: Posteromedial bowing. The angulation spontaneously corrects, but with limb-length inequality. **B:** Anterolateral bowing. This disorder eventually progresses to spontaneous tibial fracture with resistant pseudarthrosis (see text).

bowing may be evident on radiograph for 5–8 years. All patients with posteromedial bowing are left with a leg-length discrepancy. At maturity, the involved limb is relatively as much shorter than the longer limb as it was at birth, usually in the range of 4 cm. The residual limb-length discrepancy presents the greatest challenge but can usually be handled with limb-lengthening techniques. Therefore, although the angular deformity needs no treatment, long-term follow-up and treatment of limb inequality are necessary.

B. Congenital Anterolateral Bowing of Tibia and Congenital Pseudarthrosis of the Tibia

Congenital anterolateral bowing of the tibia and congenital pseudarthrosis of the tibia represent the other extreme of tibial bowing. For reasons not understood, anterolateral bowing in the tibia and fibula is associated with inevitable progressive sclerosis and atrophy of the tibial shaft underlying the deformity. The ultimate fate of this atrophic abnormal bone is spontaneous fracture, which does not heal readily as most fractures in children do (ie, pseudarthrosis). Some children with this condition are born with a tibial fracture, whereas others simply have anterolateral bowing and sclerosis at birth, with fractures occurring up to 8–10 years of age. In approximately 50% of cases, confirmed neurofibromatosis is present.

All children with variations of this disorder require treatment. Because the prognosis is worse for those whose fracture occurs at a younger age, treatment methods vary. If anterolateral bowing is present but fracture has not occurred, protective bracing may be helpful. The fracture may heal in children whose first fracture occurs at 8 years or older, using prolonged casting or surgical bone grafting (with or without internal fixation).

Bone grafting in children whose fracture occurs before 3 years of age almost always fails, although repeated attempts to graft show some success.

The dismal results with conventional treatment of congenital pseudarthrosis of the tibia in younger patients prompted some surgeons to try innovative treatments. Electrical stimulation, free microvascular transfer of the fibula, and Ilizarov transport of normal bone to the defect are all reported to improve the success of treatment. So much surgery may be required to achieve a functional result, however, that many patients eventually undergo amputation to achieve rapid return to the normal functional activities of childhood.

Feldman DS, Jordan C, Fonseca L: Orthopaedic manifestations of neurofibromatosis type 1. *J Am Acad Orthop Surg* 2010;18:346. [PMID: 20511440]

Tudisco C, Bollini G, Dungl P, et al: Functional results at the end of skeletal growth in 30 patients affected by congenital pseudarthrosis of the tibia. *J Pediatr Orthop B* 2000;9:94. [PMID: 10868385]

Vander Have KL, Hensinger RN, Caird M, Johnston C, Farley FA: Congenital pseudarthrosis of the tibia. *J Am Acad Orthop Surg* 2008;16:228. [PMID: 18390485]

KNEE DISORDERS

1. Discoid Meniscus

The normal menisci of the knee are semilunar in shape and wedge shaped in cross section. They deepen the flat tibial articular surface to allow cupping of the rounded femoral condyles. The medial meniscus is longer and narrower than the lateral meniscus.

Rarely, the lateral meniscus remains congenitally round (or discoid) instead of acquiring its normal semilunar shape (Figure 10–26). This reduces its cupping function and may cause some instability of either the lateral compartment of the knee or of the lateral meniscus itself.

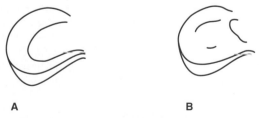

▲ **Figure 10–26.** **A:** Normal lateral meniscus. **B:** Discoid lateral meniscus, which may cause clicking, effusion, or pain.

Clinical Findings

The classic physical finding of discoid meniscus is loud clicking over the lateral meniscus during flexion and extension of the knee. This clicking is usually painless but may be accompanied by aching or effusion. Physical exam may demonstrate an extension block. Discoid meniscus may be suspected on radiograph by widening of the lateral knee compartment, a subtle increase in subchondral sclerosis laterally, and convexity of the lateral tibial articular surface. Confirmation is attained on arthrography or MRI. The abnormal mechanical function of discoid lateral meniscus makes it susceptible to tears, particularly in children older than 10 years.

Treatment

In the past, symptomatic discoid menisci were treated by total lateral meniscectomy, but the resultant late degenerative knee changes dictate a far more conservative course. Current practice is to avoid treatment unless symptoms are significant and disabling. If treatment is required, the safest approach appears to be arthroscopic removal of the central portion of the discoid shape, thus sculpting the lateral meniscus into a roughly semilunar form.

Good CR, Green DW, Griffith MH, Valen AW, Widmann RF, Rodeo SA: Arthroscopic treatment of symptomatic discoid meniscus in children: classification, technique, and results. *Arthroscopy* 2007;23:157. [PMID: 17276223]

Kramer DE, Micheli LJ: Meniscal tears and discoid meniscus in children: diagnosis and treatment. *J Am Acad Orthop Surg* 2009;17:698. [PMID: 19880680]

2. Chondromalacia and Internal Derangements of the Knee

Patellar chondromalacia and patellar subluxation are common in active adolescents, particularly in females who have small patellas and a slight exaggeration of knee valgus and quadriceps (Q) angle. Meniscal and ligament injuries are managed as in the adult, although these injuries are not as common in children.

A somewhat more conservative approach to suspect internal knee derangements is warranted in most children. The diagnostic accuracy of both physical exam and complex imaging studies (such as MRI) is surprisingly low in children. False-positive MRIs are particularly typical in children.

These disorders are described in Chapter 2, "Musculoskeletal Trauma Surgery," and Chapter 3, "Sports Medicine."

3. Osteochondritis Dissecans

Osteochondritis dissecans is a poorly understood disorder most commonly of the distal femoral condyle ossification

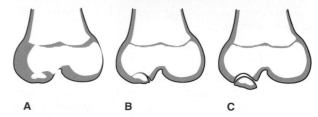

▲ **Figure 10–27.** Various forms of the osteochondritis dissecans lesion found in children. **A:** Defect in ossification center without cartilage defect. **B:** Lesion with a hinged flap. **C:** Complete separation of bone and cartilage, which can lead to loose body in the knee joint.

center, although other joints (talus, elbow) can be affected. A portion of the joint surface softens, shears, or separates through the articular cartilage and underlying bone (Figure 10–27). This disorder is common, but not exclusive, in children 8–14 years of age; however, it is an infrequent problem in the adult.

The disease appears to be caused by a combination of two factors: (1) mechanical shearing or injury from activity and (2) femoral condyle susceptibility (fragility) resulting from immature ossification of the femoral condyle (which can be quite irregular in children). The importance of each factor depends on age. Athletic trauma seems more important in older children and adults, whereas in younger children, ossification defects render the femoral condyle more susceptible to minor repetitive injury.

Clinical Findings

A. Symptoms and Signs

Symptoms and physical findings can be highly variable. Younger children may have an asymptomatic radiographic abnormality of condylar fragmentation or may simply have a vague aching after strenuous activity. Older children and adults may have pain, effusion, and locking or catching if the affected fragment actually separates and becomes a loose body in the knee joint.

B. Imaging Studies

Plain radiographs show an irregular fragment of the surface that is usually sclerotic but may be osteopenic and is usually on the lateral side of the medial condyle. It is often necessary to obtain tangential views of the condyle such as notch views. Occasionally, the defect is visible only on lateral projection. Contralateral comparison views should always be obtained. So-called ossification defects that mimic osteochondritis dissecans may be normal ossification fronts, seen to be bilateral and symmetric.

In children older than 11–12 years, MRI or arthrography is used to determine whether the underlying bone alone is involved or whether there is an actual separation of overlying cartilage. Although these studies are helpful in refining treatment strategy in this age group, they are seldom useful in younger children.

▶ Treatment

Young children with asymptomatic osteochondritis dissecans need not be treated because most of these lesions heal spontaneously. In preadolescents with symptoms or with large lesions seen on radiographs, simple immobilization with either a knee immobilizer or cylinder cast for 6 weeks frequently heals the defect and eliminates symptoms.

Sometimes immobilization is not effective, though. If the lesion is large and accompanied by cartilage separation or displacement, or if the skeleton has reached maturity, treatment may be the same as in the adult. This includes arthroscopic debridement and stabilization of the loose fragment using pins for internal fixation. Excision is less likely to result in a good result. The presence of open physes may necessitate modifications of standard adult techniques.

Gudas R, Simonaityte R, Cekanauskas E, Tamosiūnas R: A prospective, randomized clinical study of osteochondral autologous transplantation versus microfracture for the treatment of osteochondritis dissecans in the knee joint in children. *J Pediatr Orthop* 2009;29:741. [PMID: 20104156]

Kocher MS, DiCanzio J, Zurakowski D, Micheli LJ: Diagnostic performance of clinical examination and selective magnetic resonance imaging in the evaluation of intraarticular knee disorders in children and adolescents. *Am J Sports Med* 2001;29:292. [PMID: 11394597]

4. Ligament and Epiphyseal Injury

Children who have not reached skeletal maturity have far fewer major ligament injuries of the knee than do older children and adults. Smaller children tend to participate in lower impact activities and sports, and their lack of muscle bulk (which increases during adolescence) limits body acceleration and the force of collision. In addition, ligaments are relatively strong in the immature skeleton compared with bone or cartilaginous physes. Therefore, physeal fractures and bony avulsions of ligament attachments are more likely than traumatic ruptures of the ligaments themselves.

Residual instability may occur in the child's knee after varus or valgus injury. In the adult, such instability is considered clinical evidence of ligament injury. In children, however, the physis rather than the ligament may be the site of failure. Instability can be caused by a physeal fracture that hinges open rather than the joint opening (Figure 10–28). It is usually clinically obvious that fracture is present, although stress radiographs may help in questionable cases.

Major intraarticular disruptions of the knee joint (meniscal tear or cruciate ligament injury) are rare in children. Detection may be delayed because symptoms may be less severe than in the adult and their presence not given as much weight in the differential diagnosis. Meniscus injury,

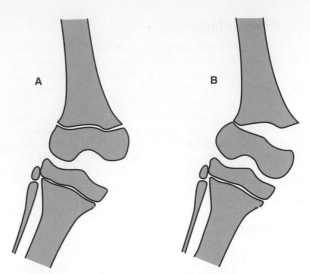

▲ **Figure 10–28.** Stress radiograph of the unstable knee in an immature patient may reveal ligament rupture **(A)** or separation of the femoral physis **(B)**.

particularly when peripheral, may lend itself to arthroscopic repair because of the excellent blood supply in children. Anterior cruciate rupture can be difficult to manage surgically in children because the anatomic sites of the tibial or femoral physes limit the options for reattachment. With the exception of cruciate injuries, most childhood knee ligament injuries are treatable by 2–4 weeks of splinting and return to function, as tolerated by pain. Physical therapy is rarely necessary in children younger than 15 years. A review of the major signs, symptoms, diagnostic procedures, and treatment options can be found in Chapter 3, "Sports Medicine."

▶ Differential Diagnosis

Not all effusions in the knee are traumatic, particularly in younger children. Because children at play are always suffering minor injuries, a history of injury may be inaccurate. The physician must remember to consider septic arthritis and pauciarticular juvenile rheumatoid arthritis in the differential diagnosis of effusion.

Beasley LS, Chudik SC: Anterior cruciate ligament injury in children: update of current treatment options. *Curr Opin Pediatr* 2003;15:45. [PMID: 12544271]

Luhmann SJ: Acute traumatic knee effusions in children and adolescents. *J Pediatr Orthop* 2003;23:199. [PMID: 12649021]

OSGOOD-SCHLATTER DISEASE

The proximal tibial physis contains a transverse component that contributes to longitudinal growth and an anterior tongue that contains the attachment of the patellar tendon.

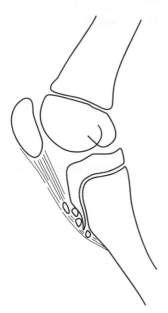

▲ **Figure 10–29.** Osgood-Schlatter disease. The radiographs would show characteristic fragmentation of the tibial tubercle apophysis, similar to diagram.

In preadolescent and adolescent children (usually boys), the distal tip of this tongue may undergo fragmentation from chronic tensile stress and enlargement from the resultant hyperemic response, which is known as Osgood-Schlatter disease. As the tibial tubercle becomes increasingly prominent, a painful bursa can form over it.

▶ **Clinical Findings**

Symptoms vary from mild aching at the tubercle to severe pain with patellar function and exaggerated bursal tenderness. Radiographs of the lateral proximal tibia show the characteristic fragmentation (Figure 10–29).

▶ **Treatment**

Treatment is symptomatic, including analgesics, knee pads to avert direct pressure, quadriceps stretching, avoidance of sports activities, and brief casting or splinting for painful cases. The disorder resolves spontaneously when the physis closes at skeletal maturity. No evidence indicates that physical activity within the limits of pain is harmful to the child with Osgood-Schlatter disease.

Adirim TA, Cheng TL: Overview of injuries in the young athlete. *Sports Med* 2003;33:75. [PMID: 12477379]

Krause BL, Williams JP, Catterall A: Natural history of Osgood-Schlatter disease. *J Pediatr Orthop* 1990;10:65. [PMID: 2298897]

SPINAL CURVATURE

Spinal curvature may occur in any age group and present with variable findings. Curvatures may be idiopathic, congenital, or accompany a wide variety of neuromuscular disorders, tumors, and infections. Curvatures may be small and nonprogressive or may worsen and require aggressive treatment. Sometimes, spinal curvature is the first clue to important underlying disease. Figure 10–30 shows the different types of spinal deformities.

▶ **Types of Curvatures**

A. Scoliosis

Scoliosis is a lateral spinal curvature in the frontal plane, best appreciated by physical examination from the patient's back and by anteroposterior radiographs. Curvatures, which may be single or multiple, are described by the direction of their convexity. In a flexible spine, the presence of a single (more rigid) curvature can lead to physiologic compensatory curvatures in the opposite direction, above and below the primary curvature. True scoliosis always includes a rotational component that may not be fully appreciated on radiograph and generally includes a lordotic component as well (see section on lordosis). Surprisingly, lateral curvature is often undetected externally. The rotation of vertebrae that accompanies scoliosis is the physical feature that allows clinical detection.

B. Kyphosis

Kyphosis is a forward (flexed) curvature of the spine in the sagittal plane, best appreciated from the side and by lateral

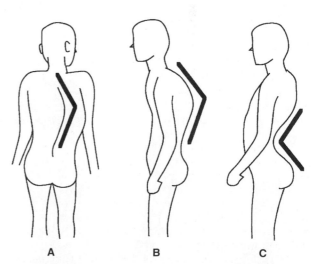

▲ **Figure 10–30.** Definitions of spinal deformities. **A:** Scoliosis. **B:** Kyphosis. **C:** Lordosis. Frequently, a combination of deformities occurs in individual patients (ie, kyphoscoliosis).

radiographs. If kyphosis is acutely angular, a posterior prominence called a gibbus may be evident in the sagittal plane.

C. Lordosis

Lordosis is a hyperextension deformity of the spine, most common in the lumbar spine but also often accompanying scoliosis. Lumbar lordosis may be secondary to flexion contracture of the hip.

▶ Detection of Curvature

Although spinal curvatures may be detected first during routine radiograph, most lesions are best diagnosed by physical examination. Spinal examination should proceed according to the following specific protocol:

1. Place the patient in the standing position (Figure 10–31).

2. Check the level of the pelvis and look for obvious asymmetry of the rib, scapula, neck, and shoulder height (leg-length inequality can cause apparent scoliosis, which disappears when the short leg is elevated on blocks).

3. Level the pelvis by seating the child on a firm surface if the pelvis cannot be leveled while standing. This is the case in children with hip contracture from neuromuscular disease.

4. Have the child bend forward, carefully noting any asymmetric prominence of the lumbar paraspinous muscle, rib cage, or scapula, which suggests the rotational portion of scoliosis. The magnitude of asymmetry corresponds to the severity of the curvature, with convexity of the curvature directed toward the most prominent side.

5. From the side, check for prominence of the spine that might indicate kyphosis, both in the upright and forward-bending position.

6. Perform a careful neurologic exam, including upper extremity reflexes and abdominal reflexes in addition to thorough lower extremity neurologic examination.

7. Use radiographs to assess type, severity, and location of the curvature and to look for underlying lesions. Because primary scoliosis and kyphosis curvatures are always stiffer than uninvolved spine segments, bending radiographs may reveal which curvatures are "structural" and which are more flexible compensations (secondary curvature). The Cobb method is usually used to measure curvatures (Figure 10–32). The degree of tilt between the most affected vertebral endplates describes curvature magnitude.

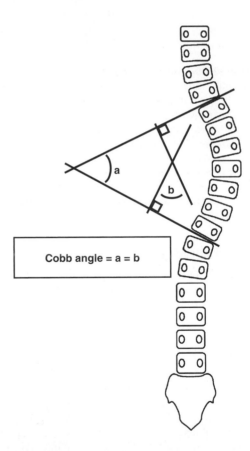

▲ **Figure 10–32.** The Cobb method of measurement is commonly used to assess spinal curvature. It measures the angle between the far (top and bottom) endplates of the most inclined vertebrae. To allow the measurement lines to fit on the radiograph, lines at 90-degree angles to the endplates are often drawn, and their relative angles measured. Geometrically, these angles are the same.

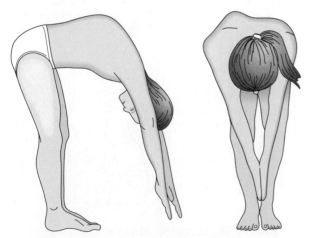

▲ **Figure 10–31.** Examination of the spine for deformity is best carried out by observing for asymmetry and deformity as the patient bends forward (see text).

▶ Scoliosis

A. Idiopathic Scoliosis

Idiopathic scoliosis has no apparent underlying cause and can be separated into adolescent (>10 years), juvenile (3–10 years), and infantile (<3 years). Adolescent idiopathic scoliosis accounts for 80% of all idiopathic scoliosis and is found most commonly in early adolescent girls, although it can be found in either gender at any age. There is typically a convex curvature to the right in the thoracic portion of the spine (right thoracic curve pattern). Patients with atypical curvature patterns, such as left thoracic curves and idiopathic curvature in younger children may require more extensive testing (eg, EMG, MRI) before the cause can be definitively designated idiopathic.

Many idiopathic curvatures progress in magnitude with growth and continue to do so until skeletal maturity. Therefore, the clinician must determine if the curvature is progressing and if the spine is still growing. Radiographs document progression, and observations of the ossification pattern of the iliac crest apophysis (Risser sign) are used to estimate skeletal maturity. This ossification pattern begins laterally at puberty and spreads medially across the ilium, capping and fusing with the bone at maturity. A variety of spinal braces are available to treat progression of idiopathic scoliosis, although there is debate about their actual effectiveness. Progressive curves in children with substantial growth potential (Risser 2), any curve of greater than 30 degrees, or patients with a curve of greater than 20–25 degrees with more than 5 degrees of documented progression should be treated. Children who mature with small curves have no symptoms and no progression in adulthood. Specifically, curves smaller than 35–40 degrees in adults generally do not progress. If a curvature progresses despite adequate bracing, surgery is the treatment of choice. Some curves are too rigid to brace effectively and can only be observed if they are relatively small. Bracing may help with curves up to 40 or 45 degrees, but for curves that exceed this magnitude, bracing is generally ineffective.

Surgery for scoliosis corrects the deformity using metal rods that can be configured to push, pull, distract, or compress portions of the spine with curvature. The involved spinal segments are then fused together using iliac or allograft bone. Typically, a posterior fusion of the laminas and facets is sufficient for many cases of idiopathic scoliosis. Severe cases may also require anterior fusion through the thorax or retroperitoneal space.

In those with juvenile scoliosis with more than a 20-degree Cobb angle, there is about a 20% prevalence of a neurologic abnormality. Therefore, workup in these children should include an MRI of the entire spine.

Lastly, infantile idiopathic scoliosis occurs more commonly in boys, with a 3 to 1 male-to-female ratio. Spinal cord abnormalities have about 20% prevalence, similar to juvenile idiopathic scoliosis. Hip dysplasia and congenital heart disease are also associated with the condition. Spontaneous correction occurs in some individuals. In others, the curves progress, and this can be predicted by the rib vertebral angle difference or the phase of the rib head. Rib overlap of the apical vertebral body or a rib vertebral angle difference of greater than 20 degrees indicates that the curve is likely to progress. Gender, family history, and age at presentation have not been found to be risk factors for progression.

B. Congenital Scoliosis

Congenital scoliosis is caused by malformations of vertebral shape. It does not refer to the age of the patient: Newborns can have idiopathic scoliosis, despite being born with spinal curvatures. Congenital vertebral malformations generally occur in early embryonic life (before 7 weeks) and are thought to represent errors in formation or segmentation of the spinal segments that originate from primitive mesenchymal condensations of embryonic cells (Figure 10–33).

Curvatures can originate when vertebral parts fail to form (eg, hemivertebrae, wedge vertebrae, butterfly vertebrae) or when embryonic somites fail to segment properly into individual vertebrae (eg, block vertebrae, unilateral unsegmented bar). Because of the embryonic timing of this process, children with congenital scoliosis frequently have abnormalities of other organ systems that form during the same embryonic period. About 60% of patients with congenital anomalies of the spine have other associated findings. The spine develops around the same time as the cardiovascular system, the genitourinary system, and the musculoskeletal system. Around 20% of patients with congenital scoliosis have an associated urologic abnormality. Approximately 25% of patients with congenital scoliosis have an associated cardiac defect. Diagnosis of congenital scoliosis must be followed by a careful cardiac examination and by ultrasound or intravenous pyelography evaluation of the kidneys. Spinal cord abnormalities may be present in as many as 30%, so evaluation of the spinal canal (MRI, EMG) may be required, especially if surgery is contemplated.

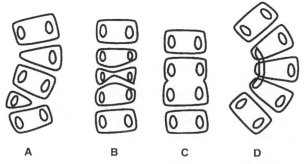

▲ **Figure 10–33.** Vertebral anomalies of congenital scoliosis. **A:** Hemivertebra. **B:** Butterfly vertebra. **C:** Block vertebra. **D:** Unilateral unsegmented bar.

Congenital scoliosis may encompass one or many deformed vertebrae, and different types of vertebral abnormalities are often seen in the same patient. Sometimes, two deforming vertebrae "cancel each other out" and no curvature is visible. For this reason, prediction of progression of the scoliosis depends on serial radiographs. If progression occurs, bracing is usually the first treatment, although surgery is indicated if progression is not halted by external means. Curvatures caused by unilateral unsegmented bars have such a strong tendency to progress that they should be treated by surgery as soon as they are detected.

C. Neuromuscular Scoliosis

Neuromuscular scoliosis includes a diverse group of curvature patterns that occur in association with various neuromuscular diseases. The cause varies with the disease. For example, scoliosis in children with cerebral palsy is usually caused by a combination of spasticity (overactivity of muscle) and weakness. Scoliosis in children with muscular dystrophy is the result of severe progressive muscle weakness that eliminates the paraspinous stability of the spinal column. Scoliosis in infants with spina bifida (myelomeningocele) is frequently congenital (see previous discussion), related to loss of posterior elements, or associated with the development of a syrinx (central cystic fluid collection) in the spinal cord, a process similar to hydrocephalus.

Patients with neuromuscular scoliosis often develop curvatures at an early age, when surgical treatment is either impossible or would result in severe stunting of spinal growth. It is common to treat such children by daytime bracing, despite the fact that bracing alone is rarely sufficient to eliminate progression or the need for later surgery. In such cases, some surgeons feel that bracing may slow progression enough to allow additional skeletal growth, and spinal correction and fusion are postponed until puberty.

D. Other Scolioses

Childhood scoliosis can be associated with benign tumors of the spine, usually osteoid osteoma and osteoblastoma. Treatment of the tumor is usually curative, although long-standing lesions may require fusion as well.

Neurofibromatosis is associated with both scoliosis and kyphosis and characteristically leads to short high-grade curvatures requiring surgical treatment. Anterior and posterior spinal fusion is required to achieve correction and fusion in neurofibromatosis.

More than 90% of preadolescent children who sustain a significant spinal cord injury subsequently develop scoliosis. Bracing has not been shown to be effective in the prevention of scoliosis in the preadolescent patient with spinal cord injury.

▶ Kyphosis

Kyphosis may be congenital, traumatic, or acquired. Some patients with kyphosis need no treatment, whereas others require immediate surgical attention.

A. Postural Kyphosis (Postural Roundback)

Postural kyphosis, a variation of normal posture, is a cosmetic problem. There is no associated underlying disease, and the spine is flexible and capable of hyperextension. Although it may be worrisome to parents, little scientific evidence indicates that it requires, or responds to, treatment.

B. Scheuermann Kyphosis

Scheuermann kyphosis is a disorder of growth of the vertebral endplates that affects adolescents, particularly boys, and produces a progressive rigid forward curvature of the thoracic spine. Less commonly, it involves the lumbar spine, causing decreased lumbar lordosis (relative kyphosis). It is often moderately painful. Radiographs show wedging of vertebral bodies, irregularity of the endplates with radiographic lucent pits known as Schmörl's nodes, and kyphosis (Figure 10–34).

Lumbar Scheuermann kyphosis responds to symptomatic treatment with nonnarcotic pain medications or a supportive lumbar corset. Thoracic involvement with pain or kyphosis of 15–20 degrees greater than normal can be

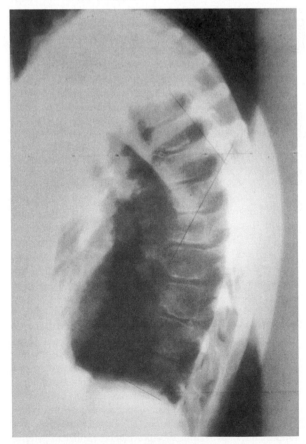

▲ **Figure 10–34.** Scheuermann kyphosis is characterized by vertebral wedging, endplate changes, and kyphosis.

managed with a Milwaukee brace. Brace treatment is usually effective in controlling pain and producing structural correction of the kyphosis, but it is very unpopular with adolescents. Braces may sometimes be used at night only so it will not have to be worn during school hours.

Scheuermann disease is the exception to the general rule that spinal bracing must be done during the active growth phase to improve deformity. Patients as old as 18 years of age show improvement with the Milwaukee brace. Severe cases (40 degrees excessive kyphosis) may require surgical correction by spinal instrumentation and fusion.

C. Congenital Kyphosis

Congenital kyphosis is a rare but important group of diseases, which, like congenital scoliosis, may be caused by failure of formation of vertebrae (hemivertebrae) or failure of embryonic segmentation (anterior unsegmented bar). In most cases, the lesion tends to cause uneven growth, so kyphosis gradually increases as the spine elongates. The risk of neurologic compromise associated with congenital kyphosis is normally secondary to risk of progression. The combination of an anterolateral bar with contralateral quadrant vertebrae has the greatest risk. Bowstringing of the spinal cord over the kyphotic prominence can occur and eventually cause paraplegia. Any progressive congenital kyphosis must be fused to prevent neurologic complications, regardless of the child's age.

D. Traumatic Kyphosis

Traumatic kyphosis is a traumatic compression of vertebrae that may lead to either cosmetic or symptomatic kyphosis. This may be prevented by early surgical stabilization of high-grade unstable traumatic spinal injuries.

E. Infectious Kyphosis

Infectious kyphosis refers to septic destruction of vertebral bodies, which can lead to severe kyphosis. In particular, tuberculous vertebral osteomyelitis can produce soft-tissue abscess, high-grade kyphosis, a sharp gibbus, and paraplegia. Bacterial infection can mimic this, although dramatic deformities are far more unusual.

Treatment includes antibiotics, surgical debridement and drainage, decompression of the spinal cord, and spinal fusion to prevent further deformity.

▶ Treatment
A. Bracing

Bracing can be used to slow progression of spinal curvatures, prevent progression, or improve underlying structural deformities. Many different types of braces are available, each with its own advocates and specific applications (Figure 10–35). When the goal is to provide postural support, slow progression, or postpone (but not prevent) surgery, a polypropylene body jacket, or so-called clamshell brace, may suffice for waking or sitting hours.

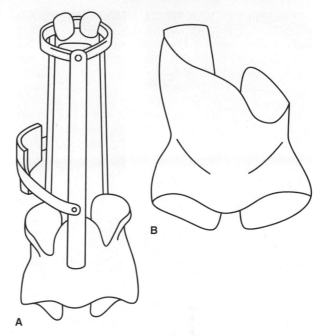

▲ **Figure 10–35.** Two popular brace styles used for the treatment of spinal deformity are the Milwaukee brace **(A)** and the low-profile (Boston-type) brace **(B)**.

Long-term braces designed to arrest progression must be custom molded for the patient, with pads placed to exert appropriate pressure to reduce deformity. Depending on the anatomic level of the curvature, they may be positioned under the arm or may extend to the neck (Milwaukee brace). This type of brace is usually worn 24 hours a day.

All braces must be modified or replaced to accommodate growth. In general, bracing is only effective with flexible curvatures in growing children.

B. Surgical Treatment

Surgical intervention is indicated for curvatures that progress despite adequate conservative treatment (usually bracing). It is also required when spinal compression is imminent (tuberculous kyphosis, congenital kyphosis) or when a curvature is so severe that bracing is impossible and future progression likely.

1. Surgical stages—Surgery involves two separate stages: correction and stabilization. After posterior exposure of the spine, correction is achieved with a variety of mechanical internal fixation devices. These are usually rods with hooks, screws, wires, or other mechanisms to distract, compress, or bend spinal segments. Correction is rarely complete because mechanical and safety considerations limit the force that can be applied. Once correction is obtained, the cortex of spine is removed and bone graft (autograft or allograft) is placed over the raw bone. Subsequently, solid fusion occurs within 6 months, permanently stabilizing the spine (Figure 10–36).

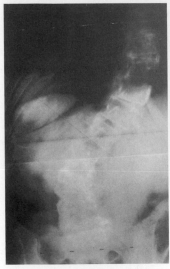
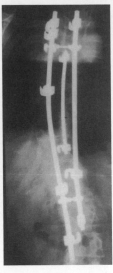

A　　　　　　　　　　　　　　B

▲ **Figure 10–36.** Treatment of a scoliotic curve by instrumentation and fusion. Preoperative view **(A)** and postoperative view **(B)**.

2. Treatment of severe curvatures—For small curvatures, posterior instrumentation and fusion are sufficient. Some large idiopathic curves and neuromuscular curves require anterior release and bone grafting to render enough acute flexibility for curvature correction and enough late stability for dependable fusion. Occasionally, fusion may fail, causing a pseudarthrosis that may be painful or may allow progression of a previously corrected curvature. In this case, fusion must be repeated.

Belmont PJ Jr, Kuklo TR, Taylor KF, et al: Intraspinal anomalies associated with isolated congenital hemivertebrae: the role of routine magnetic resonance imaging. *J Bone Joint Surg* 2004: 86-A:1704. [PMID: 15292418]

Danielsson AJ, Nachemson AL: Radiologic findings and curve progression 22 years after treatment for adolescent idiopathic scoliosis: comparison of brace and surgical treatment with matching control group of straight individuals. *Spine* 2001; 26:516. [PMID: 11242379]

Dobbs MB, Lenke LG, Szymanski DA, et al: Prevalence of neural axis abnormalities in patients with infantile idiopathic scoliosis. *J Bone Joint Surg Am* 2002;84:2230. [PMID: 12473713]

Dobbs MB, Weinstein SL: Infantile and juvenile scoliosis. *Orthop Clin North Am* 1999;30:331. [PMID: 10393759]

Feldman DS, Jordan C, Fonseca L: Orthopaedic manifestations of neurofibromatosis type 1. *J Am Acad Orthop Surg* 2010;18:346. [PMID: 20511440]

Nakahara D, Yonezawa I, Kobanawa K, et al: Magnetic resonance imaging evaluation of patient with idiopathic scoliosis: a prospective study of four hundred seventy-two outpatients. *Spine* 2011;36:E482. [PMID: 20479697]

Negrini S, Negrini F, Fusco C, Zaina F: Idiopathic scoliosis patients with curves more than 45 Cobb degrees refusing surgery can be effectively treated through bracing with curve improvements. *Spine J* 2011;11:369. [PMID: 21292562]

Richards BS, Vitale MG: Screening for idiopathic scoliosis in adolescents. An information statement. *J Bone Joint Surg Am* 2008;90:195. [PMID: 18171974]

Suh SW, Modi HN, Yang JH, Hong JY: Idiopathic scoliosis in Korean schoolchildren: a prospective screening study of over 1 million children. *Eur Spine J* 2011;20:1087. [PMID: 21274729]

Ueno M, Takaso M, Nakazawa T, et al: A 5-year epidemiological study on the prevalence rate of idiopathic scoliosis in Tokyo: school screening of more than 250,000 children. *J Orthop Sci* 2011;16:1. [PMID: 21293892]

NEUROMUSCULAR DISORDERS

▶ **Essentials of Diagnosis**

- Neuromuscular diseases may cause significant deformities (especially of feet, hips, and spine) due to muscle imbalance during growth.

- There is considerable overlap in clinical appearance associated with different diagnoses, so accurate assessment is essential.

- Treatment should be influenced by function as well as deformity.

Because muscle weakness or imbalance changes the underlying structure of a growing skeleton, neuromuscular diseases of children often require orthopedic evaluation. Treatment may be required to reverse skeletal deformity and contracture or to effect functional improvement.

Many childhood neuromuscular diseases require coordinating the services of the pediatrician, neurologist, radiologist, physiatrist, therapist, educator, social worker, nurse, and parent.

1. Cerebral Palsy

Cerebral palsy is a static encephalopathy in a growing child. Although it is often birth related, the term also includes childhood head injury, stroke, metabolic brain conditions, and degenerative neurologic conditions.

The challenges to physicians evaluating cerebral palsy are making an accurate diagnosis and detecting correctable conditions. It is essential that functional evaluation of the child's condition take into account the need for education, communication, socialization, and mobility.

▶ **Types of Cerebral Palsy**

The hallmark of most cases of cerebral palsy is alteration in motor tone (spasticity or dystonia). Spasticity is increased tone associated with stretching of muscle; dystonia is present without changing muscle length. Diagnosis of spasticity can be direct (increased tone, increased deep tendon reflexes, clasp-knife rigidity, and clonus) or inferred (shortening of muscles, contractures of joints, joint dislocations, and scoliosis). Dystonia can be confused with spasticity, but it does not generally lead to contractures.

A. Hemiplegia

Hemiplegia is spasticity involving only one side of the body. Most hemiplegia involves the pyramidal tract, especially at the cerebral cortex. It may be mild or severe and typically is more pronounced in the distal skeleton (hand and foot-ankle). Hemiplegia is usually caused by congenital loss of portions of the parietal, contralateral cerebral cortex. This loss may reflect vascular insufficiency, trauma, or porencephalic cysts.

Many patients with hemiplegia have normal development and intelligence. Children with hemiplegia frequently walk at a normal age, although sometimes with marked posturing of the involved side. Right hemiplegia (left cerebral cortex) may involve the Broca area and thus cause speech deficits. Because sensory and motor cortex areas are contiguous, hemiplegia is strongly associated with abnormalities of sensation and proprioception in the affected limbs, and particularly in the hand. This may prove more disabling than the spasticity because a child may not appreciate an insensate limb as part of overall body image.

B. Diplegia

Diplegia, or diplegic cerebral palsy, is an encephalopathy usually associated with prematurity. It is characterized by relatively symmetric involvement of the lower extremities and lesser involvement of the upper extremities. Prematurity is often accompanied by intracerebral hemorrhage and periventricular leukomalacia, which lead to edema and necrosis in the region of the trigone. This involvement of the pyramidal tract and associated basal ganglia is the main cause of diplegia.

Most diplegic children exhibit mixed patterns of spasticity with a variety of less obvious neurologic symptoms, including ataxia, rigidity, and athetosis (dystonia). Many have normal intelligence (if the cortex is spared) but may suffer developmental delays caused by damage to associative fibers in the brain. Although they may initially be hypotonic ("floppy"), most diplegic patients develop high tone (spasticity and/or dystonic rigidity) by 12–18 months of age.

Diplegia is relatively symmetric and usually more severe in the lower extremities. Many children with diplegia eventually walk, exhibiting a crouching gait characterized by flexed, internally rotated hips, flexed knees, and plantar-flexed ankles.

C. Quadriplegia

Quadriplegia (total body involvement) often occurs in children who suffer birth asphyxia, metabolic encephalopathy, or encephalitis. Severe spasticity, seizures, mental retardation,

joint contractures, and scoliosis are typical but not always individually present in this type of cerebral palsy. Children with quadriplegia are particularly susceptible to spontaneous hip dislocations (because of hip muscle imbalance) and high-grade scoliosis. Both of these conditions interfere with sitting and may require surgery. Most quadriplegic patients require wheelchair assistance and do not walk.

D. Mixed Neurologic Involvement

Mixed neurologic involvement of extrapyramidal portions of the brain can cause athetosis, dystonia, ballismus, and ataxia. Many children with cerebral palsy exhibit subtle signs of some of these disorders, in addition to spasticity. In some children, one of these signs may predominate, but spasticity is absent. In general, prognosis varies with the anatomy of involvement.

▶ Treatment

Before treating cerebral palsy, specific goals should be set for the patient. Although many important goals are not orthopedic, the surgeon may help the patient achieve them. Increased mobility, for instance, may facilitate achieving a variety of nonorthopedic goals. Especially urgent are the patient's ability to communicate, move independently, and socialize. Orthopedic treatment may improve sitting position in the wheelchair or improve walking by releasing muscles or joints.

Many children benefit from physical or occupational therapy during the first few years of life. Although the exact role of such therapy in cerebral palsy remains undefined, therapists often help parents and children deal more effectively with the complex problems presented by the disease. Therapists also help parents and children set optimistic and realistic goals for the future.

Bracing or surgery may be required to control effects of spasticity on individual joints and to decrease spasticity, correct dislocation or contracture, or control scoliosis. Surgery is ineffective in the case of extrapyramidal neurologic symptoms. A variety of nonorthopedic treatments are also used for cerebral palsy. Selective dorsal rhizotomy, a neurosurgical procedure to cut a portion of the posterior roots of the lumbar spinal cord, may reduce spasticity in selected patients by interrupting the reflex arc. Botulinum toxin injection (or phenol injection) into the motor endplate region of a muscle temporarily interrupts the myoneural junction, relaxing a spastic muscle for several months and allowing therapy or other evaluation. Oral baclofen can reduce overall spasticity. Intrathecal baclofen, delivered by a subcutaneous pump, may offer relaxation of troublesome lower extremity muscle tension in both dystonic and spastic patients.

Hip subluxation is common in quadriplegia, and pelvic radiographs in young quadriplegic patients are needed to detect early, reversible involvement. Subluxation may be treated in children younger than 3 years by adductor muscle release, which improves abduction. Rarely, the anterior obturator nerve (which innervates the adductor longus muscle) is resected to weaken the adductors. In older children, bony reconstruction by varus-derotation osteotomy and acetabular reorientation or supplementation may be necessary to correct the bone malformation that results from the force of spastic muscles on the growing skeleton. Children who develop hip subluxation often develop scoliosis as well (see section on scoliosis).

A. Adductor Release

Adductor release may be done as an open procedure (usually by myotomy or transverse sectioning of the adductor longus and a portion of the adductor brevis) or by percutaneous adductor tenotomy (section of the tendon origin of the adductor longus at the pelvis). The exact technique and amount of release is dictated by the severity of contracture and other factors. When done for hip subluxation, adductor release is most effective before 3 years of age. Release should be sufficient to allow hip abduction of 70–80 degrees on the operating table. When frank subluxation is present, some surgeons perform an anterior obturator neurectomy in addition to the adductor myotomy. This open procedure removes a segment of the obturator nerve that supplies the released adductor longus muscle, so the muscle remains loose after spontaneously reattaching after surgery.

Obturator neurectomy must be used carefully because it can cause excessive weakening of the adductors and, subsequently, late hip abduction contracture. After each of these procedures, the patient is casted in abduction for 3–4 weeks to allow muscle healing in the new elongated position.

Dynamic spasticity or joint contracture (the result of chronic spasticity) can interfere with walking in children with hemiplegia or diplegia. This may be treated by bracing involved joints in a functional position or by surgical lengthening of the muscle–tendon unit. Such muscle releases can be done by complete tenotomy, tendon Z-lengthening (common at the Achilles tendon), or lengthening of the aponeurosis of a muscle, which is often done for the iliopsoas or hamstrings (Figure 10–37).

It is convenient to combine multiple procedures for children with cerebral palsy. For example, a typical hemiplegic with a tiptoe (equinus) gait may benefit from lengthening the Achilles tendon to make the foot plantargrade. A typical diplegic patient with a crouching gait may benefit from hip flexor, hamstring, and Achilles tendon lengthenings performed bilaterally during a single operation. The exact timing and extent of surgery are controversial among experts in cerebral palsy. Three-dimensional computerized gait analysis, performed in motion laboratories, can guide the surgeon.

B. Muscle Release for Dynamic Deformity

Muscle releases for dynamic deformity may be done in several ways, depending on the specific muscle, the presence of contracture, and the surgeon's preference. The goal is to

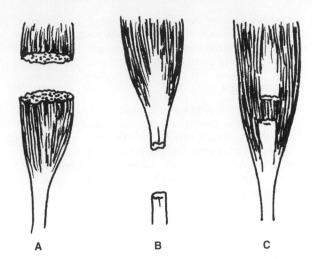

▲ **Figure 10–37.** Schematic representation of surgical options for muscle release or lengthening in cerebral palsy. **A:** Myotomy; **B:** tenotomy; **C:** aponeurotomy.

weaken spastic muscles to reduce their abnormal influence while not lengthening them so much that the opposite deformity occurs. The more common procedures are described here.

1. Achilles tendon lengthening—Achilles tendon lengthening is usually done by Z-lengthening of the distal tendon. Cuts for Z-lengthening can be either open or percutaneous. The ankle is carefully dorsiflexed just beyond neutral to allow the tendon fibers to slide into an elongated position. The surgeon must avoid overlengthening (a matter of judgment) because an excessively weakened gastrocnemius-soleus group hinders walking and can actually encourage a deeper crouching gait.

2. Gastrocnemius lengthening—Gastrocnemius lengthening is required in patients whose gastrocnemius is considerably more spastic than the soleus. In such cases, ankle dorsiflexion is limited and ankle clonus occurs when the knee is extended, but free dorsiflexion occurs when the knee is flexed. In such patients, the gastrocnemius alone may be released by approaching the musculotendinous junction in the calf and sectioning the aponeurosis or by release of the insertion of the gastrocnemius where it attaches to the soleus and Achilles tendon. This effectively recesses the muscle, selectively weakening it while retaining soleus strength for pushoff during walking.

3. Hamstring lengthening—Hamstring lengthening is indicated when the hamstrings are tight (limited straight-leg raising) and knee flexion is persistent during the stance phase of gait (crouching gait). Usually, the distal medial and lateral hamstrings are released, but procedures vary widely among surgeons. On the medial side, the gracilis and semitendinosus tendons are usually Z-lengthened or tenotomized (transversely released). The semimembranosus is lengthened by transverse incision of its aponeurosis, which allows the interior muscle fibers to stretch and lengthen. Laterally, both heads of the biceps femoris can be managed by aponeurotic lengthening as well. The procedure must be done carefully to avoid cutting or stretching the sciatic or peroneal nerves. The leg is splinted or casted in extension for 3–4 weeks to allow soft-tissue healing.

4. Iliopsoas lengthening—The hip flexors (psoas and iliacus) may be released at the insertion of the conjoined tendon into the lesser trochanter, usually done in sitters also undergoing adductor release for spastic hip subluxation. If the child is walking and less weakening of hip flexion is desired, the psoas tendon alone can be sectioned at the level of the pelvic brim, retaining the iliacus portion of the muscle for strength.

Gordon GS, Simkiss DE: A systematic review of the evidence for hip surveillance in children with cerebral palsy. *J Bone Joint Surg Br* 2006;88:1492. [PMID: 17075096]

Muthusamy K, Chu HY, Friesen RM, Chou PC, Eilert RE, Chang FM: Femoral head resection as a salvage procedure for the severely dysplastic hip in nonambulatory children with cerebral palsy. *J Pediatr Orthop* 2008;28:884. [PMID: 19034183]

Schwartz MH, Viehweger E, Stout J, Novacheck TF, Gage JR: Comprehensive treatment of ambulatory children with cerebral palsy: an outcome assessment. *J Pediatr Orthop* 2004;24:45. [PMID: 14676533]

2. Myelomeningocele (Spina Bifida)

Myelomeningocele (or meningomyelocele) is a complex birth defect affecting the spinal cord and central nervous system. Although the cause is not fully understood, there is a hereditary component. Lack of maternal folic acid is identified as a causative factor in an estimated 50–70% of cases.

▶ Embryologic Defect

The basic embryologic defect is a failure of complete tubulation and dorsal closure of the embryonic neural tube and placode, including incomplete closure of the skin over the spinal cord, resulting from lack of induction. In its mildest form, this spinal dysraphism consists of a simple spina bifida occulta or isolated meningocele (protrusion of spinal membranes, but not nerve, outside of the spinal canal, without neurologic deficit). The more severe varieties include herniation of membranes and nervous tissue through large dorsal bony and skin defects at birth and hydrocephalus with cerebral malformations (Figure 10–38).

Myelomeningocele can occur at any spinal level but usually is seen between levels T12 and S2. Because neural tissue fails to form properly, the child is paraplegic and insensate

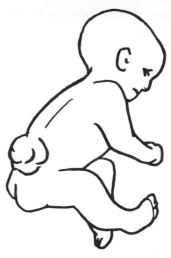

▲ **Figure 10–38.** Spina bifida (myelomeningocele). The sac includes dysplastic spinal cord and membrane elements, and it must be surgically closed in the first days of life. Hydrocephalus and congenital scoliosis are commonly associated.

below the level of the dysraphism. The clinical determination of neurologic level is most easily accomplished by describing the last muscles contracting under active voluntary motor control (Table 10–8). This may be difficult because of anatomic variability, the age of the child, and other central nervous system involvement.

Table 10–8. Muscle function at neurologic levels in myelomeningocele (spina bifida).

Neurologic Level	Functions	Muscles Active
T12	Hip flexion (weak)	Iliopsoas (weak)
L1	Hip flexion	Iliopsoas
L2	Hip adduction (weak)	Adductor longus, brevis (weak)
L3	Hip adduction Knee extension (weak)	Adductors Quadriceps (weak)
L4	Knee extension Ankle dorsiflexion	Quadriceps Anterior tibialis (variable)
L5	Knee flexion Hip abduction	Medial hamstring Tensor fascia lata
S1	Knee flexion Ankle plantar flexion	All hamstrings Gastrocnemius-soleus
S2	Toe flexion	Flexor digitorum longus

▶ Treatment of Orthopedic Problems

Orthopedic problems associated with myelomeningocele include clubfoot or congenital vertical talus, torsional deformities of the legs, contractures, hip dislocations, and scoliosis. The lack of sensation may allow extensive pressure sores to develop, or painless fractures may go undetected by patients. The health defects of children with spina bifida, in addition to their paralysis, usually include nonmusculoskeletal organ system problems such as hydrocephalus or Arnold-Chiari malformation (brain), syrinx formation or tethering (spinal cord), and neurogenic bladder or hydronephrosis (renal system). Early in life, most of these are more important than the orthopedic manifestations, and a team approach is needed to decide when and how best to coordinate management. The most pressing needs of the infant born with spina bifida are usually neural defect closure and ventricular shunting.

Orthopedic management depends on the deformities and the long-term mobility goals for the child. The level of paralysis often is helpful in determining whether the child will ultimately be able to walk (L5 or S1 function usually required) or will require a wheelchair (because of function only proximal to L4 or L5). Foot deformities such as clubfoot or congenital vertical talus usually require surgery. If foot deformities recur or progress, tethered cord should be suspected.

Spina bifida is theoretically a static neurologic disease, but many children exhibit a drifting deterioration of neurologic function as they grow; progression of foot deformities, especially during growth spurts, suggests tethering (and therefore stretching) of the cord. Hip dislocations, although dramatic on radiograph, frequently require no treatment; they are painless and tend to occur in children with neurologic involvement at L2 to L4, which precludes long-term walking.

A young child with scoliosis may require bracing until the thorax is long enough for spinal fusion. Scoliosis surgery is complicated by absent posterior neural arches. Some scoliosis seen with spina bifida is congenital (see section on scoliosis). If rapidly progressive scoliosis occurs, the physician should suspect a neurologic cause such as syrinx. Because of chronic exposure to latex materials in contact with mucous membranes and internal tissues (shunts, catheters), children with spina bifida are exceedingly susceptible to latex allergy, which can be fatal. Steps to limit latex exposure are essential in this population and must be observed by medical personnel working with them.

Bartonek A, Saraste H: Factors influencing ambulation in myelomeningocele: a cross-sectional study. *Dev Med Child Neurol* 2001;43:253. [PMID: 11305403]

Centers for Disease Control and Prevention: Spina bifida and anencephaly before and after folic acid mandate—United States, 1995–1996 and 1999–2000. *MMWR Morb Mortal Wkly Rep* 2004;53:362. [PMID: 15129193]

3. Muscular Dystrophy

Duchenne muscular dystrophy is an X-linked disorder that presents in boys 6–9 years of age. The disorder is one of progressive muscle weakness, usually first involving more proximal muscles of the limb girdles. Pseudohypertrophy caused by replacement of gastrocnemius muscles (or other muscles) with fat is a classic finding, as is Gower sign (an inability to rise from the floor without using the hands to "walk up" the body and legs). As the muscles weaken, imbalance can cause fixed flexion contractures of the hip, knee, and ankle plantar flexors, which limits walking ability. Because weakness eventually forces patients into a wheelchair, a decision to brace or correct these contractures surgically depends on estimates of remaining strength and likely duration of ambulation after treatment. Most often, progressive foot deformities (usually equinovarus) require muscle release and correction (including bracing) because use of the wheelchair also requires relatively well-positioned feet.

As weakness progresses, the child requires an electric wheelchair for mobility. At this point, scoliosis begins to appear and is usually relentlessly progressive. Attempts to control the scoliosis of muscular dystrophy by wheelchair inserts and braces are ineffective. Early surgery (before cardiorespiratory status deteriorates) is often the best answer. Chapter 12, "Rehabilitation," provides more information.

4. Myotonic Dystrophy

Myotonic dystrophy is a genetic muscle disease whose name reflects the hallmark of the disease: myotonic EMG potentials. The disease is often associated with mild-to-moderate retardation, obesity, and foot deformities. Initial diagnosis is made by identifying the characteristic myotonic face (weak perioral muscles with a distinctive pyramidal mouth), confirmed by EMG. Myotonic dystrophy worsens with each succeeding generation; genetic markers are available for diagnosis.

The most frequent foot deformity is equinovarus, often with weakness of the anterior tibialis and overactivity of the posterior tibialis. Surgery is often required, and recurrence requiring additional surgery is common. Surgical treatment of myotonic dystrophy foot deformities includes joint release (for passive correction of the deformity) and muscle transfers (for rebalancing muscle forces).

5. Spinal Muscular Atrophy

This heterogeneous group of disorders includes static and degenerative lesions of the anterior horn cell population in the spinal cord. These disorders all involve muscle weakness caused by a lower motor neuron lesion, that is, flaccid paralysis. Sensation is intact, and the major goals are mobility (with electric wheelchair), adaptive devices to aid in daily living (eg, feeding devices), and control of scoliosis, which is similar to management of scoliosis in advanced muscular dystrophy (see section on muscular dystrophy).

King WM, Ruttencutter R, Nagaraja HN, et al: Orthopedic outcomes of long-term daily corticosteroid treatment in Duchenne muscular dystrophy. *Neurology* 2007;68:1607. [PMID: 17485648]

Mercado E, Alman B, Wright JG: Does spinal fusion influence quality of life in neuromuscular scoliosis? *Spine (Phila Pa 1976)* 2007;32 (19 Suppl):S120. [PMID: 17728678]

Voisin V, de la Porte S: Therapeutic strategies for Duchenne and Becker dystrophies. *Int Rev Cytol* 2004;240:1. [PMID: 15548414]

6. Arthrogryposis (Arthrogryposis Multiplex Congenita)

Arthrogryposis is not a disease per se but rather a symptom complex that includes joint contractures or dislocations, rigid skeletal deformities (especially clubfoot), shiny skin with decreased wrinkling and subcutaneous tissue, weakness, and muscle wasting. Although many factors contribute to arthrogryposis, the common link among the symptoms appears to be decreased fetal movement during a critical period in limb development. This can be caused by neurologic lesions (congenital absence of anterior horn cells, Werdnig-Hoffman spinal muscular atrophy, myelomeningocele), myopathic lesions (myotonic dystrophy, congenital myopathies), various syndromes (Moebius syndrome), or physical restriction associated with oligohydramnios.

Arthrogrypotic infants frequently have extension or flexion contractures of knees and elbows, dislocated hips, and severe clubfeet. The contractures may partially resolve with passive ROM therapy in the first 6–12 months of life; however, they must be released surgically after that if they interfere with walking or arm use. Hip dislocations may not limit function and often are not treated. Clubfeet require surgery, which is often of limited success; multiple operations are frequently necessary. Arthrogrypotic children are generally highly resourceful in achieving mobility, and they care for themselves completely independently, despite seemingly overwhelming skeletal problems.

Bernstein RM: Arthrogryposis and amyoplasia. *J Am Acad Orthop Surg* 2002;10:417. [PMID: 12470044]

Fassier A, Wicart P, Dubousset J, Seringe R: Arthrogryposis multiplex congenita. Long-term follow-up from birth until skeletal maturity. *J Child Orthop* 2009;3:383. [PMID: 19669823]

TUMORS

Skeletal neoplasms, particularly benign ones, are fairly common in children. Common benign bone lesions of childhood include osteochondroma, osteoid osteoma, unicameral (simple) bone cysts, chondroblastoma, hemangioma, histiocytosis X (eosinophilic granuloma), and fibrous dysplasia. Malignant tumors, which are usually seen after 10 years of age, include Ewing sarcoma and osteosarcoma.

Certain systemic diseases can be manifested in childhood as apparent bone tumors (hyperparathyroidism, renal disease, leukemia). Chapter 5 offers a detailed discussion of bone tumors.

AMPUTATIONS

▶ Congenital Amputations and Absence of Segments

Congenital absence of limb segments at birth can occur sporadically, as part of a syndrome (Streeter dysplasia) or as a result of mutagens (eg, thalidomide). Absence may be terminal (eg, congenital below-knee amputation) or intercalary (eg, congenital shortening or absence of the humerus).

Although congenital amputations can be dramatic in appearance, the missing limb is not part of the child's body image. Thus, the child has a natural instinct to be mobile. Children with severe limb deficiencies at birth are almost always able to be completely independent and functional. They accept prostheses quite readily but only if the device truly improves their efficiency. For example, nearly all congenital above-elbow amputees reject artificial limbs, opting for function over appearance. Parents may harbor strong feelings of guilt over the child's condition, so the psychological issues associated with the condition are more those of the adults than the child.

It is not unusual for congenital amputations to require conversion to a level more easily fitted with a prosthesis. For example, fibular hemimelia (severe shortening of the tibia with absent fibula and foot deformity) sometimes can be most effectively treated by removing the foot and converting the limb to an ankle disarticulation level. This facilitates prosthetic fitting and simplifies management of the leg-length discrepancy, thus permitting normal function.

Boostra AM, Rijnders LJ, Groothoff JW, et al: Children with congenital deficiencies or acquired amputations of the lower limbs: functional aspects. *Prosthet Orthot Int* 2000;24:19. [PMID: 10855435]

Ephraim PL, Dillingham TR, Sector M, et al: Epidemiology of limb loss and congenital limb deficiency: a review of the literature. *Arch Phys Med Rehabil* 2003;84:747. [PMID: 12736892]

Fixsen JA: Major lower limb congenital shortening: a mini review. *J Pediatr Orthop B* 2003;12:1. [PMID: 12488764]

Klaassen Z, Shoja MM, Tubbs RS, Loukas M: Supernumerary and absent limbs and digits of the lower limb: a review of the literature. *Clin Anat* 2011;24:570. [PMID: 21204092]

▶ Traumatic Amputation

In contrast to the congenital amputee, the child with a traumatic amputation is particularly likely to be male, adolescent, rebellious, and troubled. Although pediatric traumatic amputations are often caused by inadvertent incidents, many result from high-risk behavior. These factors must be taken into account when dealing with the psychological issues of the patient and family; social, as well as medical, intervention is often appropriate.

The orthopedic management of traumatic amputees is modified in children by the presence of growth plates and the remarkable healing and rehabilitation powers of children. This must be considered during surgical completion of amputations because injury to the physis may cause severe shortening or angulation of a stump, rendering the amputation far less satisfactory than a similar amputation in the adult. The child amputee rarely has vascular problems, however, and the use of split-thickness skin grafting may allow preservation of length that would be impossible in most adults.

▶ Overgrowth of Amputation Stump

Amputations through the long bones of children exhibit the unique phenomenon of terminal overgrowth. Eventually, the distal end of the stump may develop a long, thin, sometimes painful bony prominence. Overgrowth is not physeal in origin (ie, closure of the physis by epiphysiodesis does not eliminate its formation), and it appears to be related to aggressive bone formation associated with the periosteal membrane.

Although overgrowth can occur in any bone, it is most troublesome in the tibia, fibula, and humerus. When symptomatic, overgrowth is treated by resecting the spike of bone (revision of the amputation), but the process does continue, and recurrence is common. Some pediatric amputees require two or more surgical revisions during growth. Overgrowth ceases at skeletal maturity. Various attempts at capping the overgrowing bone end (using foreign materials or free epiphyseal grafts) have met with inconsistent success.

Jeans KA, Browne RH, Karol LA: Effect of amputation level on energy expenditure during overground walking by children with an amputation. *J Bone Joint Surg Am* 2011;93:49. [PMID: 21209268]

Tenholder M, Davids JR, Gruber HE, et al: Surgical management of juvenile amputation overgrowth with a synthetic cap. *J Pediatr Orthop* 2004;24:218. [PMID: 15076611]

FRACTURES

▶ Common Pediatric Fracture Patterns

Many fractures in children are similar to their counterparts in adults. However, the added factor of growth contributes to the unique issues of fracture care in children. Pediatric bone is softer and more easily broken than adult cortical bone. Thus, the amount of energy required to produce a fracture is less in the child, even as soft-tissue injury is frequently less severe in the child than in the adult. In addition, the periosteal membrane in children is far thicker and more osteogenic

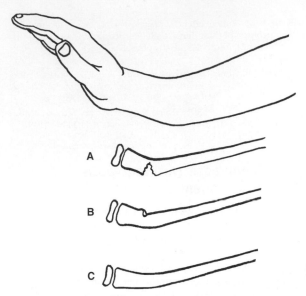

▲ **Figure 10–39.** Softer bone in children can lead to unique fracture behavior (in addition to the fracture patterns seen in adults). **A:** Greenstick fracture; **B:** torus fracture; **C:** plastic deformation.

than in adults. The periosteum is so leathery in immature humans that it frequently holds bone ends together, contributing greatly to stability and ease of manipulative reduction. The excellent osteogenic potential of pediatric periosteum permits rapid, aggressive fracture healing, so nonunions are extremely rare in children.

Less brittle pediatric bone is subject to fracture patterns unique to children (Figure 10–39). A greenstick fracture is a transverse crack that retains its continuity, just as a small moist twig breaks without actually snapping apart.

A torus fracture is a small buckle or impaction of one cortex with a slight bend on the opposite cortex. Plastic deformation is a change in the natural shape of a bone without a detectable fracture line.

Remodeling (gradual correction in alignment or size of a fractured bone back to normal) is generally far more rapid in children than in adults. Remodeling of angular deformities is particularly rapid when the deformity is in the same plane of motion as the nearest joint (Figure 10–40) or when the deformity is near a rapidly growing physis. Remodeling of rotational deformities is less reliable. Overgrowth is a singular feature of remodeling that occurs in certain fractures of the long bones, particularly the femur. It is a product of physeal stimulation by the hyperemic response to fracture and healing and may increase the length of a bone by 2 cm or more over the course of a year.

The combination of low-energy injury, rapid bone healing, and dependable remodeling of angular deformity makes

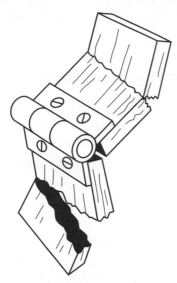

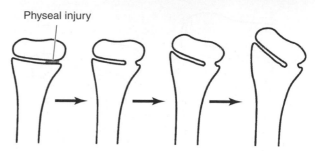

Physeal injury

▲ **Figure 10–41.** Progressive angular deformity can occur if there is asymmetric closure of the physis after fracture.

▲ **Figure 10–40.** Remodeling of bone after fracture is most rapid when it is in the plane of a nearby joint. Schematically, if the joint is thought of as a hinge, the fracture above (in the plane of the hinge) is likely to remodel faster than the fracture below the hinge (out of plane).

it possible to treat many pediatric fractures by simple closed reduction (often incomplete) and casting. Surgical management of children's fractures is rarely required. The surgeon may accept a less-than-perfect reduction if the fracture is known to remodel into satisfactory alignment.

1. Epiphyseal Fracture

The cartilage physeal plates are a region of low strength relative to the surrounding bone and are susceptible to fracture in the child. They are analogous to a scratch on a pane of glass, in which concentrated force facilitates damage. Once injury occurs, the physis usually is able to recover and resume growth. But if an offset occurs in the physeal substance, bone may grow across it (from epiphyseal bone to metaphyseal bone), forming a bridge that anchors further growth and leads to either progressive shortening or a worsening angulation (Figure 10–41).

Because physes are near joints and physeal fractures are common, children may suffer injuries to joint surfaces that require careful surgical repair and realignment. Thus, open reduction is more likely in fractures involving physes and joints than in other pediatric fractures.

Most physeal fractures propagate through the weakest region of the cartilage. Physeal cartilage begins in a dense resting zone on the epiphyseal side, and chondrocytes gradually multiply, elongate, and arrange into longitudinal columns that produce longitudinal growth. Hypertrophic, balloon-like chondrocyte columns then undergo cell death, and the remaining cell walls are calcified and eventually ossify to form metaphyseal bone.

The weakest spot is usually the interface between hypertrophic dying columns of cells and the stiff calcified cell walls beneath them; this area is highly susceptible to shearing forces. So, physeal fractures (eg, Salter-Harris fractures) typically occur through the zone of hypertrophy. Fortunately, the region also represents the boundary between the process of epiphyseal elongation (supported by the epiphyseal blood supply) and metaphyseal ossification (supported by the metaphyseal blood supply). Thus, physeal fractures do not often damage the growth potential of the physis because they do not interrupt its critical blood supply. An exception to the usual location of these fractures is the growth plate in the distal femur. It has an undulating topography, with prominences called mammillary bodies that interdigitate with other portions of the physis to provide stability at the distal femur. A typical distal femoral physeal fracture propagates through multiple layers of the growth plate. This results in displaced physeal fractures of the distal femur being at high risk for causing premature growth arrest of the involved physis and subsequent deformity.

Although physeal fractures can occur in a wide variety of configurations, certain patterns are seen frequently enough that a descriptive classification aids in understanding physeal injury (Figure 10–42). Fractures that either cross the joint or result in spatial malalignment of portions of the physis have the worst prognosis.

Physeal fractures heal rapidly, usually within 4 weeks. Careful monitoring is required to detect early posttraumatic closure of the growth plate. Occasionally, an epiphyseal–metaphyseal bony bridge forms and tethers growth. If this growth is minor, surgical removal of the bridge (epiphyseal bar resection) may successfully restore physeal growth. Otherwise, the procedures for evaluation and treatment of limb-length inequality should be followed (see previous section on limb-length inequality).

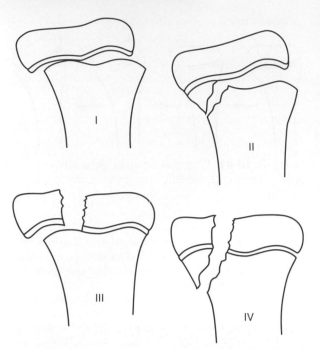

▲ **Figure 10–42.** The Salter-Harris classification of physeal fractures is widely used to describe such injuries. With some exceptions, the potential for problems with growth arrest is greater in the higher numbered patterns.

Salter RB, Harris WR: Injuries involving the growth plate. *J Bone Joint Surg Am* 1963;45:587. [No PMID]

2. Upper Extremity Fractures

▶ Clavicle Fracture

Clavicle fractures are among the most common injuries in children. They are usually closed and may be treated with a simple sling. Healing occurs rapidly with abundant callus, which leaves a lump that may concern parents. This enlargement remodels over several years of growth.

Clavicle fractures can occur at birth and heal rapidly but are sometimes accompanied by neurologic injury. Then, return of active biceps before 3 months and preservation of full passive shoulder ROM are predictors of a good outcome. Breech delivery is usually associated with preganglionic injury. Preganglionic injury can result in a Horner sign, which includes ptosis, miosis, and anhydrosis. Preganglionic injuries are unlikely to recover. The Moro reflex is elicited by dropping a baby's head a short distance and observing active elbow extension and fanning of the fingers, followed by elbow flexion and crying. Absence of the Moro reflex suggests a poor prognosis.

An extremely rare condition, atraumatic congenital pseudarthrosis of the clavicle can mimic the radiographic appearance of fracture. It may be right sided or bilateral, with little or no pain and no history of trauma. Treatment is generally unnecessary.

▶ Proximal Humerus Fracture

Proximal humerus fractures are usually epiphyseal injuries (usually Salter-Harris type II injuries) that may progress into significant varus angulation (medial deviation). Fortunately, the proximal humerus is a rapidly growing physis and shoulder motion is full in all planes, so remodeling is rapid. These fractures generally require only a sling or shoulder immobilization for 3–4 weeks, without reduction. Rarely, fractures with extreme angulation (>90 degrees) may require surgical reduction and fixation.

▶ Elbow Region Fracture

Most elbow region fractures are indirect injuries caused by a fall on the outstretched hand. Both diagnosis and treatment can be difficult in this serious group of injuries. Epiphyseal ossification is incomplete in the group that is susceptible to falls (2–10 years of age), making radiographs difficult to interpret (Figure 10–43). Swelling, if severe, can block venous or arterial structures and lead to forearm compartment syndromes. Reductions are often unstable, and operative intervention may be required. Most surgeons immobilize pediatric elbow fractures for 4 weeks after treatment. The most important fractures are listed next.

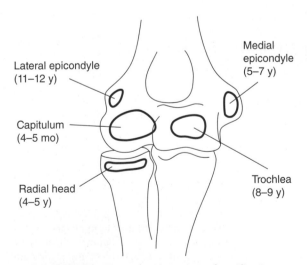

▲ **Figure 10–43.** Ages of appearance of ossification centers. The ossification centers of the elbow region emerge at different ages as indicated and can complicate the interpretation of radiographs. It is often advisable to obtain comparison radiographs of the opposite elbow if injury is suspected.

A. Supracondylar Fracture of Humerus

Supracondylar fracture of the humerus occurs at the metaphyseal bone, proximal to the elbow joint, and does not involve the growth plate (Figure 10–44). Displacement may be severe, and nerve injury, usually caused by stretching, is common. If swelling is marked, there may be interruption of the blood supply; it is not uncommon for such a distal extremity to lack a pulse.

The most appropriate treatment is rapid anatomic reduction under general anesthesia. Because the reduction is highly unstable, many surgeons prefer to fix the fracture after reduction with percutaneous wires. Once the fracture is reduced, the swelling recedes rapidly and the pulse returns. On rare occasions, the surgeon must perform vascular or nerve exploration or repair.

Some displaced supracondylar humerus fractures are incompletely reduced or lose position because of fracture instability after apparently adequate initial reduction. This progresses to a characteristic malunion with an apex-lateral angular deformity of the elbow (known as cubitus varus or so-called gunstock deformity). Although cosmetically unsightly, cubitus varus rarely has any significant functional consequences. If desired, it may be corrected by valgus osteotomy at the old fracture site.

B. Lateral Condyle Fracture

The lateral condyle fracture is an oblique shearing fracture of the lateral portion of the joint surface that occurs when the radial head drives into the capitulum of the humerus during a fall. The lack of significant ossification may obscure the fracture or give the false appearance of a benign Salter-Harris II fracture pattern, but most lateral condyle fractures are highly unstable Salter-Harris IV fractures (Figure 10–45). Because both the joint surface and the physis are displaced, they usually require open reduction and fixation using pins.

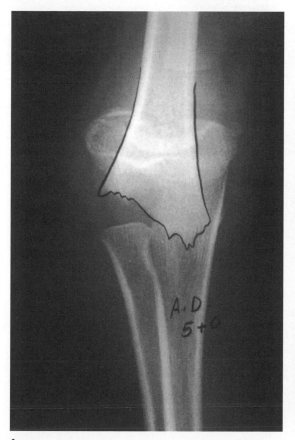
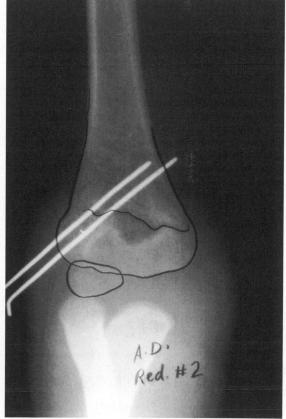

A   **B**

▲ **Figure 10–44.** Displaced supracondylar fracture of the humerus. Injury film **(A)**; after closed reduction and internal fixation using percutaneous pins **(B)**.

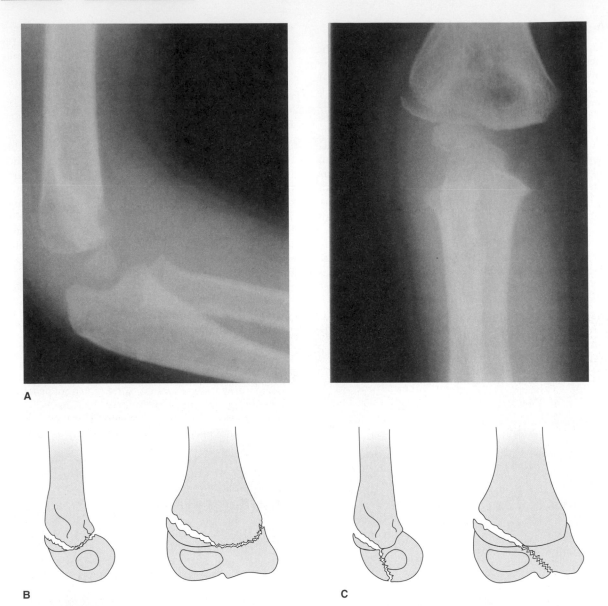

A

B

C

▲ **Figure 10–45.** Lateral condyle fracture of the humerus **(A)** can easily be mistaken for a relatively simple Salter-Harris type II injury, which carries a good prognosis **(B)**. In reality, however, it is almost always a Salter-Harris type IV injury, with a fracture pattern crossing both the joint surface and the physis **(C)**; unless it is not displaced, it requires open reduction.

C. Radial Neck Fracture

Fracture of the radial neck is similar to a lateral condyle fracture. The radial neck just distal to the joint may angulate up to 70–80 degrees, although lesser angulation is more common (Figure 10–46). It is important to determine the location of the radial head despite traumatic angulation of the radial neck. Surprisingly, angulation of 45 degrees or less usually remodels spontaneously and requires only symptomatic

treatment that permits early return to activity. Larger degrees of angulation can often respond to closed manipulation.

D. Forearm Fracture

Forearm fractures are a common result of falls. If they involve both bones, one bone may be completely displaced while the other only bends or suffers a greenstick fracture. In children, most forearm fractures that involve both bones

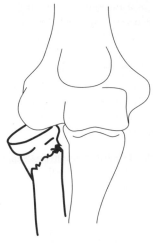

▲ **Figure 10–46.** Fracture of the radial neck may angulate greatly yet still remodel spontaneously in the younger child.

can be treated successfully by closed reduction and casting; minor angular malalignment can easily be tolerated if rotational alignment of the bone ends is accurate. In addition, the ends of fractured bones often overlap. This is not necessarily of concern if alignment is satisfactory because side-to-side bone healing and remodeling are rapid in children.

E. Monteggia Fracture

Monteggia fracture is fracture of the ulna only, with the radius remaining intact. Because two-bone systems generally must fail in two spots if they break at all, the radial head dislocates from the capitulum. In such cases, reduction must include the elbow component. As with other pediatric forearm fractures, closed reduction is usually successful, although some Monteggia fractures require open reduction. The physician should be alert to the possibility of Monteggia fracture because the fracture can lead to chronic loss of elbow motion if it is not properly reduced.

In children, Galeazzi fracture of the radius, in which the distal radioulnar joint is dislocated, is far less common than the analogous Monteggia fracture.

F. Torus Fracture of Radius

Torus fracture of the radius is a minor buckle of the dorsal cortex of the distal radius, usually 1–2 cm proximal to the distal radial physis. It occurs after a minor fall on the hand. Many torus fractures are mistaken for wrist sprains because they are stable and not as painful as unstable fractures. They heal uneventfully in 3–4 weeks, with excellent long-term results.

Mirsky EC, Karas EH, Weiner LS: Lateral condyle fractures in children: evaluation of classification and treatment. *J Orthop Trauma* 1997;11:117. [PMID: 9057147]

Price CT: The treatment of displaced fractures of the lateral humeral condyle in children. *J Orthop Trauma* 2010;24:439. [PMID: 20577076]

Wattenbarger JM, Gerardi J, Johnston CE: Late open reduction internal fixation of lateral condyle fractures. *J Pediatr Orthop* 2002;22:394. [PMID: 11961463]

Weiss JM, Graves S, Yang S, Mendelsohn E, Kay RM, Skaggs DL: A new classification system predictive of complications in surgically treated pediatric humeral lateral condyle fractures. *J Pediatr Orthop* 2009;29:602. [PMID: 19700990]

▶ Metacarpal and Phalangeal Fractures

Fractures of the metacarpals and phalanges commonly occur from crush injuries in children (eg, catching a hand or finger in a door) and are generally quite stable because the periosteum remains intact. Rarely severely angulated or rotationally malaligned, they can usually be managed by immobilization for 2–3 weeks.

3. Lower Extremity Fractures

▶ Pelvic Fracture

Pelvic fractures in children are usually seen in conjunction with major blunt trauma. Gross displacement is fairly uncommon and usually can be treated symptomatically because the intact periosteum stabilizes the large flat bones. The patient should be carefully evaluated for intraabdominal and other injuries. Properly treated pelvic fractures in an immature skeleton resolve satisfactorily.

Adolescents exhibit a special type of avulsion fracture of apophyses because aggressive pulling of muscles during sports can detach an apophysis from its parent bone. These avulsion fractures are sometimes called transitional fractures because the physes are in transition within 2 years of skeletal maturity. During this time, relatively weak cartilage physes may not be strong enough to withstand the pull of growing muscles suddenly grown powerful under the influence of hormones. Transitional avulsion fractures may occur at the iliac crest (abdominal muscles), lesser trochanter of the femur (iliopsoas muscle), or ischial tuberosity (hamstring muscle). Transitional fractures of the pelvis and femur are treated symptomatically. Although these fractures do not require reduction, they may heal with a significant bump that requires excision later.

Tsirikos AI, Spiegel PG, Laros GS: Transepiphyseal fracture-dislocation of the femoral neck: A case report and review of the literature. *J Orthop Trauma* 2003;17:648. [PMID: 14574194]

▶ Hip Fracture

Pediatric hip fractures are rare but may be serious because trauma to this area may produce significant injury. As in the adult, the fracture pattern may disrupt the blood supply of the proximal femoral head and lead to avascular necrosis of the proximal femoral epiphysis, femoral neck, or both. In older children, this can be a devastating complication; it is treated like LCP but may result in such severe collapse that hip fusion is required.

Femoral neck fractures in children are highly unstable and treated by reduction and internal fixation. The mechanical fixation may be imperfect because the surgeon must avoid injury to the proximal femoral physis. For this reason, a spica cast (body and legs) is generally used as well.

Odent T, Glorion C, Pannier S, et al: Traumatic dislocation of the hip with separation of the capital epiphysis: 5 adolescent patients with 3–9 years of follow-up. *Acta Orthop Scand* 2003; 74:49. [PMID: 12635793]

▶ Femoral Shaft Fracture

Fractures of the femoral shaft are common injuries caused by falls as well as bicycle and motor vehicle accidents. In young children, they may be the result of child abuse. Although most are closed injuries, blood loss can be significant because of bleeding into the soft tissues of the thigh. Nerve injury is rare, and the fact that the fracture is surrounded by richly nourished muscle ensures rapid solid union (usually within 6 weeks).

Longitudinal muscle pull and spasm cause femoral shaft fractures to shorten and angulate. Initial treatment requires longitudinal traction (skin traction in younger children, skeletal traction in older children) to restore length and alignment. At this point, treatment largely depends on the patient's age.

Femur fractures in children 2–10 years of age have a strong tendency to exhibit overgrowth of 1–2.5 cm because of fracture hyperemia. In this group, therefore, it may be desirable to use a cast and allow some shortening to occur. Rapid remodeling of the bone makes perfect reduction unnecessary. Most surgeons apply a spica cast immediately or within the first week.

Femoral overgrowth following fracture becomes unlikely in children older than 10 years. In these older children, the bone either must be kept to anatomic length by traction for 3–4 weeks (until sufficient callus has formed to stabilize length) or treated by intramedullary nails or other operative measures, as in the adult. The medial femoral circumflex artery supplies blood to the femoral head. Its position along the posterior-superior femoral neck places this structure at risk with intramedullary nailing of the femur. Therefore, lateral entry through the greater trochanter is preferred when intramedullary fixation is performed. Currently, flexible intramedullary nails are popular because they do not require reaming prior to insertion, and they are less likely to disrupt the precarious blood supply of the proximal femur. There is now a tendency at many centers to fix femur fractures using flexible nails in children 6 years and older.

After healing or cast removal, the child may begin walking. Limping is common in the first month after fracture because the hip girdle musculature regains its strength only slowly. No physical therapy is required, however, because normal walking permits spontaneous recovery, and long-term results of pediatric femur fractures are excellent.

▶ Epiphyseal Separation

Epiphyseal separations (fracture) of the distal femoral physis are usually Salter-Harris type I or II injuries. All are caused by significant trauma, and injury to the growth mechanism of the plate is common. As many as 50% of cases exhibit subsequent growth arrest. Major neurovascular injury can occur, as with knee dislocations. Displaced epiphyseal separations require gentle reduction under general anesthesia. Some are so unstable, however, that they require percutaneous pin fixation for several weeks until the fracture is sticky, as it were, or healed enough so displacement does not occur. If physeal closure occurs, the treatment depends on age and remaining growth potential. (See earlier discussion of limb-length inequality.)

▶ Tibial Eminence Injury

The tibial eminence (spine), located entirely on the proximal tibial epiphysis, is the site of attachment of the anterior cruciate ligament. Twisting injuries of the knee can shear off the eminence and may displace it within the joint. Most fractures occur in children ages 8 to 14 years, and they typically present with a painful hemarthrosis and refusal to bear weight. A type I fracture is minimally displaced, type II is anteriorly displaced with an intact posterior hinge, and type III is completely displaced. Long leg casting for 6 weeks, until the bone heals (Figure 10–47), is advocated for type I

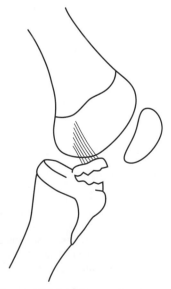

▲ **Figure 10–47.** Tibial eminence fracture usually includes an anterior cruciate avulsion component. It can be treated nonoperatively if the fragment reduces with extension of the knee.

fractures, although there is debate about whether the knee should be maintained in full extension or in 10–20 degrees of flexion. Management of type II and III fractures is much more controversial. Type II fractures can be treated closed if adequate reduction can be achieved, but if not, surgical management is indicated. Surgery is also indicated for type III fractures. In these displaced injuries, the medial meniscus can be trapped under the fragment and/or the lateral meniscus; if the anterior cruciate ligament is still attached to the avulsed fracture fragment, this may cause pulling on the fragment and therefore block reduction. Unlike many other pediatric fractures, tibial eminence injuries often lead to mild long-term knee symptoms, especially during athletic activities

▶ Tibial Tubercle Avulsion Fracture

Tibial tubercle avulsion fractures are most often seen in adolescent males (13–14 years of age) who suffer sports-related injuries. The anterior tongue of the proximal tibial epiphysis is the site of attachment of the patellar tendon. During strenuous jumping, as in basketball, the tongue may avulse and displace. Tibial tubercle avulsions are transitional fractures in that they occur immediately before physeal closure and are not seen in younger children. They are classified as follows: type I, a small fragment of the tuberosity is avulsed and is displaced upward; type II, the whole tongue formed by the anterior aspect of the tibial epiphysis is hinged upward without being completely fractured at its base; and type III, the entire tibial tuberosity is fractured at its base, with the line of fracture directed proximally and posteriorly into the articular surface. Nearly all these fractures require open reduction and internal fixation, although the surgeon need not take the usual precautions when operating near the physis because maturity follows too rapidly to permit deformity. There is a high incidence of compartment syndrome seen in type III tibial tubercle fractures. Fasciotomy should be considered at the time of initial repair. Type III tibial tubercle fractures extending through the joint are often associated with meniscal injuries, which must be repaired. Delayed complications included recurvatum and refracture.

▶ Proximal Tibial Metaphyseal Fracture

Proximal tibial metaphyseal fractures are usually undisplaced or minimally displaced. In the absence of fibular overgrowth (Figure 10–48), they can exhibit troublesome late angular deformity (valgus) caused by tibial overgrowth after fracture. The phenomenon is most pronounced at the age of maximum physiologic valgus (3–6 years). Over a number of years, the valgus has a tendency to remodel, so the best approach is observation.

▶ Tibial Shaft Fracture

Tibial shaft fractures, which are usually accompanied by fibula fractures, generally result from major trauma. An

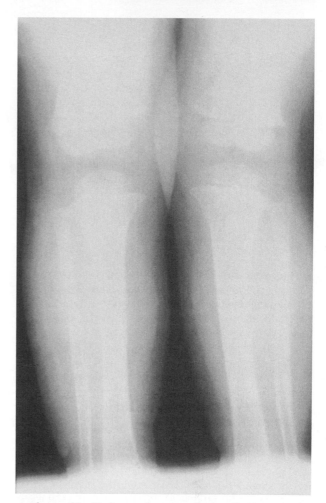

▲ **Figure 10–48.** Even when not displaced, fracture of the proximal tibial metaphysis can stimulate the tibial physis and cause progressive valgus deformity, especially in patients younger than 6 years. Long-term observation indicates that slow remodeling eventually occurs.

exception is the nondisplaced, isolated spiral tibial fracture often seen after minor trauma in children just learning to walk (toddler's fracture). In the pediatric population, open tibia fractures are fairly common. As in the adult, injury to neurovascular structures and compartment syndromes are major risks (see Chapter 2, "Musculoskeletal Trauma Surgery"). Open fractures of the tibia and fibula require surgical debridement, but because skin loss is less likely than in the adult, they can often be managed the same way as closed fractures, following lavage.

Most tibial fractures in children can be adequately aligned and immobilized in above-knee casts. Rare, unstable cases, some open fractures, or fractures in older children also may require external fixation or other devices to maintain reduction and alignment. As in the adult, pediatric tibia

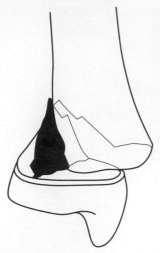

▲ **Figure 10–49.** Simple fracture of the distal tibia (and fibula) at the ankle is usually a Salter-Harris type II pattern in patients younger than 10 years.

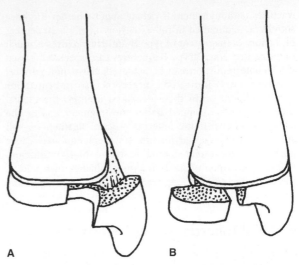

A   **B**

▲ **Figure 10–50.** The triplane **(A)** and juvenile Tillaux **(B)** fractures are variations of ankle fracture that occur in the adolescent shortly before physeal closure. Because they involve the joint surface, such fractures may require open reduction.

fractures are relatively slow to heal, frequently requiring 10–12 weeks; nonunion is rare, however.

▶ ## Ankle Fracture and Distal Tibial Fracture

Ankle fractures and distal tibial fractures in younger children are often either metaphyseal or Salter-Harris type II distal tibial physeal injuries that heal rapidly. These fractures have very little tendency to suffer growth arrest or other serious consequences (Figure 10–49). Posttraumatic physeal arrest occurs most commonly after injury in the distal medial tibia. In children 8–11 years of age, inversion injuries can push off the medial malleolus, causing an oblique Salter-Harris type IV fracture that disrupts both the joint and the growth plate. These fractures generally require open reduction for accurate realignment of the physis and articular surface. Subsequent growth arrest can cause a medial physeal bridge and produce a progressive varus deformity of the distal tibial articular surface as the lateral physis continues untethered elongation. If this occurs, either epiphyseal bar resection or corrective tibial osteotomy should be considered.

The distal tibia is the site of several distinct transitional fracture patterns. These physeal injuries occur only at the end of growth, shortly before complete distal tibial physeal closure at maturity. The distal physis begins early closure medially, with gradual lateral closure over the next year. The exact fracture pattern depends on how much of the plate is still open and on the force applied (ie, mechanism of injury). When just the medial physis is closed, a triplane fracture (ie, sagittal, transverse, and frontal) of the distal tibia occurs (Figure 10–50). This fracture contains a complex of fracture

lines and crosses the growth plate. Triplane fractures usually require open reduction, although minimally displaced injuries can be managed nonoperatively. CT scans may be necessary to define the exact fracture configuration for accurate treatment.

In slightly older patients, when only a small anterolateral segment of the physis remains open, this anterolateral fragment can be avulsed by fibers of the distal tibiofibular syndesmosis (juvenile Tillaux fracture). This is a Salter-Harris type III fracture involving the articular surface and frequently requires open reduction to restore perfect joint anatomy.

Leary JT, Handling M, Talerico M, Yong L, Bowe JA: Physeal fractures of the distal tibia: predictive factors of premature physeal closure and growth arrest. *J Pediatr Orthop* 2009;29:356. [PMID: 19461377]

Spiegel PG, Cooperman DR, Laros GS: Epiphyseal fractures of the distal ends of the tibia and fibula: a retrospective study of two hundred and thirty-seven cases in children. *J Bone Joint Surg Am* 1978;60:1046. [PMID: 721852]

INJURIES RELATED TO CHILD ABUSE

Child abuse crosses all socioeconomic boundaries and takes many forms. The musculoskeletal system is frequently the site of abuse-related injuries, but findings may be subtle or misleading. The most critical issue to consider in suspected abuse is whether the history can explain the injury adequately and believably.

The classic radiographic picture of abuse is the presence of multiple healing fractures of various ages; in the absence of a bone fragility syndrome, the diagnosis may thus be obvious (Figure 10–51). Soft-tissue injuries were found in 92% of children suspected of having been physically abused, with ecchymosis as the most common finding, increasing in incidence with age. Long bones (femur or humerus) are the bones most commonly fractured during child abuse. These fractures are transverse or oblique shaft injuries, a common pattern that is not by itself diagnostic. The history is often one of a minor fall or a limb "catching" in the side of the crib. But studies of fractures in young children disclosed that injury mechanisms of this type are almost never the cause of serious skeletal injury, and the dichotomy between story and findings is highly suggestive of abuse. A good rule of thumb is to consider any long bone fracture in a child younger than 3 years as abuse until proved otherwise.

The orthopedic management of abuse fractures is rarely complex, and simple closed methods usually suffice. Nearly all such fractures carry an excellent prognosis and heal or remodel rapidly. It is the detection of the abuse, and its subsequent social management, that are the main determinant of outcome.

McMahon P, Grossman W, Gaffney M, et al: Soft-tissue injury as an indication of child abuse. *J Bone Joint Surg Am* 1995;77:1179. [PMID: 7642662]

Oral R, Blum KL, Johnson C: Fractures in young children: are physicians in the emergency department and orthopedic clinics adequately screening for possible abuse? *Pediatr Emerg Care* 2003;19:148. [PMID: 12813297]

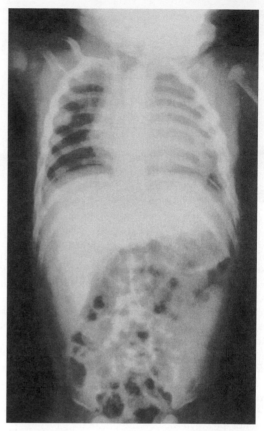

▲ **Figure 10–51.** The presence of multiple fractures of various ages as well as unexplained long-bone fracture in a young child should suggest the diagnosis of child abuse.

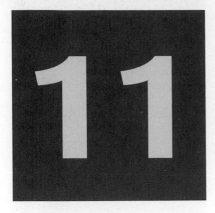

Amputations

Douglas G. Smith, MD

Harry B. Skinner, MD, PhD

Amputations are performed to remove extremities that are severely diseased, injured, or no longer functional. Although medical advances in antibiotics, trauma care, vascular surgery, and the treatment of neoplasms have improved the prospects for limb salvage, in many cases, prolonged attempts to save a limb that should be amputated lead to excessive morbidity or even death. To counsel a patient regarding amputation versus limb salvage adequately, the physician must provide sufficient information about the surgical and rehabilitative steps involved with each procedure and must also appraise the probable outcome for function realistically with each alternative. Attempting to salvage a limb is not always in the best interest of the patient.

The decision to amputate is an emotional process for the patient, the patient's family, and the surgeon. The value of taking a positive approach to amputation cannot be overemphasized. It is not a failure and should never be viewed as such. The amputation is a reconstructive procedure designed to help the patient create a new interface with the world and to resume his or her life. The residual limb must be surgically constructed with care to maintain muscle balance, transfer weight loads appropriately, and assume its new role of replacing the original limb.

For patients to achieve maximal function of the residual limb, they also need a clear understanding of what to expect for an early postoperative prosthetic fitting, a rehabilitation program, and long-term medical and prosthetic needs. For these discussions, the team approach to meeting the patient's needs can be especially rewarding. Nurses, prosthetists, physical and occupational therapists, and amputee support groups can be invaluable in providing the physical, psychological, emotional, and educational support needed in returning patients to a full and active life. Many new amputees state that a peer visitor program was one of the most helpful events during their hospitalization and rehabilitation. The Amputee Coalition of America, a not-for-profit organization, supports this peer visitor training and can help locate programs that are available throughout the country.

SPECIAL CONSIDERATIONS IN THE TREATMENT OF PEDIATRIC PATIENTS

In infants and children, amputations are frequently associated with congenital limb deficiencies, trauma, and tumors. Traumatic amputations in children in 2003 in the United States resulted in $22 million in inpatient costs for 946 cases. The majority of amputations were finger and thumb, but the highest costs were due to traumatic leg amputations. Congenital limb deficiencies are commonly described using the Birch revision of the Frantz and O'Rahilly classification system. Amelia is the complete absence of a limb; hemimelia is the absence of a major portion of a limb; and phocomelia is the attachment of the terminal limb at or near the trunk. Hemimelias can be further classified as terminal or intercalary. A terminal hemimelia is a complete transverse deficit at the end of the limb. An intercalary hemimelia is an internal segmental deficit with variable distal formation. In discussions of limb deficiencies, preaxial refers to the radial or tibial side of a limb, and postaxial refers to the ulnar or fibular side. The International Organization for Standardization (ISO) published a recommended classification for limb deficiencies in 1989 based on standard anatomic and radiologic characteristics and terminology. Although the ISO intentionally avoided the use of the terminology in the Frantz and O'Rahilly system, the older system is widely used, and the definitions and unusual language must still be understood by those caring for children with limb deficiency.

Reamputation of a congenital upper limb deficiency is rarely indicated, and even rudimentary appendages can often be functionally useful. In the lower limb, however, the ability to bear weight and the relative equality of leg lengths are mandatory for maximal function.

Reamputation may be indicated in proximal femoral focal deficiency and congenital absence of the fibula or tibia to produce a more functional residual limb and improve prosthetic placement. In fibular deficiency, outcomes were shown to be better in one study in adults who underwent lengthening procedures versus amputations, but these patients spent more of their childhood undergoing treatment.

These patients also had more residual foot rays than the initial amputation patients.

In the growing child, proportional change occurs in residual limb length from childhood to adulthood—an important concept to keep in mind when determining the surgical approach. A diaphyseal amputation in an infant or young child removes one of the epiphyseal growth centers, and the involved bone therefore does not keep proportional growth with the rest of the body. What initially appears to be a long transfemoral amputation in a small child can turn out to be a short and troublesome residual limb when the child reaches skeletal maturity. All attempts should be made to save the distal-most epiphysis by disarticulation. If this is not technically possible, the greatest amount of bone length should be saved.

Terminal overgrowth occurs in 8–12% of pediatric patients who had a surgical amputation. The growth of appositional bone at the transected end of a long bone exceeds the growth of the surrounding soft tissues. If left untreated, the appositional bone can penetrate through the skin (Figure 11–1). Terminal overgrowth of the transected bone does not occur as a result of the normal growth from the proximal physis pushing the distal end of the bone through the soft tissues, nor does it occur in limb disarticulations. Terminal overgrowth occurs most commonly in the humerus, fibula, tibia, and femur, in that order. Although numerous surgical procedures are used to manage this problem, the best approach consists of stump revision with adequate bone resection or autogenous osteochondral stump capping as originally described by Marquardt (Figure 11–2). If the stump-capping procedure is done at the time of original amputation, the graft material can be obtained from part of the amputated limb,

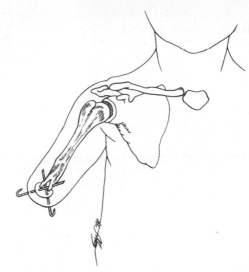

▲ **Figure 11–2.** Stump-capping procedure. The bone end was split longitudinally and the osteochondral graft fixed temporarily with K-wires.

such as the distal tibia, talus, or calcaneus. If a procedure is done later, the graft material can be obtained from the posterior iliac crest. Although techniques with nonautologous material are used, significant complications are reported. A report of using a modified Ertl osteomyoplasty to prevent terminal overgrowth in childhood limb deficiencies was not successful.

In a growing child, the fitting of a prosthesis can be challenging and requires frequent adjustments. Specialty pediatric amputee clinics can ease this process, provide family support, and make care more cost effective. The timing of prosthetic fitting should be initiated to coincide closely with normal motor skill development.

Prosthetic fitting for the upper limb should begin near the time the child gains sitting balance, usually around 4–6 months of age. A passive terminal device with blunt rounded edges is used initially. Active cable control and a voluntary opening terminal device are added when the child exhibits initiative in placing objects in the terminal device, usually in the second year of life. Myoelectric devices are usually not prescribed until the child masters traditional body-powered devices. The physical demand placed on prosthetic devices by children can often exceed the durability of current myoelectric designs, so maintenance and repair costs must be considered. The decision to prescribe a myoelectric device for a child is individual and depends on many factors, including the physical characteristics of the residual limb, the desires of the child, the training available, the proximity of prosthetic facilities for fitting and maintenance, and issues about funding.

Prosthetic fitting for the lower limb commonly begins when the child develops the ability to crawl and pull to a standing position, which is usually at 8–12 months. A child

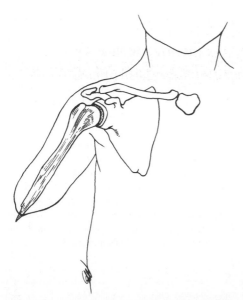

▲ **Figure 11–1.** Terminal overgrowth of the transected bone in a pediatric amputee.

with a Syme amputation or a transtibial amputation generally adapts to a prosthesis with surprising ease, and although formal gait training is not required, educational efforts are focused on teaching the parents about the prosthesis. For a child with a transfemoral amputation, control of a knee unit should not be expected immediately. The knee unit should be eliminated or locked in extension until the child is ambulating well and demonstrates proficient use of the prosthesis. The initial gait pattern used by a child with a transfemoral amputation is not a normal heel strike, midstance, toe-off gait pattern but is instead a more circumducted gait pattern with a prolonged foot flat phase. Formal gait training is seldom warranted until the child reaches 5 or 6 years of age. Attempts to force gait training too early can be frustrating for all involved. When pediatric patients are allowed to develop their own gait patterns as they grow and gain improved motor coordination, they are surprisingly adept at discovering the most efficient gait pattern without formal training.

Bernd L, Bläsius K, Lukoschek M, et al: The autologous stump plasty: treatment for bony overgrowth in juvenile amputees. *J Bone Joint Surg Br* 1991;73:203. [PMID: 2005139]

Birch JG, Walsh SJ, Small JM, et al: Syme amputation for the treatment of fibular deficiency. An evaluation of long-term physical and psychological functional status. *J Bone Joint Surg Am* 1999;81:1511. [PMID: 10565642]

Conner KA, McKenzie LB, Xiang H, et al: Pediatric traumatic amputations and hospital resource utilization in the United States, 2003. *J Trauma* 2010;68:131. [PMID: 20065768]

Drvaric DM, Kruger LM: Modified Ertl osteomyoplasty for terminal overgrowth in childhood limb deficiencies. *J Pediatr Orthop* 2001;21:392. [PMID 1137827]

Fixsen JA: Major lower limb congenital shortening: a mini review. *J Pediatr Orthop B* 2003;12:1. [PMID: 12488764]

Greene WG, Cary JM: Partial foot amputation in children: a comparison of the several types with the Syme's amputation. *J Bone Joint Surg Am* 1982;64:438. [PMID: 7061561]

International Organization for Standardization: ISO 8548-1: Prosthetics and orthotics—Limb deficiencies, Part 1: Method of describing limb deficiencies present at birth. Geneva, Switzerland: International Organization for Standardization; 1989.

Walker JL, Knapp D, Minter C, et al: Adult outcomes following amputation or lengthening for fibular deficiency. *J Bone Joint Surg Am* 2009;91:797. [PMID: 19339563]

Weber M: Neurovascular calcaneo-cutaneus pedicle graft for stump capping in congenital pseudarthrosis of the tibia: preliminary report of a new technique. *J Pediatr Orthop B* 2002;11:47. [PMID: 11866081]

GENERAL PRINCIPLES OF AMPUTATION

▶ Epidemiology

Epidemiologic data on the incidence of major amputation in the United States indicate a 38% decrease from 1998 to 2007 with a concomitant doubling in the rate of endovascular lower extremity revascularization. Nearly two thirds of amputations are performed in individuals with diabetes, even though people with diabetes represent only 6% of the population. The incidence of lower extremity amputation in 2008 was 4.5 per 1000 diabetic patients and varied by region, with high rates in Texas, Oklahoma, Louisiana, Arkansas, and Mississippi. Black patients are less likely to undergo limb salvage procedures for peripheral vascular disease and have a lower extremity amputation rate two to four times the rate in white patients.

Egorova NN, Guillerme S, Gelijns A, et al: An analysis of the outcomes of a decade of experience with lower extremity revascularization including limb salvage, lengths of stay, and safety. *J Vasc Surg* 2010;51:878. [PMID: 20045618]

Holman KH, Henke PK, Dimick JB, et al: Racial disparities in the use of revascularization before leg amputation in Medicare patients. *J Vasc Surg* 2011;54:420. [PMID: 21571495]

Margolis DJ, Hoffstad O, Nafash J, et al: Location, location, location: geographic clustering of lower-extremity amputation among Medicare beneficiaries with diabetes. *Diabetes Care* 2011;34:2363. [PMID: 21933906]

▶ Preoperative Evaluation and Decision Making

The decision to amputate a limb and the choice of amputation level can be difficult and are often subject to differences in opinion. Advances in the treatment of infection, peripheral vascular disease, replantation, and limb salvage complicate the decision-making process. The goals are to optimize a patient's function and reduce the level of morbidity.

A. Vascular Disease and Diabetes

Ischemia resulting from peripheral vascular disease remains the most frequent reason for amputation in the United States. Nearly two thirds of patients with ischemia also have diabetes. The preoperative assessment of these patients includes a physical examination and an evaluation of perfusion, nutrition, and immunocompetence. Preoperative screening tests can be helpful, but no single test is 100% accurate in predicting successful healing. Clinical judgment based on experience in examining and following many patients with vascular disease and diabetes is still the most important factor in preoperative assessment. The risk ratio of lower extremity amputation in diabetics was found to be 1.26 for each 1% increase in hemoglobin A1c.

Adler AI, Erqou S, Lima TA, et al: Association between glycated haemoglobin and the risk of lower extremity amputation in patients with diabetes mellitus: a review and meta-analysis. *Diabetologia* 2010;53:840. [PMID: 20127309]

1. Doppler ultrasound studies—The most readily available objective measurement of limb blood flow and perfusion is by Doppler ultrasound. Its use is especially valuable in the diagnosis of vascular injury associated with extremity trauma. Arterial wall calcification increases the pressure needed to compress the vessels of patients with vascular disease, and this often gives an artificially elevated reading. Low-pressure levels are indicative of poor perfusion, but normal and high levels can be confusing because of vessel wall calcification and are not predictive of normal perfusion or of wound healing. Digital vessels are not usually calcified, and blood pressure levels in the toes appear to be more predictive of healing than do those in the ankles. Maximal systolic acceleration as measured by Doppler has been found to be a sensitive, noninvasive predictor of the presence of arterial occlusive disease.

Halvorson JJ, Anz A, Langfitt M, et al: Vascular injury associated with extremity trauma: initial diagnosis and management. *J Am Acad Orthop Surg* 2011;19:495. [PMID: 21807917]

Van Tongeren RB, Bastiaansen AJ, Van Wissen RC, et al: A comparison of the Doppler-derived maximal systolic acceleration versus the ankle-brachial pressure index or detecting and quantifying peripheral arterial occlusive disease in diabetic patients. *J Cardiovasc Surg* 2010;51:391. [PMID: 20523290]

2. Transcutaneous oxygen tension measurements— Tests to measure transcutaneous partial pressure of oxygen (PO_2) are noninvasive and becoming more readily available in many vascular laboratories. These tests use a special temperature-controlled oxygen electrode to measure the PO_2 diffusing through the skin. The ultimate reading is based on several factors: the delivery of oxygen to the tissue, the utilization of oxygen by the tissue, and the diffusion of oxygen through the tissue and skin. Caution in interpreting the transcutaneous PO_2 measurements during acute cellulitis or edema is warranted because the presence of either of these disorders can increase oxygen utilization and decrease oxygen diffusion, thereby resulting in lower measurements of PO_2. Paradoxical measurements are also reported on the plantar skin of the foot. Despite these limitations, transcutaneous PO_2 and transcutaneous partial pressure of carbon dioxide (PCO_2) are both statistically accurate in predicting amputation healing, but this does not rule out false-negative results. Transcutaneous PO_2 levels of 34 mm Hg have been suggested as the threshold for revascularization in diabetics with the probability of above-the-ankle amputation of 9.7%; levels above 40 mm Hg drop the predicted amputation rate to 3 %.

Faglia E, Clerici G, Caminiti M, et al: Predictive values of the transcutaneous oxygen tension for above-the-ankle amputation in diabetic patients with critical limb ischemia. *Eur J Vasc Endovasc Surg* 2007;33:731. [PMID: 17296318]

3. Arteriography—Arteriography is not helpful in predicting successful healing of amputations, and this invasive test is probably not indicated solely for the purpose of selecting the proper level of amputation. Arteriography is indicated if the patient is truly a candidate for arterial reconstruction or angioplasty.

4. Nutrition and immunocompetence studies—Both nutrition and immunocompetence correlate directly with amputation wound healing. Many laboratory tests are available to assess nutrition and immunocompetence, but some are quite expensive. Screening tests for albumin level and total lymphocyte count are readily available and inexpensive. Several studies show increased healing of amputations in patients who have vascular disorders but have a serum albumin level of at least 3 g/dL and a total lymphocyte count exceeding 1500/mL. Nutritional screening is recommended to allow for nutritional improvement preoperatively and to help determine whether a higher level of amputation is needed.

5. Other issues—Activity level, ambulatory potential, cognitive skills, and overall medical condition must be evaluated to determine if the distal-most level of amputation is really appropriate for the patient.

For patients who are likely to remain ambulatory, the goals are to achieve healing at the distal-most level that can be fit with a prosthesis and to make successful rehabilitation possible. Newer studies of patients with vascular insufficiency and diabetes demonstrate that successful wound healing can be achieved in 70–80% of these patients at the transtibial or more distal amputation level. This is in sharp contrast to 25 years ago, when because of a fear of wound failure, surgeons elected to perform 80% of all lower extremity amputations at the transfemoral level.

For nonambulatory patients, the goals are not simply to obtain wound healing but also to minimize complications, improve sitting balance, and facilitate position transfers. Occasionally, a more proximal amputation more successfully meets these goals. For example, a bedridden patient with a knee flexion contracture might be better served with a knee disarticulation than a transtibial amputation, even if the biologic factors are present to heal the more distal amputation. Preoperative assessment of the patient's potential ability to use a prosthesis, the patient's specific needs for maintaining independent transfers, and the best weight distribution for seating can help in making wise decisions concerning the appropriate level of amputation and the most successful type of postoperative rehabilitation program.

Some nonambulatory patients do benefit from a partial foot amputation, or even transtibial amputation with prosthetic fitting, not with the goal of walking but to use that leg as a standing pivot for independent transfers. In these cases, prosthetic fitting is justified.

Sun JH, Tsai JS, Huang CH, et al: Risk factors for lower extremity amputation in diabetic foot disease categorized by Wagner classification. *Diabetes Res Clin Pract* 2012;95:358. [PMID: 22115502]

Wagner FW: The dysvascular foot: a system of diagnosis and treatment. *Foot Ankle* 1981;2:64. [PMID: 7319435]

B. Trauma

As vascular reconstruction techniques improved, more attempts to salvage limbs were initially made, often with the result that multiple surgical procedures were subsequently required. In many cases, amputation was ultimately performed after a substantial investment of time, money, and emotional energy. Current studies offer guidelines for immediate or early amputation and show the value of amputation not only in saving lives but also in preventing the emotional, marital, and financial disasters that can follow unwise and desperate limb salvage attempts. Although several scoring systems for mangled limbs are published, none can perfectly predict when an amputation should be performed. These scores can help in the decision-making process, but good clinical experience and judgment are still required.

The absolute indication for amputation in trauma remains an ischemic limb with unreconstructable vascular injury. Massively crushed muscle and ischemic tissue release myoglobin and cell toxins, which can lead to renal failure, adult respiratory distress syndrome, and even death. In two groups of high-risk patients (multiply injured patients and elderly patients with a mangled extremity), limb salvage, even though technically possible, can become life-threatening and generally should be avoided. In all patients, the decision about whether to undertake immediate or early amputation of a mangled limb must also depend on whether it is an upper extremity or lower extremity.

An upper extremity can function with minimal or protective sensation, and even a severely compromised arm can serve as an assistive limb. An assistive upper extremity often functions better than the currently available prosthetic replacements. The decision of salvage versus amputation in the upper limb should be based on the chance of maintaining some useful function, even if that function is limited.

In the lower extremity, weight bearing is mandatory. A lower limb functions poorly without sensation, and an assistive limb is not useful. A salvaged lower limb often functions worse than a modern prosthetic replacement unless the limb can tolerate full weight bearing, is relatively pain free, has enough sensation to provide protective feedback, and has durable skin and soft-tissue coverage that does not break down whenever walking is attempted. The decision to salvage a mangled lower extremity should be based on providing a limb that can tolerate the demands of walking.

Zaraca F, Ponzoni A, Stringari C, et al: Lower extremity traumatic vascular injury at a level II trauma center: an analysis of limb loss risk factors and outcomes. *Minerva Chir* 2011;66:397. [PMID: 22117207]

C. Frostbite

Exposure to cold temperatures can directly damage the tissue and cause a related vascular impairment from endothelial vessel injury and increased sympathetic tone. If the foot or hand is wet or directly exposed to the wind, cold injury can result even in temperatures above freezing. The immediate treatment involves restoring the core body temperature and then rewarming the injured body part in a water bath at a temperature of 40–44°C for 20–30 minutes. Rewarming can be painful, and the patient often requires opiate analgesia. After rewarming, the involved part should be kept dry, blisters left intact, and dry gauze dressings used. Tissue plasminogen activator administration may be helpful in reducing digital amputations after warming from frostbite. The goals are to keep the injured extremity clean and dry and to prevent maceration, especially between the digits.

The temptation to perform early amputation should be avoided because the amount of recovery can be dramatic. As the extremity recovers from frostbite, a zone of mummification (dry gangrene) develops distally, and a zone of intermediate tissue injury forms just proximal to this. Even at the time of clear demarcation, the tissue just proximal to the zone of mummification continues to heal from the cold insult, and although the outward appearance is often pink and healthy, this tissue is not totally normal. Delaying amputation can improve the chance of primary wound healing. It is not unusual to wait 2–6 months for definitive surgery. Despite having mummified tissue, infection is rare if the tissue is kept clean and dry.

Johnson AR, Jensen HL, Peltier G, et al: Efficacy of intravenous tissue plasminogen activator in frostbite patients and presentation of a treatment protocol for frostbite patients. *Foot Ankle Spec* 2011;4:344. [PMID: 21965579]

D. Tumors

Patients with musculoskeletal neoplasms face new choices in treatment with the development of limb salvage techniques and adjuvant chemotherapy and radiation therapy. If an amputation is chosen, the amputation incisions must be carefully planned to achieve the appropriate surgical margin.

Surgical margins (Figure 11–3) are characterized by the relationship of the surgical incision to the lesion, to the inflammatory zone surrounding the lesion, and to the anatomic compartment in which the lesion is located. The four types of margins are the intralesional margin, in which the surgical incision enters the lesion; the marginal margin, in which the incision enters the inflammatory zone but not the lesion; the wide margin, in which the incision enters the same anatomic compartment as the lesion but is outside of the inflammatory zone; and the radical margin, in which the incision remains outside of the involved anatomic compartment. Biopsy incisions and amputation incisions must be planned with careful consideration as to the tumor margin required.

Newer studies continue to evaluate the complex issues and outcomes of amputation versus limb-sparing procedures for patients with extremity sarcomas. Studies still suggest that functional outcomes in terms of kinesiologic

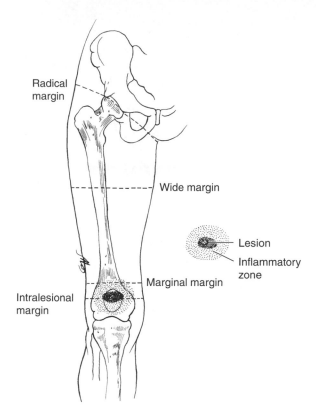

Radical margin

Wide margin

Lesion

Inflammatory zone

Marginal margin

Intralesional margin

▲ **Figure 11–3.** Surgical margins in tumors of the extremity.

parameters are comparable with either limb salvage or amputation. Both treatment groups report quality of life problems involving employment, health insurance, social isolation, and poor self-esteem. Overall survival remains comparable with either treatment. In some tumors, amputation may achieve better local disease control. These results confirm that the decision about treatment must be made on an individual basis, according to the specific lifestyle and needs of the patient.

Muramatsu K, Ihara K, Miyoshi T, et al: Clinical outcome of limb-salvage surgery after wide resection of sarcoma and femoral vessel reconstruction. *Ann Vasc Surg* 2011;25:1070. [PMID: 21831587]

▶ Surgical Definitions and Techniques

Terminology for amputation level now uses an accepted international nomenclature. *Transtibial* should be used instead of below knee, and *transfemoral* instead of above knee. In the upper extremity, the terms *transradial* and *transhumeral* replace the older terms below elbow and above elbow.

Careful surgical techniques, especially in soft-tissue handling, are more critical to wound healing and functional outcome in amputation procedures than in many other surgical procedures. The tissues are often traumatized or poorly vascularized, and the risk of wound failure is high, particularly if close attention is not paid to soft-tissue technique. Flaps should be kept thick, avoiding unnecessary dissection between the skin and subcutaneous, fascial, and muscle planes. In adults, periosteum should not be stripped proximal to the level of transection. In children, however, removing 0.5 cm of the distal periosteum may help prevent terminal overgrowth. The rounding of all bone edges and the beveling of prominences are necessary for optimal prosthetic use.

Muscle loses its contractile function when the skeletal attachments are divided during amputation. Stabilizing the distal insertion of muscle can improve residual limb function by preventing muscle atrophy, providing counterbalance to the deforming forces resulting from amputation, and providing stable padding over the end of the bone. Myodesis is the direct suturing of muscle or tendon to the bone or the periosteum. Myodesis techniques are most effective in stabilizing strong muscles needed to counteract strong antagonistic muscle forces, such as in cases involving transfemoral or transhumeral amputation and in cases involving knee or elbow disarticulation. Myoplasty involves the suturing of muscle to muscle over the end of the bone. The distal stabilization of the muscle is more secure with myodesis than with myoplasty. Care must be taken to prevent a mobile sling of muscle over the distal end of the bone, which usually results in a painful bursa.

The transection of nerves always results in neuroma formation, but all neuromas are not symptomatic. Historical attempts to diminish symptomatic neuromas include clean transection, ligation, crushing, cauterization, capping, perineural closure, and end-loop anastomosis. No technique is more effective than careful and meticulous isolation, retraction, and clean transection of the nerve. This allows the cut end to retract into the soft tissues, away from the scar, pulsating vessels, and prosthetic pressure points. Ligation of a nerve is still indicated to control bleeding from the blood vessels contained within larger nerves, such as the sciatic.

Split-thickness skin grafts are generally discouraged except as a means to save a knee or elbow joint that has a stable bone and good muscle coverage. Skin grafts do best with adequate soft-tissue support and are least durable when closely adherent to bone. New prosthetic interfaces, such as silicone-based liners, can help reduce the shear at the interface and improve durability in skin-grafted residual limbs.

An open amputation is occasionally necessary to control a severe ascending infection. The term *guillotine amputation* should be avoided because it gives the impression that the limb is transected at one level through skin, muscle, and bone. Open amputations need to be performed with careful planning and forethought as to how the amputation will eventually be closed. The surgical plan must obviously consider adequate debridement of tissue necrosis and drainage of infection but must also consider the surgical flaps and tissue needed for a functional closure of the amputation to allow prosthetic fitting.

The problem of ascending infection is seen, for example, in a diabetic patient with a severe infection of the foot and cellulitis extending upward to the calf. The open amputation removes the source of infection, provides adequate drainage, and allows the acute cellulitis to resolve. After resolution, a definitive amputation and closure can be done safely. In the case of a diabetic foot infection, an open ankle disarticulation is simple, relatively bloodless, and preserves the posterior calf flap for a definitive transtibial amputation. Occasionally, it is necessary to make a longitudinal incision to drain the posterior tibial, anterior tibial, or peroneal tendon sheaths, in which case care should be taken not to violate the posterior flap of the definitive amputation. This approach often prevents having open, transected muscle bellies that can retract and become edematous—a problem that commonly occurs if an open calf-level amputation was initially performed and one that can make the definitive amputation difficult. In more severe infections or in cases in which the level of the definitive amputation will clearly be transfemoral, an open knee disarticulation has the same advantages as the open ankle disarticulation.

▶ Postoperative Care

A. Postoperative Care and Planning

The terminal amputation allows the unique opportunity to manipulate the physical environment of the wound during healing. A variety of methods are described, including rigid dressings, soft dressings, controlled environment chambers, air splints, and skin traction. The use of a rigid dressing controls edema, protects the limb from trauma, decreases postoperative pain, and allows early mobilization and rehabilitation.

The use of an immediate postoperative prosthesis, or IPOP (Figure 11–4), is effective in decreasing the time to limb maturation and the time to definitive prosthetic fitting. In most cases involving a lower limb amputation, the surgeon has the patient start with partial weight bearing if the wound appears stable after the first cast change, which usually takes place between the fifth and tenth day after surgery. Immediate postoperative weight bearing can be initiated safely in selected patients, usually young patients in whom an amputation was performed following a traumatic injury and above the zone of injury. Rigid dressings and the IPOP need to be applied carefully, but their application is easily learned and well within the scope of interested physicians. For upper extremity amputations, an IPOP can be applied immediately. Early training with an IPOP is believed to increase the long-term acceptance and use of a prosthesis. Chapter 12 offers a detailed discussion of rehabilitation.

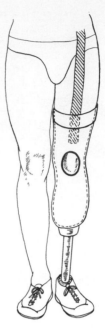

▲ **Figure 11–4.** Immediate postoperative prosthetic cast for transtibial amputation.

To counsel patients adequately, some insight into the typical surgical and postoperative course can be helpful. Many patients require inpatient hospital care for 5–8 days after a transtibial amputation. Epidural or patient-controlled analgesia is usually required for pain control. Assistance with basic mobility and emotional support are also necessary. Antibiotics can minimize the risk of infection. The cast applied at the end of the surgical procedure is changed about postoperative day 5. If the wound healing is adequate, a new cast with a foot attachment is applied, and the patient can begin ambulating with approximately 30 lb of weight on the amputated extremity. Transtibial amputees are discharged to home or a nursing facility typically 5 or 8 days after surgery. Outpatient visits are scheduled weekly to change the cast, which frequently becomes loose as edema lessens, and to monitor wound healing and allow suture removal. Active and active-assisted knee range of motion (ROM) is performed between each cast. On average, approximately six casts are applied on a weekly basis until the wound heals, edema resolves, wrinkles return to the skin, and the patient is ready for prosthetic fitting. The cast and the prosthetic foot attachment are applied and aligned by either the surgeon or the prosthetist. New prefabricated, removable postoperative prosthetic systems are alternatives to the traditional casting techniques. Unfortunately, comparison trials versus traditional techniques have not been done.

Close interaction between the patient, the physical therapist, and the prosthetist is required in the first 12–18 months.

The socket made for the first prosthesis must allow modifications as the residual limb continues to change shape during this time. Volume changes and mismatch between the shape of the socket and the evolving shape of the residual limb are treated with amputation socks and by adding pads to the socket or socket liner. Pads are usually needed in the region that contacts the anteromedial and anterolateral tibial flares, and posteriorly, in the popliteal region. Even with careful modifications, the prosthetic socket must be changed two or three times in the first 18 months. Because of these frequent prosthetic modifications, encouraging the patient to work with a prosthetic provider who is located close to the patient's residence can help tremendously in this rehabilitation phase. Many patients have an immediate desire to have the most advanced and high-tech components in their first prosthesis. But often these components are designed for higher activity levels than are typically achieved in the rehabilitation phase and are too rigid. Discussing how the prosthesis will evolve and be upgraded as the patient's activity increases can ease this process. A new prosthesis is typically required around month 18; the old components often can be turned into a shower leg.

Van Velzen AD, Nederhand MJ, Emmelot CH, et al: Early treatment of trans-tibial amputees: retrospective analysis of early fitting and elastic bandaging. *Prosthet Orthot Int* 2005;29:3. [PMID: 16180373]

Taylor L, Cavenett S, Stepien JM, et al: Removable rigid dressings: a retrospective case-note audit to determine the validity of post-amputation application. *Prosthet Orthot Int* 2008;32:223. [PMID: 18569890]

B. Prevention and Treatment of Complications

1. Failure of the wound to heal properly—Problems with wound healing, especially in diabetic and ischemic limbs, occur as the result of insufficient blood supply, infection, or errors in surgical technique. Healing failure rates are difficult to interpret because they depend so much on the level of amputation selected. Low failure rates can be achieved by doing amputations at an extremely proximal level in the majority of cases, but this sacrifices the rehabilitation potential of many patients because the ability to ambulate decreases dramatically with a transfemoral amputation. Wound healing failure that necessitates reamputation at a more proximal level occurs in approximately 5–10% of cases at centers specializing in amputee treatment.

Most surgeons prefer open wound care if the wound gap is less than 1 cm wide and prefer revision surgery if the gap is wider. If the surgical edema has resolved and some atrophy has already occurred, a wedge excision of all nonviable tissue can be performed and still allow primary closure without any tension at the original level. If it is not possible to oppose the viable tissue gently without tension, bone shortening or reamputation at a more proximal level should be performed.

In patients with small local areas of wound-healing failure, successful treatment with rigid dressings and an IPOP has been reported. The wounds are debrided weekly and packed open, and the IPOP is applied to allow some weight bearing. The stimulation of weight bearing can increase local circulation, decrease edema, and promote wound healing.

2. Infection—Infection without widespread tissue necrosis or flap failure may be seen after surgery, especially if active distal infection was present at the time of the definitive amputation or if the amputation was done near the zone of a traumatic injury. Hematomas can also predispose a wound to infection. In cases involving infection or hematomas, the wound must be opened, drained, and debrided. If the wound is allowed to remain open for an extended time, the flaps retract and become edematous, which makes delayed closure difficult or impossible without shortening the bone. One solution, which can be instituted after thorough debridement and irrigation, is to close only the central one third to one half of the amputation wound and to use open packing for the medial and lateral corners (Figure 11–5). This method provides coverage of the bone but also allows adequate drainage and open wound management for the edges. If the original problem was truly infection and not tissue failure, the open portions of the wound heal secondarily, and the result is still a residual limb suitable for prosthetic fitting.

3. Phantom sensation—Phantom sensation is the feeling that all or a part of the amputated limb is still present. This sensation is felt by nearly everyone who undergoes surgical amputation, but it is not always bothersome. Phantom sensation

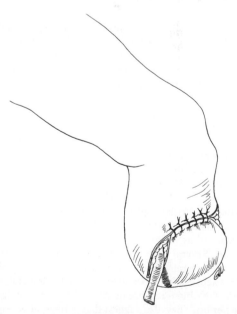

▲ **Figure 11–5.** Partial closure of the infected transtibial amputation.

usually diminishes over time, and telescoping (the sensation that the phantom foot or hand has moved proximally toward the stump) commonly occurs.

4. Pain and phantom pain—Phantom pain is defined as a bothersome, painful, or burning sensation in the part of the limb that is missing. Although from 80 to 90% of patients with acquired amputation experience some episodes of phantom pain, the episodes are often infrequent and brief. The dreaded problem of unrelenting phantom pain fortunately occurs only in a much smaller minority of patients. Surgical intervention for this problem is not very successful.

Local physical measures, including massage, cold packs, exercise, neuromuscular stimulation by external electrical currents, acupuncture, and regional sympathectomy, may under given circumstances have a place in therapy when the pain is intractable. A technique that has gained some acceptance and success is the use of transcutaneous electrical nerve stimulation (TENS), incorporated either into a prosthesis or used as an isolated unit. The TENS system can be worn by the amputee at night and even during the day with the battery pack attached to the belt or inside a pocket. We use this TENS system with moderate short-term success, but it is rare to see a patient who continues to use a TENS system for more than a year.

Pharmacologic treatment shows some success with several oral agents including gabapentin, amitriptyline, carbamazepine, phenytoin, and mexiletine. Medications can decrease the frequency of phantom pain episodes and decrease the intensity of these episodes. The appropriate use of an intravenous lidocaine challenge is predictive of a favorable response to oral mexiletine. Unfortunately, no indicators are good at predicting who will respond to treatment with gabapentin, amitriptyline, carbamazepine, or phenytoin. Psychological support can be beneficial, particularly when personality problems seem to accentuate the occurrence of pain. The individual needs patience and reassurance that the discomfort will improve with time, especially when a supportive social environment is present.

The sensations described by patients with phantom pain may be similar to the symptoms of reflex sympathetic dystrophy after an injury. Reflex sympathetic dystrophy can occur in amputated limbs and should be treated aggressively if present. Although rare, pain unrelated to the amputation can easily be overlooked. The differential diagnosis includes radicular nerve pain from proximal entrapment or disk herniation, arthritis of proximal joints, ischemic pain, and referred visceral pain.

Research has progressed in the prevention of phantom limb pain. Several authors document that the use of perioperative epidural anesthesia or intraneural anesthesia can block the acute pain associated with amputation surgery and decrease the opiate requirements in the immediate postoperative period. They also suggest that perioperative analgesia can prevent or decrease the later incidence of phantom pain, although this is difficult to document. The literature unfortunately is not conclusive on whether preemptive measures can truly reduce the frequency or severity of phantom limb pain. Some reports dispute the claims that preemptive analgesia reduces the frequency of phantom limb problems. A randomized trial by Lambert and colleagues found that perioperative epidural block started 24 hours before amputation is not superior to infusion of local anesthetic via a perineural catheter in preventing phantom pain but does give better relief in the immediate postoperative period.

Attal N, Rouaud J, Brasseur L, et al: Systemic lidocaine in pain due to peripheral nerve injury and predictors of response. *Neurology* 2004;62:218. [PMID: 14745057]

Bone M, Critchley P, Buggy DJ: Gabapentin in postamputation phantom limb pain: a randomized, double-blind, placebo-controlled, cross-over study. *Reg Anesth Pain Med* 2002;7:481. [PMID: 12373695]

Siddle L: The challenge and management of phantom limb pain after amputation. *Br J Nurs* 2004;13:664. [PMID: 15218432]

Subedi B, Grossberg GT: Phantom limb pain: mechanisms and treatment approaches. *Pain Res Treat* 2011;2011:864605. [PMID: 22110933]

5. Edema—Postoperative edema is common in patients who have undergone amputation. Rigid dressings can help reduce this problem. If soft dressings are used, they should be combined with stump wrapping to control edema, especially if the patient is a prosthetic candidate. The ideal shape of a residual limb is cylindrical, not conical. One common mistake is wrapping the stump too tightly at the proximal end, which can lead to congestion and worsening edema and also cause the residual limb to become shaped like a dumbbell. Another common mistake is not wrapping transfemoral amputations in a waist-high soft spica cast that includes the groin. If wrapped incorrectly, the limb has a narrow, conical shape, and a large adductor roll develops. Because of the difficulty in wrapping the transfemoral amputation with elastic bandages, shrinker socks with a waist belt are frequently used as a safer alternative for the transfemoral level.

Stump edema syndrome is a condition commonly caused by proximal constriction and characterized by edema, pain, blood in the skin, and increased pigmentation. The syndrome usually responds to temporary removal of the prosthesis, elevation of the residual limb, and compression.

6. Joint contractures—Joint contractures usually develop between the time of amputation and prosthetic fitting. Contractures that exist preoperatively can seldom be corrected postoperatively.

In transfemoral amputees, the deforming forces are flexion and abduction. Adductor and hamstring stabilization can oppose the deforming forces. During the postoperative period, patients should avoid propping up the residual limb on a pillow and should begin active and passive motion exercises early, including lying prone to stretch the hip.

In transtibial amputees, knee flexion contractures greater than 15 degrees can cause major prosthetic problems and failure. Long leg rigid dressings, early postoperative prosthetic fitting, quadriceps-strengthening exercises, and hamstring stretching can prevent this complication. Because contractures in below-knee amputees can seldom be corrected, their prevention is paramount.

In the upper extremity amputee, shoulder and elbow flexion contractures often follow amputation, especially with short residual limbs. Efforts should be directed at prevention, with aggressive physical therapy beginning soon after surgery.

7. Dermatologic problems—Good general hygiene includes keeping the residual limb and prosthetic socket clean, rinsed well to remove all soap residual, and thoroughly dry. Patients should avoid the application of foreign materials and be encouraged not to shave a residual lower limb. Shaving may increase the problems with ingrown hairs and folliculitis.

Reactive hyperemia is the early onset of redness and tenderness after amputation. It is usually related to pressure and resolves spontaneously.

Epidermoid cysts commonly occur at the prosthetic socket brim, especially posteriorly. These cysts are difficult to treat and commonly recur, even after excision. The best initial approach is to modify the socket and relieve pressure over the cyst. Warm heat, often with a warm tea bag; topical agents; and oral antibiotics can be required as local treatment.

Verrucous hyperplasia is a wartlike overgrowth of skin that can occur on the distal end of the residual limb. It is caused by a lack of distal contact and failure to remove normal keratin. The disorder is characterized by a thick mass of keratin, sometimes accompanied by fissuring, oozing, and infection. The infection should be addressed first, and then the limb should be soaked and treated with salicylic acid paste to soften the keratin. Topical hydrocortisone is occasionally helpful in resistant cases. Prosthetic modifications to improve distal contact must be made to prevent recurrences. Because the distal limb is often tender and prosthetic modifications are uncomfortable, an aggressive preventive approach is warranted.

Contact dermatitis sometimes occurs in amputees and can be confused with infection. The primary irritation type of dermatitis is caused by contact with acids, bases, or caustics and frequently results from failure to rinse detergents and soaps from prosthetic socks. Patients should be instructed to use mild soap and to rinse extremely well. Allergic contact dermatitis is commonly caused by the nickel and chrome in metal, antioxidants in rubber, carbon in neoprene, chromium salts used to treat leather, and unpolymerized epoxy and polyester resins in plastic laminated sockets. After infection is ruled out and contact dermatitis is confirmed, treatment begins and consists of removal of the irritant and use of soaks, corticosteroid creams, and compression with elastic wraps or shrinkers.

Superficial skin infections are common in amputees. Folliculitis occurs in hairy areas, often soon after the patient starts to wear a prosthesis. Pustules develop in the eccrine sweat glands surrounding the hair follicles, and this problem is often worse if the patient shaves. Hidradenitis, which occurs in apocrine glands in the groin and axilla, tends to be chronic and responds poorly to treatment. Socket modification to relieve any pressure in these areas can be helpful. Candidiasis and other dermatophytoses present with scaly, itchy skin, often with vesicles at the border and clearing centrally. Dermatophytoses are diagnosed with a potassium hydroxide preparation and treated with topical antifungal agents.

C. Lengthening of Residual Limbs

The ultimate function of an amputation depends on both the length of the bone and the quality of the soft-tissue envelope for the residual limb. Ilizarov techniques of distraction osteogenesis are applied to lengthen the tibia or ulna in amputees. Bone lengthening can be successful, but often issues of soft-tissue coverage remain. Although great success is described in a small series of congenital short transradial amputations, another author describes the pending necrosis of the skin over the tip of the lengthened ulna. Nonadherent, mobile soft tissue that can pad the distal end of the bone is vitally important to successful prosthetic fitting. Microsurgical techniques are also applied to use free tissue transfer to supply this type of coverage over bone in select patients, most often in trauma or tumor surgery. By using these techniques, the gracilis or latissimus dorsi muscle can be transferred to the end of the residual limb and covered with skin graft. The transposed tissues do not have sensation, and the bulk of the flap can lead to tremendous volume changes over the first 2 years. Lack of sensation and volume issues do complicate prosthetic fitting and function. These extraordinary techniques are probably best reserved for very select and unique circumstances.

Orhun H, Saka G, Bilgic E, et al: Lengthening of short stumps for functional use of prostheses. *Prosthet Orthot Int* 2003;27:153. [PMID: 14571946]

Walker JL, White H, Jenkins JO, et al: Femoral lengthening after transfemoral amputation. *Orthopedics* 2006;29:53. [PMID: 16429935]

D. Osseointegration of Prosthetic Devices

The success of the Branemark method of osseointegration of dental implants into the maxilla and mandible has been translated into the use of direct attachment of prostheses to the musculoskeletal system. This is done by implanting a titanium porous-coated stem into the medullary canal of the femur and allowing ingrowth with a closed wound. After the interface has matured (6 months), the wound is opened and the prosthesis interface is attached directly (percutaneously) to the bone implant. After a gradual rehabilitation protocol, the prosthesis is attached and the patient has a direct connection of the prosthesis to the skeletal system. The originator of this technique recently published his experience, and of 106 implants, 68 were currently using the implant with a range of follow-up of 3 months to 17.5 years. Another earlier report by another group suggests that despite improvements in comfort, function, and quality of life due to this technology, issues need to be addressed prior to general use. This technology has been approved for use in the Europe.

Hagberg K, Branemark R: One hundred patients treated with osseointegrated transfemoral amputation prostheses—rehabilitation perspective. *J Rehabil Res Dev* 2009;46:331. [PMID: 19675986]

Sullivan J, Uden M, Robinson KP, et al: Rehabilitation of the transfemoral amputee with an osseointegrated prosthesis: the United Kingdom experience. *Prosthet Orthot Int* 2003;27:114. [PMID: 14571941]

E. Control of Prostheses

Electromyography (EMG) is a commonly used method to control motorized upper extremity prostheses. The EMG signal is detected from an electrode on the skin, is optimized, and is then used to modulate the function of a motor controlling the motion of, for example, the wrist or elbow. The quality of the performance of the function of the prosthesis is highly dependent on the ability of the interface (eg, EMG signal, skin interface) to transmit information. EMG information is noisy, nonlinear with force or motion, and can be affected by intervening tissue and motion between the skin and electrode. Use of EMG signals is intuitive if the signal that controls the prosthesis function is from muscles that previously controlled that same function in the intact extremity (eg, EMG signal from the triceps and biceps used to control prosthetic elbow flexion and extension). Different signals are required for each motion of the prosthesis that is desired. One means of achieving multiple signals, or signals where there are no appropriate residual muscles from which to obtain a signal, is to use **targeted muscle reinnervation**. The concept is to implant nerves that, before amputation, went to muscles of the amputated limb into other muscles. These secondary muscles then can be directed by the brain to contract when the amputee wants a particular function, because the brain is sending messages to the same nerves that previously directed this function. The EMG signal from those muscles can be used to intuitively drive a prosthesis motion. This method was used to allow a patient with shoulder disarticulations to control two degrees of freedom of a myoelectric prosthesis with reinnervation of different portions of the pectoralis major with the median, radial, and musculocutaneous nerves. This technique makes the pectoralis muscle a source for EMG signals, which are intuitive to the functions of the extremity (eg, the EMG signal from the portion of the pectoralis muscle now innervated by

the radial nerve can be used to drive elbow extension). It is necessary to denervate the recipient muscle and implant the transplanted nerve directly at the motor point of the muscle. The technique is finding increasing popularity by surgeons working to improve amputee prosthetic function.

Corbett EA, Perreault EJ, Kuiken TA: Comparison of electromyography and force as interfaces for prosthetic control. *J Rehabil Res Dev* 2011;48:629. [PMID: 21938651]

Dumanian GA, Ko JH, O'Shaughnessy KD, et al: Targeted reinnervation for transhumeral amputees: current surgical technique and update on results. *Plast Reconstr Surg* 2009;124:863. [PMID: 19730305]

Kuiken TA, Dumanian GA, Lipschutz RD, et al: The use of targeted muscle reinnervation for improved myoelectric prosthesis control in a bilateral shoulder disarticulation amputee. *Prosthet Orthot Int* 2004;28:245. [PMID: 1565863]

Simon AE, Hargrove LJ, Lock BA, et al: Target achievement control test: evaluating real-time myoelectric pattern-recognition control of multifunctional upper-limb prostheses. *J Rehabil Res Dev* 2011;48:619. [PMID: 21938650]

F. Prescription of Prosthetic Limbs

For lower limb prostheses, the major advances include the development of new lightweight structural materials (see Chapter 1), the incorporation of elastic response ("energy-storing") designs, the use of computer-assisted design and computer-assisted manufacturing technology in sockets, and microprocessor control of the prosthetic knee joint. For upper limb use, new electronic technology has increased the success and durability of myoelectric prostheses. The surgeon who prescribes prosthetic limbs should have a basic understanding of the general features available to match optimally the components with the patient's specific needs.

A good prosthetic prescription specifies the socket type, suspension, shank construction, specific joints, and terminal device. The socket can be a hard socket with no or minimal interface, or it can incorporate a liner. For the transfemoral amputee, a wide variety of socket shapes are available and range from the traditional quadrilateral design to the newer narrow mediolateral design. The prosthesis is suspended from the body by straps, belts, socket contour, liners that roll on the limb and then lock to the socket, suction, friction, or physiologic muscle control.

Shank construction can be either exoskeletal or endoskeletal. The older exoskeletal type has a rigid outer shell that is hollow in the center. The endoskeletal type has a central pylon or pipe surrounded by a soft and lightweight cosmetic foam cover. In the past, exoskeletal systems were more durable; however, as materials technology has improved, so has the durability and cosmetic appearance of endoskeletal systems. The endoskeletal systems also allow more adjustment and fine tuning of alignment and are now considered structurally as durable as the older exoskeletal designs.

However, the cosmetic and foam covers for the endoskeletal systems are not as durable as an exoskeletal shell. Exoskeletal systems are rarely prescribed, except for very active patients without easy access to prosthetic services or for those involved in activities that would stain, tear, or destroy the endoskeletal cover. As the public's impression of disability has evolved, many active patients now decide not to cover the prosthesis and often take pride in the high-tech look of the titanium or carbon fiber components incorporated in an endoskeletal prosthesis.

A large variety of elbow, wrist, knee, and ankle joints are now available, as well as numerous terminal devices, including hands, hooks, feet, and special adaptive equipment for sports and work. The choice of an appropriate terminal device is extremely important. For an upper extremity amputee, there is no sensation in the prosthesis, and the critical feedback of touch and proprioception is missing. Initially, a hook may be a better choice than a prosthetic hand because vision must substitute for upper extremity proprioception, and a prosthetic hand blocks vision and makes dexterous use of the terminal device difficult and clumsy. In each case, the prosthetic prescription must be individualized to ensure the most efficient system for a particular patient.

Nearly all prosthetic sockets are fabricated by forming a thermoplastic or laminate socket over a plaster mold. An exact mold of the residual limb does not make a good socket for a prosthesis. The original mold must be modified to relieve the socket over areas that cannot tolerate pressure and to indent the socket over areas that can. Test sockets of clear plastic are commonly made to visualize the blanching of the skin at troublesome areas. Automated fabrication of mobility aids (AFMA) technology uses computer-assisted design and manufacturing to aid the prosthetist by digitizing the residual limb, adding the standard modifications usually applied to a mold, and allowing additional fine manipulation of the shape on the computer screen. The computer can direct the carving of the mold or fabrication of the socket. AFMA technology can decrease the time needed for the fabrication of prostheses and increase the time available for the evaluation and training of patients. The best use of AFMA is to allow fabrication of multiple sockets for one patient during the fitting process. By using computer modifications, refinements are added in each iteration, ultimately to optimize the fit and comfort of the final socket. Before AFMA, this technique was not cost effective.

Myoelectric components are exciting but should generally not be prescribed for patients until they master traditional body-powered devices and their residual limb volume is stable. Myoelectric devices are used most successfully by patients with a midlength transradial amputation. Although a long below-elbow limb has better rotation, it is less able to contain the electronics. The need for myoelectric devices is greater in patients with a more proximal upper extremity amputation, but the weight and slow speed of the myoelectric components is a deterrent for their use. Hybrid devices utilizing body power and myoelectric components can be effective.

Muscles stabilized by myodesis or myoplasty techniques seem to generate a better signal for myoelectric use.

Microprocessor control systems are applied to the knee units for transfemoral amputees. Several are available, including the Hybrid Knee (Energy Knee), Rheo Knee, and Adaptive 2 knee, but the most well-known is the C-Leg. This knee unit was shown in one study to have clear advantages in swing phase resistance and damping in terminal extension. The microprocessor control alters the resistance of the knee unit to flexion or extension appropriately by sensing the position and velocity of the shank relative to the thigh. The current microprocessor-controlled knee units still do not provide power for active knee extension that would assist in rising from the sitting position or in providing power to the amputee's gait and rise up stairs. The new microprocessor-controlled so-called intelligent knee units do offer superior control when walking at varied speeds, descending ramps and stairs, and walking on uneven surfaces. Patients report improved confidence and a decrease in the tendency for the knee unit to buckle. Despite their high cost, they should be prescribed for amputees who need stability and fall prevention, and thus, these units help less active rather than more active amputees. Some more active amputees find the microprocessor-controlled legs too slow. One transfemoral amputee credits this new technology for his survival by allowing him to descend 70 stories in the World Trade Center at a normal pace during the terrorist attacks.

Bellmann M, Schmalz T, Blumentritt S: Comparative biomechanical analysis of current microprocessor-controlled prosthetic knee joints. *Arch Phys Med Rehabil* 2010;91:644. [PMID: 20382300]

Bosse MJ, MacKenzie EJ, Kellam JF, et al: A prospective evaluation of the clinical utility of the lower-extremity injury-severity scores. *J Bone Joint Surg Am* 2001;83-A:3. [PMID: 11205855]

Brooks B, Dean R, Patel S, et al: TBI or not TBI: that is the question. Is it better to measure toe pressure than ankle pressure in diabetic patients? *Diabet Med* 2001;18:528. [PMID: 11553180]

Burgess EM, Romano FL, Zettl JH: *The Management of Lower-Extremity Amputations.* Publication TR 10-6. U.S. Washington, DC: Government Printing Office; 1969.

Hafner BJ, Willingham LL, Buell NC, et al: Evaluation of function, performance, and preference as transfemoral amputees transition from mechanical to microprocessor control of the prosthetic knee. *Arch Phys Med Rehabil* 2007;88:207. [PMID: 17270519]

Lane JM, Christ GH, Khan SN, et al: Rehabilitation for limb salvage patients: kinesiological parameters and psychological assessment. *Cancer* 2001;92(Suppl 4):1013. [PMID: 11519028]

Marks LJ, Michael JW: Science, medicine, and the future: artificial limbs. *BMJ* 2001;323:732. [PMID: 11576982]

Melzack R: Phantom limbs. *Sci Am* 1992;266:120. [PMID: 1566028]

Smith DG, Burgess EM: The use of CAD/CAM technology in prosthetics and orthotics—current clinical models and a view to the future. *J Rehabil Res Dev* 2001;38:327. [PMID: 11440264]

Smith DG, McFarland LV, Sangeorzan BJ, et al: Postoperative dressing and management strategies for transtibial amputations: a critical review. *J Rehabil Res Dev* 2003;40:213. [PMID: 14582525]

Waters RL, Perry J, Antonelli D, et al: The energy cost of walking of amputees: influence of level of amputation. *J Bone Joint Surg Am* 1976;58:42. [PMID: 1249111]

▼ TYPES OF AMPUTATION

UPPER EXTREMITY AMPUTATIONS AND DISARTICULATIONS

▶ Hand Amputation

Although microsurgical replantation techniques have reduced the incidence of hand amputations, for many patients, replantation is still not feasible or results in failure. There is considerable controversy about the best treatment for any given hand injury, and the optimal treatment takes into consideration the injured patient's occupation, hobbies, skills, and hand of dominance. The hand is a highly visible and important part of body image. Many patients with partial hand amputations can benefit tremendously from using a cosmetic partial hand prosthesis.

A. Fingertip Amputation

Fingertip injuries occur frequently, and fingertip amputation is the most common type of amputation. The treatment of choice usually depends on the geometry of the defect and whether or not bone is exposed. Although a large variety of local flap procedures are used to cover defects of different shapes and sizes, there is also a growing understanding that allowing secondary healing of fingertip injuries is the treatment least prone to complications in adults as well as in children. Even if bone is exposed, simply rongeuring back the exposed bone proximal to the soft-tissue defect and allowing secondary healing can give excellent results. The amount of the bone that can be removed is limited because at least a third of the distal phalanx must be left intact to prevent a hook deformity of the nail.

Two problems frequently result from fingertip amputations: cold intolerance and hypersensitivity. Overall, regardless of which treatment is chosen, approximately 30–50% of patients experience these problems. One criticism of the many local flap procedures used to obtain coverage and primary wound healing is that all of them involve incising and advancing uninjured tissue, which extends the area of scarring and damages the fine branches of the digital nerves. Newer studies suggest that the incidence of cold intolerance and hypersensitivity may be lower with secondary healing than with skin grafts or local flaps.

B. Thumb Amputation

The thumb, with its unique range of motion, plays the major role in all three prehensile activities of the hand: palmar grip, side-to-side pinch, and tip-to-tip pinch. Amputation of the thumb can result in the loss of virtually all hand function. Thumb amputations can involve (1) the distal third of the thumb (ie, distal to the interphalangeal joint), (2) the middle third of the thumb (ie, from the metacarpophalangeal joint to the interphalangeal joint), or (3) the proximal third of the thumb.

Thumb amputation of the distal third allows the patient to retain a tremendous amount of thumb function. Cold intolerance and hypersensitivity are frequent problems, as noted in the previous discussion of fingertip amputations. Treatment of distal third injuries should allow secondary healing of the thumb or should use relatively uncomplicated techniques for coverage.

Thumb amputation in the middle third is more complicated. The issues here are length, stability, and sensate skin coverage. More aggressive procedures may well be warranted and may consist of cross-finger flaps, volar advancement flaps, neurovascular island flaps from the dorsal index finger (radial nerve) or volar middle finger (median nerve), bone lengthening, or web space deepening.

Thumb amputation in the proximal third has a devastating impact on hand function. Local reconstruction for this degree of loss is not generally successful. Pollicization of another digit, a toe-to-hand transfer, or other complicated surgical techniques, such as osseointegration of a prosthesis, may be indicated to restore function.

Jönsson S, Caine-Winterberger K, Brånemark R: Osseointegration amputation prostheses on the upper limbs: methods, prosthetics and rehabilitation. *Prosthet Orthot Int* 2011;35:190. [PMID: 21697201]

C. Digit Amputation

Isolated amputation of a lesser digit can cause a variety of functional and cosmetic problems. Replantation of digits can often be performed but must be individualized to the patient, as function is often acceptable with an amputation and amputation will allow a quicker return to activities. Digit amputations distal to the insertion of the sublimis flexor tendon retain active flexor tendon activity and maintain useful metacarpophalangeal joint flexion. The long flexor tendon should not be sewn to the extensor tendon because it limits the excursion of both tendons and definitely limits the function of the remaining digits.

Amputations proximal to the sublimis tendon insertion retain approximately 45 degrees of proximal phalanx flexion at the metacarpophalangeal joint through the action of the intrinsic muscles. This is usually enough to keep small objects from falling through the defect and to allow the residual finger to participate to some degree in grip. If the patient uses a cosmetic finger prosthesis and wears a ring to cover the proximal edge of the prosthesis, the amputation is almost unnoticeable.

The index finger participates principally in side-to-side and tip-to-tip pinch with the thumb. After an amputation of the index finger at the metacarpophalangeal joint, the middle finger assumes this important role. The residual second metacarpal can interfere with side-to-side pinch between the thumb and the middle finger, however. Converting this amputation to a ray amputation often can improve function and cosmesis, but the drawback is that it also narrows the width of the palm and can decrease grip and torque strength significantly. Surgical decisions must be individualized, but the second metacarpal should probably be retained if the patient uses hand tools extensively, as does a carpenter or machinist.

Amputation of the middle or ring finger at the metacarpophalangeal joint can make it difficult for the patient to hold small objects because they tend to fall through the defect. Full ray resection can narrow the central defect and occasionally improve function, but narrowing the palm can decrease grip and torque strength.

Amputation of the small finger at the metacarpophalangeal joint is often cosmetically unacceptable because of the abrupt and noticeable change in contour of the hand. Although converting a fifth digital amputation to a ray amputation by including the metacarpal can improve cosmesis, it also narrows the width of the palm and can decrease grip and torque strength. Surgical decisions must be based on individual factors and concerns.

D. Carpus Amputation

Amputations through the carpus are generally discouraged. Most surgeons believe the result to have no real advantages over a wrist disarticulation or transradial amputation. There are isolated reports of patients valuing the little bit of wrist flexion and extension that allows them to hold objects against their body and to stabilize objects for two-handed grasp. The flexor and extensor carpi radialis and ulnaris tendons must be reattached to provide this limited motion. The prosthetic options are less standard and generally considered to be less functional than the traditional transradial designs.

Carpus amputations should probably be considered in bilateral cases. Although rare, more patients sustaining tissue loss from ischemia are seen in the intensive care unit after prolonged resuscitations and the use of vasopressors. Without the vasopressors, these patients would die. Unfortunately, part of the body's response to these lifesaving medications can be to shunt blood flow from the distal extremities, resulting in demarcation and dry gangrene in the hands and feet. Just as in frostbite, if infection is not present, it is worthwhile to delay any surgical intervention and allow adequate time for tissue demarcation and recovery. Partial hand amputation is occasionally necessary, and if required, the carpus level should be considered.

▶ Wrist Disarticulation

Wrist disarticulation continues to be controversial. Proponents frequently argue that it has two advantages over the shorter transradial amputation: It retains the distal radioulnar joint, which preserves more forearm rotation, and it retains the distal radial flare, which dramatically improves prosthetic suspension. Volar and dorsal fish-mouth incisions are usually best, and removal of the radial and ulnar styloids can prevent painful pressure points. Tenodesis of the major forearm motors stabilizes the muscle units and thereby improves physiologic and myoelectric performance.

Opponents of wrist disarticulation argue that prosthetic substitution after this procedure is slightly more complicated than it is after a standard transradial amputation. The prosthetic socket is more difficult to fabricate because of the bone contours. Conventional wrist units add too much length to the prosthetic arm after wrist disarticulation and therefore cannot be used. The terminal device for a wrist disarticulation also needs to be modified because of length. Myoelectric prostheses are difficult to fit because there is less space to conceal the electronics and power supply.

Despite these prosthetic concerns, wrist disarticulation patients are often excellent upper extremity prosthetic users. Some patients with an unsatisfactory hand can gain improved function by undergoing a wrist disarticulation and using a standard prosthesis. This decision must be individualized and based on contributory factors such as severity of tissue loss, pain, functional requirements, and the patient's body image.

▶ Transradial Amputation

The transradial amputation is extremely functional, and successful prosthetic rehabilitation and sustained use are achieved in 70–80% of patients who undergo amputation at this level. Forearm rotation and strength are proportional to the length retained. Surgical incisions are best with equal volar and dorsal flaps. A myodesis should be performed to prevent a painful bursa, facilitate physiologic muscular suspension, and allow for myoelectric prosthetic use. An extremely short transradial residual limb requires the use of a Muenster-type socket, which molds up around the humeral condyles for added suspension. Occasionally, side hinges and a humeral cuff are required to achieve suspension of the prosthesis. Both of these types of suspension preserve elbow flexion and extension but limit rotation.

The value of preserving the elbow joint cannot be overemphasized. Skin grafts and even composite grafts should be considered to retain the tremendous functional benefit of an elbow with some active motion. Even a limited range of elbow motion can be useful, and an ingeniously designed, geared step-up elbow hinge can convert a limited active range of elbow motion to an improved prosthetic ROM. Although body-powered prostheses are extremely functional at the transradial level of amputation, this level is also the most successful level at which to use myoelectric devices.

▶ Krukenberg Amputation

The Krukenberg kineplastic operation transforms the transradial amputation stump into radial and ulnar digits that are capable of strong prehension and have excellent manipulative

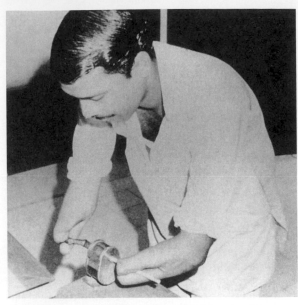

▲ **Figure 11–6.** A patient with bilateral Krukenberg hands demonstrates bimanual dexterity in sharpening a pencil. (Reproduced, with permission, from Garst RJ: The Krukenberg hand. *J Bone Joint Surg Br* 1991;73:385.)

ability because of retained sensation on the "fingers" of the forearm. The operation should not be performed as a primary amputation.

The Krukenberg amputation can be performed as a secondary procedure in a transradial amputee who has a residual limb of at least 10 cm from the tip of the olecranon, an elbow flexion contracture of less than 70 degrees, and good psychological preparation and acceptance. In this case, the amputee can become completely independent in daily activities because of the retained sensory ability of the pincers as well as the quality of the grasping mechanism (Figure 11–6). The Krukenberg amputation traditionally was indicated for blind patients with bilateral below-elbow amputations, but it also may be indicated at least unilaterally in bilateral below-elbow amputees who are able to see and in those who have limited access to prosthetic facilities.

A conventional prosthesis can be worn over the Krukenberg forearm, and myoelectric devices can be adapted to use the forearm motion. The major disadvantage is the appearance of the arm, which many people consider grotesque and do not accept. As society continues to become more understanding and accepting of disabled individuals, concerns about appearance may diminish. Intensive preoperative preparation and counseling are mandatory.

▶ Elbow Disarticulation

Elbow disarticulation can be a satisfactory amputation level and has the advantage of retaining the condylar flare to improve prosthetic suspension and allow for the transfer of humeral rotation to the prosthesis. The longer lever arm improves strength. The disadvantage is in the design of the prosthetic elbow hinge. An outside hinge is bulky and hard on clothing, whereas the conventional elbow unit provides a disproportionately long upper arm and short forearm. Whether the advantages of the elbow disarticulation outweigh the disadvantages remains controversial. Surgically, volar and dorsal flaps work best, and myodesis of the biceps and triceps tendons are needed to preserve the distal muscle attachments.

▶ Transhumeral Amputation

When transhumeral amputation is performed, efforts should be made to retain as much as possible of the bone length that has suitable soft-tissue coverage. Even if only the humeral head remains and no functional length is salvageable, an improved shoulder contour and cosmetic appearance results. Myodesis helps preserve biceps and triceps strength, prosthetic control, and myoelectric signals. In most cases of transhumeral amputation, an immediate postoperative prosthesis and rigid dressings can be used successfully. Physical therapy should focus on proximal joint and muscle function. Because the terminal prosthetic device is usually controlled by active shoulder girdle motion, early prosthetic use and therapy can prevent contracture and maintain strength.

Prosthetic suspension traditionally was incorporated in the body-powered harness, which can be somewhat uncomfortable. Among the alternative techniques are humeral angulation osteotomy (rarely used), socket-suction suspension, and the newer elastomeric roll on locking liners. Many prosthetic options are available for the transhumeral amputee. One option is a prosthesis that is totally body powered. Another is a hybrid prosthesis that uses myoelectric control of one component (either the terminal device or the elbow device) and body-powered control of the other. The transhumeral prosthesis is heavy, often considered slow, and requires much mental concentration to use effectively. These issues lead many unilateral transhumeral amputees to choose not to wear a prosthesis at all or to wear only a lightweight cosmetic prosthesis for special occasions.

Transhumeral amputation is sometimes elected to manage a dysfunctional arm following a severe brachial plexus injury. The advantages of amputation are that it unloads the weight from the shoulder and scapulothoracic joints and eliminates the problem of having a paralyzed arm that gets in the way and hinders body function. The decision to undertake shoulder arthrodesis in combination with transhumeral amputation is controversial and should be made on an individualized basis. Investigators who compared two groups of patients with transhumeral amputation because of brachial plexus injury—one group without shoulder arthrodesis and one group with it—found a somewhat better return-to-work rate in the group without shoulder arthrodesis. Prosthetic expectations in these patients should be limited because prosthetic fitting adds weight to a dysfunctional shoulder girdle, often defeating one of the original goals of the amputation.

▶ Shoulder Disarticulation and Scapulothoracic (Forequarter) Amputation

The performance of shoulder disarticulation (Figure 11–7) or scapulothoracic amputation (Figure 11–8) is rare. When either operation is performed, it is usually in cases of cancer or severe trauma. Either operation results in a loss of the normal shoulder contour and causes the patient difficulty because clothing does not fit well. Saving the humeral head, if possible, can improve the contour of a shoulder disarticulation tremendously. The scapulothoracic amputation, usually performed for proximal tumors, removes the arm, scapula, and clavicle. Dissection often extends into the neck and into the thorax.

Elaborate myoelectric prostheses are available for patients but are expensive, heavy, and require intensive maintenance. Body-powered prostheses are also heavy, hard to suspend comfortably, and difficult to use. Most patients request prosthetic help for improved cosmesis and fitting of clothes. Often a simple soft mold to fill out the shoulder meets these expectations and is an alternative to a full-arm cosmetic prosthesis.

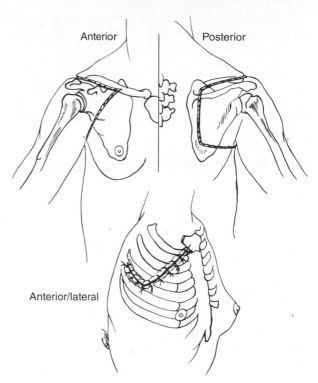

▲ **Figure 11–8.** Forequarter amputation.

▶ Postural Abnormalities After High Upper Extremity Amputation

Normally, the weight of the arm and the muscle activity associated with shoulder and arm function keep the shoulders appropriately level. Unilateral hypertrophy of an upper limb, including the shoulder girdle, occurs in certain occupations and is also seen in some sports. Some people are born with a degree of asymmetry of their shoulders, which is a relatively minor postural abnormality and does not require special clothing.

When the arm is removed and the clavicle and scapula remain, the muscles elevating the shoulder girdle are unopposed by both the weight of the arm and those muscles that pass across the shoulder and tend to depress the shoulder and arm. The consequence of this imbalance is an upward elevation described as "hiking" of the shoulder girdle. This high shoulder tends to accentuate the cosmetic loss, even when the individual is wearing a cosmetic shoulder filler or a cosmetic limb. Abnormal shoulder elevation can be countered by corrective exercises beginning as soon as they can be tolerated after the amputation. The wearing of a prosthesis with its dependent weight also diminishes shoulder hike. In most circumstances, the shoulder girdle elevation is inevitable; however, its degree can be minimized by appropriate physical measures.

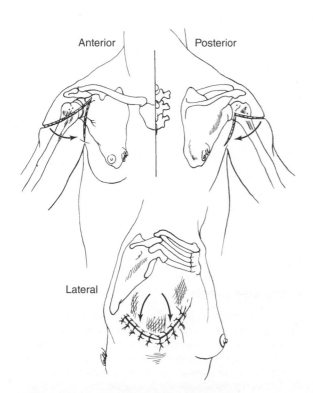

▲ **Figure 11–7.** Shoulder disarticulation.

Removal of the entire upper limb in the growing skeleton can result in a scoliosis of the spine. Muscular imbalance is considered to be the cause of the deformity. It may be seen to a slighter degree in the adult but is primarily confined to the growing skeleton. The combined postural deformity of upper dorsal spine scoliosis and elevation of the shoulder girdle produces asymmetry of the head and neck on the trunk, with the head appearing to be placed asymmetrically as the person stands.

In general, no corrective splinting or orthotic device can successfully counteract the postural changes associated with shoulder-level amputation. Neck and shoulder-girdle exercises offer the most effective prophylaxis and treatment. The postural deficits are particularly evident with forequarter amputation. Soft, light polyurethane cosmetic restoration, either as part of a cosmetic prosthesis or separately used with the empty sleeve, counters to some degree the unsightly upper body contour.

▶ Hand Transplantation

Hand transplantation and the suppression of rejections are now technically possible. Approximately 49 documented cases of hand transplantation have been performed with varying degrees of success. Protective sensory function is reported for all patients, with discriminative sensation in 82% of patients, while motor function was adequate to perform most activities. However, of the 33 patients (16 bilateral), there was one death and seven graft removals. The potential benefits for the amputee are certainly many, but they must be balanced against the real risks. In general, skin, muscle, and bone marrow appear to reject earlier and more aggressively than bone, cartilage, or tendon. Preventing this rejection is an ongoing and lasting issue, with real consequences for the individual's health and life expectancy. The current immunosuppressive drugs needed to prevent rejection of a composite hand transplant include toxic side effects, opportunistic infections, and increase in malignancies. The visibility of the hand, as compared to the internal transplanted organs, allows detection of rejection much more readily. Advances in immunology are permitting less aggressive immunoregulation instead of immunosuppression, which may improve the feasibility of this procedure.

Also, the real psychological impact following hand and other organ transplantation should not be underestimated. One study examining the issues 5 years following heart transplant showed a significant increase in emotional issues such as irritability, depression, and low self-esteem. Even for a patient with no preexisting psychological issues, living with a hand transplantation, which remains constantly in view, may not be easy.

Baumeister S, Kleist C, Dohler B, et al: Risks of allogeneic hand transplantation. *Microsurgery* 2004;24:98. [PMID: 15038013]

Crandall RC, Tomhave W: Pediatric unilateral below-elbow amputees: retrospective analysis of 34 patients given multiple prosthetic options. *J Pediatr Orthop* 2002;22:380. [PMID: 11961460]

Petruzzo P, Lanzetta M, Dubernard JM, et al: The International Registry on Hand and Composite Tissue Transplantation. *Transplantation* 2010;90:1590. [PMID: 21052038]

Schatz RL, Rosenwasser MP: Krukenberg kineplasty: a case study. *J Hand Ther* 2002;15:260. [PMID: 12206329]

Scheker LR Becker GW: Distal finger replantation. *J Hand Surg Am* 2011;36:521. [PMID: 21371629]

Sebastin SJ, Chung KC: A systematic review of the outcomes of replantation of distal digital amputation. *Plast Reconstr Surg* 2011;128:723. [PMID: 21572379]

Shores JT, Brandacher G, Schneeberger S, et al: Composite tissue allotransplantation: hand transplantation and beyond. *J Am Acad Orthop Surg* 2010;18:127. [PMID: 20190102]

Wilkinson MC, Birch R, Bonney G: Brachial plexus injury: when to amputate? *Injury* 1993;24:603. [PMID: 8288380]

LOWER EXTREMITY AMPUTATIONS AND DISARTICULATIONS

▶ Foot Amputation

A. Toe Amputation

Toe amputations can be performed with side-to-side or plantar-to-dorsal flaps to use the best available soft tissue. The bone should be shortened to a level that allows adequate soft-tissue closure without tension.

In great toe amputations, if the entire proximal phalanx is removed, the sesamoids can retract and expose the keel-shaped plantar surface of the first metatarsal to weight bearing. This often leads to high local pressure, callous formation, or ulceration. The sesamoids can be stabilized in position for weight bearing by leaving the base of the proximal phalanx intact or by performing tenodesis of the flexor hallucis brevis tendon.

An isolated amputation of the second toe commonly results in severe hallux valgus deformity of first toe (Figure 11–9). This situation may be prevented by amputation of the second ray or by fusion of the first metatarsal and phalanx. In the shorter toe amputations at the metatarsophalangeal joint level, transferring the extensor tendon to the capsule may help elevate the metatarsal head and maintain an even distribution for weight bearing. Prosthetic replacement is not required after toe amputations.

B. Ray Amputation

A ray amputation removes the toe and all or some of the corresponding metatarsal. Isolated ray amputations can be durable. Multiple ray amputations, however, especially in patients with vascular disease, can narrow the foot excessively. This increases the amount of weight that must be borne by the remaining metatarsal heads and can lead to new areas of increased pressure, callous formation, and ulceration.

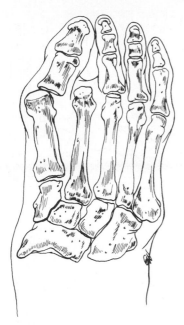

▲ **Figure 11–9.** Severe hallux valgus deformity occurring after isolated second toe amputation.

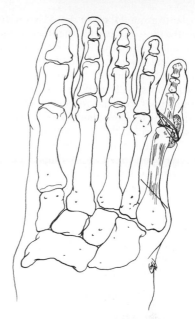

▲ **Figure 11–10.** Fifth ray amputation for fifth metatarsal head ulcer.

Surgically, it is often difficult to achieve primary closure of ray amputation wounds because more skin is usually required than is readily apparent. Instead of closing these wounds under tension, it is usually advisable to leave them open and allow for secondary healing.

The fifth ray amputation is the most useful of all the ray amputations. Plantar and lateral ulcers around the fifth metatarsal head often lead to exposed bone and osteomyelitis. A fifth ray amputation allows the entire ulcer to be excised and the wound to be closed primarily (Figure 11–10). In general, for more extensive involvement of the foot, a transverse amputation at the transmetatarsal level is more durable. Prosthetic requirements after ray amputations include extra-depth shoes with custom-molded insoles. The insole should include a metatarsal pad that loads the shafts of the metatarsal and unloads some of the pressure at the metatarsal heads.

C. Midfoot Amputation

The transmetatarsal and Lisfranc amputations are reliable and durable. The Lisfranc amputation is actually a disarticulation just proximal to the metatarsals where the cuneiform and cuboid bones are retained. Surgically, a healthy, durable soft-tissue envelope is more important than a specific anatomic level of amputation, so the length of bone to be removed should be based on the ability to perform soft-tissue closure without tension. A long plantar flap is preferable, but equal dorsal and plantar flaps work well, especially for transmetatarsal amputation in the treatment of metatarsal head ulcers (Figure 11–11).

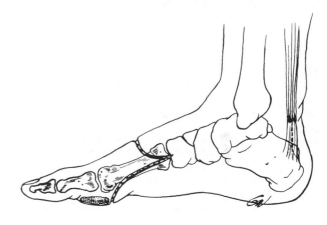

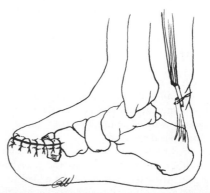

▲ **Figure 11–11.** Transmetatarsal amputation with Achilles tendon lengthening.

Muscle balance around the foot should be carefully evaluated preoperatively, with specific attention to tightness of the heel cord and strength of the anterior tibial, posterior tibial, and peroneal muscles. Midfoot amputations significantly shorten the lever arm of the foot, so lengthening of the Achilles tendon should be done if necessary. Tibial or peroneal muscle insertions should be reattached if they are released during bone resection. For example, if the base of the fifth metatarsal is resected, the peroneus brevis tendon should be reinserted into the cuboid bone. In patients with vascular disease, this can be performed with a minimal amount of dissection to prevent further compromise of the tissues.

Postoperative casting prevents deformities, controls edema, and speeds rehabilitation. Prosthetic requirements can vary widely. During the first year following amputation, many patients benefit from the use of an ankle-foot orthosis (AFO) with a long footplate and a toe filler. To prevent an equinus deformity from developing, patients should be advised to wear the orthosis except when taking a bath or shower. Later, the use of a simple toe filler combined with a stiff-soled shoe may be adequate. Cosmetic partial foot prostheses are also available.

D. Hindfoot Amputation

A Chopart amputation removes the forefoot and midfoot and saves only the talus and calcaneus. Rebalancing procedures are required to prevent equinus and varus deformities. Achilles tenotomy, transfer of the anterior tibial or extensor digitorum tendons, and postoperative casting are all usually necessary. Although tendon transfer to the talus was previously recommended, transfer to the calcaneus is now done to minimize varus positioning. Beveling the inferior, anterior surface of the calcaneus can remove a potential bone pressure point.

Two other types of hindfoot amputations are the Boyd and the Pirogoff amputations. The Boyd procedure consists of a talectomy and calcaneal-tibial arthrodesis after forward translation of the calcaneus. The Pirogoff procedure consists of a talectomy with calcaneal-tibial arthrodesis after the vertical transection of the calcaneus through the midbody and a forward rotation of the posterior process of the calcaneus under the tibia. These two types of hindfoot amputations are done mostly in children to preserve length and growth centers, prevent heel pad migration, and improve socket suspension.

Studies in which various procedures in children are compared showed that a hindfoot amputation results in better function than a Syme amputation (see section on Syme amputation) in cases in which the hindfoot is balanced and no equinus deformity has developed.

The hindfoot prosthesis requires more secure stabilization than a midfoot prosthesis to keep the heel from pistoning during gait. An anterior shell can be added to an ankle-foot prosthesis, or a posterior opening socket prosthesis can be used.

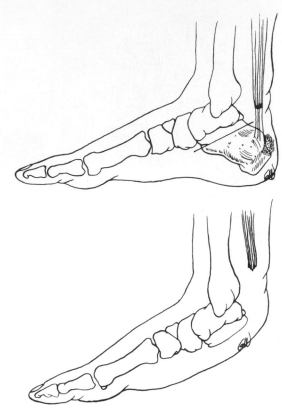

▲ **Figure 11–12.** Partial calcanectomy.

E. Partial Calcanectomy

Partial calcanectomy, which consists of excising the posterior process of the calcaneus (Figure 11–12), should be considered an amputation of the back of the foot. In selected patients with large heel ulcerations or calcaneal osteomyelitis, partial calcanectomy can be a functional alternative to transtibial amputation. The removal of the entire posterior process of the calcaneus allows for fairly large soft-tissue defects to be closed primarily. Patients must have adequate vascular perfusion and nutritional competence for wound healing to occur. As with other amputations, partial calcanectomy creates a functional and cosmetic deformity. Use of an ankle-foot prosthesis with a cushion heel is usually required to replace the missing heel and prevent further skin ulceration.

▶ Syme Amputation

In the Syme amputation, the surgeon removes the calcaneus and talus while carefully dissecting on bone to preserve the heel skin and fat pad to cover the distal tibia (Figure 11–13). The surgeon must also remove and contour the malleoli, but whether this should be done during the initial operation or of weight. Because of the ability to end-bear, the amputee can occasionally ambulate without a prosthesis in emergency situations or for bathroom activities.

The Syme prosthesis is wider at the ankle level than is a transtibial prosthesis, and this cosmetic problem can be bothersome to some patients. The surgical narrowing of the malleolar flare and the use of new materials in the prosthesis, however, can improve the appearance of the final prosthesis. Moreover, patients can now benefit from energy-storing technology provided by the newly designed lower profile elastic response feet. Sockets do not need the high contour of a patellar-tendon bearing design because of the end-bearing quality of the residual limb. The socket can be windowed either posteriorly or medially if the limb is bulbous, or a flexible socket within a rigid frame design can be used if the limb is less bulbous. Because of the tibial flare, the socket used following Syme amputation is usually self-suspending.

▶ Transtibial Amputation

Transtibial amputation is the most commonly performed major limb amputation. The long posterior flap technique (Figure 11–14) is now standard, and good results can be expected even in the majority of patients with vascular disease. Anterior and posterior flaps, sagittal flaps, and skewed flaps can be helpful in specific patients.

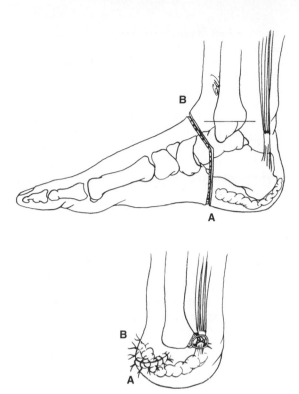

▲ **Figure 11–13.** Syme amputation with tenodesis of the Achilles tendon to the distal tibia.

6–8 weeks later remains controversial. Proponents of the two-stage procedure argue that it can improve healing in patients with vascular disease. Opponents point out that it delays rehabilitation because the patient cannot bear weight until after the second stage of the operation. One series supports the use of the one-stage procedure, even in the presence of vascular disease or diabetes. A late complication of the Syme amputation is the posterior and medial migration of the fat pad. One of these surgical procedures can be done to stabilize the fat pad: tenodesis of the Achilles tendon to the posterior margin of the tibia through drill holes; transfer of the anterior tibial and extensor digitorum tendons to the anterior aspect of the fat pad; or removal of the cartilage and subchondral bone to allow scarring of the fat pad to bone, with or without pin fixation. Careful postoperative casting can also help keep the fat pad centered under the tibia during healing. The Syme amputation is one of the most difficult amputations to perform in terms of surgical technique and achievement of primary healing and heel pad stability.

Syme amputation should be designed to allow end bearing. Retaining the smooth, broad surface of the distal tibia and the heel pad allows direct transfer of weight from the end of the residual limb to the prosthesis. A transtibial or transfemoral amputation does not allow this direct transfer

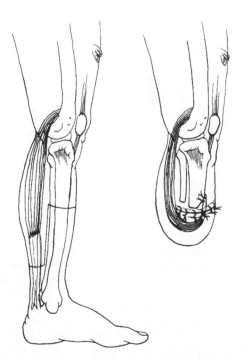

▲ **Figure 11–14.** Transtibial amputation with long posterior flap technique.

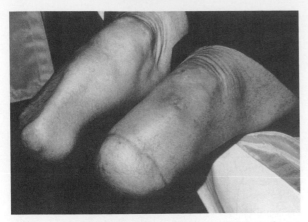

▲ **Figure 11–15.** Bilateral transtibial amputations that emphasize the benefits of the long posterior flap technique. The right limb, amputated by using equal anterior and posterior flaps, is conically shaped and atrophic. The left limb, amputated by using the long posterior flap technique, is cylindrical and well padded. (Reproduced, with permission, from Smith DG, Burgess EM, Zettl JH: Fitting and training the bilateral lower-limb amputee, in Bowker JH, Michael JW (eds): *Atlas of Limb Prosthetics Surgical, Prosthetic, and Rehabilitation Principles.* Rosemont, IL, American Academy of Orthopaedic Surgeons, 2002; pp 599–622.)

Efforts should be made to preserve as much bone length as possible between the tibial tubercle and the junction of the middle and distal thirds of the tibia, based on the available healthy soft tissues. Amputations in the distal third of the tibia should be avoided because they result in poor soft-tissue padding and are more difficult to fit comfortably with a prosthesis. The goal is a cylindrically shaped residual limb with muscle stabilization, distal tibial padding, and a nontender and nonadherent scar (Figure 11–15). The transtibial amputation is especially well suited to rigid dressings and immediate postoperative prosthetic management. The removable rigid dressing has been shown to reduce hospital stay and time to initial fitting of a prosthesis. Distal tibiofibular synostosis (Ertl procedure) should be considered for the treatment of a wide trauma-induced diastasis to improve stabilization of the bone and soft tissue. The bone–bridge procedure recently was shown to have a higher complication rate, suggesting that its use be limited. The procedure is less often indicated in the treatment of patients with vascular disease. The synostosis is developed to create a broad bone mass terminally to improve the distal end-bearing property of the limb and minimize motion between the tibia and fibula. Although there is renewed interest in these techniques, true comparison of patients with osteomyoplastic techniques versus standard techniques has not been done.

A wide variety of prosthetic designs are available for the transtibial amputee. Sockets can be designed to incorporate a liner, which offers the advantages of increased comfort and accommodation of minor changes in residual limb volume. Disadvantages include increased perspiration and a less sanitary, less comfortable feeling in hot humid weather. Hard sockets are designed to have cotton or wool stump socks of an appropriate ply or thickness as the interface between the leg and the socket. Hard sockets are easier to clean and more durable than the liners are.

The Icelandic-Swedish-New York (ISNY) socket refers to the use of a more flexible socket material that is supported by a rigid frame. The flexible socket changes shape to accommodate underlying muscle contraction. This socket style can also be useful for limbs that are scarred or difficult to fit. Open-ended sockets with side joints and a thigh corset are not used much today except by patients who wore them successfully in the past and by patients with limited access to prosthetic care. The patellar tendon-bearing shape is most commonly used for the transtibial amputee. Despite its name, the majority of the weight is borne on the medial tibial flare and laterally on the interosseus space, whereas the rest of the weight is borne on the patellar tendon area. Even the new so-called total-contact transtibial socket, which is designed to have increased contact on all areas of the residual limb, preferentially loads the tibial flare and patellar tendon regions.

Numerous types of suspension devices are available for the transtibial prosthesis. The simplest and most common is a suprapatellar strap, which wraps above the femoral condyles and patella. Sockets can be designed to incorporate a supracondylar mold or wedge to grip above the femoral condyles, but this higher profile is bulkier and less cosmetic when the patient is sitting. A waist belt and fork strap are helpful for the patient who has a very short transtibial residual limb because these devices decrease pistoning in the socket; they are also helpful for the patient whose activities require extremely secure suspension. If the patient has a limb with poor soft tissue or has intrinsic knee pain, side hinges and a thigh corset can help unload the lower leg and transfer some of the weight to the thigh.

External suspension sleeves made of latex or neoprene are still used quite frequently. Latex is more cosmetic but less durable and can be constricting. Neoprene is more durable and not as constricting but sometimes causes contact dermatitis. The newest suspension uses an elastomeric or silicone-based liner that is rolled on over the residual leg and offers an intimate friction fit. A small metal post on the distal end of the liner then locks into a catch in the prosthetic socket to suspend the socket securely to the liner. Many patients who use these elastomeric locking liners like the secure suspension and feeling of improved control of the prosthesis. The liners have the disadvantages of being less durable and requiring frequent replacement. These elastomeric locking liners can be expensive. Although elastomeric locking liners were originally touted as preventing skin problems; rashes, skin irritation, and skin breakdown remain a frequent complaint even with this new technology, however. Approximately a third of amputees cannot tolerate the forces generated at the distal part of the amputation with liners using the metal post or pin lock system. New techniques were designed to attach the elastomeric liner to the socket with vacuum pumps, clips on the side of the liner, or sealing liners and one-way socket valves to maintain a suction between the liner and the socket. Suspension must be individualized, and no system is yet proven acceptable to all amputees.

Many different designs for prosthetic feet are now available, ranging from the original solid ankle cushion heel (SACH) foot to the newer elastic response technology with a variety of keel, ankle, and pylon designs. Cost and function can vary widely, and care should be used in prescribing an appropriate prosthetic foot for an individual patient. A common error is to prescribe a foot that is either too stiff or does not get to feel flat quickly enough for an individual patient, especially in the first 12–18 months after an amputation.

▶ Knee Disarticulation

Disarticulation through the knee joint (Figure 11–16) is indicated in ambulatory patients when a below-knee amputation is not possible but suitable soft tissue is present for a knee disarticulation. These circumstances are most commonly found in cases involving traumatic injuries. In patients with vascular disease, the blood supply is such that if a knee disarticulation would heal, a short transtibial amputation would usually heal as well. The knee disarticulation is indicated in patients who have vascular problems and are nonambulatory, especially if knee flexion contractures or spasticity are present. Although sagittal flaps or the traditional long posterior flap can be used to take advantage of the best available soft-tissue coverage, newer literature supports use of the posterior flap technique when possible. The patella is retained and the patellar tendon sutured to the cruciate stumps to stabilize the quadriceps muscle complex. The biceps tendons can also be stabilized to the patellar tendon. A short section of gastrocnemius muscle can be sutured to the anterior capsule to pad the distal end. Although many techniques are described to trim the condyles of the femur, trimming is rarely necessary, and radical trimming can decrease some of the advantages of the knee disarticulation.

For ambulatory patients, the advantages of a knee disarticulation over a transfemoral amputation include improved socket suspension by contouring above the femoral condyles, the added strength of a longer lever arm, the retained muscle balance of the thigh, and most important, the end-bearing potential to transfer weight directly to the prosthesis. In the past, the objections to a bulky prosthesis and asymmetric knee-joint level led many surgeons to abandon the practice of performing knee disarticulations. New materials allow a less bulky prosthesis to be fabricated, and the four-bar linkage knee unit, which can fold under the socket, improves the appearance of the prosthesis when the patient is sitting. The four-bar linkage knee remains the prosthetic knee of choice for a knee disarticulation. It is low profile, has excellent stability, and can incorporate a hydraulic unit for control during the swing phase of gait in patients who can walk at different cadences.

For nonambulatory patients, a knee disarticulation eliminates the problem of knee flexion contractures, provides a balanced thigh to decrease hip contractures, and provides a long lever arm for good sitting support and transfers.

The Gritti-Stokes amputation is not recommended. In this operation, the patella is advanced distally and fused by arthrodesis to the distal femur, theoretically to allow direct weight bearing. The concept behind this operation is flawed because even in normal kneeling, the weight is borne on the pretibial and patellar tendon areas and not on the patella. The added length and the asymmetry of the knee joints complicate prosthetic fitting.

Transcondylar amputation can be performed, but the end-bearing comfort and improved suspension of a transcondylar amputation appear to be diminished when compared with the true knee disarticulation.

▶ Transfemoral Amputation

Transfemoral amputation is usually performed with equal anterior and posterior fish-mouth flaps. Atypical flaps can and should be used to save all possible femoral length in

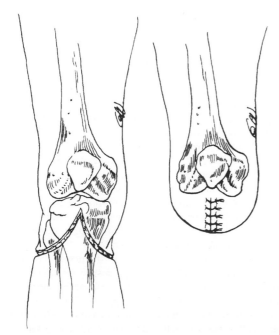

▲ **Figure 11–16.** Knee disarticulation.

cases of trauma because the amount of function is directly proportional to the length of the residual limb. Residual limb wound problems resulting in delayed ambulation with immediate postoperative prostheses should be treated, rather than revised, when possible to preserve length. One means proposed for this is the incorporation of the vacuum-assisted closure system into the fitting process. Rehabilitation is not delayed while wound healing occurs.

Muscle stabilization is more important in the transfemoral amputation than in any other major limb amputation. The major deforming force is into abduction and flexion. Myodesis of the adductor muscles through drill holes in the femur can counteract the abductors, prevent a difficult adductor tissue roll in the groin, and improve prosthetic control (Figure 11–17). Without muscle stabilization, the femur commonly migrates laterally through the soft-tissue envelope to a subcutaneous location. Newer transfemoral socket designs attempt to better control the position of the femur, but they are not as effective as muscle stabilization. Even in nonambulatory patients, muscle stabilization is helpful in creating a more durable, padded residual limb by preventing migration of the femur.

An IPOP and rigid dressings are more difficult to apply and keep positioned after a transfemoral amputation than after more distal amputations. IPOP techniques do offer the advantages of early rehabilitation and control of edema and pain, and these techniques are preferred if the expertise to use them is available. The major complaints of patients with the transfemoral IPOP are the weight of the cast and the discomfort when sitting. In many cases, only a soft compressive dressing alone is used, and in these patients, the dressing should be carried proximally around the waist as a spica to better suspend the dressing and to include the medial thigh and prevent the development of an adductor roll of tissue. Proper postoperative positioning and therapy are essential to prevent hip flexion contractures. The limb should be positioned flat on the bed, rather than elevated on a pillow, and hip extension exercises and prone positioning should be started early.

Suspension of the prosthesis is more complicated in transfemoral amputations than in more distal amputations because of the short residual limb, the lack of bony contours, and the increased weight of the prosthesis. The transfemoral amputation prosthesis can be suspended by suction, Silesian bandage, hip-joint and pelvic band, or the newer elastomeric locking liners.

Traditional socket-suction suspension works when the skin forms an airtight seal against the socket. Air is forced distally through a small one-way valve when the prosthesis is donned and with each step during gait, thus maintaining negative pressure distally in the socket. No prosthetic sock or other liner is used between the hard socket and the limb because air leaks out around the sock and prevents suction from developing. Donning a socket-suction prosthesis requires skill and exertion, and patients must have good coordination, upper extremity function, and balance to perform this task. Socket-suction systems work well for average-to-long transfemoral residual limbs that have adequate soft tissues and stable shape and volume. It is usually comfortable and the most cosmetically acceptable method of socket suspension.

A Silesian bandage is a flexible strap that attaches laterally to the prosthesis, wraps back around the waist and over the contralateral iliac crest, and then comes forward to attach to the anterior proximal socket (Figure 11–18). It provides good suspension and added rotational control of the prosthesis. A Silesian bandage is commonly used to augment suction suspension for patients who have shorter-length limbs or for patients whose activities require more secure suspension than suction alone can offer.

As with the transtibial prosthesis, the newer elastomeric locking liners can provide excellent suspension and control. An elastomeric or silicone-based liner is rolled onto the leg similar to the way a condom is applied. This liner has an intimate fit with the residual limb and avoids pistoning and rotational forces. A small metal post at the distal end of the liner locks down into a catch at the bottom of the prosthetic

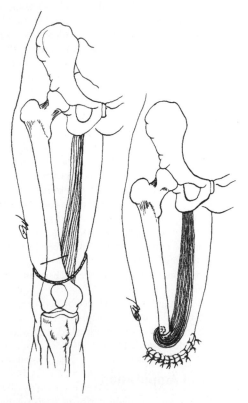

▲ **Figure 11–17.** Transfemoral amputation with adductor myodesis.

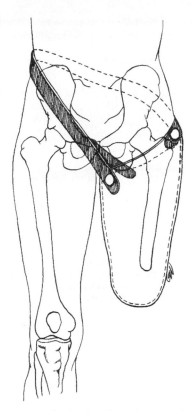

▲ **Figure 11–18.** Silesian band suspension of a transfemoral prosthesis.

socket to create a secure mechanical suspension. A small button must be pushed to disengage the lock and release the prosthesis. Many amputees express an improved sense of security and improved proprioception with these systems. The disadvantages continue to be the added cost, the need to replace the liners as they tear, and rarely, developing a contact dermatitis. As discussed with transtibial amputees, approximately a third of amputees cannot tolerate the forces generated at the distal part of the amputation with liners using the metal post or pin lock system. For these patients, new methods to attach the liner to the socket must be explored.

The hip joint and pelvic band provides extremely secure suspension and control, but the band is bulky, the least cosmetically acceptable method of suspension, and the least comfortable, especially when the patient is sitting. The pelvic band, made of metal or plastic, is thicker than a Silesian bandage. The pelvic band runs from the hip hinge, around the waist, between the contralateral iliac crest and trochanter, and back to the hip hinge. The hinge is located laterally, just anterior to the trochanter, over the anatomic axis of the hip joint. Hip joint and pelvic band suspension is indicated for very short transfemoral limbs, geriatric patients who cannot

don a suction suspension, and obese patients who cannot get adequate control with suction, silicone suspension sleeves, or Silesian band suspension.

Socket design for the transfemoral amputation has changed. The traditional quadrilateral socket has a narrow anteroposterior diameter to keep the ischium positioned back and up on top of the posterior brim of the socket for weight bearing. The anterior wall of the socket is 5–7 cm higher than the posterior wall to hold the leg back on the ischial seat. Anterior pain is a frequent complaint and should be addressed by modification of the prosthetic socket in a small local area such as over the anterior superior iliac spine. If the entire anterior wall is lowered or relieved, the ischium slips inside the socket and totally alters the load transfer and pressure areas. Even though the lateral wall is contoured to hold the femur in adduction, the overall dimensions of the quadrilateral socket are not anatomic and provide poor femoral stability in the coronal plane.

Narrow mediolateral transfemoral socket designs attempt to solve the problems of a traditional quadrilateral socket by contouring the posterior wall to set the ischium down inside the socket, not up on the brim. Weight is transferred through the gluteal muscle mass and lateral thigh instead of the ischium, which eliminates the need for anterior pressure from a high anterior wall. Attention is then focused on a narrow mediolateral contour to better hold the femur in adduction and minimize the relative motion between the limb and the socket. The normal shape and normal alignment (NSNA) socket and the contoured adducted trochanteric-controlled alignment method (CAT-CAM) socket are two of the narrow mediolateral designs available.

A socket made of flexible material with a rigid frame can also be used. The flexible material allows socket wall expansion with underlying muscle contraction. A flexible socket can be made in either the traditional quadrilateral or narrow mediolateral shapes. Advantages of this type of socket include improved comfort in walking and sitting and possibly improved muscular efficiency. One drawback is that the flexible material is less durable, and cracks can result in the loss of suction suspension and skin irritation.

Prosthetic knee joints are available in many designs to address specific patient needs. The traditional standard was the single-axis constant-friction knee. The constant-friction knee is simple, durable, lightweight, and inexpensive. The friction can be set at only one level to optimize function at one cadence, and patients have difficulty when walking at different speeds.

Outside hinges were the old standard for the knee disarticulation patient, to better approximate the center of motion of the knee. Outside hinges are cosmetically poor but still available for patients who used them successfully in the past and remain satisfied with them. For new patients, other types of knee units are used.

The term *stance control knee* has replaced the term *safety knee*. It refers to a knee unit that has weight-activated friction to increase stability and resistance to buckling as more of the amputee's body weight is applied. This unit is particularly useful for patients who are older, feel less secure, and have a very short residual limb, weak hip extensors, or hip flexion contractures.

A polycentric knee provides a changing center of rotation that is located more posteriorly than other knee joints. The posterior center of rotation offers more stability during stance and the first few degrees of flexion than other knee units do. The four-bar knee is one of many polycentric knee units available.

A hydraulic or pneumatic unit can be added to most knee joints to provide superior control of the prosthesis in swing phase by using fluid hydraulics to vary the resistance according to the speed of gait. This option is useful in active amputees who walk and run at different speeds. The variable-friction knee unit can be a less expensive way to accommodate patients who walk at different speeds. This knee changes the friction according to the degree of flexion in the knee unit and leads to an improvement in the swing phase of walking. Although a variable-friction knee is less costly and requires less maintenance than a hydraulic unit, it is not as effective in allowing the amputee to walk at different cadences.

A manual locking option can also be added to most knee units to lock the knee in full extension. Locking is helpful if the patient is blind, feels less secure, has a very short residual limb, or is a bilateral amputee.

As mentioned previously, microprocessor-controlled so-called intelligent knee units incorporate the latest technology to provide superior control of the swing and stance characteristics or the knee and respond to the amputee's speed, cadence, and accelerations. Recent studies show these knee units can improve function and assist amputees to increase their Medicare Functional Classification Level from 2 to 3 (Table 11–1). Technology has not yet advanced enough for knee units to replace the tremendous motor power lost when an amputation is done above the knee.

Specifically designed prostheses known as *stubbies* are initially recommended for bilateral knee disarticulation or transfemoral amputees, regardless of age, who have lost both legs simultaneously but are candidates for ambulation. Stubbies consist of prosthetic sockets mounted directly over rocker-bottom platforms that serve as feet. The rocker-bottom platforms have a long posterior extension to prevent the patient from falling backward, and they have a shortened anterior process that allows smooth rollover into the push-off phase of gait. These prostheses look as if the foot were positioned backward. The use of stubbies results in a lowering of the center of gravity, and the rocker bottom provides a broad base of support that teaches trunk balance, provides stability, and allows the patient to build confidence during standing and ambulation. As the patient's confidence and skills improve, periodic lengthening of the stubbies is permitted until the height becomes nearly compatible with full-length prostheses, at which time the transition is attempted.

Table 11–1. Medicare Functional Classification Level (MFCL) descriptions.

MFLC Level	MFCL Description
MFLC-0	Does not have the ability or potential to ambulate or transfer safely with or without assistance and a prosthesis does not enhance quality of life or mobility.
MFLC-1	Has the ability or potential to use a prosthesis for transfers or ambulation on level surfaces at fixed cadence. Typical of the limited and unlimited household ambulator.
MFLC-2	Has the ability or potential for ambulation with the ability to traverse low-level environmental barriers such as curbs, stairs, or uneven surfaces. Typical of the limited community ambulator.
MFLC-3	Has the ability or potential for ambulation with variable cadence. Typical of the community ambulatory who has the ability to traverse most environmental barriers and may have vocational, therapeutic, or exercise activity that demands prosthetic utilization beyond simple locomotion.
MFLC-4	Has the ability or potential for prosthetic ambulation that exceeds the basic ambulation skills, exhibiting high impact, stress, or energy levels, typical of the prosthetic demands of the child, active adult, or athlete.

Adapted from Hafner BJ, Smith DG: Differences in function and safety between Medicare Functional Classification Level-2 and -3 transfemoral amputees and influence of prosthetic knee joint control. *J Rehabil Res Dev* 2009;46:418. [PMID:19675993].

Many patients reject full-length prostheses and prefer the stability and balance afforded by the stubbies.

▶ Hip Disarticulation

Hip disarticulation (Figure 11–19) is rarely performed. Surgically, the traditional racket-shaped incision with an anterior apex is used in patients with vascular problems and in trauma-injured patients when possible. In tumor surgery, creative flaps based on the uninvolved anatomic compartments must be designed.

Prosthetic replacement can be successful in healthy young patients who required hip disarticulation because of trauma or cancer but is generally not indicated for patients with vascular disease. The standard prosthesis is the Canadian hip disarticulation prosthesis. The socket contains the involved hemipelvis and suspends over the iliac crests. Although the hip joint and other endoskeletal components are made of lightweight materials in an effort to keep the

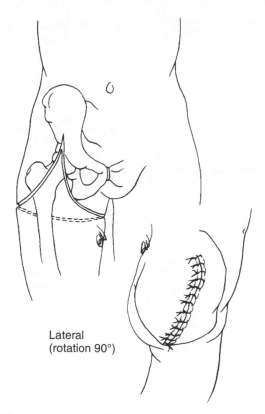

**Lateral
(rotation 90°)**

▲ **Figure 11–19.** Hip disarticulation.

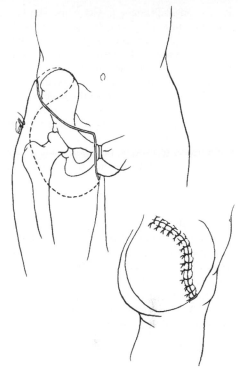

▲ **Figure 11–20.** Hemipelvectomy.

weight to a minimum, the prosthesis is still heavy and difficult to manipulate. Ambulation with the prosthesis usually requires more energy than it would take to ambulate with crutches and a swing-through gait. For this reason, many ambulatory patients use crutches and no prosthesis. The advantage of the prosthesis is that it does allow freer use of the upper extremities.

▶ Hemipelvectomy

Although a hemipelvectomy (Figure 11–20) is even less frequently required than a hip disarticulation, it is sometimes indicated for trauma injuries or cancer involving the pelvis. Use of a prosthesis after this procedure is extremely rare because the body weight must be transferred onto the sacrum and thorax. Special considerations for seating are usually required after hemipelvectomy.

▶ Prosthetic Prescription Following Amputation at or Above the Knee

To be considered a candidate for a high anatomic level prosthesis (knee disarticulation and higher), a patient must be able to transfer independently, rise from sitting to standing independently, and ambulate using one leg and a swing-through gait over a distance of 100 feet on the parallel bars or with a walker. Although these requirements seem extreme, they are necessary for the successful use of this heavy and complicated prosthesis. The use of a transtibial prosthesis can make it easier to transfer and to ambulate. But a current transfemoral prosthesis can make it much more difficult to rise from sitting to standing because the powerful motor force required to extend the knee is not present. High-level prosthetic devices can actually increase the energy required for walking compared with one-leg swing-through gait. Unfortunately, without the ability to meet the activity demands unassisted, a prosthesis acts as an anchor to decrease overall independence. We use these same activity requirements as a functional test before prescribing a prosthesis for all transfemoral, hip disarticulation, and hemipelvectomy amputees.

▶ Percutaneous Direct Skeletal Attachment of Artificial Limbs

The benefits of attaching prosthetic limbs through the skin, directly to the skeleton, were envisioned for nearly 100 years. Documentation of temporary external fixation for fractures dates to Malgaigne in 1845. During and just after World War II, independent attempts were made in Germany and the United States to attach a transtibial prosthesis directly to the tibia. Four humans were fit in May 1946 by Drummer, a general surgeon in Pinneberg, Germany. The two major hurdles continue to be the bone–implant interface, and the skin–implant interface. Breakthrough work by Branemark in Gothenburg, Sweden, advanced the use of titanium and improved design implants that led to over 30 years of successful dental and maxillofacial reconstruction with prosthetic devices directly connected to the bone of the mouth and face.

The skin of the extremities posed a larger challenge to the cutaneous–implant interface. Improvements in implant design and surgical technique, however, made it possible to implant and fit thumb, forearm, and transfemoral amputees successfully. Approximately 60 amputees have undergone surgical implantation and prosthetic fitting in Sweden, the United Kingdom, and Australia.

The early results confirm the potential promise of major improvements in attachment, proprioception, and function of osseointegrated prosthetic limbs compared with socket-style prostheses. Much work remains to be accomplished, however, especially in the skin–implant interface. A tremendous improvement in the bone–implant interface led to results that far outdistance historical attempts at directly attaching artificial limbs to the skeleton. Without true cutaneous–implant integration that provides a durable and biologic barrier, however, the risk of bacterial migration causing infection and loosening continues. It is fantastic to see this dream continue and advance.

Bowker JH, San Giovanni TP, Pinzur MS: North American experience with knee disarticulation with use of a posterior myofasciocutaneous flap. Healing rate and functional results in seventy-seven patients. *J Bone Joint Surg Am* 2000;82-A:1571. [PMID: 11097446]

Dillon MP, Barker TM: Comparison of gait of persons with partial foot amputation wearing prosthesis to matched control group: observational study. *J Rehabil Res Dev* 2008;45:1317. [PMID: 19319756]

Elsharawy MA: Outcome of midfoot amputations in diabetic gangrene. *Ann Vasc Surg* 2011;25:778. [PMID: 21514113]

Frykberg RG, Abraham S, Tierney E, et al: Syme amputation for limb salvage: early experience with 26 cases. *J Foot Ankle Surg* 2007;46:93. [PMID: 17331868]

Fuller M, Luff R, Van Den Boom M: A novel approach to wound management and prosthetic use with concurrent vacuum-assisted closure therapy. *Prosthet Orthot Int* 2011;35:246. [PMID: 21527397]

Hafner BJ, Smith DG: Differences in function and safety between Medicare Functional Classification Level-2 and -3 transfemoral amputees and influence of prosthetic knee joint control. *J Rehabil Res Dev* 2009;46:418. [PMID: 19675993]

Marfori ML, Wang EH: Adductor myocutaneous flap coverage for hip and pelvic disarticulations of sarcomas with buttock contamination. *Clin Orthop Relat Res* 2011;469:257. [PMID: 20632137]

Morse BC, Cull DL, Kalbaugh C, et al: Through-knee amputation in patients with peripheral arterial disease: a review of 50 cases. *J Vasc Surg* 2008;48:638. [PMID: 18586441]

Schade VL, Roukis TS, Yan JL: Factors associated with successful Chopart amputation in patients with diabetes: a systematic review. *Foot Ankle Spec* 2010;3:278. [PMID: 20966454]

Sherman CE, O'Connor MI, Sim FH: Survival, local recurrence, and function after pelvic limb salvage at 23 to 38 years of followup. *Clin Orthop Relat Res* 2012;470:712. [PMID: 21748513]

Smith DG, Michael JW, Bowker JH: *Atlas of Amputations and Limb Deficiencies: Surgical, Prosthetic, and Rehabilitation Principles,* 3rd ed. Rosemont, IL: American Academy of Orthopaedic Surgeons; 2004.

Stone PA, Back MR, Armstrong PA, et al: Midfoot amputations expand limb salvage rates for diabetic foot infections. *Ann Vasc Surg* 2005;19:805. [PMID: 16205848]

Taylor L, Cavenett S, Stepien JM, et al: Removable rigid dressings: a retrospective case-note audit to determine the validity of post-amputation application. *Prosthet Orthot Int* 2008;32:223. [PMID: 18569890]

Tintle SM, Keeling JJ, Forsberg JA, et al: Operative complications of combat-related transtibial amputations: a comparison of the modified burgess and modified Ertl tibiofibular synostosis techniques. *J Bone Joint Surg Am* 2011;93:1016. [PMID: 21655894]

Unruh T, Fisher DF Jr, Unruh TA, et al: Hip disarticulation: an eleven-year experience. *Arch Surg* 1990;125:791. [PMID: 2346379]

Rehabilitation

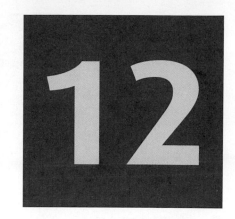

Mary Ann E. Keenan, MD
Samir Mehta, MD
Patrick J. McMahon, MD

GENERAL PRINCIPLES OF REHABILITATION

Rehabilitation involves care of the injured person with either neurologic or musculoskeletal problems. It focuses on improving function through surgical and nonsurgical management and is recognized as an important part of the care of both acute and chronic problems. Rehabilitation programs address a variety of problems, including congenital or acquired musculoskeletal problems (eg, bone deformities, arthritis, or fractures) as well as neurologic trauma or diseases that affect limb function (eg, spinal cord injury [SCI], stroke, or poliomyelitis). Rehabilitation in these patients frequently involves increasing muscle strength, maximizing motor control, training individuals to make the most effective use of residual function, and providing adaptive equipment to minimize limb deformities.

The most successful model for rehabilitation addresses all the needs of the patient, including physical and emotional needs, and is based on a team approach. Among those frequently included in the team are physicians and nurses from various medical specialties, physical and occupational therapists, speech therapists, psychologists, orthotists, and social workers as well as the patient and members of the patient's family. The shared goal of team members is to prevent barriers to rehabilitation by (1) diagnosing all current problems, (2) treating the problems adequately, (3) establishing adequate nutrition, (4) monitoring the patient for any complications that might impede progress in recovery, (5) mobilizing the patient as soon as possible, and (6) restoring function or helping the patient adjust to an altered lifestyle.

▶ Management of Common Problems in Rehabilitation

Inadequate nutrition, decubitus ulcers, urinary tract infections, impaired bladder control, spasticity, contractures, acquired musculoskeletal deformities, muscle weakness, and physiologic deconditioning are common complications that can obstruct rehabilitation efforts and cause further loss of function in an already compromised patient. Because these problems are costly in both human and financial terms, every effort should be made to prevent them.

A. Inadequate Nutrition

Good nutritional status is a basis for avoiding many complications. After trauma, a patient's nutritional requirements are markedly increased from the normal maintenance requirement of 30 kcal/kg/day. Most trauma patients have been receiving intravenous fluids with minimal nutritional benefit and so arrive at the rehabilitation center in various degrees of malnutrition. Patients with chronic illnesses commonly have poor appetites. Physically handicapped people expend much of their energy performing simple activities of daily living (ADLs) and may also have difficulty in obtaining and preparing adequate amounts of food. An often overlooked form of poor nutrition is obesity. Individuals with high body mass index (BMI) can become malnourished after trauma. Also, inactivity leads to diminished calorie need, but boredom may result in increased consumption of an unbalanced diet in which certain nutrients are lacking.

B. Decubitus Ulcers (Pressure Sores)

The combination of poor nutritional status, lack of sensation at pressure points of the body, and decreased ability to move can cause decubitus ulcers (Figure 12–1) and greatly add to a patient's discomfort and the length and cost of their hospital stay. The ulcer is a potential source of sepsis in an already compromised individual. And for a severe sacral decubitus ulcer, for example, it may be necessary to have surgery to rotate a flap graft to cover the defect. This in turn requires the patient to remain prone until the graft heals and significantly hampers the patient's participation in a rehabilitation program because mobility and ability to interact with others are hindered. Prevention is the best

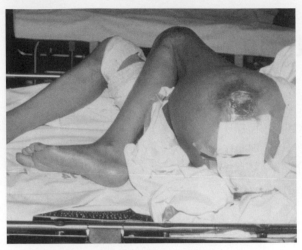

▲ **Figure 12–1.** Patient with contractures and a decubitus ulcer over the greater trochanter of the femur.

treatment. The clinical rule of protecting the patient's skin is to change position every 2 hours. No cushion alone can prevent decubitus ulcers.

C. Urinary Tract Infections and Impaired Bladder Control

Urinary tract infections are a common source of sepsis and prolonged illness. An indwelling catheter is the most frequent source. In an acutely ill or multiply injured patient, an indwelling catheter may be necessary for medical reasons but should be removed as soon as possible. Urinary incontinence is not sufficient reason for continued use of an indwelling catheter. In male patients, incontinence can be managed with a carefully applied condom catheter. Care must be taken to inspect the penis frequently for signs of skin maceration or pressure. In female patients, diapering and frequent linen changes are necessary.

Restoring bladder function to achieve adequate reflex voiding or a balanced bladder may require the use of an intermittent catheterization program. The basis of a balanced bladder program is that the volume of residual urine not exceed a third of the volume of voided urine. In general, an intermittent catheterization program is initiated if the residual volume is greater than 100 mL or if the voided volume exceeds 400 mL. The patient is catheterized every 4 hours initially and then every 6 hours for 24 hours, and the patient is reassessed. Good records are necessary throughout the program.

D. Muscle Weakness and Physiologic Deconditioning

During sustained exercise, the metabolism is mainly aerobic. The principal fuels for aerobic metabolism are carbohydrates and fats. In aerobic oxidation, the substrates are oxidized through a series of enzymatic reactions that lead to the production of adenosine triphosphate (ATP) for muscular contraction. A physical conditioning program can increase the aerobic capacity by improving cardiac output, increasing hemoglobin levels, enhancing the capacity of cells to extract oxygen from the blood, and increasing the muscle mass by hypertrophy.

Prolonged immobilization of extremities, bed rest, and inactivity lead to pronounced muscle wasting and physiologic deconditioning in a short time. Because disabled patients generally expend more energy than normal individuals in performing routine ADLs, they must be mobilized as quickly as possible to prevent unnecessary physiologic decline and subsequent decline in abilities. They should also be placed on a daily exercise program to maximize muscle strength and aerobic capacity.

E. Spasticity

Patients with spasticity exhibit an excessive response to the quick stretch of a muscle, which leads to hyperactive deep tendon reflexes and clonus. Spasticity must be managed aggressively to prevent permanent deformities and joint contractures.

1. Spasmolytic drugs—Drugs can be of some assistance in controlling spasticity associated with upper motor neuron diseases. Drugs are used when spasticity affects multiple large muscle groups in the body and when the spasticity is not severe.

Baclofen (Lioresal) can inhibit both polysynaptic and monosynaptic reflexes at the spinal cord level. It does, however, depress general central nervous system function. Use of oral baclofen should be avoided in traumatic brain-injured patients, when possible, because it may cause sedation and impede cognitive recovery. Patients with attention deficits or memory disorders may be compromised by antispastic agents, such as diazepam and clonidine, which, like baclofen, have sedating properties. Tizanidine (Zanaflex) affects the central nervous system less than other agents and may be useful. Even a drug such as dantrolene sodium, which acts peripherally, may cause drowsiness.

Baclofen pump technology has an advantage over oral drug therapy because of the small concentrations that can be introduced intrathecally. The small intrathecal doses control spasticity effectively while minimizing central nervous system side effects. The pump is placed in a subcutaneous pocket in the abdominal wall. A catheter is routed subcutaneously from the intrathecal space to the pump. The pump can be refilled by injection into the reservoir chamber. The dosage and rate of administration can be easily adjusted by using a laptop computer that sends radio signals to the pump.

Dantrolene (Dantrium), another drug that can be used to control spasticity, is the drug of choice for treating clonus. Dantrolene produces relaxation by directly affecting the contractile response of skeletal muscle at a site beyond the myoneural junction. It causes dissociation of the excitation–contraction coupling probably by interfering with the release of calcium from the sarcoplasmic reticulum. Although it does not affect the central nervous system directly, it does cause drowsiness, dizziness, and generalized weakness, which may interfere with the patient's overall function. Use of dantrolene for the control of spasticity is indicated in upper motor neuron diseases, such as SCI, cerebral palsy, stroke, or multiple sclerosis. The most serious problem with use of dantrolene is hepatotoxicity. The risk appears greatest in females, in patients older than 35 years, and in patients taking other medications. When using dantrolene, the lowest effective dose should be used, and liver enzyme functions should be monitored closely. If no effect is noted after 45 days of use, the drug should be stopped.

2. Casts—Casting temporarily reduces muscle tone and is frequently used to correct a contracture. The cast is changed weekly until the problem is corrected. If a cast must be used for a prolonged period, the patient should be placed on anticoagulant therapy to prevent deep venous thrombosis.

3. Splints—Anterior and posterior clamshell splints can be used to control joint position and still allow for active and passive range of motion (ROM) of the joints in therapy. A splint applied to only one side of an extremity is not sufficient to control excessive spasticity and may result in skin breakdown from motion against the splint. A splint can also obscure an early contracture.

4. Nerve-blocking agents—Anesthetic and phenol nerve blocks are often combined with a casting or splinting program. Anesthetic nerve blocks are commonly used to eliminate muscle tone temporarily. They can be used diagnostically to evaluate what portion of a deformity is dynamic (occurring because of muscle spasticity) and what portion is secondary to myostatic contracture. The block can also be prognostic of the likely results of surgical neurectomy or tendon lengthening. Repeated blocks of local anesthetics give a carryover effect to decrease muscle tone.

When muscle spasticity requires control for an extended period of time but the patient still has potential for spontaneous improvement, a phenol nerve block may be indicated. Phenol exerts two actions on the nerves. The first is a short-term effect, similar to the effect produced by a local anesthetic and directly proportional to the thickness of the nerve fibers. The second is a long-term effect that results from protein denaturation. Although this leads to wallerian degeneration of the axons, experimental studies in animals showed that the nerves regenerate with time. In patients, the direct injection of a nerve with a 3–5% solution of phenol after surgical exposure gives relief of spasticity for up to 6 months. Mixed nerves containing sensory fibers should not be injected because it could cause unwanted sensory loss or painful dysesthesia. Reduction of spasticity for up to 3 months can also be achieved by the percutaneous injection of muscle motor

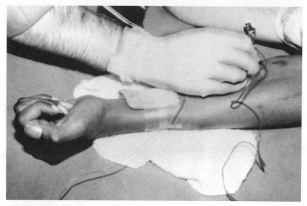

▲ **Figure 12–2.** Use of a Teflon-coated needle and nerve stimulator to locate the motor points of spastic forearm muscles for phenol injection.

points with an aqueous solution of phenol after localization using a needle and nerve stimulator (Figure 12–2).

A. BOTULINUM TOXIN—Ordinarily, an action potential propagating down a motor nerve to the neuromuscular junction triggers the release of acetylcholine (ACh) into the synaptic space. The released ACh causes depolarization of muscle membrane. Botulinum toxin type A is a protein produced by *Clostridium botulinum* that attaches to the presynaptic nerve terminal and inhibits the release of ACh at the neuromuscular junction. Botulinum toxin A is injected directly into a spastic muscle. Clinical benefit lasts 3–5 months. Current practice is to avoid administering a total of more than 400 U in a single treatment session to avoid excessive weakness or paralysis. This upper limit of 400 U may be reached rather quickly when injecting a few large muscles. A delay of 3–7 days between injection and the onset of clinical effect is typical. Because the patient does not see effects immediately, a follow-up visit is usually arranged to check the result. Because botulinum toxin A is the most potent biologic toxin known and the cost is relatively high, the smallest possible dose should be used to achieve results. Most studies report side effects in 20–30% of patients per treatment cycle. **The incidence of adverse effects varies based on the dosage used (ie, the higher the dose, the more frequent the adverse effects); however, the incidence of complications is not related to the total dose of botulinum toxin used.** Local pain at the injection site is the most commonly reported side effect. Other adverse effects such as local hematoma, generalized fatigue, lethargy, dizziness, flulike syndrome, and pain in neighboring muscles are also reported.

5. Surgical procedures—If muscle spasticity is permanent and no change in muscle tone is anticipated, definitive procedures such as dorsal rhizotomy, peripheral neurectomy, tendon lengthening or release, and tendon transfer should be considered.

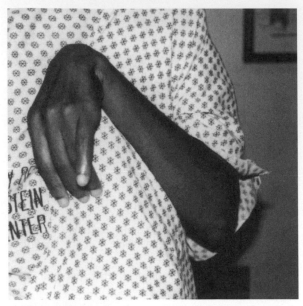

▲ **Figure 12–3.** Upper extremity contractures in a patient with untreated spasticity.

F. Joint Contractures

Inactivity and uncontrolled spasticity often lead to joint contractures (Figure 12–3), which are difficult to correct and greatly extend the needed rehabilitation program. Contractures may cause difficulties in positioning in a bed or chair or problems in using orthotic devices. They can also cause difficulties with hygiene and skin care and increase the risk of decubitus ulcers. Shoe wear may be rendered impossible because of foot deformities.

Muscle weakness is accentuated by contractures and malalignment, which cause the muscle to function at a mechanical disadvantage. Sitting and standing balance are compromised when contractures abnormally displace the center of gravity relative to the base of support. Functional use of the extremities is severely limited by lack of adequate joint motion. Joint contractures may require surgical release, which could further decrease function in an already compromised individual. Moreover, in children, joint contractures can lead to structural changes in the skeleton. Muscle growth lags behind skeletal growth, and this discrepancy in growth rates can cause increasing deformity with time.

To prevent contractures, exercises to maintain ROM must be performed several times daily. The patient, family members, therapists, and nursing personnel should all participate in this task.

Splinting can help maintain joints in a functional position when motor control is lacking. Splints should be removed regularly to inspect the skin condition and reassess their efficacy in maintaining the desired position.

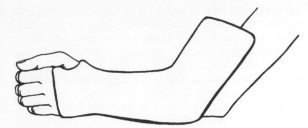

▲ **Figure 12–4.** An elbow dropout cast used to increase elbow extension while preventing flexion.

Treatment of established contractures can be time consuming and expensive. In general, if a contracture is present for less than 3 months, it may be amenable to nonsurgical methods of correction such as serial casting or electrical stimulation of the antagonist muscles. Excessive muscle tone must be treated aggressively if present because it accentuates the tendency to form contractures. An anesthetic nerve block can be given to eliminate excessive tone temporarily and provide analgesia prior to manipulation of the joint and application of a cast. Each week, the cast is removed, a nerve block is given, and a new cast is applied. When the desired limb position is obtained, a holding cast is used to maintain the position for an additional week. The cast can then be bivalved and made into anterior and posterior clamshell splints, which can be removed for ROM or other activities. Another useful technique is the application of a dropout cast (Figure 12–4), which allows for further correction of the contracture while preventing the original deformity from recurring.

When contractural deformities are long standing and fixed, surgical release is indicated. Tendons, ligaments, and joint capsules are all involved. If the deformity is severe, complete correction at the time of surgery may be impossible. Neurovascular structures must be protected from excessive traction. Serial casts or dropout casts may be necessary following surgery to gain the desired limb position.

G. Other Acquired Musculoskeletal Deformities

Paralysis or weakness of trunk muscles can lead to scoliotic deformities of the spine. When severe, these deformities can impair respiratory function and tend to cause balance problems with walking and sitting. External support in the form of bracing or seating modifications can minimize or eliminate this.

Disuse and lack of muscle tone lead to osteoporosis, which in turn predisposes patients to fractures. The fractures should be treated aggressively and in a manner that maximizes function rather than prolongs immobilization.

Peripheral nerve palsy can result from pressure secondary to decreased mobility in patients confined to a bed or chair. Pressure can also result from braces, splints, and casts, and these require careful monitoring. In patients who form heterotopic ossification (HO), the new bone formation and the accompanying inflammation may impinge on peripheral nerves, thereby causing nerve palsy.

▶ Evaluation of Impairment

A. Nerves

Many disabilities requiring rehabilitation result from diseases affecting the nervous system. The location and the extent of the primary lesion determine not only the degree of paralysis but also the extent to which motor control is impaired and spasticity is present. In injuries or diseases of the peripheral nerves, the damage is confined to the lower motor neurons. Normal motor control is preserved, spasticity is absent, and the magnitude of disability depends on the extent of paralysis and weakness (paresis). In pathologic conditions of the brain or spinal cord, the upper motor neurons are affected, which not only causes muscular weakness but also impairs motor control.

Motor activity can be considered as a hierarchic system of voluntary and involuntary neurologic mechanisms.

1. Voluntary muscle activity—Two types of voluntary muscle activity are clinically identifiable: selective and patterned movements. The highest level of motor activity, selective movement, depends on the integrity of the cerebral cortex. Selective movement is the ability to flex or extend one joint preferentially without initiating a mass flexor or extensor motion at other joints of the limb. Patterned movement (synergy) at a joint refers to the ability to move one joint by invoking a mass flexion or extension synergy involving movement at other joints of the limb. Patients with central nervous system disorders may have voluntary patterned movement but lack selective movement. Because most patients have mixtures of selective and patterned movement at different joints, however, the strength of each type of activity must be assessed at each joint. Patterned flexion and extension movements of the lower limb can provide sufficient motor control for ambulation, but patterned motion does not provide sufficient fine control for upper extremity function.

2. Involuntary muscle activity—Spasticity relates to two types of involuntary muscle activity: clonic and tonic responses. Each type depends on the sensitivity of the muscle spindle to the rate of stretch. If a muscle is quickly extended above the threshold of the velocity-sensitive receptors of the spindle, a phasic response may be elicited. If spasticity is severe, sudden stretch may trigger clonus, which consists of repeated bursts of phasic activity at 6–8 cycles per second. The phasic stretch response has practical clinical significance. For example, if an ankle equinus deformity is present and spasticity is severe, clonus of the triceps surae may be triggered in the stance phase each time the patient takes a step. A rigid ankle-foot orthosis (AFO) that blocks ankle motion and prevents the triceps surae from stretching may inhibit clonus, enabling the foot to be held in a neutral position.

An articulated or flexible AFO that allows the ankle to move and the triceps surae to stretch may not prevent clonus from being elicited and may be less effective.

If the muscle is stretched slowly below the threshold of the velocity components of the spindle, a phasic response is not triggered, but the spindle is still capable of detecting changes in length that may generate a tonic response consisting of continuous muscle hypertonus. The tonic muscle activity during slow stretch is called **clasp-knife resistance**. This tonic activity is also of practical significance. Even if the ankle is slowly dorsiflexed for a prolonged time, hypertonus may persist in the triceps surae and restrict normal motion. Consequently, it may be necessary to differentiate spasticity from myostatic contracture by performing peripheral nerve blocks.

Patients with injury involving the brainstem may exhibit severe hypertonus that is continuously present and is called either **decorticate rigidity** or **decerebrate rigidity**, depending on the posture of the limbs. In decerebrate posturing, the patient's arms are held tightly flexed while the legs are held in extension. In decorticate posturing, both the upper and lower extremities are in rigid extension. Patients with severe muscular rigidity are at extreme risk of developing contractural deformities.

When a spastic patient is sitting or standing, labyrinthine activation increases tone in the extensor muscles of the lower extremity and also increases upper limb flexion. Consequently, patients who are examined for spasticity should be evaluated in the upright rather than supine position, to elicit the maximal stretch response. Conversely, patients who are examined for maximal ROM should be evaluated in the supine position, to minimize muscle tone and enable maximal joint range. The limb posture of patients also influences the intensity of reflex and voluntary activity.

3. Sensory perception—The final steps of sensory integration occur in the cerebral cortex, where basic sensory data are integrated into the more complex sensory phenomena. When central nervous system injury involves the cerebral cortex, the patient responds to basic modalities of touch and pain. Responses to tests of more complex aspects of sensation (such as shape, texture, and proprioception) and two-point discrimination may be impaired, however. These simple tests quickly determine the patient's ability to interpret basic sensory information. Patients with absent proprioception across the major lower joints have balance abnormalities or are unable to walk. Most patients do not routinely use an affected hand unless proprioception is intact. Patients without lesions of the cerebral cortex can generally discriminate between two points less than 10 mm apart applied simultaneously to the fingers.

B. Muscles

Manual muscle testing is often useful for evaluating an individual's ability to perform functional tasks and also documents progress made in the rehabilitation program.

Table 12–1. Muscle strength.

Grade	Strength	Description
0	Absent	Muscle does not contract.
1	Trace	Muscle contracts, but no motion is generated.
2	Poor	Muscle contraction produces movement, but muscle cannot function against gravity.
3	Fair	Muscle functions against gravity.
4	Good	Muscle can overcome some outside resistance as well as gravity.
5	Normal	Muscle can overcome resistance to motion.

Several systems are currently used, but all are based on the grading system introduced by Robert Lovett in 1932. The evaluation is subjective, but the use of gravity resistance provides a measure of objective standardization (Table 12–1). A normal muscle grade as determined by manual testing does not always imply normal strength. A significant amount of weakness (a 25–30% loss of strength) must be present to be detected by this method.

C. Gait

1. Normal gait—Normal gait is the combination of postures and muscle activities that produce forward motion with minimal energy expenditure (Figure 12–5).

A. SWING PHASE—The swing phase (Figures 12–5 and 12–6) is divided into three equal periods: initial swing, midswing, and terminal swing. During the three-part phase, the pelvis rotates from backward to forward and the hip flexes 20–30 degrees. The knee flexes to 60 degrees initially and then extends in preparation for contact with the ground. The knee flexion is largely responsible for the foot clearing the ground during swing. Knee flexion occurs as the result of the forward momentum of the limb swinging and not as a result of hamstring contraction. The ankle joint initially plantarflexes 10 degrees and then assumes a neutral position during terminal swing so that the heel normally contacts the floor first.

The hip flexor muscles provide the power for advancing the limb and are active during the initial two thirds of the swing phase. The ankle dorsiflexors become active during the latter two thirds of the phase to ensure foot clearance as the knee begins to extend. The hamstring muscles decelerate the forward motion of the thigh during the terminal period of the swing phase.

B. STANCE PHASE—The stance phase (Figures 12–5 and 12–7) accounts for 60% of the gait cycle and can be divided into five distinct activities: initial contact, the loading response, midstance, terminal stance, and preswing. At initial ground contact, the ankle is in neutral position, the knee is extended,

and the hip is flexed. The hip extensor muscles contract to stabilize the hip because the body's mass is behind the hip joint. During the loading response, the knee flexes to 15 degrees, and the ankle plantarflexes to absorb the downward force and conserve energy by minimizing the up-and-down movement of the body's center of gravity. As the knee flexes and the stance leg accepts the weight of the body, the quadriceps muscle becomes active to stabilize the knee. In midstance, the knee is extended, and the ankle is in a neutral position. As the body's mass moves forward of the ankle joint, the calf muscles become active to stabilize the ankle and allow the heel to rise from the floor. In terminal stance, the heel leaves the floor, and the knee begins to flex as momentum carries the body forward. In the final portion of terminal stance, as the body rolls forward over the forefoot, the toes dorsiflex at the metatarsophalangeal joints. During preswing, the knee is flexed to 35 degrees and the ankle plantarflexes to 20 degrees. Because the opposite extremity is also in contact with the floor, the preswing is called the time of double-limb support.

Throughout the stance phase, the hip gradually extends and the pelvis rotates backward. During the first portion of the stance phase, the ankle dorsiflexors and hamstring muscles remain active. During the loading response and early midstance, the gluteus and quadriceps muscles become active to provide hip and knee stability. In midstance, the gastrocnemius and soleus muscles become active to stabilize the ankle joint and control the forward advancement of the tibia. This allows the heel to rise from the floor and the body weight to roll forward over the forefoot.

2. Abnormal gait—The study of movement (kinesiology) provides many important tools for evaluating patients with gait abnormalities. Among the areas of study are stride analysis, motion analysis (kinematics), force analysis (kinetics), and muscle activity analysis.

Three of the many specialized tools used in these studies are dynamic electromyography, force plate studies, and motion analysis. Dynamic electromyography, which records the electrical activity in multiple muscles simultaneously during functional activities, elucidates the patterns of motor control in both the upper and the lower extremities and helps in the management of spasticity and gait abnormalities. Force plate studies, which measure ground reaction forces and the fluctuations of the center of pressure, can be used to analyze gait problems and quantify balance reactions in impaired patients. Motion analysis uses multiple cameras located at different positions around the room. The cameras detect sensors placed on the patient and create a three-dimensional model of the patient moving through space.

Muscle strength can be accurately measured using torque, which can be correlated with joint position. Joint stiffness can also be assessed by measuring torque while moving the joint through a passive arc of motion. Joint powers can be calculated by multiplying joint moment times angular velocity.

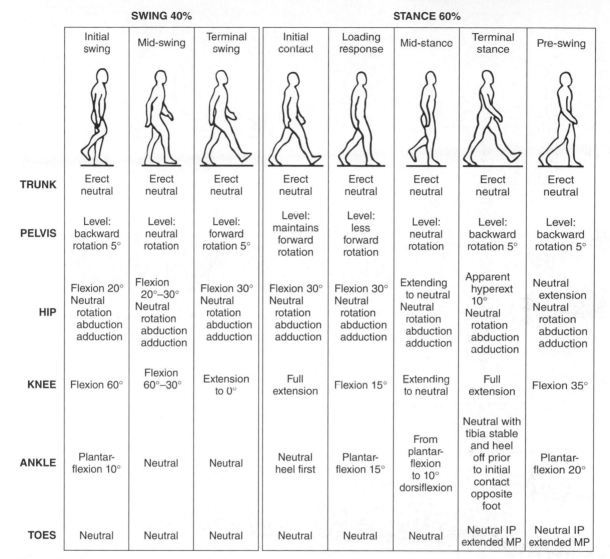

	SWING 40%			STANCE 60%				
	Initial swing	Mid-swing	Terminal swing	Initial contact	Loading response	Mid-stance	Terminal stance	Pre-swing
TRUNK	Erect neutral	Erect neutral	Erect neutral	Erect neutral	Erect neutral	Erect neutral	Erect neutral	Erect neutral
PELVIS	Level: backward rotation 5°	Level: neutral rotation	Level: forward rotation 5°	Level: maintains forward rotation	Level: less forward rotation	Level: neutral rotation	Level: backward rotation 5°	Level: backward rotation 5°
HIP	Flexion 20° Neutral rotation abduction adduction	Flexion 20°–30° Neutral rotation abduction adduction	Flexion 30° Neutral rotation abduction adduction	Flexion 30° Neutral rotation abduction adduction	Flexion 30° Neutral rotation abduction adduction	Extending to neutral Neutral rotation abduction adduction	Apparent hyperext 10° Neutral rotation abduction adduction	Neutral extension Neutral rotation abduction adduction
KNEE	Flexion 60°	Flexion 60°–30°	Extension to 0°	Full extension	Flexion 15°	Extending to neutral	Full extension	Flexion 35°
ANKLE	Plantar-flexion 10°	Neutral	Neutral	Neutral heel first	Plantar-flexion 15°	From plantar-flexion to 10° dorsiflexion	Neutral with tibia stable and heel off prior to initial contact opposite foot	Plantar-flexion 20°
TOES	Neutral	Neutral	Neutral	Neutral	Neutral	Neutral	Neutral IP extended MP	Neutral IP extended MP

▲ **Figure 12–5.** The normal gait cycle. (Reproduced, with permission, from American Academy of Orthopaedic Surgeons: Home study syllabus. In Heckman JD, ed: *Orthopaedic Knowledge Update,* I. Rosemont, IL: American Academy of Orthopaedic Surgeons; 1984.)

Measurement of velocity, stride length, cadence, and single- and double-limb support times can be combined with dynamic electromyography, force plate studies, and joint goniometric recordings to present a complete analysis of gait dysfunction. These studies can also be used to assess the influence of surgery, orthotic corrections, or prosthetic design on gait characteristics.

D. Oxygen Consumption and Aerobic Capacity

Perhaps the most important measurement for understanding the difficulties faced by disabled people comes from oxygen consumption studies. Oxygen consumption indicates the energy required to perform an activity. Measuring an individual's maximal aerobic capacity is the single best indicator of the level of physical fitness.

1. Effects of disease and aging on energy expenditure— Cardiorespiratory disease, anemia, muscle atrophy, and any other condition that restricts oxygen uptake cause a decrease in the maximal aerobic capacity. Even in a healthy person, 3 weeks of bed rest decreases maximal aerobic capacity by up to 30%.

During normal walking, the rate of energy expenditure by adults varies from approximately 30 to 45% of the

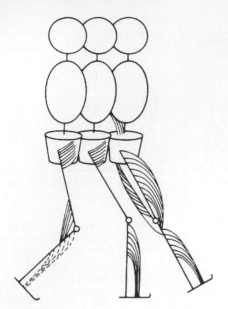

▲ **Figure 12–6.** Swing phase of gait. (Reproduced, with permission, from American Academy of Orthopaedic Surgeons: Home study syllabus. In Heckman JD, ed: *Orthopaedic Knowledge Update,* I. Rosemont, IL: American Academy of Orthopaedic Surgeons; 1984.)

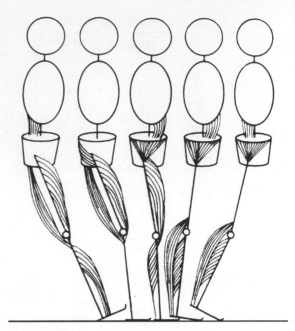

▲ **Figure 12–7.** Stance phase of gait. (Reproduced, with permission, from American Academy of Orthopaedic Surgeons: Home study syllabus. In Heckman JD, ed: *Orthopaedic Knowledge Update,* I. Rosemont, IL: American Academy of Orthopaedic Surgeons; 1984.)

maximal aerobic capacity, with the higher percentage being in people over 60 years. Because of the decline in maximal aerobic capacity with age, an older person is more susceptible than a person under 50–60 years of age to the penalties of a gait disability.

2. Effects of exercise on energy expenditure—When exercise is performed at less than 50% of an individual's maximal aerobic capacity, the exercise can be continued for prolonged periods because the ATP needed for muscle contraction is provided by aerobic pathways. Anaerobic pathways of ATP production, which do not use oxygen, increasingly come into play when exercise is performed at work rates exceeding approximately 50% of maximal aerobic capacity. The amount of energy that can be delivered by anaerobic metabolism is limited, and fatigue ensues because of the accumulation of lactate in the muscle. Consequently, the normal ADLs and work that must be performed throughout an 8-hour day, including walking, are performed below anaerobic threshold.

3. Effects of musculoskeletal impairment on energy expenditure—Gait abnormalities that interfere with efficient, coordinated limb movement can increase energy demand. Some affected patients respond to this increased demand by working harder, which increases the output of physiologic energy and is reflected in the higher-than-normal heart rate and oxygen consumption rate. Rather than increasing the rate of energy expenditure, however, most

patients slow their gait velocity in an effort to keep the power requirement from exceeding normal limits.

Among amputees, patients progressively walk slower at increasingly more proximal amputation levels. Younger patients with traumatic or congenital amputations walk faster than older dysvascular amputees because of their greater maximal aerobic capacity. Children with a Syme amputation, transtibial amputation, or knee disarticulation walk with the same speed and energy expenditure as control children. Children with bilateral amputations, unilateral transfemoral amputation, or unilateral hip disarticulation walk at a lower speed, higher heart rate, and higher energy expenditure. Patients with limited joint movement or with arthritis and painful joints also reduce their gait velocity. The heart rate and energy expenditure rate do not exceed normal in any of these groups of patients if crutches are not required.

Patients requiring crutches and exerting considerable force to support the body often have high heart rates and energy expenditure rates. A swing-through, crutch-assisted gait in a paraplegic or a patient who has a fracture and is unable to bear weight on one leg requires strenuous physical exertion, which is why few paraplegics use swing-through gait and why older patients with fractures can ambulate for only short distances. Even patients who use a reciprocal gait pattern, such as patients with low lumbar paraplegia resulting from SCI or myelodysplasia, use their arms for considerable exertion. Consequently, these types of patients may also be restricted ambulators in the community.

Patients with hip and knee flexion deformities caused by fixed or dynamic contractures require increasing muscle effort not only to walk but also to maintain an upright posture because the center of gravity during stance passes farther away from the axis of rotation of the joint. The fact that knee flexion greater than 30 degrees significantly increases the energy expenditure rate points to the importance of preventing and correcting contractures.

Children who have cerebral palsy and diplegia and who walk in a crouch gait may have energy expenditure rates that are above the anaerobic threshold. This is why these children are restricted ambulators who frequently discontinue walking when they mature and their maximal aerobic capacities decrease.

▶ Use of Orthoses

Orthotic (brace) prescription plays a vital role in rehabilitation. The physician must understand the functional needs of the patient and provide the orthotist with an exact prescription that specifies the materials, type of joints, joint position, and ROM. Brace prescriptions should not be left to the discretion of the patient and orthotist.

A temporary orthosis may be used in an early stage of illness until a definitive, custom-fitted orthosis is fabricated. Definitive orthoses for the lower extremity are the below-knee AFO and the above-knee knee-ankle-foot orthosis (KAFO).

The bichannel adjustable ankle-locking (BiCAAL) type of AFO is commonly applied as the first orthosis following stroke, head trauma, spinal injury, or other condition that causes extensive muscle imbalance about the foot and ankle (Figure 12–8). A rigid ankle is useful in controlling plantarflexion spasticity, stabilizing the ankle in a flaccid limb, and correcting a dynamic varus deformity (inversion of the foot). The adjustable ankle joint mechanism enables the clinician to determine the optimal ankle position in the acute period following onset of illness when the neurologic picture and orthotic requirement are changing. Once neurologic recovery stabilizes, a plastic (polypropylene) orthosis often becomes the treatment of choice (Figure 12–9).

The use of plastic materials in lower extremity orthotics is now widespread. Orthoses fabricated from plastics are lighter, more comfortable, and more attractive. A plastic AFO can be rigid or can be flexible, allowing motion at the ankle. Polypropylene is presently the most practical plastic material. Skillful fitting is critical because of the close skin and bone contact.

A. Ankle-Foot Orthosis

1. Types—Of several currently available orthoses classified as limited-motion ankle joint orthoses, two are commonly

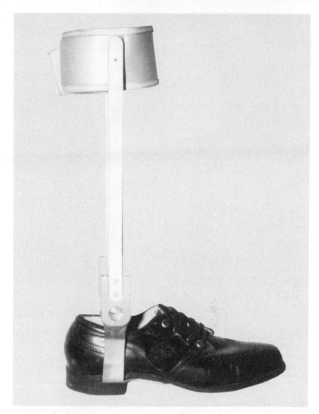

▲ **Figure 12–8.** The bichannel adjustable ankle-locking (BiCAAL) type of ankle-foot orthosis.

used: the conventional metal, double-upright, single-adjustable ankle joint with dorsiflexion spring assist (Klenzak) and the molded plastic posterior shells made from 116-inch polypropylene. The use of plastic materials makes the latter design preferable for most patients. When a greater restriction of ankle motion is desired, rigidity can be attained in several ways: by using a thicker sheet of polypropylene, by extending the lateral trim lines farther anteriorly at the ankle to serve as side struts, by adding an anterior shell to the posterior shell and totally enveloping the ankle, or by stiffening the posterior shell with the use of carbon fiber or lamination techniques. The trim lines may be reinforced with metal or additional layers of plastic. The foot plate of the orthosis extends just proximal to the metatarsal heads. Total circumferential orthoses combining anterior and posterior shells require exceptionally careful fitting to avoid excessive skin pressure over bony prominences. They are not recommended for routine use.

Insertion of a polypropylene orthosis inside a shoe generally requires a shoe size that is a half size larger and wider than that previously worn by the patient. To eliminate the need to purchase two pairs of shoes of different sizes, an inlay can be inserted in the shoe of the sound limb to prevent

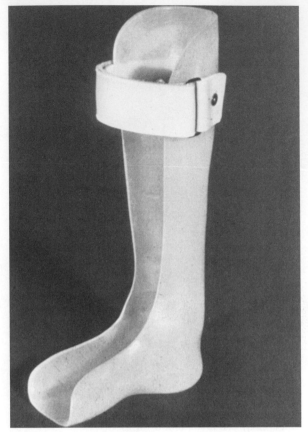

▲ **Figure 12–9.** The molded polypropylene ankle-foot orthosis.

excessive looseness once a shoe is fitted on the polypropylene side. The ankle position of the polypropylene orthosis should be assessed with the patient wearing his or her shoe with the normal heel height.

2. Indications—The primary requirement for orthotic support is that all joints must be passively capable of being positioned in adequate alignment. An orthosis cannot correct a fixed bony deformity or fixed joint contracture.

A. INADEQUATE DORSIFLEXION FOR FOOT CLEARANCE DURING SWING—An AFO is indicated for inadequate toe clearance (footdrop) during the midswing phase of gait. This problem may result from inadequate ankle dorsiflexion caused by weakness of the dorsiflexors or by the inability of dorsiflexors to overcome spasticity of the triceps surae. A lightweight, flexible polypropylene orthosis is indicated if inadequate dorsiflexion is the only problem at the ankle. A flexible orthosis can also be used for a mild swing-phase varus deformity (foot inversion). A rigid orthosis is needed in patients who have excessive plantarflexion resulting from

severe spasticity and in patients who initiate a strong extensor pattern activity prior to heel strike.

B. INADEQUATE DORSIFLEXION FOR INITIAL CONTACT—A patient with inadequate dorsiflexion, from any cause, contacts the ground with the forefoot or with the foot flat and the tibia extended backward. This problem is commonly combined with varus deformity, and weight bearing is on the lateral edge of the foot. The results are a backward thrust to the limb, which decreases forward momentum and produces excessive hyperextension forces on the knee, which leads to knee instability in the patient who is a functional walker. A rigid AFO in the neutral position results in heel strike for the patient who has full-knee extension and allows the tibia to rotate forward during stance.

C. MEDIAL-LATERAL SUBTALAR INSTABILITY DURING STANCE—Varus deformity is more common than valgus deformity. The patient walks on the lateral border of the foot and is hesitant to accept weight on the leg. A rigid orthosis can correct the varus deformity unless spasticity is severe. To correct a mild varus deformity, a limited ankle orthosis may be used. No orthosis is effective in controlling the severe spastic varus deformity.

D. INADEQUATE TIBIAL STABILITY DURING STANCE—Some patients have inadequate strength or control of the plantarflexors for maintenance of normal tibial position and alignment during stance. Early after midstance, this problem is manifested by excessive dorsiflexion and accompanying knee flexion. Whether or not the limb collapses during weight bearing depends on the amount of quadriceps muscle control and strength. Patients with sufficient proprioception learn to compensate by locking the knee in hyperextension as the foot contacts the floor, which keeps the knee from buckling. A rigid orthosis that prevents both dorsiflexion and plantarflexion is indicated to provide vertical tibial alignment during midstance. Its use prevents tibial collapse during terminal stance as a substitution for adequate calf control.

A knee extension thrust, caused by inadequate calf control as described earlier, may result also from severe plantarflexion tone or fixed equinus deformity resulting from contracture. At foot strike, the forefoot strikes the floor first, resulting in a knee extension or hyperextension thrust. A rigid AFO with a plantarflexion block prevents the development of knee instability and pain.

A T-strap (a leather T-shaped strap attached to the brace at the ankle and applied around the ankle to hold the foot from either an inverted or everted position) is usually not desirable for correction of severe varus deformity in patients fitted with metal orthoses. If a T-strap is applied with sufficient force to provide significant control to prevent foot twisting, it usually causes excessive pressure over the lateral malleolus in the patient with severe spasticity. This problem can be treated better by the use of a split anterior tibial tendon transfer or by the addition of a lateral wedge and flare to the shoe of the nonsurgical candidate.

B. Knee-Ankle-Foot Orthosis

A KAFO may be used if quadriceps muscle weakness or hamstring muscle spasticity is present. A knee immobilizer may be used as a training aid before having a KAFO fabricated. A KAFO is more difficult to don than a below-knee brace, and most patients with a central nervous system disease such as stroke or cerebral palsy have difficulty walking with a KAFO. Consequently, if hamstring spasticity rather than quadriceps spasticity necessitates external support to align the knee in extension, it is preferable to perform hamstring tenotomy or tendon lengthening, thereby eliminating the need for knee support.

Most patients with lower extremity quadriceps paresis resulting from SCI lack sufficient proprioception to walk with a free-knee mechanism (unlocked knee joint mechanism) when a KAFO is prescribed for quadriceps paresis. Then, it is necessary to determine if the knee will be locked while walking or if it will be freely movable to allow knee flexion in swing. When a KAFO is prescribed because of knee instability or because of varus or valgus instability, a polycentric joint (a joint in which the center of rotation moves following the anatomic instantaneous center of rotation) permits flexion extension movement but blocks medial and lateral angulation. A posterior stop added to the knee mechanism prevents excessive hyperextension.

If proprioception is intact, as is the case with poliomyelitis, even patients with considerable quadriceps weakness may be able to walk with an unlocked knee using an offset knee joint. This is accomplished by careful orthotic alignment. The center of rotation of the orthosis is positioned anterior to the center of rotation of the knee. As long as the patient can fully extend the knee in the swing stage preparatory to limb loading, the resulting movement caused by vertical loading acts to extend the knee against the posterior stop, thereby locking the knee in extension. This requires at least fair (grade 3) hip flexor strength (see Table 12–1) to provide sufficient forward momentum of the leg to position the knee in full extension.

The substitution of plastic components, such as a pretibial shell, has led to significantly improved fit and reduced weight in KAFOs.

Chumanov ES, Heiderscheit BC, Thelen DG: Hamstring musculotendon dynamics during stance and swing phases of high-speed running. *Med Sci Sports Exerc* 2011:43:525. [PMID: 20689454]

Hosalkar H, Pandya NK, Hsu J, Keenan MA: What's new in orthopaedic rehabilitation. *J Bone Joint Surg Am* 2011;93-A:1367. [PMID: 21792505]

Hsu JD: Rancho Los Amigos Medical Center. A unique orthopaedic resource and teaching institution. *Clin Orthop* 2000;374:125. [PMID: 10818973]

Jeans KA, Browne RH, Karol LA: Effect of amputation level on energy expenditure during overground walking by children with an amputation. *J Bone Joint Surg* 2011;93:49. [PMID: 21209268]

Kaelin DL, Oh TH, Lim PA, et al: Rehabilitation of orthopedic and rheumatologic disorders. 4. Musculoskeletal disorders. *Arch Phys Med Rehabil* 2000;81(3 Suppl 1):S73. [PMID: 10721764]

Pearson OR, Busse ME, van Deursen RW, et al: Quantification of walking mobility in neurological disorders. *QJM* 2004;97:463. [PMID: 15256604]

Schmalz T, Blumentritt S, Jarasch R: Energy expenditure and biomechanical characteristics of lower limb amputee gait: the influence of prosthetic alignment and different prosthetic components. *Gait Posture* 2002;16:255. [PMID: 12443950]

Ulkar B, Yavuzer G, Guner R, et al: Energy expenditure of the paraplegic gait: comparison between different walking aids and normal subjects. *Int J Rehabil Res* 2003;26:213. [PMID: 14501573]

SPINAL CORD INJURY

Trauma to the spinal cord causes dysfunction of the cord, with nonprogressive loss of sensory and motor function distal to the injury. Approximately 400,000 people have spinal cord damage in the United States, and the incidence is about 10,000 per year. The leading causes of SCI are motor vehicle accidents, gunshot wounds, falls, sports (especially diving) injuries, and water injuries.

Patients are generally categorized into three groups. The first consists predominantly of younger individuals who sustained their injury from a motor vehicle collision or other high-energy traumatic accident. The second consists of individuals over 50 years of age with cervical spinal stenosis caused by congenital narrowing or spondylosis. Patients in this second group often sustained their injury from minor trauma and commonly have no vertebral fracture. The third group consists of people with gunshot wounds, which are now the leading cause of spinal injury in many urban centers in the United States. With the benefits of an organized program of medical care, the life expectancy of survivors of SCI is now approaching normal.

▶ Terminology

A. Tetraplegia

The term *tetraplegia* (preferred to *quadriplegia*) refers to loss or impairment of motor or sensory function (or both) in the cervical segments of the spinal cord with resulting impairment of function in the arms, trunk, legs, and pelvic organs.

B. Paraplegia

Paraplegia refers to loss or impairment of motor or sensory function (or both) in the thoracic, lumbar, or sacral segments of the spinal cord. Arm function is intact but, depending on the level of the cord injured, impairment in the trunk, legs, and pelvic organs may be present.

C. Complete Injury

The term *complete injury* refers to an injury with no spared motor or sensory function in the lowest sacral segments.

D. Incomplete Injury

Incomplete injury refers to an injury with partial preservation of sensory or motor function (or both) below the neurologic level and includes the lowest sacral segments.

▶ Neurologic Impairment and Recovery

A. Neurologic Examination

The neurologic examination is critical to the classification and treatment of spinal injuries because it determines the patient's potential level of recovery. The neurologic level of the lesion refers to the highest neural segment having normal motor and sensory function. Patients are further subdivided according to whether they have complete or incomplete spinal cord function. This is determined by the absence or presence of motor or sensory function in the most distal part of the spinal cord innervating the sacral nerves. The presence of sacral nerve function is critical because patients with incomplete injuries have the potential to recover normal neurologic function over a time span of up to 2 years even if paralysis is initially complete.

1. Spinal shock—The diagnosis of complete SCI cannot be made until the period of spinal shock is over, as evidenced by the return of the bulbocavernosus reflex. To elicit this reflex, the clinician examines the patient's rectum digitally, feeling for contraction of the anal sphincter while squeezing the glans penis or clitoris. The concept of spinal shock is important and can be understood on the basis of the monosynaptic stretch reflex. At a given neural segment of the spinal cord, afferent sensory fibers enter the spinal cord and anastomose with the anterior motor neurons at the same level. If trauma to the spinal cord causes complete injury, reflex activity at the site of injury will not return because the reflex arc is permanently interrupted. When spinal shock disappears, however, reflex activity does return in the distal segments below the level of injury. In a patient with complete SCI, spinal shock may last for as little as several hours or as long as several months. Patients with complete SCI who have recovered from spinal shock have a negligible chance for any useful motor return.

2. Sacral reflexes—The presence or absence of sacral function determines the completeness of the injury. Sacral motor function is assessed by testing contraction of the external anal sphincter (graded as present or absent). Sacral sensation is tested at the anal mucocutaneous junction. Additionally, testing of the external anal sphincter is performed by assessing perceived deep sensation as present or absent when the examiner's finger is inserted.

B. Spinal Cord Syndromes

1. Anterior cord syndrome—Anterior cord syndrome commonly results from direct contusion to the anterior cord by bone fragments or from damage to the anterior spinal artery. Depending on the extent of cord involvement, only posterior column function (proprioception and light touch) may be present. The ability to respond to pain (tested by discriminating sharp and dull) and to light touch (tested with a wisp of cotton) signifies that the entire posterior half of the cord has some intact function and thus offers a better prognosis for motor recovery. If there is no recovery of motor function and pain sensation 4 weeks after injury, the prognosis for significant motor return is poor.

2. Central cord syndrome—Central cord syndrome can be understood on the basis of the spinal cord anatomy. The gray matter in the spinal cord contains nerve cell bodies and is surrounded by white matter consisting primarily of ascending and descending myelinated tracts. The central gray matter has a higher metabolic requirement and is therefore more susceptible to the effects of trauma and ischemia. Central cord syndrome often results from a minor injury such as a fall in an older patient with cervical spinal canal stenosis. The overall prognosis for patients with central cord syndrome is variable. Most patients are able to walk despite severe paralysis of the upper extremity.

3. Brown-Séquard syndrome—Brown-Séquard syndrome is caused by a complete hemisection of the spinal cord, resulting in a greater ipsilateral proprioceptive motor loss and a greater contralateral loss of pain and temperature sensation. Affected patients have an excellent prognosis and can usually ambulate.

4. Mixed syndrome—Mixed syndrome is characterized by a diffuse involvement of the entire spinal cord. Affected patients have a good prognosis for recovery. As with all incomplete SCI syndromes, early motor recovery is the best prognostic indicator.

▶ Management

A. Acute Management

Most patients with SCIs have associated injuries. In this setting, assessment and treatment of airway, respiration, and circulation take precedence. The patient is best treated initially in the supine position.

Airway management in the setting of SCI, with or without a cervical spine injury, is complex and difficult. The cervical spine must be maintained in neutral alignment. Clearing of oral secretions and/or debris is essential to maintain airway patency and to prevent aspiration. Failure to intubate emergently when indicated because of concerns regarding the instability of the patient's cervical spine is a potential pitfall.

Hypotension may be hemorrhagic and/or neurogenic in acute SCI. Because of the vital sign confusion in acute SCI and the high incidence of associated injuries, a diligent search for occult sources of hemorrhage must be made. The most common causes of occult hemorrhage are chest, intraabdominal, or retroperitoneal injuries and pelvic or long bone fractures. Appropriate investigations, including radiography or computed tomography (CT) scanning, are required.

Once occult sources of hemorrhage are excluded, initial treatment of neurogenic shock focuses on fluid resuscitation. Judicious fluid replacement with isotonic crystalloid solution to a maximum of 2 L is the initial treatment of choice.

Associated head injury occurs in approximately 25% of SCI patients. A careful neurologic assessment for associated head injury is compulsory. The presence of amnesia, external signs of head injury or basilar skull fracture, focal neurologic deficits, associated alcohol intoxication or drug abuse, and a history of loss of consciousness mandate a thorough evaluation for intracranial injury, starting with noncontrast head CT scanning.

Ileus is common. Placement of a nasogastric tube is essential. Aspiration pneumonitis is a serious complication in the SCI patient with compromised respiratory function. Antiemetics should be used aggressively.

Current neuroprotective treatments for SCI remain controversial. The National Acute Spinal Cord Injury Studies (NASCIS) II and III, a Cochrane review of all randomized clinical trials and other published reports, revealed there to be significant improvement in motor function and sensation in patients with complete or incomplete SCIs who were treated with high doses of methylprednisolone within 8 hours of injury. The treatment protocol is to start steroid within 3 hours as follows: methylprednisolone 30 mg/kg bolus over 15 minutes and an infusion of methylprednisolone at 5.4 mg/kg/hour for 23 hours beginning 45 minutes after the bolus. However, the risks of steroid therapy are not inconsequential. An increased incidence of avascular necrosis and infectious complications such as pneumonia, urinary tract infections, and wound infections are documented. A recent study evaluating steroid use for SCI using the NASCIS II protocol found no difference in function and more complications with high-dose steroids.

The NASCIS III study evaluated methylprednisolone 5.4 mg/kg/hour for 24 or 48 hours versus tirilazad 2.5 mg/kg every 6 hours for 48 hours. (Tirilazad is a potent lipid preoxidation inhibitor. High doses of steroids or tirilazad are thought to minimize the secondary effects of acute SCI.) All patients received a 30 mg/kg bolus of methylprednisolone intravenously. The study found that in patients treated earlier than 3 hours after injury, the administration of methylprednisolone for 24 hours was best. In patients treated 3–8 hours after injury, the use of methylprednisolone for 48 hours was best. Tirilazad was equivalent to methylprednisolone for 24 hours.

B. Lower Extremities

Prevention of contractures and maintenance of ROM are important in all patients with SCI and should begin immediately following the injury. Teaching the patient to sleep in the prone position is the most effective means of preventing hip and knee flexion contractures. Passive stretching of the hamstring muscles with the knee extended is initiated to prevent shortening of these muscles secondary to spasticity. For patients to be able to dress the lower parts of their body independently, they must be able to flex the lumbar spine and hip 120 degrees with the knee extended.

Patients with extensive paralysis of the lower extremity need strength in both arms to manipulate crutches and bring the body to a standing position. Patients who lack at least fair (grade 3) strength in their quadriceps muscles (see Table 12–1) require KAFOs to stabilize the knee and also require the knee to be locked in extension while walking. Patients who have bilateral KAFOs commonly use a swing-through, crutch-assisted gait rather than a reciprocal gait. Because strenuous upper extremity exertion is required and the rate of energy expenditure is extremely high when crutches are used, nearly all patients prefer to use a wheelchair. In contrast, patients who have fair (grade 3) or greater strength in their hip flexors and knee extensors are able to walk with unlocked (free) knees and only require AFOs to stabilize their feet and ankles. These patients also usually require crutches because of absent or impaired hip extensor and adductor muscles, but they are able to achieve a reciprocal gait pattern and can walk for a limited duration outside the home. Most of them prefer a wheelchair when they must ambulate over long distances.

Because most ambulatory patients with SCI have impaired hip extensor support, they learn to hyperextend the lumbar spine so the center of gravity of the trunk is posterior to the hip joint in the stance phase of gait. This prevents forward collapse and decreases the demand on the arms during crutch use. Spine stabilization procedures that decrease the flexibility of the lower lumbar spine or reduce the amount of lordosis deprive the patient of an important gait maneuver.

C. Upper Body and Extremities

1. C4 level function—Patients with cervical lesions above C4 may have impairment of respiratory function, depending on the extent of injury, and may require a tracheostomy and mechanical ventilatory assistance.

Phrenic nerve stimulation via implanted surgical electrodes enables patients to use their own diaphragm and ventilate without mechanical assistance if the cause of their diaphragm paralysis is upper motor neuron injury. With training, these patients should be able to achieve a vital capacity that is 50–60% of normal using only the diaphragm.

Patients with high tetraplegia can use chin or tongue controls to operate an electric wheelchair with attached respiratory equipment. Mouth sticks that are lightweight rods attached to a dental bite plate enable patients to perform desktop skills, operate push-button equipment, and pursue vocational and recreational activities.

2. C5 level function—At the C5 level, the key muscles are the deltoid and biceps muscles, which are used for shoulder abduction and elbow flexion. If these muscles are weak, the patient benefits from mobile arm supports attached to the wheelchair and balanced to exert a vertical force to counteract gravity. This enables the patient with poor muscle strength to feed independently and perform other functional tasks with the hands. A ratchet wrist-hand orthosis (WHO) with a fixed wrist joint and a passively closing mechanism attached to the thumb and fingers enables the patient to grasp objects between the thumb and fingers.

Surgery can further enhance upper extremity function. The goals of surgery are to provide active elbow and wrist extension and to restore the ability to pinch the thumb against the index finger (key pinch or lateral pinch). Transferring the posterior deltoid to the triceps muscle provides active elbow extension, and another option is to transfer the biceps to the triceps. One option is to transfer the brachioradialis to the extensor carpi radialis brevis to provide active wrist extension and attach the flexor pollicis longus tendon to the distal radius and fuse the interphalangeal joint of the thumb to provide for key pinch by tenodesis when the wrist is extended.

3. C6 level function—At the C6 level, the key muscles are the wrist extensors, which enable the patient to propel a wheelchair manually, transfer from one position to another, and even live independently.

If wrist extensor strength is poor, an orthosis is indicated. A WHO with a free wrist joint and a rubber-band extensor-assist mechanism enables the patient to complete wrist extension. A wrist-driven WHO with a flexor hinge mechanism that causes the metacarpophalangeal joint to flex when the wrist is extended enables the patient to grasp actively between the fingers and thumb. Some patients develop a natural tenodesis of their thumb and finger flexor muscles because of myostatic contracture or spasticity, and this tenodesis enables them to grasp without an orthosis.

Most patients with good wrist extensor strength are able to operate a manual wheelchair but may require an electric wheelchair for long distances. These patients may also be able to transfer independently if they have no elbow flexion contractures and they can lock their elbows passively in extension while transferring.

The goals of surgery in the C6 patient are the restoration of lateral pinch and active grasp. Lateral pinch can be restored either by tenodesis of the thumb flexor or by transfer of the brachioradialis to the flexor pollicis longus. Active grasp can be restored by transfer of the pronator teres to the flexor digitorum profundus.

4. C7 level function—At the C7 level, the key muscle is the triceps. All patients with intact triceps function should be able to transfer and live independently if no other complications are present. Despite their ability to extend the fingers, these patients may also require a WHO with a flexor hinge mechanism.

The goals of surgery in the C7 tetraplegic patient are active thumb flexion for pinch, active finger flexion for grasp, and hand opening by extensor tenodesis. Transfer of the brachioradialis to the flexor pollicis longus provides active pinch. Transfer of the pronator teres to the flexor digitorum profundus allows for active finger flexion and grasp. If the finger extensors are weak, tenodesis of these tendons to the radius provides hand opening with wrist flexion.

5. C8 level function—At the C8 level, the key muscles are the finger and thumb flexors, which enable a gross grasp. The functioning flexor pollicis longus enables patients to obtain lateral pinch between the thumb and the side of the index finger. Intrinsic muscle function is lacking, and clawing of the fingers is usually present. A capsulodesis of the metacarpophalangeal joints corrects the clawing and improves hand function. Active intrinsic function can be gained by splitting the superficial finger flexor tendon of the ring finger into four slips and transferring these tendons to the lumbrical insertions of each finger.

D. Skin

Maintaining skin integrity is crucial to spinal injury care. From the moment the patient enters the emergency room, preventive measures are instituted to avoid skin breakdown even while critical diagnostic procedures and lifesaving measures are performed. Only 4 hours of continuous pressure on the sacrum is sufficient to cause full-thickness skin necrosis. Turning the patient from side to back to side every 2 hours avoids skin ulceration, a problem that greatly prolongs the cost and length of rehabilitation. Following the simple procedures outlined here usually obviates the need for flotation devices, Stryker frames, cyclically rotating beds, and similar equipment.

Once the patient is allowed to sit, a progressive program to increase the time of sitting tolerance is undertaken. Paraplegics with normal upper extremity function are taught to perform raises automatically in the wheelchair and decompress the skin for approximately 15 seconds every 15 minutes. Tetraplegics who are unable to perform raises can lean to either side or lean forward for 1-minute intervals every hour. Those patients unable to perform decompressive maneuvers require assistance from another person or may use an electric wheelchair with a powered recliner that enables them to assume a supine posture every hour.

All patients must be taught to inspect their skin at least twice a day, when dressing and undressing. Mirrors attached to a rod enable paraplegics to examine their skin over the sacrum and ischia independently. Tetraplegics usually require assistance with skin inspection.

If there is evidence of chronic skin inflammation over bony prominences or if redness persists 30 minutes after removal of pressure, action must be taken to avoid incipient pressure necrosis. Pressure transducers placed under the bony prominences determine if pressure exceeds acceptable levels. Up to 40 mm Hg is well tolerated by most patients. If pressures exceed this amount, a custom-fitted foam cushion with appropriate cutouts is prescribed.

Development of any open areas in the skin over the ischia or sacrum, even superficial areas, is an indication to discontinue sitting temporarily. The patient must remain in a prone or side-lying position to avoid pressure until the lesion is healed. Failure to take aggressive steps to eliminate pressure and allow healing leads to chronic inflammation, scarring, and a loss of elasticity, creating a vicious cycle that further increases susceptibility to pressure necrosis.

Excessive hip and knee flexor spasticity that prevents patients from assuming the prone position or lying supine and requires them constantly to assume a side-lying posture when in bed can lead to excessive pressure over the greater trochanters. Flexor spasticity or contracture that prevents continuous turning should be corrected medically prior to development of pressure sores and must be performed before skin flap placement. Failure to correct flexion deformities inevitably decreases the likelihood of successful skin closure. Surgical tenotomy and myotomy of hip and knee flexors is the most effective surgical method for correcting the problem when nonoperative measures fail. Neurosurgical procedures such as myelotomy or rhizotomy are usually less effective and run the risk of interfering with reflex bladder emptying and penile erections.

In the neglected patient with a full-thickness pressure sore, surgery is necessary. The initial phase consists of debridement of all infected soft tissue and bone as well as treatment of spasticity and contractures that may have predisposed the patient to pressure sores. Once all wounds have a clean granulating base and the patient is able to remain prone 24 hours a day, he or she becomes a candidate for a rotational flap. The gluteus maximus, the tensor fasciae latae, and other types of musculocutaneous flaps give the surgeon a superior and reliable method of providing skin coverage. Sitting tolerance must be carefully reestablished following flap surgery. Because most pressure sores in patients with chronic SCI are the result of failure to relieve pressure by appropriate measures, patient education is the key element of a successful rehabilitation outcome.

Ischial or trochanteric pressure sores commonly lead to septic arthritis of the hip. In such cases, femoral head and neck resection is required. In the paraplegic with an intact hip joint, the passive weight of the limbs cantilevered about the posterior thigh exerts an upward force on the pelvis, which decompresses the ischia. Consequently, approximately 30% of the body weight is supported on the thigh. Femoral head and neck resection disrupts the bony leg of the femur to the pelvis and results in a greater concentration of pressure on the ischia, thereby increasing the chance of recurrence even after successful flap closure.

Pressure sores affecting the ankle commonly occur over the heel or malleolus. After initial debridement, wound healing can nearly always be obtained by placing the patient in a short leg cast that protects the wound from any external pressure. The cast is changed every 1 or 2 weeks until healing occurs. Rotational flaps are rarely needed.

E. Bladder Function

Intermittent catheterization is the factor most responsible for the nearly normal life span of patients with SCIs. In this group, urinary tract infection is no longer the leading cause of death. Most patients who have intact sacral reflex activity following complete injury are able to obtain reflex bladder emptying. Some patients with complete SCI are able to trigger reflex bladder emptying by tapping the suprapubic area, stroking the thighs, or using the Credé method (applying external pressure on the bladder to induce emptying) or the Valsalva maneuver (forcibly exhaling against the closed glottis). These patients require an external condom catheter for men or diapering for women. Patients with nonreflex bladders void by the application of pressure on the bladder by the Valsalva maneuver or Credé method. Not all so-called reflex bladders empty reflexively, and some, despite reflex emptying, have an excessive amount of residual urine. Anticholinergic medications to decrease bladder neck spasm of the smooth muscle of the internal sphincter or spasmolytic medications to decrease tone in the striated muscle of the external sphincter may improve bladder emptying. Some patients require surgical sphincterotomy.

Bladder diversion using an ileal conduit as a primary means of achieving bladder drainage is contraindicated. This procedure leads to a chronic acid–base imbalance, osteoporosis, and, ultimately, renal failure from secondary infection. The suprapubic catheter also is to be avoided as a means of primary treatment for the same reasons that permanent indwelling catheters are contraindicated. The constant presence of an indwelling catheter leads to bladder constriction and increases the risks of renal calculi, infection, and death from renal failure. For male patients, the external condom catheter is the treatment of choice. For female patients, padding or diapering is the preferred treatment, although some women prefer an indwelling catheter despite the risks of a shortened life span.

F. Sexual Function

Women with or without intact reflex activity can perform coitus and deliver normal children. Approximately 90% of men with complete SCI and sacral reflex activity can be expected to have reflex erections. Most of these men are able to perform coitus; however, fewer than half can ejaculate. Sacral sparing plays a great role in prognosticating sexual potential in the male patient. Those able to distinguish pain (discrimination of sharp and dull) are usually able to achieve psychogenic erections.

G. Autonomic Dysreflexia

Splanchnic outflow conveying sympathetic fibers to the lower body exits at the T8 region. Patients with lesions above T8 are prone to autonomic dysreflexia. They are subject to bouts of hypertension that may be heralded by dizziness, sweating, and headaches. A plugged catheter is the most common precipitating cause of dysreflexia. The catheter should be carefully checked and the bladder irrigated. Other frequent causes of dysreflexia include calculi or infections in any portion of the urinary system, fecal impaction, and pressure sores. If the patient's blood pressure does not lower in response to treatment of the causative agent, management with antihypertensive medication is begun.

▶ Recovery

The *International Standards for Neurological and Functional Classification of Spinal Cord Injury,* published by the American Spinal Injury Association (ASIA) and the International Medical Society of Paraplegia (IMSOP), represent the most reliable instrument for assessing neurologic status in SCI. These standards provide a quantitative measure of sensory and motor function.

Neurologic recovery is assessed by determining the change in ASIA Motor Score (AMS) between successive neurologic examinations. The AMS is the sum of strength grades for each of the 10 key muscles tested bilaterally that represent neurologic segments from C5 to T1 and L2 to S1. In a neurologically intact individual, the total possible AMS is 100 points.

The most important prognostic indicator of recovery is completeness of injury using the sacral-sparing definition. Using completeness and level of injury (tetraplegia or paraplegia), patients are divided into four groups: complete tetraplegia, incomplete tetraplegia, complete paraplegia, and incomplete paraplegia. The rate of motor recovery in all groups declines rapidly in the first 6 months following injury with minimal further changes after this time (Figure 12–10).

A. Complete Paraplegia

Patients with paraplegia that remains complete 1 month after injury have a 96% chance of remaining complete. Thirty-eight percent of those with injuries at or below T9 recover some lower extremity function. No patients with a neurologic level above T9 regain volitional lower extremity motor function. Only 5% of muscles with a strength of 0/5 at 1 month recover to 3/5 or greater strength 1 year after injury. Furthermore, only 5% of individuals become independent community ambulators at 1 year.

B. Incomplete Paraplegia

Motor recovery is better in individuals with incomplete injuries. Between 1 month and 1 year after injury, the AMS increases by an average of 12 points regardless of the level

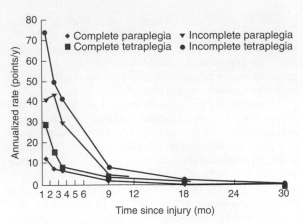

▲ **Figure 12–10.** Recovery rates of ASIA Motor Score for persons with incomplete and complete paraplegia and tetraplegia. (Reproduced, with permission, from Waters RL, Adkins R, Yakura J, Sie I: Functional and neurological recovery following acute SCI. *J Spinal Cord Med* 1998;21:195.)

of injury. Additionally, these patients have a 76% chance of becoming community ambulators.

C. Complete Tetraplegia

Ninety percent of individuals with complete tetraplegia 1 month after injury remain complete. Among the 10% who undergo late conversion to incomplete status, lower extremity motor recovery is minimal and inadequate for ambulation. Recovery of AMS points is independent of neurologic level. Waters and colleagues reported that with the exception of the triceps muscle, all upper extremity muscles with a grade of at least 1/5 1 month after injury recover to at least 3/5 1 year after injury.

D. Incomplete Tetraplegia

In patients with incomplete tetraplegia, motor recovery of upper and lower extremity muscles occurs concurrently. Nearly all muscles with at least 1/5 strength 1 month after injury recover to at least 3/5 1 year after injury. Forty-six percent of the patients examined by Waters and colleagues attained independent community ambulation status 1 year after injury. The number of individuals with incomplete tetraplegia who can attain independent community ambulation is less than for individuals with incomplete paraplegia and comparable lower extremity function. This is because upper extremity function may be insufficient to allow crutch-assisted ambulation in the former group, whereas those with incomplete paraplegia have normal upper extremity strength. Regaining hand and arm function is a high priority for those with tetraplegia, and this requires adequate shoulder ROM and strength. Patients do better when they participate in a rehabilitation program focused on shoulder stretching and strengthening as well as training in optimizing

Table 12–2. Community ambulators at 1 year postinjury.

ASIA Lower Extremity Motor Score[a] (at 30 days postinjury)	Complete Paraplegia (%)	Incomplete Paraplegia (%)	Incomplete Tetraplegia (%)
0	<1	33	0
1–9	45	70	2
10–19		100	63
20 or greater		100	100
Total	5	76	46

[a]Score based on five key muscles.
Total possible 50 points for both lower extremities for normals.
Reprinted, with permission, from Waters RL, Adkins R, Yakura J, et al: Functional and neurological recovery following acute SCI. *J Spinal Cord Med* 1998;21:195.

transfers, raises from a sitting position, and wheelchair propulsion.

Taken as a whole, a minority of individuals with SCI can ambulate independently after injury. The proportion of patients who can ambulate does, however, vary with the level and completeness of the injury. The lower extremity motor score (LEMS), which is the sum of the strength grades of the bilateral key lower extremity muscles, can be used to predict successful ambulation (Table 12–2). The motor groups are as follows: L2, hip flexors (iliopsoas); L3, knee extensors (quadriceps); L4, ankle dorsiflexors (tibialis anterior); L5, long toe extensors (extensor hallucis longus); and S1, ankle plantarflexors (gastrocnemius, soleus). In an individual with no deficit, the total possible LEMS is 50 points. The LEMS at 30 days is used to predict the chance of successful ambulation in incomplete tetraplegics, incomplete paraplegics, and complete paraplegics. All individuals with an LEMS of at least 20 and an incomplete injury are expected to be community ambulators 1 year after injury.

American Spinal Injury Association, International Medical Society of Paraplegia: *International Standards for Neurological Classification of Spinal Cord Injury* (revised). Atlanta, GA: American Spinal Injury Association; 2000.

Bracken MB: Methylprednisolone and acute spinal cord injury: an update of the randomized evidence. *Spine* 2001;26(Suppl 24):S47. [PMID: 11805609]

Bracken MB, Holford TR: Neurological and functional status 1 year after acute spinal cord injury: estimates of functional recovery in National Acute Spinal Cord Injury Study II from results modeled in National Acute Spinal Cord Injury Study III. *J Neurosurg Spine* 2002;96:259. [PMID: 11990832]

Burns AS, Ditunno JF: Establishing prognosis and maximizing functional outcomes after spinal cord injury: a review of current and future directions in rehabilitation management. *Spine* 2001;26:S137. [PMID: 11805621]

Hosalkar H, Pandya NK, Hsu J, Keenan MA: What's new in orthopaedic rehabilitation. *J Bone Joint Surg Am* 2011;93-A(14):1367. [PMID: 21792505]

Ito Y, Sugimoto Y, Tomioka M, Kai N, Tamaka M: Does high dose methylprednisone sodium succinate really improve neurological recovery in patients with acute spinal cord injury? A prospective study of neurological recovery and early complications. *Spine* 2009;34:2121. [PMID: 19713878]

Keith MW, Hoyen H: Indications and future directions for upper limb neuroprostheses in tetraplegic patients: a review. *Hand Clin* 2002;18:519, viii. [PMID: 12474601]

Kirshblum SC, O'Connor KC: Levels of spinal cord injury and predictors of neurologic recovery. *Phys Med Rehabil Clin North Am* 2000;11:1, vii. [PMID: 10680155]

Kozin SH, D'Addesi L, Chafetz RS, Answorth S, Mulcahey MJ: Biceps-to-triceps transfer for elbow extension in persons with tetraplegia. *J Hand Surg Am* 2010;35:968. [PMID: 20513578]

Lee TT, Green BA: Advances in the management of acute spinal cord injury. *Orthop Clin North Am* 2002;33:311. [PMID: 12389277]

Little JW, Burns S, James J, et al: Neurologic recovery and neurologic decline after spinal cord injury. *Phys Med Rehabil Clin North Am* 2000;11:73. [PMID: 10680159]

Macciocchi SN, Bowman B, Coker J, et al: Effect of co-morbid traumatic brain injury on functional outcome of persons with spinal cord injuries. *Am J Phys Med Rehabil* 2004;83:22. [PMID: 14709971]

McKinley WO, Seel RT, Gadi RK, et al: Nontraumatic vs. traumatic spinal cord injury: a rehabilitation outcome comparison. *Am J Phys Med Rehabil* 2001;80:693. [PMID: 11523972]

Mulroy SJ, Thompson L, Kemp B, et al: Physical Therapy Clinical Research Network (PTClinResNet). Strengthening and optimal movements for painful shoulders (STOMPS) in chronic spinal cord injury: a randomized controlled trial. *Phys Ther* 2011;91:305. [PMID: 21292803]

Nockels RP: Nonoperative management of acute spinal cord injury. *Spine* 2001;26(24 Suppl):S31. [PMID: 11805606]

Pollard ME, Apple DF: Factors associated with improved neurologic outcomes in patients with incomplete tetraplegia. *Spine* 2003;28:33. [PMID: 12544952]

Salisbury SK, Choy NL, Nitz J: Shoulder pain, range of motion, and functional motor skills after acute tetraplegia. *Arch Phys Med Rehabil* 2003;84:1480. [PMID: 14586915]

Van der Putten JJ, Stevenson VL, Playford ED, et al: Factors affecting functional outcome in patients with nontraumatic spinal cord lesions after inpatient rehabilitation. *Neurorehabil Neural Repair* 2001;15:99. [PMID: 11811258]

von Wild KR: New development of functional neurorehabilitation in neurosurgery. *Acta Neurochir Suppl (Wien)* 2003;87:43. [PMID: 14518522]

Waters RL, Sie IH: Spinal cord injuries from gunshot wounds to the spine. *Clin Orthop* 2003;408:120. [PMID: 12616048]

STROKE

Stroke (cerebrovascular accident or brain attack) occurs when thrombosis, embolism, or hemorrhage interrupts cerebral oxygenation and causes the death of neurons in the brain. This leads to deficits in cognition and in motor and sensory function.

In the United States, where cerebrovascular accidents are the leading cause of hemiplegia in adults and the third leading cause of death, 2 million people have permanent neurologic deficits from stroke. The annual incidence of stroke is 1 in 1000, with cerebral thrombosis causing nearly three fourths of the cases. More than half of stroke victims survive and have an average life expectancy of approximately 6 years. Most survivors have the potential for significant function and useful lives if they receive the benefits of rehabilitation.

▶ Neurologic Impairment and Recovery

Infarction of the cerebral cortex in the region of the brain supplied by the middle cerebral artery (MCA) or one of its branches is most commonly responsible for stroke. It supplies the area of the cerebral cortex responsible for hand function; the anterior cerebral artery supplies the area responsible for lower extremity motion (Figure 12–11). The typical clinical picture following MCA stroke is contralateral hemianesthesia (decreased sensation), homonymous hemianopia (visual field deficit), and spastic hemiplegia with more paralysis in the upper extremity than in the lower extremity. Because hand function requires relatively precise motor control, even for activities with assistive equipment, the prognosis for the functional use of the hand and arm is considerably worse than for the leg. Return of even gross motor control in the lower extremity may be sufficient for walking.

Infarction in the region of the anterior cerebral artery causes paralysis and sensory loss of the opposite lower limb and, to a lesser degree, the arm.

Patients who have cerebral arteriosclerosis and suffer repeated bilateral infarctions are likely to have severe cognitive impairment that limits their general ability to function even when motor function is good.

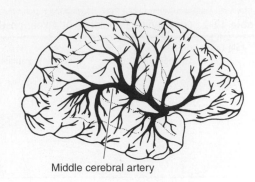

Middle cerebral artery

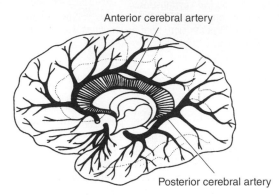

Anterior cerebral artery

Posterior cerebral artery

▲ **Figure 12–11.** Cerebral artery circulation.

After stroke, motor recovery follows a fairly typical pattern. The size of the lesion and the amount of collateral circulation determine the amount of permanent damage. Most recovery occurs within 6 months, although functional improvement may continue as the patient receives further sensorimotor reeducation and learns to cope with disability.

Initially after a stroke, the limbs are completely flaccid. Over the next few weeks, muscle tone and spasticity gradually increase in the adductor muscles of the shoulder and in the flexor muscles of the elbow, wrist, and fingers. Spasticity also develops in the lower extremity muscles. Most commonly, there is an extensor pattern of spasticity in the leg, characterized by hip adduction, knee extension, and equinovarus deformities of the foot and ankle (Figure 12–12). In some cases, however, a flexion pattern of spasticity occurs, characterized by hip and knee flexion.

Whether the patient recovers the ability to move one joint independently of the others (selective movement) depends on the extent of the cerebral cortical damage. Dependence on the more neurologically primitive patterned movement (synergy) decreases as selective control improves. The extent to which motor impairment restricts function varies in the upper and lower extremities. Patterned movement is not functional in the upper extremity, but it may be useful in the lower extremity, where the patient uses the flexion synergy

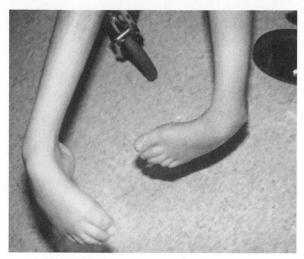

▲ **Figure 12–12.** Equinovarus deformities of the feet in a patient with spasticity.

to advance the limb forward and the mass extension synergy for limb stability during standing.

The final processes in sensory perception occur in the cerebral cortex, where basic sensory information is integrated to complex sensory phenomena such as vision, proprioception, and perception of spatial relationships, shape, and texture. Patients with severe parietal dysfunction and sensory loss may lack sufficient perception of space and awareness of the involved segment of their body to ambulate. Patients with severe perceptual loss may lack balance to sit, stand, or walk. A visual field deficit further interferes with limb use and may cause patients to be unaware of their own limbs.

▶ Management

A. Acute Management

Medical intervention in the treatment of a stroke is most effective when initiated within 3 hours from the onset of symptoms. However, pharmacologic intervention may play a role, although limited, if administered within 24 hours of onset.

1. Thrombolytics

A. TISSUE PLASMINOGEN ACTIVATOR (T-PA) (ALSO KNOWN AS RECOMBINANT T-PA OR RECOMBINANT TISSUE-TYPE PLASMINOGEN ACTIVATOR [RT-PA])—The efficacy of intravenous t-PA was established in two randomized, double-blind, placebo-controlled studies published in combination by the National Institute of Neurological Disorders and Stroke (NINDS). At 3 months after stroke, approximately 12% more patients in the t-PA group experienced a cure of symptoms relative to those who did not receive it. The risk of intracerebral hemorrhage in the t-PA group was 6% (50% of which were fatal), compared to 0.6% in the placebo group.

Despite the differences in hemorrhage rates, there were no differences in mortality (17% in the t-PA group versus 21% in the placebo group).

Key points about the administration of thrombolytic agents include the following:

1. They must be administered within 3 hours of symptom onset. The time of onset in patients who wake up with symptoms or those who cannot describe accurately the time of their symptom onset is when they were last known to be well.

2. An imaging study of the head (CT scan or magnetic resonance imaging [MRI]) must be performed prior to treatment to rule out hemorrhage as a cause of symptoms.

3. Blood pressure should be lower than 185 systolic and 110 diastolic. Agents such as labetalol may be used to lower the blood pressure for the purposes of treatment.

4. Blood must be tested for platelet count (should be >100,000), international normalized ratio (INR) (many recommend it be <1.6), partial thromboplastin time (PTT) (many recommend <40), and glucose (should be 50–400). INR has particular relevance because individuals properly treated with warfarin to diminish the incidence of stroke (eg, those with atrial fibrillation) may not be candidates for thrombolytic treatments.

B. PROUROKINASE (ALSO KNOWN AS RECOMBINANT PROUROKINASE, OR R-PRO-UK)—This intraarterial therapy requires the involvement of a skilled interventionist. The time window is 6 hours from symptom onset. In addition, and in contrast to the NINDS t-PA study, patients with a CT scan showing over a third involvement of the MCA territory as seen on CT scan are not eligible for treatment. The absolute percentage increase in patients with slight or no disability at 3 months was 15% in the prourokinase group compared with the placebo group. The hemorrhage rate in the prourokinase group was 10% versus 2% in subjects who received placebo. No difference was noted, however, in mortality (25% in the prourokinase group versus 27% in the placebo group).

This therapy may be especially useful for patients who arrive later than 3 hours from symptom onset and who have less than a third involvement of the MCA territory on initial scan.

2. Antiplatelet agents

A. ASPIRIN—The Chinese Acute Stroke Trial (CAST) and the International Stroke Trial (IST) are two large studies evaluating the use of aspirin (160–300 mg/day) within 48 hours of ischemic stroke symptom onset. Compared to no treatment, there was approximately a 1% absolute reduction in stroke and death in the first few weeks. At further time points (eg, 6 months), there was a similar absolute reduction of approximately 1% in death or dependence.

B. **Abciximab**—An ongoing phase III study of the efficacy of abciximab (ReoPro) in acute stroke is being conducted. A phase II study of 400 patients found an 8% absolute reduction in poor outcomes at 3 months ($P < 0.05$). Symptomatic intracranial hemorrhage occurred in 3.6% of patients on abciximab and in 1.0% of patients on placebo.

3. Anticoagulants

A. **Warfarin**—No studies have evaluated use of warfarin for the acute treatment of stroke.

B. **Heparin and heparinoids**—At this time, only one randomized trial showed benefit for heparins or heparinoids in acute ischemic stroke. In that study, no benefit was seen at 10 days or 3 months, only at 6 months. Other large studies failed to find benefit of heparin or heparinoids, either intravenous or subcutaneous, at 3 months. An exploratory post hoc analysis of one intravenous low-molecular-weight heparin randomized study suggested benefit in patients with severe large vessel (eg, carotid) atherosclerosis; however, the authors conclude that these findings need to be properly evaluated in a prospective randomized trial.

B. Lower Extremities

1. Hemiplegia—To walk independently, the hemiplegic patient requires intact balance reactions, hip flexion to advance the limb, and stability of the limb for standing. If a patient meets these criteria and has acceptable cognition, the clinician can restore ambulation in most cases by prescribing an appropriate lower extremity orthosis and an upper extremity assistive device such as a cane. Orthopedic surgery to rebalance the muscle forces in the leg can greatly enhance ambulation.

Except for the correction of severe contractures in non-ambulatory patients, surgical procedures should be delayed for at least 6 months to allow spontaneous neurologic recovery to occur and the patient to learn how to cope with the disability. After this time, surgery may safely be performed to improve usage in the functional limb.

In the nonfunctional limb, surgery may be performed to relieve pain or correct severe hip and knee flexion contractures caused by spasticity. Most severe contractural deformities in the nonfunctional limb, however, are the result of an ineffective program of daily passive ROM, splinting, and limb positioning.

Most hemiplegics with motor impairment have hip abductor and extensor weakness. A quad cane (cane with four feet to provide more stability) or a hemiwalker is prescribed to provide better balance. Because of paralysis in the upper extremity, the hemiplegic patient is unable to use a conventional walker.

2. Limb scissoring—Scissoring of the legs caused by overactive hip adductor muscles is a common problem. This gives the patient an extremely narrow base of support while standing and causes balance problems. When no fixed contracture

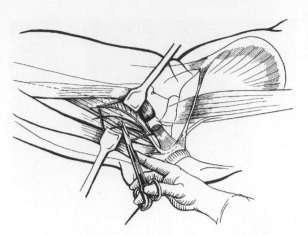

▲ **Figure 12–13.** Release of the hip adductor tendons and neurectomy of the anterior branches of the obturator nerve to correct the problem of limb scissoring. (Illustration by Anthony C. Berlet. Reproduced, with permission, from Keenan MAE, Kozin SH, Berlet AC: *Manual of Orthopaedic Surgery for Spasticity.* Philadelphia, PA: Raven; 1993.)

of the hip adductor muscles is present, transection of the anterior branches of the obturator nerve denervates the adductors and allows the patient to stand with a broader base of support. If a contracture of the adductors occurs, surgical release of the adductor longus, adductor brevis, and gracilis muscles should be performed (Figure 12–13).

3. Stiff-knee gait—Patients with a stiff-knee gait are unable to flex the knee during the swing phase of gait. The deformity is a dynamic one, meaning that it only occurs during walking. Passive knee motion is not restricted, and the patient does not have difficulty sitting. Usually the knee is maintained in extension throughout the gait cycle. Toe drag, which is likely in the early swing phase, may cause the patient to trip. Thus, balance and stability are also affected. The limb seems to be longer than the other side, but this is only functional. Circumduction of the involved limb, hiking of the pelvis, or contralateral limb vaulting may occur as compensatory maneuvers.

A gait study with dynamic electromyography (EMG) should be done preoperatively to document the activity of the individual muscles of the quadriceps. Dyssynergic activity is commonly seen in the rectus femoris from pre-swing through terminal swing throughout the gait cycle. Abnormal activity is also common in the vastus intermedius, vastus medialis, and vastus lateralis muscles. If knee flexion is improved with a block of the femoral nerve or with botulinum toxin injection of the quadriceps, the rationale for surgical intervention is strengthened. Any equinus deformity of the foot should be corrected prior to evaluation of a stiff-knee gait because equinus causes a knee extension force during stance. Because the amount of knee flexion

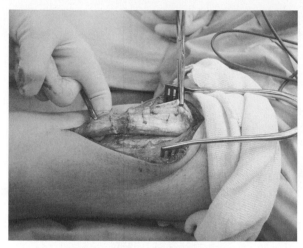

▲ **Figure 12–14.** Selective lengthening of the rectus femoris tendon to correct a stiff-knee gait abnormality.

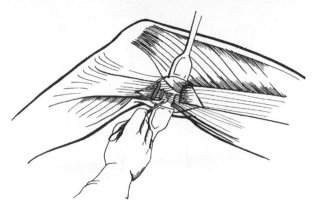

▲ **Figure 12–15.** Distal release of the hamstring tendons to correct a knee flexion contracture. (Illustration by Anthony C. Berlet. Reproduced, with permission, from Keenan MAE, Kozin SH, Berlet AC: *Manual of Orthopaedic Surgery for Spasticity.* Philadelphia, PA: Raven; 1993.)

during swing is directly related to the speed of walking, the patient should be able to ambulate with a reasonable velocity to benefit from surgery. Hip flexion strength is also needed for a good result because the forward momentum of the leg normally provides the inertial force to flex the knee. In the past, a selective release of the rectus femoris or both the rectus femoris and vastus intermedius was done to remove their inhibiting knee flexion. On average, a 15-degree improvement in peak knee flexion is seen after surgery. Transfer of the rectus femoris to a hamstring tendon not only removes it as a deforming muscle force, it also converts the rectus into a corrective flexion force. This procedure provides improved knee flexion over selective release. When any of the vasti muscles are involved, they can be selectively lengthened at their myotendinous junction (Figure 12–14), and knee flexion improves.

4. Knee flexion deformity—A knee flexion deformity increases the physical demand on the quadriceps muscle, which must continually fire to hold the patient upright. Knee flexion often leads to knee instability and causes falls. It is most often caused by spasticity of the hamstring muscles. A KAFO can be used to hold the knee in extension on a temporary basis as a training aid in physical therapy. Such an orthosis, however, is difficult for the stroke patient to don and wear for permanent usage.

Surgical correction of the knee flexion deformity is the most desirable treatment. Hamstring tenotomy (Figure 12–15) eliminates the dynamic component of the deformity and generally results in a 50% correction of the contracture at the time of surgery. The residual joint contracture is then corrected by serial casting done weekly after surgery. Hamstring function posterior to the knee joint is not necessary for ambulation. In fact, ambulation may only be feasible in patients with knee flexion deformities of greater than 30 degrees if a hamstring release is done.

5. Equinus or equinovarus foot deformity—Surgical correction of an equinus deformity is indicated when the foot cannot be maintained in the neutral position with the heel in firm contact with the sole of the shoe in a well-fitted, rigid AFO. Despite a wide variety of surgical methods designed to decrease the triceps surae spasticity, none is more effective than Achilles tendon lengthening. In this procedure, triple hemisection tenotomy is performed via three stab incisions, with the most distal cut based medially to alleviate varus pull of the soleus muscle (Figure 12–16).

An anesthetic block of the posterior tibial nerve can be a valuable tool in preoperative assessment of the patient with equinus deformity because it demonstrates the potential benefits of Achilles tendon lengthening if the deformity is a result of increased muscle tone.

Surgical release of the flexor digitorum longus and brevis tendons at the base of each toe (Figure 12–17) is done prophylactically at the time of Achilles tendon lengthening because increased ankle dorsiflexion following heel cord tenotomy increases tension on the long toe flexor and commonly leads to excessive toe flexion (toe curling). The flexor hallucis longus and flexor digitorum longus tendons can be transferred to the os calcis to provide additional support to the weakened calf muscles.

Surgical correction of varus deformity is indicated when the problem is not corrected by a well-fitted orthosis. It is also indicated to enable the patient to walk without an orthosis when varus deformity is the only significant problem. The tibialis anterior, tibialis posterior, extensor hallucis longus, flexor hallucis longus, flexor digitorum, and soleus pass medial to the axis of the subtalar joint and are potentially responsible for varus deformity. EMG studies demonstrate that the peroneus longus and peroneus brevis are generally inactive, and the tibialis posterior is also usually inactive or minimally active.

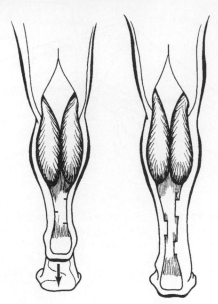

▲ **Figure 12–16.** Hoke triple hemisection Achilles tendon lengthening to correct an equinus foot deformity. (Illustration by Anthony C. Berlet. Reproduced, with permission, from Keenan MAE, Kozin SH, Berlet AC: *Manual of Orthopaedic Surgery for Spasticity*. Philadelphia, PA: Raven; 1993.)

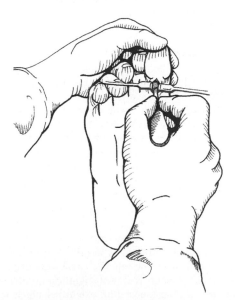

▲ **Figure 12–17.** Release of the flexor digitorum longus and brevis tendons to correct the problem of toe curling. (Illustration by Anthony C. Berlet. Reproduced, with permission, from Keenan MAE, Kozin SH, Berlet AC: *Manual of Orthopaedic Surgery for Spasticity*. Philadelphia, PA: Raven; 1993.)

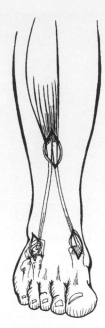

▲ **Figure 12–18.** Split anterior tibial tendon transfer to correct a spastic varus foot deformity. (Illustration by Anthony C. Berlet. Reproduced, with permission, from Keenan MAE, Kozin SH, Berlet AC: *Manual of Orthopaedic Surgery for Spasticity*. Philadelphia, PA: Raven; 1993.)

The tibialis anterior is the key muscle responsible for varus deformity, and in most patients, this can be confirmed by visual examination or palpation while the patient walks. A procedure known as the split anterior tibial tendon transfer (Figure 12–18) diverts the inverting deforming force of the tibialis anterior to a corrective force. In this procedure, half of the tendon is transferred laterally to the os cuboideum. When the extensor hallucis longus muscle is overactive, it can be transferred to the middorsum of the foot as well.

Treatment of equinovarus deformity consists of simultaneously performing the Achilles tendon lengthening procedure and the split anterior tibial tendon transfer. At surgery, the tibialis anterior is secured and held sufficiently taut to maintain the foot in a neutral position. After healing, 70% of patients are able to walk without an orthosis.

C. Upper Extremities

1. Spasticity—The first objective in treating the spastic upper extremity is to prevent contracture. Severe deformities at the shoulder, elbow, and wrist are seen in the neglected or noncompliant patient. Assistive equipment can be used to position the upper extremity, to aid in prevention of contractures, and to support the shoulder. Positioning extends spastic muscles but does not subject them to sudden postural changes that trigger the stretch reflex and aggravate spasticity. Brief periods should be scheduled when the upper extremity is not suspended and time can be devoted to ROM therapy and hygiene.

Most hemiplegics do not use their hand unless some selective motion is present at the fingers or thumb. Thumb opposition begins with opposition of the thumb to the side of the index finger (lateral or key pinch) and proceeds by circumduction to oppose each fingertip. In most stroke patients with selective thumb–finger extension, proximal muscle function is comparatively intact. Hence, orthotic stabilization of proximal joints is rarely necessary in the patient with a functional hand.

An overhead suspension sling attached to the wheelchair is used for patients with adductor or internal rotator spasticity of the shoulder. An alternative is an arm trough attached to the wheelchair.

It is usually not possible to maintain the wrist in neutral position with a WHO when wrist flexion spasticity is severe or when the wrist is flaccid. With minimal to moderate spasticity, either a volar or dorsal splint can be used. The splint should not extend to the fingers if the finger flexor spasticity is severe because slight motion and sensory contact of the fingers or palm may elicit the stretch reflex or grasp response, causing the fingers to jack-knife out of the splint.

2. Shoulder or arm pain—The hemiplegic shoulder deserves special attention because it is a common source of pain. A variety of different factors contribute to the painful shoulder: reflex sympathetic dystrophy, inferior subluxation, spasticity with internal rotation contracture, adhesive capsulitis, and degenerative changes about the shoulder. If early ROM exercises are performed and the extremity is properly positioned with a sling to reduce subluxation, severe or chronic pain at the shoulder can usually be prevented or minimized.

The classic clinical signs of reflex sympathetic dystrophy (swelling and skin changes) may not be apparent in the hemiplegic patient. If the patient complains that the arm is painful and no cause is apparent, a technetium bone scan assists in establishing the diagnosis (Figure 12–19).

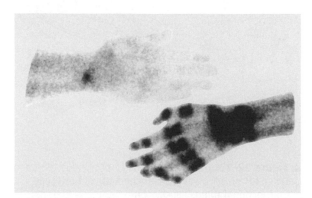

▲ **Figure 12–19.** Technetium bone scan showing the periarticular increase in activity characteristic of reflex sympathetic dystrophy.

Treatment should be instituted immediately, and the patient should be given positive psychological reinforcement. The use of narcotics must be avoided. Treatment options include the use of medications, such as corticosteroids, amitriptyline, or gabapentin (Neurontin), physical therapy, or nerve blocks (stellate ganglion blocks, brachial plexus blocks, or Bier IV regional blocks). Each of these techniques is successful with some patients; however, none is reliable for all patients.

3. Shoulder contracture—Contracture of the shoulder can cause pain, hygiene problems in the axilla, and difficulty in dressing and positioning. Shoulder adduction and internal rotation are caused by spasticity and myostatic contracture of four muscles: the pectoralis major, the subscapularis, the latissimus dorsi, and the teres major.

When the deformity is not fixed, lengthening of the pectoralis major, latissimus, and teres major at their myotendinous junction provides satisfactory correction of the deformity. In a nonfunctional extremity, surgical release of all four muscles (Figure 12–20) is usually necessary to resolve the deformity. Release of the subscapularis muscle is performed without violating the glenohumeral joint capsule. The joint capsule should not be opened because instability or intraarticular adhesions may result. A Z-plasty of the axilla may be needed if the skin is contracted. After the wound heals, an aggressive mobilization program is instituted. Gentle ROM exercises are employed to correct any remaining contracture. Careful positioning of the limb in abduction and external rotation is necessary for several months to prevent recurrence.

4. Elbow flexion contracture—Persistent spasticity of the elbow flexors causes a myostatic contracture and flexion deformity of the elbow. Frequent accompanying problems include skin maceration, breakdown of the antecubital space, and compression neuropathy of the ulnar nerve.

Surgical release of the contracted muscles and gradual extension of the elbow correct the deformity and decrease the ulnar nerve compression. The brachioradialis muscle and biceps tendon are transected. The brachialis muscle is fractionally lengthened at its myotendinous junction by transecting the tendinous fibers on the anterior surface of the muscle while leaving the underlying muscle intact (Figure 12–21). Complete release of the brachialis muscle is not performed unless a severe contracture was present for several years. An anterior capsulectomy is not needed and should be avoided because of the associated increased stiffness and intraarticular adhesions that occur postoperatively. Anterior transposition of the ulnar nerve may be necessary to further improve ulnar nerve function.

Approximately 50% correction of the deformity can be expected at surgery without causing excessive tension on the contracted neurovascular structures. Serial casts or dropout casts can be used to obtain further correction over the ensuing weeks.

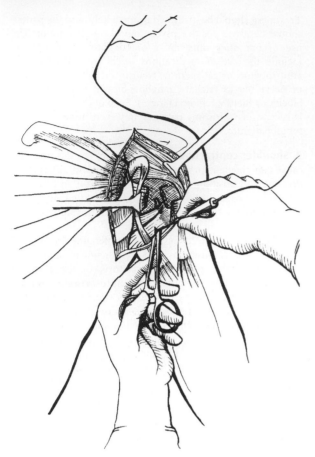

▲ **Figure 12–20.** Release of the pectoralis major, sub-scapularis, latissimus dorsi, and teres major to correct an internal rotation and adduction contracture of the shoulder. (Illustration by Anthony C. Berlet. Reproduced, with permission, from Keenan MAE, Kozin SH, Berlet AC: *Manual of Orthopaedic Surgery for Spasticity.* Philadelphia, PA: Raven; 1993.)

5. Clenched-fist deformity—A spastic clenched-fist deformity in a nonfunctional hand causes palmar skin breakdown and hygiene problems. Recurrent infections of the fingernail beds are also common.

Adequate flexor tendon lengthening to correct the deformity cannot be attained by fractional or myotendinous lengthening without causing discontinuity at the musculotendinous junction. Transection of the flexor tendons is not recommended because any remaining extensor muscle tone may result in an unopposed hyperextension deformity of the wrist and digits. The recommended procedure is a superficialis-to-profundus tendon transfer (Figure 12–22), which provides sufficient flexor tendon lengthening with preservation of a passive tether to prevent a hyperextension deformity. The wrist deformity is corrected by release of the wrist

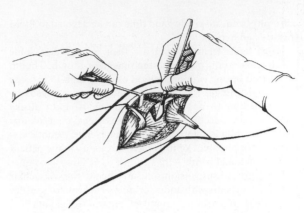

▲ **Figure 12–21.** Surgery of the brachioradialis muscle, biceps tendon, and brachialis muscle to correct an elbow flexion contracture in a nonfunctional arm. (Illustration by Anthony C. Berlet. Reproduced, with permission, from Keenan MAE, Kozin SH, Berlet AC: *Manual of Orthopaedic Surgery for Spasticity.* Philadelphia, PA: Raven; 1993.)

flexors. A wrist arthrodesis is done to maintain the hand in a neutral position and to eliminate the need for a permanent splint. Because intrinsic muscle spasticity is always present in conjunction with severe spasticity of the extrinsic flexors, a neurectomy of the motor branches of the ulnar nerve in the Guyon canal should be routinely performed along with the superficialis-to-profundus tendon transfer to prevent the postsurgical development of an intrinsic plus deformity.

After surgery, the wrist and digits are immobilized for 4 weeks in a short arm cast extended to the fingertips.

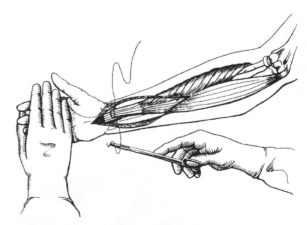

▲ **Figure 12–22.** The superficialis-to-profundus tendon transfer to correct a severe clenched-fist deformity in a nonfunctional hand. (Illustration by Anthony C. Berlet. Reproduced, with permission, from Keenan MAE, Kozin SH, Berlet AC: *Manual of Orthopaedic Surgery for Spasticity.* Philadelphia, PA: Raven; 1993.)

Botte MJ, Bruffey JD, Copp SN, et al: Surgical reconstruction of acquired spastic foot and ankle deformity. *Foot Ankle Clin* 2000; 5:381. [PMID: 11232236]

Fuller DA, Keenan MA, Esquenazi A, et al: The impact of instrumented gait analysis on surgical planning: treatment of spastic equinovarus deformity of the foot and ankle. *Foot Ankle Int* 2002;23:738. [PMID: 12199388]

Hansen AP, Marcussen NS, Klit H, Andersen G, Finnerup NB, Jensen TS: Pain following stroke: A prospective study. *Eur J Pain* 2012;16:1128. [PMID: 22407963]

Keenan MA: The management of spastic equinovarus deformity following stroke and head injury. *Foot Ankle Clin* 2011;16:499. [PMID: 21925364]

Massie CL, Fritz S, Malcolm MP: Elbow extension predicts motor impairment and performance after stroke. *Rehabil Res Pract* 2011;2011:381978. [PMID: 22110974]

Mayer NH: Choosing upper limb muscles for focal intervention after traumatic brain injury. *J Head Trauma Rehabil* 2004;19:119. [PMID: 15247823]

Namdari S, Horneff JG, Baldwin K, Keenan MA: Muscle releases to improve passive motion and relieve pain in patients with spastic hemiplegia and elbow flexion contractures. *J Shoulder Elbow Surg* 2012;21:1357. [PMID: 22217645]

Pollock A, Baer G, Pomeroy V, et al: Physiotherapy treatment approaches for the recovery of postural control and lower limb function following stroke. *Cochrane Database Syst Rev* 2003;2:CD001920. [PMID: 12804415]

Tilson JK, Wu SS, Cen SY, et al: Characterizing and identifying risk for falls in the LEAPS study: a randomized clinical trial of interventions to improve walking poststroke. *Stroke* 2012;43:446. [PMID: 22246687]

GERIATRIC ORTHOPEDICS

▶ General Principles

A major challenge facing society is the aging of the population. By 2020, 52 million Americans will be older than 65 years. By 2040, 68 million people will be older than 65 years. Both the absolute numbers and proportion of elderly people is increasing dramatically. People are living longer and have higher expectations for a good quality of life. Despite this trend, proportionally less disability occurs among the elderly now than in the past.

Although the passage of time, chronological age, is the convenient measure used, it is not necessarily the most precise marker of aging. A more sensitive marker would be to consider the person's functional age, but this is often difficult to define and measure. Age 65 is generally considered the beginning of old age. The young elderly are those individuals 65 to 75 years of age. These people are usually functionally intact. They have isolated orthopedic problems, such as mild osteoporosis, osteoarthrosis, overuse injuries (sports), and occasionally cancer.

The frail, very elderly are those persons older than 80 years. These people tend to have multiple musculoskeletal impairments such as advanced osteoporosis, generalized muscle weakness, multiple organ diseases, and dementia.

1. Disability

The leading causes of death in the elderly are heart disease, malignant neoplasms, and cerebrovascular disease. The overall leading causes of disability in the elderly are cancer, heart disease, dementia, and musculoskeletal disorders. The leading causes of disease-related disability before death are arthritis, hypertension, hearing impairment, heart disease, and orthopedic conditions. Despite the increasing incidence of disability with aging, only 5% of Americans live in nursing homes.

When evaluating the elderly, five functional domains of disability need to be considered:

1. *Physical ADLs* include activities such as bathing, dressing, eating, and walking.

2. *Instrumental ADLs* are home management tasks such as shopping, meal preparation, money management, using the telephone, and performing light housework.

3. *Cognitive functioning* is particularly important in the elderly. Dementia is one of the four leading causes of disability in the elderly and a principal reason for institutionalization.

4. *Affective function* is important. Secondary depressions are common in the elderly, and suicide is a more frequent cause of death in the elderly than in the young.

5. *Social functioning* is less of a problem. Only 1% of the elderly rate their social interactions as inadequate.

Disability in basic ADLs is common among community-dwelling older persons, with prevalence rates ranging from 7% in those 65–74 years of age to 24% in those 85 years of age or older. Restricted activity, defined as staying in bed for at least half a day and/or cutting down on usual activities because of an illness, injury, or other problem, is common among community-living older persons, regardless of risk for disability, and it is usually attributable to several concurrent health-related problems. Although disability in older persons is often thought to be progressive or permanent, previous research shows it is a dynamic process, with individuals moving in and out of states of disability. To set realistic goals and plan for appropriate care, disabled older persons, along with their families and clinicians, need accurate information about the likelihood and time course of recovery. Prevention of functional decline and disability includes not only management of acute episodes of disability and promotion of recovery, but also ongoing evaluation and management of key risk factors for disability and use of preventive interventions. The high likelihood of recurrent disability among older persons suggests that those who recently recovered from an episode of disability are an important target population for preventive interventions. Although some interventions designed to prevent recurrent disability may be disease specific (eg, anticoagulation after embolic stroke), others may be broadly applicable regardless of the specific precipitant of disability (eg, exercise-based programs).

2. Challenges for the Orthopedic Surgeon

When working with the elderly, the orthopedic surgeon becomes a member of a multidisciplinary team. The people making up this team include internists, geriatricians, rehabilitation specialists, psychiatrists, psychologists, social workers, nutritionists, skin care specialists, physical and occupational therapists, and the so-called young elderly children of the patient. Osteoporosis, fractures, arthritis, foot disorders, stroke, and amputations are the most frequent causes of musculoskeletal impairment.

3. Osteoporosis

Osteoporosis is an age-related disorder characterized by decreased bone mass and increased fracture risk in the absence of other recognizable causes of bone loss. Osteoporosis can occur either as a primary disorder or secondary to other diseases.

A. Primary Osteoporosis

Primary osteoporosis, the most common form of the disease, occurs in people from 51 to 65 years of age with a female-to-male ratio of 6:1. Primary osteoporosis can be further subdivided into two types. Type I, postmenopausal osteoporosis, results from decreased circulating levels of estrogen. It is seen in postmenopausal women and affects the majority of persons older than 70 years. Bone loss is rapid. There is swift trabecular bone loss up to 8% per year. Type I osteoporosis causes primarily trabecular bone loss with only 0.5% cortical bone loss per year. Fractures occur in locations of trabecular bone loss such as the distal radius and vertebrae. The cause of primary osteoporosis is a changing hormonal milieu.

Type II, senile osteoporosis, is a consequence of aging. It causes a more global bone loss affecting cortical and cancellous bone such as in the femoral neck. Type II osteoporosis is seen in persons older than 70 years. The female-to-male ratio is 2:1. The bone loss occurs in both the trabecular and cortical bone and averages 0.3–0.5% per year. Fractures occurring as the result of type II osteoporosis typically involve the hip, pelvis, humerus, tibia, and vertebral bodies. The causes of senile osteoporosis are those seen with aging and include calcium deficiency, decreased vitamin D, and increased parathormone activity.

B. Secondary Osteoporosis

Secondary osteoporosis results from a variety of causes. The most common are chronic or prolonged corticosteroid use and endocrine disorders. The endocrine disorders associated with osteoporosis are hyperthyroidism, hyperparathyroidism, diabetes, Cushing disease, and euplastic disorders.

▶ Prevention Strategies

Restoration of bone is difficult. It is therefore imperative to maximize peak bone mass during skeletal growth and then to maintain it during maturity. This requires adequate dietary calcium and vitamin D intake. The recommended amounts for adults are 1200 mg/day of calcium and 400 mg of vitamin D. For postmenopausal women, 1500 mg/day of calcium is recommended. Impact exercise is effective in maintaining bone mass. It is also important to avoid those factors that promote osteoporosis such as the use of tobacco products and excessive alcohol consumption.

▶ Diagnosis

Osteoporosis is a clinical diagnosis often made following a fracture. Radiographic findings include osteopenia (seen with >30% mineral loss); loss of horizontal trabeculae in vertebral bodies; thoracic wedge fractures; lumbar spine endplate fractures; stress fractures of the pelvis; and fractures of humerus, wrist, hip, supracondylar femur, and tibial plateau. Quantification of bone mass is done for confirmation and follow-up. Dual-energy x-ray absorptiometry (DEXA) is used to quantify bone mass. The following criteria for diagnosis are based on the DEXA scan:

> Normal: within 1 standard deviation (SD) of young adult reference
>
> Osteopenia: between 1.0 and 2.4 SDs below reference
>
> Osteoporosis: 2.5 or more SDs below reference
>
> Severe osteoporosis: 2.5 plus one or more fragility fractures

▶ Treatment

Weight-bearing exercise is useful in maintaining bone mass. Adequate daily calcium replacement is also helpful. Calcium and vitamin D alone do not prevent bone loss but may reduce the risk of hip fractures if given in combination. In late menopause (>6 years), calcium replacement does reduce bone loss.

Hormone therapy in postmenopausal women has been controversial. Current evidence supports the use of hormone therapy to prevent osteoporosis in women at high risk of fracture. Estrogen therapy has a more favorable benefit-risk profile for long-term use compared to estrogen-progestogen therapy, which has increased breast cancer risk.

Bisphosphonates, teriparatide, and denosumab have been shown to be effective in reducing the risk of fragility fractures. While there are few robust long-term studies of their use, these osteoporosis treatments are safe (with the possible exception of atypical subtrochanteric fractures associated with long-term bisphosphonates) and generally maintain bone mineral density over time.

Bisphosphonates are a class of compounds similar to pyrophosphate that are readily adsorbed by bone mineral surfaces. Once bound, they inhibit the bone absorption activity of osteoclasts. Bisphosphonates currently available for clinical use include alendronate sodium (Fosamax) and risedronate sodium (Actonel). Teriparatide (Forteo) is a recombinant form of parathyroid hormone, a primary regulator of calcium and phosphate metabolism in bone and kidney. Intermittent exposure to parathyroid hormone activates osteoblasts more than osteoclasts, and once-daily injection injections of teriparatide are thought to have a net effect of stimulating new bone formation leading to increased bone mineral density. Denosumab (Prolia) is a human monoclonal antibody that targets RANKL, a protein that acts as the primary signal to promote bone removal. Raloxifene (Evista) is a selective estrogen receptor modulator that has estrogenic effects on bone and thus is used in prevention of osteoporosis in women.

▶ Exercise

The ability to walk safely is vital for independent living. Both strength and endurance determine the capacity for independent movement. Muscle strength is associated with the capacity to perform ADLs. A reduction in strength with age is attributed to these factors:

1. A loss of muscle mass because of smaller and fewer fibers
2. A loss of motor neurons (anterior horn cells)
3. Changes in muscle architecture
4. A defect in the excitation-contraction mechanism
5. Psychosocial changes leading to reduced capacity to activate motor units

Strength training can lead to major functional improvements in the elderly. The plasticity of the motor system to adapt to a training load appears to be maintained into the 10th decade of life. Strength training has no effect on the central determinants of aerobic capacity such as maximum heart rate, blood pressure, hemoglobin concentration, and blood volume.

Aerobic exercise does lead to increased endurance and functional capacity. Endurance is the time a person can maintain either a static force or a power level involving a combination of concentric or eccentric muscular contractions. The stress that exercise imposes on a person and the tolerance or endurance for that exercise intensity depends on how much energy is needed to perform the task in relation to the person's maximal capacity. With training, activities become easier to perform. The person has increased endurance for submaximal exercise. Improvements in movement can lower the energy cost of an activity.

4. Arthritis

Osteoarthritis is very prevalent in the elderly. Total joint arthroplasty has dramatically improved the mobility and quality of life for the elderly. A variety of studies confirm the appropriateness and effectiveness of both total hip and total knee arthroplasty in the elderly with low complication rates. The elderly patient is more likely to require the use of an upper extremity assistive device for ambulation following joint replacement.

5. Fractures

A. General Considerations

One of the most compelling reasons to determine the etiology of a fracture and provide appropriate treatment is that a previous low-energy fracture is one of the strongest risk factors for new fractures. Specifically, patients with a low-energy fracture of the wrist, hip, proximal humerus, or ankle have nearly a two- to fourfold greater risk for future fractures than individuals who have never experienced a fracture. Furthermore, up to half of patients with a prior vertebral fracture experience additional vertebral fractures within 3 years, many within the first year. Indeed, compared to individuals with no history of fracture, a patient with a prior vertebral fracture has nearly a fivefold increased risk of future vertebral fractures and up to a sixfold increased risk of hip and other nonvertebral fractures. Taken together, these data indicate that patients with a history of any type of prior fracture have a two- to sixfold increased risk of subsequent fractures compared to those without a previous fracture.

These findings emphasize that optimal care of fragility fracture patients includes not only management of the presenting fracture, but also evaluation, diagnosis, and treatment of the underlying cause(s) of the fracture, including low bone density or other medical conditions. In this regard, supplementation with calcium and vitamin D lowers fracture risk in the elderly. In addition, several pharmacologic agents reduce the risk of future fracture by as much as 50% in patients with existing fractures. Nonpharmacologic interventions, such as fall prevention programs and individually tailored exercise programs, reduce falls among the elderly, which may decrease the incidence of fractures. In addition, trochanteric padding dramatically reduces hip fractures among those at highest risk. Thus, initiating interventions soon after a fragility fracture occurs may significantly reduce the incidence and severity of subsequent fractures.

In the elderly, fractures result from low-energy injuries. Falls in the home most frequently result in fractures of the hip, distal radius, pelvis, proximal humerus, and ribs. Approximately 90% of fractures of the pelvis, hip, and forearm result from a fall. Only 3–5% of falls result in fractures.

Many of the risk factors for fracture are also risk factors for falls. Risk factors can be divided into categories. Risk factors associated with aspects of aging include primary osteoporosis, impaired vision or balance, gait abnormalities, and loss of muscle and fat padding the bones. Environmental risk factors consist of uneven surfaces; slippery surfaces; obstacles such as throw rugs, pets, and steps; poor lighting; and lack of railings or other supports for balance. Fall prevention programs include home safety measures such as the installation of safety bars in the bathtub and shower, elimination of heavily waxed floors and slippery rugs, and the use of rubber sole shoes with low wide heels that provide more stability.

Genetic factors are seen in both gender and race. Women sustain more fractures than men. Whites have more fractures than African Americans. Illnesses commonly associated with fractures include stroke, syncope, hypotension, secondary osteoporosis, Parkinson disease, dementia, and paraparesis. The use of medications such as benzodiazepines, tricyclic antidepressants, antipsychotics, corticosteroids, and barbiturates is connected with fractures. Lifestyle factors include exercise, nutrition, alcohol or other substance abuse, immobilization, and shoe style.

Other factors contribute to the risk of traumatic fractures occurring in falls. The first is the orientation of the fall. A fall that happens while standing still or walking very slowly imparts little or no forward momentum, so the point of impact is near the hip. Gait velocity slows with aging, putting the hip more at risk of injury in a fall. Protective responses during a fall decrease with age. Local shock absorbers, muscle and fat, that surround the bone decrease with age. Bone strength is less secondary to the osteoporosis associated with aging.

B. Hip Fractures

Fractures of the hip are classified by location and severity. The basic considerations are whether the fracture occurs in the intracapsular or extracapsular area and the stability of the fracture pattern. Intracapsular fractures occur along the neck of the femur. When they are displaced, the blood supply to the femoral head is likely disrupted, which increases the possibility of osteonecrosis.

Treatment of hip fractures is operative whenever possible because nonoperative treatments involve months of bed rest and sometimes traction. It requires excellent nursing care to avoid decubitus ulcers and respiratory dysfunction. Fracture malunion, limb-length inequality, pain, and higher mortality rates are common with nonoperative care. The chances for eventual ambulation are only 55% compared with 76% for patients treated operatively. Nonoperative treatment of hip fractures is very occasionally chosen for patients at high medical risk and is also sometimes recommended for demented nonambulatory patients.

The basic principles of treatment of hip fractures are well established. Nondisplaced fractures of the femoral neck are usually treated with multiple pins or screws. Displaced fractures of the femoral neck are usually treated with a hemiarthroplasty because of the high incidence of avascular necrosis. Stable intertrochanteric fractures are generally treated with a sliding screw and either a side plate or intramedullary rod. Unstable intertrochanteric fractures may require additional measures to gain adequate medial support. In very osteoporotic bone, it may be necessary to add methyl methacrylate bone cement to gain sufficient fixation and stability. A patient with prior hip arthritis may be treated with a total hip arthroplasty.

The postoperative rehabilitation of the elderly patient is critical to a successful outcome. Non–weight-bearing ambulation is extremely difficult and more often impossible for elderly patients. Every effort should be made in the operative treatment to gain enough stability of the fracture to allow weight bearing as tolerated. The patient should be mobilized on the first or second day after surgery to prevent the many complications of immobility. Pain management is important to allow mobilization while minimizing oversedation. When a prosthesis has been placed, dislocation must be avoided. The elderly patient may not remember the precautions. Use of elevated chairs and toilet seats helps avoid the excessive hip flexion associated with posterior dislocation. A knee immobilizer splint while in bed prevents knee flexion that in turn results in flexion of the hip. It is sometimes prudent to place the patient in a hip brace, which limits flexion and adduction while soft-tissue healing occurs.

C. Fractures of the Pelvis

A common pelvic classification is based on whether or not the ring of the pelvis is disrupted because this indicates the amount of energy involved with the initial trauma. A fracture that does not disrupt the pelvic ring such as a pubic ramus fracture is a low-energy injury. Formerly, pelvic fractures were associated with high-energy trauma, were displaced, and occurred in patients less than 40 years old. With the aging of America, now more than 50% of fractures occur in those older than 60 years, with a preponderance occurring in women. The majority of pelvis fractures in the elderly are low-energy injuries and can be treated nonoperatively with analgesia and bed rest. Early mobilization is desirable to prevent the complications of immobility. Full weight bearing is allowed. A walker or other assistive device is useful to decrease pain and increase stability during walking. Stool softeners are often helpful. Fractures of the coccyx and sacrum are treated in a similar manner.

D. Fractures of the Distal Femur

The management of distal femur fractures in the elderly patients must be individualized. Advanced age in itself is not a contraindication to surgery. The objects of surgical treatment of the distal femur are anatomic reduction and stable fixation. In the presence of severe osteopenia, stable fixation is difficult. The addition of methyl methacrylate or long-stem knee replacement can help with stability. Occasionally, a postoperative cast brace is needed to supplement the internal fixation.

E. Fractures of the Forearm

Most fractures of the distal radius (Colles fracture) can be treated by closed reduction and casting. Significant loss of radial height and dorsal comminution can occur in osteoporotic bone even after lower energy injuries. In this situation, most surgeons would agree that external fixation and bone grafting of the fracture are warranted to obtain and maintain a more anatomic reduction. Early ROM exercises for both the shoulder and the fingers should be encouraged to avoid stiffness.

F. Fractures of the Proximal Humerus

Fractures of the proximal humerus account for 4–5% of all fractures and occur most commonly in the elderly. Humeral fractures in the elderly are minimally displaced 80% of the time. In these cases, sling immobilization is used to control pain. Pendulum exercises are begun within 2 weeks after injury to prevent excessive stiffness. Limited external rotation of the shoulder predisposes to a future spiral fracture of the humerus while dressing. Unstable, displaced fractures are best treated with open reduction and internal fixation, and those involving the humeral head and/or prone to avascular necrosis are best treated with hemiarthroplasty. In the frail elderly, a reverse total shoulder arthroplasty is also an option.

6. Stroke

As detailed earlier, stroke is a common cause of disability in the elderly.

7. Foot Disorders

The foot tends to widen with age as the transverse arch support weakens and abnormal bony alignments of the foot become common. Surgical reconstruction of foot deformities may be contraindicated in the frail elderly patient, particularly because of peripheral vascular disease. Nonoperative treatment consists of active and passive ROM exercises of the foot to maximize flexibility. Strengthening exercises of the lower extremity can be useful to improve the overall gait pattern. The patient should try to optimize body weight to eliminate excessive forces on the foot. Functional orthoses of a semirigid material with little or no posting may improve the foot position and provide symptomatic relief. Accommodative orthoses of a soft material may also be used. These soft orthoses are designed to control foot posture and eliminate areas of pressure, but they are not intended to correct the foot position. Orthoses are used in combination with soft extra-depth shoes that provide more clearance for deformities of the toes. Flat shoes are helpful for forefoot deformities because they prevent the foot sliding forward in the shoe. A shoe with a low heel is desirable for patients with a severe pronation deformity because the Achilles tendon is commonly tight. Placing the heel cord on stretch only increases the pronation forces on the foot.

8. Amputation

The majority of all amputations done in a civilian population are of the lower extremity. Most amputations are done in the sixth decade of life or later and are the result of vascular insufficiency. Posttraumatic amputations largely result from blunt trauma, with motor vehicle collisions and machinery accidents being the most common etiologies. Most are of the lower extremity, and about two thirds are amputations of one or more digits. In these patients, multiple limb amputation is an independent risk factor for death, whereas a single limb amputation is not.

The issues associated with amputation are discussed in Chapter 11.

Bamparas G, Inaba K, Tiexeria PG, et al: Epidemiology of post-traumatic limb amputation: a National Trauma Databank analysis. *Ann Surg* 2010;76:1214. [PMID: 21140687]

Cooper C, Reginster JY, Cortet B, et al: Long-term treatment of osteoporosis in postmenopausal women: a review for the European Society for Clinical and Economic Aspects of Osteoporosis and Osteoarthritis (ESCEO) and the International Osteoporosis Foundation (IOF). *Curr Med Res Opin* 2012;28:475. [PMID: 22356012]

Gill TM, Allore HG, Holford TR, et al: Hospitalization, restricted activity, and the development of disability among older persons. *JAMA* 2004;292:2115. [PMID: 15523072]

Hardy SE, Gill TM: Factors associated with recovery of independence among newly disabled older persons. *Arch Intern Med* 2005;165:106. [PMID: 15642885]

Horwitz DS, Kubiak EN: Surgical treatment of osteoporotic fractures about the knee. *Instr Course Lect* 2010;59:511. [PMID: 20415402]

Iwamoto J, Satrao Y, Takenda T, Matsumoto H: Efficacy of antiresorptive agents for preventing fractures in Japanese patients with an increased risk of fracture: review of the literature. *Drugs Aging* 2012;29:191. [PMID: 22372723]

Murad MH, Drake MT, Mullan RJ, et al: Comparative effectiveness of drug treatments to prevent early fragility fractures: a systematic review and network meta-analysis. *J Clin Endocrinol Metab* 2012;97:1871. [PMID: 22466336]

North American Menopause Society: The 2012 hormone therapy position of the North American Menopause Society. *Menopause* 2012;19:257. [PMID: 22367731]

Roux C, Wyman A, Hooven FH, et al: Burden of non-hip, nonvertebral fractures on quality of life in postmenopausal women: the Global Longitudinal Study of Osteoporosis in Women (GLOW). *Osteoporos Int* 2012;23:2863. [PMID: 22398855]

BRAIN INJURY

Brain injury resulting from trauma to the head is a leading cause of death and disability. Head injury is at least twice as common in males as in females and occurs most often in people 15–24 years of age. Approximately half of the injuries result from motor vehicle accidents. In the United States, 410,000 new cases of traumatic brain injury can be expected each year, with each case presenting a challenge to the team of health care providers involved in providing emergency treatment and long-term management.

▶ Neurologic Impairment and Recovery

The Glasgow Coma Score (Table 12–3) is frequently used to evaluate eye opening, motor response, and verbal response

Table 12–3. The Glasgow Coma Score.

Response	Description	Numerical Value
Eye opening	Spontaneous response	4
	Response to speech	3
	Response to pain	2
	No response	1
Motor response	Obeying response	6
	Localized response	5
	Withdrawal	4
	Abnormal flexion	3
	Extension	2
	No response	1
Verbal response	Oriented conversation	5
	Confused conversation	4
	Inappropriate words	3
	Incomprehensible sounds	2
	No response	1

Adapted, with permission, from: Teasdale G, Jennett B: Assessment of coma and impaired consciousness. A practical scale. *Lancet* 1974;2:81.

of patients with impaired consciousness. Analysis of scores from patients in several countries sheds light on the chances for survival and neurologic recovery. According to the data, approximately 50% of patients with impaired consciousness survived. Six months after injury, moderate or good neurologic recovery was seen in 82% of patients with initial (24-hour) Glasgow scores of 11 or higher, 68% of patients with initial scores of 8–10, 34% with initial scores of 5–7, and 7% with initial scores of 3 or 4. Age was an important factor related to neurologic outcome, with 62% of patients younger than 20 years and 46% of patients between 20 and 29 years of age showing moderate or good recovery.

The incidence of good recovery declines not only with advancing age but also with advancing duration of coma. Patients recovering from coma within the first 2 weeks of injury have a 70% chance of good recovery. The recovery rate drops to 39% in the third week and to 17% in the fourth week. Decerebrate or decorticate posturing indicates a brainstem injury and is indicative of a poor prognosis.

▶ Management

The rehabilitation process has three distinct phases: the acute injury period, the subacute period of neurologic recovery, and the residual period of functional adaptation. Health care workers from a variety of disciplines are involved in each phase.

A. Phases of Patient Care and Rehabilitation

1. Acute injury phase—The initial phase of rehabilitation begins as soon as the patient reaches the acute-care hospital.

Brain injury is frequently the result of a high-velocity accident. Diagnosis is problematic because multiple injuries are common, resuscitation and other lifesaving efforts make a complete examination difficult, and the patient who is comatose or disoriented cannot assist in the history or physical examination.

Under the circumstances, three important principles should be followed. The first is to make an accurate diagnosis based on a thorough examination. Fractures or dislocations are missed in 11% of patients, and peripheral nerve injuries are missed in 34%. The second is to assume that the patient will make a good neurologic recovery. Basic treatment principles should not be waived on the erroneous assumption that the patient will not survive. The third principle is to anticipate uncontrolled limb motion and lack of patient cooperation. The patient often goes through a period of agitation as neurologic recovery progresses. Traction and external fixation devices are best avoided for extremity injuries. Open reduction and internal fixation of fractures and dislocations diminishes complications, requires less nursing care, allows for earlier mobilization, and results in fewer residual deformities.

2. Subacute phase of neurologic recovery—During the subacute phase, when the patient is generally in a rehabilitation facility, spontaneous neurologic recovery occurs. During this recovery period, which may last from 12 to 18 months, spasticity is frequently present, and HO may develop. Management is aimed at preventing limb deformities, maintaining a functional arc of motion in the joints, and meeting both the physical and the psychological needs of the patient.

3. Residual phase or period of functional adaptation—When neurologic recovery reaches a plateau, the third phase of rehabilitation begins. Medical and surgical management is aimed at correction of residual limb deformities and excision of HO while specialists from various disciplines continue moving toward the goals planned for the individual patient.

B. The Team Approach to Patient Care and Rehabilitation

Members of the rehabilitation team are involved in setting short-term goals, which are meant to be accomplished by the time of discharge from the rehabilitation program, and long-term goals, which will take an extended period of time to achieve. The identification of needs and the setting of goals are performed independently by health care workers from each discipline. The team members then meet to discuss their goals and draw up a coordinated plan.

1. Medical management—General medical goals are usually straightforward. Because most patients with traumatic brain injuries are younger persons, chronic premorbid illnesses are uncommon. Prevention and treatment of infections are important goals, especially while shunts, tubes, and catheters are in place. If seizures are present, controlling them without causing sedation is vital.

In patients with decreased ROM in a joint, the cause of the problem should be explored. Possible causes include increased muscle tone, pain, myostatic contracture, periarticular HO, an undetected fracture or dislocation, and lack of patient cooperation secondary to diminished cognition. Peripheral nerve blocks with local anesthetics are useful in distinguishing between severe spasticity and fixed contractures.

Phenol blocks or botulinum toxin injections are used to decrease spasticity only during the period of potential neurologic recovery. The rationale for phenol injection is that by the time the nerve regenerates, the patient will have recovered more control of the affected muscle.

The technique for administering the phenol block depends on the anatomic accessibility and composition of the nerve; the direct injection of a peripheral nerve gives the most complete and long-lasting block. If a peripheral nerve has a large sensory component, however, direct injection is not recommended because loss of sensation is undesirable and some patients may develop painful hyperesthesia. In some cases, it is necessary to dissect surgically the individual motor branches of a nerve that runs to a muscle and inject each branch separately. In other cases, the motor points of the muscles can be localized using a needle electrode and nerve stimulator and then injected. Motor point injections do not completely relieve spasticity but can be helpful in reducing muscle tone. The duration of motor point blocks is approximately 2 months, and the blocks can be repeated as necessary.

Botulinum toxin is injected directly into the muscle belly. The onset of action is delayed but lasts for approximately 3 months. The injections can be repeated as needed and do not result in any scarring of the muscle. The limitation of botulinum toxin is the total dose tolerated at a given time and its high cost relative to phenol.

2. Nursing care—Nursing goals concentrate on basic bodily needs such as nutrition, hygiene, and handling of secretions. Removal of tubes at the earliest possible time is a desirable goal.

Tracheostomy tubes are commonly used in patients with brain injury. General principles of care include changing an uncuffed tube as soon as possible to prevent pressure necrosis of the trachea, adding mist if necessary to provide moisture to the artificial airway, establishing suctioning procedures to prevent trauma and infection, and eliminating the dressing once the tracheostomy incision is healed because the dressing can be a source of infection. The size of the tube is gradually reduced, and the tube is then plugged to tolerance. When continual plugging is tolerated for 3 consecutive days, the tube can be removed.

Feeding tubes are also commonly used. If oral feeding is not anticipated in the near future, a percutaneous endoscopic gastrostomy tube is recommended. If oral feeding is anticipated soon, a nasogastric tube is inserted, cleaned daily, and changed once a week. Instituting and carrying out an oral feeding program requires the combined efforts of the nursing and physical therapy staffs. Head and trunk control are necessary to provide alignment of swallowing structures. The presence of a cough reflex indicates some measure of laryngeal control and the ability to clear the airway. The presence of a swallowing reflex indicates inherent coordination of swallowing structures. The gag reflex, although protective, is not necessary for functional swallowing. Oral feeding should be started with thickened liquids and pureed foods, which provide more oral stimulus and allow time to initiate swallowing. Thin liquids are more easily aspirated.

The ability to inhibit voiding is generally a cognitive function. Restoring continence in the brain-injured patient requires a consistent routine with repeated instructions and positive feedback. Bowel programs should be initiated as soon as the patient begins taking nourishment via the gastrointestinal tract. Again, a consistent routine is most successful.

3. Cognitive and neuropsychological management—The return of cognitive abilities follows the same sequence of stages that normal cognitive development follows, with each new level of cognitive function stemming from the previous level. Table 12–4 shows the eight levels. Cognitive and behavioral management focuses on providing stimulation for patients with a level II or III response; providing structure for patients with a level IV, V, or VI response; and encouraging community activities for patients with a level VII or VIII response.

Memory loss and diminished cognitive function are frequently the most pervasive limitations to overall function. Cognitive retraining is an essential part of the rehabilitation process at every stage. As cognition increases and the patient becomes more aware of the injury, he or she also becomes increasingly aware of the possible consequences of the injury and requires counseling and psychological support.

Table 12–4. Cognitive function.

Level	Description
I	No response
II	Generalized response
III	Localized response
IV	Confused, agitated response
V	Confused, inappropriate response
VI	Confused, appropriate response
VII	Automatic, appropriate response
VIII	Purposeful, appropriate response

Adapted from Malkmus D: *Rehabilitation of the Head-Injured Adult. Comprehensive Cognitive Management.* Downey, CA: Professional Staff Association of Rancho Los Amigos Hospital; 1980.

4. Speech therapy—After traumatic brain injury, patients may have temporary or permanent physical handicaps that prevent them from communicating effectively. In communicating with nonverbal patients, a variety of methods and devices can be used, ranging from yes-and-no signals to communication boards and electronic devices. Patients need to acquire at least a minimal level of attentional, memory, and organizational skills to facilitate use of such communication devices. In verbal patients, language disorders may be present because of an underlying cognitive disruption following head trauma. The most frequent residual language disorders are those seen in the areas of work retrieval and auditory processing. Language therapy in patients with these long-term disorders should be directed toward reorganization of the cognitive process.

5. Physical therapy—Areas of concern in physical therapy include patient positioning, mobility, and performance of daily activities. Making it possible for bedridden patients to sit can significantly improve the quality of life and greatly enhance the opportunities to interact with other people. In some patients, casts or orthotic devices may be required to maintain the desired limb positions. Aggressive joint ROM exercises are necessary to prevent contractures.

Among the factors that influence whether a patient can walk are limb stability, motor control, good balance reactions, and adequate proprioception. Equipment and devices to aid in movement (canes, walkers, wheelchairs, etc.) should always be of the least complex design to accomplish the goal and should be chosen on the basis of the individual patient's cognitive and physical level of function.

In developing appropriate exercises and activities for a patient, the physical therapist should consider factors such as the joint ROM, muscle tone, motor control, and cognitive functions of the patient. Even the confused and agitated patient may respond to simple, familiar functional activities such as washing the face and brushing the teeth. Patients with higher cognitive function should be encouraged to carry out hygiene, grooming, dressing, and feeding activities.

6. Surgical management of residual musculoskeletal problems—After neurologic recovery stabilizes, surgical procedures may be indicated to correct residual limb deformities and to excise HO.

A. CORRECTION OF LIMB DEFORMITIES IN THE LOWER EXTREMITIES—In functional lower limbs, surgery is most often directed at correcting the equinovarus deformity of the foot (see Figure 12–12). The procedures needed for correction of the deformity are determined by clinical evaluation combined with laboratory assessment using dynamic poly-electromyography (poly-EMG). Commonly, several procedures are done simultaneously: lengthening of the Achilles tendon (see Figure 12–16); release of the flexor digitorum longus, flexor hallucis longus, and flexor brevis tendons (see Figure 12–17); a split anterior tibial tendon transfer (see Figure 12–18); and transfer of the flexor digitorum longus

tendon to the heel. The object of surgery is to provide a plantigrade foot for standing and walking, and the surgery is highly successful in this goal. Seventy percent of patients are able to ambulate without a brace after surgery.

A stiff-knee gait is a common deformity that causes the patient to hike the pelvis and circumduct the leg for clearance of the foot during the swing phase of walking. Inappropriate activity in the quadriceps muscle at this time prevents knee flexion. If the vasti muscles of the quadriceps muscle are firing out of phase, the affected head or heads can be lengthened surgically (see Figure 12–14) to allow knee flexion while retaining quadriceps function. Transfer of the rectus femoris muscle to the sartorius or gracilis muscle provides active knee flexion during swing.

In nonfunctional lower limbs, surgery commonly consists of releasing contractures of the hips and knees.

B. CORRECTION OF LIMB DEFORMITIES IN THE UPPER EXTREMITIES—In functional upper limbs, surgery is frequently needed to correct problems of the wrist, fingers, and thumbs. If active hand opening is restricted by flexor spasticity, lengthening of the extrinsic finger flexors (Figure 12–23) weakens the overactive flexors and improves hand function while preserving the ability of the patient to grasp objects. In cases in which spastic thenar muscles cause thumb-in-palm deformity, a procedure consisting of proximal release of the thenar muscles (Figure 12–24) corrects the problem while preserving function of the thumb. In some patients, adequate placement of the hand for functional activities is impaired by elbow spasticity, although triceps function is generally normal. In these patients, lengthening the elbow

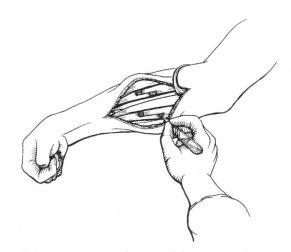

▲ **Figure 12–23.** Lengthening of the extrinsic finger flexors to correct the problem of flexor spasticity and improve hand function while preserving the ability to grasp objects. (Illustration by Anthony C. Berlet. Reproduced, with permission, from Keenan MAE, Kozin SH, Berlet AC: *Manual of Orthopaedic Surgery for Spasticity.* Philadelphia, PA: Raven; 1993.)

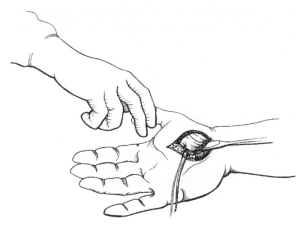

▲ **Figure 12–24.** Proximal release of the thenar muscles to correct a thumb-in-palm deformity while preserving function of the thumb. (Illustration by Anthony C. Berlet. Reproduced, with permission, from Keenan MAE, Kozin SH, Berlet AC: *Manual of Orthopaedic Surgery for Spasticity.* Philadelphia, PA: Raven; 1993.)

flexors (Figure 12–25) enhances the ability to extend the elbow smoothly while preserving active flexion.

In nonfunctional upper limbs, common procedures consist of releasing various contractures and performing neurectomies to eliminate muscle spasticity. The problems of shoulder contracture, elbow contracture, and clenched-fist deformity are discussed in the section on stroke (see previous discussion), and the surgical procedures used in their treatment are shown in Figures 12–20, 12–21, and 12–22.

C. Excision of heterotopic ossification—Surgical measures for treatment of this problem are discussed later in this chapter.

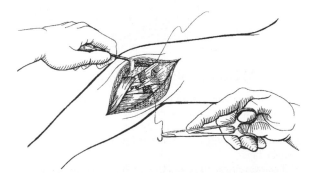

▲ **Figure 12–25.** Lengthening of the elbow flexors to correct flexor spasticity and improve movement of the elbow. (Illustration by Anthony C. Berlet. Reproduced, with permission, from Keenan MAE, Kozin SH, Berlet AC: *Manual of Orthopaedic Surgery for Spasticity.* Philadelphia, PA: Raven; 1993.)

D. Occupational therapy and social services—Before patients are released from the hospital or rehabilitation facility, both they and their families must be informed about social service agencies, support groups, and special programs that can be of help. Social adjustment and the resumption of occupational pursuits and leisure activities depend on the recovery of mental factors first, personality status second, and physical factors third. Physical factors are more responsive to rehabilitation than are mental, personality, or social factors. Mental impairment, however, interferes the most with independence in ADLs.

7. Inpatient rehabilitation—Changes in the rules governing inpatient rehabilitation hospitals and units, particularly the implementation of the new prospective payment system for inpatient rehabilitation facilities by the Centers for Medicare and Medicaid Services (CMS), complicate the admission of patients with rehabilitation goals to an inpatient setting.

Physicians generally agree on the circumstances that justify a medical or surgical patient's hospitalization. In addition, in some cases, an admission to a rehabilitation hospital or to the rehabilitation service of a short-term hospital can be justified on essentially the same medical or surgical grounds. In other cases, however, a patient's medical or surgical needs alone may not warrant inpatient hospital care, but hospitalization may nevertheless be necessary because of the patient's need for rehabilitative services.

Patients needing rehabilitative services require a hospital level of care if they need a relatively intense rehabilitation program that requires a multidisciplinary coordinated team approach to upgrade their ability to function (eg, patients with traumatic brain injury or SCI after corrective extremity surgery). Two basic requirements must be met for inpatient hospital stays for rehabilitation care to be covered:

1. The services must be reasonable and necessary (in terms of efficacy, duration, frequency, and amount) for the treatment of the patient's condition.

2. It must be reasonable and necessary to furnish the care on an inpatient hospital basis, rather than in a less intensive facility such as a skilled nursing facility (SNF), or on an outpatient basis.

To meet the requirements just cited, the following basic components must be met:

1. Close medical supervision by a physician with specialized training or experience in rehabilitation

2. The patient requires the 24-hour availability of a registered nurse with specialized training or experience in rehabilitation

3. The general threshold for establishing the need for inpatient hospital rehabilitation services is that the patient must require and receive at least 3 hours a day of physical and/or occupational therapy

4. A multidisciplinary team (usually includes, at minimum, a physician, rehabilitation nurse, and one therapist)

Esquenazi A, Mayer NH, Keenan MA: Dynamic polyelectromyography, neurolysis, and chemodenervation with botulinum toxin A for assessment and treatment of gait dysfunction. *Adv Neurol* 2001;87:321. [PMID: 11347237]

Gardner MJ, Ong BC, Liporace F, et al: Orthopedic issues after cerebrovascular accident. *Am J Orthop* 2002;31:559. [PMID: 12405561]

HETEROTOPIC OSSIFICATION

HO is commonly detected 2 months after traumatic brain injury or SCI and is characterized by increasing pain and decreasing ROM about a joint. The problem affects adults but is virtually unheard of in children. Although the cause of HO is unknown, a genetic predisposition is suspected. Unidentified humoral factors that enhance osteogenesis are demonstrated in the sera of patients with brain injury. Other contributing factors include soft-tissue trauma and spasticity.

▶ Clinical Findings

Clinically significant HO is seen in 20% of adults with traumatic brain injuries or SCIs and may affect one joint or multiple joints. The overall rate of joint ankylosis is 16%. In affected patients, the bone forms in association with spastic muscles, and the alkaline phosphatase level is elevated. Bone scans may aid in early diagnosis, and the diagnosis is most commonly confirmed by radiographs.

In 27% of patients with HO, shoulder involvement is found inferomedial to the glenohumeral joint. Although ankylosis of the joint in these cases is unusual, motion may be sufficiently restricted to require surgical resection. Elbow involvement is seen in 26% of patients with HO and in 89% of those who suffered a fracture or dislocation about the elbow. When ossification forms posterior to the elbow joint, pressure neuritis of the ulnar nerve is common. Anterior transposition of the ulnar nerve is frequently required to prevent entrapment, and this procedure also facilitates later bone resection. Joint ankylosis is a common complication in patients with elbow involvement. Hip involvement is seen in 44% of patients who form ectopic bone. Bilateral hip involvement and joint ankylosis are common in these patients. HO in the knee joint is less common but significantly impedes both flexion and extension of the joint.

▶ Management

A. Early Measures

Aggressive treatment of spasticity is necessary because this problem appears to play an etiologic role in mechanically stimulating bone formation. To eliminate spasticity in the muscle groups adjacent to the bone formation, phenol blocks are administered. To prevent the deposition of calcium crystals in the collagen matrix of the periarticular connective tissue, etidronate disodium (Didronel) is used. When the HO is detected very early, the use of intravenous etidronate sodium,

300 mg for 3 days, followed by oral therapy is very effective. The recommended dosage is 20 mg/kg/day orally in a single dose, and the drug should be taken on an empty stomach for proper absorption. Anti-inflammatory medications are also used to control the intense inflammatory reaction that occurs during the formation of HO. The most commonly documented medication is indomethacin, 75–150 mg daily, but in theory, other nonsteroidal anti-inflammatory drugs are equally effective. Physical therapy is aimed at providing gentle ROM to the joint to prevent ankylosis. Forceful joint manipulation is not advised because it can cause fractures or soft-tissue damage with contracture formation.

B. Definitive Treatment

Surgical excision is the definitive treatment for HO. Following surgery, physical therapy and radiation therapy (800 rads) and/or medications should be used to diminish recurrence.

Banovac K, Sherman AL, Estores IM, et al: Prevention and treatment of heterotopic ossification after spinal cord injury. *J Spinal Cord Med* 2004;27:376. [PMID: 15484668]

Burd TA, Lowry KJ, Anglen JO: Indomethacin compared with localized irradiation for the prevention of heterotopic ossification following surgical treatment of acetabular fractures. *J Bone Joint Surg Am* 2001;83-A:1783. [PMID: 11741055]

Dahners LE, Mullis BH: Effects of nonsteroidal anti-inflammatory drugs on bone formation and soft-tissue healing. *J Am Acad Orthop Surg* 2004;12:139. [PMID: 15161166]

Hamid N, Ashraf N, Bosse MJ, et al: Radiation therapy for heterotopic ossification prophylaxis acutely after elbow trauma: a prospective randomized study. *J Bone Joint Surg Am* 2010;92:2032. [PMID: 20810853]

Kaplan FS, Glaser DL, Hebela N, et al: Heterotopic ossification. *J Am Acad Orthop Surg* 2004;12:116. [PMID: 15089085]

Park MJ, Chang MJ, Lee YB, Kang HJ: Surgical release for posttraumatic loss of elbow flexion. *J Bone Joint Surg Am* 2010;92:2692. [PMID: 21084579]

van Kuijk AA, Geurts AC, van Kuppevelt HJ: Neurogenic heterotopic ossification in spinal cord injury. *Spinal Cord* 2002;40:313. [PMID: 12080459]

RHEUMATOID ARTHRITIS

Rheumatoid arthritis (RA) is a chronic systemic disease that affects connective tissue and results in chronic inflammatory synovitis, usually with bilateral joint involvement. It is discussed in Chapter 6, so only the aspects pertinent to rehabilitation are described here.

The systemic nature of RA and its variable clinical pattern make it difficult to devise a precise system for describing the overall functional ability of the patient. The most commonly employed scale is the functional classification devised by the American Rheumatism Association (Table 12–5). In addition, patient-reported outcome measures are effective in rating disease activity.

Table 12–5. American Rheumatism Association classification of function in patients with rheumatoid arthritis.

Class	Description
I	Complete function; able to perform usual duties without handicap.
II	Adequate function for normal activities, despite handicap of pain or limited range of motion in one or more joints.
III	Limited function; able to perform few or none of the duties of usual occupation or self-care.
IV	Largely or wholly incapacitated; bedridden or confined to a wheelchair; able to perform little or no self-care.

▶ Management

A. The Team Approach to Patient Care and Treatment

Optimal management requires an interdisciplinary team approach involving many specialists, including a liaison nurse, rheumatologist, orthopedic surgeon, physical therapist, occupational therapist, psychologist, and social worker. The patient and family are also important members of the team. Because the disease is an ongoing and progressive process, the goal of management is to prevent deformities and maintain function for the patient over a lifetime.

1. Nursing care and patient education—The liaison nurse functions as the coordinator of the team. The nurse provides the critical link between the inpatient medical and surgical management of the disease and the continuation of treatment in the outpatient environment.

Much of the responsibility for patient education in the daily care of the disease rests with the nurse, who explains the techniques for protecting joints; advises patients about the need to perform exercises for maintaining joint ROM and optimizing failing muscle strength; cautions patients that exercising too vigorously can damage weakened joints and ligaments; and reminds patients that because the disease tends to decrease their physical activity, they will need regular periods of rest during the day and good nutrition to maximize their general health and to prevent obesity.

2. Medical and surgical management—The rheumatologist is commonly the team leader and in charge of medical management, which is directed toward the control of synovitis, the relief of pain, and the prevention or treatment of other organ involvement by the disease. The medications used for treatment include aspirin, nonsteroidal anti-inflammatory drugs (NSAIDs), corticosteroids, immunosuppressive drugs, and suppressive agents. A local injection of corticosteroids can be useful in controlling an acute inflammatory process in a specific joint.

The orthopedic surgeon should be involved early in the course of the patient's disease and not merely be called on when medical management fails to be effective. Knowledge of biomechanics, gait dynamics, and energy requirements can be useful in preserving function for the patient. The orthopedist can often recommend orthotic supports, walking aids, and shoe wear that minimize unwanted stress on joints and maximize strength.

In selected situations, early surgical intervention may prevent excessive deterioration of joint structure and function. Synovectomy is effective in preventing tendon rupture in the hand, whereas arthroscopic synovectomy of the knee and shoulder show promise for preventing joint destruction. Fusion of an unstable cervical spine can prevent the disastrous effect of an SCI.

Most surgical procedures are reconstructive. Because relief of pain is the most consistent result of reconstructive surgery, pain is the primary indication for surgery. Restoration of motion and function and the correction of deformity are additional indications for surgical intervention but are more difficult goals to achieve. Preoperative assessment is a painstaking process. In addition to performing a physical examination and reviewing radiographic findings, the surgeon must attempt to elicit sufficient information from the patient, family, and therapists to ascertain which deformities are causing the greatest functional losses. The patient can only tolerate a finite number of surgical procedures, and these must be carefully staged to obtain the maximal result.

3. Physical therapy—The physical therapist uses modalities such as heat and ultrasound to decrease joint stiffness and relieve pain. An exercise program is essential for preserving the functional abilities of the patient. The exercise should gently put all joints through their full arc of motion to maintain this range.

Patients with joint effusions and synovitis automatically assume positions that minimize intraarticular pressure and therefore minimize pain. These positions are usually not optimal for function and can result in flexion deformities. An abnormal position may be reversible if discovered early. Daily joint ROM exercises are central to preventing unwanted contractures.

Muscles weakened by the concomitant myopathy need strengthening but are susceptible to damage from overuse or from an excessively vigorous exercise program. Orthotics may be indicated to support weakened ligaments and provide a means of joint protection and support for functional activities such as walking. Upper extremity walking aids may be useful to give the patients additional support. These aids often require modification to meet the specific needs of the individual. Forearm troughs allow the patient to use the entire arm for support when the hands and wrists are weak or deformed. They are also useful for protecting the hands from excessive stress. A rolling walker, which does not require the patient to lift the walker for advancement, may be useful in patients with limited strength.

4. Occupational therapy—The occupational therapist evaluates and instructs the patient in modified techniques for performing ADLs, such as grooming, dressing, and meal preparation. Because of the weakness and deformities imposed by the arthritis, adaptive equipment and alternative methods are commonly needed. Modifications in clothing, such as larger fasteners for ease of manipulation, Velcro strips at seams or on shoes, and front openings, can all facilitate dressing. Upper extremity splints can be used to provide joint protection and stabilization and to prevent further deformity from occurring. The splints must be lightweight and easily donned by the patient.

5. Psychological counseling—It is not uncommon for patients or their family members to have feelings of anxiety, denial, anger, or depression. The psychologist provides assistance in dealing with these feelings and coping with alterations in lifestyle and self-image. Comprehensive care involves an understanding of how patients respond to weakness, fatigue, altered physical appearance, progressive disability, diminished independence, and the financial burdens of chronic illness. Coping skills are needed to deal with these problems as well as with pain, which becomes an everyday occurrence and may interfere with both intellectual and emotional functioning.

6. Social services—A variety of modifications in lifestyle accompany chronic illness with RA. Occupational changes may be necessary, or the patient may no longer be able to work at all. Additional assistance may be needed in the home for housework and the preparation of meals. In more advanced stages, the patient may require help for personal care. Transportation needs become more complex, and the patient finds it increasingly difficult to leave the home. The social worker becomes an invaluable team member in helping families with the numerous practical arrangements required for everyday existence and for locating financial aid to help defray the mounting costs.

Beasley J: Osteoarthritis and rheumatoid arthritis: conservative therapeutic management. *J Hand Ther* 2012;25:163. [PMID: 22326361]

Durmus B, Altay Z, Baysal O, et al: Can the patient-reported outcome instruments determine disease activity in rheumatoid arthritis? *Bratisl Lek Listy* 2011;112:555. [PMID: 21954539]

POLIOMYELITIS

Poliomyelitis is caused by an enterovirus that attacks the anterior horn cells of the spinal cord. Infection can lead to a variety of clinical findings, ranging from minor symptoms to paralysis. The last major epidemics in the United States occurred during the early 1950s. Immunization programs are effective and safe but parental concerns persist and ought to be acknowledged. Acute poliomyelitis is now rare in the United States and other developed nations of the world.

Nevertheless, orthopedic surgeons today are frequently called on to treat patients with postpoliomyelitis syndrome.

▶ Classification

Four stages of poliomyelitis are recognized.

A. Acute Poliomyelitis

All of the anterior horn cells are attacked during the acute stage, which accounts for the diffuse and severe paralysis seen with the initial infection. The anterior horn cells control the skeletal muscle cells of the trunk and limbs. Clinically, the infection is characterized by the sudden onset of paralysis and the presence of fever and acute muscle pain, often accompanied by stiff neck. Paralysis of the respiratory muscles is life-threatening in the acute stage. When the shoulder muscles are involved, respiratory compromise should be suspected because of the close proximity of the anterior horn cells controlling each in the spinal cord. Mechanical support of ventilation may be required.

A variable number of anterior horn cells survive the initial infection. The treatment in the acute stage of the disease consists of providing the needed respiratory support, decreasing muscle pain, and performing regular ROM exercises to prevent the formation of joint contractures.

B. Subacute Poliomyelitis

Anterior horn cell survival, axon sprouting, and muscle hypertrophy occur in the subacute phase and provide three mechanisms for regaining strength. An average of 47% (range of 12–94%) of the anterior horn cells in the spinal cord survive the initial attack. Because cell survival occurs in a random fashion, the distribution of paralysis is variable and depends on which anterior horn cells were destroyed. Each anterior horn cell innervates a group of muscle cells. When a group of muscle cells is orphaned, as it were, by the death of the anterior horn cell that supports it, a nearby nerve cell can sprout additional axons and adopt some of the orphaned cells. By means of this process, a motor unit (defined as a nerve cell and the muscle cells it innervates) can expand greatly. Moreover, muscle cells in the unit enlarge, and this hypertrophy provides additional strength for the patient.

C. Residual Poliomyelitis

It is only after 16–24 months following onset that the ultimate extent of poliomyelitis can be determined and procedures to restore lost function and provide structural stability can be instituted.

D. Postpoliomyelitis Syndrome

Patients who had acute poliomyelitis during childhood often complain of increased muscle weakness 30–40 years later. This weakness is not a result of infectious spread of the earlier disease but, rather, is caused by the overuse of muscles that were originally affected, whether or not they were known to have been affected at the onset of the disease. Studies show that a muscle must lose from 30 to 40% of its strength for weakness to be detected using manual muscle testing. Studies of gait also demonstrate that the ADLs require more muscle strength and stamina than were previously appreciated. The traditional program, which encouraged patients to work harder to regain strength and was based on the concept of "no pain, no gain," proved detrimental because it encouraged chronic overuse of muscles and resulted in further deterioration of function.

The diagnosis of postpoliomyelitis syndrome is based on a history of poliomyelitis; a pattern of increased muscle weakness that is random and does not follow any nerve root or peripheral nerve distribution; and the presence of additional symptoms such as muscle pain, severe fatigue, muscle cramping or fasciculations, joint pain or instability, sleep apnea, intolerance to cold, and depression. No pathognomonic tests for the syndrome are currently available. Electromyography can demonstrate the presence of large motor units resulting from the previous axon sprouting. This finding is supportive but not diagnostic of poliomyelitis.

▶ Management

A. Acute Poliomyelitis

When the shoulder muscles are involved, respiratory compromise should be suspected, and mechanical support of ventilation should be instituted. Other measures are aimed at decreasing muscle pain and preventing complications. Regular ROM exercises prevent the formation of joint contractures.

B. Subacute Poliomyelitis

During the subacute stage, which may last as long as 24 months, the emphasis is on preventing deformities and preserving function. Splints and braces are often helpful for maintaining joint position and supplementing function.

C. Residual Poliomyelitis

Patients with compromised function of the diaphragm can be taught glossopharyngeal breathing. This method, in which air is swallowed into the lungs, provides sufficient air exchange for the patient to perform light activities in the sitting position. Mechanical support of ventilation may still need to be continued while the patient sleeps. It is during the residual stage that orthopedic surgery is commonly performed to restore lost function and provide structural stability. If the patient is still growing, it is important to prevent the formation of skeletal deformities that result from muscle imbalance. Before any surgery that requires general anesthesia or significant sedation is performed, the vital capacity should be assessed to determine the patient's need for respiratory support.

D. Postpoliomyelitis Syndrome

Treatment is directed at preserving current muscle strength and preventing further weakness from occurring. Generally, strength cannot be restored in a muscle that was weakened by poliomyelitis. Some gain in strength can be seen, however, when chronic overuse is corrected.

General management strategies consist of modifying lifestyle to prevent chronic overuse of weak muscles; instituting a limited exercise program that incorporates frequent rest periods to prevent disuse atrophy and weakness; providing lightweight orthotic support of the limbs to protect joints and substitute for muscle function; and performing orthopedic surgery to correct limb or trunk deformities.

Specific management strategies depend on the areas of disease involvement.

1. Spine—Back pain is a common complaint and usually results from postural strain caused by excessive lumbar extension in patients who have weak or paralyzed hip extensor muscles. Neck pain, like back pain, is a common complaint associated with slowly increasing weakness. Both complaints can be treated by the use of external supports. Patient education is imperative because many patients are reluctant to don braces again, after having passed decades without using them. Patients should be instructed in methods to relieve excess strain on the neck muscles and prevent further deterioration. Tilting the chair seat 10 degrees backward is often sufficient to relieve the fatigue of the posterior cervical muscles from supporting the head.

Paralysis of the cervical spine musculature can result in the inability to maintain the head erect and can interfere with the performance of a vast number of functions, including ambulation. Surgical fusion of the cervical spine corrects the problem.

Scoliosis is common in patients with muscle imbalance caused by paralysis. The condition is particularly pronounced in patients with leg-length discrepancies. External supports can be used to hold the spine in position, but these often interfere with respiration if the patient depends on the use of accessory muscles for breathing. Posterior spinal fusion may be needed to control the spine adequately. After fusion is performed, prolonged immobilization must be avoided. Segmental spine fixation may be helpful.

2. Lower extremities—Full ROM of the hip and knee joints is needed for function. Contractures should be corrected when possible to permit more effective bracing. In iliotibial band contractures, which are common deformities, the hip assumes a position of flexion, external rotation, and abduction; the knee assumes a valgus alignment; and the tibia is externally rotated on the femur. Release or lengthening of the iliotibial band corrects the deformity.

A patient with flailing lower extremities can stand using crutches and a KAFO with the knees locked in extension and the ankles in slight dorsiflexion by hyperextending the hips and using the strong anterior hip capsule for support.

Flexion contractures of the hips or knees prevent this alignment. If trunk support and upper extremity strength are adequate, the patient could ambulate with a swing-through gait for short distances. This gait has high-energy demands. With time, the posterior knee joint capsule becomes stretched, and the knee develops a recurvatum deformity that is painful and can lead to arthritic degeneration of the knee. A KAFO protects the knee and provides improved stability for walking. If there is fair (grade 3) strength in the hip flexor muscles (see Table 12–1) and passive full-knee extension, then the knee joints can be left unlocked for walking. In this case, a posteriorly offset knee joint is used to stabilize the knee, and ankle dorsiflexion is limited to minus 3 degrees of neutral dorsiflexion to provide a hyperextension moment to the knee for stability. Thus, at stance phase, the net ankle plantarflexion locks the knee in hyperextension, restrained by posterior capsular static structures.

Quadriceps muscle strength is not essential for ambulation. A strong gluteus maximus and good calf strength can substitute by keeping the knee locked in extension. If the calf strength is inadequate to control the forward motion of the tibia in mid to late stance, an AFO is needed. It is not necessary to fix the ankle in mild plantarflexion to provide knee stability, and such a position could cause a recurvatum deformity in any case. An equinus position of the foot inhibits forward momentum and limits step length by preventing body weight from rolling over the forefoot prior to contact of the contralateral extremity with the ground. When good hamstring function is present, the biceps femoris and the semitendinosus can be transferred anteriorly to the quadriceps tendon to provide dynamic knee stability.

Muscle imbalances in the foot can lead to deformity. When muscle imbalances exist, tendon releases or transfers should be considered prior to the development of fixed deformities.

Equinus contracture of the ankle is a common problem and results in genu recurvatum. Accommodating the equinus posture by using an elevated heel places excessive stress on the calf muscles to control the leg. A surgical procedure to lengthen the Achilles tendon is frequently needed to correct the equinus contracture of the ankle and to permit adequate bracing.

A cavus foot deformity causes forefoot equinus, which also limits bracing. If no fixed bony abnormalities are present, then release of the plantar fascia is sufficient to correct the deformity. If the cavus deformity is caused by bony abnormalities, then a closing wedge osteotomy is needed. A triple arthrodesis of the hindfoot can also be used to correct deformities and provide a stable base of support.

The long-standing muscle imbalances, patterns of muscle substitution, and resulting joint and ligament strains often lead to degenerative arthritis. Total joint replacement can be performed, but several special considerations are needed. In patients with postpoliomyelitis syndrome, osteoporosis is common because of prolonged lack of muscle action on the bone. Joint contractures must be corrected at the time of surgery to prevent excessive forces on the prosthetic components because these forces might lead to loosening of the prosthesis. Weak muscles must be supported with the appropriate orthoses after surgery. The rehabilitation program is lengthy because it takes an extended period to regain joint motion and muscle function. Continuous passive motion devices and frequent joint ROM must be used to gain joint mobility after surgery. Because the hip joint is difficult to brace, there must be at least fair (grade 3) strength (see Table 12–1) in the hip extensors, abductors, and flexors to provide stability to the hip after surgery. Surgery can be expected to weaken the surrounding muscles, which must be taken into account before total hip arthroplasty is undertaken to prevent chronic dislocation.

3. Upper extremities

A. Shoulders—The shoulder is important for placing the hand in the desired position for use. The shoulder totally depends on muscle strength for active mobility. In patients who use a wheelchair, weak muscles about the shoulder can be made more functional with the use of mobile arm supports on the wheelchair. These supports allow the patient a greater arc of motion with less muscle strength. Shoulder stability is more important in the ambulatory patient who requires upper extremity aids. A glenohumeral fusion may be helpful if the patient has sufficient strength in the scapulothoracic muscles. When the shoulder is fused, scapulothoracic motion is maintained, allowing use of the extremity for tabletop activities. Glenohumeral fusion does restrict the ability of the patient to position the hand for bathroom hygiene, so it is undesirable to perform the procedure on both shoulders.

Preservation of shoulder strength should be a priority of treatment. Rotator cuff tears are a common problem in postpolio patients. Surgical repair of the torn rotator cuff should be done when possible. In large tears that cannot be repaired, arthroscopic debridement offers significant relief of pain. Shoulder weakness is found in 95% of patients with postpoliomyelitis syndrome and correlates closely with the amount of lower extremity weakness present. Patients with weak legs use their arms to push up from a chair and pull themselves up stairs. They also lean heavily on upper extremity aids while walking. It is therefore important to remove as many unnecessary strains from the shoulders as possible with the use of elevated seats, motorized lift chairs, elevators or motorized stair chair glides, and optimal lower extremity bracing. In minimally ambulatory or nonambulatory patients, an electric wheelchair or motorized scooter should be prescribed to prevent excessive strain on the shoulder muscles caused by propelling a manual wheelchair.

B. Elbows—The elbow requires sufficient flexor strength to lift an object against gravity for function. A mobile arm support can maximize the effectiveness of the muscle strength for the patient. Tendon transfers, such as those involving the deltoid and biceps muscles, may also be useful in restoring active flexion.

C. WRISTS AND HANDS—Opponens paralysis is common in the hand and results in a 50% loss of hand function. A splint used during the acute and recovery phases is useful in preventing an adduction contracture. Opponens function can be restored by tendon transfer. The most common muscle transferred is the flexor digitorum superficialis of the ring finger.

Paralysis of the intrinsic muscles of the hand interferes with function. A lumbrical bar orthosis prevents hyperextension of the metacarpophalangeal joints and allows the long extensors to extend the fingers and open the hand. Surgical capsulodesis to limit metacarpophalangeal joint extension accomplishes the same result.

Paralysis of the finger flexors and extensors can be overcome with the use of a flexor hinge orthosis if wrist extensor function is present. Tendon transfers can provide the same result, allowing the tenodesis effect to provide grasp and pinch functions.

Boyer FC, Tiffreau V, Rapin A, et al: Post-polio syndrome: Pathophysiological hypotheses, diagnosis criteria, drug therapy. *Ann Phys Rehabil Med* 2010;53:34. [PMID: 20093102]

Chatterjee A, O'Keefe C: Current controversies in the USA regarding vaccine safety. *Expert Rev Vaccines* 2010;9:497. [PMID: 20450324]

Gonzalez H, Olsson T, Borg K: Management of postpolio syndrome. *Lancet Neurol* 2010;9:634. [PMID: 20494327]

Koopman FS, Uegaki K, Gilhus NE, et al: Treatment for postpolio syndrome. *Cochrane Database Syst Rev* 2011;2:CD007818. [PMID: 21328301]

Nollet F: Postpolio syndrome: unanswered questions regarding cause, course, risk factors, and therapies. *Lancet Neurol* 2010; 9:561. [PMID: 20494317]

CEREBRAL PALSY (STATIC ENCEPHALOPATHY)

Cerebral palsy is a nonprogressive and nonhereditary disorder of impaired motor function. The onset may be prenatal, perinatal, or postnatal. An exact cause is not always known, but the impairment is sometimes associated with prematurity, perinatal hypoxia, cerebral trauma, or neonatal jaundice. In the United States, more than 500,000 people are affected by cerebral palsy. The degree of neurologic impairment is severe in a third of patients and mild in approximately a sixth.

▶ Classification

Because of the diversity of neurologic findings seen in patients with cerebral palsy, a classification system is essential. The disease can be classified by the types of movement disorder and by the patterns of neurologic deficit.

A. Types of Movement Disorder

Three types of disorder are seen.

1. Spastic disorders—These are characterized by the presence of clonus and hyperactive deep tendon reflexes. Patients with spastic movement can be helped by orthopedic intervention.

2. Dyskinetic disorders—Among the conditions classified as dyskinetic disorders are athetosis, ballismus, chorea, dystonia, and ataxia. For practical purposes, these conditions are grouped together because they are not amenable to surgical correction.

3. Mixed disorders—These usually consist of a combination of spasticity and athetosis with total body involvement.

B. Patterns of Neurologic Involvement

1. Monoplegia—With single-limb involvement, the disorder is usually spastic in nature. Because monoplegia is rare, it is advisable to test the patient before making the diagnosis. The stress of performing an activity such as running at a fast pace often uncovers spasticity in another limb.

2. Hemiplegia—Spasticity affects the upper and lower extremities ipsilaterally. Equinovarus posturing is common in the lower extremity. The upper extremity is usually held with the elbow, wrist, and fingers flexed and the thumb adducted. The major problem interfering with upper extremity function, however, is a loss of proprioception and stereognosis. Surgery for the upper extremity is aimed at making the hand assistive and at improving cosmesis. An arm that is involuntarily held in severe flexion while walking can be a major social disadvantage for the patient.

3. Paraplegia—In paraplegia, neurologic deficits involve only the lower extremities. Because paraplegia is rare in patients with spastic cerebral palsy, the presence of a high spinal cord lesion that could also be responsible for the neurologic findings must be ruled out. Bladder problems coexist with spastic paralysis that affects the lower extremities and is secondary to spinal cord damage.

4. Diplegia—Spastic diplegia, seen in 50–60% of cerebral palsy patients in the United States, is the most common neurologic pattern. It is characterized by major involvement in both lower extremities with only minor incoordination in the upper extremities. Findings in the lower extremities include marked spasticity, particularly about the hips, hyperactive deep tendon reflexes, and a positive Babinski sign. The hips are commonly held in a position of flexion, adduction, and internal rotation secondary to the spasticity. The knees are in the valgus position and may have excessive external rotation of the tibia. The ankles are held in the equinus position, with a valgus attitude of the feet. Speech and intellectual functions are usually normal or only slightly impaired. Esotropia and visual perception problems are common.

5. Total body involvement—Sometimes referred to as quadriplegia, total body involvement is characterized by impairments affecting all four extremities, the head, and the trunk. Sensory deficits are typical, and speech and swallowing are commonly impaired. The most serious deficit is often the inability to communicate with others. Although mental retardation is found in approximately 45% of patients, intelligence is often masked by communication dysfunction. Ambulation is not usually a goal because the equilibrium reactions of affected patients are severely impaired or absent. Sitting may require braces or adaptive supportive devices. Scoliosis, contractures, and dislocated hips are common orthopedic problems and may interfere with sitting.

▶ Management

Because cerebral palsy in children is discussed elsewhere (see Chapter 10), the following discussion concentrates on the needs of the adult with cerebral palsy.

A. Special Considerations in Adult Patients

1. Musculoskeletal problems—Long-standing deformities may be rigid. Bony deformities are common and may preclude surgery for soft-tissue rebalancing unless concomitant osteotomies are done. In comparison with the young patient, the adult patient has a greater body mass to support and therefore has increased energy demands. Spastic muscles are weak and frequently further compromised by the chronic overuse of muscles to compensate for contractural deformities.

2. Mobility—The patient who can sit independently has good balance and may propel a wheelchair. It may be easier to propel the wheelchair backward, using the feet to push. A self-propped sitter may require some external support to remain erect, whereas a propped sitter needs a straight spine and flexible hips to remain erect with support.

Ambulation can be divided into four categories: community ambulation, household ambulation, physiologic ambulation (exercise), and wheelchair ambulation. A patient categorized as a community ambulator is able to maneuver independently and safely around obstacles normally encountered in the community. Orthotics or upper extremity walking aids may be required. A household ambulator is able to walk independently for short distances but requires assistance to negotiate obstacles such as stairs or curbs and requires a wheelchair for long distances. A physiologic ambulator is someone who is capable of walking for short distances with assistance or walks as a means of exercise but finds it impractical to walk for normal activities. The energy requirements for walking determine the category to which a patient belongs and also determine the types of equipment that are recommended. It is unreasonable to expect patients to expend all their energy in merely transporting themselves from one location to another.

B. Treatment of Patients with Lower Extremity Problems

1. Hips—An adduction and internal rotation deformity of the hip is sometimes seen during ambulation. Release of the hip adductor tendons (see Figure 12–13) may be needed to correct this tendency.

A crouch gait and lumbar lordosis are evidence of hip flexion deformity. In patients with cerebral palsy, gait studies with dynamic poly-EMG demonstrated dysphasic activity of the iliopsoas, which is the main hip flexor muscle. Gait studies with poly-EMG should be undertaken to evaluate the activity of the iliopsoas and pectineus and to aid in surgical decision making. If release of the iliopsoas is indicated, the tendon is cut distally and allowed to retract proximally to the point where it reattaches to the anterior hip capsule (Figure 12–26). Release of the pectineus muscle is often also necessary.

2. Knees—Correction of a knee flexion deformity in a patient with a crouch gait may be necessary. Attention should first be paid to the hip deformity. Weakness of the gastrocnemius and soleus muscles and inability to maintain the position of the tibia may also contribute to a crouch posture and should be considered prior to performing any knee surgery. Gait electromyograms are useful in determining which muscles are responsible for the abnormal posture. Release of the offending hamstring tendons (see Figure 12–15) or hamstring lengthening may be useful.

3. Feet—Equinus posturing of the ankle is common. If no fixed contracture is present, an AFO controls the position of the foot. If the deformity is the result of an equinus contracture, Achilles tendon lengthening (see Figure 12–16) should

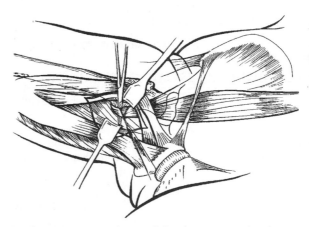

▲ **Figure 12–26.** Release of the iliopsoas tendon from its insertion on the lesser trochanter of the femur to correct a hip flexion deformity. (Illustration by Anthony C. Berlet. Reproduced, with permission, from Keenan MAE, Kozin SH, Berlet AC: *Manual of Orthopaedic Surgery for Spasticity.* Philadelphia, PA: Raven; 1993.)

be performed to bring the foot to a neutral position. The foot should be held in a short leg walking cast for 6 weeks following surgery. An AFO is then used to maintain the position of the foot and support the tibia during walking.

Equinovarus posturing of the ankle is also common. Although the anterior tibial muscle is the primary varus force in patients with stroke or traumatic brain injuries, it is equally likely that the posterior tibial muscle may be causing equinovarus posturing in patients with cerebral palsy. Therefore, in order to find the cause and make the correct decision concerning surgery, it is important to make dynamic EMG recordings while the patient walks.

If the anterior tibial muscle is overactive, Achilles tendon lengthening should be accompanied by a split anterior tibial tendon transfer (see Figure 12–18). If the posterior tibial muscle is overactive, it is advisable to lengthen the posterior tendon. If the EMG studies show that the posterior tibial muscle is active only during the swing phase of gait, it may be more logical to transfer the posterior tendon through the interosseous membrane to the dorsum of the foot, rather than performing a split anterior tibial tendon transfer. After surgery is performed, a short leg cast that allows weight bearing is worn for 6 weeks, and the leg is then supported with an AFO. If hallux valgus subsequently develops, management consists of correcting the subtalar deformity and realigning the first digital ray.

A pes cavus deformity of the foot is occasionally seen in patients with spasticity of the intrinsic muscles. If the problem is detected early, it can be corrected by plantar fasciotomy and release of the flexor origins from the os calcis. If the problem is detected late and a concomitant bony deformity is present, a wedge osteotomy of the midtarsal bones should be performed.

C. Treatment of Patients with Upper Extremity Problems

Function of the upper extremities depends on a variety of factors, including cognition, intact sensation, and the ability to place the hand in space. The amount of spasticity present also affects the ability to control movement of the arm and hand. Surgery can influence hand placement and modify spasticity, but a successful outcome requires the ability to cooperate with postoperative therapy programs. Mental impairment, motion disorders, and poor sensation are relative contraindications to surgery in the functional arm and hand.

1. The functional upper extremity—In patients with problems involving the functional hand, treatment begins with careful clinical evaluation of motor and sensory deficits. Dynamic EMG is extremely useful in determining which muscles should be lengthened or transferred to improve function. The least severely involved hands exhibit a minor degree of spasticity in the flexor carpi ulnaris and a resulting mild flexion deformity of the wrist. In this case, all that is required to improve hand function and position is surgical lengthening of the flexor carpi ulnaris tendon.

In some patients, release of objects from the hand is a problem. In this case, the synergistic action of the finger extensors and wrist flexors causes difficulty with finger extension when the wrist is extended. This resembles the tenodesis effect seen in paralytic hands, but the mechanism is a dynamic one. Selective lengthening of the overactive finger flexors (see Figure 12–23) improves hand function.

Transfer of a wrist flexor to a wrist extensor should be done with caution. Often a patient flexes the wrist to adjust the dynamic balance between the finger flexors and extensors. Holding the wrist in extension can rob the patient of this important method of compensation.

The thumb-in-palm deformity is treated by proximal release of the thenar muscles (see Figure 12–24) and lengthening of the flexor pollicis longus tendon. Distal release of the thenar muscles is not recommended because it may cause a hyperextension deformity of the metacarpophalangeal joint of the thumb.

2. The nonfunctional upper extremity—Surgery may be indicated in the nonfunctional upper extremity to prevent skin breakdown, to improve hygiene or cosmesis, or to make dressing easier. The problems of shoulder contracture and elbow contracture are discussed in the section on stroke, and the surgical procedures used in their treatment are shown in Figures 12–20 and 12–21. Patients who have a flexed wrist with flexed fingers and a thumb-in-palm deformity should be treated because severe wrist flexion can cause median nerve compression against the proximal edge of the transverse carpal ligament. An arthrodesis of the wrist in neutral position, combined with a superficialis-to-profundus tendon transfer (see Figure 12–22), reliably corrects the wrist deformity and also improves skin care. Management of the thumb deformity consists of lengthening the flexor pollicis longus tendon, fusing the interphalangeal joint, and performing a proximal release of the thenar muscles (see Figure 12–24).

D. Treatment of Patients with Total Body Involvement

Patients with total body involvement are rarely functional ambulators, although they may transfer from one position to another either independently or with assistance. They frequently have a combination of spasticity and motion disorders such as athetosis, and they spend most of their time in a chair. Flexible hips and a straight spine are needed for functional sitting.

Occasionally, knee flexion deformities require distal hamstring release or lengthening to allow for greater flexibility in positioning the patient. Rigid extension contractures of the knee are sometimes seen and interfere with sitting tolerance. Lengthening of the quadriceps tendon (Figure 12–27) allows the knee to flex.

Foot deformities in the spastic patient are extremely common and require treatment to allow shoe wear and to

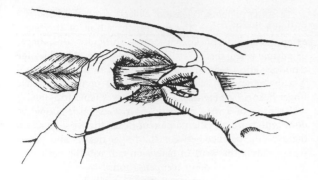

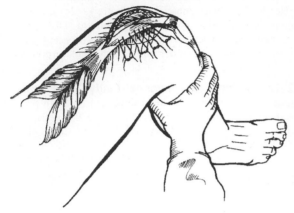

▲ **Figure 12–27.** The dV-Y incision (*top*) and lengthening (*bottom*) of the quadriceps tendon to correct a rigid extension contracture of the knee and allow improved sitting. (Illustration by Anthony C. Berlet. Reproduced, with permission, from Keenan MAE, Kozin SH, Berlet AC: *Manual of Orthopaedic Surgery for Spasticity.* Philadelphia, PA: Raven; 1993.)

prevent skin breakdown. Sitting balance is improved when the feet can be positioned on the leg support of a wheelchair.

The spine is of major concern in patients with total body involvement because scoliosis is common. Adaptive seating or orthotics are useful in supporting the spine and helping the patient maintain an erect posture while seated. Spinal fusion with instrumentation is indicated for treatment of progressive scoliosis. Obliquity of the pelvis greatly interferes with sitting. When this problem is present, fusion should include the sacrum.

Aisen ML, Kerkovich D, Mast J, et al: Cerebral palsy: clinical care and neurological rehabilitation. *Lancet Neurol* 2011;10:844. [PMID: 21849165]

Koman LA: Cerebral palsy: past, present, and future. *J South Orthop Assoc* 2002;11:93. [PMID: 12741589]

Moran CG, Tourret LJ: Recent advances: orthopaedics. *BMJ* 2001;322:902. [PMID: 11302907]

Novak I: Effective home programme intervention for adults: a systematic review. *Clin Rehabil* 2011;25:1066. [PMID: 21831927]

Ryan SE: An overview of systematic reviews of adaptive seating interventions for children with cerebral palsy: where do we go from here? *Disabil Rehabil Assist Technol* 2012;7:104. [PMID: 21877900]

Sussman MD, Aiona MD: Treatment of spastic diplegia in patients with cerebral palsy. *J Pediatr Orthop B* 2004;13:S1. [PMID: 15076595]

Wright PA, Durham S, Ewins DJ, Swain ID: Neuromuscular electrical stimulation for children with cerebral palsy: a review. *Arch Dis Child* 2012;97:364. [PMID: 22447997]

NEUROMUSCULAR DISORDERS

The neuromuscular disorders represent a diverse group of chronic diseases characterized by the progressive degeneration of skeletal musculature, which results in weakness, atrophy, joint contractures, and increasing disability. These disorders are best classified as motor unit diseases because the primary abnormality may involve the motor neuron, the neuromuscular junction, or the muscle fiber. Two broad categories are considered. Myopathies are diseases of the muscle fibers. Neuropathies are disorders in which muscle degeneration is seen secondary to lower motor neuron disease. Most of the neuromuscular disorders are hereditary (Table 12–6), although point mutations may result in spontaneous cases. Early diagnosis is important not only for initiation of appropriate therapy but also for genetic counseling. Treatment programs are aimed at symptomatic and supportive care. Appropriate orthopedic intervention can significantly increase the functional capacity of patients with neuromuscular disorders.

▶ Diagnosis

A. History and Physical Examination

A careful genetic history is important. The clinical history and physical examination delineate the onset and pattern of muscle involvement. Neuropathies generally present with distal involvement. Muscle fasciculation and spasticity are common, and muscle atrophy is in excess of the weakness. Myopathies usually display weakness of the proximal limb musculature initially. Fasciculations and spasticity are not seen. The weakness is more pronounced than the atrophy. Disorders of neuromuscular transmission, such as myasthenia gravis, present with fatigue and ptosis.

B. Muscle Enzyme Studies

Serum levels of muscle enzymes are elevated in myopathies but normal in neuropathies. The enzymes studied include creatine phosphokinase (CPK), lactate dehydrogenase (LDH), aldolase, aspartate aminotransferase (AST, SGOT), and alanine aminotransferase (ALT, SGPT). CPK levels are the most elevated in the Duchenne type of muscular

Table 12–6. Classification of the more commonly encountered neuromuscular disorders.

Disorder	Inherited	Creatine Phosphokinase Level	Electromyographic Pattern	Nerve Conduction	Biopsy Pattern
Muscular dystrophies					
Duchenne (pseudohypertrophic) type	Yes	Markedly elevated	Myopathic	Normal	Myopathic
Facioscapulohumeral type	Yes	Normal or elevated	Myopathic	Normal	Myopathic
Limb-girdle type	Yes	Elevated	Myopathic	Normal	Myopathic
Spinal muscular atrophy					
Werdnig-Hoffmann and Kugelberg-Welander types	Yes	Normal or slightly elevated	Neuropathic	Normal	Neuropathic
Hereditary motor and sensory neuropathies					
Type I (Charcot-Marie-Tooth disease)	Yes	Normal	Neuropathic	Markedly decreased	Neuropathic
Type II	Yes	Normal	Neuropathic	Decreased or normal	Neuropathic
Type III	Yes	Normal	Neuropathic	Decreased	Neuropathic
Type IV	Yes	Normal	Neuropathic		Neuropathic
Type V	Yes	Normal	Neuropathic	Normal	Neuropathic
Myopathies					
Central core, nemaline, minicore, mitochondrial, myotubular, and other types	Often	Often normal	Normal or mildly myopathic	Usually normal	Myopathic
Poliomyelitis	No		Neuropathic	Normal	Neuropathic
Guillain-Barré syndrome	No	Normal	Neuropathic	Slow in acute phase	Neuropathic
Polymyositis	No	Normal or elevated	Myopathic	Normal	Myopathic
Myotonic diseases	Usually	Usually normal	Diagnostic	Normal	
Myasthenia gravis	Sometimes		Diagnostic		

Data compiled by Irene Gilgoff, MD, Rancho Los Amigos Medical Center, Downey, CA.

dystrophy and less elevated in the more slowly progressive disease forms. In Duchenne-type muscular dystrophy, the highest enzyme levels are seen at birth and during the first few years of life, before the disease is clinically apparent. As the disease progresses and the muscle mass deteriorates, the enzyme levels decrease.

C. Electromyography and Nerve Conduction Studies

EMG and nerve conduction studies differentiate between primary muscle diseases and neuropathies (see Table 12–6). EMG is useful in differentiating among muscle diseases, peripheral nerve disorders, and anterior horn cell abnormalities. A myopathic pattern on EMG is characterized by (1) increased frequency, (2) decreased duration, and (3) decreased amplitude of action potentials. In addition, increased insertional activity, short polyphasic potentials, and a retained interference pattern are evident. A neuropathic pattern on EMG is characterized by the opposite constellation of findings: (1) decreased frequency, (2) increased duration, and (3) increased amplitude of action potentials. In addition, frequent fibrillation potentials, a group polyphasic

potential, and a decreased interference pattern can be seen. In myasthenia gravis and the myotonic diseases, the patterns on EMG are diagnostic. In myasthenia gravis, the fatigue phenomenon is exhibited. In myotonia, the EMG is characterized by positive waves and trains of potentials that fire at high frequency and then wax and wane until they slowly disappear.

D. Muscle Biopsy

To gain the maximal amount of information from muscle biopsy, the clinician should choose a muscle that has mild to moderate involvement and was not recently traumatized by electrodes during EMG. Muscle biopsy can be used to differentiate myopathy, neuropathy, and inflammatory myopathy. The biopsy, however, cannot be used to determine prognosis. Histochemical staining further distinguishes the congenital forms of myopathy.

Histologically, myopathies are characterized by muscle fiber necrosis, fatty degeneration, proliferation of the connective tissue, and an increased number of nuclei, some of which have migrated from their normal peripheral position to the center of the muscle fiber.

Neuropathies display small, angulated muscle fibers. Bundles of atrophic fibers are intermingled with bundles of normal fibers. There is no increase in the amount of connective tissue.

Biopsy findings in polymyositis include prominent collections of inflammatory cells, edema of the tissues, perivasculitis, and segmental necrosis with a mixed pattern of fiber degeneration and regeneration.

1. Duchenne-Type Muscular Dystrophy

Duchenne-type muscular dystrophy, which is also called **pseudohypertrophic muscular dystrophy**, is a progressive disease that affects males. It is inherited in an X-linked recessive manner and has its onset in early childhood. Generally, affected children have a normal birth and developmental history. But by the time they reach 3–5 years of age, sufficient muscle mass has been lost to impair function.

▶ Clinical Findings

Early signs of disease include pseudohypertrophy of the calf, which is the result of the increase in connective tissue; planovalgus deformity of the feet, which is secondary to heel cord contracture; and proximal muscle weakness. Muscle weakness in the hips may be exhibited by the Gower sign, in which the patient uses the arms to support the trunk while attempting to rise from the floor. Other signs are hesitance when climbing stairs, acceleration during the final stage of sitting, and shoulder weakness.

Weakness and contractures prevent independent ambulation in approximately 45% of patients by 9 years of age and in the remainder by 12 years of age. It is common for patients to have difficulty first in rising from the floor, next in ascending the stairs, and then in walking. Cardiac involvement is seen in 80% of patients. Findings generally include posterobasal fibrosis of the ventricle and electrocardiographic changes. In patients with a decreased level of activity, clinical evidence of cardiomyopathy may not be obvious. Pulmonary problems are common in the advanced stages of the disease and are found during periodic evaluations of pulmonary function. Mental retardation, noted in 30–50% of patients, is present from birth and not progressive.

▶ Management

Efforts are made to keep patients ambulating for as many years as possible to prevent the complications of obesity, osteoporosis, and scoliosis. The hip flexors, tensor fasciae latae, and triceps surae develop ambulation-limiting contractures. With progressive weakness and contractures, the base of support decreases and the patient cannot use normal mechanisms to maintain upright balance. The patient walks with a wide-based gait, hips flexed and abducted, knees flexed, and the feet in equinus and varus position. Lumbar lordosis becomes exaggerated to compensate for the hip flexion contractures and weak hip extensor musculature.

Equinus contractures of the Achilles tendon occur early and are caused by the muscle imbalance between the calf and pretibial muscles. Initially, this problem can be managed by heel cord stretching exercises and night splints. A KAFO may be needed to control foot position and substitute for weak quadriceps muscles. When contractures are worse, serial casting is often effective. Stretching exercises and pronation can be employed to treat early hip flexion contractures.

Surgical intervention is directed toward the release of ambulation-limiting contractures. Early postoperative mobilization is important to prevent further muscle weakness. Anesthetic risks are increased in these patients because of their limited pulmonary reserve and because the incidence of malignant hyperthermia is higher than normal in patients with muscle disease.

The triceps surae and tibialis posterior are the strongest muscles in the lower extremity of the patient with muscular dystrophy. These muscles are responsible for equinus and varus deformities. Management that consists of releasing the contracted tensor fasciae latae, lengthening the Achilles tendon, and transferring the tibialis posterior muscle anteriorly is indicated and prolongs walking for approximately 3 years. Postoperative bracing is required.

Scoliosis is common in nonambulatory patients confined to a wheelchair. Adaptive seating devices that hold the pelvis level and the spine erect are useful in preventing deformity. Alternatively, a rigid plastic spinal torso orthosis may be used for support. When external support is not effective, scoliosis develops rapidly. Spinal fusion is occasionally indicated. Blood loss during surgery is high, and the incidence of pseudarthrosis is increased. Postoperative immobilization is to be avoided; therefore, segmental spinal stabilization is often the preferred technique of internal stabilization.

Fractures in patients with myopathies occur secondary to osteoporosis from the inactivity and the loss of muscle tension. No abnormalities of bone mineralization are present. The incidence of fracture increases with the severity of the disease. Most fractures are metaphyseal in location, show little displacement, cause minimal pain, and heal in the expected time without complication.

Bushby K, Finkel R, Birnkrant DJ, et al: Diagnosis and management of Duchenne muscular dystrophy, part 1: diagnosis, and pharmacological and psychosocial management. *Lancet Neurol* 2010;9:77. [PMID: 19945913]

Bushby K, Finkel R, Birnkrant DJ, et al: Diagnosis and management of Duchenne muscular dystrophy, part 2: implementation of multidisciplinary care. *Lancet Neurol* 2010;9:177. [PMID: 19945914]

Glanzman AM, Flickinger JM, Dholakia KH, Bönnemann CG, Finkel RS: Serial casting for the management of ankle contracture in Duchenne muscular dystrophy. *Pediatr Phys Ther* 2011;23:275. [PMID: 21829124]

Jung IY, Chae JH, Park SK, et al: The correlation analysis of functional factors and age with Duchenne muscular dystrophy. *Ann Rehabil Med* 2012;36:22. [PMID: 22506232]

Markert CD, Ambrosio F, Call JA, Grange RW: Exercise and Duchenne muscular dystrophy: toward evidence-based exercise prescription. *Muscle Nerve* 2011;43:464. [PMID: 21404285]

Roberto R, Fritz A, Hagar Y, et al: The natural history of cardiac and pulmonary function decline in patients with Duchenne muscular dystrophy. *Spine (Phila Pa 1976)* 2011;36:E1009. [PMID: 21289561]

Sussman M: Duchenne muscular dystrophy. *J Am Acad Orthop Surg* 2002;10:138. [PMID: 11929208]

2. Spinal Muscular Atrophy

Spinal muscular atrophy is a neuropathic disorder in which fewer anterior horn cells are present in the spinal cord congenitally. The severe infantile form of the disease is called **Werdnig-Hoffmann paralysis**. The disorder is inherited in an autosomal-recessive pattern.

Approximately 20% of patients with spinal muscular atrophy are ambulatory, and 1% are totally dependent. Fractures are common in these patients and occur secondary to decreased mobility and function.

The goal of orthopedic intervention is to prevent collapse of the spine and contractures. Orthotic support is often needed to stabilize the spine. In the nonambulatory patient, adaptive seating devices or orthotics may be used. If collapse of the spine occurs, spinal fusion is indicated, but progression can occur even with after fusion. Skeletal immaturity and length of posterior instrumentation may influence curve progression and should be considered during preoperative planning.

McElroy MJ, Shaner AC, Crawford TO, et al: Growing rods for scoliosis in spinal muscular atrophy: structural effects, complications, and hospital stays. *Spine (Phila Pa 1976)* 2011;36:1305. [PMID: 21730818]

Wadman RI, Bosboom WM, van der Pol WL, et al: Drug treatment for spinal muscular atrophy types II and III. *Cochrane Database Syst Rev* 2012;4:CD006282. [PMID: 22513940]

Zebala LP, Bridwell KH, Baldus C, et al: Minimum 5-year radiographic results of long scoliosis fusion in juvenile spinal muscular atrophy patients: major curve progression after instrumented fusion. *J Pediatr Orthop* 2011;31:480. [PMID: 21654453]

3. CHARCOT-MARIE-TOOTH DISEASE

Charcot-Marie-Tooth disease is the most common of the hereditary degenerative myopathies affecting at least 1 in 2500 persons. It is generally inherited in an autosomal-dominant pattern. Over the past few decades, there have been significant advances in elucidating the molecular basis of Charcot-Marie-Tooth disease with more than 30 causative genes now described. EMG studies show a neuropathic pattern, and the nerve conduction velocity of the involved nerves is markedly decreased. Muscle enzyme levels are normal. Clinical onset of the disease is between 5 and 15 years of age.

The peroneal muscles are affected early in the course of the disease. For this reason, Charcot-Marie-Tooth disease is sometimes referred to as **progressive peroneal muscular atrophy**. The intrinsic muscles of the feet and hands are affected later. Patients usually present with progressive clawtoe and cavus deformities of the feet. In the skeletally immature patient, release of the plantar fascia is done to correct the cavus deformity. This is often combined with transfer of the extensor digitorum longus tendon to the neck of the metatarsal and fusion of the proximal interphalangeal joints of the toes to correct the clawtoe deformities. If the tibialis posterior muscle is active during swing phase, it can be transferred through the interosseous membrane to the lateral cuneiform bone. Triple arthrodesis is often necessary in the adult to correct the deformity.

The intrinsic minus hand deformity causes difficulty in grasping objects. An orthosis with a lumbrical bar to hold the metacarpophalangeal joints flexed improves hand use. A capsulodesis of the volar portion of the metacarpophalangeal joints accomplishes the same objective. To restore active intrinsic muscle function in the hand, the flexor digitorum superficialis tendon of the ring finger can be divided into four slips and transferred through the lumbrical passages to the proximal phalanx.

Reilly MM, Murphy SM, Laurá M: Charcot-Marie-Tooth disease. *J Peripher Nerv Syst* 2011;16:1. [PMID: 21504497]

Sapienza A, Green S: Correction of the claw hand. *Hand Clin* 2012;28:53. [PMID: 22117924]

Yagerman SE, Cross MB, Green DW, Scher DM: Pediatric orthopedic conditions in Charcot-Marie-Tooth disease: a literature review. *Curr Opin Pediatr* 2012;24:50. [PMID: 22189393]

PARKINSON DISEASE

A. Epidemiology

Parkinson disease (PD) is a progressive neurodegenerative disorder associated with a loss of dopaminergic nigrostriatal neurons. PD is recognized as one of the most common neurologic disorders, affecting approximately 1–2% of individuals older than 65 years. The incidence and prevalence of PD increase with age, and PD affects 4–5% of those over 85 years of age. The average age of onset is approximately 60 years. Onset in persons younger than 40 years is relatively uncommon.

B. Pathophysiology

The major neuropathologic findings in PD are a loss of pigmented dopaminergic neurons in the substantia nigra and the presence of Lewy bodies. The loss of dopaminergic neurons occurs most prominently in the ventral lateral substantia nigra. Approximately 60–80% of dopaminergic neurons are lost before clinical symptoms of PD emerge.

C. History

Onset of PD is typically asymmetric, with the most common initial finding being an asymmetric resting tremor in an upper extremity. Approximately 20% of patients first experience clumsiness in one hand. Over time, patients notice symptoms related to progressive bradykinesia, rigidity, and gait difficulty. The initial symptoms of PD may be nonspecific and include fatigue and depression.

D. Physical Examination

The three cardinal signs of PD are resting tremor, rigidity, and bradykinesia. Of these cardinal features, two of three are required to make the clinical diagnosis. Postural instability is the fourth cardinal sign, but it emerges late in the disease, usually after 8 years or more.

E. Medical Care

The goal of medical management of PD is to provide control of signs and symptoms for as long as possible while minimizing adverse effects. Medications (eg, levodopa) usually provide good symptomatic control for 4–6 years. After this, disability progresses despite best medical management, and many patients develop long-term motor complications including fluctuations and dyskinesia. Additional causes of disability in late disease include postural instability (balance difficulty) and dementia.

F. Neurosurgical Care

When medical management is exhausted, neurosurgical interventions include deep brain stimulation, thalamotomy, and pallidotomy.

G. Orthopedic Care

Treatment of orthopedic problems in patients with PD can be problematic and include failure of fixation or prosthetic dislocation. Despite successful pain relief, the functional results of total joint arthroplasty in patients with PD are less predictable and complications are more frequent. Satisfactory outcomes can be obtained with appropriate medical management of PD after orthopedic intervention.

Macaulay W, Geller JA, Brown AR, Cote LJ, Kiernan HA: Total knee arthroplasty and Parkinson disease: enhancing outcomes and avoiding complications. *J Am Acad Orthop Surg* 2010;18:687. [PMID: 21041803]

Moon SH, Lee HM, Chun HJ, et al: Surgical outcome of lumbar fusion surgery in patients with Parkinson disease. *J Spinal Disord Tech* 2012;25:351. [PMID: 21685805]

Queally JM, Abdulkarim A, Mulhall KJ: Total hip replacement in patients with neurological conditions. *J Bone Joint Surg Br* 2009;91:1267. [PMID: 19794158]

BURNS

More than 2 million people sustain burns of sufficient severity each year in the United States to require medical attention. Of these, 50,000 individuals remain hospitalized for more than 2 months, attesting to the serious nature of their injuries.

Thermal burns affect the skin most directly but can also involve the underlying muscles, tendons, joints, and bones. Scar contractures cause the greatest limitation to later function and the greatest deformity. Rehabilitation efforts ideally should begin when the patient first enters the hospital, immediately following acute resuscitation and continuing through the reconstruction process.

▶ Classification

Burn wounds are traditionally classified as first, second, or third degree, depending on the depth of the damage. Currently, it is thought to be more useful to simply divide burns into two categories: partial thickness (involving part of the dermis) and full thickness (involving the entire dermis). In children, a burn size of roughly 60% total body surface area is a crucial threshold for postburn morbidity and mortality.

First-degree burns damage only the epidermis. They cause erythema, minor edema, and pain. The skin surface remains intact, and healing occurs uneventfully in 5–10 days, without residual scar formation.

Second-degree burns involve the epidermis and a variable amount of the underlying corium. The depth of damage to the corium determines the outcome of healing. In the more superficial second-degree burns, blister formation is prominent and occurs secondary to the osmotic gradient formed by particles in the vesicle fluid. Superficial second-degree burns heal in 10–14 days, with minimal scarring. Deep dermal burns are characterized by either a reddish appearance or by the presence of a white tissue that is barely perceptible and adheres to the underlying viable dermis. These wounds may advance to a full-thickness loss if infection occurs. They heal with a fragile epithelial covering. Healing occurs over 25–30 days, and dense scar formation is common.

Third-degree burns are full-thickness injuries that damage the epidermis and the entire corium. Because of the loss of pain receptors, which are normally found within the corium, pain is absent. The burns have a thick leathery surface of dead tissue.

▶ Management
A. Techniques for Maintaining Functional Position

Burn scars contract and become rigid, so it is critical to maintain the head, trunk, and extremities in a functional position. Contractures, if allowed to form, severely limit later function. The location of the burns determines which techniques are useful in preventing deformity.

To prevent deformities of the neck and jaw in patients with burns of the neck or upper torso, molded splints should be applied early to maintain the head and neck in a neutral position or in slight extension. Patients with burns in the shoulder region are at risk for contractures characterized by a protracted scapula with an adducted arm. Placing a roll between the scapulae and providing support with a firm mattress help prevent scapula protraction. To keep the arms abducted 75–80 degrees and the shoulder flexed 20–30 degrees, axillary foam pads are used and can be held in position with a figure-of-8 wrapping, which maintains the glenohumeral joint in a functional position. Untreated contractures not only limit limb motion but also can result in joint subluxation from extremes in positioning.

When the burns involve the torso, the goal is to maintain a straight spine in the face of contracting scar tissue. Burns involving only one side of the trunk sometimes result in scoliosis. This should be corrected by scar excision and splinting. If left uncorrected, the scoliosis becomes structural, with resultant bony changes. Burns in the groin area tend to cause flexion and adduction contractures of the hip. To prevent this, the patient should be positioned with the hips extended and in 15–20 degrees of abduction. If the patient is lying on a soft mattress, mild flexion deformities of the hips may be masked. Daily pronation is useful in maintaining the extension range of the hips.

Regardless of the location of burn wounds on the extremities, the knees and elbows tend to develop flexion contractures. Custom-molded thermoplastic splints can be applied over dressings or skin grafts to maintain the extremities in extension. The splints should be removable to allow for daily wound care. Burns in the ankle area result in equinus contractures with inversion of the foot. Splints can be used here also to maintain the foot in a neutral position, but care must be taken to ensure the splint is holding the foot adequately and not merely obscuring a deformity. Custom-molded splints applied to the anterior and posterior surfaces in a clamshell fashion are more effective in maintaining the desired position. They also assist in the control of edema and can be removed for wound care and motion exercises. Burns on the dorsum of the foot cause hyperextension deformities of the toes. Early grafting and toe traction are useful.

Burns of the hands present special problems. Scar contracture results in a flexion deformity of the wrist and a clawhand position similar to that seen with loss of the intrinsic musculature. The hand should be splinted with the wrist in neutral or in a slightly extended position. The metacarpophalangeal joints should be flexed 60–75 degrees and the interphalangeal joints extended. The thumb should be held with the metacarpal in abduction and flexion, the metacarpophalangeal joint in mild flexion, and the interphalangeal joint in the extended position.

B. Skeletal Traction and External Suspension

In patients with circumferential burns on an extremity, the use of skeletal traction or external fixators and suspension is efficacious and has several advantages. It permits access to all surfaces, elevates the limb to decrease edema, and maintains the extremity in the desired position while allowing joint motion. Traction can be used to correct contractures. In addition, traction still allows for daily hydrotherapy. Generally, traction is only employed for a 2-week period because longer use may result in a pin tract infection with formation of sequestra.

Special splints are fabricated for use in the hand. The traction frame is secured proximally with a pin inserted through the distal radius. Pins are also placed through the distal phalanges of the fingers and thumb by drilling through the nail bed from the dorsal to the volar surface. Traction is applied to the fingers in the desired direction by attaching rubber bands from the distal pins to the outrigger frame. The frame can be modified for use in the foot to apply traction to the toes. In this case, the traction frame is secured proximally with a pin inserted through the calcaneus.

C. Pressure Dressings

Consistent pressure of 25 torr applied evenly aids in the prevention of hypertrophic scar formation and contracture. Elastic wraps applied over splints are used early after the injury and following grafting because they can be adjusted for changes in the amount of edema present. Later, when the amount of swelling shows little fluctuation, custom elastic garments are employed. Pressure must be continued for as long as the scar tissue is biologically active. When the skin is soft and flat and returns to normal color, the pressure can be discontinued. Pressure dressings should be employed for a minimum of 6 months and may be necessary for as long as a year. The daily application of lanolin relieves the dryness of grafted skin or substitutes for the loss of sebaceous gland secretions in deep burns.

D. Mobilization

Early motion is desirable for burned and uninvolved extremities. Splints should be removed frequently to allow for ROM exercises. If the patient is being treated with skeletal traction, motion exercises can be performed on the extremities. If the patient is receiving hydrotherapy for the burn wounds, the motion exercises are facilitated with the extremities supported in the fluid environment.

Patients with burns of the lower extremities can begin to stand or walk before skin grafts are performed, provided the legs are wrapped with elastic supports to control edema. Ambulation should be resumed after skin grafting as soon as the grafts are stable. Early mobilization not only preserves joint motion but also decreases the incidence of sequelae such as osteoporosis, physiologic deconditioning, muscle atrophy, and heterotopic ossification.

E. Treatment of Special Problems

1. Fractures—If fractures occurred at the time of the burn, they can be treated with the use of skeletal traction or external supports such as splints. Diagnosis may be delayed if the fractures do not result in any obvious deformity. If fractures occur secondary to disuse osteoporosis, they are usually minimally displaced and heal uneventfully. Pathologic fractures are less common with early mobilization.

2. Osteomyelitis—Osteomyelitis is not a common complication, despite the high incidence of sepsis associated with burns. Prolonged exposure of bone sometimes results in the formation of a tangential sequestrum in the devitalized cortex. Exposed bone surfaces can be drilled to promote the formation of a granulation tissue bed for skin grafting without an increased risk of infection. The prolonged use of pins for skeletal traction causes infection in 5% of patients who require traction. The use of threaded traction pins minimizes the motion of the pin in the bone. Pins should be removed as soon as possible.

3. Exposed joints—Children and adolescents with exposed joint surfaces may retain some function after healing, but adults often develop joint ankylosis or deformities that require arthrodesis at a later date. To maintain the joint in the desired position, traction can be used. The joint should be irrigated with hypochlorite solution daily and debrided as necessary. The exposed bone surfaces can be drilled to promote the formation of granulation tissue. When the bed of tissue covers the joint, skin grafting is performed.

4. Heterotopic ossification—Heterotopic ossification is the presence of lamellar bone in nonskeletal tissue. Periarticular bone formation is seen in 2–3% of patients with severe burns. Although the cause is unknown, predisposing factors include full-thickness burns involving more than 30% of the body surface, prolonged immobilization, and superimposed trauma. The location of the HO is not determined by the

distribution of the burns. Ossification can occur in any of the major joints. In adults, the elbow is the joint most frequently affected; the hip is rarely affected. In children, the hip and elbow are common sites; the shoulder is an uncommon site.

HO can continue to form as long as open granulating wounds are present. If joint ankylosis does not occur, the ossification gradually diminishes after the burns heal. In children, it may disappear completely. If joint ankylosis occurs, surgical resection is indicated and usually restores a functional arc of motion, particularly when the articular surface is not damaged. This may be done with multiple small incisions without raising cutaneous flaps. Early mobilization of patients with burns decreases the incidence and severity of heterotopic ossification.

Disseldorp LM, Nieuwenhuis MK, Van Baar ME, Mouton LJ: Physical fitness in people after burn injury: a systematic review. *Arch Phys Med Rehabil* 2011;92:1501. [PMID: 21878221]

Kraft R, Herndon DN, Al-Mousawi AM, et al: Burn size and survival probability in paediatric patients in modern burn care: a prospective observational cohort study. *Lancet.* 2012;379:1013. [PMID: 22296810]

Maender C, Sahajpal D, Wright TW: Treatment of heterotopic ossification of the elbow following burn injury: recommendations for surgical excision and perioperative prophylaxis using radiation therapy. *J Shoulder Elbow Surg* 2010;19:1269. [PMID: 20850996]

Schneider JC, Qu HD, Lowry J, Walker J, Vitale E, Zona M: Efficacy of inpatient burn rehabilitation: a prospective pilot study examining range of motion, hand function and balance. *Burns* 2012;38:164. [PMID: 22119446]

Shakirov BM: Evaluation of different surgical techniques used for correction of post-burn contracture of foot and ankle. *Ann Burns Fire Disasters* 2010;23:137. [PMID: 21991213]

Index

NOTE: Page numbers followed by *f* or *t* indicate figures or tables, respectively.